SEVENTH EDITION

NEONATOLOGY

Management, Procedures, On-Call Problems, Diseases, and Drugs

Editor

TRICIA LACY GOMELLA, MD
Part-Time Assistant Professor of Pediatrics
Johns Hopkins University School of Medicine
Baltimore, Maryland

Associate Editors

M. DOUGLAS CUNNINGHAM, MD
Professor of Pediatrics/Neonatology
Interim Chief of the Division of Neonatology, Department of Pediatrics
College of Medicine
University of Kentucky
Lexington, Kentucky
Clinical Professor of Pediatrics/Neonatology
Department of Pediatrics, School of Medicine
University of California, Irvine
Irvine, California

FABIEN G. EYAL, MD
Professor of Pediatrics
Chief and Louise Lenoir Locke Professor of Neonatology
Medical Director, Intensive Care Nurseries
University of South Alabama Children's and Women's Hospital
Mobile, Alabama

Consulting Editor

DEBORAH J. TUTTLE, MD
Assistant Professor of Pediatrics
Jefferson Medical College
Thomas Jefferson University
Philadelphia, Pennsylvania
Director, Performance Improvement
Christiana Care Health System
Director, Milk Bank
Attending Neonatologist
Christiana Care Health System
Newark, Delaware

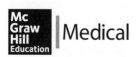
Medical

New York   Chicago   San Francisco   Lisbon   London   Madrid   Mexico City
Milan   New Delhi   San Juan   Seoul   Singapore   Sydney   Toronto

Neonatology: Management, Procedures, On-Call Problems, Diseases, and Drugs, Seventh Edition

Copyright © 2013 by McGraw-Hill Education LLC. All rights reserved. Printed in the United States of America. Except as permitted under the United States Copyright Act of 1976, no part of this publication may be reproduced or distributed in any form or by any means, or stored in a data base or retrieval system, without the prior written permission of the publisher.

7 8 9 10   LCR   19 18 17

ISBN 978-0-07-176801-6
MHID 0-07-176801-7
ISSN 0697-6295

This book was set in Minion Pro by Cenveo® Publisher Services.
The editors were Alyssa K. Fried and Harriet Lebowitz.
The production supervisor was Sherri Souffrance.
Project management was provided by Arushi Chawla, Cenveo Publisher Services.
The text was designed by Eve Siegel.
RR Donnelley was printer and binder.

This book is printed on acid free paper.

McGraw-Hill Education books are available at special quantity discounts to use as premiums and sales promotions, or for use in corporate training programs. To contact a representative please e-mail us at bulksales@mcgraw-hill.com.

International Edition ISBN 978-0-07-181699-1; MHID 0-07-181699-2. Copyright © 2013. Exclusive rights by The McGraw-Hill Companies, Inc., for manufacture and export. This book cannot be re-exported from the country to which it is consigned by McGraw-Hill. The International Edition is not available in North America.

International Editorial Board

To my twin sons, Leonard and Patrick, and singletons Andrew and Michael.

Contents

Contributors

Irfan Ahmad, MD
Assistant Clinical Professor of Pediatrics
University of California, Irvine
Neonatologist
Children's Hospital of Orange County
Orange, California
*Necrotizing Enterocolitis; Spontaneous
Intestinal Perforation*

Marilee C. Allen, MD
Professor of Pediatrics
Department of Pediatrics, Division of
Neonatology
Johns Hopkins University School of Medicine
Co-Director of the NICU Developmental
Clinic, Kennedy-Kreiger Institute
Baltimore, Maryland
*Follow-Up of High-Risk Infants; Counseling
Parents Before High-Risk Delivery*

Gad Alpan, MD, MBA
Professor of Clinical Pediatrics
Department of Pediatrics, Division of
Newborn Medicine
New York Medical College
Maria Fareri Children's Hospital
Westchester Medical Center
Valhalla, New York
*Infant of a Substance-Abusing Mother;
Patent Ductus Arteriosus; Persistent
Pulmonary Hypertension of the
Newborn*

Hubert O. Ballard, MD, FAAP
Associate Professor of Pediatrics
Medical Director of ECMO
Department of Pediatrics, Division of
Neonatology
Kentucky Children's Hospital
University of Kentucky
Lexington, Kentucky
Newborn Screening

Fayez Bany-Mohammed, MBBS, FAAP
Clinical Professor of Pediatrics
Director, Neonatal Perinatal Medicine
Fellowship Program
Department of Pediatrics
University of California, Irvine
Irvine, California
*Chlamydial Infection; Cytomegalovirus;
Gonorrhea; Hepatitis; Herpes Simplex
Viruses; Human Immunodeficiency
Virus; Meningitis; Methicillin-Resistant
Staphylococcus aureus Infections;
Parvovirus B19 Infection; Respiratory
Syncytial Virus; Rubella; Sepsis;
Syphilis; TORCH Infections;
Toxoplasmosis; Ureaplasma Infections;
Varicella-Zoster Infections*

Daniel A. Beals, MD, FACS, FAAP
Associate Professor of Surgery and Pediatrics
Chief, Division of Pediatric Surgery
University of South Alabama
Mobile, Alabama
Neonatal Bioethics

Vincenzo Berghella, MD
Professor of Obstetrics and Gynecology
Director of Maternal Fetal Medicine
Department of Obstetrics and Gynecology
Thomas Jefferson University
Philadelphia, Pennsylvania
Fetal Assessment

**Dilip R. Bhatt, MD, FAAP, FACC,
FACMQ**
Clinical Assistant Professor of Pediatrics
Loma Linda University
Loma Linda, California
Neonatologist and Pediatric Cardiologist
Kaiser Permanente
Fontana, California
Isolation Guidelines

Michael B. Bober, MD, PhD
Associate Professor
Department of Pediatrics
Jefferson Medical College
Thomas Jefferson University
Philadelphia, Pennsylvania
Co-Director, Skeletal Dysplasia Program
Division of Medical Genetics
Nemours/Alfred I. duPont Hospital for
   Children
Wilmington, Delaware
*Common Multiple Congenital Anomaly
   Syndromes*

Gary E. Carnahan, MD, PhD
Director of Transfusion Medicine,
   Coagulation, and Clinical Chemistry
Department of Pathology
College of Medicine
University of South Alabama
Director of Pathology and Clinical
   Laboratories
University of South Alabama Children's and
   Women's Hospital
Mobile, Alabama
Blood Component Therapy

Daniel Casella, MD
Resident in Urology
Department of Urology
University of Pittsburgh
Pittsburgh, Pennsylvania
*Surgical Diseases of the Newborn: Urologic
   Disorders; Urinary Tract Infection*

Leslie Castelo-Soccio, MD, PhD
Assistant Professor of Pediatrics and
   Dermatology
Department of Pediatrics, Division of
   Dermatology
The Children's Hospital of Philadelphia
Philadelphia, Pennsylvania
Rash and Dermatologic Problems, Images

Pik-Kwan Chow, MSN, NNP-BC
Neonatal Nurse Practitioner
Department of Pediatrics, Division of
   Neonatology
Christiana Care Health System
Newark, Delaware
Laryngeal Mask Airway

Carol M. Cottrill, MD
Professor Emerita
Department of Pediatrics
Post-Retirement Director, Division of
   Community Cardiology
University of Kentucky College of
   Medicine
Lexington, Kentucky
*Defibrillation and Cardioversion; Arrhythmia;
   Congenital Heart Disease*

M. Douglas Cunningham, MD
Professor of Pediatrics/Neonatology
Interim Chief of the Division of Neonatology,
   Department of Pediatrics
College of Medicine
University of Kentucky
Lexington, Kentucky
Clinical Professor of Pediatrics/Neonatology
Department of Pediatrics, School of
   Medicine
University of California, Irvine
Irvine, California
Fluid and Electrolytes

Jennifer L. Das, MD
Pediatrics Resident
Department of Pediatrics
The University of Toronto
Toronto, Ontario, Canada
Myasthenia Gravis (Transient Neonatal)

Nirmala S. Desai, MBBS FAAP
Professor of Pediatrics
Department of Pediatrics, Division of
   Neonatology
Kentucky Children's Hospital
University of Kentucky Medical
   Center
Lexington, Kentucky
Pain in the Neonate; Ostomy Care

Steven G. Docimo, MD
Professor of Surgery
Department of Urology
Children's Hospital of Pittsburgh of UPMC
University of Pittsburgh School of
   Medicine
Pittsburgh, Pennsylvania
*Surgical Diseases of the Newborn: Urologic
   Disorders; Urinary Tract Infection*

John M. Draus Jr., MD
Assistant Professor of Surgery and
  Pediatrics
Department of Surgery, Division of Pediatric
  Surgery
Kentucky Children's Hospital
University of Kentucky
Lexington, Kentucky
Surgical Diseases of the Newborn: Abdominal
  Masses; Surgical Diseases of the
  Newborn: Abdominal Wall Defects;
  Surgical Diseases of the Newborn:
  Alimentary Tract Obstruction; Surgical
  Diseases of the Newborn: Diseases
  of the Airway, Tracheobronchial Tree,
  and Lungs; Surgical Diseases of the
  Newborn: Retroperitoneal Tumors

Kevin Dysart, MD
Associate Medical Director, Newborn/Infant
  Intensive Care Unit
Children's Hospital of Philadelphia
Clinical Associate, Perelman School of
  Medicine
University of Pennsylvania
Philadelphia, Pennsylvania
Infant of a Diabetic Mother

Omar Elkhateeb, MBChB
Fellow in Neonatology
Section of Neonatology
University of Manitoba
Winnipeg, Manitoba, Canada
Intracranial Hemorrhage

Fabien G. Eyal, MD
Professor of Pediatrics
Chief and Louise Lenoir Locke Professor of
  Neonatology
Medical Director, Intensive Care Nurseries
University of South Alabama Children's and
  Women's Hospital
Mobile, Alabama
Temperature Regulation; Blood Component
  Therapy; Sedation and Analgesia;
  Anemia; Coagulation Disorders

Catherine A. Finnegan, MS, NNP-BC
Neonatal Nurse Practitioner
Department of Neonatology
Johns Hopkins Bayview Medical Center
Baltimore, Maryland
Venous Access: Percutaneous Central Venous
  Catheterization

Maria A. Giraldo-Isaza, MD
Maternal Fetal Medicine Fellow
Department of Obstetrics and Gynecology
Jefferson Medical College of Thomas
  Jefferson University
Philadelphia, Pennsylvania
Fetal Assessment

Andrew Gomella, BS
Intramural Research Training Associate
Lab of Imaging Physics
National Heart, Lung, and Blood Institute
National Institutes of Health
Bethesda, Maryland
Graphics, Imaging, and IT Assistant

Tricia Lacy Gomella, MD
Part-Time Assistant Professor of Pediatrics
Johns Hopkins University School of Medicine
Baltimore, Maryland
Gestational age and Birthweight Classification; Newborn Physical Examination; Arterial Access: Arterial Puncture (Radial Artery Puncture); Arterial Access: Percutaneous Arterial Catherization (Radial Arterial Line); Arterial Access: Umbilical Artery Catheterization; Bladder Aspiration (Suprapubic Urine Collection); Bladder Catheterization; Chest Tube Placement; Endotracheal Intubation and Extubation; Gastric and Transpyloric Intubation; Heelstick (Capillary Blood Sampling); Lumbar Puncture (Spinal Tap); Paracentesis (Abdominal); Pericardiocentesis; Transillumination; Venous Access: Intraosseous Infusion; Venous Access: Peripheral Intravenous Catheterization; Venous Access: Umbilical Vein Catheterization; Venous Access: Venipuncture (Phlebotomy); Abnormal Blood Gas; Apnea and Bradycardia ("A's and B's"); Bloody Stool; Cyanosis; Death of an Infant; Eye Discharge and Conjunctivitis; Gastric Aspirate (Residuals); Gastrointestinal Bleeding from the Upper Tract; Hyperbilirubinemia, Conjugated; Hyperbilirubinemia, Unconjugated; Hyperglycemia; Hyperkalemia; Hypertension; Hypoglycemia; Hypokalemia; Hyponatremia; Hypotension and Shock; No Stool in 48 Hours; No Urine Output in 24 Hours; Pneumoperitoneum; Pneumothorax; Polycythemia; Poor Perfusion; Postdelivery Antibiotics; Pulmonary Hemorrhage; Seizure Activity; Traumatic Delivery; Vasospasms and Thromboembolism; Abbreviations Used in Neonatology; Apgar Scoring; Blood Pressure Determinations; Chartwork; Temperature Conversion Table; Weight Conversion Table

Janet E. Graeber, MD
Associate Professor Emerita
Department of Pediatrics
West Virginia University
Morgantown, West Virginia
Retinopathy of Prematurity

George W. Gross, MD
Professor of Radiology
Department of Diagnostic Radiology
University of Maryland School of
   Medicine
Director, Division of Pediatric
   Radiology
University of Maryland Medical
   Center
Baltimore, Maryland
Imaging Studies

Olga E. Guzman, RN, BSN, CIC
Infection Control Preventionist
Department of Infection Control
Kaiser Permanente Medical Center
Fontana, California
Isolation Guidelines

Wayne Hachey, DO, MPH
Executive Secretary
Defense Health Board
Department of Defense Medical
   Headquarters
Falls Church, Virginia
Meconium Aspiration

Janell F. Hacker, NNP-BC, ARNP
Neonatal Nurse Practitioner
Kentucky Children's Hospital
University of Kentucky
Lexington, Kentucky
Ostomy Care

Charles R Hamm Jr., MD
Professor and Vice Chair of Pediatrics
Department of Pediatrics, Division of
   Neonatology
University of South Alabama College of
   Medicine
Mobile, Alabama
Respiratory Management

Pip Hidestrand, MD
Fellow in Pediatric Cardiology
Instructor in Pediatrics
Department of Pediatrics, Division of
    Pediatric Cardiology
Children's Hospital of Wisconsin/Medical
    College of Wisconsin
Milwaukee, Wisconsin
Defibrillation and Cardioversion

H. Jane Huffnagle, DO, FAOCA
Clinical Professor of Anesthesiology
Director of Obstetric Anesthesia
Department of Anesthesiology
Thomas Jefferson University Hospital
Philadelphia, Pennsylvania
Obstetric Anesthesia and the Neonate

Musaddaq Inayat, MD, FAAP
Consultant Neonatologist
Shifa International Hospital
Assistant Professor
Shifa College of Medicine
Shifa Tameer-e-Millat University
Islamabad, Pakistan
*Calcium Disorders (Hypocalcemia,
    Hypercalcemia); Magnesium Disorders
    (Hypomagnesemia, Hypermagnesmia)*

Joseph A. Iocono, MD
Associate Professor of Surgery and Pediatrics
Division Chief, Pediatric Surgery
Department of Surgery
Kentucky Children's Hospital
University of Kentucky
Lexington, Kentucky
*Surgical Diseases of the Newborn: Abdominal
    Masses; Surgical Diseases of the
    Newborn: Abdominal Wall Defects;
    Surgical Diseases of the Newborn:
    Alimentary Tract Obstruction; Surgical
    Diseases of the Newborn: Diseases of
    the Airway, Tracheobronchial Tree, and
    Lungs; Surgical Diseases of the Newborn:
    Retroperitoneal Tumors*

Kathy B. Isaacs, MSN, RNC-NIC
Patient Care Manager, Neonatal Intensive
    Care Unit
Department of Pediatrics, Division of
    Neonatology
Kentucky Children's Hospital University of
    Kentucky
Lexington, Kentucky
Pain in the Neonate

Shamin Jivabhai, MD
Fellow
Department of Pediatrics, Division of
    Neonatology
University of California, Irvine
Orange, California
*Enteroviruses and Parechoviruses; Lyme
    Disease*

Jamieson E. Jones, MD
Neonatologist
Department of Neonatology
Desert Regional Medical Center
Palm Springs, California
*Complementary and Alternative Medical
    Therapies in Neonatology*

Genine Jordan, APRN, NNP-BC
Neonatal Nurse Practitioner
Department of Pediatrics, Division of
    Neonatology
University of Kentucky
Kentucky Children's Hospital
Lexington, Kentucky
*Management of the Extremely Low
    Birthweight Infant During the First Week
    of Life*

David E. Kanter, MD
Neonatologist
Division of Newborn Medicine
Herman and Walter Samuelson Children's
    Hospital at Sinai
Sinai Hospital of Baltimore
Baltimore, Maryland
Is the Infant Ready for Discharge?

Kathy Keen, MSN, NNP-BC
Neonatal Nurse Practitioner
Christiana Care Health System
Neonatal Nurse Practitioner Service
Newark, Delaware
*Peripheral IV Extravasation and Infiltration:
    Initial Management*

**Christoph U. Lehmann, MD, FAAP,
FACMI**
Professor, Pediatrics and Biomedical
    Informatics
Vanderbilt University
Nashville, Tennessee
Studies for Neurologic Evaluation

William G. Mackenzie, MD
Chairman of Orthopedic Surgery
Department of Orthopedic Surgery
Nemours/Alfred I. duPont Hospital for
   Children
Wilmington, Delaware
Orthopedic and Musculoskeletal Problems

Barbara McKinney, PharmD
Neonatal Clinical Pharmacist
Christiana Hospital
Newark, Delaware
*Medications Used in the Neonatal Intensive
   Care Unit; Effects of Drugs and
   Substances on Lactation and Infants*

Prasanthi Koduru Mishra, MD
Fellow in Neonatology
Department of Pediatrics, Division of
   Neonatology
University of California, Irvine
Orange, California
Perinatal Asphyxia; Pertussis; Tuberculosis

Solomonia Nino, MD
Fellow in Neonatology
Department of Pediatrics, Division of
   Neonatology
University of Kentucky
Lexington, Kentucky
*Air Leak Syndromes; Hydrocephalus and
   Ventriculomegaly*

Paul H. Noh, MD, FACS, FAAP
Director, Minimally Invasive Surgery
Assistant Professor of Surgery
Division of Pediatric Urology
Cincinnati Children's Hospital Medical
   Center
Cincinnati, Ohio
*Hematuria; Renal Failure, Acute (Acute
   Kidney Injury)*

Murali Mohan Reddy Palla, MD
Fellow in Neonatology
Department of Pediatrics, Division of
   Neonatology
University of Kentucky
Lexington, Kentucky
*Exchange Transfusion; Apnea; Thyroid
   Disorders*

Ambadas Pathak, MD
Assistant Professor Emeritus
Department of Pediatrics
John Hopkins University School of Medicine
Clinical Associate Professor
Department of Pediatrics
University of Maryland School of Medicine
Baltimore, Maryland
Seizures

David A. Paul, MD
Professor of Pediatrics
Department of Pediatrics
Jefferson Medical College
Philadelphia, Pennsylvania
Associate Director
Division of Neonatology
Director, Neonatal Research
Christiana Care Health System
Newark, Delaware
Multiple Gestation

Stephen A. Pearlman, MD, MSHQS
Clinical Professor of Pediatrics
Department of Pediatrics
Fellowship Director in Neonatology
Jefferson Medical College
Philadelphia, Pennsylvania
Attending Neonatologist
Christiana Care Health System
Newark, Delaware
Management of the Late Preterm Infant

Keith J. Peevy, JD, MD
Professor of Pediatrics and Neonatal
   Medicine
Department of Pediatrics, Division of
   Neonatology
University of South Alabama College of
   Medicine
Mobile, Alabama
Polycythemia and Hyperviscosity

Valerie D. Phebus, PA-C
Neonatal Physician Assistant
Department of Pediatrics, Division of
   Neonatology
University of Kentucky
Lexington, Kentucky
*Management of the Extremely Low
   Birthweight Infant During the First Week
   of Life*

Judith Polak, DNP, NNP-BC
Clinical Assistant Professor
School of Nursing
West Virginia University
Morgantown, West Virginia
Eye Disorders of the Newborn

Rakesh Rao, MD
Assistant Professor of Pediatrics
Department of Pediatrics, Division of
Newborn Medicine
Washington University in St. Louis
St. Louis, Missouri
*Nutritional Management; Intrauterine Growth
Restriction (Small for Gestational Age);
Osteopenia of Prematurity*

Katie Victory Shreve, RN, BSN, MA
Assistant Patient Care Manager
Neonatal Intensive Care Unit
Kentucky Children's Hospital
Lexington, Kentucky
Pain in the Neonate

Jack Sills, MD
Clinical Professor of Pediatrics
Department of Pediatrics
University of California, Irvine
Orange, California
Pediatric Subspecialty Faculty
Children's Hospital of Orange County
Orange, California
Perinatal Asphyxia

Kendra Smith, MD
Clinical Associate Professor of Pediatrics
Department of Pediatrics, Division of
Neonatology
University of Washington and Seattle
Children's Hospital
Seattle, Washington
Extracorporeal Life Support in the Neonate

Ganesh Srinivasan, MD, DM, FAAP
Assistant Professor of Pediatrics and Child
Health
Department of Pediatrics, Division of
Neonatology
Director Neonatal-Perinatal Medicine
Fellowship Program
University of Manitoba
Winnipeg, Manitoba, Canada
Thyroid Disorders

Theodora A. Stavroudis, MD
Assistant Professor of Pediatrics
Department of Pediatrics
University of Southern California Keck School
of Medicine
Children's Hospital of Los Angeles
Los Angeles, California
Studies for Neurologic Evaluation

Thomas P. Strandjord, MD
Associate Professor of Pediatrics
Department of Pediatrics, Division of
Neonatology
University of Washington
Seattle, Washington
Resuscitation of the Newborn

Wendy J. Sturtz, MD
Director, Neonatal Transport
Medical Director, IMPACT
Attending Neonatologist
Christiana Care Health System
Newark, Delaware
Infant Transport

Outi Tammela, MD
Adjunct Professor in Neonatology
Pediatric Research Center
Tampere University Hospital
Tampere, Finland
Respiratory Distress Syndrome

Arjan te Pas, MD PhD
Associate Professor of Pediatrics
Division of Neonatology
Leiden University Medical Center
Leiden, The Netherlands
Transient Tachypnea of the Newborn

Ahmed M. Thabet, MD
Former Fellow, Department of
Orthopedics
Nemours/Alfred I. duPont Hospital for
Children
Wilmington, Delaware
Lecturer of Orthopedics
Department of Orthopedics
Banha University Medical School
Banha, Egypt
Orthopedic and Musculoskeletal Problems

Christiane Theda, MD, PhD, MBA
Neonatologist and Medical Geneticist
Royal Women's Hospital
University of Melbourne
Murdoch Children's Research Institute
Newborn Emergency Transport Service
Royal Children's Hospital
Melbourne, Australia
*Disorders of Sex Development; Inborn
    Errors of Metabolism with Acute Neonatal
    Onset; Neural Tube Defects*

**Christopher Tomlinson, MBChB,
BSc, PhD**
Assistant Professor of Pediatrics
Department of Pediatrics
University of Toronto
Staff Physician
Neonatal Intensive Care Unit
Hospital for Sick Children
Toronto, Ontario, Canada
Myasthenia Gravis (Transient Neonatal)

Deborah J. Tuttle, MD
Assistant Professor of Pediatrics
Jefferson Medical College
Thomas Jefferson University
Philadelphia, Pennsylvania
Director, Performance Improvement
Christiana Care Health System
Director, Milk Bank
Attending Neonatologist
Christiana Care Health System
Newark, Delaware
Immunization Tables

Cherry Uy, MD
Clinical Professor
Department of Pediatrics, Division of
    Neonatology
University of California, Irvine
Orange, California
*Therapeutic Hypothermia; Hyperbilirubinemia,
    Direct (Conjugated Hyperbilirubinemia);
    Hyperbilirubinemia, Indirect
    (Unconjugated Hyperbilirubinemia)*

Richard M. Whitehurst Jr., MD
Associate Professor of Pediatrics
Department of Pediatrics, Division of
    Neonatology
Assistant Professor of Pharmacology
Department of Pharmacology
University of South Alabama
Mobile, Alabama
ABO Incompatiblity; Rh Incompatiblity

Tiffany N. Wright, MD
General Surgery Resident
Department of Surgery
University of Kentucky Medical Center
Lexington, Kentucky
*Surgical Diseases of the Newborn: Abdominal
    Masses; Surgical Diseases of the
    Newborn: Abdominal Wall Defects;
    Surgical Diseases of the Newborn:
    Alimentary Tract Obstruction; Surgical
    Diseases of the Newborn: Diseases of
    the Airway, Tracheobronchial Tree, and
    Lungs; Surgical Diseases of the Newborn:
    Retroperitoneal Tumors*

Michael Zayek, MD
Professor of Pediatrics
Department of Pediatrics, Division of
    Neonatology
University of South Alabama
Mobile, Alabama
*Bronchopulmonary Dysplasia/Chronic
    Lung Disease; Thrombocytopenia and
    Platelet Dysfunction*

Preface

I am pleased to present the seventh edition of *Neonatology*, the 25th anniversary silver edition. The first edition was published in 1988 and was started during my neonatology fellowship at University of Kentucky Medical Center in Lexington. The origins of the manual were fairly simple and started as a series of handouts designed to help students and residents get through their NICU rotation. Because of a complicated twin pregnancy during my fellowship, I had to delay my training and finish my required neonatology fellowship at Johns Hopkins University. Therefore, the roots of this manual began at University of Kentucky while I was a fellow with Dr. Doug Cunningham's program, but it was ultimately completed while I was finishing my fellowship at Johns Hopkins University and working at the Bayview campus under Dr. Fabien Eyal. This has made the book somewhat unique since it was originally written from the perspective of two programs. Over the years this fact, along with the addition of other authors from around the United States and the world, helps to diversify our contributors and provide a more varied overview of the field.

In this seventh edition we reformatted the table of contents to make it more user friendly and hopefully more logical. Section I includes "Fetal Assessment," "Obstetric Anesthesia and the Neonate," "Resuscitation of the Newborn," and "Infant Transport." Section II encompasses basic assessment and management of a newborn. Section III includes advanced management such as the evolving areas of complementary and alternative medical therapies and bioethics in neonatology. Section IV includes all the basic and advanced procedures commonly used in neonatology, and new chapters include "Transillumination," "Therapeutic Hypothermia," "Laryngeal Mask Airway," "Peripheral IV Extravasation and Infiltration: Initial Management," and "Transpyloric Intubation" was added to the "Gastric Intubation" chapter. One of the most popular sections of the book, the On-Call Problems section, now includes a total of 34 common neonatal problems. "Hematuria" was added as a new on-call problem. Section VI, Diseases and Disorders, covers all the common and a few not so common, but clinically important, diseases of the neonate. We have added new chapters on coagulation disorders, transient neonatal myasthenia gravis, pertussis, and tuberculosis. The section on neonatal pharmacology includes significant updates of medications for neonates. We believe it to be the most comprehensive list of medications found in a manual such as ours. The "Effects of Drugs and Substances on Lactation and Infants" chapter has been revised to include the most common medications that might be used by a breast-feeding mother. The appendices include other useful reference tables and information. A hallmark of our book has been noting areas that are **controversial**, and this edition continues that tradition.

In addition to completely updating each chapter we have added several new clinically important areas such as pain management in the neonate. Several years ago, the concept of neonatal pain was occasionally mentioned, but definitive treatment plans did not exist. Since the American Academy of Pediatrics (AAP) has produced pain management guidelines for certain procedures, we have also added pain management in each procedure where appropriate. This addition provides AAP recommendations and also covers some recommendations from other countries. We have also added a chapter on "Pain in the Neonate" in Section III. The chapter "Sedation and Analgesia" goes over pain and sedation issues when on call. Also new to this edition are 21 color plates of common and not so common pictures of neonatal rashes and disorders. This corresponds to our chapter, "Rash and Dermatologic Problems."

Another exciting ongoing aspect of this manual is its global reach. As we have a growing number of readers all over the world, we have added an international editorial board of physicians. They are from Poland, the Netherlands, the Philippines, Finland, Japan, India, Canada, and Australia. These physicians, along with our many international contributors, help to make the manual a useful reference worldwide. The manual has been translated into 12 different languages over the last 25 years. These translations include Russian, Spanish,

Portuguese, Polish, Chinese (short and long form), Turkish, Greek, Yugoslavian (now Serbian), Italian, Hungarian, and Korean.

I would like to thank Drs. Doug Cunningham and Fabien Eyal, my valued mentors and associate editors; Dr. Deborah Tuttle, my consulting editor; Dr. Barbara McKinney, who put together an excellent pharmacology and breast-feeding section; and all the contributors to this and previous editions of the book. In addition to their long-term commitment to this manual, the associate editors have brought together outstanding authors from all over the United States and the international community. Dr. Deborah Tuttle's extensive clinical experience brings unique perspectives from a different neonatal unit. I also express appreciation to Louise Bierig, Alyssa Fried, Harriet Lebowitz, and the editorial and production staff at McGraw-Hill and their colleagues abroad (especially Arushi Chawla) for their extensive assistance during the 2-year journey to complete this new edition. A special thanks to my husband, Lenny, who helped me extensively concerning matters of editorial content, and my awesome children, Leonard, Patrick, Andrew, and Michael, who helped troubleshoot computer issues and tolerated many sacrifices while I worked on the book. Michael often served as our "house chef" for many nights when the book required work into late hours. Andrew provided a level of expertise concerning graphics, imaging, and IT issues. Patrick provided advice from a medical student perspective. Leonard provided moral support by Skype from China.

Please visit our web site, www.neonatologybook.com, for additional information on this book and for links to enhanced online content for images in this edition, indicated by the symbol [✿]. Any suggestions and comments about this manual are always welcome.

Tricia Lacy Gomella, MD
editor@neonatologybook.com

1 Fetal Assessment

PRENATAL DIAGNOSIS

Prenatal diagnosis refers to those testing modalities used during pregnancy to screen and diagnose fetal aneuploidies and anomalies.

I. **Nuchal translucency (NT).** An ultrasound measurement of the amount of fluid behind the neck of the fetus, best done between 10 3/7 and 13 6/7 weeks. An increase in the NT correlates with an elevated risk for chromosomal abnormalities such as trisomy 21 or 18. In addition, those gestations with increased NT have an elevated risk of adverse pregnancy outcomes, including fetal cardiac defects and intrauterine fetal demise, even when karyotype is normal. A measurement of NT alone has a low detection rate for trisomy 18 and 21; therefore, it is not recommended as a sole screening test for aneuploidy.

II. **Combined first-trimester screening.** Nuchal translucency combined with a measurement of the maternal serum markers, free beta human chorionic gonadotropin (free β-hCG) and pregnancy-associated plasma protein A (PAPP-A), is used to calculate the risk for trisomies 18 and 21. It is performed between 10 3/7 and 13 6/7 weeks' gestation. It is an effective screening tool, with a detection rate of 82–87% for trisomy 21 at a 5% false-positive screen rate. Free β-hCG is elevated and PAPP-A is decreased in a pregnancy affected by Down syndrome.

III. **Second-trimester screening.** The quadruple screen (Quad screen) involves analyzing levels of maternal serum alpha fetoprotein (MSAFP), total hCG, unconjugated estriol, and inhibin A between 15 and 21 weeks' gestation to calculate the risk for trisomies 18 and 21. In addition, it provides a risk assessment for open neural tube defects. For patients who present after 13 6/7 weeks or choose not to undergo first-trimester screening, the Quad screen is an option. In a pregnancy affected by Down syndrome, both MSAFP and unconjugated estriol are low and hCG and inhibin A are elevated. The Quad screen has a detection rate of 81% for Down syndrome at a 5% false-positive rate. Like first-trimester screening, the Quad screen requires an invasive test to confirm the diagnosis of a chromosomal abnormality (ie, amniocentesis or chorionic villous sampling [CVS]). For those patients who chose to undergo first-trimester screening and/or CVS, neural tube defect screening in the form of a second-trimester MSAFP level should be offered. The MSAFP is elevated in the presence of an open neural tube defect. Evidence exists that focused ultrasound during the second trimester is an effective tool for detecting an open neural tube defect.

IV. **Integrated screening and sequential screening (independent, step wise, and contingent).** These options involve a combination of first- and second-trimester screening.

   A. **Integrated screen.** The NT and maternal serum levels of PAPP-A are obtained in the first trimester, and the Quad screen is obtained in the second trimester. When the test does not include an NT measurement it is called **serum integrated**. With both full-integrated screening and serum screening the results are reported when all the tests are completed, yielding a detection rate for Down syndrome of 94% and 87%, respectively, at a 5% false-positive rate.

   B. **Sequential screening.** NT, PAPP-A, and free β-hCG are measured in the first trimester followed by a Quad screen in the second trimester. With the **independent approach**, results are given after the first trimester, and women with an increased risk are offered invasive testing. If there's a low risk, a second-trimester screening is completed and interpreted independently of first-trimester results with a high false-positive rate of 11% at a detection rate of 94%. With the **step-wise approach**, those patients determined to be at high risk after the first-trimester screenings are offered invasive testing. Otherwise, the second-trimester portion is completed and the results are given and combined with those in the first trimester. The detection rate is 95% at a 5% false-positive rate. The **contingent approach** does the first-trimester portion of the sequential testing and follows with the Quad screen when an elevated risk is noted. Those at intermediate risk complete the second portion. However, those at low risk do not undergo further testing. **The contingent sequential screening has an excellent detection rate and a low false-positive rate, and it is the most cost-effective screening tool for trisomy 21.**

V. **Ultrasound testing.** Uterine ultrasound examination is used in the following circumstances:

  A. **Determination of pregnancy viability.** Fetal heart motion can be detected at 6 weeks' gestation by an abdominal scan and a few days earlier by transvaginal ultrasound. Once the **crown-rump length (CRL)** is ≥5 mm, fetal heart motion should be seen. Ultrasound is also used in the case of a suspected fetal demise later in pregnancy.

  B. **Calculation of gestational age.** Measurement of the **CRL between 6 and 14 weeks' gestation allows for the most accurate assessment of gestational age,** to within 5 days. After the first trimester, a combination of biparietal diameter, head circumference, abdominal circumference, and femur length is used to estimate gestational age and fetal weight. Measurements in the second trimester are accurate to within ~10–14 days and in the third trimester to within 14–21 days. See also Chapter 5.

  C. **Diagnosis of multiple pregnancy and determination of chorionicity and amnionicity.** The determination of chorionicity and amnionicity is made by ultrasound examination of the fetal membranes and is best done as early as possible in the first trimester but after 6 weeks' and prior to 14 weeks' gestation.

  D. **Anatomic survey.** A large number of congenital anomalies can be diagnosed reliably by ultrasonography, including anencephaly, hydrocephalus, congenital heart defects, gastroschisis, omphalocele, spina bifida, renal anomalies, diaphragmatic hernia, cleft lip and palate, and skeletal dysplasia. Identification of these anomalies before birth can help determine the safest method of delivery and the support personnel needed at delivery. Ultrasonography can also aid in determining fetal gender for patients in whom this determination impacts the likelihood of a known X-linked genetic disorder.

  E. **Visual guidance.** Ultrasound is used for guidance during procedures such as amniocentesis, CVS, percutaneous umbilical blood sampling (PUBS), and some fetal surgeries (eg, placement of bladder or chest shunts).

  F. **Assessment of growth and fetal weight.** Ultrasonography is useful to detect and monitor both intrauterine growth restriction (IUGR; defined as an estimated fetal weight <10%) and fetal macrosomia (estimated fetal weight >4500 g). Evidence is accumulating that maternal physical size and race should be considered in customizing the fetal weight for determination of IUGR. Estimation of fetal weight is also important in counseling patients regarding expectations after delivering a premature infant. Ultrasound assessment for fetal weight by an experienced sonographer is accurate within 10–20% of actual weight.

  G. **Assessment of amniotic fluid volume.** Amniotic fluid volume may be assessed objectively with ultrasound by measuring the **maximum vertical pocket (MVP) or amniotic fluid index** (**AFI**: total of cord-free deepest vertical pockets in four quadrants) in centimeters.

    1. **Oligohydramnios.** Defined as an AFI of <5 cm, AFI <10% for gestational age, or MVP <2 cm. Oligohydramnios is associated with increased fetal morbidity, and mortality with spontaneous rupture of membranes as the most common cause.

Other causes include placental insufficiency, chronic hypertension, postdates gestation, and fetal anomalies such as renal agenesis, bladder outlet obstruction, cardiac disease, and karyotypic abnormalities.

2. **Polyhydramnios.** Defined as an AFI >25 cm, AFI >95% for gestational age, or MVP >8 cm. Causes of polyhydramnios include diabetes, multiple gestation with twin-twin transfusion syndrome, nonimmune hydrops, and fetal anomalies such as open neural tube defects, cardiac diseases, and gastrointestinal obstruction. Most cases of polyhydramnios are idiopathic; however, the risk for fetal anomalies increases with the severity of the polyhydramnios.

H. **Assessment of placental location and presence of retroplacental hemorrhage.** This is useful in suspected cases of placenta previa or accreta. Most cases of abruptio placentae are not diagnosed by ultrasonography because abruption is a clinical diagnosis.

I. **Assessment of fetal well-being**

1. **Biophysical profile.** Ultrasonography is used to assess fetal movements, fetal breathing, fetal tone, and amniotic fluid volume. See biophysical profile under antepartum tests of fetal well-being (Table 1–1).

2. **Doppler studies.** Doppler ultrasonography of fetal vessels, particularly the **umbilical artery**, is a useful adjunct in the management of high-risk pregnancies, especially those complicated by IUGR. Changes in the vascular Doppler pattern (ie, increased systolic/diastolic ratios and absent or reversed end-diastolic flow in the umbilical artery) signal elevations in placental vascular resistance. These abnormalities correlate with an increased risk for perinatal morbidity and mortality. In high-risk pregnancies, assessment of the **middle cerebral artery** is useful for evaluating for the presence of fetal anemia, and Doppler assessment of the uterine artery may be useful in the prediction and evaluation of preeclampsia. The overall use of Doppler ultrasonography has been associated with a 29% decrease in perinatal mortality and fewer inductions of labor and cesarean deliveries in high-risk pregnancies; however, no benefit in using this technique has been demonstrated in screening a low-risk population.

VI. **Amniocentesis.** Amniotic fluid can be analyzed for prenatal diagnosis of karyotypic abnormalities, genetic disorders (for which testing is available), fetal blood type and hemoglobinopathies, fetal lung maturity, and monitoring the degree of isoimmunization by measurement of the content of bilirubin in the fluid, and for the diagnosis of chorioamnionitis. Testing for karyotypic abnormalities is usually done at 16–20 weeks' gestation. A sample of amniotic fluid is removed under ultrasound guidance. Fetal cells in the fluid can be grown in tissue culture for genetic study. With visual guidance from the ultrasound, the pregnancy loss rate related to amniocentesis is usually quoted at between 1 per 200 and 1 per 1600. Early amniocentesis (before 14 weeks) is generally not recommended because it is associated with a significantly higher rate of fetal loss

Table 1–1. BIOPHYSICAL PROFILE

Variable	Normal Response (2 points)
Fetal breathing	≥1 episode of continuous breathing movement of at least 30 seconds
Fetal gross body movements	≥3 body or limb movements
Fetal tone	≥1 extension of fetal extremity or spine with return to flexion, or opening of fetal hand
Amniotic fluid	≥1 pocket of amniotic fluid of >2 cm in two perpendicular planes
Nonstress test	Reactive

and limb deformities. Indications for amniocentesis include women at an increased risk of aneuploidy, either by history or abnormal first- or second-trimester screening tests; women with prior children with a chromosomal abnormality; suspected X-linked disorder; autosomal recessive disorders when both parents are carriers of the trait in question; and evaluation of inborn errors of metabolism.

VII. **Chorionic villus sampling.** CVS is usually performed between 10 and 12 weeks' gestation. Chorionic villi are withdrawn from the placenta, either through a needle inserted through the abdomen or through a trans-cervical catheter, and the cells obtained are grown and analyzed. Indications are the same as those for amniocentesis. Pregnancy loss rates after CVS are similar to those for amniocentesis but are highly operator dependent. CVS is generally not recommended prior to 10 weeks' gestation due to the increased rate of limb anomalies reported.

VIII. **Percutaneous umbilical blood sampling.** Under ultrasound guidance, a needle is placed transabdominally into the fetal umbilical artery or vein. Samples of fetal blood can be obtained for karyotype, viral studies, fetal blood type, hematocrit, or platelet count. This also provides a route for in utero transfusion of red blood cells or platelets. PUBS is most often used in cases of severe hemolytic disease of the fetus with or without hydrops, such as that due to Rh or atypical antibody isoimmunization.

ANTEPARTUM TESTS OF FETAL WELL-BEING

Antepartum testing refers to those testing modalities used during pregnancy to assess fetal health and identify fetuses at risk for poor pregnancy outcome.

I. **Nonstress test (NST).** The nonstress test is a simple noninvasive test used to check fetal well-being by measuring the heart rate in response to fetal movements. Fetal well-being is confirmed if the baseline heart rate is normal and there are periodic accelerations in the fetal heart rate. The following guidelines can be used, although there may be variations between institutions.

   A. **Reactive NST.** In a 20-minute monitoring period, there are ≥2 accelerations of the fetal heart rate 15 beats/min above the baseline, each lasting at least 15 seconds. In a fetus <32 weeks' gestation, the accelerations must reach 10 beats/min above the baseline and last at least 10 seconds. The perinatal mortality within 1 week after a reactive NST is ~1.9 per 1000.

   B. **Nonreactive NST.** Fetal heart rate does not meet the established criteria during a prolonged period of monitoring (usually at least 1 hour). There are many causes of a nonreactive NST besides fetal compromise, including fetal sleep cycle, chronic maternal smoking, and exposure to medications such as central nervous system depressants and propranolol. Because of this low specificity (the false-positive rate is ~75–90%), a nonreactive NST should be followed by more definitive testing such as a biophysical profile or a contraction stress test.

II. **Biophysical profile (BPP).** The biophysical profile is another test used to assess fetal well-being. It involves performing an NST to assess fetal heart rate and ultrasound over 30 minutes to assess fetal breathing movements, gross body movements, tone, and amniotic fluid index (AFI).Two points are given for each variable if present and zero if absent during the observation period (see Table 1–1). A score of 8–10 is considered normal, 6 is equivocal and warrants a repeat BPP in 24 hours, and 0–4 is abnormal with delivery usually indicated. Changes in the BPP parameters are due to fetal hypoxemia. Caution is needed since it can also be affected by other factors such as gestational age, medications, and improper technique. The BPP is widely used among institutions to monitor high-risk pregnancies. However, evidence from randomized clinical trials does not support its use to monitor complicated pregnancies. Institutional variation exists regarding gestational age for performance of BPP, starting as low as 24 weeks, even when its utility has only been studied at higher gestational ages.

   Modified biophysical profile. The BPP scoring system has been modified to shorten testing time. The most common combination includes an evaluation of only an NST and AFI. In some cases, the modified BPP is used as an initial test and if abnormal, it is followed by additional testing including a full BPP. The stillbirth rate within 1 week of a normal BPP or a modified BPP is the same at 0.8 per 1000.

III. **Contraction stress test (CST).** The CST is used to assess a fetus at risk for uteroplacental insufficiency. The fetal heart rate and uterine contractions are continuously monitored. An adequate test consists of three 40- to 60-second contractions within a period of 10 minutes. If sufficient contractions do not occur spontaneously, oxytocin or nipple stimulation may be used. If oxytocin is needed to produce contractions for the CST, it is called the **oxytocin challenge test (OCT)**. If late decelerations occur during or after contractions, uteroplacental insufficiency may be present. The CST may be contraindicated in patients with placenta previa, those who have had a previous cesarean section with a vertical incision, and those with high-risk factors for preterm delivery (eg, premature rupture of membranes or cervical insufficiency). Test results are interpreted as follows:

A. **Negative (normal) test.** No late decelerations occur. This result is associated with a very low perinatal mortality rate of 0.3 per 1000 in the week following the test.

B. **Positive (abnormal) test.** Late decelerations occur with at least 50% of the contractions. This result is associated with an increased risk of perinatal morbidity or mortality and indicates that delivery is usually warranted.

C. **Equivocal (suspicious) test.** Late decelerations occur but with <50% of the contractions. Prolonged fetal monitoring is usually recommended, and the CST should be repeated in 24 hours.

IV. **Doppler studies.** See Doppler studies under prenatal diagnosis section.

V. **Fetal movement counting.** Maternal perception of fetal movement has been proposed as a tool to evaluate fetal well-being. Different methods have been evaluated including "the count to 10," which involves counting 10 fetal movements over 2 hours during maternal rest. Other approaches include counts for some period of time each day or some days per week. However, results from different studies in the literature are mixed, and the utility of maternal kick counts to predict stillbirth is *controversial*. Maternal reports of abnormal fetal counting warrants further evaluation.

INTRAPARTUM TESTS OF FETAL WELL-BEING

Intrapartum testing refers to those testing modalities used during labor to identify fetuses at risk for acidosis, adverse neonatal outcome, or death.

I. **Electronic fetal heart rate monitoring (EFM).** Although EFM has become widely used, its benefits over intermittent auscultation of the fetal heart rate have been *controversial*. It was not until recently that EFM was associated with a decrease in early infant and neonatal mortality, a decreased risk for Apgar scores <4 at 5 minutes, and a decreased risk of neonatal seizures. EFM is associated with an increase in the rates of both cesarean sections and operative vaginal deliveries. Fetal heart rate monitoring may be **internal**, with an electrode attached to the fetal scalp, or **external**, with a monitor attached to the maternal abdomen. The nomenclature and interpretation of EFM are based on the 2008 National Institute of Child Health and Human Development (NICHD) workshop report:

A. **Baseline fetal heart rate.** The baseline fetal heart rate (FHR) is the rate maintained for at least 2 minutes apart from periodic variations, rounded to the nearest 5 beats/min over a 10-minute period. The normal FHR is 110–160 beats/min. Fetal tachycardia is present at >160 beats/min and fetal bradycardia at <110 beats/min. Causes of fetal tachycardia include maternal or fetal infection, fetal hypoxia, thyrotoxicosis, and maternal use of drugs such as parasympathetic blockers or β-mimetic agents. Causes of bradycardia include hypoxia, complete heart block, and maternal use of drugs such as β-blockers.

B. **Variability.** In the normal mature fetus there are rapid fluctuations in the baseline FHR. This variability indicates a functioning sympathetic–parasympathetic nervous system interaction and is the most sensitive indicator of fetal well-being. An amplitude range from peak to trough of 6–25 beats/min indicates moderate variability and suggests the absence of fetal hypoxia. Marked variability occurs when >25 beats/min is noted. **Minimal variability** is quantified as <5 beats/min; **absent variability** refers to an amplitude range that is undetectable. **Decreased variability** may be caused by severe hypoxia, anencephaly and other fetal neurologic abnormalities, complete heart block, and maternal use of drugs such as narcotics or magnesium sulfate. In addition, variability is decreased during normal fetal sleep cycles.

C. **Accelerations.** Accelerations are often associated with fetal movement and are an indication of fetal well-being. The presence of accelerations suggests the absence of any acidosis.

D. **Decelerations.** There are three types of decelerations (Figure 1–1).

1. **Early decelerations.** Early decelerations result from physiologic head compression and occur secondary to an intact vagal reflex tone, which follows minor,

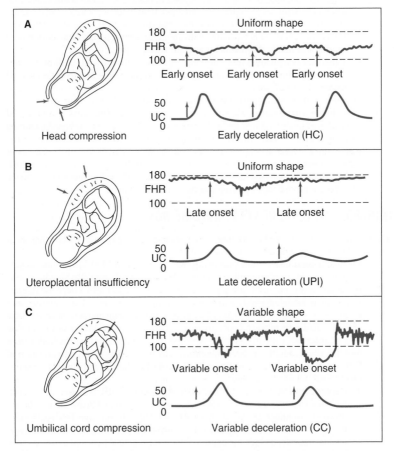

FIGURE 1–1. Examples of fetal heart rate monitoring. CC, cord compression; FHR, fetal heart rate (beats/min); HC, head compression; UC, uterine contraction (mm Hg); UPI, uteroplacental insufficiency. (*Modified and reproduced, with permission, from McCrann JR, Schifrin BS. Fetal monitoring in high-risk pregnancy.* Clin Perinatol. *1974;1:149. Copyright Elsevier Science.*)

transient fetal hypoxic episodes. These are benign and are not associated with fetal compromise. They appear as mirror images of the contraction pattern.

2. **Late decelerations.** Late decelerations are a result of uteroplacental insufficiency (UPI) and indicate the presence of fetal hypoxia. Potential causes include maternal hypotension, sometimes as a result of supine positioning or regional anesthesia, as well as uterine hypertonicity. More chronic causes of UPI, such as hypertension, postdate gestation, and preeclampsia may predispose a fetus to the development of late decelerations. Although by themselves they reflect only a decreased oxygen tension for the fetus, their persistence may lead to the development of fetal acidemia and eventual compromise. The nadir occurs after the contraction peaks, with the shape demonstrating a gradual decrease and slow return to baseline.

3. **Variable decelerations.** Variable decelerations result from abrupt compression of the umbilical cord. They can also be seen as a consequence of cord stretch, as in phases of rapid fetal descent, and with a cord prolapse. Variable decelerations tend to increase in the setting of oligohydramnios. The majority of these decelerations are benign and not predictive of an acidemic fetus. However, severe variable decelerations (those lasting >60 seconds), especially in the setting of decreased variability and/or tachycardia, may portend a compromised fetus. They have a V or W nonuniform shape with a rapid descent and return to baseline: time from baseline to the nadir of the deceleration is 30 seconds.

E. **Interpretation of electronic fetal monitoring.** FHR patterns can be classified in one of 3 categories: I (Normal), II (Indeterminate), or III (Abnormal).

1. **Category I FHR pattern.** This has 4 characteristics: normal baseline rate (110–160 beats/min), moderate variability (6–25 beats/min), absence of late or variable decelerations, and absence or presence of early decelerations or accelerations. In the setting of these findings, there is a high likelihood of a normally oxygenated fetus.

2. **Category III FHR pattern.** Conversely, there are 4 FHR patterns predictive of abnormal fetal acid-base status grouped in category III.

   a. **Sinusoidal pattern.** These include a sinusoidal heart rate, defined as a pattern of regular variability resembling a sine wave, with fixed periodicity of 3–5 cycles/min and amplitude of 5–40 beats/min. A sinusoidal pattern may indicate fetal anemia caused by fetomaternal hemorrhage or alloimmunization.

   b. **Baseline FHR variability is absent.** The other three abnormal FHR patterns in category III are diagnosed when **baseline FHR variability is absent** and any one of the following is present:
      i. **Recurrent late decelerations**
      ii. **Recurrent variable decelerations**
      iii. **Bradycardia**

3. **Category II.** Comprises all FHR patterns not in category I or III. Category II tracings are not predictive of abnormal fetal acid-base status. When a category II tracing is identified, a fetal scalp stimulation test may help identify fetuses in which acid-base status is normal.

II. **Fetal scalp blood sampling.** FHR had been used during labor to determine the fetal acid-base status when the FHR tracing was nonreassuring or equivocal. Many practitioners have little experience in obtaining the sample, and noninvasive methods (vibroacoustic and fetal scalp stimulation) provide similar reassurance. Therefore, it is not commonly used in clinical care.

III. **Scalp stimulation/vibroacoustic stimulation.** An acceleration in FHR in response to either manual stimulation of the fetal presenting part or vibroacoustic stimulation through the maternal abdomen has been associated with a fetal pH of >7.20. These tests are often used in labor to determine fetal well-being; however, a lack of fetal response to stimulation is not predictive of acidemia.

IV. **Fetal pulse oximetry.** This technique was designed as an adjunct to FHR monitoring in labor and involves the placement of a fetal pulse oximeter transcervically next to the fetal cheek. Normal fetal oxygen saturation as measured by pulse oximetry (**Spo$_2$**) is 30–70%. Due to the lack of clinical significance it is currently not recommended.

TESTS OF FETAL LUNG MATURITY

I. **Testing strategies.** Fetal lung maturity testing is recommended when considering delivery at <39 weeks unless clinically indicated for maternal/fetal reasons. Testing at <32 weeks is not recommended since most likely it will be immature. A mature result from any fetal lung maturity test indicates a very low likelihood of neonatal respiratory distress syndrome (RDS). The positive predictive value of all of the tests is poor, ranging from 30 to 60%, implying that an immature result does not correlate well to the presence of RDS. The choice and availability of tests for fetal lung maturity are institution dependent.

II. **Lecithin-sphingomyelin (L-S) ratio.** Lecithin is a phospholipid that can be measured specifically in amniotic fluid. It is a principal active component of surfactant and is manufactured by type II alveolar cells. Sphingomyelin is a phospholipid found predominantly in body tissues other than the lungs. The L-S ratio compares levels of lecithin, which gradually increase after 28 weeks, to levels of sphingomyelin, which remain constant. **An L-S ratio ≥2:0 is considered mature.**

Some disorders are associated with delayed lung maturation including diabetes mellitus and Rh isoimmunization complicated by fetal hydrops. Acceleration of fetal lung maturity is seen in sickle cell disease, maternal narcotic addiction, prolonged rupture of membranes, chronic maternal hypertension, IUGR, and smoking. Differences may also occur in various racial groups. The L-S ratio measurement can be affected by the presence of blood or meconium. In addition, the L-S ratio is costly, difficult to perform, and time-consuming compared with other available tests.

III. **Phosphatidylglycerol (PG).** Phosphatidylglycerol appears in amniotic fluid at ~35 weeks, and levels increase at 37–40 weeks. This substance is a useful marker for lung maturation late in pregnancy because it is the last surfactant to appear in the fetal lung. It is reported as either **present or absent**, and its presence is a strong marker that RDS will not occur. PG levels are not affected by blood or meconium contamination and can also be performed on vaginal pool specimens from patients who have ruptured membranes.

IV. **Surfactant/albumin ratio by TDx fetal lung maturity (TDx FLM II).** This test (Abbott Laboratories, Abbott Park, IL) measures the relative concentrations of surfactant and albumin (milligrams of surfactant per gram of albumin) in amniotic fluid, which increases with increasing lung maturity. Like the L-S ratio, blood and meconium can interfere with the results. **A value ≤39 mg/g is considered immature, 40–54 mg/g is indeterminate, and ≥55 mg/g is mature.** TDx FLM II has several advantages over the L-S ratio: less technical expertise is required, it is performed more easily, and results are available quicker. Unfortunately, this test will no longer be available since it has been discontinued by the manufacturer.

V. **Lamellar body count (LBC).** After its secretion by type II pneumocytes, surfactant is packaged into storage granules called lamellar bodies. This test uses a standard hematologic cell counter to count these lamellar bodies. **A count >50,000 per microliter suggests lung maturity.** Like the TDx FLM II, this test provides quicker results and is easier to perform than the L-S ratio at an equal or better sensitivity. Both blood and meconium can affect the interpretation of this test.

CORD BLOOD BANKING

Stem cells from the umbilical cord are collected after the baby is born and are stored by private or public cord blood banks. The family is given a collection kit to bring on the day of delivery. The delivering provider typically collects the blood after the baby is delivered. After the umbilical cord has been clamped, the blood is drawn with a needle that transfers the blood into a bag that is sealed after the collection is completed. The sample is then taken to the cord blood bank. Parents can opt for cord blood banking, understanding the benefits and limitations; however, it is not universally recommended. Private cord blood banking should be considered when there is a family member with a known condition that can be treated with a hematopoietic transplant. The cells can potentially be used to treat some diseases with an estimated chance of an individual using his or her own cells of 1:2700. However, some diseases including inborn errors of metabolism and genetic diseases cannot be treated in the same individual since the cells contain the mutation.

Selected References

Alfirevic Z, Stampalija T, Gyte GM. Fetal and umbilical Doppler ultrasound in high-risk pregnancies. *Cochrane Database Syst Rev.* 2010;1:CD007529.

American College of Obstetricians and Gynecologists. ACOG Committee Opinion, No. 399: Umbilical cord blood banking. *Obstet Gynecol.* 2008;111:475–477.

American College of Obstetricians and Gynecologists. ACOG Practice Bulletin, No. 9: Antepartum fetal surveillance. *Obstet Gynecol.* 1999;93(2):285–291.

American College of Obstetricians and Gynecologists. ACOG Practice Bulletin, No. 70: Intrapartum fetal heart rate monitoring: nomenclature, interpretation, and general management principles. *Obstet Gynecol.* 2005;106:1453–1460.

American College of Obstetricians and Gynecologists. ACOG Practice Bulletin, No. 97: Fetal lung maturity. *Obstet Gynecol.* 2008;112(3):717–726.

Ball RH, Caughey AB, Malone FD, et al. First- and second-trimester evaluation of risk for Down syndrome. *Obstet Gynecol.* 2007;110:10–17.

Chen HY, Chauhan SP, Ananth CV, Vintzileos AM, Abuhamad AZ. Electronic fetal heart rate monitoring and its relationship to neonatal and infant mortality in the United States. *Am J Obstet Gynecol.* 2011;204(6):491.e1–491.e10.

Lalor JG, Fawole B, Alfirevic Z, Devane D. Biophysical profile for fetal assessment in high-risk pregnancies. Review. *Cochrane Database Syst Rev.* 2008;2:CD000038.

Macones GA, Hankins GD, Spong CY, Hauth J, Moore T. The 2008 National Institute of Child Health and Human Development workshop report on electronic fetal monitoring: update on definitions, interpretation, and research guidelines. *Obstet Gynecol.* 2008;112:661–666.

Malone FD, Canick JA, Ball RH, et al. First-trimester or second-trimester screening, or both, for Down's syndrome. *N Engl J Med.* 2005;353:2001–2011.

2 Obstetric Anesthesia and the Neonate

During birth, the status of the fetus can be influenced by obstetric analgesia and anesthesia. Care in choosing analgesic and anesthetic agents can often prevent respiratory depression in the newborn, especially in high-risk deliveries.

I. Placental transfer of drugs. Drugs administered to the mother may affect the fetus via placental transfer or may cause a maternal disorder that affects the fetus (eg, maternal drug-induced hypotension producing fetal hypoxia). All anesthetic and analgesic drugs cross the placenta to some degree. Flow-dependent passive diffusion is the usual mechanism.

Most anesthetic and analgesic drugs have a high degree of lipid solubility, low molecular weight (<500), and variable protein-binding and ionization capabilities.

These characteristics lead to rapid placental transfer. Local anesthetics and narcotics (lipid-soluble, unionized) cross the placenta easily; neuromuscular blocking agents (highly ionized) do not.

II. **Analgesia in labor**

A. **Inhalation analgesia.** Inhalation analgesia is rarely used in the United States as a result of the wide availability of regional anesthesia (**Note:** Entonox, a mixture of 50% oxygen and 50% nitrous oxide, is used outside the United States). In addition, several problems associated with inhalational anesthesia limit its routine use:

1. **The need for specialized vaporizers**
2. **Potential pollution of the labor and delivery environment** with waste anesthetic gases
3. **Incomplete analgesia**
4. **Maternal childbirth amnesia**
5. **Possible loss of maternal protective airway reflexes** and pulmonary aspiration of gastric contents

B. **Pudendal block and paracervical block.** Paracervical blocks are rarely used today because they may precipitate severe fetal bradycardia or increased uterine activity or cause a direct vasoconstrictive effect of the local anesthetic, resulting in decreased uteroplacental/fetoplacental perfusion. If a paracervical block is performed, the fetal heart rate (FHR) must be monitored. Paracervical blocks are effective in the first stage of labor, and pudendal blocks are effective during the second stage. Pudendal blocks have little direct effect on the fetus; however, seizures have been reported after both.

C. **Opioids.** All intravenously administered opioids are rapidly transferred to the fetus and cause dose-related respiratory depression and alterations in Apgar and neurobehavioral scores.

1. **Meperidine.** Meperidine can cause severe neonatal depression (measured by Apgar scoring) if the drug is administered 2–3 hours before delivery as a result of maximum fetal uptake. Depression is manifested as respiratory acidosis, decreased oxygen saturation, decreased minute ventilation, and increased time to sustained respiration. Fetal normeperidine, a long-acting meperidine metabolite and significant respiratory depressant, accumulates after multiple doses or a prolonged dose-delivery interval.
2. **Morphine.** Morphine has a delayed onset of action and may generate greater neonatal respiratory depression than meperidine.
3. **Butorphanol and nalbuphine.** These are agonist-antagonist narcotic agents that may be safer than morphine because they demonstrate a ceiling effect for respiratory depression with increasing doses. Unlike butorphanol, maternal administration of nalbuphine can result in decreased FHR variability, sinusoidal FHR patterns, fetal tachycardia, and fetal bradycardia.
4. **Fentanyl and remifentanil.** These are synthetic opioids, best administered via patient-controlled analgesia during labor. Both are short acting and have no active metabolites. Fentanyl may cause low 1-minute Apgar scores, but neonatal neurobehavioral scores are normal. Remifentanil requires careful monitoring and one-on-one maternal nursing care.

D. **Opioid antagonist (naloxone).** Naloxone should *never* be administered to neonates of women who have received *chronic* opioid therapy because it may precipitate acute withdrawal symptoms. It can be used to reverse respiratory depression caused by *acute* maternal opioid administration during labor.

E. **Sedatives and tranquilizers**

1. **Barbiturates.** Barbiturates cross the placenta rapidly and can have pronounced neonatal effects (somnolence, flaccidity, hypoventilation, failure to feed) that may last for days. Effects are intensified if opioids are used simultaneously. This is rarely an issue when barbiturates are used to induce general anesthesia for an emergent cesarean delivery. Barbiturates rapidly redistribute into maternal

tissues before placental transfer and, when they cross the placenta, are preferentially uptaken by the fetal liver.

2. **Benzodiazepines (diazepam, lorazepam, and midazolam).** These agents promptly cross the placenta and equilibrate within minutes after intravenous administration. Fetal levels are often higher than maternal levels. Diazepam given in low doses (<10 mg) may cause decreased beat-to-beat variability and tone, but has little effect on Apgar scores and blood gas levels. Larger doses of diazepam may persist for days and can result in hypotonia, lethargy, poor feeding, and impaired thermoregulation. Benzodiazepines are not frequently administered during labor because they induce maternal childbirth amnesia.

3. **Phenothiazines.** Phenothiazines are rarely used today because they may produce hypotension via central α-blockade, but are sometimes combined with a narcotic (neuroleptanalgesia).

4. **Ketamine.** Ketamine induces dissociative analgesia. Doses >1 mg/kg may cause uterine hypertonia, neonatal depression (low Apgar scores), and abnormal neonatal muscle tone. Doses normally used in labor (0.1–0.2 mg/kg) are relatively safe, producing minimal maternal or neonatal effects.

F. **Lumbar epidural analgesia.** Lumbar epidural analgesia is the most frequently used neuraxial anesthetic technique for childbirth. Maternal pain and catecholamine levels are reduced, decreasing maternal hyperventilation and improving fetal oxygen delivery (excessive catecholamines can cause prolonged incoordinate labor and decreased uterine blood flow). Vasospasm of uterine arteries, common in preeclampsia, may be lessened. Labor epidural analgesia lasting >4 hours is associated with benign maternal temperature increases of up to 1°C. Unfortunately, this may lead to unnecessary neonatal sepsis evaluations.

Local anesthetic (eg, bupivacaine, ropivacaine) is injected incrementally and/or infused continuously through an epidural catheter placed in a lumbar (L2–3, L3–4, L4–5) interspace to block the T10–L1 and S2–S4 spinal cord segments. Small doses of an opioid may be added as well; these have little effect on the neonate. Maternal hypotension caused by sympathetic blockade is easily treated with fluid administration and/or intravenous ephedrine.

G. **Intrathecal opioid analgesia/combined spinal epidural.** Intrathecal opioids (sufentanil or fentanyl ± morphine) provide rapid labor analgesia with minimal motor and sympathetic blockade. They are usually administered in combination with an epidural (combined spinal epidural; CSE) via a "needle-through-needle" technique (spinal needle through epidural needle, opioid injected, epidural catheter placed). When intrathecal analgesia recedes, epidural analgesia takes over. Indications include early first-stage labor (opioid alone) or when labor is very advanced (opioid + bupivacaine). Transient FHR changes occur in 10–15% of cases, usually without adverse neonatal outcomes.

H. **Caudal epidural analgesia.** Caudal epidural analgesia blocks the sacral nerve roots and provides excellent pain relief in the second stage of labor. Use is limited during the first stage because the larger doses of local anesthetic needed increase pelvic muscle relaxation and impair fetal head rotation. Fetal intracranial local anesthetic injection can occur also.

I. **Continuous spinal analgesia.** A catheter is placed directly into the spinal space either through or over the top of an introducer needle. Usually the introducer is large, making the incidence of spinal headache unacceptably high. An infusion of opioid (fentanyl or sufentanil) ± bupivacaine is maintained throughout labor. The catheter may be readily dosed for emergent cesarean delivery.

J. **Local anesthetics.** All of the neuraxial anesthetic/analgesic techniques (eg, epidural, spinal) and local blocks (eg, pudendal, paracervical) depend on the use of local anesthetic agents.

1. **Lidocaine.** Placental transfer of lidocaine is significant, but Apgar scores are not affected in healthy neonates. Acidotic fetuses accumulate larger amounts of lidocaine through pH-induced ion trapping.

2. **Bupivacaine.** Bupivacaine is theoretically less harmful than lidocaine for the fetus because it has a higher degree of ionization and protein binding. Maternal toxicity leading to convulsions and cardiac arrest has been reported after inadvertent intravascular injection. Bupivacaine, in very low concentrations, is the most commonly used local anesthetic agent for continuous labor analgesia because it provides excellent sensory analgesia with minimal motor blockade.

3. **2-Chloroprocaine.** After systemic absorption, 2-chloroprocaine is rapidly broken down by pseudocholinesterase; therefore, very little reaches the placenta or fetus. However, because of its short duration and significant motor blockade, 2-chloroprocaine is not useful for continuous labor analgesia.

4. **Ropivacaine.** Ropivacaine is similar to bupivacaine but produces less motor block and maternal cardiotoxicity. The Neonatal Neurologic and Adaptive Capacity Score (NACS) is slightly better in infants whose mothers received epidural ropivacaine compared with bupivacaine for labor analgesia.

5. **Levobupivacaine.** Levobupivacaine is the purified levorotary enantiomer of racemic bupivacaine. Like ropivacaine, it has less potential for cardiotoxicity than bupivacaine.

K. **Psychoprophylaxis.** The **Lamaze technique** of prepared childbirth involves class instruction for prospective parents. The process of childbirth is explained, and exercises, breathing skills, and relaxation techniques are taught to relieve labor pain. However, the popular assumption that the neonate benefits if the mother receives no drugs during childbirth may not be true. Pain and discomfort may cause psychological stress and hyperventilation in the mother, which can negatively impact the neonate. Approximately 50–70% of women who have learned the Lamaze method request medications or an anesthetic during labor. Other analgesic techniques include transcutaneous electric nerve stimulation (TENS), hypnosis, and acupuncture.

III. **Anesthesia for cesarean delivery.** Aortocaval compression may decrease placental perfusion if the mother is positioned supine; the bed must be tilted left side down or a wedge placed under the right hip. Regional anesthesia is chosen for most cesarean deliveries because it is usually safer for mother and baby. If immediate delivery is indicated, general anesthesia is often used because it has the shortest induction time.

A. **Spinal anesthesia.** Spinal anesthesia (injection of local anesthetic directly into cerebrospinal fluid) requires one-tenth of the drug needed for epidural anesthesia. Maternal and fetal drug levels are low. Hypotension occurs rapidly but can be attenuated by administering 1.5–2.0 L of a balanced salt solution intravenously and treated with intravenous ephedrine or phenylephrine. Better quality anesthesia, more rapid placement, and faster onset make spinal preferred over epidural anesthesia for cesarean delivery. Abnormalities in neurobehavioral scores are more common after general anesthesia than spinal.

B. **Lumbar epidural anesthesia.** Placental transfer of local anesthetics occurs to a small degree, but drug effects can only be detected by neurobehavioral testing. Maternal hypotension may also occur, as with spinal anesthesia, but more slowly and to a lesser extent.

C. **Combined spinal epidural.** If a cesarean delivery of prolonged duration is anticipated, a CSE may be used. Rapid, good-quality spinal anesthesia is obtained with the ability to initiate epidural anesthesia when the spinal wanes.

D. **General anesthesia.** General anesthesia is used in the following circumstances: strong patient preference, emergency delivery (eg, maternal hemorrhage, fetal bradycardia), and contraindications to regional anesthesia (eg, maternal coagulopathy, neurologic problems, sepsis, infection). After induction, anesthesia is maintained with a combination of nitrous oxide in oxygen and low doses of inhaled halogenated agents or intravenous drugs. Opioids or benzodiazepines are rarely necessary before the cord is clamped.

1. **Agents used in general obstetric anesthesia**
   a. **Premedication.** Cimetidine or ranitidine (H_2 receptor antagonists) may be administered to help prevent aspiration pneumonitis by decreasing gastric volume and increasing gastric pH; metoclopramide speeds gastric emptying. The neonate is not affected by these agents. Premedications traditionally used in surgery (eg, atropinics, opioids, benzodiazepines) are rarely given.
   b. **Propofol.** Propofol (2–2.5 mg/kg), another induction agent, is currently not approved for use in pregnancy, as well-controlled studies in humans have not been done. It rapidly crosses the placenta and distributes into the fetus. Most investigators have reported no difference in Apgar scores or NACS of infants exposed to propofol alone or with other anesthetic agents.
   c. **Ketamine.** Ketamine (1 mg/kg) is typically reserved for induction in severe asthmatics because of its bronchodilator properties and in patients with mild to moderate hypovolemia when cesarean delivery is emergent. Neonatal neurobehavioral scores after ketamine administration are similar to those after thiopental.
   d. **Muscle relaxants.** Muscle relaxants, which are highly ionized, cross the placenta only in small amounts and have little effect on the neonate.
      i. **Succinylcholine.** Succinylcholine crosses the placenta in minimal amounts. In twice-normal doses, it is detectable in the fetus, but no respiratory effects are seen until the dose is 5 times normal or both mother and fetus have abnormal pseudocholinesterase levels or activity.
      ii. **Atracurium, cisatracurium, vecuronium, and rocuronium.** These are medium-duration nondepolarizing muscle relaxants. In clinical doses, an insufficient amount of drug crosses the placenta to affect the neonate.
      iii. **Pancuronium.** Pancuronium is a long-duration muscle relaxant that does not affect the neonate when administered in clinical doses.
   e. **Nitrous oxide.** Nitrous oxide has rapid placental transfer. Prolonged administration of high (>50%) concentrations of nitrous oxide can result in low Apgar scores because of neonatal anesthesia and diffusion hypoxia. Concentrations of up to 50% are safe, but neonates may need supplemental oxygen after delivery.
   f. **Halogenated anesthetic agents (isoflurane, enflurane, sevoflurane, desflurane, and halothane).** These are used to maintain general anesthesia. Beneficial effects include decreased maternal catecholamines, increased uterine blood flow, and improved maternal anesthesia compared with nitrous oxide alone. Low concentrations of these agents rarely cause neonatal anesthesia and are readily exhaled. High concentrations may decrease uterine contractility. The lowest effective concentration is chosen, and the agent is usually discontinued after delivery to decrease uterine atony and prevent excessive blood loss.
2. **Neonatal effects of general anesthesia.** Maternal hypoxia resulting from aspiration or failed endotracheal intubation can cause fetal hypoxia. Maternal hyperventilation ($Paco_2$ <20 mm Hg) decreases placental blood flow and shifts the maternal oxyhemoglobin curve to the left, which can also lead to fetal hypoxia and acidosis.
3. **Interval between incision of the uterus and delivery.** Incision and manipulation of the uterus produces reflex uterine vasoconstriction, which may result in fetal asphyxia. Long intervals between uterine incision and delivery (>90 seconds) are associated with significant lowering of Apgar scores. If the interval is >180 seconds, low Apgar scores and fetal acidosis could result. Regional anesthesia decreases reflex vasoconstriction, so the incision-to-delivery interval is less important. The interval may be prolonged with a breech, multiple gestation, or preterm delivery; uterine scarring; or a large fetus.

4. **Regional versus general anesthesia**
   a. **Apgar scores.** Early studies showed that neonates were less depressed at 1- and 5-minute Apgar scores when regional rather than general anesthesia was used. New general anesthetic techniques lower Apgar scores at 1 minute only. This represents transient sedation (temporary neonatal general anesthesia), not asphyxia. If the interval between induction and delivery is short, the difference between regional and general anesthesia is less, but regional anesthesia is preferred if a prolonged delivery time is anticipated. However, low Apgar scores from sedation do not have the negative prognostic value that low Apgar scores from asphyxia do, provided the neonate is adequately resuscitated.
   b. **Acid-base status.** The differences in acid-base status are minimal and probably not significant. Infants of diabetic mothers may be less acidotic with general than with regional anesthesia because regional anesthesia-induced hypotension may exacerbate any existing uteroplacental insufficiency.
   c. **Neurobehavioral examinations.** These are used to detect subtle changes in the neonate during the first few hours after birth. The goal is to detect central nervous system depression from drugs and to differentiate it from effects associated with birth trauma and perinatal asphyxia. Neonates are complex, and using only one assessment tool (Apgar score, acid-base balance, neurobehavioral testing) cannot predict developmental outcome.
      i. **The Brazelton Neonatal Behavioral Assessment Scale (NBAS).** Developed in 1973, this scale consists of 47 individual tests; 27 evaluate behavior, and 20 evaluate elicited responses. The NBAS evaluates the ability of the newborn to perform complex motor behaviors, to alter its state of arousal, and to suppress meaningless stimuli. However, it requires at least 45 minutes, an experienced examiner, and does not generate a single number indicating a depressed neonate; it is rarely used in the immediate postnatal setting.
      ii. **The Scanlon Early Neonatal Neurobehavioral Scale (ENNS).** Developed in 1974, this scale includes 15 observations of muscle tone, primary reflexes, and decrement response to stimulation; 11 observations on states of consciousness; and one general assessment of neurobehavioral status. It uses noxious stimuli (repeated pin-prick and Moro maneuvers), is complicated, and although faster to perform than the NBAS, still does not yield a single number signifying a depressed neonate.
      iii. **The Neonatal Neurologic and Adaptive Capacity Score (NACS).** This score was developed in 1982 by Amiel-Tison, Barrier, and Shnider and is used worldwide to examine neonatal effects of peripartum medications. The NACS includes 20 criteria to evaluate 5 areas: adaptive capacity (response to sound, habituation to sound, response to light, habituation to light, consolability), passive tone (scarf sign, recoil of elbows, popliteal angle, recoil of lower limbs), active tone (active contraction of neck flexors, active contraction of neck extensors), primary reflexes (palmar grasp, response to traction, supporting reaction, automatic walking, placing reaction, sucking, Moro reflex), and general neurologic status (alertness, crying, motor activity). A single number is generated that immediately identifies a depressed or vigorous neonate. It is rapid (3–15 minutes), simple, and avoids the use of noxious stimuli.

Selected References

Aucott SW, Zuckerman RL. Neonatal assessment and resuscitation. In: Chestnut DH, ed. *Obstetric Anesthesia: Principles and Practice.* 4th ed. Philadelphia, PA: Elsevier; 2009:175–177.

Fernando R, Jones T. Systemic analgesia: parenteral and inhalational agents. In: Chestnut DH, ed. *Obstetric Anesthesia: Principles and Practice.* 4th ed. Philadelphia, PA: Elsevier; 2009:415–427.

Macarthur A, Riley ET. Obstetric anesthesia controversies: vasopressor of choice for postspinal hypotension during cesarean delivery. *Int Anesthesiol Clin.* 2007;45:115–132.

Nelson KE, Rauch T, Terebuh V, D'Angelo R. A comparison of intrathecal fentanyl and sufentanil for labor analgesia. *Anesthesiology.* 2002;96:1070–1073.

Pan PH, Eisenach JC. The pain of childbirth and its effect on the mother and the fetus. In: Chestnut DH, ed. *Obstetric Anesthesia: Principles and Practice.* 4th ed. Philadelphia, PA: Elsevier; 2009:387–403.

Tsen LC. Anesthesia for cesarean delivery. In: Chestnut DH, ed. *Obstetric Anesthesia: Principles and Practice.* 4th ed. Philadelphia, PA: Elsevier; 2009:521–554.

Viscomi CM, Manullang T. Maternal fever, neonatal sepsis evaluation, and epidural labor analgesia. *Reg Anesth Pain Manage.* 2000;25:549–553.

Wong DA. Epidural and spinal analgesia/anesthesia for labor and vaginal delivery. In: Chestnut DH, ed. *Obstetric Anesthesia: Principles and Practice.* 4th ed. Philadelphia, PA: Elsevier; 2009:429–492.

3 Resuscitation of the Newborn

About 10% of all newborns require some assistance to begin breathing after birth, and ~1% require extensive resuscitation efforts. Newborn resuscitation cannot always be anticipated in time to transfer the mother before delivery to a facility with specialized neonatal support. Therefore, every hospital with a delivery suite should have an organized, skilled resuscitation team and appropriate equipment available (Table 3–1).

   I. **Normal physiologic events at birth.** Normal transitional events at birth begin with initial lung expansion, generally requiring large negative intrathoracic pressures, followed by a cry (expiration against a partially closed glottis). Umbilical cord clamping is accompanied by a rise in systemic blood pressure and massive stimulation of the sympathetic nervous system. With onset of respiration and lung expansion, pulmonary vascular resistance decreases, followed by a gradual transition (over minutes to hours) from fetal to adult circulation, with closure of the foramen ovale and ductus arteriosus.

  II. **Abnormal physiologic events at birth.** The asphyxiated newborn undergoes an abnormal transition. Acutely with asphyxiation the fetus develops **primary apnea**, during which spontaneous respirations can be induced by appropriate sensory stimuli. If the asphyxial insult persists about another minute, the fetus develops deep gasping for 4–5 minutes, followed by a period of **secondary apnea**, during which spontaneous respirations cannot be induced by sensory stimulation. Death occurs if secondary apnea is not reversed by vigorous ventilatory support within several minutes. Because one can never be certain whether an apneic newborn has primary or secondary apnea, resuscitative efforts should proceed as though secondary apnea is present.

 III. **Preparation for high-risk delivery.** Preparation for a high-risk delivery is often the key to a successful outcome. Cooperation between the obstetric, anesthesia, and pediatric staff is important. Knowledge of potential high-risk situations and appropriate interventions is essential (Table 3–2). It is useful to have an estimation of weight and gestational age (Table 3–3), so that drug dosages can be calculated and the appropriate endotracheal tube (see Table 29–1) and umbilical catheter size (page 316) can be chosen. While waiting for the infant to arrive, it is useful to think through potential problems, steps that may be undertaken to correct them, and which member of the team will handle each step. Provided there is both time and opportunity, resuscitative measures should be discussed with the parents. This is particularly important when the fetus is at the limit of viability or when life-threatening anomalies are anticipated.

Table 3–1. EQUIPMENT FOR NEONATAL RESUSCITATION

Standard equipment setup
Radiant warmer
Stethoscope
Compressed air and oxygen source
Oxygen blender
Manometer
Pulse oximeter
Suction source, suction catheter, and meconium "aspirators"
Nasogastric tubes
Apparatus for bag-and-mask ventilation, or T-piece resuscitator
Ventilation masks
Laryngoscope (handles, No. 00, 0, and 1 blades; extra batteries)
Endotracheal tubes (2.5, 3.0, 3.5, and 4.0 mm)
Epinephrine (1:10,000 solution)
Volume expanders (normal saline, lactated Ringer's solution, 0-negative packed red blood cells
    [cross-matched against the mother's blood])
Clock (Apgar timer)
Syringes, hypodermic needles, and tubes for collection of blood samples
Equipment for umbilical vessel catheterization (see page 316)
Warm blankets

Additional recommended equipment
Pressure manometer for use during ventilation
Micro–blood gas analysis availability
Blood gas laboratory immediately available
Plastic bags or polyethylene plastic wrap for infants <29 weeks' gestation
Portable warming pad for placement under infant

IV. **Assessment of the need for resuscitation.** The Apgar score (Appendix B) is assigned
at 1, 5, and, occasionally, 10–20 minutes after delivery. It gives a fairly objective retrospective idea of how much resuscitation a term infant required at birth and the
infant's response to resuscitative efforts. **It is, however, not useful during resuscitation.** During resuscitation, simultaneous assessment of respiratory activity and heart
rate provides the quickest and most accurate evaluation of the need for continuing
resuscitation.
   A. **Respiratory activity.** Respiratory activity is assessed by observing chest movement
      or listening for breath sounds. If there is no respiratory effort or the effort is poor,

Table 3–2. SOME HIGH-RISK SITUATIONS FOR WHICH RESUSCITATION MAY BE ANTICIPATED

High-Risk Situation	Primary Intervention
Preterm delivery	Intubation, lung expansion
Thick meconium	Endotracheal suction
Acute fetal or placental hemorrhage	Volume expansion
Hydrops fetalis	Intubation, paracentesis, or thoracentesis
Polyhydramnios: gastrointestinal obstruction	Nasogastric suction
Maternal diabetes	Early glucose administration

Table 3–3. **EXPECTED BIRTHWEIGHT (50TH PERCENTILE) AT 24–38 WEEKS' GESTATION**

Gestational Age (wk)	Birthweight (g)
24	700
26	900
28	1100
30	1350
32	1650
34	2100
36	2600
38	3000

Based on data published in Battaglia FC, Lubchenco LO. A practical classification of newborn infants by weight and gestational age. *J Pediatr.* 1967;71:159.

the infant needs respiratory assistance by either manual stimulation or positive-pressure ventilation.
  B. Heart rate. The heart rate is typically evaluated by listening to the apical beat or feeling the pulse by lightly grasping the base of the umbilical cord. The evaluator should tap out each beat so that all team members can hear it. If no heart rate can be heard or felt, ventilatory efforts should be halted for a few seconds so that another team member can verify this finding. Pulse oximetry is also useful for monitoring heart rate during resuscitation.
V. Technique of resuscitation. The American Heart Association (AHA) and American Academy of Pediatrics' (AAP) *Textbook of Neonatal Resuscitation* (6th ed., 2011) provides a widely used standard of care used in most delivery services for the resuscitation of newborns (Figure 3–1).
  A. Ventilatory resuscitation
    1. General measures
      a. Suctioning. Oropharyngeal and nasal secretions should be partially removed with a brief period of suctioning using either a bulb syringe or a suction catheter if there are signs of airway obstruction or before initiation of positive-pressure ventilation.
      b. Positive-pressure ventilation. Most infants can be adequately ventilated with a **bag and mask** provided that the mask is the correct size with a close seal around the mouth and nose, and there is an appropriate flow of gas to the bag (Figure 3–2). A **T-piece resuscitator** is an alternative method to provide positive-pressure ventilation that controls peak pressure and positive end-expiratory pressure (PEEP), or continuous positive airway pressure (CPAP) (Figure 3–3). Respiratory rate should be 40–60 breaths/min, or 30 breaths/min if accompanying chest compressions. Peak pressures of 20–25 cm H_2O are usually sufficient, but initial pressures as high as 30–40 cm H_2O may be required. The stomach should be emptied during and after prolonged bag-and-mask ventilation by orogastric suctioning. The AAP and AHA recommend that blended gas be used for positive-pressure ventilation and oxygen concentration be adjusted to meet the preductal (right wrist) pulse-oximetry goals based on the age after birth (Table 3–4).
      c. Endotracheal intubation. Endotracheal intubation should be performed when indicated. However, multiple unsuccessful attempts at intubation by inexperienced persons may make a difficult situation worse. In these cases, it may be best to continue mask ventilation until experienced help arrives. An alternative to endotracheal intubation when intubation attempts are unsuccessful

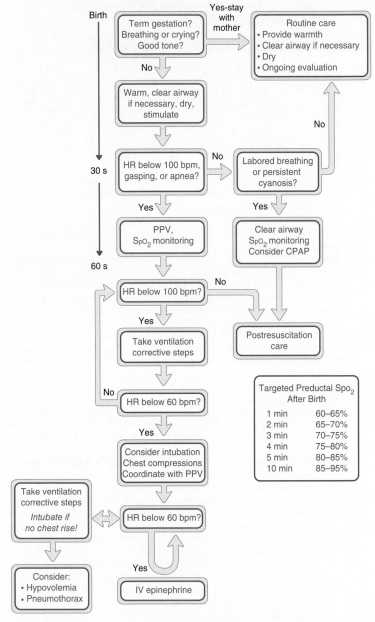

FIGURE 3–1. American Academy of Pediatrics Neonatal Resuscitation Program algorithm. bpm, beats/min; HR, heart rate; CPAP, continuous positive airway pressure; PPV, positive pressure ventilation. (*Reproduced, with permission from Kattwinkel J, Perlman JM, Aziz K, et al. Neonatal resuscitation: 2010 American Heart Association guidelines for cardiopulmonary resuscitation and emergency cardiovascular care. Circulation. 2010;122:S909–S919.*)

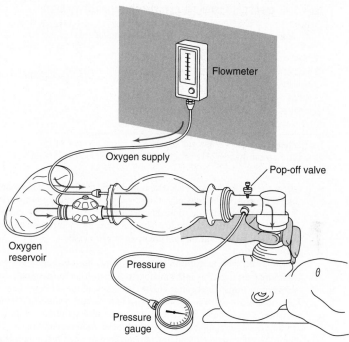

FIGURE 3–2. Bag-and-mask ventilation of the neonate.

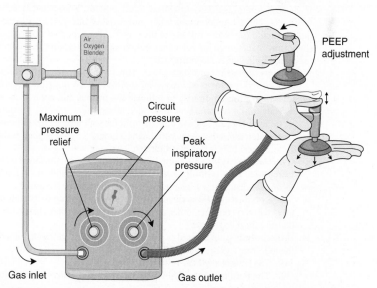

FIGURE 3–3. T-piece resuscitator. PEEP, positive end-expiratory pressure. (*Reproduced, with permission, from Kattwinkel J.* Textbook of Neonatal Resuscitation. *6th ed. Elk Grove, Illinois, IL: American Academy of Pediatrics and American Heart Association; 2011.*)

Table 3–4. **TARGETED PREDUCTAL OXYGEN SATURATION AFTER BIRTH**

Age	Oxygen Saturation
1 minute	60–65%
2 minutes	65–70%
3 minutes	70–75%
4 minutes	75–80%
5 minutes	80–85%
10 minutes	85–95%

From Kattwinkel J. *Textbook of Neonatal Resuscitation.* 6th ed. Elk Grove Village, Illinois, IL: American Academy of Pediatrics and American Heart Association; 2011.

and mask ventilation is not effective is placement of a **laryngeal mask airway** (see Chapter 34). Absolute indications for aggressive ventilatory support with endotracheal intubation are difficult to list here because institutional guidelines and clinical situations vary widely. The procedure for endotracheal intubation and some general guidelines are discussed in Chapter 29.

2. Specific measures
   a. **Term infant with meconium staining.** Infants born through thick meconium may aspirate this inflammatory material in utero (gasping), during delivery, or immediately after birth. The sickest of these infants have usually aspirated in utero and generally also have reactive pulmonary vasoconstriction. Gregory and associates (1974) were among the first to show that endotracheal suctioning at birth was beneficial. More recently, the AAP and the AHA recommended endotracheal suctioning when meconium is present in the amniotic fluid and the infant is not vigorous (eg, without good muscle tone, good respirations, and heart rate >100 beats/min). **Clinical judgment** is always important in deciding whether or not aggressive endotracheal suctioning is necessary. (Meconium aspiration is discussed in detail in Chapter 108.) A randomized multicenter trial of intrapartum suctioning (ie, suctioning before delivery of the chest) of the hypopharynx has not shown any reduction in the risk of meconium aspiration syndrome, and this procedure is no longer recommended.
      i. In nonvigorous infants (heart rate <100, poor tone, or poor respiratory effort), perform endotracheal suctioning. Do not stimulate the infant but proceed directly to intubate the trachea and apply suction directly to the endotracheal tube. Suctioning with a negative pressure of 100 mm Hg can be done directly from the wall unit via a connector (meconium aspirator) to the endotracheal tube. Suction is applied as the endotracheal tube is slowly withdrawn.
      ii. If meconium has been suctioned "below the cords," suctioning should be repeated after reintubation. Prolonged or repeated suctioning is not recommended, as it will exacerbate the preexisting asphyxia insult.
      iii. The procedures just described may be continued for up to 2 minutes after delivery, but then other resuscitative measures (particularly ventilation) must be started.
      iv. If meconium-stained fluid is reported at <34 weeks' gestation, one of the following situations should be suspected:
         (a) The fetus is a growth-restricted term infant.
         (b) The fluid may actually be purulent (consider *Listeria* or *Pseudomonas* species).
         (c) The fluid may actually be bile stained (consider proximal intestinal obstruction).

b. **Term infant with perinatal asphyxia**
   i. Initially all infants without meconium-stained amniotic fluid should be dried and have their oropharynx suctioned. If the infant is not vigorous (strong cry, good tone), a brief period of tactile stimulation by rubbing the back and/or tapping the soles of the feet can be used. Follow immediately by evaluating respirations and heart rate.
   ii. A term infant with a heart rate of <100 beats/min or no spontaneous respiratory activity requires positive-pressure ventilation. If brief tactile stimulation fails to stimulate adequate respirations, positive-pressure ventilation should be initiated at 40–60 breaths/min. If this is not successful in stimulating spontaneous respiratory effort or an improved heart rate, airway patency and positioning of the mask should be confirmed and then peak-inflating pressures should be adjusted as necessary to expand the lungs. If bag-and-mask ventilation is ineffective or prolonged positive-pressure ventilation is necessary, endotracheal intubation or placement of a laryngeal mask airway is indicated. (See Chapters 29 and 34.)

c. **Preterm infant.** Preterm infants weighing <1200 g often require immediate lung expansion in the delivery room.
   i. Mask continuous positive airway pressure (CPAP), administered with a T-piece resuscitator or a flow-inflating bag-and-mask system, providing a pressure of 4–6 cm water, may be sufficient to expand the lungs of a preterm infant and improve ventilation.
   ii. If intubation is required, a smaller (2.5- or 3-mm internal diameter) endotracheal tube is selected.
   iii. Although high peak-inflating pressures may initially be needed to expand the lungs, as soon as the lungs "open up" the pressure should be quickly decreased to as low as 20–25 cm H_2O by the end of the resuscitation if the clinical course permits.
   iv. If available, one of several forms of surfactant may be administered intratracheally as prophylaxis for respiratory distress syndrome. (See Chapters 8 and 124.) However, surfactant is not considered a resuscitative medication and should be administered only to a stable neonate with a correctly placed endotracheal tube.

B. **Cardiac resuscitation.** During delivery room resuscitation, efforts should be directed first to assisting ventilation and providing supplemental oxygen. A sluggish heart rate usually responds to these efforts.
   1. If the heart rate continues to be <60 beats/min in spite of 30 seconds of positive-pressure ventilation, chest compression should be initiated. The thumbs are placed on the lower third of the sternum, between the xiphoid and the line drawn between the nipples (Figure 3–4). Alternatively, the middle and ring fingers of one hand can be placed on the sternum while the other hand supports the back. The sternum is compressed a third of the anteroposterior diameter of the chest at a regular rate of 90 compressions/min while ventilating the infant at 30 breaths/min, synchronized such that every 3 compressions are followed by 1 breath. The heart rate should be checked periodically and chest compression discontinued when the heart rate is >60 beats/min.
   2. An infant with no heart rate (a true Apgar of 0) who does not respond to ventilation and oxygenation may be considered stillborn. Prolonged resuscitative efforts are a matter for ethical consideration. The American Academy of Pediatrics and American Heart Association state that **if there is no heart rate after 10 minutes of adequate resuscitation efforts, discontinuation of resuscitation efforts may be appropriate.**

C. **Drugs used in resuscitation.** (See also Emergency Medications and Therapy for Neonates, inside the front and back covers, and Chapter 148 for more details.) The *Textbook of Neonatal Resuscitation*, 6th ed., recommends giving medications if the

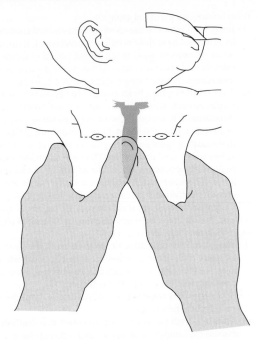

FIGURE 3–4. Technique of external cardiac massage (chest compression) in the neonate. Note the position of the thumbs on the lower third of the sternum, between the xiphoid and the line drawn between the nipples.

heart rate remains <60 beats/min despite adequate ventilation and chest compression for a minimum of 30 seconds.

1. **Route of administration**
   a. **The umbilical vein** is the preferred route for rapid drug administration in the delivery room. A 3.5 or 5F umbilical catheter should be inserted just until blood is easily withdrawn (usually 2–4 cm); this should avoid inadvertent placement in the hepatic or portal vein. Formal umbilical vein catheterization is discussed in Chapter 44.
   b. **The endotracheal tube** is an alternative route for administration of epinephrine in the delivery room while vascular access is being obtained, but absorption is variable. This route may be used while vascular access is being obtained. See Chapter 29 for medications that can be administered by this route.
   c. **Alternate routes** of administration include **peripheral venous** (see Chapter 43) and **intraosseous** routes (see Chapter 41).
2. **Medications commonly used in neonatal resuscitation**
   a. **Epinephrine.** Epinephrine may be necessary during resuscitation when adequate ventilation, oxygenation, and chest compression have failed and the heart rate is still <60 beats/min. This drug causes peripheral vasoconstriction, enhances cardiac contractility, and increases heart rate. **The dose is 0.1–0.3 mL/kg of 1:10,000 solution given intravenously or 0.5–1 mL/kg of 1:10,000 if given by the endotracheal tube.** This may be repeated every 3–5 minutes.

b. **Volume expanders.** Hypovolemia should be suspected in an infant requiring resuscitation when there is evidence of acute blood loss with extreme pallor despite adequate oxygenation, poor peripheral pulse volume despite a normal heart rate, long capillary refill times, or poor response to resuscitative efforts. **Appropriate volume expanders include normal saline, lactated Ringer's solution, or O-negative packed red blood cells (cross-matched against the mother's blood). All are given 10 mL/kg intravenously over 5–10 minutes.**

c. **Naloxone.** Naloxone is a narcotic antagonist and can be administered to an infant with respiratory depression unresponsive to ventilatory assistance whose mother has received narcotics within 4 hours before delivery. The initial corrective action is positive-pressure ventilation. One major contraindication to the use of naloxone is the newborn infant of a mother chronically exposed to narcotics. These infants should never receive naloxone because acute withdrawal symptoms may develop. **The intravenous or intramuscular dosage for naloxone is 0.1 mg/kg.** Two concentrations of naloxone are available: 0.4 mg/mL and 1.0 mg/mL. The dose may be repeated every 5 minutes as necessary. It should be emphasized that the half-life of naloxone is shorter than that of narcotics.

d. **Sodium bicarbonate.** Sodium bicarbonate is usually not useful during the acute phase of neonatal resuscitation. Without adequate ventilation and oxygenation, it will not improve the blood pH and may worsen cerebral acidosis. After prolonged resuscitation, however, sodium bicarbonate may be useful in correcting documented metabolic acidosis. **Give 1–2 mEq/kg intravenously at a rate of 1 mEq/kg/min or slower.**

e. **Atropine and calcium.** Although previously used during resuscitation of the asphyxiated newborn, **atropine and calcium are no longer recommended** by the AAP or the AHA during the **acute phase** of neonatal resuscitation. These medications are used sometimes in special circumstances in resuscitation (such as atropine for severe reflex bradycardia after repeated attempts of suction or intubation resulting in a vagal response with prolonged bradycardia).

D. **Other supportive measures**

1. **Temperature regulation.** Although some degree of cooling in a newborn infant is desirable because it provides a normal stimulus to respiratory effort, excessive cooling increases oxygen consumption and exacerbates acidosis. This is a problem especially for preterm infants, who have thin skin, decreased stores of body fat, and increased body surface area. Heat loss may be prevented by the following measures.

   a. **Dry the infant thoroughly immediately after delivery.**

   b. **Maintain a warm delivery room.**

   c. **Place the infant under a prewarmed radiant warmer.** (See Chapter 7.) Cover extremely preterm infants (<1500 g) with plastic wrap or a plastic bag up to the neck, and place a portable warming pad under the layers of towel on the resuscitation table.

2. **Preparation of the parents for resuscitation.** Initial resuscitation usually occurs in the delivery room with one or both parents present. It is helpful to prepare the parents in advance, if possible. Describe what will be done, who will be present, who will explain what is happening, where the resuscitation will take place, where the father should stand, why crying may not be heard, and where the infant will be taken after stabilization. (See Chapter 50.)

3. **Withholding or discontinuing resuscitation.** A consistent and coordinated approach by the obstetric and neonatal teams with prenatal involvement of parents is important in making decisions regarding potentially withholding resuscitation efforts. In situations where functional survival is highly unlikely, it is reasonable not to initiate resuscitation. Examples include extreme prematurity

(<22 weeks or birthweight <400 g) or major chromosomal abnormalities, such as trisomy 13. Regional outcomes must be taken into account when making decisions regarding withholding resuscitation. When a newborn infant has no detectable heart rate, it is appropriate to consider stopping resuscitation efforts after 10 minutes.

Selected References

Battaglia FC, Lubchenco LO. A practical classification of newborn infants by weight and gestational age. *J Pediatr.* 1967;71(2):159–163.

Gregory GA, Gooding CA, Phibbs RH, Tooley WH. Meconium aspiration in infants—a prospective study. *J Pediatr.* 1974;85(6):848–852.

Kattwinkel J. *Textbook of Neonatal Resuscitation.* 6th ed. Elk Grove, Illinois, IL: American Academy of Pediatrics and American Heart Association; 2011.

Kattwinkel J, Perlman JM, Aziz K, et al. Neonatal resuscitation: 2010 American Heart Association guidelines for cardiopulmonary resuscitation and emergency cardiovascular care. *Pediatrics.* 2010;126(5):e1400–e1413.

Merril JD, Ballard RA. Resuscitation in the delivery room. In: Taeusch HW, Ballard RA, Gleason CA, eds. *Avery's Diseases of the Newborn.* 8th ed. Philadelphia, PA: Elsevier Saunders; 2005:349–363.

Rabi Y, Rabi D, Yee W. Room air resuscitation of the depressed newborn: a systematic review and meta-analysis. *Resuscitation.* 2007;72:353–363.

Singh A, Duckett J, Newton T, Watkinson M. Improving neonatal unit admission temperatures in preterm babies: exothermic mattresses, polyethylene bags or a traditional approach? *J Perinatol.* 2010;30:45–49.

Vain NE, Szyld EG, Prudent LM, Wiswell TE, Aguilar AM, Vivas NI. Oropharyngeal and nasopharyngeal suctioning of meconium-stained neonates before delivery of their shoulders: multicentre, randomised controlled trial. *Lancet.* 2004;364(9434):597–602.

Watkinson M. Temperature control of premature infants in the delivery room. *Clin Perinatol.* 2006;33(1):43–53.

Wiswell TE, Gannon CM, Jacob J. Delivery room management of the apparently vigorous meconium-stained neonate: results of the multicenter, international collaborative trial. *Pediatrics.* 2000;105(1 Pt 1):1–7.

4 Infant Transport

I. **General principles.** A seamless transport of infants from a referring hospital to a higher level neonatal intensive care unit (NICU) enables each patient to benefit from the regionalization and specialization of critical care personnel and services. Clear guidelines and a transport algorithm must be established regarding transport procedures, personnel, and necessary equipment. The goals of an infant transport are:
   A. **Provide early stabilization and initiation of advanced care** at a referring institution.
   B. **Continue critical care therapies and monitoring** during transport to ensure safety and a positive neonatal outcome.
II. **Predeparture assessment and preparation**
   A. **Procedures.** Policies and procedures reflect the unique characteristics of each region (size, geography, and level of medical services). Lines of communication must always be open between the referring hospital and the NICU at all levels

(ie, administrators, physicians, nurses) and with ambulance or air services. On receiving a request for a transport, an intake record should be completed, documenting the referring physician and hospital contact information and patient information. A predeparture assessment of the patient may determine transport team composition and guide the referring hospital with management.

B. **Personnel.** The team may include physicians, nurses, neonatal nurse practitioners or advanced practice nurses, respiratory therapists, and perhaps emergency medical technicians. Limited research supports similar outcomes from transport teams with and without the direct presence of a transport physician. Team members should have received special training regarding issues and equipment specific to transport and have the ability to contact the medical command at any time during transport.

C. **Equipment.** Each transport team should be self-sufficient (ie, be a mobile NICU). Special emphasis is placed on having the necessary equipment to enable maximal stabilization of the infant at the referring hospital to facilitate an uneventful transport. Medications and equipment can be chosen according to published lists. Well-calibrated monitoring equipment is necessary given the added noise and vibration during transport, which often compromise auditory and visual monitoring. An instant camera is an important consideration to provide pictures of the infant to the family.

D. **Transport mode.** Clear guidelines should be established regarding the indications for air versus ground transport based on distance, time of day, geography, weather, location of landing sites, and severity and stability of the patient's condition. The most critical factor in determining mode of transport is the safety of the team and patient. Decisions regarding flight safety should be made according to weather and other flight conditions and not be influenced by patient status. Follow instructions from the flight crew regarding loading and unloading of the aircraft. Transport personnel should be restrained in safety harnesses throughout every transport.

III. **Patient assessment and stabilization at the referring hospital**

A. **General procedures.** Unless active resuscitation is underway, the team's first task at the referring hospital is to listen to the history and assessment of the infant's status. Team members should conduct themselves as professional representatives of the NICU, avoiding situations of conflict or criticism with the staff. A complete physical assessment should be performed, as well as review of all laboratory values and radiographic studies. Obtain copies of the medical record and radiographic studies if possible. The accepting NICU should be given an expected arrival time and update on the infant's status.

B. **General stabilization.** Attention to the details of stabilization is important! In most cases, an infant is not ready for transport until basic neonatal needs are met: acceptable cardiac and respiratory function, establishment of vascular access, acceptable blood gas and glucose levels, and thermal stabilization. Catheters and tubes should be appropriately placed and positions confirmed. Infants at risk for sepsis should have antibiotic therapy initiated after blood cultures are obtained.

C. **Respiratory stabilization**

1. **Surfactant administration.** Surfactant administration to premature infants before transport is associated with a low incidence of complications and is generally considered safe and beneficial in the initial respiratory management. There is no consensus on timing of transport after surfactant administration, but most agree on ~30 minutes or after respiratory parameters are stabilized.

2. **Inhaled nitric oxide.** Inhaled nitric oxide (iNO) used for the treatment of hypoxic respiratory failure in term and near-term infants with pulmonary hypertension may be continued or initiated during transport. An infant who is already receiving iNO therapy must be transported by a team capable of continuing iNO because abrupt discontinuation may result in deleterious effects.

3. **Elective intubation.** Elective intubation of otherwise stable infants receiving a prostaglandin infusion who are at risk for apnea may not be necessary. However, consultation with cardiology is recommended to weigh the risks of transport complications after intubation with possible benefits of prophylactic intubation before the transport of such infants.

D. **Gastric intubation.** If the infant has a gastrointestinal disorder (eg, an ileus or a diaphragmatic hernia) or if positive airway pressure is administered, venting of the stomach with a nasogastric or orogastric tube is indicated before departure, especially if air transport is used. See Chapter 32.

E. **Temperature control and fluid balance.** Special attention to temperature and fluid balance is required for infants with open lesions (eg, myelomeningocele or omphalocele) or premature infants at risk of excessive insensible water loss. A dry or moist protective dressing over an open defect can be covered by thin plastic wrap to reduce evaporative heat loss. An occlusive plastic wrap may be used in very low birthweight infants after birth to minimize evaporative losses. Infants at risk of hypoxic ischemic encephalopathy who may be candidates for head cooling should not be warmed and may be passively cooled by turning off active heating devices. Attention to continuous central temperature monitoring is important to avoid excessive cooling.

F. **Family support.** Keep parents updated by outlining the initial medical concerns and potential hospital course. The parents should be offered to see and touch the infant before transport and if possible be provided with pictures. Contact information and directions to the accepting hospital should be supplied. Obtain consents for transport and admission. After transfer is completed, the team should update the parents and referring physician.

IV. **Transport**

A. **Monitoring.** During transport, monitoring of respiratory rate, heart rate, blood pressure, and pulse oximetry should continue to assess changes in the infant's status. The infant's status, vital signs, assessment, and interventions performed should be documented until arrival at the accepting hospital.

B. **Special considerations during air transport.** In helicopters and unpressurized aircraft, **dysbarism** (imbalance between air pressure in the atmosphere and the pressure of gases within the body) causes predictable problems. Partial pressures of inspired gases decrease as altitude increases (Dalton's law), so infants require an increased concentration of inspired oxygen. Trapped free air in the thorax or intestines expands in volume (as pressure decreases; Boyle's law) and may cause significant pulmonary compromise or intraabdominal changes. A **cuffed tube** or **catheter** should be **evacuated** before takeoff. **Gastric venting** should be performed before transport because the air trapped in the gastrointestinal tract will expand in volume as atmospheric pressure decreases. Because blood pressure varies with changing gravitational force, fluctuations noted during climbing or descent should not be cause for alarm. Hearing protection should be worn by the transport team and patient because of excessive noise.

V. **Quality improvement**

A. **Outreach education.** Transport team members should regularly meet with professionals from each referring hospital. Such a forum for discussion of transport issues and specific transported patients provides mutual feedback and stimulates interhospital protocol decision making as well as quality improvement processes.

B. **Evaluation of transports.** Each transport should have a scoring system that reflects the "before" and "after" status of the infant. This system provides quality control of transports and is useful in outreach education to convey constructive criticism to referring hospitals. It is also important to regularly review team response time, referring hospital satisfaction, difficult transports, safety updates, team credentialing, medical protocols, and so forth as part of quality assurance and safety evaluation.

Selected References

American Academy of Pediatrics Task Force on Inter-hospital Transport. *Guidelines for Air and Ground Transport of Neonatal and Pediatric Patients.* 3rd ed. Elk Grove, IL: American Academy of Pediatrics; 2007.

Biniwale M, Kleinman M. Safety of surfactant administration before transport of premature infants. *Air Med J.* 2010;29:170–177.

Hallberg B, Olson L, Bartocci M, Edqvist I, Blennow M. Passive induction of hypothermia during transport of asphyxiated infants: a risk of excessive cooling. *Acta Paediatr.* 2009;98:942–946.

King BR, King TM, Foster RL, McCans KM. Pediatric and neonatal transport teams with and without a physician: a comparison of outcomes and interventions. *Pediatr Emerg Care.* 2007;23:77–82.

Lee JH, Puthucheary J. Transport of critically ill neonates with cardiac conditions. *Air Med J.* 2010;29:320–322.

Meckler GD, Lowe C. To intubate or not to intubate? Transporting infants on prostaglandin E1. *Pediatrics.* 2009;123:e25–e30.

5 Gestational Age and Birthweight Classification

Gestation is the period of fetal development from the time of conception to birth. **Gestational age** (or menstrual age), as defined by the American Academy of Pediatrics (AAP), is the "time elapsed between the first day of the last menstrual period and the day of delivery." Gestational age is expressed in completed weeks (26-week and 4-day-old fetus is expressed as a 26-week fetus). Gestational age assessment is important for the obstetrician for obstetric care and management. Gestational age assessment is extremely important for the neonatologist for evaluation of the infant and to anticipate high-risk infants and complications. Gestational age and birthweight classification helps the neonatologist to categorize infants, guide treatment, and assess risks for morbidity and mortality. Neonates can be classified based on **gestational age** (preterm, late preterm, term, post term), **birthweight** (extremely low birthweight [ELBW], very low birthweight [VLBW], low birthweight [LBW], etc.), and **gestational age and birthweight combined** (small for gestational age [SGA], appropriate for gestational age [AGA], large for gestational age [LGA]). **The AAP recommends that all newborns be classified by birthweight and gestational age.**

I. Gestational age assessment. Gestational age can be determined prenatally and postnatally.

   A. Prenatal gestational age assessment. Determined by maternal history, clinical examination, and ultrasound examination. Based on these, the obstetrician is able to give his/or her "best estimate" of gestational age, since variability as much as 2 weeks can occur.

   1. Maternal history

      a. Date of last menstrual period. Reliable if dates remembered. The first day of the last menstrual period is about 2 weeks before ovulation and about 3 weeks before blastocyst implantation.

      b. Assisted reproductive technology. In vitro fertilization pregnancies have a known date of conception and can accurately predict gestational age within 1 day. If pregnancy was achieved by using assisted reproductive technology, the gestational age is calculated by adding 2 weeks to the chronological age (time elapsed from birth). Intrauterine insemination may have a few days' delay.

      c. Quickening. Date of first reported fetal activity by the mother (18–20 weeks for a primigravida, 15–17 weeks for a multipara).

   2. Clinical examination

      a. Pelvic examination. Uterine size by bimanual examination in the first trimester can be accurate within 2 weeks.

      b. Symphysis pubis fundal height. This is accurate up to 28–30 weeks' gestation. In resource-poor countries, gestational age can be estimated from serial measurements of symphysis pubis fundal height. It is only accurate within 4 weeks. One centimeter is equal to 1 week from the 18th to 20th weeks of gestation. At 20 weeks the fundus is at the umbilicus, and at term it is at the xiphoid process.

      c. Ultrasound examination

         i. First fetal heart tones by Doppler ultrasound heard at 8–10 weeks.

         ii. Fetal heart motion/beat by ultrasound. Cardiac activity on ultrasound is detectable at 5.5–6.5 weeks by vaginal ultrasound, and 6.5–7 weeks by fetal ultrasound.

  iii. **First trimester examination**
    (a) **Gestational sac mean diameter** is obtained by the average of 3 measurements and then the gestational age is obtained from a table. It is accurate within 1 week.
    (b) **Crown-rump length** measures the embryo at the tip of the cephalic pole to the tip of the caudal pole and is the most reliable measurement of gestational age. It is used to date pregnancy between 6 and 14 weeks. It is accurate within 5 days.
  iv. **Second- and third-trimester examination.** There are many parameters used to date gestational age in the second and third trimesters. The most common is the **biparietal diameter, and it is measured from the leading outer edge to the inner edge of the calvarium bone.** It determines gestational age with 95% confidence within 7 days if done between 14 and 20 weeks of gestation. Other parameters used are head circumference, abdominal circumference, femur length, fetal foot length, cranial ultrasound assessment, cerebellar dimension assessment, fetal scapular length, corpus callosum measurements, head and mid-arm circumference, and epiphyseal ossification centers. Measurements in the second trimester are generally accurate within 10–14 days and in the third trimester within 14–21 days.
B. **Postnatal gestational age assessment.** Usually done because prenatal estimates are not always accurate. Four approaches have been used: physical criteria alone, neurologic examination alone, physical criteria and neurologic examination together, and direct ophthalmoscopy. Physical criteria alone are more accurate than neurological criteria alone, with the combination being the best estimate of gestational age. Dubowitz and Dubowitz originally described a method that included a total of 21 physical and neurologic assessments. The test was widely used, but because of the time and difficulty in performing the assessment it was shortened and replaced by the **Ballard examination.** Both the Dubowitz and Ballard examinations were inaccurate at assessing gestational age in preterm neonates <1500 g and overestimated gestational age. Ballard and associates later refined and expanded their test to include the assessment of extremely premature infants, called the **New Ballard Score (NBS).** Postnatal gestational assessment discussed here includes the rapid assessment in the delivery room, NBS, and the direct ophthalmoscopy examination.
  1. **Rapid assessment of gestational age in the delivery room.** There are multiple methods for rapid assessment of gestational age. Most include some of the following physical characteristics: skin texture, skin color, skin opacity, edema, lanugo hair, skull hardness, ear form, ear firmness, genitalia, breast size, nipple formation, and plantar skin creases. One method for rapid gestational age assessment includes the **most useful clinical signs in differentiating among premature, borderline mature, and full-term infants, which are as follows (in order of utility):** creases in the sole of the foot, size of the breast nodule, nature of the scalp hair, cartilaginous development of the earlobe, and scrotal rugae and testicular descent in males. These signs and findings are listed in Table 5–1.
  2. **New Ballard Score.** The score spans from 10 (correlating with 20 weeks' gestation) to 50 (correlating with 44 weeks' gestation). It is best performed at <12 hours of age if the infant is <26 weeks' gestation. If the infant is >26 weeks' gestation, there is no optimal age of examination up to 96 hours.
    a. **Accuracy.** The examination is accurate whether the infant is sick or well to within 2 weeks of gestational age. It overestimates gestational age by 2–4 days in infants between 32 and 37 weeks' gestation.
    b. **Criteria.** The examination consists of 6 neuromuscular and 6 physical criteria. The neuromuscular criteria are based on the understanding that passive tone is more useful than active tone in indicating gestational age.
    c. **Procedure.** The examination is administered twice by 2 different examiners to ensure objectivity, and the data are entered on the chart (Figure 5–1). This form is

Table 5-1. **CRITERIA FOR RAPID GESTATIONAL ASSESSMENT AT DELIVERY**

Feature	36 Weeks and Earlier	37–38 Weeks	39 Weeks and Beyond
Creases in soles of feet	One or two transverse creases; posterior three-fourths of sole smooth	Multiple creases; anterior two-thirds of heel smooth	Entire sole, including heel, covered with creases
Breast nodule[a]	2 mm	4 mm	7 mm
Scalp hair	Fine and woolly; fuzzy	Fine and woolly; fuzzy	Coarse and silky; each hair single stranded
Earlobe	No cartilage	Moderate amount of cartilage	Stiff earlobe with thick cartilage
Testes and scrotum	Testes partially descended; scrotum small, with few rugae	?	Testes fully descended; scrotum normal size with prominent rugae

[a]The breast nodule is not palpable before 33 weeks. Underweight full-term infants may have retarded breast development.
Usher R, McLean F, Scott KE. Judgment of fetal age: II. Clinical significance of gestational age and objective measurement. *Pediatr Clin North Am.* 1966;13:835. Modified and reproduced with permission from Elsevier Science.

available in most nurseries. The examination consists of 2 parts: neuromuscular maturity and physical maturity. The 12 scores are totaled, and the **maturity rating** is expressed in weeks of gestation (**gestational age**), estimated by using the chart provided on the form.

  i. **Neuromuscular maturity**
    (a) **Posture.** Score **0** if the arms and legs are extended, and score +1 if the infant has beginning flexion of the knees and hips, with arms extended; determine other scores based on the diagram.
    (b) **Square window.** Flex the hand on the forearm between the thumb and index finger of the examiner. Apply sufficient pressure to achieve as much flexion as possible. Visually measure the angle between the hypothenar eminence and the ventral aspect of the forearm. Determine the score based on the diagram.
    (c) **Arm recoil.** Flex the forearms for 5 seconds then grasp the hand and fully extend the arm and release. If the arm returns to full flexion, give a score of +4. For lesser degrees of flexion, score as noted in the diagram.
    (d) **Popliteal angle.** Hold the thigh in the knee-chest position with the left index finger and the thumb supporting the knee. Then extend the leg by gentle pressure from the right index finger behind the ankle. Measure the angle at the popliteal space and score accordingly.
    (e) **Scarf sign.** Take the infant's hand and try to put it around the neck posteriorly as far as possible over the opposite shoulder and score according to the diagram.
    (f) **Heel to ear.** Keeping the pelvis flat on the table, take the infant's foot and try to put it as close to the head as possible without forcing it. Grade according to the diagram.
  ii. **Physical maturity.** These characteristics are scored as shown in Figure 5-1.
    (a) **Skin.** Carefully look at the skin and grade according to the diagram. Extremely premature infants have sticky, transparent skin and receive a score of +1.
    (b) **Lanugo hair.** Examine the infant's back and between and over the scapulae.

Name _____ Date/Time of birth _____ Sex _____

Hospital No. _____ Date/Time of exam _____ Birthweight _____

Race _____ Age when examined _____ Length _____

Apgar score: 1 minute _____ 5 minutes _____ 10 minutes _____ Head circ. _____

Examiner _____

SCORE

Neuromuscular _____

Physical _____

Total _____

Maturity rating

Score	Weeks
-10	20
-5	22
0	24
5	26
10	28
15	30
20	32
25	34
30	36
35	38
40	40
45	42
50	44

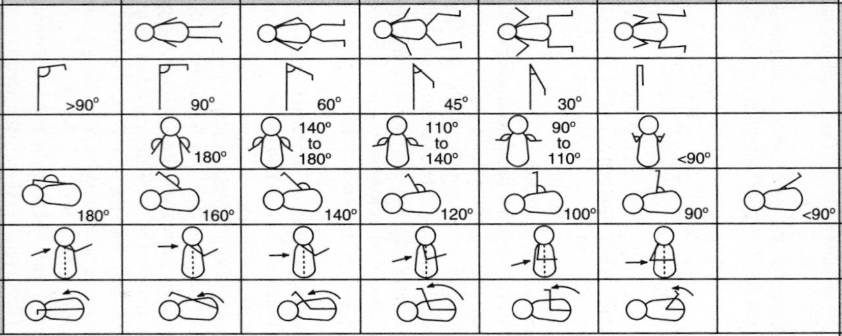

Neuromuscular maturity

Neuromuscular maturity sign	Score							Record score here
	-1	0	1	2	3	4	5	
Posture								
Square window (wrist)	>90°	90°	60°	45°	30°	0°		
Arm recoil		180°	140° to 180°	110° to 140°	90° to 110°	<90°		
Popliteal angle	180°	160°	140°	120°	100°	90°	<90°	
Scarf sign								
Heel to ear								
						Total neuromuscular maturity score		

FIGURE 5–1. Maturational assessment of gestational age (New Ballard Score). (*Reproduced, with permission, from Ballard JL, Khoury JC, Wedig K, Wang L, Elters-Walsman BL, Lipp R. New Ballard Score, expanded to include extremely premature infants. J Pediatr. 1991;119:417.*)

Physical maturity

Physical maturity sign	Score							Record score here
	−1	0	1	2	3	4	5	
Skin	sticky friable transparent	gelatinous red translucent	smooth pink visible veins	superficial peeling &/or rash, few veins	cracking pale areas rare veins	parchment deep cracking no vessels	leathery cracked wrinkled	
Lanugo	none	sparse	abundant	thinning	bald areas	mostly bald		
Plantar surface	heel-toe 40–50 mm: −1 <40 mm: −2	>50 mm no crease	faint red marks	anterior transverse crease only	creases ant. 2/3	creases over entire sole		
Breast	imperceptible	barely perceptible	flat areola no bud	stippled areola 1–2 mm bud	raised areola 3–4 mm bud	full areola 5–10 mm bud		
Eye/ear	lids fused loosely: −1 tightly: −2	lids open pinna flat stays folded	sl. curved pinna; soft slow recoil	well curved pinna; soft but ready recoil	formed and firm, instant recoil	thick cartilage ear stiff		
Genitals (male)	scrotum flat, smooth	scrotum empty, faint rugae	testes in upper canal rare rugae	testes descending few rugae	testes down good rugae	testes pendulous deep rugae		
Genitals (female)	clitoris prominent & labia flat	prominent clitoris & small labia minora	prominent clitoris & enlarging minora	majora & minora equally prominent	majora large minora small	majora cover clitoris & minora		

Total physical maturity score

Gestational age (weeks)

By dates _____
By ultrasound _____
By exam _____

FIGURE 5–1. (*Continued*)

33

   (c) **Plantar surface.** Measure foot length from the tip of the great toe to the back of the heel. If the results are <40 mm, give a score of –2. If it is between 40 and 50 mm, assign a score of –1. If the measurement is >50 mm and no creases are seen on the plantar surface, give a score of 0. If there are creases, score accordingly.

   (d) **Breast.** Palpate any breast tissue and score.

   (e) **Eye and ear.** This section has been expanded to include criteria that apply to the extremely premature infant. Loosely fused eyelids are defined as closed, but gentle traction opens them (score as –1). Tightly fused eyelids are defined as inseparable by gentle traction. Base the rest of the score on open lids and the examination of the ear.

   (f) **Genitalia.** Score according to the diagram.

3. **Direct ophthalmoscopy.** Another method for determination of gestational age uses direct ophthalmoscopy of the lens. It is based on the normal embryological process of the gradual disappearance of the anterior lens capsule vascularity between 27 and 34 weeks of gestation. Before 27 weeks, the cornea is too opaque to allow visualization; after 34 weeks, atrophy of the vessels of the lens occurs. Therefore, this technique allows for accurate determination of gestational age at 27–34 weeks only. This method is reliable to ±2 weeks. The pupil must be dilated under the supervision of an ophthalmologist, and the assessment must be performed within 48 hours of birth before the vessels atrophy. This method is highly accurate and is not affected by alert states or neurological deficits. The following grading system is used, as shown in Figure 5–2.

   a. **Grade 4 (27–28 weeks).** Vessels cover the entire anterior surface of the lens or the vessels meet in the center of the lens.

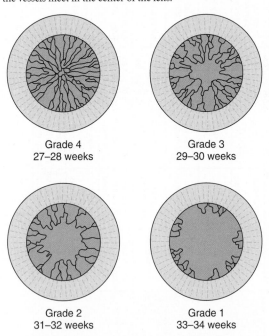

Grade 4
27–28 weeks

Grade 3
29–30 weeks

Grade 2
31–32 weeks

Grade 1
33–34 weeks

FIGURE 5–2. Grading system for assessment of gestational age by examination of the anterior vascular capsule of the lens. (*Reproduced, with permission, from Hittner HM, Hirsch NJ, Rudolph AJ. Assessment of gestational age by examination of the anterior vascular capsule of the lens. J Pediatr. 1977;91:455.*)

       b. Grade 3 (29–30 weeks). Vessels do not meet in the center but are close. Central portion of the lens is not covered by vessels.

       c. Grade 2 (31–32 weeks). Vessels reach only to the middle-outer part of the lens. The central clear portion of the lens is larger.

       d. Grade 1 (33–34 weeks). Vessels are seen only at the periphery of the lens.

   C. Newborn classification based on gestational age. Infants can be classified based on their gestational age. This classification categorizes the infant as **preterm, late preterm, term (early term or late term),** or **post term.** It is based on the weeks of gestation or completed weeks of gestation or days (see Table 5–2 for a full description).

  II. Birthweight classification. Infants can be classified by birthweight; some of the classifications used are noted in the following.

   A. Micropreemie. <800 g or 1.8 lb.

   B. Extremely low birthweight (ELBW). <1000 g or 2.2 lb.

   C. Very low birthweight (VLBW). <1500 g or 3.3 lb.

   D. Low birthweight (LBW). <2500 g or 5.5 lb.

   E. Normal birthweight (NBW). 2500 g (5.5 lb) to 4000 g (8.8 lb).

   F. High birthweight (HBW). 4000 g (8.8 lb) to 4500 g (9.9 lb).

   G. Very high birthweight (VHBW). >4500 g (9.9 lb).

 III. Classification by birthweight and gestational age combined. Newborns can be classified by assessing their gestational age and obtaining their birthweight and plotting these against standardized intrauterine growth charts. This allows categorization as SGA, AGA, or LGA. These refer to the size of the infant at birth and not fetal growth.

   A. How to decide if the infant is SGA, AGA, or LGA? Plot gestational assessment against weight, length, and head circumference on one of the intrauterine growth charts to determine whether the infant is small, appropriate, or large for gestational age.

Table 5–2. **DEFINITIONS OF PRETERM, LATE-PRETERM, TERM, AND POST-TERM INFANTS**

	Weeks of Gestation (number of weeks after the first day of the mother's last menstrual period)	Completed Weeks (number of 7-day intervals after the first day of the mother's last menstrual period)	Days (common medical terminology)
Preterm	<37 weeks	On or before the end of the last day of the 37th week	≤259 days
Late preterm	34 0/7 to 36 6/7 weeks	On or after the first day of the 35th week through the end of the last day of the 37th week	239–259 days
Term (**early term:** 37 0/7 to 38 6/7 weeks; **full term:** 39 0/7 to 41 6/7 weeks)	37 0/7 to 41 6/7 weeks	On or after the first day of the 38th week through the end of the last day of the 42nd week	260–294 days
Post term	42 0/7 weeks or more	On or after first day of the 43rd week	≥295 days

Definitions of postnatal gestational age are based on conventional medical definition (day of birth counted as day 1) by the American Academy of Pediatrics, the American College of Obstetricians and Gynecologists, and the World Health Organization definitions.

Based on Engle WA, Tomashek KM, Wallman C; Committee on Fetus and Newborn, American Academy of Pediatrics. Late preterm infants: a population at risk. *Pediatrics.* 2007;120:1390–1401. Reaffirmed May 2010.

There are multiple intrauterine growth charts available. The most commonly used ones that involve weight, length, and head circumference are Lubchenco (1966), Usher and McLean (1969), Beeby (1996), Niklasson (1991), Fenton (2003), and now Olsen (2010). **Which chart to use?** The original charts were the Lubchenco charts (Figure 5–3). The Fenton chart (which is the updated Babson and Benda chart) includes premature infants at 22 weeks (Figure 5–4). New gender-specific intrauterine growth charts are now available from Olsen (Figure 5–5). The Olsen charts include more infant sizes and more accurately represent the current diverse U.S. population. Deciding which chart to use usually depends on the preference of the neonatal intensive care unit.

B. **Definitions and characteristics of AGA, SGA, and LGA**
   1. **Appropriate for gestational age (AGA).** Defined as a birthweight between the 10th and 90th percentiles for the infant's gestational age.
   2. **Small for gestational age (SGA).** Defined as a birthweight 2 standard deviations below the mean weight for gestational age or below the 10th percentile for gestational age (see also Chapter 105). SGA refers to the size of the infant at birth and not fetal growth. SGA is associated with **maternal factors** (chronic disease, malnutrition, multiple gestation, high altitude, or conditions affecting the blood flow and oxygenation in the placenta [hypertension, preeclampsia, or smoking]), **placental factors** (infarction, previa, abruption, anatomic malformations, etc.), **fetal factors** (usually symmetric, birthweight, length, and head circumference all depressed the same), congenital infections (TORCH, see Chapter 141), chromosomal abnormalities, and congenital malformations (dysmorphic syndromes and other congenital anomalies, fetal diabetes mellitus, familial causes, multiple gestation constitutional). **IUGR** (intrauterine growth restriction) and **constitutionally small fetus** should be included when discussing SGA infants.
      a. **Intrauterine growth restriction (fetal growth restriction).** (See Chapter 105.) IUGR is a reduction in the expected fetal growth of an infant. The failure to obtain optimal intrauterine growth is due to an in utero insult. There is no standard definition, but a fetus <10th weight percentile for age or a ponderal index <10% is sometimes used to classify an infant as IUGR. *Note:* SGA and IUGR are related but not synonymous. All infants born SGA may not be small as a result of IUGR. All infants born IUGR may not be SGA. SGA is a clinical finding and IUGR is an ultrasound finding.
      b. **Constitutionally small infants.** Include 70% of infants with a birthweight below the 10th percentile. They are constitutionally small, are anatomically normal, have no increased obstetrical or neonatal risks, are well proportioned, and have normal development. They grow parallel to the lower percentiles throughout pregnancy. Mothers are usually slim, petite women. The infants are small because of constitutional reasons: maternal ethnicity, female sex, body mass index, and others. They are not high-risk infants.
   3. **Large for gestational age (LGA).** Defined as a birthweight 2 standard deviations above the mean weight for gestational age or above the 90th percentile for gestational age. LGA can be seen in infants of diabetic mothers (maternal or gestational), infants with Beckwith-Wiedemann syndrome and other syndromes, constitutionally large infants with large parents, postmature infants (gestational age >42 weeks), and infants with hydrops fetalis. LGA infants are also associated with increased maternal weight gain in pregnancy; multiparity; male sex; congenital heart disease, especially transposition of the great arteries ("happy chubby blue male infant"); islet cell dysplasias; and certain ethnicities (Hispanic). Large-for-gestational-age infants are sometimes referred to as infants with "**macrosomia.**"
      a. **Macrosomia** means "large body." Hispanic women have a higher risk of fetal macrosomia when compared to Asian, African American, and white women. Because males weigh more at birth, it is also more common in males.

Name _____

Hospital No. _____

Race _____

Date of birth _____

Date of exam _____

Sex _____

Birthweight _____

Length _____

Head circ. _____

Gestational age _____

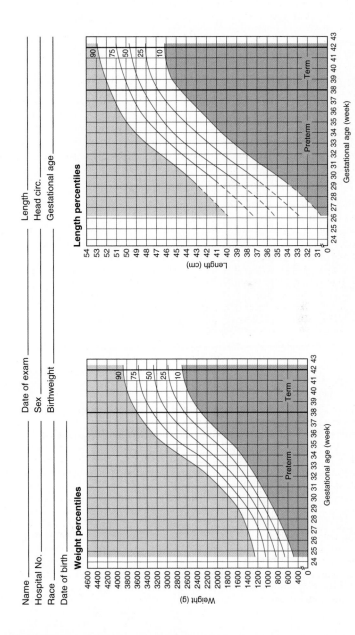

FIGURE 5–3. Classification of newborns (both sexes) by intrauterine growth and gestational age. (Reproduced, with permission, from Battagli FC, Lubchenco LO. *A practical classification for newborn infants by weight and gestational age.* J Pediatr. 1967;71:159; and Lubchenco LO. Hansman C, Boyd E. *Intrauterine growth in length and head circumference as estimated from live births at gestational ages from 24 to 42 weeks.* Pediatrics. 1966;37:403. Courtesy of Ross Laboratories, Columbus, Ohio 43216.)

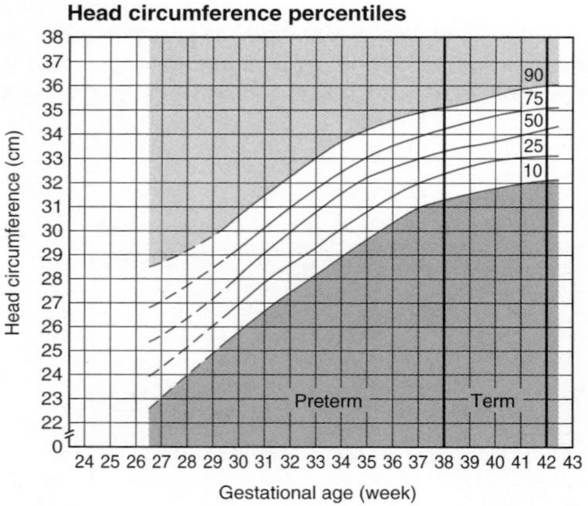

Head circumference percentiles

Head circumference (cm): 38 37 36 35 34 33 32 31 30 29 28 27 26 25 24 23 22

90 75 50 25 10

Preterm — Term

0 24 25 26 27 28 29 30 31 32 33 34 35 36 37 38 39 40 41 42 43

Gestational age (week)

FIGURE 5-3. (*Continued*)

Classification of infant*	Weight	Length	Head circ.
Large for gestational age (LGA) (>90th percentile)			
Appropriate for gestational age (AGA) (10th to 90th percentile)			
Small for gestational age (SGA) (<10th percentile)			

*Place an "X" in the appropriate box (LGA, AGA, or SGA) for weight, for length, and for head circumference.

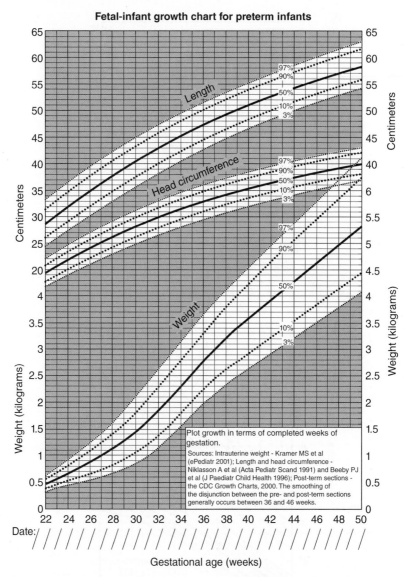

Fetal-infant growth chart for preterm infants

Plot growth in terms of completed weeks of gestation.

Sources: Intrauterine weight - Kramer MS et al (ePediatr 2001); Length and head circumference - Niklasson A et al (Acta Pediatr Scand 1991) and Beeby PJ et al (J Paediatr Child Health 1996); Post-term sections - the CDC Growth Charts, 2000. The smoothing of the disjunction between the pre- and post-term sections generally occurs between 36 and 46 weeks.

Gestational age (weeks)

FIGURE 5–4. Growth chart for preterm infants. (*From Fenton TR. A new growth chart for preterm babies: Babson and Benda's chart updated with recent data and a new format.* BMC Pediatrics. *2003,3:13. http://www.biomedcentral.com/1471-2431/3/13. Accessed October 24, 2012.*)

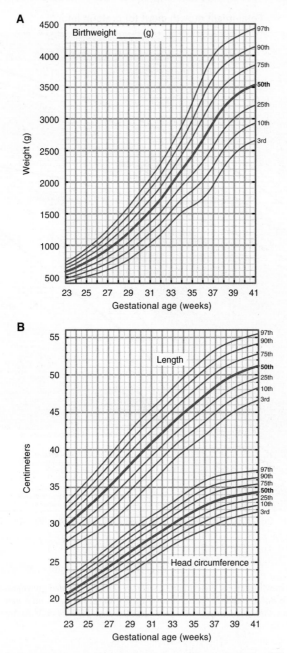

FIGURE 5–5. Intrauterine growth curves for males and females including (A) girls weight for age, (B) girls length and HC for age, (C) boys weight for age, and (D) boys length and HC for age. (*Based on Olsen IE, Groveman SA, Lawson ML, Clark RH, Zemel BS. New intrauterine growth curves based on United States data. Pediatrics. 2010;125;e214; originally published online, January 25, 2010. DOI:10.1542/peds. 2009-0913.*)

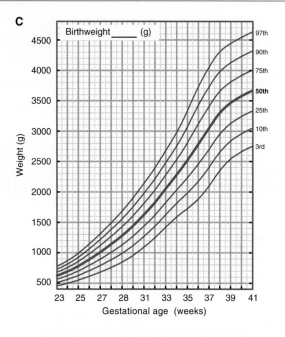

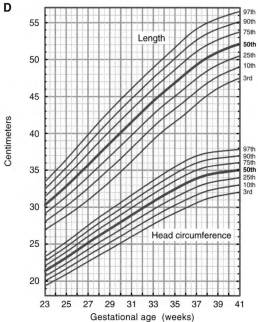

FIGURE 5–5. (*Continued*)

It is associated with diabetes (gestational and maternal), maternal obesity, and a longer duration of gestation. It has multiple definitions in the literature.

    i. **Birthweight** >4000 g or >4500 g regardless of gestational age.

    ii. **Large for gestational age (LGA).** Birthweight ≥90% for gestational age.

    iii. **Weight is above a defined limit** at any gestational age.

IV. Other age terminology (recommended by the AAP) used to describe the age and gestation of an infant:

    A. **Chronological age (or postnatal age).** The time elapsed since birth. It is expressed in days, weeks, months, or years.

    B. **Postmenstrual age.** Gestational age plus chronological age. It is expressed in weeks and is the preferred term to describe premature infants in the perinatal period.

    C. **Corrected age (or adjusted age; only used in children born preterm <3 years old).** The chronological age minus the number of weeks born before 40 weeks' gestation and is the preferred term after the perinatal period. It is expressed in weeks or months. **Corrected age** is the preferred term.

Selected References

American Academy of Pediatrics Policy Statement. Age terminology during the perinatal period. *Pediatrics.* 2004;114(5):1362–1364; reaffirmed October 2007.

Amiel-Tison C. Neurological evaluation of the maturity of newborn infants. *Arch Dis Child.* 1968;43:89.

Ballard JL, Khoury JC, Wedig K, Wang L, Elters-Walsman BL, Lipp R. New Ballard Score, expanded to include extremely premature infants. *J Pediatr.* 1991;119:417.

Ballard JL, Novak KK, Driver M. A simplified score for assessment of fetal maturation of newly born infants. *J Pediatr.* 1979;95:769.

Dodd V. Gestational age assessment. *Neonatal Netw.* 1996;15:1.

Dubowitz LM, Dubowitz V, Goldberg C. Clinical assessment of gestational age in the newborn infant. *J Pediatr.* 1970;77:1.

Engle WA, Tomashek KM, Wallman C; Committee on Fetus and Newborn, American Academy of Pediatrics. Late preterm infants: a population at risk. *Pediatrics.* 2007;120:1390–1401.

Farr V, Kerridge DF, Mitchell RG. The definition of some external characteristics used in the assessment of gestational age in the newborn infant. *Dev Med Child Neurol.* 1966;8:657.

Fleischman AR, Oinuma M, Clark SL. Rethinking the definition of "term pregnancy." *Obstet Gynecol.* 2010;116(1):136–139.

Fletcher MA. *Physical Diagnosis of Neonatology.* Philadelphia, PA: Lippincott Raven; 1998: 55–66.

Hittner HM, Hirsch NJ, Rudolph AJ. Assessment of gestational age by examination of the anterior vascular capsule of the lens. *J Pediatr.* 1977;91:455.

Olsen IE, Groveman SA, Lawson ML, Clark RH, Zemel BS. New intrauterine growth curves based on United States data. *Pediatrics.* 2010;125:e214; originally published online, January 25, 2010. DOI:10.1542/peds. 2009-0913.

Parkin JM, Hey EN, Clowes JS. Rapid assessment of gestational age at birth. *Arch Dis Child.* 1976;51:259–263.

Usher R, McLean F, Scott KE. Judgment of fetal age: II. Clinical significance of gestational age and objective measurement. *Pediatr Clin North Am.* 1966;13:835.

6 Newborn Physical Examination

Newborns are examined immediately after birth to check for major abnormalities and to help ensure that the transition to extrauterine life is without difficulty. The newborn infant should undergo a complete physical examination within 24 hours of birth. Perform the examinations that cause the least amount of disturbance first. It is easier to listen to the heart and lungs first when the infant is quiet. Warming the stethoscope before use decreases the likelihood of making the infant cry.

I. Vital signs

A. Temperature. Indicate whether the temperature is rectal (which is usually 1° higher than oral), oral, or axillary (which is usually 1° lower than oral). Axillary temperature is usually measured in the neonate, with rectal temperature done if the axillary is abnormal.

B. Respirations. The normal respiratory rate in a newborn is 40–60 breaths/min. Periodic breathing (≥3 apneic episodes lasting >3 seconds within a 20-second period of otherwise normal respirations) is normal and common in newborns.

C. Blood pressure. Blood pressure correlates directly with gestational age, postnatal age of the infant, and birthweight. (For normal blood pressure curves, see Appendix C.)

D. Heart rate. The normal heart rate is 100–180 beats/min in the newborn (usually 120–160 beats/min when awake, 70–80 beats/min when asleep). In the healthy infant, the heart rate increases with stimulation. See Table 48–1.

E. Pulse oximetry. Useful for screening for critical congenital cyanotic heart disease. The goal is to identify infants with structural heart defects associated with hypoxia that could have significant morbidity and mortality in the newborn period. These include hypoplastic left heart syndrome, pulmonary atresia, tetralogy of Fallot, tricuspid atresia, transposition of the great arteries, truncus arteriosus, and total anomalous pulmonary venous return. Routine screening for all newborns has been endorsed by the American College of Cardiology Foundation, American Heart Association, and American Academy of Pediatrics (AAP). These criteria may need to be modified in high-altitude areas. Recommendations include the following:

1. Screen all healthy newborn infants. Best to screen when alert.
2. Use a motion tolerant pulse oximeter.
3. Screen at 24–48 hours of age or as late as possible for early discharge.
4. Obtain oxygen saturation in the right hand and one foot
   a. Negative screen
      i. Results. Pulse oximetry reading of ≥95% in either extremity and a ≤3% difference between the right hand and foot.
      ii. Plan. No further testing or treatment necessary.
   b. Positive screen is any of the following:
      i. Results. Any of the following:
         (a) Pulse oximetry <90%. In either right hand or foot.
         (b) Pulse oximetry 90 to <95%. In right hand and foot on 3 different measures, each separated by an hour.
         (c) Pulse oximetry >3% difference. Between the right hand and foot on 3 different measures, each separated by an hour.
      ii. Plan. Perform a comprehensive evaluation for hypoxia. Rule out other reasons for hypoxia (respiratory, sepsis, and others). If no obvious cause is found, a diagnostic echocardiogram is done, and consider pediatric cardiology consultation.

II. Head circumference, length, weight, chest circumference, abdominal circumference, and gestational age. (For intrauterine growth charts, see Figures 5-3, 5-4, and 5-5). For standard infant/child growth charts based on Centers for Disease Control and World Health Organization data from birth to 36 months, see http://www.cdc.gov/growthcharts/.

   A. Head circumference and percentile. Place the measuring tape around the front of the head (above the brow [the frontal area]) and the occipital area. The tape should be above the ears. This is known as the occipital-frontal circumference, which is normally 32–37 cm at term.

   B. Length and percentile. Normal length is 48–52 cm.

   C. Weight and percentile. See details in Chapter 5.

   D. Chest circumference. With the infant supine, measure the circumference of the chest at the level of the nipples during normal breathing. This is a good indicator of low birthweight. Normal is 30–35 cm (head circumference is 2 cm larger than chest circumference).

   E. Abdominal circumference. Measure the distance around the abdomen at the umbilicus. A baseline is valuable because if there is a question of abdominal distension, one will have a measurement to compare. Increases of abdominal circumference of <1.5 cm occur normally and should not be a cause of concern, especially if there are no other abnormal clinical signs. An increase in abdominal girth >2 cm is abnormal.

   F. Gestational age and birthweight classification. Access gestational age by using the Ballard examination and classify as preterm, late preterm, etc. Classify by birthweight, if ELBW, LBW, etc. Determine if small, appropriate, or large for gestational age based on weight and gestational age (see Chapter 5).

III. General appearance. Observe the infant and record the general appearance (eg, activity, skin color, obvious congenital abnormalities). Are the general movements normal? Is the skin tone normal? Abnormal odors suggest inborn error of metabolism: odor of maple syrup or burnt sugar: maple syrup urine disease, odor of sweaty feet: isovaleric acidemia, glutaric acidemia type II, odor of cat urine: HMG-CoA lyase deficiency.

IV. Skin. See also Chapter 75.

   A. Color

      1. Plethora (deep, rosy red [ruddy] color). Plethora is more common in infants with polycythemia but can be seen in an over-oxygenated or overheated infant. It is best to obtain a central hematocrit on any plethoric infant.

      2. Jaundice (yellowish color if secondary to indirect hyperbilirubinemia, greenish color if secondary to direct hyperbilirubinemia). With jaundice, bilirubin levels are usually >5 mg/dL. This condition is abnormal in infants <24 hours of age and may signify Rh incompatibility, sepsis, and TORCH (toxoplasmosis, other, rubella, cytomegalovirus, and herpes simplex virus) infections. After 24 hours, it may result either from these diseases or from such common causes as ABO incompatibility or physiologic causes.

      3. Pallor (washed-out, whitish appearance). Pallor may be secondary to anemia, birth asphyxia, shock, or patent ductus arteriosus (PDA). Ductal pallor is the term sometimes used to denote pallor associated with PDA.

      4. Excessive pigmentation. Infants with more melanin can have increased pigment in the following places: in the axilla, over the scrotum or labia, over the helices of the ear, base of the nails, and around the umbilicus. The skin color of the parents and maternal hormones in utero will affect the pigmentation of the infant. The linea nigra (dark line down the middle of the abdomen) is from exposure of maternal hormone.

5. Cyanosis (desaturation of >3–5 g/dL of hemoglobin is usually necessary for one to note a bluish color)
   a. **Central cyanosis (bluish skin, including the tongue, mucosal membranes, and lips).** Caused by low oxygen saturation in the blood. Rule out cardiac, lung, central nervous system (CNS), metabolic, or hematologic diseases.
   b. **Peripheral cyanosis (bluish skin with pink lips and tongue).** Best noted in the nail beds and can be caused by all the common causes of central cyanosis. Peripheral cyanosis may be associated with methemoglobinemia (hemoglobin oxidized from the ferrous to the ferric form; is incapable of transporting oxygen or carbon dioxide); the blood actually can have a chocolate hue. This disorder can be caused by exposure to certain drugs or chemicals (eg, nitrates or nitrites) or may be hereditary (eg, nicotinamide adenine dinucleotide methemoglobin reductase deficiency or hemoglobin M disease [treated with methylene blue]).
   c. **Acrocyanosis (bluish hands and feet only).** Peripheral cyanosis of the extremities. This may be normal: immediately after birth or within the first few hours after birth or with cold stress. Spasm of smaller arterioles can cause this (up to 24–48 hours of life). In a normothermic older infant, consider hypovolemia.
   d. **Perioral cyanosis (bluish color around the lips and philtrum [nose to upper lip]).** Common after birth. This is due to the close proximity of the blood vessels to the skin (infants have a superficial perioral venous plexus around the mouth). It is not a sign of peripheral or central cyanosis and usually resolves after 48 hours.
   e. **Differential cyanosis. The prerequisite for this is the presence of a right to left shunt through the PDA.** There are two types:
      i. **Differential cyanosis (most common).** Occurs in infants with a patent ductus arteriosus with a right to left shunt. The preductal part of the body (upper part) is pink, and the postductal part (lower body) is cyanotic. Oxygen saturation in the right hand is greater than in the foot. Seen in severe coarctation of aorta or interrupted aortic arch or in a newborn with a structurally normal heart, it can occur with severe persistent pulmonary hypertension with right to left shunting through the ductus arteriosus.
      ii. **Reverse differential cyanosis.** This is a **newborn cardiac emergency**. The preductal part of the body (upper part) is cyanotic (blue), and the postductal part (lower part) is pink. This occurs when oxygen saturation is lower in the upper extremity (right hand) than in the lower extremity (foot). This occurs with complete transposition of the great arteries with PDA and persistent pulmonary hypertension or in transposition of the great arteries with PDA and preductal coarctation or aortic arch interruption and supracardiac total anomalous pulmonary venous connection. The ductus allows saturated blood to perfuse the lower body.
   f. Asphyxia stages after birth (historical degrees of severity)
      i. **Asphyxia livida (early stage).** The phase during asphyxia when primary apnea occurs (heart rate decreases, respiratory efforts may be present, blood pressure rises then drops, $Paco_2$ and pH increases). The infant is **cyanotic**, has some muscle tone, and has adequate circulation.
      ii. **Asphyxia pallida (late stage).** The phase during asphyxia when secondary apnea occurs (heart rate and blood pressure drop, circulatory collapse, shock, low Pao_2, increased $Paco_2$, low pH). The infant has **pale gray/white skin** and is limp; reflexes are absent and respiratory efforts are absent.

g. **Stages of shock**
  i. Warm shock (early stage of shock). **Extremities are warm,** with loss of vascular tone, peripheral vasodilation, tachycardia, bounding peripheral pulses, increase in systemic blood flow, and a decrease in blood pressure.
  ii. Cold shock (late stage of shock). **Extremities are cold and mottled,** with a prolonged capillary refill time (>2 seconds), decreased peripheral pulses, increase in vascular tone, vasoconstriction, decrease in systemic blood flow, and decrease in blood pressure.

6. Extensive bruising (ecchymoses). May be associated with a prolonged and difficult delivery and may result in early jaundice. Facial bruising can occur with a tight nuchal cord or difficult delivery. This can be confused with cyanosis. **Petechiae (pinpoint hemorrhages)** can be limited to one area and are usually of no concern. If they are widespread and progressive, then they are of concern, and a workup for coagulopathy should be considered. Upper body petechiae can be seen in pertussis.

7. "Blue on pink" or "pink on blue." Whereas some infants are pink and well perfused and others are clearly cyanotic, some do not fit in either of these categories. They may appear bluish with pink undertones or pink with bluish undertones. This coloration may be secondary to poor perfusion, inadequate oxygenation, inadequate ventilation, or polycythemia.

8. Harlequin sign/coloration. A clear line of demarcation between an area of redness and an area of normal coloration. This is a vascular phenomenon and the cause is usually unknown, but may be due to immaturity of the hypothalamic center that controls the dilation of peripheral blood vessels. The coloration can be benign and transient (a few seconds to <30 minutes) or can be indicative of shunting of blood (persistent pulmonary hypertension or coarctation of the aorta). There can be varying degrees of redness and perfusion. The demarcating line may run from the head to the belly, dividing the body into right and left halves, or it may develop in the dependent half of the body when the newborn is lying on one side. The dependent half is usually deep red, and the upper half is pale. This occurs most commonly in lower birthweight infants. It can also occur in 10% of full-term infants and usually occurs on the second to fifth day of life. (*Note:* This is not **Harlequin fetus;** see page 47).

9. Cutis marmorata. Reticular mottling, lacy red pattern of the skin, marbled, purplish skin discoloration.
   a. Physiologic cutis marmorata. May be seen in healthy infants and in those with cold stress, hypovolemia, shock, or sepsis. It can be caused by an instability or immaturity of the nerve supply to the superficial capillary blood vessels in the skin. Physiologic dilatation of capillaries and venules occurs in response to cold stimulus. In hypovolemia, shock, and sepsis, it occurs because of insufficient perfusion of the skin, and mottling can occur. It is usually in a symmetric pattern and can be seen on the extremities but also on the trunk. It is most pronounced when the skin is cooled. It disappears with rewarming.
   b. Persistent cutis marmorata. Occurs in infants with Down syndrome, Cornelia de Lange syndrome, homocystinuria, Menkes disease, familial dysautonomia, trisomy 13, trisomy 18, Divry-Van Bogaert syndrome, and in hypothyroidism, cardiovascular hypertension, and CNS dysfunction.
   c. Cutis marmorata telangiectatica congenita. A rare congenital cutaneous vascular malformation. The marbling is persistent, and 20–80% have another congenital abnormality with skin atrophy and ulceration. Asymmetry of the lower extremities is the most common extracutaneous finding. The mottling does not disappear with warming. It can be associated with

body asymmetry, glaucoma, retinal detachment, neurologic anomalies, and other vascular anomalies (Plate 1).

10. **Lanugo.** Downy hair seen in infants (more common in premature infants but can be seen in term infants).

11. **Vernix caseosa.** This greasy white substance covers the skin until the 38th week of gestation. Its purpose is to provide a moisture barrier and is completely normal.

12. **Collodion infant.** The skin resembles parchment, and there can be some restriction in growth of the nose and ears. This may be a normal condition or can be a manifestation of another disease.

13. **Dry skin.** Infants can have a dry flaky skin, and postdate or postmature infants can exhibit excessive peeling and cracking of the skin. Congenital syphilis and candidiasis can present with peeling skin at birth.

14. **Harlequin fetus.** The most severe form of congenital ichthyosis. Affected infants have thickening of the keratin layer of skin that causes thick scales. Survival of these infants has improved with supportive care.

15. **Aplasia cutis congenita.** Absence of some or all the layers of the skin. Most common is a solitary area on the scalp (70%). The prognosis is excellent, but if the area is large, surgical repair may be necessary (Plate 3).

16. **Subcutaneous fat necrosis.** A reddish lesion with a firm nodule in the subcutaneous tissue that is freely mobile. It is more common in difficult deliveries, perinatal asphyxia, and cold stress. They are usually benign unless there are extensive lesions, in which case calcium levels should be monitored (Plate 9).

17. **Abnormal fat distribution.** Seen with congenital disorders of glycosylation.

18. **Constriction rings around digits, arms, legs.** Occurs in amniotic band syndrome (Plate 2).

19. **Decreased pigmentation.** Seen in phenylketonuria.

B. Rashes

1. **Milia.** A rash in which tiny sebaceous retention (of keratin) cysts are seen. The whitish yellow pinhead-size concretions are usually on the chin, nose, forehead, and cheeks without erythema. These are seen in ~33% of infants, and these benign cysts disappear within a few weeks after birth. **Miliaria** occurs from sweat retention from incomplete closure of the eccrine structures. **Miliaria crystallina** usually are on the head, neck, and trunk and are from superficial eccrine duct closure. **Miliaria rubra** (heat rash) involves a deeper area of sweat gland obstruction. **Pearls** are large single milia or inclusion cysts that can occur on the newborn's palate **(Epstein pearls)**, on buccal or lingual mucosa **(Bohn nodules)**, or dental lamina cysts (on crests of alveolar ridges), genitalia **(penile pearls)**, and areola (Plate 6).

2. **Sebaceous hyperplasia.** In contrast to milia, these raised lesions are more yellow and are sometimes referred to as "miniature puberty of the newborn." The cause is maternal androgen exposure in utero; they are benign and resolve spontaneously within a couple of weeks.

3. **Erythema toxicum (erythema neonatorum toxicum).** Consists of numerous small areas of red skin with a yellow-white papule in the center. Lesions are most noticeable 48 hours after birth but may appear as late as 7–10 days. Wright staining of the papule reveals eosinophils. This benign rash, which is the most common rash, resolves spontaneously. If suspected in an infant <34 weeks' gestation, rule out other causes because this rash is more common in term infants (Plate 4).

4. *Candida albicans* rash ("diaper rash"). Appears as erythematous plaques with sharply demarcated edges. Satellite bodies (pustules on contiguous areas of skin) are also seen. Usually the skin folds are involved. Gram stain of a smear or 10% KOH prep of the lesion reveals budding yeast spores, which are easily treated with nystatin ointment or cream applied to the rash 4 times daily for 7–10 days.

5. **Transient neonatal pustular melanosis.** A benign, self-limiting condition that requires no specific therapy. The rash starts in utero and is characterized by 3 stages of lesions, which may appear over the entire body: pustules, ruptured vesicopustules with scaling/typical halo appearance, and hyperpigmented macules. These remain after the pustules have resolved (Plate 5).

6. **Infantile seborrheic dermatitis.** A common rash usually occurring on the scalp "cradle cap," face, neck, and diaper area that is erythematous and with greasy scales. A self-limiting condition.

7. **Acne neonatorum.** Lesions are typically seen over the cheeks, chin, and forehead and consist of comedones and papules. The condition is usually benign and requires no therapy; however, severe cases may require treatment with mild keratolytic agents (Plate 8).

8. **Herpes simplex.** Seen as pustular vesicular rash, vesicles, bullae, or denuded skin. The rash is most commonly seen at the fetal scalp monitor site, occiput, or buttocks (presentation site at time of delivery). Tzanck smear reveals multinucleated giant cells (Plate 12).

9. **Sucking blisters.** Solitary lesions that can be intact blisters or can appear as flat, scabbed areas on the hand or forearm. They are only in areas accessible by the mouth. They are benign and resolve spontaneously.

C. **Nevi** can be pigmented, present at birth, brown or black to bluish (see Chapter 75), or vascular.

1. **Nevus simplex (fading macular stain; "stork bites," "angel kiss," "salmon patch").** A macular stain is a common capillary malformation normally seen on the occipital area, eyelids, and glabella. They are called "angel kisses" when located on the forehead or eyelids and "stork bites" when on the back of the neck. The lesions disappear spontaneously within the first year of life. Occasionally lesions on the nape of the neck may persist as a medial telangiectatic nevus.

2. **Port-wine stain (nevus flammeus).** Usually seen at birth, does not blanch with pressure, and does not disappear with time. If the lesion appears over the forehead and upper lip, then **Sturge-Weber syndrome** (port-wine stain over the forehead and upper lip, glaucoma, and contralateral Jacksonian seizures) must be ruled out (Plate 20).

3. **Mongolian spots are the most common birthmark.** These are dark blue or purple bruise-like macular spots usually located over the sacrum. Usually present in 90% of blacks and Asians, they occur in <5% of white children and disappear by 4 years of age (Plate 10).

4. **Cavernous hemangioma.** Usually appears as a large, red, cyst-like, firm, ill-defined mass and may be found anywhere on the body. The majority of these lesions regress with age, but some require corticosteroid therapy. In more severe cases, surgical resection may be necessary. If associated with thrombocytopenia, **Kasabach-Merritt syndrome** (thrombocytopenia associated with a rapidly expanding hemangioma) should be considered. Transfusions of platelets and clotting factors are usually required in patients with this syndrome.

5. **Strawberry hemangioma (macular hemangioma).** Strawberry hemangiomas are flat, bright red, sharply demarcated lesions that are most commonly found on the face. Spontaneous regression usually occurs (70% disappearance by 7 years of age).

V. **Head.** Note the general shape of the head. Some amount of molding is normal in all infants. Inspect for any cuts or bruises secondary to forceps or fetal monitor leads. Check for microcephaly or macrocephaly. Transillumination can be done for severe hydrocephalus and hydranencephaly. Bruising of the vertex of the head is common after birth. Look for unusual hair growth (**hair whorls**). Multiple hair whorls or hair whorls in unusual locations can signify abnormal brain growth. **Abnormal hair** can also be seen in some inborn errors of metabolism: argininosuccinic acidemia, lysinuric protein intolerance, Menkes kinky hair syndrome. Swelling may represent **caput succedaneum, a cephalohematoma, or a subgaleal hemorrhage.** Examine the occipital, parietal, and frontal bones and the suture lines. The fontanelles should be soft when palpated.

A. Macrocephaly. Occipitofrontal circumference is >90th percentile. May be normal or be secondary to hydrocephaly, hydrencephaly, or a neuroendocrine or chromosomal disorder.

B. Microcephaly. Occipitofrontal circumference is <10th percentile. Brain atrophy or decreased brain size can occur.

C. Anterior and posterior fontanelles. The anterior fontanelle usually closes by 24 months (median age ~13 months) and the posterior fontanelle by 2 months. Normal size of anterior fontanelle is 0.6–3.6 cm (African American: 1.4–4.7 cm). Posterior fontanelle size is 0.5 cm (African American: 0.7 cm). A **large anterior fontanelle** can be a normal variation or can be seen in congenital hypothyroidism and may also be found in infants with skeletal disorders such as achondroplasia, hypophosphatasia, and chromosomal abnormalities such as Down syndrome and in those with intrauterine growth restriction. A **bulging fontanelle** may be associated with increased intracranial pressure, meningitis, or hydrocephalus. **Depressed (sunken) fontanelles** are seen in newborns with dehydration. A **small anterior fontanelle** may be associated with hyperthyroidism, microcephaly, or craniosynostosis.

D. Cephalic molding. A temporary asymmetry of the skull resulting from the birth process. Most often seen with prolonged labor and vaginal deliveries, it can be seen in cesarean deliveries if the mother had a prolonged course of labor before delivery. A normal head shape is usually regained within 1 week. Rarely it may be associated with other abnormalities. If it persists, then intracranial hypertension can occur.

E. Caput succedaneum. A diffuse edematous swelling of the soft tissues of the scalp that may extend across the suture lines but usually is unilateral. It does not increase after birth. It is secondary to the pressure of the uterus or vaginal wall on areas of the fetal head bordering the caput. Elicit the characteristic pitting edema by putting firm constant pressure in one area. Usually, it resolves within several days (Figure 6–1).

F. Cephalhematoma. A subperiosteal hemorrhage that *never extends across the suture* line and can be secondary to a traumatic delivery or forceps delivery. It increases after birth. Radiographs or computed tomography scans of the head should be obtained if an underlying skull fracture is suspected (<5% of all cephalhematomas). Hematocrit and bilirubin levels should be monitored. Most cephalhematomas resolve in 2–3 weeks. Aspiration of the hematoma is rarely necessary (see Figure 6–1).

G. Subgaleal hematoma/hemorrhage. The subgaleal area is the area between the scalp and the skull and is a very large space. Hemorrhage occurs between the epicranial aponeurosis and the periosteum, and when pressure is placed, a fluid wave can be seen. It can cross over the suture line and onto the neck or ear. It progresses after birth. It may be necessary to replace blood volume lost and correct coagulopathy if present and can be life-threatening. It can be caused by asphyxia, vacuum extraction, forceps delivery, or coagulopathy (see Figure 6–1).

H. Increased intracranial pressure. The increased pressure may be secondary to hydrocephalus, hypoxic-ischemic brain injury, intracranial hemorrhage, or subdural hematoma. The following signs are evident in an infant with increased intracranial pressure:

1. Bulging anterior fontanelle
2. Separated sutures
3. Paralysis of upward gaze ("setting-sun sign")

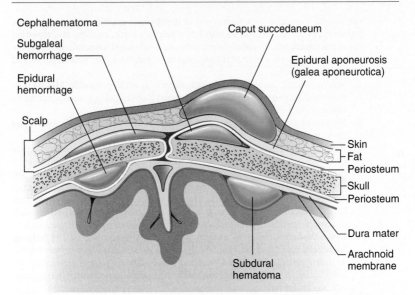

FIGURE 6–1. Types of extradural fluid collections seen in newborn infants. (*Modified from Volpe JJ. Neurology of the Newborn, 4th ed. Philadelphia, PA: WB Saunders; 2001.*)

    4. Prominent veins of the scalp
    5. Increasing macrocephaly
  I. **Craniosynostosis.** The premature closure of ≥1 sutures of the skull; must be considered in any infant with an asymmetric skull. On palpation of the skull, a bony ridge over the suture line may be felt, and inability to move the cranial bones freely may occur. Radiographs of the head should be performed, and surgical consultation may be necessary.
  J. **Craniotabes.** A benign condition, craniotabes is a congenital softening or thinness of the skull that usually occurs around the suture lines (top and back of head) and disappears within days to a few weeks after birth. It can also be associated with rickets, osteogenesis imperfecta, syphilis, and subclinical vitamin D deficiency in utero.
  K. **Plagiocephaly.** An oblique shape of a head, which is asymmetric and flattened. It can be seen in preemies and infants whose heads stay in the same position. Anterior plagiocephaly can be due to premature fusion of the coronal or lambdoidal sutures.
  L. **Brachycephaly.** This is caused by premature closure of the coronal suture and causes the head to have a short broad appearance. It can be seen in trisomy 21 or Apert syndrome.
  M. **Anencephaly.** The anterior neural tube does not close and the brain is malformed. Most of these infants are stillborn or die shortly after.
  N. **Acrocephaly.** The coronal and sagittal sutures close early. The skull has a narrow appearance with a cone shape at the top. This can be seen in Crouzon and Apert syndromes.
  O. **Dolichocephaly/scaphocephaly.** The sagittal suture closes prematurely and there is a restriction of lateral growth of the skull, resulting in a long, narrow head.
  VI. **Neck.** Eliciting the rooting reflex (see page 63) causes the infant to turn the head and allows easier examination of the neck. Palpate the sternocleidomastoid for a hematoma and the thyroid for enlargement, and check for thyroglossal duct cysts.

A. **Short neck.** Seen in Turner, Noonan, Down, and Klippel-Feil syndromes.

B. **Webbed neck (with redundant skin).** Seen in Turner, Noonan, Down, and Klippel-Feil syndromes.

C. **Brachial cleft cysts.** Firm, <1 cm cysts that can be on the lateral aspects of the neck, along the anterior margin of the sternomastoid muscle. If dimples are seen here, they are brachial cleft sinuses.

D. **Cystic hygroma.** The most common neck mass. It is a fluctuant mass that can be transilluminated and is usually found laterally or over the clavicles.

E. **Goiter.** May be a result of maternal thyroid disorders or neonatal hyperthyroidism.

F. **Thyroglossal duct cyst.** Rarely seen in neonates. They are subcutaneous structures in the midline of the anterior neck at the level of the larynx.

G. **Torticollis ("wry neck").** A shortening of the sternocleidomastoid muscle that causes the head to go toward the affected side. Treated initially with physical therapy.

VII. **Face.** Observe for obvious abnormalities. Note the general shape of the nose, mouth, and chin. Look for unequal movement of the mouth and lips. **Coarse facies** can be seen in lysosomal disorders. Flat facial profile can be seen in Down syndrome. The presence of **hypertelorism** (eyes widely separated) or **low-set ears** should be noted. If delivered by **forceps, a forceps mark** may be present. It is usually a semicircular mark on the cheek that will resolve spontaneously. **Micrognathia** is a small lower jaw that can interfere with feeding. It is most commonly seen in Pierre Robin sequence but can also be seen in other genetic syndromes.

A. **Low set ears (melotia).** See Section VIII on ears.

B. **Micrognathia.** A small lower jaw that can interfere with feeding. It is most commonly seen in Pierre Robin sequence but can also be seen in some genetic syndromes.

C. **Hypertelorism.** See page 53.

D. **Facial nerve injury.** Unilateral branches of the facial (seventh) nerve are most commonly involved. There is facial asymmetry with crying, the corner of the mouth droops, and the nasolabial fold is absent in the paralyzed side. The infant may be unable to close the eye or move the lip and drools on the side of the paresis. If the palsy is secondary to trauma, most symptoms disappear within the first week of life, but sometimes resolution may take several months. If the palsy persists, absence of the nerve should be ruled out.

VIII. **Ears.** Evaluate for an unusual shape or an abnormal position. Confirm that structures of the ear are all present: helix, antihelix, tragus, antitragus, scaphoid/triangular fossa, and external auditory canal. Genetic syndromes are frequently associated with abnormal ear shapes. Assess gross hearing when an infant blinks in response to loud noises. The normal position of ears is determined by drawing an imaginary horizontal line from the inner and outer canthi of the eye across the face, perpendicular to the vertical axis of the head. If the helix of the ear lies below this horizontal line, the ears are designated as **low set.** An otoscopic examination is usually not done on the first examination because the ear canal is usually full of amniotic debris.

A. **Low-set ears (melotia).** Seen with many congenital anomalies, most commonly Treacher-Collins, Down, triploidy, and trisomy 9 and 18 syndromes, fetal aminopterin effects, and trisomy 13 and 21.

B. **Preauricular skin tags (papillomas).** Benign, common, and usually inherited.

C. **Ear pits (preauricular pits).** May be unilateral or bilateral and are usually located at the superior attachment of the pinna. They are more common in the Asian population (10%).

D. **Hairy ears.** Seen in infants of diabetic mothers.

E. **Anotia.** Complete absence of the pinna of the ear. It is associated with thalidomide and retinoic acid embryopathy. Bilateral anotia is sometimes seen in infants of consanguineous parents.

F. **Microtia (small ears).** Used to describe small pinnae, it is a misshaped dysplastic ear that can be associated with other abnormalities such as middle ear abnormalities. Approximately 50% of infants with microtia will have an underlying congenital syndrome. Pediatric ear, nose, and throat (ENT) evaluation and hearing evaluation are required. Renal ultrasound is also recommended. Small ears are seen in trisomy 21, as well as trisomy 18 and 13 triploidy and thalidomide and retinoic acid embryopathy.

G. **Macrotia (large ears).** The auricle is large and the scaphoid fossa is the most exaggerated part. It is usually bilateral and symmetric. It can be autosomal dominant and can also be associated with Marfan syndrome, fragile X syndrome, De Lange type 2 syndrome, and others.

H. **Lop ear (folded down superior edge of the helix) and cup ear or prominent ear (ear stands away from the head).** Plastic surgery consultation can be obtained. A **hypoplastic ear** may be an indicator of internal ear abnormalities.

I. **Satyr ear ("Spock ear").** Characterized by a flattened scaphoid fossa and a flat helix at the superior pole and a third crus into the helix. This is only a cosmetic concern, and molding in the first week of life can be done. Plastic surgery consultation is recommended.

IX. **Eyes.** Most infants have some degree of eyelid edema after birth, which usually resolves after the first few days of life. The eyes can still be gently opened and examined. The sclera, which is normally white, can have a bluish tint if the infant is premature because the sclera is thinner in these infants than in term infants. Check for the following: **scleral hemorrhages, exudates** (suggest conjunctivitis), and **yellow sclera (icterus)** indicative of hyperbilirubinemia. Is there a **cherry red spot** in the macula of the eye (lipidosis, or occlusion of the central retinal artery)? Check the pupil size bilaterally (if not the same size, rule out tumor or vascular abnormality) and reactivity, and evaluate eye movements. Check the red reflex with an ophthalmoscope. If a red reflex cannot be obtained, or if the pupil is white or cloudy, immediate evaluation by a pediatric ophthalmologist is required. See also Chapter 93.

A. **Leukocoria (opacification of the lens).** A white pupil with loss of a red light reflex. Opacity behind the pupil is sometimes seen without an ophthalmoscope. Evaluate further for:

1. **Congenital cataracts.** If suspected, emergency referral of a pediatric ophthalmologist is necessary for early intervention and to preserve sight. Infants with congenital cataracts should be evaluated for an underlying metabolic, genetic, or infectious cause, and 20% will have an identifiable cause. This can be seen in galactosemia and Zellweger syndrome. An **oil drop cataract** can be seen with galactosemia, and on retinoscopy one sees a classic "oil droplet" against a red reflex due to accumulation of dulcitol within the lens.

2. **Glaucoma.** Infant can present with corneal opacities.

3. **Retinoblastoma.** Tumor requires emergency ophthalmology consultation.

4. **Retinal detachment.** Most commonly occurs from retinopathy of prematurity.

5. **Peters anomaly.** Abnormal cleavage of the anterior chamber occurs from anterior segment dysgenesis. There is a central or para central or a complete corneal opacity.

B. **Osteogenesis imperfecta.** Sclera is deep blue.

C. **Coloboma.** A key-shaped defect in the iris.

D. **Brushfield spots.** Salt-and-pepper speckling of the iris or white or yellow spots on the iris. Often seen with Down syndrome or may be normal.

E. **Subconjunctival hemorrhage.** Occurs in 5% of newborns as a result of rupture of small conjunctival capillaries and can occur normally but is more common after a traumatic delivery. Petechiae on the forehead may be associated. It is asymptomatic and resolves in a few days.

F. **Conjunctivitis.** Suspected if a discharge is present. (See Chapter 53.)

G. **Epicanthal folds.** May be normal or may occur in infants with Down syndrome. This is a skin fold of the upper eyelid covering the inner corner of the eye.

H. **Dacryocystoceles.** Obstructions of both the superior and inferior ends of the nasolacrimal duct. Presents as bluish nodules inferior to the medial canthi of both eyes. If bilateral, ENT consult should be obtained to evaluate nasal obstruction.

I. **Dacryostenosis.** The nasolacrimal ducts are too narrow to drain tears properly. Tears may pool on the eyelids and eyelashes. Usually resolves within the first week of life for ~50% of infants. Others it resolves in several weeks to a few months.

J. **Hypertelorism (widely spaced eyes).** The interorbital distance is greater than normal. Normal interorbital distance is 20 mm at birth. This can occur alone or with other congenital deformities.

K. **Nystagmus.** This is an involuntary usually rapid eye movement that can be horizontal, vertical, or mixed. Can be normal if occasional, but if persistent, it needs to be evaluated.

L. **Ptosis.** A drooping of an upper eyelid caused by third cranial nerve paralysis or weakness in the levator muscle. Ptosis and ophthalmoparesis can be seen in transient neonatal myasthenia gravis.

M. **Dysconjugate eye movements.** During the first months of life, infants will have dysconjugate eye movements, where eyes appear to move independently of each other. They may even appear crossed. Transient movements are normal, especially if this occurs when the infant falls asleep or awakes. If the movement is fixed, a consult with a pediatric ophthalmologist should be obtained.

X. **Nose.** Check the appearance of the nose. Sometimes due to a positional deformity, the nose will be asymmetric. If unilateral or bilateral choanal atresia is suspected, verify the patency of the nostrils with gentle passage of a nasogastric tube. **Infants are obligate nose breathers**; therefore, if they have **bilateral choanal atresia,** they will have cyanosis and severe respiratory distress at rest.

A. **Nasal flaring.** Indicative of respiratory distress.

B. **Sniffling/snuffles and discharge.** Typical of congenital syphilis.

C. **Sneezing.** This can be a response to bright light or drug withdrawal.

D. **Dislocated nasal septum.** Four percent incidence. Vertical axis of the nose is deviated, and the septum is not straight. Immediate pediatric ENT evaluation is needed, as correction in the first few days of life can prevent a permanent deformity.

XI. **Mouth.** Examine the hard and soft palates for evidence of a cleft palate and submucosal and partial clefts that can be easily missed.

A. **Cleft lip/palate.** Secondary to midline fusion failure. Unilateral clefts are usually an isolated finding; midline clefts are often associated with midline defects in the brain.

B. **Bifid uvula.** The uvula is larger than normal and has two halves and is associated with a submucous cleft.

C. **Positional deformity of the jaw.** Causes asymmetry of the chin, and gums are not parallel to each other, usually due to utero molding. Resolution occurs without treatment.

D. **Epstein pearl.** A small white papule usually in the midline of the palate. Common and benign, it is secondary to epithelial tissue that is trapped during palatal fusion.

E. **Alveolar cysts.** Oral mucosal cysts located on alveolar ridge.

F. **Teeth.** Primary teeth usually begin to erupt at 6–8 months of age. **Natal teeth** are teeth that are present at birth. **Neonatal teeth** are teeth that erupt during the first 30 days after birth. **Infancy teeth** are teeth that erupt after 30 days. **Supernumerary teeth** are extra teeth. Teeth in newborns are uncommon (incidence 1:1000 to 1:30,000). Etiology is unknown, but the most common accepted theory is based on hereditary factors. Other causes include infection, endocrine disturbances, nutritional deficiency, maternal fever, environmental factors, and position of the tooth germ. Eighty-five percent of natal or neonatal teeth erupt in the mandibular incisor area. Radiographs are sometimes needed to differentiate if the teeth are supernumerary or have a normal deciduous dentition. Clinically, teeth can be classified as mature or immature. Pediatric dentistry consultation is recommended.

1. **Natal teeth (more common).** Erupt most commonly in pairs and are usually poorly attached to the bony structure and have a poorly developed root system. They are associated with Ellis-van Creveld syndrome, Jadassohn-Lewandowski syndrome, Hallermann Streiff syndrome, Soto syndrome, and Pierre Robin syndrome. It is best to leave these teeth in the mouth to avoid future space management issues unless symptomatic (highly mobile, cause pain for mom during breast feeding, or cause irritation and injury to infant's tongue); then they can be extracted after birth. If loose, it is very important to remove the teeth to decrease the risk of aspiration.

2. **Neonatal teeth.** These have a firm root structure and are more securely anchored. If mature they have a good prognosis for maintenance.

G. **Bohn nodules.** Appear as white bumps on the gum (may look like teeth) or periphery of the palate and are secondary from heterotrophic salivary glands or from remnants of the dental lamina. Benign and will resolve without treatment.

H. **Ranula.** Cystic swelling in the floor of the mouth. Most disappear spontaneously.

I. **Mucocele.** This small lesion on the oral mucosa is secondary to trauma to the salivary gland ducts. It is usually benign and subsides spontaneously.

J. **Macroglossia.** Enlargement of the tongue can be congenital or acquired. Localized macroglossia is usually secondary to congenital hemangiomas. Macroglossia can be seen in **Beckwith syndrome** (macroglossia, gigantism, omphalocele, and severe hypoglycemia), **Pompe disease** (type II glycogen storage disease), GM 1 gangliosidosis, and hypothyroidism.

K. **Glossoptosis.** Downward displacement/retraction of the tongue. It can be seen in Pierre Robin sequence and Down syndrome.

L. **Ankyloglossia (short lingual frenulum, "tongue tied").** Occurs in 4% of newborns. Often a frenotomy will be indicated if tongue mobility and feeding are an issue.

M. **Frothy or copious saliva.** Commonly seen in infants with an esophageal atresia with tracheoesophageal fistula.

N. **Thrush.** Oral thrush, common in newborns, is a sign of *C. albicans.*

O. **Micrognathia (small jaw).** An underdeveloped jaw that is seen in **Pierre Robin syndrome;** other genetic syndromes should be considered.

XII. **Chest**

A. **Observation.** Note the shape and symmetry of the chest. An asymmetric chest may signify a space- or air-occupying lesion such as tension pneumothorax. Tachypnea (increased respiratory rate), sternal subcostal and intercostal retractions, nasal flaring, and grunting on expiration indicate respiratory distress. *Note:* **Grunting, nasal flaring, and intercostal or subcostal retractions indicate increased work of breathing**.

1. **Grunting.** Occurs when the glottis is closed during expiration. This improves oxygenation by increasing the end expiratory pressure in the lungs. Occasional grunting is acceptable; grunting with every breath is abnormal.

2. **Nasal flaring.** Widening of the nostrils on inspiration; occurs with respiratory distress.

3. **Retractions.** Can be subcostal or intercostal and represent muscles sucked in between the ribs to increase air flow. One sees a shadow at the lower margin of the rib cage with subcostal retractions ("rib shadows"). Mild retractions, usually subcostal, may be normal.

4. **Phonatory abnormalities.** Depend on the level of abnormality or obstruction. Phonation is a primary function of the larynx, and an abnormality of this causes no cry or a weak cry. Laryngeal obstruction can be supraglottic, glottic, or subglottic. A **muffled cry and inspiratory stridor** occurs with supraglottic obstruction; a **high-pitched or absent cry** is associated with glottic abnormalities (laryngeal web or atresia). Subglottic stenosis can present with **hoarse or weak cry, stridor,** and obstructive breathing.

   a. **Stridor.** A high-pitched sound on inspiration heard without a stethoscope. It can be normal if it occurs occasionally and there are no other signs of respiratory distress. If the stridor is persistent, **laryngomalacia is the most common cause.** Other causes include congenital subglottic stenosis, vocal cord paresis, double aortic arch, and other congenital anomalies. **Inspiratory stridor with cyanotic attacks with feeding with aspiration** and pulmonary infections that reoccur can occur with laryngeal and laryngotracheoesophageal clefts.

   b. **Intermittent hoarseness, dyspnea, weak cry, or aphonia** can be seen in saccular cysts.

   c. **High-pitched inspiratory stridor and inspiratory cry.** Bilateral vocal cord paralysis.

   d. **Weak cry,** usually no serious airway obstruction, occasional breathy, feeding problems. Unilateral vocal cord paralysis.

   e. **Mild hoarseness, little airway obstruction.** Thin anterior laryngeal web.

   f. **Weaker voice, increased airway obstruction.** Thicker laryngeal webs (>75% glottic involvement causes aphonia and severe airway obstruction).

   g. **Muffled or absent cry.** Laryngeal web or pharyngeal obstruction.

   h. **Weak cry, weak sucking, aphonia, lethargy** can be seen from medications in pregnancy (selective serotonin reuptake inhibitor–induced neonatal abstinence syndrome).

   i. **Weak but high-pitched cry** resembling a cat. Cri du chat syndrome.

   j. **Whistling noise** can occur with a blockage in the nostril.

   k. **Weak cry.** Hypoglycemia.

   l. **Weak cry, mild respiratory distress.** Transient neonatal myasthenia gravis.

   m. **High-pitched cry.** Neonatal abstinence syndrome or hypoglycemia.

   n. **Hiccups.** Nonketotic hyperglycinemia.

B. **Breath sounds.** Listen for the presence and equality of breath sounds. A good place to listen is in the right and left axillae. Absent or unequal sounds may indicate pneumothorax or atelectasis. Absent breath sounds with the presence of bowel sounds plus a scaphoid abdomen (flat abdomen relative to the chest) suggest diaphragmatic hernia; an immediate radiograph and emergency surgical consultation are recommended.

C. **Fractured clavicle.** Palpate both clavicles; if can not be palpated easily and crepitus is felt over the clavicle, the infant may have a fractured clavicle. No treatment is necessary. Note that a healed clavicle fracture will have a firm lump (as new bone develops) in the area.

D. **Pectus excavatum (funnel chest).** A sternum that is depressed in shape. Usually, this condition is of no clinical concern but may be associated with Marfan and Noonan syndromes.

E. **Pectus carinatum (pigeon chest).** Caused by a protuberant sternum. May be associated with Marfan and Noonan syndromes.

F. **Prominence of the xiphoid process.** A firm lump at the end of the sternum; it is a benign finding.

G. **Barrel chest.** Occurs when there is an increased anteroposterior diameter of the chest. It can be secondary to mechanical ventilation, pneumothorax, pneumonia, or space-occupying lesions.

H. **Breasts in a newborn.** Usually 1 cm in diameter in term male and female infants and may be abnormally enlarged (3–4 cm) secondary to the effects of maternal estrogens. This effect, which lasts <1 week, is of no clinical concern. A usually white discharge, commonly referred to as "neonatal milk" or **"witch's milk,"** may be present and is normal. It is seen in full-term infants with larger than average breast nodules and may continue for up to 2 months of age. **Supernumerary nipples (polythelia)** are extra nipples along the mammary line ("milk line") and occur as a normal variant; the association with renal disorders is *controversial*. They can occur singularly or be multiple and can be unilateral or bilateral. Skin tags on the nipple area are usually small and do not need to be removed. **Inverted nipples** can be seen in congenital disorders of glycosylation.

XIII. **Heart.** Observe for heart rate (normal 110–160 beats/min awake, may drop to 80 beats/min during sleep), rhythm, quality of heart sounds, active precordium, and presence of a murmur. The position of the heart may be determined by auscultation. Abnormal situs syndromes and other physical manifestations of congenital heart disease are discussed in Chapter 89.

A. **Murmurs.** May be associated with the following conditions:

1. **Ventricular septal defect.** The most common heart defect, this accounts for ~25% of congenital heart disease. Typically, a loud, harsh, blowing pansystolic murmur is heard (best heard over the lower left sternal border). It is not heard at birth but often on day 2 or day 3 of life. Symptoms such as congestive heart failure usually do not begin until after 2 weeks of age and typically are present from 6 weeks to 4 months. The majority of these defects close spontaneously by the end of the first year of life.

2. **Patent ductus arteriosus.** A harsh, continuous, machinery-type, "washing machine like" or "rolling thunder" murmur that usually presents on the second or third day of life, localized to the second left intercostal space. It may radiate to the left clavicle or down the left sternal border. It can be heard loudest along the left sternal border. A hyperactive precordium is also seen. Clinical signs include wide pulse pressure and bounding pulses.

3. **Coarctation of the aorta.** A systolic ejection murmur that radiates down the sternum to the apex and to the interscapular area. It is often loudest in the back.

4. **Peripheral pulmonic stenosis.** A systolic murmur is heard bilaterally in the anterior chest, in both axillae, and across the back. It is secondary to the turbulence caused by disturbed blood flow because the main pulmonary artery is larger than the peripheral pulmonary arteries. This usually benign murmur may persist up to 3 months of age. It may also be associated with rubella syndrome.

5. **Hypoplastic left heart syndrome.** A short midsystolic murmur usually presents anywhere from day 1 to 21. A gallop is usually heard.

6. **Tetralogy of Fallot.** Typically a loud, harsh systolic or pansystolic murmur best heard at the left sternal border. The second heart sound is single.

7. **Pulmonary atresia**
   a. **With ventricular septal defect.** An absent or soft systolic murmur with the first heart sound is followed by an ejection click. The second heart sound is loud and single.
   b. **With intact intraventricular septum.** Most frequently, there is no murmur, and a single second heart sound is heard.

8. **Tricuspid atresia.** A pansystolic murmur along the left sternal border with a single second heart sound is typically heard.

9. **Transposition of the great vessels.** More common in males than females.
   a. **Isolated (simple).** Cardiac examination is often normal, but cyanosis and tachypnea are present along with a normal chest radiograph and electrocardiogram.

b. **With ventricular septal defect.** The murmur is loud and pansystolic and is best heard at the lower left sternal border. The infant typically has congestive heart failure at 3–6 weeks of life.

10. **Ebstein disease.** A long systolic murmur is heard over the anterior portion of the left chest. A diastolic murmur and gallop may be present.

11. **Truncus arteriosus.** A systolic ejection murmur, often with a thrill, is heard at the left sternal border. The second heart sound is loud and single.

12. **Single ventricle.** A loud systolic ejection murmur with a loud single second heart sound is heard.

13. **Atrial septal defects**
    a. **Ostium secundum defect.** Rarely presents with congestive heart failure in infancy. A soft systolic ejection murmur is best heard at the upper left sternal border.
    b. **Ostium primum defect.** Rarely occurs in infancy. A pulmonary ejection murmur and early systolic murmur are heard at the lower left sternal border. A split second heart sound is heard.
    c. **Common atrioventricular canal.** Presents with congestive heart failure in infancy. A harsh systolic murmur is heard all over the chest. The second heart sound is split if pulmonary flow is increased.

14. **Anomalous pulmonary venous return**
    a. **Partial anomalous pulmonary venous return.** Findings are similar to those for ostium secundum defect.
    b. **Total anomalous pulmonary venous return.** With a severe obstruction, no murmur may be detected on examination. With a moderate degree of obstruction, a systolic murmur is heard along the left sternal border, and a gallop murmur is heard occasionally. A continuous murmur along the left upper sternal border over the pulmonary area may also be audible.

15. **Congenital aortic stenosis.** A coarse systolic murmur with a thrill is heard at the upper right sternal border and can radiate to the neck and down the left sternal border. If left ventricular failure is severe, the murmur is of low intensity. Symptoms that occur in infants only when the stenosis is severe are pulmonary edema and congestive heart failure.

16. **Pulmonary stenosis (with intact ventricular septum).** If the stenosis is severe, a loud systolic ejection murmur is audible over the pulmonary area and radiates over the entire precordium. Right ventricular failure and cyanosis may be present. If the stenosis is mild, a short pulmonary systolic ejection murmur is heard over the pulmonic area along with a split-second heart sound.

B. **Palpate the pulses (femoral, pedal, radial, and brachial).** Bounding pulses can be seen with PDA. Absent or delayed femoral pulses are associated with coarctation of the aorta.

C. **Check for signs of congestive heart failure.** Signs may include hepatomegaly, gallop, tachypnea, wheezes and rales, tachycardia, and abnormal pulses.

XIV. **Abdomen.** See also Chapters 132, 133, and 134.

A. **Observation.** Obvious defects may include an **omphalocele,** in which the intestines are covered by peritoneum and the umbilicus is centrally located; **gastroschisis,** in which the intestines are not covered by peritoneum (the defect is usually to the right of the umbilicus); or **exstrophy of the bladder,** in which the bladder protrudes out.

B. **Auscultation.** Listen for bowel sounds.

C. **Palpation.** Check the abdomen for distention, tenderness, or masses. The abdomen is most easily palpated when the infant is quiet or during feeding. In normal circumstances, the liver can be palpated 1–2 cm below the costal margin and the spleen tip at the costal margin. Hepatomegaly can be seen with congestive heart failure, hepatitis, some inborn errors of metabolism (storage disorders, urea cycle defects), or sepsis.

Splenomegaly is found with cytomegalovirus or rubella infections or sepsis. The lower pole of both kidneys can often be palpated. Kidney size may be increased with polycystic disease, renal vein thrombosis, or hydronephrosis. Abdominal masses are more commonly related to the urinary tract.

D. **Linea nigra.** See page 44.

E. **Diastasis rectus abdominis.** A protrusion (vertical bulge) from the xiphoid to the umbilicus because of the weakness of the fascia between the two rectus abdominis muscles, which causes a separation of the muscles. It can be seen when intraabdominal pressure increases. It is a benign finding in newborns and typically will disappear with time.

F. **Scaphoid abdomen.** A sunken abdomen that can be seen with a congenital diaphragmatic hernia. The abdomen looks flat relative to the chest.

G. **Prune belly syndrome.** Usually seen in males (97%) and of unknown genetic origin, it consists of a large, thin, wrinkled abdominal wall, genitourinary malformations, and cryptorchidism. Surgery may be required, and survival rate has improved.

XV. **Umbilicus.** Normally, the umbilicus has 2 arteries and 1 vein. The absence of 1 artery occurs in 5–10 of 1000 singleton births and in 35–70 of 1000 twin births. The presence of **only 2 vessels** (1 artery and 1 vein) could indicate renal or genetic problems (commonly trisomy 18). If there is a **single umbilical artery**, there is an increased prevalence of congenital anomalies (40%) and intrauterine growth restriction and a higher rate of perinatal mortality. If it occurs without any other abnormalities, it is usually benign. **If the umbilicus is abnormal, ultrasonography of the abdomen is recommended.** In addition, inspect for any discharge, redness, or edema around the base of the cord that may signify a **patent urachus or omphalitis.** Some amount of periumbilical erythema is considered normal with separation of the cord. The cord should be translucent; a **greenish yellow color** suggests meconium staining, usually secondary to fetal distress. **Dark stripes** in the cord are intravascular clots and are a normal finding. A normal umbilical cord sloughs off at ~7–10 days of age.

A. **Omphalitis.** Infection of the cord. This is a very serious condition, can be fatal, and requires immediate treatment. Therefore, any redness of the cord should be promptly evaluated. (See Chapter 75.)

B. **Patent urachus.** Communication between the bladder and the umbilicus occurs, resulting in urine coming from the umbilicus. Workup to rule out lower urinary tract obstruction.

C. **Umbilical hernias.** Result from a weakness in the muscle of the abdominal wall or umbilical ring and usually resolve during the first year of life without treatment.

D. **Umbilical hematomas.** From rupture of the umbilical vessels, usually the vein from birth or trauma or a spontaneous occurrence. Risk factors include traction on the cord, chorioamnionitis, cord prolapse cord torsion, velamentous insertion, short cord, or thinning of the cord from a postdate delivery. They are rare (1:5000) and usually resolve with no treatment.

E. **Umbilical hemangiomas.** Rare but can be very serious.

F. **Wharton jelly cyst.** Where liquefaction of the jelly has occurred. The cord appears translucent and cystic, and 20% of infants will have other abnormalities.

XVI. **Genitalia.** Any infant with a disorder of sex development (presence of genitalia that do not fit into a male or female classification, formerly "ambiguous genitalia") should not undergo gender assignment until a formal endocrinology and urologic evaluation has been performed (see Chapter 91). *Note:* **A male with any question of a penile abnormality should not be circumcised until he is evaluated by a urologist or pediatric surgeon.**

A. **Male genital examination.** Observe the color of the scrotum. Pigment in the scrotum varies depending on the ethnicity and hormonal influence. It can also be hyperpigmented from adrenogenital syndromes. A **bluish color** may suggest testicular torsion or trauma and requires immediate urologic/surgical consultation. Infants will have well-developed scrotal rugae at term; a smooth scrotum suggests prematurity. **Examine the penis**; newborn males always have a marked **phimosis** and the foreskin may not be easily retracted. Verify that the testicles are in the scrotum and examine for groin hernias and masses. If born breech by vaginal delivery, the infant can have bruised and swollen genitals from pressure on the cervix.

1. Determine the site of the meatus. **Hypospadias** is abnormal location of the urethral meatus on the ventral surface of the penis, **epispadias** is abnormal location of the urethral meatus on the dorsal surface of the penis, **dorsal hood** (foreskin that is incompletely formed that covers the dorsal or top of the penis) is associated with hypospadias, and **chordee** is a dorsal or ventral curvature of the penis. **Megalourethra** is congenital dilation of the urethra usually caused by abnormal development of the corpus spongiosum and will require surgical correction.

2. Check the size of the penis. Normal stretched penile length at birth is at least 2 cm. **Micropenis** is a penis 2 standard deviations below the mean length and width for age.

3. Priapism. Persistent erection of the penis is an abnormal finding and can be seen in polycythemia, but the most common reason is idiopathic.

4. Webbed penis. Penoscrotal web can occur and is a contraindication for circumcision.

5. Buried penis. Rare congenital penile deformity where the penis appears buried in the tissues surrounding it. Do not circumcise.

6. Penile pearls. Similar to Epstein pearls on palate and can be present on the tip of the foreskin and will resolve with time.

7. Penile torsion. Check to see position of the penis and if it is toward the midline. If it is facing the thigh, torsion may be present. Also check the position of the median raphe. It should start and end at the midline of the scrotum and the tip of the penis. Mild torsion of <60 degrees is normal. High degrees of torsion will need to be surgically corrected.

8. Hypoplastic urethra. Infants will have thinning of the foreskin on the ventral side and a penile raphe that is not straight. If a feeding tube through the urethra is visible through the skin, then a hypoplastic urethra is present and circumcision is contraindicated. A pediatric urology consult should be obtained.

9. Undescended testicles. More common in premature infants. Sometimes term infants will have one testicle that has not descended from the abdomen to the scrotum. Palpation of the inguinal canal will verify that the testicle is there. **Unilateral undescended testicle is common** and should be followed by routine physical examinations over time. **Bilateral undescended testicles are considered a disorder of sex development.** An ectopic testicle passes through the inguinal ring and then goes off in another location (perineum, femoral canal, superficial inguinal pouch, or the other hemiscrotum).

10. Hydroceles. Hydroceles are common and usually disappear by 1 year of age unless associated with a hernia. Palpation or transillumination will assist in the diagnosis.

11. Testicular torsion. Infants present with an acute color change (usually bluish) with no signs of pain (in contrast to older patients). The torsed testicle is smaller in size, and this is a surgical emergency.

12. Antenatal testicular torsion. Usually the appearance is normal. The torsed testicle can be larger in size and feel more mass-like in texture. A Doppler ultrasound should be done to verify blood flow. The torsed testicle must be removed and the other side fixed to prevent torsion since it is at an increased risk.

13. Inguinal hernia. Presents as a fullness in the inguinal area. Premature infants have a higher risk for inguinal hernias.

B. **Female genital examination**
   1. **Examine the labia majora and minora and clitoris.** Labia majora of term infants are enlarged and frequently reddish in color. If the labia are fused and the clitoris is enlarged, adrenal hyperplasia should be suspected.
   2. **Clitoromegaly (a large clitoris).** This can be normal in a premature infant or can be associated with maternal drug ingestion (excess androgens during fetal life) or a disorder of sex development. Normal newborn clitoral length is <7 mm and mean length is 4 mm.
   3. **Mucosal/vaginal tag.** Commonly attached to the wall of the vagina. It is of no clinical significance.
   4. **Discharge from the vagina.** Common and is often clear, thick, and white or blood tinged. It usually only lasts a few days. If bloody discharge, it is normal and secondary to maternal estrogen withdrawal.
   5. **Vaginal mass.** Seen with crying or from increased abdominal pressure. Imaging studies are required.
   6. **Paraurethral cyst (rare).** Interlabial spherical cystic mass that is yellowish in color and can cover both urethral meatus and orifice of the vagina. Surgery is usually not necessary as many resolve spontaneously.
   7. **Perineal groove (failure of midline fusion).** Rare. This has three major features: moist perineal cleft between the anus and the posterior fourchette, hypertrophy of the labial tails, and normal vagina and urethra. Check anus, as some may have an ectopically placed anus. Conservative management is recommended.
   8. **Prolapsed ureterocele.** This is a urologic emergency.

XVII. **Anus and rectum.** Check for patency of the anus to rule out **imperforate anus** (absence of a normal anal opening). Insert a small feeding tube not >1 cm or observe for passage of meconium. Check the position of the anus. Meconium should pass within 48 hours of birth for term infants. Premature infants are usually delayed in passing meconium.

XVIII. **Lymph nodes.** Palpable lymph nodes, usually in the inguinal and cervical areas, are found in ~33% of normal neonates.

XIX. **Extremities.** Examine the arms and legs, paying close attention to the digits and palmar creases. (See also Chapter 115.) Most infants have 2 major creases on the palm. A single transverse palmar crease is associated with Down syndrome. Edematous hands and feet can be associated with Turner syndrome. Was the infant born breech? If the infant was born frank breech (baby buttocks aimed at birth canal with legs sticking straight up in front with feet near the head), the legs may maintain this position for days after birth.
   A. **Syndactyly.** Abnormal fusion of the digits; most commonly involves the third and fourth fingers and the second and third toes. A strong family history exists. Surgery is performed when the neonates are older. Severe syndactyly can involve all 4 digits being fused together.
   B. **Polydactyly.** Supernumerary digits on the hands or the feet. The most common is postaxial polydactyly. This condition is associated with a strong family history. Preaxial polydactyly is less common and may have an underlying medical condition. A radiograph of the extremity is usually obtained to verify whether any bony structures are present in the digit. If there are no bony structures, a suture can be tied around the digit until it falls off. If bony structures are present, surgical removal is necessary. Axial extra digits are associated with heart anomalies. **Polysyndactyly** involves more than normal amount of digits with fusion of some of them.
   C. **Brachydactyly.** This is a shortening of ≥1 digits. It is usually benign if an isolated trait.
   D. **Camptodactyly.** This usually involves the little finger and is a flexion deformity that causes it to be bent.

E. **Arachnodactyly.** This is spiderlike fingers that can be seen in Marfan syndrome and homocystinuria.

F. **Clinodactyly.** This usually involves the little finger, is usually benign, and is usually a slight medial incurvation, a radial or ulnar deviation. Can be associated with Down syndrome and other genetic disorders.

G. **Finger or toe hypoplasia.** Nail hypoplasia usually accompanies this. This can be seen in association with maternal teratogens, chorionic villus sampling, chromosome abnormalities, and malformation syndromes, or there can be no cause.

H. **Digit or thumb aplasia.** Amniotic bands can cause missing digits. A workup for genetic and chromosomal causes should be done.

I. **Overlapping toes.** Usually a positional deformity that has no significance if an isolated finding. If other abnormal physical findings are seen, a genetic workup may need to be done.

J. **Nail deformities.** Hypoplastic nails can be seen in Turner syndrome, Edward syndrome (with overlapping digits), nail-patella syndrome, and fetal phenytoin exposure. Hyperconvex nails can be seen in Patau syndrome.

K. **Arthrogryposis multiplex congenita.** A persistent contracture of the joints of the fingers. Can be associated with oligohydramnios.

L. **Positional deformities of the feet.** Positional deformities of the foot are usually from in utero position, and there is resolution without treatment.

M. **Simian crease.** A single transverse palmar crease is most commonly seen in Down syndrome but is occasionally a normal variant seen in 5% of newborns.

N. **Clubfoot (Talipes equinovarus).** More common in males. The foot is turned downward and inward, and the sole is directed medially. If this problem can be corrected with gentle force, it will resolve spontaneously. If not, orthopedic treatment and follow-up are necessary.

O. **Metatarsus varus.** A defect in which the forefoot rotates inward (adduction). This condition usually corrects spontaneously.

P. **Metatarsus valgus.** A defect in which the forefoot rotates outward.

Q. **Rocker bottom feet.** Usually seen with trisomy 13 and 18, it involves an arch abnormality that causes a prominent calcaneus with a rounded bottom of the sole.

R. **Tibial torsion.** This is an inward twisting of the tibia bone that causes the feet to turn in. It is most commonly caused by the position in the uterus and resolves spontaneously.

S. **Genu recurvatum.** The knee is able to be bent backward. This abnormal hyperextensibility can be secondary to joint laxity or trauma and is found in Marfan and Ehlers-Danlos syndromes.

T. **Congenital amputation of arms, legs, digits.** Think amniotic band syndrome or maternal substance use.

XX. **Trunk and spine.** Check for any gross defects of the spine. An increased amount of hair on the lower back can be normal in those infants who have an increase in pigmentation. Any abnormal pigmentation, swelling, or hairy patches over the lower back should increase the suspicion that an underlying vertebral or spinal abnormality exists. A sacral or pilonidal dimple may indicate a small meningocele or other anomaly. **Sacral dimples** below the line of the natal cleft are benign. If they are above the natal cleft, an ultrasound is indicated to check for a track to the spinal cord. Congenital midline vascular lesions may raise suspicion about occult spinal dysraphism, and if the lesions appear with other abnormal findings, then imaging studies should be done.

A. **Simple dimple.** This dimple is within 2.5 cm of the anus and has a visible base and no other abnormalities on physical examination. These require no further examination.

B. **Coccygeal pits.** A simple dimple in which the base cannot be seen. These are benign.

      C. **Sacral skin tags.** Require spinal ultrasound examination to rule out spinal dys-
         raphism. They may also represent a residual tail.

      D. **Meningomyelocele.** A neural tube defect in which there is incomplete closure of
         the posterior spine; the lumbar spine is the most common location.

XXI. **Hips.** (See also Chapter 115.) The US Preventive Services Task Force does not recommend routine screening for **developmental dysplasia of the hip (DDH)**. AAP
recommends screening for DDH, but states the net benefits of screening are unclear:
serial clinical examinations of the hips of both sexes are recommended. DDH occurs
in ~1.5–20 per 1000 births, 1 in 100 newborns have evidence of instability (most
resolve spontaneously), and 1–1.5 cases of dislocation occur per 1000 newborns. It is
a condition in which the femoral head has an abnormal relationship to the acetabulum (exact definition is *controversial*). It can include frank dislocation (luxation),
partial dislocation (subluxation), dysplastic hips, instability involving the femoral
head going in and out of the socket, and other abnormalities on radiographs that
show inadequate formation of the acetabulum. The earlier it is detected, the simpler and more effective is the treatment. More common in white females (9:1), this
condition is more likely to be unilateral and to involve the left hip. It is also more
common if there is a positive family history or breech presentation and in infants
with a neuromuscular disorder. Three clinical signs of dislocation are asymmetry
of the skin folds on the dorsal surface, shortening of the affected leg, and limited
abduction. Screening is *controversial*, as most cases of neonatal hip instability and
dysplasia resolve spontaneously.

    A. **AAP recommendations**

      1. **Screen all newborns by physical examination.** Ultrasonography of all new-
         borns not recommended.

      2. **Orthopedic referral.** Recommended with a positive Ortolani or Barlow test.
         Ultrasonography is not recommended in infants with positive findings, nor is
         radiographic examination of the pelvis and hips.

      3. **Use of triple diapers.** Not recommended in infants with presumed DDH.

      4. **Equivocal findings.** Soft click, mild asymmetry, no Ortolani or Barlow sign;
         perform follow-up hip examination at 2 weeks of age.

      5. **Positive Ortolani or Barlow test.** If positive at the 2-week examination, ortho-
         pedic referral is urgent but not an emergency.

      6. **Negative Ortolani or Barlow test.** If negative at the 2-week examination, but
         physical findings raise the suspicion of DDH, orthopedic referral or ultraso-
         nography at age 3–4 weeks recommended.

      7. **Negative examination at 2 weeks of age.** Routine follow-up recommended.

      8. **Negative newborn hip examination.** Consider any risk factors for DDH.
         These include female sex, a family history of DDH, and breech presentation.

         a. **Females.** Increased risk (DDH 19 per 1000). Reevaluate at 2 weeks if nega-
            tive or equivocal.

         b. **Family history.** When positive, the newborn DDH risk is 9.4 per 1000 (boys)
            and 44.0 per 1000 for girls. When the newborn examination is negative or
            equivocally positive in boys with a family history, reevaluation of the hips
            at 2 weeks of age is recommended. In girls with a family history, perform
            ultrasound at 6 weeks of age or radiographic examination of the pelvis and
            hips at 4 months of age.

         c. **Breech presentation.** The newborn DDH risk is 26 per 1000 (boys) and
            120 per 1000 for girls born breech. For girls, follow family history guide-
            lines; for boys with negative or equivocal newborn examination, periodic
            follow-up is recommended. Ultrasonographic evaluation is an option in all
            children born breech.

    B. **Evaluate for DDH by using the Ortolani and Barlow maneuvers.** Place the
      infant in the frog-leg position. Abduct the hips by using the middle finger to
      apply gentle inward and upward pressure over the greater trochanter (**Ortolani**).

Adduct the hips by using the thumb to apply outward and backward pressure over the inner thigh **(Barlow)**. (Some clinicians suggest omitting the Barlow maneuver because this action may contribute to hip instability by stretching the capsule unnecessarily.) A "clunk" of reduction and a "clunk" of dislocation are elicited in infants with hip dislocation (positive examination). Signs of DDH include:

1. **Asymmetric skin folds of the inguinal, buttock, thigh, or gluteal folds/ creases.** Normal inguinal folds do not extend beyond the anus.
2. **Limb length discrepancy.** Finding a true short leg can be a warning sign.
3. **Limited abduction.** Restricted movement can be a significant sign. Normal findings: abduction to 75 degrees, adduction to 30 degrees in a supine infant with stable pelvis.

C. **Galeazzi test (Allis sign).** This test can be done on an older infant (8–12 weeks) since the Ortolani and Barlow maneuver is no longer useful in decreased capsule laxity. With the infant supine, bend the knees and place both feet on the table and observe the symmetry of the height of the knees. If the height is unequal, then the sign is positive, and it suggests a unilaterally dislocated hip. A bilateral dislocation will be symmetric.

D. **Imaging DDH.** Real-time ultrasonography is the imaging of choice in the first few months. It is recommended as an adjunct to clinical evaluation. Radiographs have limited value since femoral heads are all cartilage and findings are often undetectable.

XXII. **Nervous system.** Observe the infant for any abnormal movement (eg, seizure activity, bicycling, jitteriness) or excessive irritability. Jitteriness can be stopped if the extremity is held (unlike seizures, which cannot be stopped) and can be normal or be secondary to hypoglycemia (most common), hypocalcemia, or drug withdrawal. Remember, neurologic symptoms of hypotonia, lethargy, poor sucking, seizures, and coma can be seen with some inborn errors of metabolism. (See Chapter 101.) Then evaluate the following parameters:

A. **Muscle tone**
   1. **Hypotonia.** Observe the posture and activity of the infant. Pick the infant up and see that the arms fall back and almost feel like a ragdoll. In ventral suspension, the head drops very low, and there is an exaggerated convex curvature of the spine. Floppiness and head lag are seen.
   2. **Hypertonia.** Increased resistance is apparent when the arms and legs are extended. Hyperextension of the back and tightly clenched fists are often seen.

B. **Reflexes.** The following reflexes are normal for a newborn infant. Primary reflexes reflect normal brainstem activity. CNS depression should be suspected if they cannot be elicited, and their persistence beyond a certain age can suggest damage of cortical functioning.
   1. **Protective reflex.** If the nose and eyes are covered with something, the infant will arch and make efforts to move the item away.
   2. **Rooting reflex.** Stroke the lip and the corner of the cheek with a finger and the infant will turn in that direction and open the mouth.
   3. **Babkin reflex.** If both thumbs are pressed equally against the palms, there is a reflex opening of the mouth and a twist of the head on the vertical axis until the median line, and at the same time the head is bowed forward. Normal in the first 10 weeks of life, persistence after 12 weeks suggests spastic-motor development disorder.
   4. **Glabellar reflex (blink reflex).** Tap gently over the forehead and the eyes will blink.
   5. **Grasp reflex (Palmar grasp).** Place a finger or object in the palm of the infant's hand and the infant will grasp the finger (flexion of the fingers will occur). This reflex is also present in the feet of a newborn. Stroke up the middle of the foot and the toes will curl under as if to grasp the examiner. It is present until 2–3 months of age.

6. Galant reflex. Suspend the infant in a prone position. Stroke the back in a cephalocaudal direction. The infant should respond by moving the hips toward the stimulated side.
7. Neck-righting reflex. Turn the infant's head to the right or left, and movement of the contralateral shoulder should be obtained in the same direction.
8. Asymmetric tonic neck reflex (fencing reflex). With the infant in a supine position, turn the infant's head to one side, and the arm and leg on the side of the head that is turned will extend outward, and there will be flexion of the limbs on the opposite side. It is the fencing position.
9. Moro reflex (startle reflex). Support the infant behind the upper back with one hand, and then drop the infant back ≥1 cm to, but not on, the mattress. This should cause symmetrical abduction of both arms and extension of the fingers followed by flexion and adduction of the arms. Asymmetry may signify a fractured clavicle, hemiparesis, or brachial plexus injury. An absent Moro reflex is of concern and may signify CNS pathology.
10. Plantar grasp. When one strokes the ball of the foot, the toes will curl.
11. Placing reflex. Hold the infant upright and place the dorsum of the foot by the edge of the bed; the infant places the foot on the surface. Disappears by 5 months of age.
12. Stepping/walking reflex. Hold the infant upright under his arms while supporting his head, have his feet touch a flat surface, the infant will appear to take a step and walk.
13. Positive support reflex. Hold the infant under the arms with head support, have the feet bounce on a flat surface, and the infant will extend the legs for 20 seconds and then flex the legs into a sitting position.
14. Swimming reflex. Place an infant abdomen down in a pool of water and the infant will paddle and kick in a swimming motion up to 6 months of age.

C. Cranial nerves. Note the presence of gross nystagmus, the reaction of the pupils, and the ability of the infant to follow moving objects with his or her eyes.

D. Movement. Check for spontaneous movement of the limbs, trunk, face, and neck. A fine tremor is usually normal. Clonic movements are not normal and may be seen with seizures.

E. Peripheral nerves
1. Brachial plexus injuries. These involve damage to the spinal nerves that supply the arm, forearm, and hand. Etiology is multifactorial.
   a. Erb-Duchenne paralysis (upper arm paralysis). Involves injury to the fifth and sixth cervical nerves and is the most common brachial plexus injury. There is adduction and internal rotation of the arm. The forearm is in pronation, the power of extension is retained, the wrist is flexed, and the Moro reflex is absent. This condition can be associated with diaphragm paralysis.
   b. Klumpke paralysis (lower arm paralysis). Involves the seventh and eighth cervical nerves and the first thoracic nerve. The hand is flaccid with little or no control. If the sympathetic fibers of the first thoracic root are injured, ipsilateral ptosis, enophthalmos, and miosis (**Horner syndrome**) can rarely occur.
   c. Paralysis of the entire arm. The entire arm is limp and cannot move. The reflexes are absent.
2. Facial nerve palsy. Intrauterine position or forceps can cause compression of the seventh cranial nerve. This results in ptosis, unequal nasolabial folds, and asymmetry of facial movement. Differentiate it from **asymmetric crying facies,** which is a congenital deficiency of the depressor anguli oris muscle, which controls the downward motion of the lip. The eye and forehead muscles are not affected in this condition. Asymmetric crying facies can be associated with cardiac, renal, respiratory defects or 22q11 deletion.

3. **Phrenic nerve injury.** This can occur secondary to a brachial plexus injury. It causes paralysis of the diaphragm, leading to respiratory distress.

F. **General signs of neurologic disorders**
   1. **Symptoms of increased intracranial pressure.** Bulging anterior fontanelle, dilated scalp veins, separated sutures, and setting-sun sign. (See page 49.)
   2. **Hypotonia or hypertonia.**
   3. **Irritability or hyperexcitability.**
   4. **Poor sucking and swallowing reflexes.**
   5. **Shallow, irregular respirations.**
   6. **Apnea.**
   7. **Apathy.**
   8. **Staring.**
   9. **Seizure activity.** Sucking or chewing of the tongue, blinking of the eyelids, eye rolling, and hiccups.
   10. **Absent, depressed, or exaggerated reflexes.**
   11. **Asymmetric reflexes.**

Selected Reference

American Academy of Pediatrics. Committee on Quality Improvement, Subcommittee on Developmental Dysplasia of the Hip. Clinical practice guideline: early detection of developmental dysplasia of the hip. *Pediatrics.* 2000;105:896–905.

7 Temperature Regulation

The chance of survival of neonates is markedly enhanced by the successful prevention of excessive heat loss. The newborn infant must be kept under a **neutral thermal environment**. This is defined as the external temperature range within which metabolic rate and hence oxygen consumption are at a minimum while the infant maintains a normal body temperature (Figures 7–1 and 7–2 and Table 7–1). The **normal skin temperature** in the neonate is 36.0–36.5°C (96.8–97.7°F) and the **normal core (rectal) temperature is** 36.5–37.5°C (97.7–99.5°F). **Axillary temperature** may be 0.5–1.0°C lower (95.9–98.6°F). A normal body temperature implies only a balance between heat production and heat loss and should not be interpreted as the equivalent of an optimal and minimal metabolic rate and oxygen consumption.

I. **Hypothermia and excessive heat loss.** Preterm infants are predisposed to heat loss because they have a high ratio of surface area to body weight (5 times more than the adult), little insulating subcutaneous fat, and reduced glycogen and brown fat stores. In addition, their hypotonic ("frog") posture limits their ability to curl up to reduce the skin area exposed to the colder environment.

A. **Mechanisms of heat loss in the newborn include the following:**
   1. **Radiation.** Heat loss from the infant (warm object) to a colder nearby (not in contact) object.
   2. **Conduction.** Direct heat loss from the infant to the surface with which he or she is in direct contact.
   3. **Convection.** Heat loss from the infant to the surrounding air.
   4. **Evaporation.** Heat loss by water evaporation from the skin of the infant. Immediately after delivery, evaporative heat loss may contribute to more than 50% of

evaporation loss is compensated for only when additional humidity is added to the incubator. One disadvantage of incubators is that they make it difficult to closely observe a sick infant or to perform any type of procedure. Body temperature changes associated with sepsis may be masked by the automatic temperature control system of closed incubators. Such changes will hence be expressed in the variations in the incubator's environmental temperature. An infant can be weaned from the incubator when his or her body temperature can be maintained at an environmental temperature of <30.0°C (usually when the body weight reaches 1600–1800 g). Enclosed incubators maintain a neutral thermal environment by using one of the following devices:

  i. **Servocontrolled skin probe attached to the abdomen of the infant.** If the temperature falls, additional heat is delivered. As the target skin temperature (36.0–36.5°C) is reached, the heating unit turns off automatically. A potential disadvantage is that overheating may occur if the skin sensor is detached from the skin or the reverse if the infant is lying on the probe-attached side.

  ii. **Air temperature control device.** The temperature of the air in the incubator is increased or decreased depending on the measured temperature of the infant. Use of this mode requires constant attention from a nurse and is usually used in older infants.

  iii. **Air temperature probe.** This probe hangs in the incubator near the infant and maintains a constant air temperature. There is less temperature fluctuation with this kind of probe.

  b. **Radiant warmer.** Typically used for very unstable infants or during the performance of medical procedures. Heating is provided by radiation and therefore does not prevent convective and evaporative heat loss. The temperature can be maintained in the "servo mode" (ie, by means of a skin probe) or the "nonservo mode" (also called the "manual mode"), which maintains a constant radiant energy output regardless of the infant's temperature. Serious overheating can result from mechanical failure of the controls, from dislodgment of the sensor probe, or from manual operation without careful monitoring. Deaths are associated with hyperthermia-induced radiant warmers. On manual mode, such as in the delivery room, they should be used only for a limited period. Insensible water loss may be extremely large in the very low birthweight (VLBW) infant (up to 8 mL/kg/h). Covering of the skin with semipermeable dressing or the use of a water-based ointment (eg, Aquaphor) may help reduce insensible transepidermal water loss.

2. **Temperature regulation in the healthy term infant (weight >2500 g).** Studies have shown that a healthy term infant can be wrapped in warm blankets and placed directly into the mother's arms without any significant heat loss.
  a. **Place the infant** under a preheated radiant warmer immediately after delivery.
  b. **Dry the infant completely** to prevent evaporative heat loss.
  c. **Cover the infant's head with a cap.**
  d. **Place the infant,** wrapped in blankets, in a crib.
3. **Temperature regulation in the sick term infant.** Follow the same procedure as that for the healthy term infant, except place the infant under a radiant warmer with temperature servoregulation.
4. **Temperature regulation in the premature infant (weight 1000–2500 g)**
  a. For an infant who weighs 1800–2500 g with no medical problems, use of a crib, cap, and blankets is usually sufficient.
  b. For an infant who weighs 1000–1800 g
    i. A well infant should be placed in a closed incubator with servo-control.
    ii. A sick infant should be placed under a radiant warmer with servo-control.

5. **Temperature regulation in the extremely low birthweight (ELBW) infant (weight <1000 g).** See Chapter 12.
   a. **In the delivery room.** Considerable evaporative heat loss occurs immediately after birth. Consequently, speedy drying of the infant has been emphasized as a very important aspect of the management of the ELBW infant. A more efficient and different approach has been advocated whereby the infant is placed in a plastic bag from feet to shoulders, without drying, immediately at birth.
   b. **In the nursery.** Either the radiant warmer or the incubator can be used, depending on the institutional preference. More recently hybrid devices such as the Versalet Incuwarmer (Hill-Rom Air-Shields, Batesville, IN) and the Giraffe Omnibed (Datex-Ohmeda; GE Medical Systems, Finland) have become available. They offer the combined features of radiant warmer and incubator with controllable humidity in a single device, allowing for seamless conversion between modes as deemed clinically necessary.
      i. **Radiant warmer**
         (a) **Use servo-control** with the temperature for abdominal skin set at 36.0–36.5°C.
         (b) **Cover the infant's head with a cap.**
         (c) **To reduce convective heat loss,** place plastic wrap (eg, Saran Wrap) loosely over the infant. Prevent this wrap from directly contacting the infant's skin. Avoid placing the warmer in a drafty area.
         (d) **Maintain an inspired air temperature** of the hood or ventilator of ≥34.0–35.0°C.
         (e) **Place under the infant** a heating pad (K-pad) that has an adjustable temperature within 35.0–38.0°C. To maintain thermal protection, it can be set between 35.0 and 36.0°C. If the infant is hypothermic, the temperature can be increased to 37.0–38.0°C (*controversial*).
         (f) **If the temperature cannot be stabilized,** move the infant to a closed incubator (in some institutions).
      ii. **Closed incubator.** Excessive humidity and dampness of the clothing and incubator can lead to excessive heat loss or accumulation of fluid and possible infections.
         (a) **Use servo-control,** with the temperature for abdominal skin set at 36.0–36.5°C.
         (b) **Use a double-walled incubator** if possible.
         (c) **Cover the infant's head** with a cap.
         (d) **Keep the humidity level** at ≥40–50% (as high as 89% if needed).
         (e) **Keep the temperature** of the ventilator at ≥34.0–35.0°C.
         (f) **Place under the infant** a heated mattress (K-pad) that has an adjustable temperature within 35.0–38.0°C. For thermal protection, the temperature can be set between 35.0 and 36.0°C. For warming a hypothermic infant, it can be set as high as 37.0–38.0°C.
         (g) **If the temperature is difficult to maintain,** try increasing the humidity level or use a radiant warmer (in some institutions).

II. **Hyperthermia.** Defined as a temperature that is greater than the normal core temperature of 37.5°C.
   A. **Differential diagnosis**
      1. **Environmental causes.** Some causes include excessive environmental temperature, overbundling of the infant, placement of the incubator in sunlight, a loose skin temperature probe with an incubator or radiant heater in servo-control mode, or a servo-control temperature set too high.
      2. **Infection.** Bacterial or viral infections (eg, herpes).
      3. **Dehydration.**
      4. **Maternal fever in labor.**
      5. **Maternal epidural analgesia during labor.**

6. **Drug withdrawal.**
7. **Unusual causes**
   a. **Hyperthyroid crisis or storm**
   b. **Drug effect** (eg, prostaglandin E_1)
   c. **Riley-Day syndrome** (periodic high temperatures secondary to defective temperature regulation)
B. **Consequences of hyperthermia.** Hyperthermia, like cold stress, increases metabolic rate and oxygen consumption, resulting in tachycardia, tachypnea, irritability, apnea, and periodic breathing. If severe, it may lead to dehydration, acidosis, brain damage, and death.
C. **Treatment**
   1. **Defining the cause of the elevated body temperature is the most important initial issue.** Determine whether the elevated temperature is the result of a hot environment or increased endogenous production, such as is seen with infections. In the former case, one may find a loose temperature probe, an elevated incubator air temperature, and the temperature of the extremities of the infant as high as the rest of the body. In the case of "true fever," one expects a low incubator air temperature as well as cold extremities secondary to peripheral vasoconstriction.
   2. **Other measures.** Turn down any heat source and remove any excessive clothing.
   3. **Additional measures for older infants with significant temperature elevation:**
      a. **A tepid water sponge bath.**
      b. **Acetaminophen** (5–10 mg/kg per dose, orally or rectally, every 4 hours).
      c. **Water-filled cooling blanket such as the Blanketrol system.** (See Figure 39–1.) Cincinnati Sub Zero, Cincinnati, OH.

Selected References

Baumgart S. Iatrogenic hyperthermia and hypothermia in the neonate. *Clin Perinatol.* 2008;35:183.

Bissinger RL, Annibale DJ. Thermoregulation in very low-birth-weight infants during the golden hour. *Adv Neonatal Care.* 2010;10:230.

Cramer K, Wiebe N, Hartling L, Crumley E, Vohra S. Heat loss prevention: a systematic review of occlusive skin wrap for premature neonates. *J Perinatol.* 2005;25:763.

Sarman I, Can G, Tunell R. Rewarming preterm infants on a heated, water-filled mattress. *Arch Dis Child.* 1989;64:687.

Sauer PJJ, Dane HJ, Visser HK. New standards for neutral thermal environment of healthy very low birthweight infants in week one of life. *Arch Dis Child.* 1984;59:18.

Scopes J, Ahmed I. Range of initial temperatures in sick and premature newborn babies. *Arch Dis Child.* 1966;41:417.

Tafari N, Gentz J. Aspects on rewarming newborn infants with severe accidental hypothermia. *Acta Paediatr Scand.* 1974;63:595.

8 Respiratory Management

The management of infants with respiratory distress has long been a basic function of neonatal intensive care. Today, death from acute respiratory failure is uncommon, even among the extremely premature, but significant morbidity from mechanical ventilation persists. Current trends in neonatal ventilation focus on reducing ventilator-induced lung injury, and noninvasive support is preferred. When mechanical ventilation is needed, new ventilators cede as much control as possible to the patient. Optimal treatment continues to be difficult to define, and considerable variability exists in assessing the risk–benefit ratio of various management strategies. This chapter provides an overview of current techniques used for neonatal respiratory support.

I. **Assessing and monitoring respiratory status**
   A. **Physical examination.** The presence of the following signs may be useful in recognizing respiratory distress and evaluating the response to treatment. The absence of signs may be secondary to neurologic depression rather than absence of pulmonary disease.
      1. **Nasal flaring.** One of the earliest signs of respiratory distress, nasal flaring may be present in intubated, ventilated patients as well.
      2. **Grunting.** Commonly seen early in respiratory distress syndrome (RDS) and transient tachypnea, grunting is a physiologic response (partial closure of the glottis during expiration) to end-expiratory alveolar collapse. Grunting helps maintain functional residual capacity (FRC) and therefore oxygenation.
      3. **Retractions.** Intercostal, subcostal, and sternal retractions are present in conditions of decreased lung compliance or increased airway resistance and may persist during mechanical ventilation if support is inadequate.
      4. **Tachypnea.** A respiratory rate >60/min implies the inability to generate an adequate tidal volume and may persist during mechanical ventilation.
      5. **Cyanosis.** Central cyanosis indicates hypoxemia. Cyanosis is difficult to appreciate in the presence of anemia. Acrocyanosis is common shortly after birth and is not a reflection of hypoxemia.
      6. **Abnormal breath sounds.** Inspiratory stridor, expiratory wheezing, and rales should be appreciable. Unfortunately, unilateral pneumothorax may escape detection on auscultation.
   B. **Blood gases.** Management of ventilation, oxygenation, and changes of acid-base status is most accurately determined by **arterial blood gas studies.**
      1. **Arterial blood gas studies.** The most standardized and accepted measure of respiratory status, especially for the oxygenation of low birthweight infants. They are considered invasive monitoring and require arterial puncture or an indwelling arterial line. Access is now considered routine by the umbilical artery or peripherally in the radial or posterior tibial artery.
      2. **Normal arterial blood gas values.** May not be the same as target values for particular patients, nor acceptable values. Table 8–1 lists examples of normal values for infants.
      3. **Calculated arterial blood gas indexes.** For determining progression of respiratory distress and are as follows:
         a. **Alveolar-to-arterial oxygen gradient (AaDO$_2$).** Greater than 600 mm Hg for successive blood gases over 6 hours is associated with high mortality in most infants if treatment and ventilation do not become effective. The formula for **AaDO$_2$** is

$$A - aDO_2 = \left[(FIO_2)(Pb - 47) - \frac{Paco_2}{R} \right] - Pao_2$$

where Pb = barometric pressure (760 mm Hg at sea level), 47 = water vapor pressure, Paco$_2$ is assumed to be equal to alveolar Pco$_2$, and R = respiratory quotient (usually assumed to be 1 in neonates).

Table 8–1. NORMAL RANGE OF ARTERIAL BLOOD GAS VALUES FOR TERM AND PRETERM INFANTS AT NORMAL BODY TEMPERATURE AND ASSUMING NORMAL BLOOD HEMOGLOBIN CONTENT[a]

Gestational Age	Pao_2 (mm Hg)	$Paco_2$ (mm Hg)	pH	HCO_3 (mEq/L)	BE/BD
Term	80–95	35–45	7.32–7.38	24–26	±3.0
Preterm (30–36 weeks' gestation)	60–80	35–45	7.30–7.35	22–25	±3.0
Preterm (<30 weeks' gestation)	45–60	38–50	7.27–7.32	19–22	±4.0

HCO_3, bicarbonate; BE, base excess; BD, base deficit.
[a]Values for Pao_2, $Paco_2$, and pH are measured directly by electrodes. HCO_3 and BE/BD values are calculated from nomograms of measured values at normal (14.8–15.5 mg/dL) hemoglobin content and body temperature (37°C) and assuming hemoglobin saturation of ≥88%.

      b. **Arterial-to-alveolar oxygen ratio (a/A ratio).** Also an index for effective respiration. The a/A ratio is the most often used index for evaluation of response to surfactant therapy and is used as an indicator for inhaled nitric oxide therapy for pulmonary hypertension. The formula for the a/A ratio is

$$a/A = Pao_2 \Big/ \left[(Fio_2)(Pb - 47) - \frac{Paco_2}{R} \right]$$

    4. **Venous blood gases.** Determination of values is the same as for arterial blood gases, but the interpretation is different. The pH values are slightly lower, and $Pvco_2$ values are slightly higher, whereas Pvo_2 values are of no value in assessing oxygenation.

    5. **Capillary blood gases.** Arterializing of capillary blood is done by warming the infant's heel just before sampling. The pH value is usually slightly lower, and the Pco_2 is usually slightly higher than arterial values, but this may vary considerably depending on the sampling technique. Po_2 data are of no value.

  C. **Noninvasive blood gas monitoring.** Use of these technologies is strongly encouraged. They allow for continuous monitoring and can dramatically reduce the frequency of blood gas sampling, reducing iatrogenic blood loss, and decreasing cost. Blood gas sampling is still necessary for calibrating noninvasive measures, determining acid-base status, and detecting hyperoxia.

    1. **Pulse oximetry.** The pulse oximeter measures the relative absorption of light by saturated and unsaturated hemoglobin, which absorbs light at different frequencies. The ratio changes in response to the rapid influx of arterial blood during the upstroke of the pulse. Through the detection of the peak of the ratio, the oximeter is able to determine the pulse rate and the percentage of arterial oxygen saturation. Sao_2 is arterial oxygen saturation by direct measurement, Spo_2 is arterial oxygen saturation by pulse oximetry.

      a. **Limitations.** Include poor correlation of Sao_2 to Pao_2 at upper and lower Pao_2 values. Sao_2 of 88–93% corresponds to Pao_2 of 40–80 mm Hg. For infants with high or low saturations, arterial blood gas correlation is needed.

      b. **Advantages.** Include minimal damage to the skin and no required manual calibration. Sao_2 by pulse oximetry is less affected by skin temperature and perfusion than transcutaneous oxygen.

      c. **Disadvantages.** Include the tendency of patient movement and excessive external lighting to interfere with readings and the lack of correction for abnormal hemoglobin (eg, methemoglobin).

2. **Transcutaneous oxygen (tcPo$_2$) monitoring.** Measures the partial pressure of oxygen from the skin surface by an electrochemical sensor. Contact is maintained through a conducting electrolyte solution and an oxygen-permeable membrane.
   a. **Limitations.** Include the need for daily recalibration, relocation to different skin sites every 4–6 hours, and irritation or injury to a premature infant's skin secondary to adhesive rings and thermal burns. Poor skin perfusion caused by shock, acidosis, hypoxia, hypothermia, edema, or anemia may prevent accurate measurements.
   b. **Advantages.** tcPo$_2$ is noninvasive and *may* provide indication of excessively high Pao$_2$ (>100 mm Hg).
3. **Transcutaneous carbon dioxide monitoring (tcPco$_2$).** Usually accomplished simultaneously by a single lead enclosed with a tcPo$_2$ electrode.
4. **End-tidal Co$_2$ monitoring (ETco$_2$ or Petco$_2$).** Expired breath analysis by infrared spectroscopy for Co$_2$ content gives close correlation to Paco$_2$. This technique is increasingly available for neonates. It gives rapid information about changes in CO$_2$, unlike the slow response time of tcPco$_2$.
   a. **Limitations.** An adapter to the endotracheal tube is required, which may significantly increase the dead space of the patient's circuit. Accuracy is limited when the respiratory rate is >60 breaths/min or if the humidity of inspired air is excessive. Current devices are of limited use for premature infants.
   b. **Advantages.** It is a noninvasive technique that may correlate well with arterial Paco$_2$.
D. **Monitoring mechanical ventilation.** Modern mechanical ventilators measure and display many variables.
   1. **Inspired oxygen.** Fraction of inspired oxygen (Fio$_2$) is a percentage of oxygen available for inspiration. It is expressed either as a percentage (21–100%) or as a decimal (0.21–1.00).
   2. **Airway pressure.** Measured either at the endotracheal tube connector or within the ventilator, depending on the specific machine. The ventilator may display set and/or measured pressures for mechanical and/or spontaneous breaths. Pressures of common interest are:
      a. **Peak inspiratory pressure (PIP).** The maximum pressure reached during inspiration. The need for high PIP reflects poor pulmonary compliance or the use of excessively large Vτ.
      b. **Positive end-expiratory pressure (PEEP).** The pressure maintained between breaths. A PEEP of 3–4 cm H$_2$O is considered physiologic. Lung compliance is often improved by increasing PEEP to 5–6 cm H$_2$O in RDS.
      c. **Mean airway pressure (P$\overline{aw}$).** Average of the proximal pressure applied to the airway throughout the entire respiratory cycle (Figure 8–1).

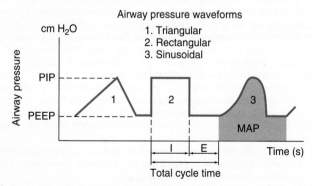

FIGURE 8–1. Graphic representation of ventilator airway pressure waveforms and other ventilator terminology. See Glossary (page 88) for explanations.

    i. $\overline{Paw}$ correlates well with mean lung volume for a given mode and strategy of mechanical ventilation.

    ii. $\overline{Paw} > 10\text{-}15$ cm H_2O during conventional ventilation is associated with an increased risk of air leaks (pneumothorax or pulmonary interstitial emphysema).

    iii. $\overline{Paw}$ of high-frequency ventilation is *not* strictly comparable with the $\overline{Paw}$ of conventional mechanical ventilation.

3. **Tidal volume (VT).** A function of PIP during mechanical ventilation, is integrated from flow (mL/s) and measured as milliliters per breath. By convention, VT is expressed as breath volume adjusted to body weight as milligrams per kilogram. Newer infant ventilators allow setting desired VT and will adjust PIP automatically in certain modes.

4. **Minute volume (MV).** The respiratory rate and VT combine to give MV as

$$MV = Rate \times VT$$
Example: 40 breaths/min $\times$ 6.5 mL/kg = 260 mL/kg/min.

5. **Pressure-volume (P-V) and flow-volume (F-V) loops.** A visualization of breath-to-breath dynamics. Flow, volume, and pressure signals combine to give P-V and F-V loops. Loops give inspiratory and expiratory limits of the breath cycle. F-V loops provide information regarding airway resistance, especially restricted expiratory breath flow. P-V loops illustrate changing lung dynamic compliance.

6. **Compliance (C_L).** Values of <1.0 cm H_2O/mL are consistent with interstitial or alveolar lung disease such as RDS. Lung compliance of 1.0–2.0 mL/cm H_2O reflects recovery, as in postsurfactant therapy.

7. **Resistance (R_L).** Value of >100 cm H_2O/L/s is suggestive of airway disease with restricted airflow such as in bronchopulmonary dysplasia or the need for airway suctioning.

8. **Time constant (K_T).** The product of $C_L \times R_L$ (in seconds). Normal values are 0.12–0.15 seconds. K_T is a measure of how long it takes for alveolar and proximal airway pressures to equilibrate. At the end of 3 time constants, 95% of the VT has entered (during inspiration) or left (during expiration) the alveoli. To avoid gas trapping, the measured expiratory time should be >3 times K_T (0.36–0.45 seconds).

E. **Chest radiographs.** Chest radiographs (see Chapter 11) are essential to the diagnosis of lung disease, in the management of respiratory support, and in the investigation of any acute change in respiratory status.

II. **Types of respiratory support.** Infants with respiratory distress may need only supplemental oxygen, whereas those with respiratory failure and apnea require mechanical ventilatory support. This section reviews the spectrum of available means for ventilatory support, with the exception of high-frequency ventilation (see Section V). Mechanical ventilatory support offers great benefits but also incurs significant risks. There continues to be considerable ***controversy*** concerning the proper use of any mode or strategy of assisted ventilation. Current practice utilizes the capabilities of ventilators to automatically coordinate support with patient effort with the goal of maintaining consistent ventilation with minimal risk for mechanical lung injury.

A. **Oxygen supplementation without mechanical ventilation.** Hypoxic infants able to maintain adequate minute ventilation are assisted with free-flow oxygen or air-oxygen mixtures. Continuous pulse oximetry is useful to monitor adequate oxygenation. Maintaining Spo_2 between 95% and 98% reduces the need for frequent arterial blood gases to prevent hypoxia.

1. **Oxygen hoods.** Provide an enclosure for blended air-oxygen supply, humidification, and continuous oxygen concentration monitoring. Hoods are easy to use and provide access to and visibility of the infant.

2. **Mask oxygen.** Usually not as well tolerated or controlled as nasal cannula oxygen delivery.

Table 8–2. **NASAL CANNULA CONVERSION TABLE**

Flow Rate (L/min)	Fio_2			
	100%	80%	60%	40%
0.25	34%	31%	26%	22%
0.50	44%	37%	31%	24%
0.75	60%	42%	35%	25%
1.00	66%	49%	38%	27%

General guideline only; numbers are not exact.

3. **Nasal cannulas.** Well suited for infants needing low concentrations of oxygen. Delivery can be controlled by flow meters delivering as little as 0.025 L/min. Flow rates of >1 L/min impart distending airway pressure. Table 8–2 gives approximate percentages of nasal cannula oxygen based on flow rates of 0.25–1.0 L/min at blended Fio_2 settings of 40–100%.

B. **Continuous positive airway pressure (CPAP).** A nasal mask, nasal prongs, or an endotracheal tube can be used to apply CPAP to improve Pao_2 by stabilizing the airway and allowing alveolar recruitment. CO_2 retention may result from excessive distending airway pressure.

1. **CPAP devices** can be broadly divided into 2 types according to their use of flow for CPAP delivery: **continuous or variable flow.**

a. **Continuous-flow CPAP devices**

i. **Bubble CPAP.** A warmed humidified gas is continuously provided through the inspiratory limb using a blender and a flow meter. CPAP is created by submersing the expiratory limb of the respiratory tubing into a water chamber to the depth of the desired cm H_2O CPAP level. A sufficient flow of gas through the system creates continuous bubbling in the water chamber. Benefits to gas exchange and lung recruitment due to the high-frequency oscillatory content of the bubbling have been hypothesized and disputed. The bubbly bottle CPAP pressure-generating system has the advantage that the adequacy of flow can be seen and heard. However, the pressure at the nares is often higher than the predicted positive pressure based on the set immersion depth. The advantages of bubble CPAP lies mostly in its ease of application and its low cost. Little clinical data are available to infer its superiority over other CPAP devices. Its resurgence in popularity relates to the report of a remarkably low incidence of bronchopulmonary dysplasia (BPD) in a single medical center using this form of CPAP.

ii. **Ventilator-derived CPAP.** Infant ventilators are used to provide a continuous flow of a blended gas. CPAP is modulated by varying the ventilator's expiratory orifice size. The expiratory valve works in conjunction with other controls, such has flow control and pressure transducers, to maintain the CPAP at the desired level. It is thus less likely than bubble CPAP to be influenced by the presence of a variable leak from the intermittent opening of the oral cavity. It also allows for rapid and simple transition to noninvasive positive pressure ventilation when required.

b. **Variable flow CPAP.** These devices (such as Infant Flow SiPAP System) use a dedicated driver and generator with unique fluidic mechanics that adjust and redirect gas flow throughout the respiratory cycle. The expiratory limb of the device is open to the atmosphere. Such devices may assist spontaneous breathing and reduce the work of breathing by reducing expiratory resistance and maintaining a stable airway pressure throughout respiration. It requires specially designed nasal prongs.

2. **CPAP modes of delivery**
   a. **Nasal Mask CPAP.** Requires the proper size mask and a good seal on the face to be effective. Although more cumbersome than nasal prongs, a mask reduces risk of injury to the nasal septum.
   b. **Nasal CPAP (nCPAP).** Nasal prongs are the most commonly applied means of delivering CPAP and are used for respiratory assistance in an infant with mild RDS. The prongs are also used postextubation to maintain airway and alveolar expansion in the process of weaning from mechanical ventilation and recovery from respiratory diseases. This treatment maintains upper airway patency and, as such, is useful in infants with apnea of infancy. nCPAPs may range from 2 to 8 cm H_2O, although 2–6 cm H_2O is most often used. Overdistention of the airway can lead to excessive CO_2 retention or air leak (pneumothorax). Gastric distention may be a complication of nCPAP, and an orogastric tube for decompression should be used. Infants can be fed by nasogastric tube during nasal CPAP therapy with close monitoring of abdominal girth.
   c. **Nasopharyngeal CPAP.** An alternative to nasal prongs. An endotracheal tube or long binasal prongs are passed nasally and advanced to the nasopharynx. A ventilator or CPAP device is used to deliver continuous distending pressure as with nasal prongs. This approach is slightly more secure in active infants and may cause less trauma to the nasal septum.
   d. **Endotracheal tube CPAP.** Rarely used or indicated in neonates.
C. **Noninvasive ventilation.** This refers to any technique that uses constant or variable pressure to provide ventilatory support, but without tracheal intubation. Sometimes this term includes CPAP techniques described previously. Common examples are nasal intermittent positive pressure ventilation (**NIPPV**) that combines nCPAP with superimposed ventilator breaths, which may be synchronized (**SNIPPV**) with patient breathing movements. (CPAP [PEEP] ranges from 3 to 6 cm H_2O, whereas PIP is set 10 cm H_2O above CPAP. Inspiratory time ranges from 0.3 to 0.5 seconds and respiratory rate from 10 to 60 breaths/min.) It may be assumed that the pressure delivered is variable and frequently lower than the set PIP, mostly because of leakage at the nose and mouth. For SNIPPV, a technically unsolved problem is the reliable identification of spontaneous breathing efforts in preterm infants to synchronize the NIV. **NIPPV** may be used as a primary mode of respiratory support in preterm infants with RDS but is more often used as a method to decrease the risk of postextubation failure/need for reintubation. Nasal ventilation seems to be particularly helpful in managing apnea. NIPPV may lead to abdominal distension and possibly gastrointestinal perforation. Nasal trauma and leak around the prongs are commonly seen; therefore, careful selection of prong size and monitoring of position are important.
D. **Mechanical ventilation.** The decision to initiate mechanical ventilation is complex. The severity of respiratory distress, severity of blood gas abnormalities, natural history of the specific lung disease, and degree of cardiovascular and other physiologic instabilities are all factors to be considered. **Because mechanical ventilation may result in serious complications, the decision to intubate and ventilate should not be taken lightly.**
   1. **Bag-and-mask or bag-to-endotracheal tube handheld assemblies.** These allow for emergency ventilatory support. Portable manometers are always required for monitoring peak airway pressures during hand-bag ventilation. Bags may be self-inflating or flow-dependent, anesthesia-type bags. All handheld assemblies must have pop-off valves to avoid excessive pressures to the infant's airway (see Figure 3–2).
   2. **Conventional infant ventilators.** Conventional mechanical ventilation delivers physiologic tidal volumes at physiologic rates via an endotracheal tube. Modern microprocessor-controlled ventilators provide numerous modes of ventilation, which vary in the degree to which patient effort controls the ventilator. These modes are critically dependent on the function of flow and/or pressure sensors

for accurate performance. The very rapid respiratory rates and small tidal volumes encountered in some neonates may prevent the use of patient-triggered or controlled ventilator modes.

a. **Ventilator settings.** Various modes of mechanical ventilation are determined by the parameters that are set by the clinician to determine the characteristics of the mechanical breath and the circumstances under which it is delivered. Not all modes are available on every ventilator, and subtle differences between the same modes may exist between different manufacturers. The characteristics of each breath are as follows:

   i. **Length of breath** (T_i). Either set by the clinician and machine controlled or patient controlled.

     (a) **Time cycled.** Each mechanical breath lasts for a machine-controlled set time, 0.2–0.3 seconds for extremely low birthweight (ELBW), up to 0.5–0.6 seconds for term.

     (b) **Flow cycled.** Each mechanical breath lasts until inspiratory flow falls below a threshold (when the patient reaches end inspiration). The T_i will vary, usually in response to changes in patient effort.

   ii. **Size of breath** (VT)

     (a) **Volume limited.** Each mechanical breath is the same volume; the pressure used may vary in response to patient effort. Historically, volume ventilators were very difficult to use safely in neonates.

     (b) **Pressure limited.** A set pressure is reached with each mechanical breath; the VT delivered will vary with patient effort.

     (c) **Volume assurance/guarantee.** The clinician sets both a maximum PIP and a desired VT (target volume) for mechanical breaths. Once the target VT is reached, the ventilator cuts the inspiration short. Some ventilators will decrease PIP for a breath if previous breaths have been cut short. If subsequent breaths are below target VT, the ventilator increases PIP until the set maximum PIP is reached. Ideally, volume assurance/guarantee delivers consistent VT, even with varying patient effort and/or variable lung pulmonary mechanical characteristics.

   iii. **Frequency of mechanical breaths**

     (a) **IMV (intermittent mandatory ventilation).** Breaths are delivered at set intervals without regard to patient effort.

     (b) **SIMV (synchronized IMV).** The set rate determines time frames during which the ventilator will deliver a breath in response to a patient trigger or will deliver a mandatory breath if no trigger is sensed. The minimum and maximum ventilator rates are equal.

     (c) **A/C (assist/control).** Each patient trigger results in a ventilator breath. If no trigger is sensed, a minimum set rate is delivered. Maximum rate may be much higher than minimum. Excessive trigger sensitivity may lead to autocycling and much greater rates than needed.

     (d) **Support or assist.** Each patient trigger results in a breath. No mandatory backup rate.

   iv. **Patient triggers.** The advanced patient-regulated ventilation modes available with modern microprocessor-controlled ventilators depend on reliable detection of patient respiratory effort. In the smallest premature infants, it is difficult to separate flow or pressure changes due to inspiratory effort from those due to measurement error or leaks.

     (a) **Flow determinations by Pneumotach or mass airflow sensors.** Sensors at the patient airway are often more reliable.

     (b) **Pressure.** Pressure triggers may be confused by ringing within the circuit, especially with rainout in the tubing.

     (c) **Neural.** Using a bipolar esophageal lead placed at the level of the diaphragm, phrenic nerve impulses to the diaphragm can be detected and used to trigger mechanical breaths. Flow and pressure sensors trigger during a breath. Neural sensors potentially allow for the onset of a mechanical breath to match onset of the spontaneous effort. This promising technology has yet to be fully evaluated in neonates.

  v. The preceding sets of parameters are often combined to yield the following modes. *Note:* Volume assurance/guarantee may be added to pressure-limited modes.

  (a) **IMV.** Refers to nontriggered, usually pressure-limited, time-cycled ventilation. **Use:** In absence of reliable patient trigger.

  (b) **SIMV.** May be either volume or pressure limited, time cycled. Synchronized pressure-limited, time-cycled ventilation (**PLV**) has been the standard mode of ventilation. **Use:** Prevents hyperventilation from autocycling. Provides no support for patient breathing above the set rate.

  (i) **SIMV + pressure support.** Patient breaths above the SIMV rate are supported with pressure-limited, flow-cycled breaths. The PS pressure is usually set well below the SIMV PIP. **Use:** Decrease the work of breathing. May facilitate weaning.

  (ii) **Volume-targeted SIMV.** Rapidly being adopted as the new standard mode. Expected benefits are decreased variability in delivered breath size resulting in more stable Pco_2 and less chance for intermittent overdistension. Limitations include poor sensor function from air leaks, condensation in the ventilator tubing, or extremely small flows/pressure in ELBW infants.

  (c) **Pressure control.** Pressure-limited (usually with a decreasing flow rate during inspiration), time-cycled, A/C. May be volume-targeted. **Use:** Provides well-tolerated support in patients with easily sensed respiratory effort.

  (d) **Volume control.** Volume-limited, time-cycled, A/C. **Use:** As in pressure control, but may result in more consistent Vt.

  (e) **Pressure support.** Pressure-limited, flow-cycled support. May be volume targeted. **Use:** In addition to SIMV, especially during weaning.

III. **Pharmacologic respiratory support and surfactant.** Numerous medications are available for improvement of respiration. They represent a broad range of therapeutics, of which the bronchodilators and anti-inflammatory drugs are the oldest and most common. The use of mixtures of inhaled gases such as helium and nitric oxide are recent forms of treatment. Sedatives and paralyzing agents remain *controversial* in neonatal respiratory management. Finally, surfactant replacement therapy has rapidly become a major adjunct in the care of preterm infants, and its use has expanded to disease states other than RDS (hyaline membrane disease), for which it was originally intended. All medications are discussed with regard to dosage and side effects in Table 8–3, but they are briefly reviewed here for the purpose of incorporating their use into respiratory management strategies.

  A. **Bronchodilators (inhaled agents).** Most of these drugs are sympathomimetic agents that stimulate β_1, β_2, or α-adrenergic receptors. They have both inotropic and chronotropic effects and provide bronchial smooth muscle and vascular relaxation. Albuterol is probably the most commonly used aerosolized bronchodilator. Other bronchodilators are presented in Table 8–3. Two anticholinergic agents (atropine and ipratropium) are also used as inhaled bronchodilators for inhibition of acetylcholine at lung receptor sites and bronchial smooth muscle relaxation. All are used to minimize airway resistance and allow decreased $\overline{Paw}$ needed for mechanical ventilation.

  B. **Bronchodilators (systemic).** Aminophylline (parenteral) and theophylline (enteral) are methylxanthines with considerable bronchial dilating action. Neonatal use includes bronchodilation and, more often, stimulation of respiratory efforts.

Table 8–3. **AEROSOL THERAPY IN NEONATES, INDICATING DOSING, RECEPTOR EFFECTS, AND COMMON SIDE EFFECTS**

Drug	Receptors	Side Effects
Albuterol (Salbutamol, Ventolin): 0.1 –0.15 mg/kg per dose Dilute with NS to 3 mL Dose: every 4–6 hours	β_2: Long lasting (duration, 3–8 hours) Fewer side effects than metaproterenol	Tachycardia (potentiated by methylxanthines) Hypertension Hyperglycemia Tremor
Metaproterenol: 0.5–1 mg/kg per dose Dilute with NS to 3 mL Dose: every 6 hours	β_2: Less specific for airways than albuterol	Tachycardia Arrhythmias Hypertension Hyperglycemia Tolerance, tremor Excessive smooth muscle relaxation = airway collapse Cardiac arrhythmias potentiated by hypoxia
Cromolyn (Intal): 20 mg Dilute with NS to 3 mL Dose: every 6–8 hours	Anti-inflammatory by stabilizing mast cells	Anaphylaxis Caution in patients with liver or renal disease Bronchospasm from inflammatory response Upper airway irritation
Terbutaline (Brethine): 0.01–0.02 mg/kg per dose Dilute IV solution with NS to 3 mL Dose: every 4–6 hours Minimum dose: 0.1 mg	β_2: Peripheral dilation	Hypertension Hyperglycemia Tachycardia
Atropine: 0.025–0.05 mg/kg per dose (maximum dose 2.5 mg) Dilute IV solution with NS to 2.5 mL Dose: every 6–8 hours	Vagolytic	Tachycardia Arrhythmia Hypotension Ileus, airway dryness If thick secretions: Suggest use in combination with albuterol
Ipratropium (Atrovent): Neonates: 25 mcg/kg per dose Infants: 125–250 mcg per dose Dilute with NS to 3 mL Dose: every 8 hours	Antagonizes acetylcholine at parasympathetic sites	Nervousness Dizziness Nausea, blurred vision Cough, palpitations Rash, urinary difficulties
Epinephrine, racemic: 0.05 mL/kg (maximum dose 0.5 mL) Dilute in 2 mL NS Dose: every 30 minutes, maximum 4 doses (Racemic epinephrine, 2 mg = L-Epinephrine, 1 mg) L-Epinephrine 1:1000: 0.5 mL/kg Dilute with NS to 3 mL Dose: every 30 minutes, maximum 4 doses	α receptor	Tachycardia Tremor Hypertension
Levalbuterol (Xopenex): 0.31–1.25 mg every 4–6 hours as needed for bronchospasm (NHLBI asthma 2007 guidelines)	β_2: R(-)enantiomer of racemic albuterol: little effect on heart rate	Nervousness, tremor, tachycardia, hypertension, hypokalemia. Paradoxical bronchospasm may occur, especially with first use

NHLBI, National Heart, Lung, and Blood Institute; NS, normal saline.
Neonate, birth to 28 days postnatal age; **infant**, >28 days to 1 year of age.

C. Anti-inflammatory agents
   1. Steroid therapy. This has been used to treat or prevent chronic lung disease. Although steroid therapy results in significant short-term improvement in pulmonary function, long-term benefit remains unproved. The substantial adverse effects of steroid therapy with dexamethasone have led the **American Academy of Pediatrics (AAP) and the Canadian Pediatric Society to issue a joint recommendation against the routine use of steroid therapy.** Hydrocortisone may provide similar pulmonary benefits without the adverse effects of dexamethasone.
   2. Cromolyn. Prevents mast cells from releasing histamine and leukotriene-like substances. Its actions are slow but progressive over 2–4 weeks. Indications for its use in neonates have not been established.
D. Inhaled gas mixtures
   1. Heliox (helium, 78–80%; oxygen, 20–22%). Produces an inspired gas less dense than nitrogen-oxygen mixtures or oxygen alone. Use of heliox reduces the increased resistive load of breathing, improves distribution of ventilation, and creates less turbulence in narrow airways. Limited neonatal use has indicated that heliox is associated with lower inspired oxygen requirements and shorter duration of mechanical ventilatory support.
   2. Inhaled nitric oxide (iNO). A potent gaseous vasodilator produced by endothelial cells. NO is rapidly bound by hemoglobin, limiting its action to the site of production or administration. Delivered in the ventilatory gas, iNO produces vasodilation only in the vascular bed of well-ventilated regions of the lung, thereby reducing intrapulmonary shunt as well as pulmonary vascular resistance. Furthermore, there is no systemic effect.
      a. Actions. iNO diffuses rapidly across alveolar cells to vascular smooth muscle, where it causes an increase in cyclic GMP, resulting in smooth muscle relaxation.
      b. Dosage. iNO is administered at low concentration, 2–40 parts per million (ppm). The dose is titrated to effect (improved oxygenation being the most common). Rarely do concentrations >20–40 ppm yield additional benefit.
      c. Administration. iNO is blended into the ventilatory gases, preferably close to the patient connector to avoid excessive dwell time with high oxygen concentrations, which may result in excessive NO_2 concentrations. Inline sensors are used to measure delivered NO and NO_2 concentrations. Techniques for use with high-frequency ventilators have also been developed. **Co-oximetry measurement of methemoglobin is required.** The NO dose should be decreased if methemoglobin is >4% or if the NO_2 concentration is >1–2 ppm.
      d. Indications for use. iNO is indicated for hypoxic respiratory failure of term and near-term newborns. Recommendations have been made by the AAP for care and referral of these infants. It is currently under investigation for use in a variety of lung diseases in which inappropriate pulmonary vascular constriction adversely affects oxygenation. The resultant vasodilation may decrease pulmonary vascular resistance in general, thereby reducing right-to-left shunting, or may result in less intrapulmonary shunt, or both. Use in cases of severe respiratory failure suggests that iNO may reduce the need for extracorporeal membrane oxygenation (ECMO) in 30–45% of eligible patients. Use of inhaled NO in premies with RDS decreases the incidence of chronic lung disease and death. Routine use of iNO early in the course of RDS in extreme premature infants may improve long-term outcome.
      e. Adverse effects. Systemic vascular effects are *not* seen with iNO use. NO_2 poisoning and methemoglobinemia are the most likely complications.
E. Other medications
   1. Sildenafil. An oral phosphodiesterase 5 inhibitor, sildenafil reduces pulmonary vascular resistance and is approved in adults for pulmonary hypertension. Its use is attractive in patients with bronchopulmonary dysplasia (BPD), with further study required before use in newborns.

　　2. Prostacyclin (PGI$_2$). A potent pulmonary vasodilator given as an aerosol or intravenous drip. Hypotension may develop. Use with iNO has been reported.

　　3. Bosentan. An oral endothelin 1 receptor blocker, bosentan reduces pulmonary vascular resistance. Its use in neonates is as yet undefined.

F. Sedatives and paralyzing agents. Agitation is a common problem for infant mechanical ventilation. Infants may have interrupted respiratory cycles and respond by "bucking" or "fighting" the ventilator breaths. The agitation that results is often associated with hypoxic episodes. Sedation or muscle relaxation by paralysis may be required. It should be noted, however, that with the use of ventilators with either flow-sensed or patient-triggered synchronized ventilation (SIMV), much less sedation is required and paralysis is rarely needed. "Fighting" the respirator may indicate inadequate respiratory support because of changes in lung compliance/airway resistance. Careful assessment for possible remedial causes for those changes (ie, obstructed or mis/malpositioned endotracheal tube, pneumothorax) needs to be performed before any pharmacological intervention.

　　1. Sedatives. Include lorazepam, phenobarbital, fentanyl, or morphine. Each agent has advantages and side effects. (See Chapter 76.)

　　2. Paralyzing agents. Include pancuronium and vecuronium. Prolonged muscle relaxation by paralysis results in considerable body fluid accumulation with the development of pulmonary and skin edema.

G. Surfactant replacement therapy. The availability of surfactant treatment has dramatically changed the care of infants with RDS (formally known as hyaline membrane disease). Surfactant administration early in the course of RDS restores pulmonary function and prevents tissue injury that otherwise results from ventilation of surfactant-deficient lungs. As a result, mortality from RDS has decreased dramatically.

　　1. Composition. Currently available surfactants are all of animal origin: beractant (Survanta) and calfactant (Infasurf) are derived from bovine lung and lung lavage, respectively. Poractant alfa (Curosurf) is derived from porcine lung. Lucinactant (Surfaxin) is a new synthetic form approved in 2012. All contain the hydrophobic surfactant proteins, SpB and SpC, although at different concentrations. Calfactant and poractant alfa contain surfactant phospholipids. In beractant, additional phospholipid is added to the minced lung extract to increase the ratio of surfactant to membrane phospholipids. Synthetic surfactants that equal the in vivo actions of the natural surfactants have been on the horizon for several years.

　　2. Actions. All surfactant preparations are intended to replace the missing or inactivated natural surfactant of the infant. Surface tension reduction and stabilization of the alveolar air–water interface are the basic functions of surfactant compounds. Air–water interface stability imparts lower alveolar surface tension and prevents atelectasis, or alternating areas of atelectasis and hyperinflation.

　　3. Dosage and administration. Each preparation has specific dosage and dosing procedures. Direct tracheal instillation is involved in all preparations. Surfactants are given both by continuous infusion via side port on the endotracheal tube adapter and mostly by aliquots via a catheter placed through the endotracheal tube. Changes in body position during dosing aid in more uniform delivery of surfactant. The relative advantages of these methods of administration are currently being studied (see Chapter 148 for detailed information on each medication).

　　　a. Prophylactic dosing at birth. This form of treatment is used less often and only when resuscitation and surfactant administration can be safely pursued simultaneously. Current practice prefers use of CPAP in the delivery room.

　　　b. Administration of surfactant preparations after respiratory distress is established. Currently, surfactant therapy occurs once the patient has been stabilized and the diagnosis of RDS has been established.

　　　c. Repeat dosing. May follow at 6- to 12-hour intervals. Repeat doses should follow loss of response after initial improvement has been seen. Repeat dosing after the second dose is *controversial*.

   d. **Airway obstruction.** May occur during surfactant administration because of the viscosity of the surfactant preparations. Increased mechanical support may be required until the surfactant is spread from the airways to the alveoli.
4. **Efficacy.** Efficacy of surfactant treatment can be observed for both immediate and long-term clinical conditions.
   a. **Early effects.** Include a reduction of FIO_2 need and improved PaO_2, $PaCO_2$, and a/A ratio. Likewise, improved VT and compliance should be noted with improved lung function and decreased ventilator PIPs.
   b. **Long-term effects.** Should result in decreased necessity for mechanical ventilation and less severe chronic lung disease of infancy. Complications of patent ductus arteriosus, necrotizing enterocolitis, and intraventricular hemorrhage have not been significantly influenced by surfactant therapy to date.
5. Side effects
   a. Small risk of pulmonary hemorrhage.
   b. Secondary pulmonary infections.
   c. Air leak (pneumothorax) following bolus administration of surfactant compounds. Rapid changes in VT require immediate reduction of PIPs. Failure to do so while also decreasing FIO_2 may lead to air leaks.
6. **Surfactant therapy for diseases other than RDS.** Encouraging preliminary reports of surfactant therapy have been noted in cases of pneumonia, meconium aspiration syndrome, persistent pulmonary hypertension, pulmonary hemorrhage, and adult respiratory distress syndrome (ARDS), but no protocols for treatment are available at this time. Dilute surfactant solutions are being studied for use as lung lavage fluids for meconium aspiration.

IV. Strategies of neonatal respiratory support
   A. **General approach.** Although use of the tools and techniques discussed in this section are essential to neonatal intensive care, their use is not without peril. One general approach is to provide the minimal support necessary for adequate gas exchange, unless a more aggressive intervention may change the course of the pulmonary disease, such as early intubation for the delivery of surfactant in RDS. Noninvasive nasal CPAP or ventilation is preferable to intubation and mechanical ventilation. Patient-triggered ventilation modes are usually better tolerated by patients and may result in less need for support. Meta-analysis of volume-targeted ventilation in neonates reveals a decrease in death and BPD/CLD as compared with classic pressure-limited ventilation. The optimal use of the myriad modes of assisted ventilation has yet to be determined, but the trend is to use ventilator modes that allow the patient more control. The decision to initiate or escalate ventilatory support should always take into account the risk of ventilator-induced lung injury and systemic effects of poorly controlled ventilation.
   1. Mechanisms of lung injury
      a. **Oxygen toxicity.** Risk factor for BPD/CLD and retinopathy of prematurity (ROP) and may be reduced by careful monitoring and the setting of gestational age appropriate SpO_2 targets.
      b. **Inflammation and infection.** Result from intubation. Use of noninvasive ventilation and early extubation are desired.
      c. **Barotrauma/volutrauma.** Results from over-inflation of the lung or stress from repeated reopening of collapsed lung units or from shear between adjacent lung units. Maintenance of FRC using appropriate PEEP and the use of small VT to prevent overdistension help limit injury.
   2. Adverse effects of poorly controlled ventilation
      a. **Hyperoxia (high PO_2)** is associated with an increased risk for ROP.
      b. **Hypoxemia (low PO_2)** has been recently associated with increased risk of mortality.
      c. **Over-ventilation (low PCO_2)** causes a decrease in cerebral blood flow that increases the risk for periventricular white matter injury and cerebral palsy.

    d. Hypercapnia (high Pco_2) may increase the risk for poor neurodevelopmental outcome.

    e. Over-inflation may impair venous return and cardiac output to the point of systemic hypotension.

B. **Initiation of mechanical ventilation for respiratory distress.** See Chapter 46 for more detail on management of ventilators.

  1. Indications

    a. Failure to maintain adequate Po_2 and Pco_2 with supplemental oxygen and nasal CPAP or nasal ventilation.

    b. Worsening RDS is an indication for early intubation for surfactant administration with subsequent mechanical ventilation.

  2. Ventilator settings. *Note:* Refer to the operating manual for your specific ventilator to understand the specific modes available.

    a. Classic pressure-limited ventilation (PLV). Preferably with synchronization and VT measurement.

      i. PEEP 4–5 cm H_2O.

      ii. Ti 0.3 seconds.

      iii. PIP to yield VT of 4–5 mL/kg. If VT measurement is unavailable, limit PIP so that chest rise is barely perceptible on breaths without patient effort.

      iv. Rate 30–40 per minute SIMV. Higher rates and/or A/C ventilation may result in initial hyperventilation.

      v. Trigger sensitivity setting requires specific machine knowledge. Refer to ventilator manual.

      vi. Evaluate response with clinical examination, noninvasive monitors, and blood gases and chest radiograph as necessary. Adjust PIP and rate as required. See later for managing ventilation.

    b. Volume targeted ventilation (VTV)

      i. PEEP 4–5 cm H_2O.

      ii. Ti 0.3 seconds.

      iii. Set volume target to 4–5 mL/kg. Set PIP limit high enough for ventilator to meet target.

      iv. Rate 30–40 per min SIMV. Higher rates and/or A/C ventilation may result in initial hyperventilation.

      v. Evaluate response with clinical examination, noninvasive monitors and blood gases and chest radiograph as necessary. Adjust PIP and rate as required. See later for managing ventilation.

      vi. Large air leaks around the endotracheal tube interfere with volume-targeted ventilator modes. In such cases either switch to PLV or reintubate with a larger tube.

C. **Fine-tuning mechanical ventilation.** (See also Chapter 46.) Adequate gas exchange must be determined for each patient because goals vary depending on diagnosis, patient's gestational age, and level of support required.

  1. Low Po_2. Usually caused by poor matching of ventilation and perfusion (low V/Q ratio). Support beyond the use of supplemental oxygen is directed either at improving aeration in the lung or influencing the distribution of perfusion. To improve oxygenation:

    a. Maintain lung expansion. Maintain lung expansion at end expiration by the use of PEEP and the use of surfactant in RDS. Preventing collapse also reduces lung injury from reopening alveoli.

    b. Recruit collapsed lung by the use of adequate VT and PIP.

    c. iNO selectively decreases vascular resistance in well-ventilated regions of the lung, improving oxygenation. Extrapulmonary shunt due to persistent pulmonary hypertension may respond to prostacyclin in addition to iNO.

    d. Consider the use of HFO. To maintain high mean lung volume in cases of severe, uniform alveolar disease (RDS, ARDS).

2. **High P_{CO_2}.** Results from inadequate minute volume.
   a. **Pa_{CO_2} is decreased by increasing MV.** If V_T is adequate ($\sim$5 mL/kg), an increase in rate is preferable. Special attention is required when adjusting patient-triggered ventilation modes to insure that a real increase in rate results from an increase in the ventilator set rate.
   b. **Increasing V_T requires increasing PIP.** Although a high PIP itself does not necessarily produce lung injury, high-frequency ventilation should be considered if a PIP >20–25 cm H_2O is required in a premature infant or >30 cm H_2O in a term infant.
   c. **When using patient-triggered ventilation modes,** set the ventilator rate high enough to prevent hypoventilation should the patient become apneic.
3. **Neonatal lung disease.** Rarely static, necessitating frequent adjustments to ventilator parameters.

D. **Weaning from mechanical ventilation and extubation.** As lung function improves with disease resolution, mechanical support should be decreased as quickly as tolerated. Most patients do not need to be "weaned" from mechanical support; they need support decreased to match their need. Continuous monitoring with pulse oximetry and tcP_{CO_2} aids in weaning and limits the need for blood gas sampling. A reduced oxygen requirement and improved compliance (decrease in PIP to maintain V_T) usually herald the weaning phase. Although *controversial, pretreatment of infants with aminophylline is believed by some clinicians to enhance infant response to progressive weaning efforts.* Disease state, gestational age, and caloric support influence response to weaning process.
   1. **PIP.** Usually weaned first because overinflation injury is more deleterious than providing a greater rate than necessary. Volume-targeted ventilation modes may adequately decrease PIP as the lungs heal and provide a somewhat automatic wean.
   2. **F_{IO_2}.** Weaned whenever possible as determined by pulse oximetry or blood gases. Decreases in PIP decrease $\overline{Paw}$ and may transiently increase oxygen requirements during weaning.
   3. **Progressive rate wean (does not apply to assist/control modes).** Rate settings should be decreased frequently. Infants ready to be weaned tolerate the rate wean and do not require more F_{IO_2}. An infant should be able to maintain adequate minute ventilation without developing hypercarbia or apnea. When the ventilator rate is <10–20 breaths/min, the infant should be extubated. Some infants may require several hours to wean, whereas others need several days to a week or more.
   4. **Weaning assist/control ventilation.** Because all spontaneous breaths are mechanically supported by this mode of ventilation, reduction of the rate below the patient's spontaneous rate has no effect on the level of support. Weaning is accomplished by successive decreases in PIP. When adequate ventilation is maintained with minimal PIP (10–15 cm H_2O), extubation may be attempted.

E. **Care after extubation.** Continued monitoring of blood gases, respiratory effort, and vital signs is required. Additional oxygen support is often needed in the immediate postextubation period.
   1. **Supplemental oxygen.** May be given by hood or by nasal cannula. The oxygen concentration may be increased by >5% over the last oxygen level obtained while the infant was on the ventilator.
   2. **Nasal CPAP.** May be especially helpful in preventing reintubation secondary to postextubation atelectasis.
   3. **Chest radiograph.** If the infant has had an increasing oxygen requirement or has clinically deteriorated, a chest radiograph should be obtained at 6 hours postextubation to monitor for atelectasis.

V. **Overview of high-frequency ventilation.** High-frequency ventilation refers to a variety of ventilatory strategies and devices designed to provide ventilation at rapid rates and very low V_Ts. The ability to provide adequate ventilation in spite of reduced V_T (equal to or less than dead space) may reduce the risk of barotrauma. Rates during high-frequency ventilation are often expressed in hertz (Hz). A rate of 1 Hz (1 cycle/s) is equivalent to 60 breaths/min. All methods of high-frequency ventilation should be administered with the assistance of well-trained respiratory therapists and after comprehensive education of the nursing staff. Furthermore, because rapid changes in ventilation or oxygenation may occur, continuous monitoring is highly recommended. Optimal use of these ventilators is evolving, and different strategies may be indicated for a particular lung disease.

A. **Definitive indications for high-frequency ventilation support**
   1. **Pulmonary interstitial emphysema (PIE).** A multicenter trial has demonstrated high-frequency jet ventilator (HFJV) to be superior to conventional ventilation in early PIE as well as in neonates who fail to respond to conventional ventilation.
   2. **Severe bronchopleural fistula.** In severe bronchopleural fistula not responsive to thoracostomy tube evacuation and conventional ventilation, HFJV may provide adequate ventilation and decrease fistula flow.
   3. **Respiratory distress syndrome (RDS).** High-frequency ventilation has been used with success. It is usually implemented at the point of severe respiratory failure with maximal conventional ventilation (a rescue treatment). Earlier treatment has been advocated. No advantages have yet been demonstrated for a very early intervention (in the first hours of life) when infants are pretreated with surfactant.
   4. **Patients qualifying for ECMO/ECLS (extracorporeal life support).** Pulmonary hypertension with or without associated parenchymal lung disease (eg, meconium aspiration, pneumonia, hypoplastic lung, or diaphragmatic hernia) can result in intractable respiratory failure and high mortality unless the patient is treated by ECMO/ECLS. The prior use of high-frequency ventilation among ECMO/ECLS candidates has been successful and eliminated the need for ECMO/ECLS in 25–45% of cases.

B. **Possible indications.** High-frequency ventilation has been used with success in infants with other disease processes. Further study is needed to develop clear indications and appropriate ventilatory strategies before this treatment can be recommended for routine use in infants with these diseases.
   1. Pulmonary hypertension
   2. Meconium aspiration syndrome
   3. Diaphragmatic hernia with pulmonary hypoplasia
   4. Postoperative Fontan procedures

C. **High-frequency ventilators, techniques, and equipment.** Two types of high-frequency ventilators in the United States are the high-frequency jet ventilator (HFJV) and the high-frequency oscillatory ventilator (HFOV).
   1. **High-frequency jet ventilator.** The HFJV injects a high-velocity stream of gas into the endotracheal tube, usually at frequencies between 240 and 600 breaths/min and V_{T}s equal to or slightly greater than dead space. During HFJV, expiration is passive. The only HFJV approved by the US Food and Drug Administration is the Life Pulse (Bunnell, Inc., Salt Lake City, UT) ventilator, discussed here.
      a. **Indications.** Mostly used for PIE, the Life Pulse HFJV has been used for the other indications described for all types of high-frequency ventilation.
      b. **Equipment**
         i. **Bunnell Life Pulse ventilator.** The inspiratory pressure (PIP), jet valve "on time," and respiratory frequency are entered into a digital control panel on the jet. PIPs are servo-controlled by the Life Pulse from the pressure port. The ventilator has an elaborate alarm system to ensure safety and to help detect changes in pulmonary function. It also has a special humidification system.
         ii. **Conventional ventilator.** A conventional ventilator is needed to generate PEEP and sigh breaths. PEEP and background ventilation are controlled with the conventional ventilator.

c. Procedure
   i. Initiation. **Close observation** is required at all times, especially during initiation.
      (a) Replace the endotracheal tube adapter with a jet adapter
      (b) Settings on the jet ventilator
         i. Default jet valve "on time." 0.020 seconds.
         ii. Frequency of jet. 420 per minute.
         iii. PIP on the jet. 2–3 cm H_2O below what was on the conventional ventilator. Frequently, infants require considerably less PIP during high-frequency jet ventilation.
      (c) Settings on the conventional ventilator
         i. PEEP. Maintain at 3–5 cm H_2O.
         ii. Rate. As the jet ventilator comes up to pressure, the rate is decreased to 5–10 breaths/min.
         iii. PIP. Once at pressure, the PIP is adjusted to a level at least 1–3 cm H_2O below that on the jet (low enough not to interrupt the jet ventilator).
d. Management. Management of high-frequency jet ventilation is based on the clinical course and radiographic findings.
   i. Elimination of CO_2. Alveolar ventilation is much more sensitive to changes in VT than in respiratory frequency during high-frequency ventilation. As a result, the **delta pressure** (PIP minus PEEP) is adjusted to attain adequate elimination of CO_2, whereas jet valve "on time" and respiratory frequency are usually not readjusted during HFJV.
   ii. Oxygenation. Oxygenation is often better during HFJV than during conventional mechanical ventilation in neonates with PIE. However, if oxygenation is inadequate and if the infant is already on 100% oxygen, an increase in P̄aw usually results in improved oxygenation. It can be accomplished by:
      (a) Increasing PEEP
      (b) Increasing PIP
      (c) Increasing background conventional ventilator (either rates or pressure)
   iii. Positioning of infants. Positioning infants with the affected side down may speed resolution of PIE. In bilateral air leak, alternating placement on dependent sides may be effective. Diligent observation and frequent radiographs are necessary to avoid hyperinflation of the nondependent side.
e. Weaning. When weaning, the following guidelines are used.
   i. PIP is reduced as soon as possible (Paco$_2$ <35–40 mm Hg). Because elimination of CO_2 is very sensitive to changes in VT, PIP is weaned 1 cm H_2O at a time.
   ii. Oxygen concentration. Weaned if oxygenation remains good (Pao$_2$ >70–80 mm Hg).
   iii. Jet valve "on time" and frequency. Usually kept constant.
   iv. Constant attention is paid to the infant's clinical condition and radiographs to detect early atelectasis or hyperinflation.
   v. Air leaks are resolved. Continuation of HFJV occurs until the air leak has been resolved for 24–48 hours, which often corresponds to a dramatic drop in ventilator pressures and oxygen requirement.
   vi. In case of no improvement in the condition. A trial of conventional ventilation is used after 6–24 hours on jet ventilation.
f. Special considerations
   i. Airway obstruction. This problem can usually be recognized quickly. Chest wall movement is decreased, although breath sounds may be adequate. The servo pressure (driving pressure) is usually very low.

    ii. **Inadvertent PEEP (air trapping).** In larger infants, the flow of jet gases may result in inadvertent PEEP. Decreasing the background flow on the conventional ventilator may correct the problem, or it may be necessary to decrease the respiratory frequency to allow more time for expiration.

2. **High-frequency oscillatory ventilator.** The HFOV generates V_T less than or equal to dead space by means of an oscillating piston or diaphragm. This mechanism creates active exhalation as well as inspiration. The SensorMedics 3100B HFOV (CareFusion Corporation, San Diego, CA) is currently approved by the US Food and Drug Administration for use in neonates.

  a. **Indications. Respiratory failure:** high-frequency oscillatory ventilation is indicated when conventional ventilation does not result in adequate oxygenation or ventilation or requires the use of very high airway pressures. Like other forms of high-frequency ventilation, success is more likely when increased airway resistance is not the dominant pulmonary pathophysiology. Best results are seen when parenchymal disease is homogeneous. Some clinicians advocate high-frequency oscillatory ventilation as the primary method of assisted ventilation in premature infants with RDS.

  b. **Equipment.** HFOV is used without a conventional ventilator. The user-defined parameters are frequency, $\overline{Paw}$, and power applied for piston displacement.

  c. **Procedure**

    i. **Initiation**

      (a) Conventional ventilator is discontinued.

      (b) **Settings**

        i. **Frequency.** Usually set at 15 Hz for premature infants with RDS. Larger infants, or those with a significant component of increased airway resistance (meconium aspiration), should be started at 5–10 Hz.

        ii. **$\overline{Paw}$.** Set higher (2–5 cm H_2O) than on the previous conventional ventilation. If overdistention or air leaks were present before initiation of high-frequency oscillatory ventilation, a lower $\overline{Paw}$ should be considered.

        iii. **Amplitude.** Analogous to PIP on conventional ventilation and is regulated by the power of displacement of the piston. This power is increased until there is visible chest wall vibration.

      (c) After high-frequency oscillatory ventilation has been initiated, careful and frequent assessment of lung expansion and adequate gas exchange are necessary. Air trapping is a continuous potential threat in this form of treatment. Signs of overdistention, such as descended and flat diaphragms and small heart shadow, are monitored with frequent chest radiographs.

  d. **Management**

    i. **Low Pao_2.** An increase in $\overline{Paw}$ may be necessary. Chest radiographs may be helpful in determining the adequacy of lung expansion.

    ii. **High $Paco_2$**

      (a) Oxygenation is also poor. The $\overline{Paw}$ may be too high or too low, resulting in either hyperinflation or widespread collapse, respectively. Again, chest radiographs are necessary to differentiate between these two conditions.

      (b) Oxygenation is adequate. The amplitude (power) should be increased. Decreasing the rate may be an alternative if hypercapnia is associated with evidence of lung hyperinflation.

  e. **Weaning**

    i. **In the absence of hyperinflation.** Fio_2 is weaned before $\overline{Paw}$ for adequate Pao_2. Below 40% Fio_2, wean $\overline{Paw}$ exclusively.

ii. $P\overline{aw}$. Should be weaned as the lung disease improves with the goal of maintaining optimal lung expansion. Excessively aggressive early weaning of $P\overline{aw}$ may result in widespread atelectasis and the need for significant increases in $P\overline{aw}$ and FIO_2.

iii. Amplitude. Should be weaned for acceptable $Paco_2$.

iv. Frequency. Usually not adjusted during weaning. A decrease in frequency is necessary when signs of lung overdistention cannot be eliminated by a reduction in $P\overline{aw}$.

v. The neonate may be switched to conventional ventilation at a low level of support or may be extubated directly from HFOV.

f. Complications. Hyperinflation with compromise of cardiac output. Frequent evaluation with CXR is advised.

GLOSSARY OF TERMS USED IN RESPIRATORY MANAGEMENT

Arterial-to-alveolar ratio (a/A ratio). See Section I.B.3b.

Assist. A setting at which the infant initiates the mechanical breath, triggering the ventilator to deliver a preset VT or pressure.

Assist/control. The same as assist, except that if the infant becomes apneic, the ventilator delivers the number of mechanical breaths per minute set on the rate control.

Continuous positive airway pressure (CPAP). A spontaneous mode in which the ambient intrapulmonary pressure that is maintained throughout the respiratory cycle is increased.

Control. A setting at which a certain number of mechanical breaths per minute is delivered. The infant is unable to breathe spontaneously between mechanical breaths.

End-tidal CO_2 ($Etco_2$ or $Petco_2$). A measure of the Pco_2 of end expiration.

Expiratory time (ET). The amount of time set for the expiratory phase of each mechanical breath.

Flow rate. The amount of gas per minute passing through the ventilator. It must be sufficient to prevent rebreathing (ie, 3 times the minute volume) and to achieve the PIP during T_i. Changes in the flow rate may be necessary if changes in the airway waveform are desired. The normal range is 6–10 L/min; 8 L/min is commonly used.

Fraction of inspired oxygen (FIO_2). The percentage of oxygen concentration of inspired gas expressed as decimals (room air = 0.21).

I:E ratio. Ratio of inspiratory time to expiratory time. The normal values are 1:1, 1:1.5, or 1:2.

Inspiratory time (T_i). The amount of time set for the inspiratory phase of each mechanical breath.

Intermittent mechanical ventilation. Mechanical breaths are delivered at intervals. The infant breathes spontaneously between mechanical breaths.

Minute ventilation. VT (proportional to PIP) multiplied by rate.

Oxygen index (OI). MAP × FIO_2 × $100/Pao_2$.

Oxyhemoglobin dissociation curve. A curve showing the amount of oxygen that combines with hemoglobin as a function of Pao_2 and $Paco_2$. The curve shifts to the right when oxygen takeup by the blood is less than normal at a given Po_2, and it shifts to the left when oxygen takeup is greater than normal.

Pao_2. Partial pressure of arterial oxygen.

PAP. The total airway pressure. In the Siemens Servo 900-C, it is the PIP plus the PEEP.

$P\overline{aw}$. The average proximal pressure applied to the airway throughout the entire respiratory cycle.

Pco_2. Carbon dioxide partial pressure.

Peak inspiratory pressure (PIP). The highest pressure reached within the proximal airway with each mechanical breath. *Note:* In the Siemens Servo 900-C, the PIP is defined as the inspiratory pressure above the PEEP.

Po_2. Oxygen partial pressure.

Positive end-expiratory pressure (PEEP). The pressure in the airway above ambient pressure during the expiratory phase of mechanical ventilation.

Rate. Number of mechanical breaths per minute delivered by the ventilator.

SaO$_2$. Oxygen saturation of arterial blood measured by direct measurement (arterial blood gas).

Tidal volume (VT). The volume of gas inspired or expired during each respiratory cycle.

Selected References

Brown MK, DiBlasi RM. Mechanical ventilation of the premature neonate. *Respir Care.* 2011;56:1298–1311.

Donn SM, Sinha SK. *Neonatal Respiratory Care.* 3rd ed. Philadelphia, PA: Mosby; 2012.

Goldsmith JP, Karotkin E. *Assisted Ventilation of the Neonate.* 5th ed. Philadelphia, PA: WB Saunders; 2011.

Gupta S, Sinha SK, Donn SM. Myth: mechanical ventilation is a therapeutic relic. *Semin Fetal Neonatal Med.* 2011;16:275–278.

Keszler M. State of the art in conventional mechanical ventilation. *J Perinatol.* 2009;29:262–275.

Klingenberg C, Wheeler KI, Davis PG, Morley CJ. A practical guide to neonatal volume guarantee ventilation. *J Perinatol.* 2011;31:575–585.

Tobin M. *Principles and Practice of Mechanical Ventilation.* New York, NY: McGraw-Hill; 2006.

Wheeler K, Klingenberg C, McCallion N, Morley CJ, Davis PG. Volume-targeted versus pressure-limited ventilation in the neonate. *Cochrane Database Syst Rev.* 2010;CD003666.

9 Fluid and Electrolytes

An assessment of body water metabolism and electrolyte balance plays an important role in the early medical management of preterm infants and sick term infants coming to neonatal intensive care. Intravenous or intra-arterial fluids given during the first several days of life are a major factor in the development, or prevention, of morbidities such as intraventricular hemorrhage (IVH), necrotizing enterocolitis (NEC), patent ductus arteriosus (PDA), and bronchopulmonary dysplasia. Clinicians must pay close attention to the details of maintaining and monitoring body water and serum electrolytes, and the management of fluid infusion therapies.

Bodily fluid balance is a function of the distribution of water in the body, water intake, and water losses. Body water distribution gradually changes with increasing gestational age of the fetus. At birth these gestational changes in body water are reflected in the developing maturity of renal function, trans-epidermal insensible water losses, and neuroendocrine adaptations. One must account for these variables when deciding the amount of infusion fluids to administer to an infant.

I. **Body water**

    A. **Total body water (TBW).** Water accounts for nearly 75% of the body weight in term infants and as much as 85–90% of body weight of preterm infants. TBW is divided into 2 basic body water compartments: intracellular water (ICW) and extracellular water (ECW). ECW is composed of intravascular and interstitial water. For the fetus there is a gradual decrease in ECW to 53% at 32 weeks' gestation and a gradual increase in ICW. Thereafter the proportions remain fairly constant until 38 weeks of gestation when increasing body mass of protein and fat stores reduce ECW further by ~5%.

        At birth there begins a further contraction of the ECW as a function of the normal transition from intrauterine to extra-uterine life. A diuresis occurs that reduces body weight proportionally to gestational age. For the very low birthweight preterm infant body, weight losses of 10–15% can be expected, whereas full-term infants usually lose 5% of body weight. These losses are largely accounted for as water and, to a lesser extent, body fat stores.

B. **TBW balance in the newborn**

1. **Renal.** Fetal urine flow steadily increases from 2–5 mL/h to 10–20 mL/h at 30 weeks' gestation. At term, fetal urine flow reaches 25–50 mL/h and then drops to 8–16 mL/h (1–3 mL/kg/h). These volume changes illustrate the large exchange of body water during fetal life and the abrupt changes forcing physiologic adaptation at birth. Despite marked fetal urine flow in utero, glomerular filtration rates (GFRs) are low. At birth, GFR remains low but steadily increases in the newborn period under the influence of increasing systolic blood pressure, increasing renal blood flow, and increasing glomerular permeability. Infant kidneys are able to produce dilute urine within limits dependent on GFR. The low GFR of preterm infants is the result of low renal blood flow but increases considerably after 34 weeks' postconceptional age. Term infants can concentrate urine up to 800 mOsm/L compared to the 1500 mOsm/L of older children and adults. The preterm infant kidney is less able to concentrate urine secondary to a relatively low interstitial urea concentration, an anatomically shorter loop of Henle, and a distal tubular and collecting system that is less responsive to antidiuretic hormone (ADH). In extreme prematurity, urine osmolarity can be as low as 70 mOsm/L. Although limitations exist, healthy preterm infants with constant sodium intake but variable fluid infusion between 90 and 200 mL/kg/d are able to concentrate or dilute urine to maintain a balance of body water.

   Against the backdrop of changing GFR and variable urine concentrating ability, all infants undergo a diuresis and a natriuresis in the days immediately following birth. Newborn diuresis is a contraction of the ECW and the initiation of body water conservation as the adaptation from an aquatic intrauterine existence to the less humidity and free water-dependent newborn state. The diuresis is facilitated by limited ADH responsiveness but is diminished by increasing serum osmolality (>285 mOsm/kg) and decreasing intravascular volume. Natriuresis is the result of increasing levels of atrial natriuretic peptide and decreased renal sodium absorption; infant kidneys also have decreased secretion of bicarbonate, potassium, and hydrogen ion.

2. **Insensible water loss (IWL).** Evaporation of body water occurs largely through the skin and mucous membranes (two-thirds) and the respiratory tract (one-third). A most important variable influencing IWL is the maturity of the infants' skin. The greater IWL in preterm infants results from body water evaporation through an immature epithelial layer. The stratum corneum is not well developed until 34 weeks' gestation. Throughout the third trimester the stratum corneum and epidermis thicken. Keratinization of the stratum corneum forms the principal barrier to water loss. Keratinization begins early in the second trimester and continues throughout the third trimester. Additionally, IWL is related to a larger skin surface area–to–body weight ratio in preterm infants and relatively greater skin vascularity.

   IWL through the respiratory tract is related to the respiratory rate and the water content of the inspired air or air-oxygen mix (humidification). Table 9–1 lists other factors for IWL in newborn infants.

   In general, for healthy premature infants weighing 800–2000 g cared for in double-walled incubators, IWL increases linearly as body weight decreases (Table 9–2).

   However, for sick infants of similar weight cared for under a radiant warmer and undergoing ventilator respiratory support, IWL increases exponentially as body weight decreases.

   Phototherapy may increase IWL by way of increasing body temperature and increasing peripheral blood flow. Generally, recommended fluid increases for preterm infants have been 10–20 mL/kg/d. This may not be necessary with newer

Table 9–1. **FACTORS IN THE NICU ENVIRONMENT THAT AFFECT INSENSIBLE WATER LOSS**

Body weight	Inversely proportional to maturity
Radiant warmer use during procedures	IWL increase by 50–100% over incubator care (see also Chapter 12)
Phototherapy	IWL *controversial*; may be minimal for term infants, but appreciable for preterm infants (up to 25%)
Ambient humidity and temperature in double- walled humidified incubators	High ambient humidity and a thermal neutral environment conserve TBW
High body temperature	May increase loss by 30–50%
Tachypnea	Variable depending on respiratory support
Skin breakdown	Most often from removal of adhesives denuding skin
Congenital absence of normal skin covering	Large omphaloceles, neural tube defects, or skin losses as in epidermolysis bullosa

IWL, insensible water loss; NICU, neonatal intensive care unit; TBW, total body water.

phototherapy lights using light emitting diodes (LEDs) because they generate very little heat. Moreover, term infants receiving adequate fluid intake and with no other increased body water loss may not need added fluid intake. Occasionally, phototherapy induces loose stools and IWL would need to be reconsidered.

3. Neuroendocrine. TBW balance is also influenced by hypothalamic osmo-receptors and carotid baroreceptors. Serum osmolarity >285 mOsm/kg stimulates the hypothalamus and ADH is released to affect free water retention. Additionally, volume diminution affects carotid bodies and baroreceptors to further stimulate ADH secretion to retain free water at the level of the collecting ducts of the distal nephrons. Collectively the osmo-receptors and the baroreceptors seek to maintain TBW with adequate intravascular volume at normal serum osmolarity. In the neonate, hypoxia with acidemia and hypercarbia are potent stimulators of ADH. An excessive secretion of ADH can follow one or more insults such as intracranial hemorrhage, sepsis, and/or hypotension. Conversely, excessive ADH secretion can occur in the absence of hyperosmolarity or volume depletion. Thus a phenomenon known as the syndrome of inappropriate ADH secretion (SIADH) can occur. It is manifested as hyponatremia, hypo-osmolar serum, dilute urine, and low blood urea nitrogen. Because ADH secretion begins early in fetal development, SIADH can occur as readily in preterm infants as in term infants.

Table 9–2. **ESTIMATES OF INSENSIBLE WATER LOSS IN PRETERM INFANTS DURING FIRST WEEK OF LIFE IN A THERMAL NEUTRAL ENVIRONMENT**

Birthweight (g)	Insensible Water Loss (mL/kg/d)
<750	100–200
750–1000	60–70
1001–1250	50–60
1251–1500	30–40
1501–2000	20–30
>2000	15–20

Adapted from Dell KM, Davis ID. Fluid and electrolyte management. In: Martin RJ, Fanaroff AA, Walsh MC, eds. *Fanaroff and Martin's Neonatal-Perinatal Medicine: Diseases of the Fetus and Infant.* 8th ed. Philadelphia, PA: Mosby Elsevier; 2006:695–703.

C. **Monitoring TBW balance**
1. **Body weight.** Using in-bed scales, body weight should be recorded daily for all infants undergoing intensive care, and twice daily for very low birthweight and extremely low birthweight infants. **Expected weight loss** during the first 3–5 days of life is 5–10% of birthweight for term infants and 10–15% of birthweight for preterm infants. A loss of >15% of birthweight during the first week of life should be considered excessive and body water balance carefully reevaluated. If weight loss is <2% in the first week of life, maintenance infusion fluid administration may be excessive.
2. **Physical examination.** Edema or loss of skin turgor, moist or dry mucous membranes, sunken or puffy periorbital tissues, and full or sunken anterior fontanel have been time-honored sites to examine for dehydration or overhydration. They may be helpful when observing newborn infants but are unreliable in low birthweight infants. They must be observed within the context of all other TBW points of monitoring.
3. **Vital signs**
   a. **Blood pressure** can be an indicator of altered intravascular volume, but usually is later rather than earlier. Pressure changes and trends are needed in the overall assessment of TBW balance.
   b. **Pulse volumes,** decreased in dehydration with tachycardia, are somewhat sensitive indicators of early intravascular volume loss.
   c. **Tachypnea** can be an early sign of metabolic acidosis accompanying inadequate intravascular volume.
   d. **Capillary refill time (CRT)** has been a reliable and time-honored observation. CRT of >3 seconds in term infants is suspect for decreased intravascular volume, whereas a CRT of barely 3 seconds in a preterm infant should be equally suspected.
4. **Hematocrit (Hct).** Increases or decreases of central Hct (venous or arterial) from accepted normal values suggest changes in intravascular volume as it relates to TBW. Apart from obvious hemorrhage, changes in Hct may reflect overhydration or dehydration and must be considered in the assessment of TBW for fluid therapy in the first week of life.
5. **Serum chemistries**
   a. **Sodium** values of 135–140 mEq/L are indicative of TBW and sodium balance. Values above or below are suggestive of hyper- or hypo-osmolarity. A sodium value of ≤130 mEq/L strongly suggests that SIADH may be a factor.
   b. **Serum osmolarity** of 285 mOsm/L (±3 mOsm) is the standard for TBW balance; values above or below must be considered indicative of over- or underhydration. If serum osmolarity is <280 mOsm/L, SIADH must also be considered in any preterm or sick full-term infant.
6. **Acid-base status**
   a. **Hydrogen ion (pH).** A less than normal pH (7.28–7.35) is indicative of metabolic acidosis and will be accompanied by other factors, suggesting a contracted intravascular volume and hyperosmolarity.
   b. **Base deficit.** An increasing base deficit (ie, metabolic acidosis with deficit >5.0) with decreased urine output, decreased blood pressure, and a prolonged CRT strongly suggests hypovolemia.
   c. **Chloride ion, carbon dioxide (CO_2) content, and bicarbonate (HCO_3).** These determinations are important for calculating anion gap and overall acid-base status.
   d. **Anion gap.** The anion gap is a unifying determination for identifying metabolic acidosis in the face of dehydration. It is the sum of the serum sodium and potassium ions *minus* the sum of the serum chloride and bicarbonate ions. The normal range for anion gap is 8–16. Values for an anion gap >16 are indicative of an organic acidemia. In the face of dehydration with decreased intravascular volume, lactic acidemia follows poor tissue perfusion and is reflected as a widening anion gap. See Chapter 46.

7. Urine

   a. Urine output should be 1–3 mL/kg/h by the third day of life in all newborn infants with normal kidneys. Preterm infants have limited urine formation on day 1 of life, but should begin to increase urine production throughout day 2.

   b. Urine specific gravity of 1.005–1.012 is consistent with TBW balance.

   c. Urine electrolytes and urine osmolarity offer additional information as to renal concentrating ability. Term infants can concentrate urine to 800 mOsm/kg, whereas preterm infants are limited to 600 mOsm/kg.

D. Maintenance of TBW. Infusion fluid therapy for newborn infants (term and preterm) must be calculated to allow for normal ECW losses and body weight losses while avoiding dehydration from excessive IWL. The consequences of dehydration are hypotension, hypernatremia, and acidosis. Conversely, excessive infusion fluid therapy is associated with clinically significant patent ductus arteriosus and may aggravate respiratory distress. Given careful monitoring for TBW as detailed earlier, the following infusion fluid therapy guidelines are offered for maintenance of TBW balance in term and preterm infants (with the exception of infusion fluid therapy for extremely low birthweight infants; see Chapter 12).

1. Term infants in need of infusion fluid therapy

   a. Day 1. Give dextrose 10% in water (D10W) at a rate of 60–80 mL/kg/d. This provides 6–7 mg/kg/min of glucose in support of energy needs while providing limited hydration during the immediate postnatal adaptation period. Neither sodium nor potassium supplementation are needed unless unusual body fluid losses are known.

   b. Days 2–7. Once tolerance of infusion fluid therapy has been established and confirmed by TBW monitoring (eg, urine output of 1–2 mL/kg/h), the rate and composition of fluid therapy can be modified. The goals of infusion fluid therapy include expected weight loss of 5% body weight, confirmed normal serum electrolyte values, and continued urine output of 2–3 mL/kg/h. Specifics of fluid therapy are as follows:

      i. Infusion fluid volume 80–120 mL/kg/d. May increase to 120–160 mL/kg/d by week's end as tolerated, or to meet needs per monitoring.

      ii. Glucose to be provided to maintain serum glucose values >60 mg/dL; may increase to 8–9 mg/kg/min infusion as D10W or D12.5W.

      iii. Sodium requirement daily is 2–4 mEq/kg/d per monitoring of serum (target values, 135–140 mEq/L).

      iv. Potassium daily requirements are 1–2 mEq/kg/d per monitoring of serum (target values, 4.0–5.0 mEq/L). Potassium supplementation is not begun until the second or third day, and only when normal renal function is confirmed by adequate urine output and normal serum electrolyte values have been established.

      v. Nutrition. Infusion fluid glucose does not meet all energy needs for basal metabolism, growth, and activity. Enteral feeds must be started as soon as possible; however, if the patient is unable to take formula by mouth or only in limited amount then total parenteral nutrition (TPN) becomes necessary. As enteral feeds increase, infusion fluids or TPN can be progressively decreased, but keeping total volume intake at 120–160 mL/kg/d.

2. Preterm infants

   a. Day 1. During the immediate postnatal period, critically ill premature infants may require volume resuscitation for shock or acidosis. Fluids administered during stabilization should be considered when planning subsequent fluid management.

   b. Days 1–3. Infusion fluid therapy is aimed at allowing a 10–15% body weight loss through the first week while maintaining TBW balance and electrolyte balance.

      i. Infusion fluid volumes. Preterm low birthweight infants (>1500 g) require 60–80 mL/kg/d. Preterm very low birthweight infants (1000–1500 g) require

80–100 mL/kg/d. Preterm extremely low birthweight infants (<1000 g) require a range of fluid volumes from 50–80 mL/kg/d if cared for in double-walled humidified (80%) incubators. If cared for under a radiant warmer or in incubators without humidity, fluid requirements may be 100–200 mL/kg/d (see Table 12–1 for breakdown into 100-g birthweight increments).

   ii. **Glucose supplementation.** Best achieved by using D5W or D7.5W infusion fluids to avoid hyperglycemia. Because of the high fluid requirements in the smallest infants, glucose utilization may not be sufficient to prevent buildup of serum glucose and a hyperosmolar state secondary to hyperglycemia. If allowable, reduced glucose maintenance is preferred, but extremes of hyperglycemia (>150 mg/dL) may require insulin therapy.

   iii. **Sodium.** During the first week of life, fluid therapy should be managed by increments or decrements of 20–40/mL/kg/d depending on weight changes and serum sodium values, while attempting to keep serum sodium at 135–140 mEq/L. Sodium supplementation is not usually required in the first 2–3 days of life. Sodium supplementation is begun on the basis of body weight losses (postnatal isotonic contraction of ECW compartment, a physiologic diuresis). Usually by day 3–5, weight loss and a slight serum sodium decrease from baseline dictate the need to start sodium supplementation by way of the infusion fluids. Judicious restriction of sodium intake during the first 3–5 days of life facilitates a trend for normal serum osmolarity throughout the first week of life for preterm infants.

   iv. **Potassium.** Supplementation follows that of term infants, meaning that well-established renal function with good urine output is required before supplementation at 1–2 mEq/kg/d.

   v. **Nutrition.** Caloric needs to provide for the relative hypermetabolic state of low birthweight infants can be met through TPN fluid therapy. Initiation of TPN after the first 24 hours of life is desirable (see Chapters 10 and 12).

  c. **Days 3–7.** Infusion fluid and electrolyte management is dictated by the monitoring parameters as already given. Infusion fluids should be advanced or decreased as the transition period progresses. Excessive weight loss suggests increased IWL losses and the threat of dehydration. Likewise, edema and minimal or no weight loss suggests excessive fluid administration or decreasing renal function and decreased urine output. All preterm infants should be cared for whenever possible in double-walled incubators for a more stable humidity control and less IWL.

3. **Other infusion fluid calculations and considerations**

  a. **Environmental**

   i. **Radiant warmers.** Infusion fluid volume recommendations as outlined earlier are for assumed double-walled incubator care. If radiant warmer exposure is to be maintained, fluid therapy must be increased by 50–100%. Plastic sheeting limits increased needs to 30–50%.

   ii. **Phototherapy.** If infant is full term, increased fluid therapy may not be needed. If infant is low birthweight, most likely 10–20 mL/kg/d will be needed to minimize IWL while phototherapy lights are in use.

  b. **Glucose.** The normal glucose requirement is 6–8 mg/kg/min, and intake can be slowly increased to 10–12 mg/kg/min as needed, but with careful monitoring for hyperglycemia and glucosuria to avoid an osmotic diuresis. Calculations for glucose supplementation are

$$\text{Glucose requirements (mg/kg/min)} = \frac{(\text{Percentage of glucose} \times \text{Rate[mL/h]} \times 0.167)}{\text{Weight (kg)}}$$

Table 9–3. **GLUCOSE CONCENTRATION IN COMMONLY USED INTRAVENOUS INFUSION FLUIDS**

Solution	Glucose Concentration (mg/mL)
Dextrose 5% water	50
Dextrose 7.5% water	75
Dextrose 10% water	100
Dextrose 12.5% water	125
Dextrose 15% water	150

An alternate method is

$$\text{Glucose requirement (mg/kg/min)} = \frac{(\text{Amount of glucose/mL [from Table 9–3]} \times \text{Total fluids})}{\text{Weight (kg)/(60 min)}}$$

   c. **Sodium.** The normal sodium requirement for infants is 2–3 mEq/kg/d. The following calculations can be used to determine the amount of sodium (Na^+) per day that an infant will receive from a given saline infusion fluid:

Amount of Na^+/mL (from Table 9–4) × Total fluids/d =

Amount of Na^+/d

$$\frac{\text{Amount of } Na^+/d}{\text{Weight (kg)}} = \text{Amount of } Na^+ \text{ (kg/d)}$$

   d. **Potassium.** The normal potassium requirement for infants is 1–2 mEq/kg/d. Potassium supplementation should not begin until adequate urine output is established.

II. **Electrolyte disturbances**

  A. **Sodium.** Serum values of 135–145 mEq/L represent homeostatic sodium balance. The wide range of 131–149 mEq/L is the lower and upper limit for sodium (Na^+) balance. Values above or below are clinical indicators of either hyper- or hyponatremia.

   1. **Hypernatremia**

    a. **Decreased ECW with Na^+ of ≥150 mEq/L**

     i. **Causes.** Include increased renal free water losses and/or increased IWL, primarily through skin, especially very low birthweight and extremely low birthweight infants.

     ii. **Clinical findings.** Weight loss, low blood pressure, tachycardia, decreased or absent urine output, and increased urine specific gravity.

Table 9–4. **SODIUM CONTENT OF COMMONLY USED INFUSION FLUIDS**

Solution	Sodium Concentration (mEq/mL)
3% normal saline	0.500
Normal saline	0.154
0.50% normal saline	0.075
0.25% normal saline	0.037
0.125% normal saline	0.019

    iii. Treatment. Requires careful infusion fluid management. **Replacing free water is the first goal, and maintaining Na⁺ balance is the second goal.** Both goals need to be accomplished without precipitating rapid ICW and ECW shifts of water or sodium, especially within the central nervous system (CNS). **Excessively rapid correction of hypernatremia can result in seizures.** Hypernatremic dehydration does not represent a deficit of body sodium. Infusion therapy should be guided to reduce serum Na⁺ by not more than 0.5 mEq/L/kg/h, or less, with a target of total correction time of 24–48 hours. Consider using D5W 0.25 normal saline (NS) as an initial infusion fluid for correction.

  b. Increased ECW and hypernatremia

    i. Causes. Include excessive administration of normal saline or sodium bicarbonate as in resuscitation efforts or postresuscitation treatment for perinatal asphyxia with metabolic acidosis and hypotension.

    ii. Clinical findings. Increased weight gain and edema. If cardiac output has been compromised, findings of edema and weight gain increase. Depending on cardiac status, heart rate, blood pressure, and urine output will be within normal limits or decreased.

    iii. Treatment. Involves identification of cardiac status. Identify infusion fluid excesses and establish maintenance infusion fluid limits; thereafter, restrict sodium until serum Na⁺ values return to normal range.

2. Hyponatremia. See also Chapter 64.

  a. Increased ECW as increased intravascular water and increased third space interstitial water

    i. Causes. Increased ECW with serum Na⁺ <130 mEq/L, which most likely represents excessive infusion fluid administration, and increased third space (interstitial) water secondary to sepsis, shock, and capillary leakage. It may also be secondary to cardiac failure or pharmacologic neuromuscular paralysis during mechanical ventilation. More frequently it occurs in newborn infants as SIADH following CNS trauma, intracranial hemorrhage, meningitis, perinatal asphyxia, or pneumothorax.

    ii. Clinical findings. Result from inadvertent excessive infusion fluid administration: body weight is increased with edema, serum Na⁺ is decreased, and urine output is increased with decreased urine osmolarity and specific gravity. Conversely, if SIADH is the root cause of increased ECW and hyponatremia, the clinical findings reveal increased body weight, variable presence of edema, decreased serum Na⁺, decreased urine output, and increased urine specific gravity. Some cases of SIADH do not reflect increased ECW but rather manifest simply as hyponatremia with decreased urine output and urine specific gravity.

    iii. Treatment. In both situations is free water restriction allowing serum Na⁺ to concentrate to normal levels. If serum Na⁺ is <120 mEq/L and neurologic symptoms are present, consider titrating with infusion of 3% saline solution boluses. Consultation by a nephrologist is recommended.

  b. Decreased ECW with hyponatremia

    i. Causes. Include excessive diuretic therapy, glycosuria with an osmotic diuresis, vomiting, diarrhea, and third space fluid with necrotizing enterocolitis.

    ii. Clinical findings. Include decreased body weight, signs of dehydration with sunken fontanel, loss of skin turgor, dry mucous membranes, increased blood urea nitrogen (BUN), metabolic acidosis, decreased urine output, and increased urine specific gravity.

    iii. Treatment. Involves replacing sodium and water while minimizing any ongoing sodium losses.

c. Isotonic losses may occur and present as hyponatremia. Such losses may be cerebrospinal fluid from drainage procedures, thoracic as in chylothorax, nasogastric drainage, or peritoneal fluid (ascites).

Normal saline for fluid replacement usually suffices, or normal saline plus colloid as fresh-frozen plasma or human albumin may facilitate intravascular volume and restore serum saline.

B. Potassium

1. Hyperkalemia. Represented by serum K^+ values >5.5 mEq/L. Some infants do not manifest symptoms until serum levels reach 7–8 mEq/L. Hyperkalemia can be caused by or related to renal failure, hemolysis, blood transfusions, exchange transfusions, or inadvertent excessive administration of a potassium solution (eg, KCl). Cardiac conduction is the most immediate concern, and electrocardiographic monitoring is essential until treatment corrects serum K^+ levels. For a detailed discussion of hyperkalemia and treatment, see Chapter 60.

2. Hypokalemia. Potassium levels <4.0 mEq/L suggest impending hypokalemia, and values <3.5 mEq/L require treatment to correct. Meanwhile, cardiac conduction abnormalities may occur, and monitoring electrocardiographically, as in hyperkalemia, is essential until hypokalemia is corrected. For a detailed discussion of hypokalemia and treatment, see Chapter 63.

C. Chloride. See also Chapter 46, section on metabolic alkalosis.

1. Hypochloremia. Serum values of 97–110 mEq/L are taken as normal in most newborn infants. Serum values <97 mEq/L are indicative of low chloride and suggest either inadequate supplementation during infusion fluid therapy or, more commonly, chloride ion losses. Typically, chloride ion accompanies Na^+ and K^+ as NaCl or KCl solutions in maintenance infusion solutions. Chloride losses independent of Na^+ or K^+ occur usually from excessive gastrointestinal fluid losses, particularly gastric hydrochloric acid losses. Chloride losses lead to increased bicarbonate reabsorption and metabolic alkalosis.

2. Hyperchloremia. Uncommon in the newborn period but may be found when inadvertent concentrations of Cl^- ion are given in parenteral nutrition solutions. Occasionally increased Cl^- ion is reflective of excessive renal conservation of Cl^- during correction of alkalosis when forming alkaline urine.

Selected References

Dell KM. Fluid, electrolyte and acid-base homeostasis. In: Martin RJ, Fanaroff AA, Walsh MC, eds. *Fanaroff and Martin's Neonatal-Perinatal Medicine: Diseases of the Fetus and the Infant.* 9th ed. Philadelphia, PA: Elsevier Mosby; 2011:669–684.

Elstgeest LE, Martens SE, Lopriore E, Walther FJ, te Pas AB. Does parenteral nutrition influence electrolyte and fluid balance in preterm infants in the first days after birth? *PLoS One.* 2010;5(2):e9033. DOI:10.1371/journal.pone.0009033.

Gawlowski Z, Aladangady N, Coen PG. Hypernatremia in preterm infants born at less than 27 weeks' gestation. *J Paediatr Child Health.* 2006;42:771–774.

Hartnoll G. Basic principles and practical steps in the management of fluid balance in the newborn. *Semin Neonatol.* 2003;8:307–313.

Maisels MJ, McDonagh AF. Phototherapy for neonatal jaundice. *N Engl J Med.* 2008; 358:920–928.

Sung MK, Lee EY, Chen J, Ringer SA. Improved care and growth outcomes by using hybrid humidified incubators in very preterm infants. *Pediatrics.* 2010;125:e137–e145.

Verma RP, Shibli S, Fang H, Komaroff E. Clinical determinants and utility of early postnatal maximum weight loss in fluid management of extremely low birth weight infants. *Early Human Dev.* 2009;85:59–64.

10 Nutritional Management

GROWTH ASSESSMENT OF THE NEONATE

   I. **Anthropometrics.** Serial measurements of weight, length, and head circumference allow for evaluation of growth patterns.
       A. **Weight.** Birthweight is reflective of maternal, placental, and fetal environment. During the first week of life, weight loss of 10–20% of birthweight is expected because of changes in body water. Preterm infants lose more weight and regain birthweight slower than term infants. Weight gain generally begins by the second week of life. Average daily weight gain based on normal intrauterine growth is 10–20 g/kg/d (1–3% of body weight/d).
       B. **Length.** Length is a better indicator of lean body mass and long-term growth and is not influenced by fluid status. Weekly assessment is recommended. Average length gain in preterm infants is 0.8–1.0 cm/wk, whereas term infants average 0.69–0.75 cm/wk.
       C. **Head circumference.** Intrauterine head growth is 0.5–0.8 cm/wk and is an indicator of brain growth. Premature infants exhibit catch-up growth in head circumference that may exceed normal growth rate, but an increase in head circumference >1.25 cm/wk may be abnormal and associated with hydrocephalus or intraventricular hemorrhage. Average head circumference growth is 0.9 cm/wk in very low birthweight (VLBW) infants. Head circumference is correlated with long-term neurodevelopment.
       D. **Weight for length.** This can be used to determine symmetry of growth. Current weight expressed as a percentage of ideal weight for length can identify infants at risk for under or over nutrition. Catch-up growth occurs faster if only weight is lagging compared with length and head circumference. Weight gain is slower in large for gestational age infants.
  II. **Classification**
       A. **Measurements.** Measurements of weight, length, and head circumference are plotted on growth charts to facilitate comparison with established norms. This can help to identify special needs.
       B. **Growth charts.** Provide longitudinal assessment of an infant's growth. Growth charts for term boys and girls are available from the Centers for Disease Control (CDC) (www.cdc.gov/growthcharts) and from the World Health Organization (WHO). The CDC growth charts are population-based growth **reference charts,** whereas the WHO charts are **growth standards**. The WHO charts are based on infants breast-fed from healthy women growing in an ideal socioeconomic environment. Postnatal growth differs between breast-fed and formula-fed infants. The two charts are now merged; the WHO centiles are used before 2 years and the CDC after 2 years (www.who.int/childgrowth/standards/en).
            Two types of charts exist for VLBW infants: those based on intrauterine growth and those based on postnatal growth. Intrauterine growth charts provide reference standards. Variations exist in the reference populations for the various growth charts. Intrauterine growth charts are found in Chapter 5. Postnatal growth charts are limited as they do not show the "catch-up growth" or the growth velocity relative to the fetus. Assessment of postnatal growth failure is better reflected on postnatal growth charts. Normal growth customarily falls between the 10th and 90th percentiles when adjusted for gestational age. Recently, population-specific customized growth charts have been developed to determine term optimal birthweight and to identify fetal growth restriction (www.gestation.net).

NUTRITIONAL REQUIREMENTS IN THE NEONATE

I. **Calories**
   A. **To maintain weight.** Give 50–60 kcal/kg/d (60 nonprotein kcal/kg/d).
   B. **To induce weight gain.** Give 100–120 kcal/kg/d to a term infant (gain: 15–30 g/d) and 110–140 kcal/kg/d to a premature infant (70–90 nonprotein kcal/kg/d). Growth in premature infants is assumed to be adequate when it approximates the intrauterine rate (ie, 15 g/kg/d).

II. **Carbohydrates.** Approximately 10–30 g/kg/d (7.5–15 g/kg/d) are needed to provide 40–50% of total calories. Lesser amounts of carbohydrates should provide total energy requirements in infants with chronic lung disease.

III. **Proteins.** Adequate protein intake has been estimated at 2.25–4.0 g/kg/d (7–16% of total calories, or 2–3 g/100 kcal for efficient utilization). Protein intake in extremely low birthweight infants should not exceed 4.4 g/kg/d.

IV. **Fats.** Fat requirements are 5–7 g/kg/d (limit: 40–55% of total calories or ketosis may result). Preterm infants may need 6.2–8.4 g/kg/d. To meet essential fatty acid requirements, 2–5% of nonprotein calories should be in the form of linoleic acid and 0.6% in the form of linolenic acid (together comprising 3% of total energy requirements). Linoleic and linolenic acids are precursors for arachidonic acid (ARA) and docosahexanoic acid (DHA), important in neural and retinal maturation. Breast milk contains long-chain polyunsaturated fatty acids (LCPUFAs), but concentrations vary over the world (0.1–1.4%). LCPUFAs are transferred predominantly through the placenta in the third trimester. LCPUFA-enriched formulas are associated with improved retinal sensitivity and visual acuity but have no effect on short-term morbidities such as bronchopulmonary dysplasia (BPD), necrotizing enterocolitis (NEC), and retinopathy of prematurity (ROP). The long-term benefits of LCPUFA supplementation in formula-fed infants are not clear. The effects on growth and anthropometric parameters are conflicting, although some long-term benefits on development are reported in preterm infants. In breast-fed preterm infants, LCPUFA may be neuroprotective and improve cognitive development, particularly in girls.

V. **Vitamins and minerals.** Vitamin and mineral requirements for preterm infants are not clearly established. Guidelines are provided in Tables 10–1 through 10–3 for low birthweight infants. Caution is required with vitamin supplementation because toxicity may occur with both water-and fat-soluble vitamins as a result of immature renal and hepatic function. Vitamin supplementation may be needed with certain types of infant formulas (see Table 10–4).
   A. **Vitamin A.** May be useful in attenuating chronic lung disease in VLBW infants at a dose of 5000 IU intramuscularly 3 times/wk for 12 doses.
   B. **For infants with osteopenia of prematurity.** Various amounts of calcium, phosphorus, and vitamin D may be supplemented.
   C. **For infants receiving recombinant human erythropoietin therapy (rHuEpo).** Additional iron supplementation is necessary. Although recommended doses vary, it is generally agreed that a dose in excess of maintenance therapy is needed. These doses may approach 6–10 mg/kg/d. Iron can also be added to parenteral nutrition. For infants receiving high doses of iron, monitoring for hemolytic anemia is important, and vitamin E supplementation (15–25 IU/d) may be required. rhEPO use is associated with increased risk of ROP.
   D. **Iron deficiency.** Associated with short-term and long-term neurodevelopmental deficits, delayed maturation of the auditory brainstem responses, and abnormalities of memory and behavior. Iron supplementation of term infants at risk of iron deficiency is associated with improved neurodevelopmental outcomes. Preterm infants are more susceptible to iron deficiency due to small iron stores at birth, high growth velocity, and phlebotomy losses. However, blood transfusions provide a rich source of iron; 1 mL of packed red blood cells provides 0.5–1.0 mg of iron, and iron overload may be a risk with multiple transfusions. Delayed cord

Table 10–1. **DAILY ENTERAL VITAMIN AND MINERAL REQUIREMENTS FOR TERM AND STABLE PRETERM LOW BIRTHWEIGHT INFANTS**

Nutrient	Term Infant (per day)	Stable Preterm Low Birthweight Infant (dose/kg)
Vitamins		
Vitamin A (with lung disease)	700 mcg	700–1500 mcg
Vitamin D	400 IU	400 IU
Vitamin E	7 IU	6–12 IU
Vitamin K	200 mcg	8–10 mcg
Vitamin C	80 mg	18–24 mg
Thiamine	1.2 mg	0.18–0.24 mg
Riboflavin	1.4 mg	0.25–0.36 mg
Niacin	17 mg	3.6–4.8 mg
Pyridoxine	1.0 mg	0.15–0.20 mg
Vitamin B$_{12}$	1.0 mcg	0.3 mcg
Folic acid	140 mcg	25–50 mcg
Biotin	20 mcg	3.6–6.0 mcg
Pantothenate	5 mg	1.2–1.7 mg
Choline	125 mg	14.4-28 mg
Minerals		
Calcium	250 mg	120–330 mg
Phosphorus	150 mg	60–140 mg
Magnesium	20 mg	7.9–15 mg
Sodium	1–2 mEq/kg	2.0–3.0 mEq
Potassium	2–3 mEq/kg	2.0–3.0 mEq
Iron	1 mg/kg	2–3 mg
Copper	20 mcg/kg	120–150 mcg
Zinc	2.5–5.0 mg/d	1000 mcg
Manganese	5 mcg/100 kcal	0.75–7.5 mcg
Molybdenum	0.75–7.5 mcg	0.3 mcg
Selenium	2 mcg/kg	1.3–3.0 mcg
Chromium	0.20 mcg/kg	0.1–0.5 mcg
Iodide	1 mcg/kg	30–60 mcg
Linoleic acid		600–1680 mg/kg
Linolenic acid		0.7–2.1% calories
Docosahexaenoic acid (DHA)		>18 mg
Arachidonic acid (ARA)		>24 mg

clamping improves iron stores in both term and preterm infants. Stable preterm infants should receive iron supplementation (2–4 mg/kg/d; maximum 15 mg/d) starting 4–8 weeks of age (some studies have suggested as early as 2 weeks) and continued until 12–15 months. Formula-fed infants require less iron supplementation than breast-fed infants. A rising reticulocyte count may indicate need for starting iron supplementation.

VI. **Fluids.** See Chapter 9 for fluid requirements.

PRINCIPLES OF INFANT FEEDING

I. **Criteria for initiating infant feeding.** Term healthy infants should be breast-fed as soon as possible within the first hour. The following criteria should usually be met before initiating infant feedings.

Table 10–2. **DAILY PARENTERAL REQUIREMENTS FOR VITAMINS AND MINERALS IN TERM, PRETERM, AND STABLE PRETERM INFANTS**

Nutrient	Term Infant (per day)	Preterm Infant (dose/kg)	Stable Preterm Infant (dose/kg)
Vitamins			
Vitamin A (with lung disease)	700 mcg	500 mcg	700–1500 mcg
Vitamin D	400 IU	160 IU	40–160 IU
Vitamin E	7 mg	2.8 mg	3.5 mg
Vitamin K	200 mcg	80 mcg	8–10 mcg
Vitamin C	80 mg	25 mg	15–25 mg
Thiamine	1.2 mg	0.35 mg	0.2–0.35 mg
Riboflavin	1.4 mg	0.15 mg	0.15–0.20 mg
Niacin	17 mg	6.8 mg	4.0–6.8 mg
Pyridoxine	1.0 mg	0.18 mg	0.15–0.20 mg
Vitamin B_{12}	1.0 mcg	0.3 mcg	0.3 mcg
Folic acid	140 mcg	56 mcg	56 mcg
Biotin	20 mcg	6 mcg	5–8 mcg
Pantothenate	5 mg	2 mg	1–2 mg
Minerals			
Calcium		75–90 mcg	
Phosphorus		48–67 mcg	
Magnesium		6–10.5 mcg	
Sodium	1–2 mEq/kg	2.5–3.5 mEq <1.5 kg: 4–8 mEq	
Potassium	2–3 mEq/kg	2–3 mEq	
Iron		2–4 mcg (after 6–8 weeks)	
Copper[a]	20 mcg/kg	20 mcg	
Zinc	250 mcg/kg	1200–1500 mcg	
Manganese	1 mcg/kg	10–20 mcg	
Molybdenum	0.25 mcg	0.3 mcg	
Selenium[b]	2 mcg/kg	2 mcg	
Chromium	0.20 mcg/kg	0.2 mcg	
Iodide	1 mcg/kg	1 mcg	

[a]Omit in cholestatic jaundice.
[b]Start supplementation at 2–4 weeks. Omit in renal dysfunction.

Table 10–3. **CONDITIONALLY ESSENTIAL NUTRIENTS**

Nutrients[a]	Supplementation/100 kcal
Cystine	225–395 mmol
Taurine	30–60 mmol
Tyrosine	640–800 mmol
Inositol	150–375 mmol
Choline	125–225 mmol

[a]Nutrients normally synthesized by humans but for which premature infants may have a reduced synthetic capability to produce.

Table 10–4. **INFANT FORMULA INDICATIONS AND USES**

Formula	Indications	Vitamins and Mineral Supplement[a]
Human milk	All infants	Vitamin D 400 IU/d; iron
Breast milk fortifiers	Preterm infant (<1500 g and <34 weeks)	Vitamin D 400 IU/d; iron; MV
Term formulas (iso-osmolar)		
Enfamil Premium	Full-term infants: as supplement to breast milk	MV if <32 oz/d
Similac Advance		(approx 1 L/d)
Preterm formulas (iso- and hyperosmolar)		
Enfamil Premature 24	Preterm infants: for infants on fluid restriction	
Similac Special Care 24 and 30	or who cannot handle required volumes of 20-cal formula to grow	
Soy formulas (**Note:** Soy formulas not recommended in infants <1800 g)		
ProSobee (lactose and sucrose free)	Term infants: milk sensitivity, galactosemia, carbohydrate intolerance	MV if <32 oz/d (approx 1 L/d)
Gerber Good Start Soy	Term infants; hydrolyzed soy proteins	
Soy Isomil (lactose free)	*Do not use in preterm infants. Phytates can bind calcium and cause rickets.*	
Protein hydrolysate formulas (casein predominant)		
Nutramigen with Enflora LGG (Probiotic LGG)	Term infants: hypoallergenic, hydrolyzed casein with lactose, galactose, and sucrose free for gut sensitivity to proteins, galactosemia, multiple food allergies, persistent diarrhea, colic due to cow's milk allergy	MV if <32 oz/d (approx 1 L/d)
Nutramigen AA	Amino acid based hypoallergenic for cow's milk protein allergy	
Pregestimil	Preterm and term infants: disaccharidase deficiency, fat malabsorption, diarrhea, GI defects, cystic fibrosis, food allergy, celiac disease, transition from TPN to oral feeding	
Alimentum	Term infants: lactose-free formula; protein sensitivity, pancreatic insufficiency, diarrhea, allergies, colic, carbohydrate, and fat malabsorption	
Protein hydrolysate formulas (whey predominant)	Partially hydrolyzed to small peptides. Not truly hypoallergenic, but less expensive and more available; iron fortified	
Gerber Good Start	Term infants: whey protein; moderate mineral content; may be more palatable	
Enfamil Gentlease Similac Sensitive	Term infants; to reduce fussiness or gas	

Table 10–4. **INFANT FORMULA INDICATIONS AND USES (*CONTINUED*)**

Formula	Indications	Vitamins and Mineral Supplement[a]
Free amino acid elemental formulas	100% amino acids as protein source (not hydro-lyzed), hypoallergenic. Used in cow's milk allergy, food protein intolerance, short bowel, eosinophilic esophagitis	
Neocate	Term infants: cow's milk protein allergies; contains 100% free amino acids (elemental formula)	
EleCare	Elemental formula containing amino acids indicated for malabsorption, protein maldigestion, short bowel syndromes	
Special formulas		
Similac PM 60/40	Preterm and term infants: problem feeders on standard formula; infants with renal, cardiovascular, or digestive diseases that require decreased protein and mineral levels; breast-feeding supplement; initial feeding	MV and Fe if standard formula weight >1500 g
Enfamil AR	Rice starch added for thickening after ingestion (pH sensitive). Used for simple reflux. Not indicated for preterm infants.	
Similac Sensitive for Spit-Up	Contains rice starch. Not for use in galactosemia.	
Enfaport	For infants with chylothorax and LCHAD deficiency	
Premature formulas (low osmolality)		
Similac Special Care 20 Enfamil Premature 20	Premature infants (<1800–2000 g) who are growing rapidly. These promote growth at intrauterine rates. Vitamin and mineral concentrations are higher to meet the needs of growth. Usually started on 20 cal/oz and advanced to 24 cal/oz as tolerated.	
Premature formulas (iso-osmolar)		
Similac Special Care 24	Same as for low-osmolality premature formulas	
Similac Special Care 24 with high protein	Contains 3.3 g protein/100 calories	
Enfamil Premature 24	Preterm infants >1800 g. Promotes catch-up growth and improved bone	
Discharge or transitional formulas		
EnfaCare Similac Expert Care NeoSure	Preterm infants; increased protein, calcium, phosphorous, Vitamins A and D, promotes better mineralization. Can also be used to fortify human milk feedings. Use up to 6–9 months corrected age	
Metabolic formulas	Special metabolic formulas are available for infants with inherited metabolic disorders www.meadjohnson.com www.abottnutrition.com	

Fe, iron; GI, gastrointestinal; MV, multivitamin; TPN, total parenteral nutrition.
[a]Such as Poly-Vi-Sol (Mead Johnson).

A. Absence of excessive oral secretions, vomiting, or bilious-stained gastric aspirate.

B. **Nondistended, soft abdomen, with normal bowel sounds.** If the abdominal examination is abnormal, an abdominal radiograph should be obtained.

C. **Respiratory rate.** Should be <60 breaths/min for oral feeding and <80 breaths/min for gavage feeding. Tachypnea increases the risk of aspiration.

D. **Prematurity.** Feedings should be initiated and advanced to full enteral feeds as soon as clinically possible. Early enteral feedings are associated with better endocrine adaptation, enhanced immune functions, and earlier discharge. Institutional practices may vary. Parenteral nutrition, including amino acids and lipids, should be initiated within 24 hours to provide adequate protein and caloric intake. Early parenteral nutrition is also associated with better weight gain.

   1. **For the stable, larger premature neonate (>1500 g).** The first feeding may be given within the first 24 hours of life. Early feeding may allow the release of enteric hormones, which exert a trophic effect on the intestinal tract.

   2. **Feeding caution should be exercised.** In the presence of perinatal asphyxia, hemodynamic instability, sepsis, absent end-diastolic flow, indomethacin or ibuprofen therapy, and hemodynamically significant patent ductus arteriosus due to continuing clinical concerns in many institutions for NEC in extremely low birthweight (ELBW) and VLBW infants.

E. **Feeding cautions.** Should also be extended to term infants with perinatal depression, polycythemia, and congenital heart disease, who are also at risk of developing NEC.

II. **Feeding guidelines and choice of formula.** Human milk is preferred for feeding term, preterm, and sick infants. If a commercial infant formula is chosen, generally no special considerations apply to healthy, full-term newborn infants. Preterm infants may require more careful planning. Many different, highly specialized formulas are available. Iron-fortified formula has become the formula of choice for term infants because its use has contributed to a decreased rate of anemia. Most term formulas are now fortified with oligosaccharides and nucleotides that are also found in breast milk. Some term formulas are also fortified with probiotics. Formulas are available as ready-to-feed liquids or as powders that can be reconstituted before feeding. Table 10–4 outlines indications for various formulas. The compositions of commonly used infant formulas and breast milk can be found in Table 10–5.

A. **Formulas**

   1. **Hypo or iso-osmolar formulas (<300 mOsm/kg water).** The majority of term and preterm infant formulas are iso-osmolar or mildly hypo-osmolar to improve tolerance and decrease risk of NEC in preterm infants. Premature formulas that contain 24 cal/oz are also iso-osmolar.

   2. **Hyperosmolar formulas (>300 mOsm/kg water).** These are 30 cal/oz formulas. Formulas such as Similac 30 are hypercaloric formulas designed to provide a greater percentage of the calories as protein and to provide increased mineral concentrations. They are used to provide nutritional needs for infants that require fluid restriction. It is important to monitor renal solute load.

   3. **Transitional formulas.** Preterm infants continue to need nutritional supplementation after discharge. These have higher protein and mineral contents *but not higher caloric density* than term formulas. Infants discharged on special formulas (eg, NeoSure, EnfaCare; see Table 10–5) have better somatic growth, weight gain, and bone mineralization. Supplementation should be continued until a corrected age of 9 months.

   4. **Organic formulas.** Some formulas with organically derived components are available. No studies to date have demonstrated any advantages over nonorganic formulas.

B. **General guidelines**

   1. **Initial feedings.** Use maternal breast milk for initiating feedings. In the absence of maternal breast milk, donor breast milk (see later discussion of

breast milk) may be used in VLBW infants (after obtaining parental consent) to initiate feeds. The use of formula feeds is associated with a 6–10 times higher incidence of NEC in preterm low birthweight (LBW) infants than breast milk and 3 times higher when breast milk and formulas are used together versus breast milk alone.

2. **Subsequent feedings.** Feedings should be advanced gradually if the initial feeds are tolerated. There are no fixed guidelines. Feedings are advanced once to twice a day. Increments range between 10 and 35 mL/kg/d in various studies. Caution should be exercised when advancing rapidly, particularly with formula feeds, due to risk of NEC. Some clinicians advance feeds in small volumes with each feeding. Particular care should be taken in IUGR infants, those with absent end-diastolic flow on antenatal Doppler ultrasonography, and those at risk for NEC (see prior discussion of NEC). Formula or breast milk should not be diluted.

3. **Continuous versus bolus feeds.** Although no clear advantage has been shown for either method, infants with short gut syndromes or gastroesophageal reflux and ELBW infants may benefit from continuous feeds. Institutional practices may vary. If using breast milk, the infusion syringe should be placed vertically to allow fats to be delivered.

4. **Minimal enteral feedings ("trophic feeding").** Trophic feeds are subnutritional quantities of milk feeds, based on the concept of minimal enteral feedings. This practice—also called hypocaloric, trophic, trickle feedings, low-volume enteral substrate, or gastrointestinal priming—is characterized by a small-volume feeding to supplement parenteral nutrition. Studies have focused on use in infants <1500 g at birth. This method has been accepted because of benefits such as improved feeding tolerance, prevention of gastrointestinal atrophy, and facilitation of gastrointestinal tract maturation leading to a shorter time required for attaining full enteral feedings. Other benefits include decreased incidences of cholestasis, nosocomial infections, metabolic bone disease, and decreased hospital stay without an increase in the incidence of NEC. There is no standard method of minimal enteral feeding, and a wide variety of feeding techniques and formulas exist. Mother's breast milk should be preferred over donor breast milk or preterm formula for trophic feedings. Start trophic feeds as soon as possible if infant is clinically stable.

   a. **Type of feeds.** Breast milk is the preferred feeding; however, positive results have been achieved using preterm infant formulas. Enteral solution patterned after human amniotic fluid have also been used.

   b. **Feeding method.** Orogastric or nasogastric routes are used for feeding. Nasogastric tubes in small infants may increase airway resistance. Both continuous and bolus feedings have been used. The most effective method remains to be identified, but a trend exists toward bolus feedings. Enteral feedings should be advanced as clinically tolerated.

   c. **Volume.** Volumes studied have varied from 0.1–24 mL/kg/d.

   d. **Minimal enteral feedings for ELBW infants** (<1000 g, <28 weeks). Should start at 10–20 mL/kg/d divided as every 2–3 hour feeds, advanced as tolerated. Alternatively, start at 0.5–2 mL every 6 hours; advance to every 4 hours and then every 2 hours. If continuous feeds are used, up to 0.5–1 mL/kg/h volume may be used.

5. **Weight-specific guidelines are based on birthweight and gestational age as presented in this section.** For an infant presumed to be at risk for NEC, the rate of enteral feeding advancement should not exceed 20 mL/kg/d and 10 cal/kg/d. Protocols vary by institution.

   a. **VLBW infants <1000 g. Gavage feeding** through an orogastric or nasogastric tube is appropriate. Gavage feeding typically involves passing a 5F (<1000 g) to 8F feeding tube into the abdomen and verifying its position by injecting a few milliliters of air and listening for a characteristic "whoosh"

Table 10–5. COMPOSITION OF SELECTED INFANT FORMULAS

Characteristics	Mature Human Breast Milk	Enfamil Premium and Enfamil Premium Infant	Similac Advance	Similac Advance Organic (Organic Iron-Fortified Formula)	Similac Special Care 20 (With Iron)
Calories/100 mL	68	67	67.6	67.6	67.6
Osmolality (mOsm/kg H$_2$O)	290	300	310	225	235
Osmolarity (mOsm/L)	255	270	270		211
Protein					
Grams/100 mL	1.05	1.41	1.4	1.4	2.02
% Total calories	6	8.5	8	8	12
Source	Nonfat milk, whey	Nonfat milk, whey (whey:casein = 60:40)	Nonfat milk, whey protein	Organic nonfat dry milk	Nonfat milk, whey concentrate
Fat					
Grams/100 mL	3.9	3.55	3.65	3.65	3.67
% Total calories	52	48	49	49	47
Source[a]		Palm olein, soy, coconut, high-oleic sunflower, DHAI- and ARA-rich oil blend	High-oleic safflower, soy, and coconut oils (0.15% DHA, 0.40% ARA)	Organic high-oleic sunflower, soy, and coconut oils (0.15% DHA, 0.40% ARA)	MCTs, soy, and coconut oils vegetable oils, (0.25% DHA, 0.40% ARA)
Oil ratio		44:19.5:19.5:14.5:2.5	40:30.29	40:30.29	
Linoleic acid (mcg) (mg)	374	573.3 (56.6)	675.7	581.6	473
DHA (mg)	0.32% ± 0.22%	11.3 (*Crypthecodinium cohnii* oil)			
ARA (mg)		22.7 (*Montrierella alpina* oil)			
Carbohydrates					
Grams/100 mL	7.2	7.4	7.57	7.37	6.97
% Total calories	42	43.5	43	43	41
Source	Lactose	Lactose	Lactose, galacto-oligosaccharides	Organic corn maltodextrin, lactose, sugar, FOS (44:27:26.3)	Lactose, corn syrup solids (50:50)
Minerals (mg/100 mL)					
Calcium (mg) (mEq)	28	52.0	52.8 (2.63)	52.8 (2.63)	121.7 (6.0)
Phosphorus (mg)	14	28.6	26.3	28.4	67.6
Iodine (mcg)	11	10.0	4.1	4.1	4.1
Iron (mg)	0.03	1.20	1.2	1.22	1.2

Magnesium (mg)	3.5	5.3	4.1	4.1	8.1
Sodium (mg) (mEq)	18	18	16.2 (7.1)	16.2 (7.1)	29.1 (1.26)
Potassium (mg) (mEq)	52	72.0	71 (1.81)	71 (1.81)	87.2 (2.23)
Chloride (mg) (mEq)	42	42.0	44 (1.24)	43.9 (1.24)	54.8 (1.55)
Zinc (mg)	0.12	0.66	0.51	0.51	1.01
Copper (mcg)	25	50.0	60.9	60.9	169.1
Manganese (mcg)	0.6	10	3.4	3.4	8.1
Selenium (mcg)	1.5	1.87	1.22	1.22	1.2
Vitamins/100 mL					
Vitamin A (IU)	223	200	202	202	845
Vitamin D (IU)	2	50	40.6	40.6	101
Vitamin E (IU)	0.3	1.3	1.0	1.0	2.7
Vitamin K (mcg)	0.2	6.0	5.4	5.4	8.1
Thiamine/B_1 (mcg)	21	53.3	67.6	67.6	169
Riboflavin/B_2 (mcg)	35	93.3	101.4	101.4	419
Niacin/B_3 (mcg)	150	666.6	710.1	710.1	3381
Vitamin B_6 (mcg)	20	40	40.6	40.6	169
Vitamin B_{12} (mcg)	0.05	0.20	0.17	0.17	0.37
Folic acid (mcg)	5	10.7	10.1	10.1	25
Vitamin C (mg)	4.1	8.0	6.1	6.1	25
Pantothenic acid (mcg)	180	333.3	304.3	304.3	1285
Biotin (mcg)	0.4	2.0	2.9	2.9	25
Choline (mg)	9.2	16	10.8	10.8	6.8
Inositol (mg)	15	4.0	3.2	3.2	27
Carnitine (mg)		1.34			
Taurine (mg)		4.0			
Prebiotic	Galacto-oligosaccharides, polydextrose		Galacto-oligosaccharide	FOS	
Nucleotides	++	++		+	
Potential renal solute load (mOsm/L)	97.6	129	126.7	126.7	188.2

(Continued)

Table 10–5. COMPOSITION OF SELECTED INFANT FORMULAS (*CONTINUED*)

Characteristics	Enfamil Premature (With Iron)	Similac Special Care 24 (With Iron)	Enfamil Premature LIPIL 24 (With Iron)	Similac Special Care 30 (With Iron)	Similac Soy Isomil
Calories/100 mL	67	81.2	81	101.4	67.6
Osmolality (mOsm/kg H₂O)	240	280	300	325	200
Osmolarity (mOsm/L)	220	246	260		
Protein					
Grams/100 mL	2	2.43	2.4	3.0	1.65
% Total calories	12	12	12	12	10
Source	Nonfat milk, whey concentrate	Nonfat milk, whey concentrate	Nonfat milk, whey concentrate	Nonfat milk, whey concentrate	Soy protein isolate, L-methionine
Fat					
Grams/100 mL	3.4	4.40	4.1	6.7	3.69
% Total calories	44	47	44	57	49
Source[a]	MCTs, soy, high-oleic vegetable oils, single-cell oil blend rich in DHA and ARA	MCTs, soy, and coconut oils (0.25% DHA, 0.40% ARA)	MCTs, soy, high-oleic vegetable oils, single-cell oil blend rich in DHA and ARA	MCTs, soy, and coconut oils (0.21% DHA, 0.33% and ARA)	High-oleic safflower, soy, and coconut oils (41:30:29)
Oil ratio		50:30:18.3		50:30:18.3	
Linoleic acid (mcg) (mg)	540 (60)	568.1	642.8 (71.4)	710.1	676.3
ARA (mg)	22.6		26.9		
DHA (mg)	11.3		13.5		
Carbohydrates					
Grams/100 mL	7.3	8.36	8.9	7.8	6.9
% Total calories	44	41	44	31	41
Source	Lactose, corn syrup solids	Lactose, corn syrup solids (50:50)	Lactose, corn syrup solids	Lactose, corn syrup solids (50:50)	Corn syrup solids, sugar, FOS (78:19:3)

Minerals (mg/100 mL)

Calcium (mg) (mEq)	110	146.1 (7.3)	130.9	182.6 (9.1)	71 (3.54)
Phosphorus (mg)	55.3	81.2	65.9	101.4	50.7
Iodine (mcg)	16.6	4.9	19.8	6.1	10.0
Iron (mg)	1.22	1.46	1.42	1.83	1.22
Magnesium (mg)	6.0	9.7	7.14	12.2	5.1
Sodium (mg) (mEq)	38.6	34.9(1.52)	46	43.6 (1.9)	29.8 (1.29)
Potassium (mg) (mEq)	65.3	104.7 (2.7)	77.7	130.8 (3.35)	73 (1.87)
Chloride (mg) (mEq)	60	65.7 (1.8)	71.4	82.1 (2.32)	41.9 (1.18)
Zinc (mg)	1.0	1.21	1.19	1.52	0.50
Copper (mcg)	80	9.7	5.0	12.2	16.9
Manganese (mcg)	4.2	202.9	95.2	253.6	50.7
Selenium (mcg)	1.9	1.46	2.2	1.83	1.22

Vitamins/100 mL

Vitamin A (IU)	833.3	1014	992.1	1268.1	202.9
Vitamin D (IU)	160	121.7	190.5	152.2	40.6
Vitamin E (IU)	4.2	3.2	5.0	4.06	1.01
Vitamin K (mcg)	5.3	9.7	6.3	12.2	7.4
Thiamine/B_1 (mcg)	133.3	202.9	158.7	253.6	40.6
Riboflavin/B_2 (mcg)	200	503.2	238.1	629.0	60.9
Niacin/B_3 (mcg)	2666.6	4057.8	3174.6	5072.2	913
Vitamin B_6 (mcg)	100	202.9	119.0	253.6	40.6
Vitamin B_{12} (mcg)	0.17	0.44	0.20	0.56	0.3
Folic acid (mcg)	26.6	30	31.7	37.5	10.1
Vitamin C (mg)	13.3	30	15.8	37.5	6.1
Pantothenic acid (mcg)	800	1541.9	952.3	1927.4	507.2
Biotin (mcg)	2.7	30	3.2	37.5	3
Choline (mg)	13.3	8.1	15.9	10.1	8.1
Inositol (mg)	29.3	32.5	34.9	40.6	3.38
Carnitine (mg)	1.6		1.9	3.38	
Taurine (mg)			4.7		
Potential renal solute load (mOsm/L)	184	225.8	220	282.3	154.5
Oligosaccharides	+				

(Continued)

Table 10–5. COMPOSITION OF SELECTED INFANT FORMULAS (*CONTINUED*)

Characteristics	Enfamil ProSobee 20 cal/oz	Enfamil Gentlease 20 cal/oz	Similac Expert Care NeoSure 22	EnfaCare[c] 22 cal/oz	Similac PM 60/40	EleCare[d]
Calories/100 mL	68	68	74.4	74	67.6	67.6
Osmolality (mOsm/kg H$_2$O)	200	230	250	250 (liquid); 260 (powder)	280	350
Osmolarity (mOsm/L)	180	210	224	220 (liquid); 230 (powder)	250	
Protein						
Grams/100 mL	1.69	1.53	2.08	2.15	1.5	2.0
% Total calories	10	9	11	11	9	15
Source	Soy protein isolates (14%)	Partially hydrolyzed whey protein concentrate solids (soy), nonfat milk	Nonfat milk, whey concentrate	Nonfat milk, whey concentrate	Whey, sodium caseinate	Free L-amino acids
Fat						
Grams/100 mL	3.6	3.5	4.1	3.9	3.79	3.2
% Total calories	48	48	49	47	50	42
Source[a]	Palm olein, soy, coconut, and high-oleic sunflower oils, single-cell oil blend rich in DHA and ARA	Palm olein, soy, coconut, and high-oleic sunflower oils, single-cell oil blend rich in DHA and ARA	Soy, high oleic-safflower, coconut, MCT oils (28:27:25:18.6) (01.5% DHA, 0.40% ARA)	MCT, high-oleic vegetable, soy coconut, single-cell oil blend rich in DHA and ARA	High-oleic safflower, soy, and coconut oils (41:30:29)	High-oleic safflower oil, MCTs, soy oil (39:33:28)
Oil ratio				20:34:14:29:<2		
Linoleic acid (mcg) (mg)	573.3	573.3	557.9	700 (63.3)	676.3	568.0 (56.8)
ARA (mg)	22.6	22.6		25.1		
DHA (mg)	11.3	11.5		12.5		
Carbohydrates						
Grams/100 mL	7.2	7.2	7.51	7.7	6.9	7.2
% Total calories	42	4.3	40	42	41	43
Source	Corn syrup solids (55%)	Corn syrup solids	Lactose, corn syrup solids (50:50)	Maltodextrin, lactose, corn syrup solids	Lactose	Corn syrup solids

Minerals/100 mL

Calcium (mg) (mEq)	70	54.6	78.1 (3.9)	37.9 (1.89)	78.1 (3.9)
Phosphorus (mg)	46	30.6	46.1	18.9	56.8
Iodine (mcg)	10.0	10.0	11.2	4.1	5.6
Iron (mg)	1.2	1.2	1.34	0.47	0.99
Magnesium (mg)	7.4	5.3	6.7	4.06	5.6
Sodium (mg) (mEq)	24	24	24.5 (1.07)	16.2 (7.1)	30.5 (1.3)
Potassium (mg) (mEq)	80	72	105.6 (2.7)	54.1 (1.38)	101 (2.6)
Chloride (mg) (mEq)	54	42	5.58 (1.57)	39.9 (1.13)	40.5 (1.1)
Zinc (mg)	0.80	0.67	0.89	0.51	0.57
Copper (mcg)	50	50	89.3	60.9	71.0
Manganese (mcg)	16.7	10	7.4	3.4	56.8
Selenium (mcg)	1.87	1.87	1.7	1.22	1.56

Vitamins/100 mL

Vitamin A (IU)	200	200	260.4	202.9	184.6
Vitamin D (IU)	40	40	52.1	40.6	40.6
Vitamin E (IU)	1.3	1.3	2.68	1.01	1.4
Vitamin K (mcg)	5.4	5.4	8.18	5.4	4.0
Thiamine/B_1 (mcg)	53.3	53.3	130.2	67.6	142.0
Riboflavin/B_2 (mcg)	60	93.3	111.6	101.4	71.0
Niacin/B_3 (mcg)	666.7	666.7	1450.6	710	1140.0
Vitamin B_6 (mcg)	40	40	74.4	40.6	56.8
Vitamin B_{12} (mcg)	0.2	0.2	0.29	0.17	0.28
Folic acid (mcg)	10.7	10.7	18.6	10.1	19.9
Vitamin C (mg)	8.0	8.0	11.2	6.1	6.1
Pantothenic acid (mcg)	333.3	333.3	595.1	304.3	284.0
Biotin (mcg)	2	2	6.7	3.0	2.8
Choline (mg)	16.0	16.0	11.9	8.1	6.4
Inositol (mg)	4.0	4.0	26.0	16.2	3.4
Carnitine (mg)	1.3	1.3	1.48		
Potential renal solute load (mOsm/L)	156	140	187.4	124.1	187.0

(Continued)

Table 10–5. COMPOSITION OF SELECTED INFANT FORMULAS (*CONTINUED*)

Characteristics	Expert Care Alimentum	Enfamil A.R. 20 cal/oz	Gerber Good Start 20 cal/oz	Enfamil Nutramigen with AA/Enflora LGG 20 cal/oz	Pregestimil 20 cal/oz	Pregestimil 24 cal/oz
Calories/100 mL	67.6	68	67	68	68	81
Osmolality (mOsm/kg H$_2$O)	370	240 (liquid); 230 (powder)		270 (liquid); 300 (powder)	280 (liquid); 330 (powder)	330
Osmolarity (mOsm/L)		220 (liquid); 210 (powder)		240 (liquid); 270 (powder)	250 (liquid); 300 (powder)	290
Protein						
Grams/100 mL	1.86	1.69	1.47	1.87	1.89	2.3
% Total calories	11	10		11	11	11
Source	Casein hydrolysate, L-cysteine, L-tyrosine, L-tryptophan	Nonfat milk	Whey protein concentrate	Casein hydrolysate (17%), amino acids	Casein hydrolysate, amino acids	Casein hydrolysate, amino acids
Fat						
Grams/100 mL	3.75	3.4	3.42	3.53	3.8	4.5
% Total calories	48	46		48	48	48
Source[a]	Safflower, MCTs, soy oil (0.15% DHA, 0.40% ARA) (38:33:28)	Palm olein, soy, coconut, and high-oleic sunflower oils single-cell blend rich in DHA and ARA	Palm olein, soy, high-oleic safflower, coconut	Palm olein, soy, coconut, and high-oleic sunflower oils, single-cell blend rich in DHA and ARA	MCT, soy, and high-oleic safflower oils	MCT, soy, and high-oleic safflower oils
Oil ratio					55:35:7.5 and 2.5% oil rich in DHA and ARA (liquid) 55:25:10:[e] 7.5 and 2.5% oil rich in DHA and ARA (powder)	
Linoleic acid (mcg) (mg)	1285	573.3 (56.6)	603 (67)	573.3 (56.6)	626.6 (80 [liquid]/63.3 [powder])	746.0 (95.2)

ARA (mg)	22.6			22.6	22.6	26.8
DHA (mg)	11.3			11.3	11.3	13.4

Carbohydrates

	Col 1	Col 2	Col 3	Col 4	Col 5	Col 6
Grams/100 mL	7.3	7.5	7.5	6.9	6.9	8.3
% Total calories	44			41	41	41
Source	Sugar, modified tapioca starch (70:30)	Lactose, rice starch, maltodextrin	Lactose, corn maltodextrin	Corn syrup solids (45%), modified corn starch (7%)	Corn syrup solids, modified corn starch, dextrose	Corn syrup solids, modified corn starch

Minerals/100 mL

	Col 1	Col 2	Col 3	Col 4	Col 5	Col 6
Calcium (mg) (mEq)	71 (3.54)	43.3	44.6	62.7	62.6	74.6
Phosphorus (mg)	50.7	35.3	25.3	34.6	34.6	41.2
Iodine (mcg)	10.1	6.7	8.0	10.0	10.0	11.9
Iron (mg)	1.2	1.2	1.0	1.2	1.2	1.42
Magnesium (mg)	5.1	5.3	4.7	5.3/7.3	5.3	8.7
Sodium (mg) (mEq)	29.8 (1.29)	26.6	18.0	31.3	31.3	37.3
Potassium (mg) (mEq)	79.8 (2.03)	72	72.0	73.3	73.3	87.3
Chloride (mg) (mEq)	54.1 (1.55)	50	43.3	57.3	57.3	68.2
Zinc (mg)	0.5	0.67	0.53	0.67	0.67	0.89
Copper (mcg)	50.7	50	53.3	50	50	59.5
Manganese (mcg)	5.4	10.0	10.0	16.6/40.0	16.7	19.8
Selenium (mcg)	1.22	1.87	2.0	1.87	1.87	2.2

Vitamins/100 mL

	Col 1	Col 2	Col 3	Col 4	Col 5	Col 6
Vitamin A (IU)	202.9	200	200	200	233.3	301
Vitamin D (IU)	30.4	40	40.2	33.3	33.3	39.6
Vitamin E (IU)	2.03	1.33	1.34	1.3	2.7	3.2
Vitamin K (mcg)	10.1	5.3	5.36	6/5.3	8.0	9.52
Thiamine/B_1 (mcg)	40.6	53.3	66.7	53.3	53.3	63.5
Riboflavin/B_2 (mcg)	60.9	93.3	93.3	60	60	71.4

(Continued)

Table 10–5. COMPOSITION OF SELECTED INFANT FORMULAS (*CONTINUED*)

Characteristics	Expert Care Alimentum	Enfamil A.R. 20 cal/oz	Gerber Good Start 20 cal/oz	Enfamil Nutramigen with AA/Enflora LGG 20 cal/oz	Pregestimil 20 cal/oz	Pregestimil 24 cal/oz
Niacin/B_3 (mcg)	913	666.7	700	666.7	666.7	793.6
Vitamin B_6 (mcg)	40.6	40	50.0	40	40	47.6
Vitamin B_{12} (mcg)	0.30	0.2	0.22	0.2	0.2	0.24
Folic acid (mcg)	10.1	10.7	10.0	10.7	10.7	12.7
Vitamin C (mg)	6.1	8.0	6.7	8.0	8.0	9.5
Pantothenic acid (mcg)	507.2	333.3	300	333.3	333.3	396.8
Biotin (mcg)	3.0	2	2.95	2	2	2.4
Choline (mg)	8.1	16.0	16.0	8.0	16	19.0
Taurine (mg)		4.0		4	4.0	4.76
Inositol (mg)	3.4	4.0	4.0	11.3	11.3	13.4
Carnitine		1.3	+	1.35	1.3	1.58
Potential renal solute load (mOsm/L)	171.3				169	200
Probiotic			B. lactis			
Nucleotides[b]			++			

ARA, arachidonic acid; DHA, docosahexanoic acid; FOS, fructo-oligosaccharide.
[a] Similac and Enfamil products: C. cohnii oil, source of DHA; M. Alpina oil, source of ARA.
[b] Nucleotides: Adenosine 5'-monophosphate, cytidine 5'-monophosphate, disodium guanosine 5'-monophosphate, disodium uridine 5'-monophosphate.
[c] Concentration of some nutrients vary depending on powder or liquid concentrate
[d] Contains molybdenum and chromium.
[e] Corn oil.

(see Chapter 32). The stomach contents are aspirated and if <20% of previous feed or <2 mL, the contents may be fed again. Small amounts of feeding are placed in the tube under gravity using the open end of the syringe. Typically 2–3 mL/min are infused.

    i. Initial feeding. Breast milk, donor breast milk (see later discussion), or preterm infant formulas.

    ii. Maintenance feeding. Breast milk (with or without human milk fortifier; see indications presented later) or preterm formulas (20 or 24 cal/oz). Donor breast milk should not be used for maintenance because it does not provide adequate proteins and minerals for long-term growth. Our practice is to transition to formula feeds once infant is between 1000 and 1200 g (around 6–8 weeks).

    iii. Subsequent feedings

      (a) Volume. Bolus feeds, 10–20 mL/kg/d in divided volumes every 2–3 hours. Advance feeds by 10–20 mL/kg/d. Alternatively, give 0.5–1.0 mL/h continuously and increase by 0.5–1.0 mL every 12–24 hours. When 10 mL/h is tolerated, change feedings to every 2 hours and advance as tolerated.

      (b) Strength. Use expressed breast milk or preterm formula. Once full feedings of 20 cal/oz are tolerated, consider advancing to 24 cal/oz feedings or adding human milk fortifier to breast milk. Some institutions start with 24 cal/oz formulas.

  b. LBW <1500 g. Gavage feeding (see earlier discussion) through a nasogastric tube should be used.

    i. Initial feeding. Give breast milk or preterm formula every 2–3 hours.

    ii. Subsequent feedings

      (a) Volume. Bolus feeds, 10–20 mL/kg/d in divided volumes, every 3 hours. Advance feeds by 10–20 mL/kg/d. Alternatively, give 2 mL/kg every 2 hours, and increase by 1 mL every 12 hours up to 20 mL every 2 hours. Then change to feedings every 3 hours.

      (b) Strength. Use breast milk or preterm formulas. Once full feedings of 20 cal/oz formula are tolerated, advance to 24 cal/oz if desired or add human milk fortifier (22 or 24 cal/oz). Some institutions start with 24 cal/oz formulas.

  c. Weight: 1500 to 2500 g. Use gavage feeding through an orogastric or nasogastric tube. Breast-feeding or bottle-feeding can be attempted if the infant is >1600 g, >34 weeks' gestation, and neurologically intact. Initiation of early nursing is associated with earlier time to achieve full enteral feeds.

    i. Initial feeding. Use expressed breast milk or preterm infant formulas. For infants >1800 g (35–36 weeks), term infant formulas are frequently used. Breast milk or preterm infant formula should be used. In stable infants, starts feeds at 80 mL/kg/d, and then advance 10–20 mL/kg/d.

  d. Weight: >2500 g. Breast-feed or use a bottle if the infant is neurologically intact. Stable infants can be fed ad libitum with breast milk or term formula.

III. Management of feeding intolerance. If feeding is initiated but not tolerated, a complete abdominal examination should be performed. Preterm infants <32 weeks may not establish antegrade peristalsis. In the absence of other clinical signs, bilious aspirate by itself is not a contraindication for feedings in VLBW infants. Increasing feeding volume or continuing feeds may be helpful in improving tolerance. Presence of bilious aspirates, emesis, blood in stool, abdominal distension, or other systemic signs such as apnea and bradycardia should be closely evaluated. Aspirate volumes >2 mL in infants <750 g and >3 mL in infants 751–1000 g (or greater than a fifth of the feed volume) in the absence of other signs should not limit feeding. Consider abdominal radiographs if the physical findings are suspicious. If the abdominal evaluation is normal:

A. **Attempt continuous feedings with a nasogastric or orogastric tube.** Check the gastric aspirate, and follow the recommendations presented in Chapter 54.

B. **Use breast milk preferably or special formula (eg, Pregestimil).** These may be better tolerated.

IV. **Nutritional supplements.** Supplements are sometimes added to feedings, primarily to increase caloric intake (Table 10–6). They provide additional energy supplies with no concomitant increase in fluid volume. Protein supplementation results in an increase in short-term weight gain, linear growth, and head growth. Long-term effects on growth and neurodevelopment are not conclusive. There are insufficient data to evaluate the effects of carbohydrate or fat supplementation on long-term growth and development in preterm infants.

Some clinicians strongly believe that any necessary caloric supplementation should be given as a high-calorie formula (ie, 24 kcal/oz) instead of as a supplement because all nutrients in such a formula are in proportion to one another and allow maximum absorption. Nutritional supplements are often used in infants with BPD who are not gaining weight and need additional calories with no increase in protein, fat, or water intake.

V. **Postnatal growth failure and catch-up growth in preterm infants.** Preterm birth deprives the fetus of nutrient transfer that takes place in the third trimester, particularly of amino acids, fats, and minerals. Preterm birth is therefore associated with significant nutritional deficits a priori. Postnatally, low amino acid and high glucose intake and delayed enteral feedings result in poor weight gain and extrauterine growth failure by as much as 20% by the time of discharge. Many infants remain at <10th percentile of the intrauterine growth charts at time of discharge that can persist for up to 18 months. A longer time to regain birthweight and total protein intake, particularly enteral protein intake, influences long-term neurodevelopmental outcomes. The expected weight gain once birthweight is regained is 10–20 g/d for infants <27 weeks gestational age and 20–30 g/d for infants >27 weeks.

Attempts have been made to reduce postnatal growth failure and to provide "catch-up" growth by 2–3 months of age in VLBW and LBW infants by initiating early parenteral and enteral nutrition. The use of aggressive parenteral nutrition including high proteins and lipids has been found to be safe, and it is associated with a shorter time to regain birthweight and a trend toward lower risks of late-onset sepsis without any increased risk of NEC or BPD. Protein intake of 3 g/kg/d results in weight gain is similar to that seen in utero. Use of specialized preterm formulas can also help in catch-up growth and can overcome mineral deficits.

However, caution must be exercised in promoting aggressive growth in the form of weight gain because rapid growth results predominantly in fat deposition and may be associated with subsequent development of obesity, insulin resistance, diabetes, and cardiovascular disease. Improvement in lean body mass and use of maternal milk results in better outcomes.

Nutrition during the first few days impacts morbidity and mortality. Sicker infants tend to receive more fluid and less energy initially. Lower initial energy (and protein) intake are associated with increased risks of BPD, higher mortality, and worse developmental outcomes. Slower growth velocity is also associated with higher risks of retinopathy of prematurity.

BREAST-FEEDING

I. Advantages

A. **Protein quality.** The predominance of whey and the mixture of amino acids are compatible with the metabolic needs of LBW infants.

B. **Digestion and absorption.** Improved with breast milk.

Table 10–6. NUTRITIONAL SUPPLEMENTS USED IN INFANTS

Supplement	Nutrient Content	Calories	Indications and Contraindications	Amount to Use
Carbohydrate				
Polycose	Glucose polymers from hydrolyzed cornstarch	3.8 kcal/g powder; 2 kcal/mL liquid	Calorie supplementation[a] (lactose and gluten free) Contains Na, K, Ca, Cl, and P	**Powder:** 0.5 g/oz of 20-cal formula = 22 cal/oz; 1 g/oz of 20-cal formula = 24 cal/oz **Liquid:** 1 mL to 1 oz of 20-cal formula = 22 cal/oz
Infant rice cereal	Rice	15 cal/tbsp	Thickens feedings	1 tsp/4 oz of formula or milk
Fat				
Medium-chain triglyceride	Lipid fraction of coconut oil	8.3 kcal/g, 7.7 cal/mL	Limit to 50% calories from fat to prevent keto-sis; may cause diarrhea; do not use in BPD because of risk of aspiration pneumonia[b]	0.5 mL/4 oz of formula = 21 cal/oz; 1 mL/4 oz of formula = 22 cal/oz; 1 mL/2 oz of formula = 22 cal/oz
Vegetable oil	Soy, corn oil	9.0 cal/g (120 cal/tbsp)	To increase calories if fat absorption is normal[c]	0.5 mL/4 oz of formula = 21 cal/oz; 1 mL/4 oz of formula = 22 cal/oz
Microlipid	Safflower oil Soy lecithin Ascorbic acid Linoleic acid	4.5 cal/mL 5.9 g/tbsp	To increase caloric density, fluid restriction[d]	1 mL/2 oz of formula = 22 cal/oz

(Continued)

117

Table 10–6. **NUTRITIONAL SUPPLEMENTS USED IN INFANTS** (*CONTINUED*)

Supplement	Nutrient Content	Calories	Indications and Contraindications	Amount to Use
Protein				
Beneprotein	Whey protein iso-late/soy lecithin	4.1 cal/g (6 g of protein/packet[e]) Calcium = 30 mg/scoop Sodium = 15 mg/scoop Potassium = 35 mg/scoop Phosphorus = 15 mg/scoop Calories = 25/scoop	Useful for protein and calorie supplementation	Clinical experience is limited

BPD, bronchopulmonary dysplasia.

[a]Limiting formula intake while increasing calories may compromise protein, vitamin, and mineral intake, which may also lead to hyperglycemia and diarrhea.
[b]Always mix with formula to avoid the possibility of lipid aspiration or pneumonia.
[c]Vitamin E may need to be increased to at least 1 IU/g of linoleic acid.
[d]See text.

[e]1 packet = 1 scoop = 1 ½ tablespoon = 7 g.

Caution: **Microlipid can induce the formation of hydroxyperoxides when mixed with human milk.** Preterm milk with Microlipid can abolish the enterocyte barrier function and can result in degradation of enterocyte transepithelial electrical resistance, suggesting that stored milk mixed with Microlipid may increase the risk of gut infections. Attempts have been made to supplement milk with immunoglobulins to decrease incidence of NEC with no significant benefits. Some benefit, however, has been noted with arginine supplementation.

C. **Immunologic benefits.** Breast-feeding provides immunologic protection against bacterial and viral infections (particularly upper respiratory tract and gastrointestinal infections). Studies of infants breast-fed for >6 months show that they have a decreased incidence of asthma and cancer.

D. **Promotion of bonding.** Breast-feeding promotes bonding between the mother and her infant.

E. **Lower renal solute load.** This facilitates better tolerance.

F. **Other advantages.** Breast-feeding in preterm infants is associated with a decreased risk for NEC and a significantly higher intelligence quotient (IQ) at the age of 8 years. The risk of breast and ovarian cancers in the mother also appears to be lower. Human milk feedings are associated with beneficial effects on visual, cognitive, psychomotor, and neurodevelopmental outcomes that persist in childhood. Breast milk contains omega-3 fatty acids, that is, α-linolenic acid (ALA), from which other essential LCPUFAs, DHA, and ARA are produced. These play an important role in retinal and neurologic development. Most formulas are now supplemented with DHA and ARA. Partial breast milk (>50 mL/kg) feedings are associated with decreased risk of late-onset sepsis and NEC in preterm infants. The volume of breast milk intake during an infant's stay in the NICU may directly impact later neurodevelopmental scores.

II. **Contraindications and disadvantages.** *Note:* Temporary problems in the mother, such as sore or cracked nipples that resolve with treatment or mastitis treated with antibiotics, do not preclude nursing.

A. **Active tuberculosis in the mother.**

B. **Certain viral and bacterial infections in the mother.** For specific recommendations, see Appendix F. Issues in HIV-infected mothers are discussed in Chapter 97.

C. **Use of medications that are passed in significant amounts in the breast milk, which may harm the infant.** For the effects of drugs and substances on lactation and breast-feeding, see Chapter 149.

D. **Galactosemia.**

E. **Infant with a cleft lip or palate.** Such infants may have difficulty in nursing. Expressed breast milk can be fed to the infant using specially designed bottles (relative contraindication).

F. **IUGR infants (<1500 g).** May require greater amounts of protein, sodium, calcium, phosphorus, and vitamin D than unfortified breast milk contains. These requirements should be monitored routinely and supplemented as necessary.

G. **Breast-feeding in drug-dependent woman.** Breast-feeding can be considered in infants with in utero exposure to illicit substance if mothers are (a) enrolled in and are compliant in treatment programs, (b) abstinent from illicit drug use for 90 days before delivery, and (c) have negative toxicology screen at delivery. Methadone treatment alone is not a contraindication for breast-feeding. The effect of buprenorphine treatment on breast-feeding is not clear but appears to be safe.

III. **Donor breast milk (Human Milk Banking Association of North America [http://www.hmbana.org]).** The use of donor breast milk is both regional and *controversial.* Historically, donor breast milk was used for centuries; however, current practice tends toward limited use. In recent years, a concern regarding transmission of infections such as HIV, cytomegalovirus, and tuberculosis has led to questions regarding the safety of its use. If donor breast milk or milk banks are to be used, donor screening, heat treatment (pasteurization) of the milk, and parental counseling on these potential risks are recommended. *Unpasteurized donor breast milk is used in some Scandinavian countries with rigorous protocols and donor testing.*

    Pasteurization and refrigeration result in loss of milk components. However, other components such as human milk oligosaccharides (HMO); vitamins A, D, and E; and LCPUFAs are preserved. HMO and LCPUFAs are important in immune function. Donor milk is deficient in protein, minerals, and calories to meet long-term requirements of preterm infants for growth and development. A recent meta-analysis showed that formula feeds compared with donor milk are associated with increased weight gain and growth but also with increased risk of NEC (relative risk, 2.5; 95% CI, 1.2–5.1). Use of fortified donor milk versus formula is associated with slower weight gain. When compared with mother's own milk, donor breast milk may offer an advantage over formula in decreasing risks of infections, NEC, and length of stay. At our institution, we initiate enteral feedings with donor milk in infants <1000 g if no maternal milk is available and subsequently transition to formula. Prolonged donor milk feeds are associated with postnatal growth failure. Fortified donor milk feeds have also been attempted (see later).

IV. **Storage.** Breast milk can be stored frozen at –20°C for up to 6 months and refrigerated at 4°C for up to 24 hours.

V. **Breast milk fortifiers (supplements).** These are designed as a supplement to mother's milk for rapidly growing premature infants (Table 10–7). Use of human milk beyond the second and third weeks in preterm infants may provide insufficient amounts of protein, calcium, phosphorus, and possibly copper, zinc, and sodium. Clinical experience has shown that the addition of human milk fortifier to a preterm mother's milk resulted in nitrogen retention, increased blood urea levels, and increased somatic and linear growth related to increased protein and energy intake. There is no effect on serum alkaline phosphatase levels. Effect on bone mineral content beyond 1 year of age is not known. One study in LBW infants comparing unfortified breast milk versus fortified breast milk up to 4 months after discharge noted no differences in growth parameters at 1 year of age. Periodic monitoring of urine osmolality, serum blood urea nitrogen, creatinine, and calcium is required. Table 10–7 shows some of the fortifiers currently available in the United States.

A. **Indications.** Breast milk fortifiers are indicated for those premature infants who tolerate unfortified human milk at full feedings, usually at 2–4 weeks of age, up to the time of discharge or at a weight of 3600 g. Criteria for use include <34 weeks' gestation at birth and <1500 g at birth. In addition, breast milk fortifiers are indicated for fluid-restricted infants who require an increase in calories. Fortifiers can be added when 100 mL/kg/d of enteral feeding is reached, although practices may vary. Iron-enriched fortifiers are well tolerated and may decrease the need for late blood transfusions. Fortification of fresh breast milk is not associated with increased bacterial growth for up to 6 hours. The fortifiers available in the United States are shown on the next page.

1. **Enfamil human milk fortifier (EHMF)** (has been replaced by liquid fortifier, see later)

   a. **Composition.** The predominant source of energy is fat. The fat is 70% medium-chain triglyceride (MCT) and 30% soy with linoleic and linolenic acid providing 1 g/4 packets. Fats also reduce the osmolar load. The protein is 60% whey protein and 40% casein, which is similar to breast milk. Four packets provide 1.1 g of protein. The carbohydrate is corn syrup solids, mineral salts, and trace amounts of lactose and galactose. This fortifier comes in powder form.

   b. **Calories.** One packet of fortifier added to 50 mL of human milk provides an additional 2 cal/fl oz. Once the powder is added to the milk, the container should be capped and mixed well. It can be covered and stored under refrigeration (2–4°C) but should be used within 24 hours. It should be used within 4 hours after mixing at room temperature. Do not reuse if it is not refrigerated for >2 hours after mixing. Agitate before each use. *Do not microwave to heat.*

   c. **Hypercalcemia.** This has been reported in some ELBW (<1000 g) infants receiving fortified breast milk. For these infants, serum calcium must be monitored. Fortification of breast milk should start beyond 2 weeks' postnatal age at a ratio not exceeding 1 packet/25 mL of breast milk.

Table 10–7. COMPOSITION OF PRETERM HUMAN MILK[a] AND COMMERCIALLY AVAILABLE BREAST-MILK FORTIFIERS

Variable	Preterm Human Milk[a]	Enfamil HMF[b]	Enfamil HMF Acidified Liquid[d]	Similac HMF[c]
Volume	100 mL	4 packets/ 100 mL	1 vial (5 mL)/ 100 mL	4 packets/ 100 mL
Total calories	67	81		79 (24 cal/oz)
Osmolality (mOsm/ kg H_2O)	290	325	+36	385
Osmolarity	255			
Calories	67	81		79
Protein (g)	1.4	2.5	4	2.3
Fat (g)	3.9	4.9	6	4.1
Linoleic acid (mg)	369	140	730	359
Linolenic acid (mg)		17	60	
Carbohydrates (g)	6.6	<0.4	8.1	8.2
Minerals /100 mL				
Calcium (mg)	24.8	90	145	138
mEq	1.24			6.9
Chloride (mg)	55	13	89	90
mEq	1.6			2.5
Copper (mcg)	64.4	44	101	228
Iron (mg)	0.12	1.44	1.91	0.45
Magnesium (mg)	3.1	1	5.3	9.8
Phosphorus (mg)	12.8	50	80	77
Potassium (mg)	57	29	98	116
mEq	1.5			2.9
Sodium (mg)	24.8	16	57	38
mEq	1.1			1.7
Zinc (mg)	0.34	0.72	1.37	1.3
Iodine (mcg)	10.7		18.4	10.5
Manganese (mcg)	0.6	10	10.7	7.6
Selenium (mcg)	1.5		2.5	1.9
Vitamins/100 mL				
Vitamins A (IU)	389	950	1250	984
Vitamin B_1 (mcg)	20.8	150	200	247
Vitamin B_2 (mcg)	48.3	220	300	453
Vitamin B_6 (mcg)	14.8	115	151	219
Vitamin B_{12} (mcg)	0.04	0.18	0.68	0.67
Vitamin C (mg)		12	21	34
Vitamin D (IU)	2	150	210	118
Vitamin E (IU)	1.1	4.6	6.2	4.1
Vitamin K (mcg)	0.2	4.4	7.9	8.3
Folic acid (mcg)	3.3	25	35	25
Niacin (mcg)	150.3	3000	4000	3622
Pantothenic acid (mcg)	180.5	730	1190	1636
Biotin (mcg)	0.4	2.7	4	25
Choline (mg)	9.4			10
Inositol (mg)	14.7			18

[a]Represents mature preterm human milk.
[b]Enfamil HMF: Data provided per 4 packets.
[c]4 packets per 100 mL human milk provides 24 cal/oz.
[d]Based on EHMFAL + preterm milk to provide 100 cal.

2. **Enfamil human milk fortifier–acidified liquid**
   a. **Composition.** Whey protein hydrolysate, MCT oil, and vegetable oil (soy and high oleic sunflower oils). The fortifier is available as a *sterile* concentrated liquid solution with higher concentration of DHA and ARA.
   b. **Calories.** When mixed with human milk, it provides 4 g protein/100 cal, and its pH is 4.3–4.7. Each vial (5 mL) + 25 mL breast milk provides an additional 4 cal/fl oz. Monitor the volume of feeds. Use the fortified breast milk within 2 hours of mixing at room temperature or within 24 hours of mixing if stored at 2–4°C.
   c. **Use of >25 vials/d** can result in hypervitaminosis A and D.
3. **Similac human milk fortifier (SHMF)**
   a. **Composition.** The protein is from nonfat milk, whey protein concentrate. There is <2% soy lecithin. The carbohydrate is lactose and corn syrup solids. The fat is predominantly coconut oil (MCT).
   b. **Calories.** The fortifier provides 24 kcal/fl oz, when added in the ratio of 1 packet/25 mL of breast milk. Each packet (0.9 g) provides 3.5 calories, 0.25 g protein, 0.45 g carbohydrate, and 0.09 g fat. Each packet provides ~29.2 mg calcium and 16.8 mg phosphorous.
   c. **Use until infant reaches a weight of 3600 g** or as directed.
4. **Human milk fortifier.** Recently, a human milk fortifier has become commercially available (Prolacta + H^2MF) that is made from 100% pasteurized donor human breast milk. Concentrated up to 2–10 times, it is fortified with essential minerals and offers protein delivery up to 2.3–3.7 g/100 mL and an additional 4–10 cal/oz of fortified milk, respectively (www.prolacta.com). A recent trial suggested that preterm infants fed human milk fortified with donor human milk fortifier had lower rates of medical and surgical NEC compared with those fed either formula or human milk supplemented with bovine fortifier. Bovine-based human milk fortifiers are associated with metabolic acidosis, altered weight gain, and decreased bone mineral content.

VI. **Probiotics and milk.** Recent studies have shown a beneficial effect of supplementing milk with *Bifidobacter* and other probiotics in decreasing the risk of NEC, nosocomial infections, and mortality in VLBW infants. Beneficial effects have also been reported on decreasing intestinal permeability, improvements in growth and head circumference, and improved feeding tolerance. *Bifidobacter* is present in human milk. The optimal doses, organism, timing of supplementation, and long-term benefits, however, remain unclear.

Concerning **prebiotics and human milk**, oligosaccharides such as inulin, galactose, and fructose enhance the growth of beneficial intestinal microbiome such as *Bifidobacter* and potentially decrease risks of NEC and nosocomial infections. Formula supplemented with nonhuman milk oligosaccharides have been shown to improve enteral feed tolerance, but not to decrease intestinal permeability. Long-term benefits are not yet known.

VII. **Organic formulas.** Several organic milk formulas are available that are produced without the use of pesticides, antibiotics, or growth hormones. Organic soy formulas are also available. Concerns have been raised about the presence of high sugar content in some of these formulas and the risk for later childhood obesity and for injury to developing tooth enamel. The increased cost of organic formulas is considerable. There are currently no clinical trials comparing benefits, or lack of, for organic formulas to proprietary infant formulas.

VIII. **Feeding in short gut.** Short gut syndrome is a frequent complication after bowel resection in infants following NEC and other congenital malformations. The loss of the ileocecal valve, bacterial overgrowth, deconjugation of bile salts, cholestatic liver disease, and vitamin B_{12} and mineral deficiency can occur. Total parenteral nutrition (TPN) toxicity can be a complication due to excess lipids (phytosterols causing liver damage), excess amino acids, and manganese and copper toxicity (*controversial*).

Adequate zinc supplementation is needed to compensate for losses through stomas. Careful attention should also be placed on fluid and electrolyte balance. Refeeding through mucous fistulas, continuous feeds, pectin, elemental amino acid formulas, and initiating early enteral feedings postoperatively have all been tried in an attempt to decrease liver disease.

TOTAL PARENTERAL NUTRITION

TPN is the intravenous administration of all nutrients (fats, carbohydrates, proteins, vitamins, and minerals) necessary for metabolic requirements and growth. **Parenteral nutrition (PN)** is supplemental intravenous administration of nutrients. **Enteral nutrition (EN)** is oral or gavage feedings. The optimal amount of energy intake remains unclear, but no additional benefit in protein balance has been shown with energy intake beyond 70–90 kcal/kg/d. Protein accretion is improved with increasing protein intake at energy intakes of 30–50 kcal/kg/d.

I. **Intravenous routes used in PN**
   A. **Central PN.** Central PN is usually reserved for patients requiring long-term (>2 weeks) administration of most calories. Basically, this type of nutrition involves infusion of a hypertonic nutrient solution (15–30% dextrose, 5–6% amino acids) into a vessel with rapid flow through an indwelling catheter whose tip is in the vena cava just above or beyond the right atrium. Disadvantages include increased risk of infection and complications from placement. Two methods are commonly used for placement.
      1. **Percutaneous inserted central catheter (PICC).** Positioned in the antecubital, temporal, external jugular vein, or saphenous vein and is advanced into the superior or inferior vena cava. This technique avoids surgical placement and results in fewer complications (see Chapter 42).
      2. **Central catheter (Broviac).** Placed through a surgical cutdown in the internal or external jugular, subclavian vein, or femoral vein. The proximal portion of the catheter (which has a polyvinyl cuff to promote fibroblast proliferation for securing the catheter) is tunneled subcutaneously to exit some distance from the insertion site, usually the anterior chest. This protects the catheter from inadvertent dislodgement and reduces the risk of contamination by microorganisms. The anesthesia and surgery needed for placement of the catheter are disadvantages to this method.
      3. **Photoprotection of parenteral nutrition.** Helps decrease vitamin loss and oxidative damage to amino acids, decrease generation of hydrogen peroxides and free radicals, limit alterations in vasomotor tone via generation of lipid peroxides and decreased nitric oxide production, and improve tolerance to minimal EN. Vitamins, trace elements, and iron should *not* be added together in the parenteral solution to decrease the risks of lipid peroxidation. Increased lipid peroxidation products may adversely influence neurodevelopment.
   B. **Peripheral PN.** The use of a peripheral vein may also be used in the neonatal intensive care unit and is usually associated with fewer complications. The concentration of the amino acids and the dextrose solution limit the amount of solution that can be infused. The maximum concentration of dextrose that can be administered is 12.5%; the maximum concentration of amino acids is 3.5%.
   C. **Umbilical catheters.** PN can be given through an **umbilical artery catheter** but it is not preferred and should be used with caution. Maximum dextrose in UAC is 15%. PN can be given via **umbilical venous catheter** after ensuring the catheter is central in the right atrium and not in the liver. Hyperosmolar infusion in the hepatic vessels is associated with portal venous thrombosis and portal hypertension.

II. **Indications.** PN is used as a supplement to enteral feedings or as a complete substitution (TPN) when adequate nourishment cannot be achieved by the enteral route. Common indications in neonates include congenital malformation of the gastrointestinal tract, gastroschisis, meconium ileus, short bowel syndrome, NEC, paralytic ileus, respiratory distress syndrome, extreme prematurity, sepsis, and malabsorption. PN, particularly amino acids, should be started on the first day of life, and as soon as possible in sick infants. In preterm ELBW and VLBW infants, 2.5 g/kg/d of amino acids should be started on day 1 and is associated with better linear growth and neurodevelopmental outcomes. Term infants who are likely to have delayed initiation of enteral nutrition should be started on 1.5 gm/kg/d of proteins.

III. **Caloric concentration.** Caloric densities of various energy sources are as follows:
   A. **Dextrose (anhydrous).** 3.4 kcal/g.
   B. **Protein.** 4 kcal/g.
   C. **Fat.** 9 kcal/g.

IV. **Composition of PN solutions**
   A. **Carbohydrates**
      1. **The only commercially available carbohydrate source is dextrose (glucose).** A solution of 5.0–12.5 g/dL is used in peripheral PN and up to 25 g/dL in central PN. Dextrose concentrations should be calculated as milligrams per kilograms per minute. Dextrose is provided to maintain blood sugar between 45 mg/dL and 125 mg/dL. Providing glucose alone in the absence of proteins results in negative nitrogen balance that can be reversed by providing 1.1–2.5 g/kg/d of protein with energy intake as low as 30 kcal/kg/d. Provide 25–40 kcal nonprotein energy/g of protein to optimize protein deposition (see Proteins later).
      2. **To allow for an appropriate response of endogenous insulin and to prevent the development of osmotic diuresis secondary to glucosuria, neonates should not routinely be started on >6–8 mg/kg/min of dextrose.** Endogenous gluconeogenesis in preterm ELBW infants may be independent of glucose infusion or of concentrations of glucose or insulin. Peripheral uptake and utilization of glucose is improved with simultaneous amino acid infusion. Infusion rates can be increased by 0.5–1 mg/kg/min each day as tolerated up to 10–12 mg/kg/min to achieve adequate caloric intake in the presence of stable blood sugar levels. This also allows adequate glucose for protein deposition. Endogenous glucose requirements decrease with increasing gestational age. In the presence of hyperglycemia, glucose infusion rate should not be reduced below 4 mg/kg/min. Insulin may be required to maintain adequate blood glucose levels, although its routine use is not recommended (see earlier). See Chapter 9 for calculating the amount of glucose (mg/kg/min) an infant is receiving.
   B. **Proteins.** Inadequate protein intake may result in failure to thrive, hypoalbuminemia, and edema. Excessive protein can cause hyperammonemia, serum amino acid imbalance, metabolic acidosis, and cholestatic jaundice. Early addition of amino acids to PN may also stimulate endogenous insulin secretion. Postnatal protein loss is inversely proportional to gestational age. LBW infants lose 1% of endogenous protein daily unless supplemented. Glutathione, an antioxidant, concentrations rise with early amino acid administration.
      1. **Crystalline amino acid solutions.** These are available as nitrogen sources. The standard solutions originally designed for adults are not ideal because they contain high concentrations of amino acids (eg, glycine, methionine, and phenylalanine) that are potentially neurotoxic in premature infants. Pediatric crystalline amino acid solutions (eg, TrophAmine, Aminosyn PF) are available that contain less of those potentially neurotoxic amino acids as well as additional tyrosine, cystine, and taurine. These pediatric solutions also have a lower pH to allow for the addition of sufficient quantities of calcium (2 mEq/dL) and phosphorus (1–2 mg/dL) to meet daily requirements. Conditionally essential amino acids are arginine, tyrosine, cysteine, glutamine, glycine and proline.
      2. **Amino acids.** Early protein intake of 3 g/kg/d within the first 24 hours is safely tolerated in VLBW infants and improves nitrogen balance because of an

increased ability to synthesize protein (see earlier). Early amino acid supplementation may help decrease hyperglycemia and hyperkalemia in the ELBW infants by promoting insulin secretion. In term infants, the starting rate can be 1.5 g, with increases of 1 g/kg/d. To avoid hyperammonemia and acidosis, total proteins should not exceed 4 g/kg/d in preterm infants. At most institutions, amino acid solutions are prepared in 1%, 2%, and 3% concentrations.

3. **Cysteine hydrochloride.** Often added to TPN solutions because cysteine is unstable over time and is omitted from amino acid solutions. The premature infant lacks the ability to convert methionine to cysteine; thus it is conditionally essential. Cysteine is also converted to cystine and to glutathione, an antioxidant. Addition of cysteine into TPN lowers the pH of the solution, resulting in acidosis. Additional acetate may be required. It may also decrease hepatic cholestasis. The recommended dose is 40 mg of cysteine per gram of protein (72–85 mg/kg/d); however, cysteine is not considered essential in enterally fed infants.

4. **Glutamine.** Glutamine has been identified as a key amino acid, as respiratory fuel for rapidly proliferating cells like enterocytes and lymphocytes, in acid-base balance, and as a nucleotide precursor. Glutamine may play a role in maintaining gut integrity and may decrease the incidence of sepsis. It also attenuates gut atrophy in fasting states. Vernix is a rich source of glutamine. Glutamine supplementation does not have significant effect on mortality or neonatal morbidities including invasive infection, NEC, time to achieve full enteral nutrition, or duration of hospital stay. Glutamine may affect somatic growth and decrease incidence of atopic dermatitis.

C. **Fats.** Fats are essential for normal body growth and development, in cell structure and function, and in retinal and brain development. Because of their high caloric density, intravenous fat solutions provide a significant portion of daily caloric needs. Most lipid solutions are derived from soybean, but newer combination oils with olive oil, MCT, and fish oil are now available (eg, Intralipid, Liposyn II, Nutrilipid, Soyacal, Omegavan, Lipoplus, and SMO Flipid). Omegavan is exclusively fish oil and rich in omega-3 fatty acids. Most intravenous fat solutions are isotonic (270–300 mOsm/L), and therefore they are not likely to increase the risk of infiltration of peripheral lines. Lipid emulsions contain linoleic and α-linolenic acid; the latter can be converted into DHA. DHA is accumulated in the third trimester, and preterm infants have limited capacity to convert α-linolenic acid to DHA. Delay in initiating lipids can result in biochemical and clinical evidence of essential fatty acid deficiency within 3 days and increase susceptibility to oxidant injury. Intravenous lipids at 0.25g/kg/d are needed to prevent essential fatty acid deficiency. When administering fat solutions to neonates with unconjugated hyperbilirubinemia, caution may be needed because of the competitive binding between bilirubin and nonesterified fatty acids on albumin, which may increase significantly with high infusion rates. Increased risks of coagulase-negative staphylococci, release of thromboxanes and prostaglandins, and increased pulmonary vascular resistance have also been noted.

1. **Concentrations.** Lipid emulsions are usually supplied either as 10 or 20% solutions providing 10 or 20 g of triglyceride, respectively. Starting lipids at 0.5–1 g/kg/d within 24–30 hours of birth is safe. Advance by 0.5–1.0 g/kg/d as tolerated up to 3.0 g/kg/d. The infusion is given continuously over 20–24 hours, and the rate should not exceed 0.12–0.15 g/kg/h. Use of 20% lipid emulsion is associated with decreased levels of cholesterol, triglycerides, and phospholipids because of its lower phospholipids-to-triglycerides ratio and lower liposomal contents than 10% lipid emulsions. Lipids should be administered separately from proteins as amino acid solutions are acidic to maintain calcium and phosphorous solubility. Adding lipids to protein solutions increases the pH and precipitates calcium/phosphorus.

2. **Complications.** Fat intolerance (hyperlipidemia) may be seen. Periodic determination of blood triglyceride levels is recommended. Levels should be <150 mg/dL when the infant is jaundiced and <200 mg/dL otherwise. The infusion of fats should be decreased or stopped when these levels are exceeded. Advance cautiously in infants with respiratory distress due to risk of hypoxemia and increased pulmonary vascular resistance.

3. **Carnitine supplementation** (*controversial*). Carnitine synthesis and storage are not well developed in infants <34 weeks' gestation. Carnitine is a carrier molecule necessary for oxidation of long-chain fatty acids. An exogenous source of carnitine is available from human milk and infant formulas; however, studies have shown that preterm infants on TPN become deficient in 6–10 days. Carnitine can be added to TPN solutions at a safe initial dose of 10 mg/kg/d. Carnitine-deficient infants may experience hypotonia, nonketotic hypoglycemia, cardiomyopathy, encephalopathy, and recurrent infections.

D. **Vitamins.** Vitamins are added to intravenous solutions in the form of a pediatric multivitamin suspension (MVI Pediatric) based on recommendations by the Nutritional Advisory Committee of the American Academy of Pediatrics. The dose of parenteral vitamins for preterm infants should be 2 mL/kg of the 5-mL reconstituted MVI Pediatric sterile lyophilized powder. Vitamin A delivery is hampered by binding to plastic tubing.

E. **Trace elements.** Trace elements are added to the solution based on weight and total volume: 0.5 mL/kg/wk for infants on short-term TPN and 0.5 mL/kg/d for those on long-term TPN. Increased amounts of zinc (1–2 mg/d) are often given to help promote healing in patients who require gastrointestinal surgery. At many institutions, a prepared solution is available. For recommended doses of trace elements, see Table 10–8.

F. **Electrolytes.** Electrolytes can be added according to specific needs, but for LBW infants, requirements are usually satisfied by standard amino acid solution formulations that contain electrolytes (Table 10–9).

G. **Heparin.** Heparin should be added to PN (0.5–1 U/mL TPN) to maintain catheter patency. In addition, there is a decreased risk for phlebitis and an increase in lipid clearance as a result of release of lipoprotein lipase.

V. **Monitoring of PN.** Hyperalimentation can cause many alterations in biochemical function. Thus compulsive anthropometric and laboratory monitoring is essential for all patients. Recommendations are given in Table 10–10.

Table 10–8. **RECOMMENDATIONS FOR TRACE ELEMENT SUPPLEMENTATION IN TOTAL PARENTERAL NUTRITION SOLUTIONS FOR NEONATES**

Element (mcg/kg/d)	Full Term	Premature
Zinc	250	400
Copper	20	20
Chromium[a]	0.2	0.2
Manganese[a]	1	1
Fluoride	500[b]	—
Iodine	1	1
Molybdenum[a]	0.25	0.25
Selenium	2.0	2.0

TPN, total parenteral nutrition.
[a]For TPN >4 weeks.
[b]Not well defined in the premature infant. Indicated only in prolonged TPN therapy (eg, >3 months).

Table 10–9. **COMPOSITION OF AMINO ACID SOLUTIONS FOR LOW BIRTHWEIGHT INFANTS (STANDARD FORMULATION)**

Electrolytes (mEq/L)	Amino Acid Concentration					
	1.0%		2.0%		3.0%	
	A	T	A	T	A	T
Na^+	20	20	20	20	20	20
Cl^-	20	20	20	20	20	20
K^+	15	15	15	15	15	15
Mg^{2+}	11	11	11	11	11	11
Ca^{2+}	15	15	15	15	15	15
Acetate	7.6	9.3	15.3	18.6	22.8	27.9
Phosphorus (mmol/L)	10	10	10	10	10	10

A, Aminosyn PF; T, TrophAmine.

Table 10–10. **SUGGESTED MONITORING SCHEDULE FOR NEONATES RECEIVING PARENTERAL NUTRITION**

Measurement	Baseline Study	Frequency of Measurement
Anthropometric		
Weight	Yes	Daily
Length	Yes	Weekly
Head circumference	Yes	Weekly
Intake and output	Daily	Daily
Metabolic		
Glucose	Yes	2–3 times per day initially; then as needed
Calcium, phosphorus, and magnesium	Yes	2–3 times per week initially; then every 1–2 weeks
Electrolytes (Na, Cl, K, CO_2)	Yes	Daily initially, then 2–3 times per week. More frequently in ELBW infants <1000 g
Hematocrit	Yes	Every other day for 1 week; then weekly
BUN and creatinine	Yes	2–3 per week; then every 1–2 weeks
Bilirubin	Yes	Weekly
Ammonia	Yes	Weekly if using high protein
Total protein and albumin	Yes	Every 2–3 weeks
AST/ALT	Yes	Every 2–3 weeks
Triglycerides	Yes	1–2 weekly
Vitamins and trace minerals		As indicated
Urine		
Specific gravity and glucose	Yes	1–3 times per day initially; then as needed (*controversial*)

ALT, alanine aminotransferase; AST, aspartate aminotransferase; BUN, blood urea nitrogen; ELBW, extremely low birthweight; VLBW, very low birthweight.

VI. **Complications of PN.** Most complications of PN are associated with the use of central hyperalimentation and primarily involve infections and catheter-related problems. Metabolic difficulties can occur with both central and peripheral TPN. The major complication of peripheral hyperalimentation is accidental infiltration of the solution, which causes sloughing of the skin.

A. **Infection.** Sepsis can occur in infants receiving central hyperalimentation. The most common organisms include coagulase-positive and coagulase-negative *Staphylococcus, Streptococcus viridans, Escherichia coli, Pseudomonas* spp, *Klebsiella* spp, and *Candida albicans.* Contamination of the central catheter can occur as a result of infection at the insertion site or use of the catheter for blood sampling or administration of blood. It is best not to open the catheter.

B. **Catheter-associated problems.** Complications associated with placement of central catheters (specifically in the subclavian vein) occur in ~4–9% of patients. Complications include pneumothorax, pneumomediastinum, hemorrhage, and chylothorax (caused by injury to the thoracic duct). Thrombosis of the vein adjacent to the catheter tip, resulting in "superior vena cava syndrome" (edema of the face, neck, and eyes), may be seen. Pulmonary embolism may occur secondary to thrombosis. Malpositioned catheters may result in collection of fluid in the pleural cavity, causing hydrothorax, or the pericardial space, causing tamponade.

C. **Metabolic complications**

1. **Hyperglycemia.** Results from excessive intake or change in metabolic rate, such as infection or glucocorticoid administration. Routine insulin infusion to prevent hyperglycemia is not recommended and is associated with increased risks of retinopathy of prematurity, mortality and hypoglycemia.

2. **Hypoglycemia.** Results from sudden cessation of infusion (secondary to intravenous infiltration).

3. **Azotemia.** Results from excessive protein (nitrogen) uptake; however, aggressive protein intake is safe (see earlier).

4. **Hyperammonemia.** All currently available amino acid mixtures contain adequate arginine (>0.05 mmol/kg/d). Therefore, if there is an increase in blood ammonia, symptomatic hyperammonemia does not occur.

5. **Abnormal serum and tissue amino acid pattern.**

6. **Mild metabolic acidosis.**

7. **Cholestatic liver disease.** With prolonged administration of intravenous dextrose and protein and absence of enteral feeding, cholestasis usually occurs. The incidence ranges from as high as 80% in VLBW infants receiving TPN for >30 days (with no enteral feeding) to ≤15% in neonates weighing >1500 g receiving TPN for >14 days. Monitoring for abnormalities in liver function and the development of direct hyperbilirubinemia is important in long-term TPN. IUGR infants are at high risk of developing cholestasis. Prolonged TPN, particularly lipid use, is associated with cholestasis. Fish oil–based lipid emulsions (Omegavan) have been used in prevention and treatment of TPN-induced cholestasis. At our institution, we cycle lipids at 1 g/kg/d 2 times a week when TPN cholestasis is anticipated, such as in patients with short gut syndromes. Interestingly, fish oil–based lipid emulsions may decrease the risk of retinopathy of prematurity. See Chapters 57 and 99.

   a. **Bacterial infection.** May play a significant role in the occurrence of cholestatic liver disease.

   b. **Amino acid mixtures.** Use of amino acid mixtures designed to maintain normal plasma amino acid patterns and early starting (as soon as possible) of enteral feedings in small amounts may help alleviate this problem.

   c. **TPN may be cycled over 10–18 hours** as opposed to a continuous 24-hour infusion. This facilitates a short period of decreased circulating insulin levels, which in turn facilitates mobilization of fat and glycogen stores, decreasing the risk of fatty infiltration of the liver and hepatic dysfunction.

This practice is reserved for infants who are stable on TPN and who are expected to remain in need of long-term TPN.

d. **Trace elements copper and manganese.** These should be withheld in the presence of hepatic dysfunction.

8. **Complications of fat administration.** Infusion of fat emulsion is associated with several metabolic disturbances, hyperlipidemia, platelet dysfunction, acute allergic reactions, deposition of pigment in the liver, and lipid deposition in the blood vessels of the lung. Most metabolic problems apparently occur with rapid rates of infusion and are not seen at infusion rates of <0.12 g/kg/h.

Exposure of lipids to light, especially phototherapy, may cause increased production of toxic hydroperoxides. Addition of multivitamins and use of protective/dark delivery tubings decrease peroxide formation and limit vitamins loss. Steroids cause elevated triglyceride levels. In sepsis, there is decreased peripheral use of lipids. Free fatty acids produced from lipid breakdown compete with bilirubin for binding with albumin, resulting in elevated free bilirubin. Lipid infusion should not exceed 0.5–1 g/kg/d with plasma bilirubin >8–10 mg/dL and albumin levels 2.5–3.0 g/dL. Additional complications include thrombocytopenia, increased risk of sepsis, alteration in pulmonary functions, and hypoxemia.

9. **Deficiency of essential fatty acids (EFAs).** Associated with decreased platelet aggregation (thromboxane A_2 deficiency), poor weight gain, scaling rash, sparse hair growth, and thrombocytopenia. EFA deficiency can occur within 72 hours in preterm infants if exogenous fatty acids are not supplemented. Use of only safflower oil to provide lipid emulsions may result in deficiency omega-3 LCPUFAs. EFAs are essential to the developing eyes and brain of the human neonate.

10. **Mineral deficiency.** Most minerals are transferred to the fetus during the last trimester of pregnancy. The following problems may occur.
    a. **Osteopenia, rickets, and pathologic fractures.** See Chapter 116.
    b. **Zinc deficiency.** Occurs if zinc is not added to TPN after 4 weeks. Cysteine and histidine in TPN solution increases urinary losses. Infants with this deficiency can have poor growth, diarrhea, alopecia, increased susceptibility to infection, and skin desquamation surrounding the mouth and anus (acrodermatitis enteropathica). Zinc losses are increased in patients with an ileostomy or colostomy.
    c. **Copper deficiency.** Infants with copper deficiency have osteoporosis, hemolytic anemia, neutropenia, and depigmentation of the skin.
    d. **Manganese, copper, selenium, molybdenum, and iodine deficiency.** May occur if not supplemented after 4 weeks.

CALORIC CALCULATIONS

An infant should receive 100–120 kcal/kg/d for growth. (Infants require fewer calories [70–90 cal/kg/d] if receiving TPN only.) Some hypermetabolic infants may require >120 kcal/kg/d. For maintenance of a positive nitrogen balance, oral intake of 70–90 nonprotein kcal/kg/d is necessary. Equations for calculating the caloric intake for oral formula and TPN follow (Table 10–11).

I. **Infant formulas.** Most standard infant formulas are 20 cal/oz and contain 0.67 kcal/mL. Specific caloric concentrations of formulas are given in Table 10–5. To calculate total daily calories, use the following equation:

$$\text{kcal/kg/d} = \frac{\text{Total mL of formula} \times \text{kcal/mL}}{\text{Wt (kg)}}$$

Table 10–11. TOTAL PARENTERAL NUTRITION CALCULATIONS

Amino acids:	$\% \text{ Amino acids} = \dfrac{\text{Wt(kg)} \times (\text{g/kg/d}) \times 100}{\text{Vol in 24 h}}$
Dextrose: glucose utilization rate (mg/kg/min):	$\dfrac{\text{Rate(mL/h)} \times \% \text{ Dextrose}}{\text{Wt(kg)} \times 6}$
Lipids:	$\text{Rate(mL/h)}: \dfrac{\text{g/kg/d} \times 5 \times \text{Wt(kg)}}{24}$
Nonprotein calories/kg/d:	$(\text{mL lipid/24 h} \times 2 \text{ cal/mL}^a) + \dfrac{\text{mL TPN/24 h} \times \% \text{Dextrose} \times 0.034}{\text{kg}}$

TPN, total parenteral nutrition.
^{a}For 20% lipids only.

II. **Carbohydrates.** If only dextrose infusion is given, the total daily caloric intake is calculated as follows. (For caloric concentration of common solutions, see Table 10–12.)

$$kcal/kg/d = \frac{\text{mL of solution/h} \times 24 \text{ h} \times \text{kcal in solution}}{\text{Wt (kg)}}$$

III. **Proteins.** Use the prior formula given for carbohydrates and the caloric concentrations given in Table 10–12.

IV. **Fat emulsions.** A 10% fat emulsion (Intralipid) contains 1.1 kcal/mL; a 20% emulsion, 2 kcal/mL. Use the following formula to calculate daily caloric intake supplied by Intralipid 20%.

$$kcal/kg/d = \frac{\text{Total mL/d of solution} \times 2 \text{ kcal/mL}}{\text{Wt (kg)}}$$

Table 10–12. CALORIC CONCENTRATIONS OF VARIOUS PARENTERAL SOLUTIONS

Dextrose Solutions (anhydrous)	% Concentration	Caloric Concentration (kcal/mL)
D_5	5	0.17
$D_{7.5}$	7.5	0.255
D_{10}	10	0.34
$D_{12.5}$	12.5	0.425
D_{15}	15	0.51
D_{20}	20	0.68
D_{25}	25	0.85
Protein Solutions (g/d)		
0.5	0.5	0.02
1.0	1	0.04
1.5	1.5	0.06
2.0	2.0	0.08
2.5	2.5	0.10
3.0	3.0	0.12

A 0.5% solution, if given 100 mL/d = 0.5 g of protein/d.

MATERNAL NUTRITIONAL STATUS AND FETAL AND POSTNATAL GROWTH

Maternal nutritional status may be an important role in fetal and postnatal growth. Maternal body-mass index (BMI) and prepregnancy weight, as well as excessive weight gain during pregnancy, increase the risk of fetal adiposity and subsequent obesity. Conversely, increased weight loss in prepregnancy in healthy nonoverweight mothers (normal BMI) increases the risk of small for gestational age infants.

Maternal diet supplemented with LCPUFA, particularly omega-3 fatty acids, may improve birthweight, length, and length of gestation. Antenatal maternal micronutrient (eg, iron, folic acid) supplementation may influence fetal growth, fetal weight, and length of gestation and decrease infant morbidity. Cord blood vitamin D status is inversely correlated with respiratory infections and childhood wheezing.

Rapid weight gain in neonates starting as early as 6 weeks of age may increase risk of obesity. Accelerated weight gain even in IUGR infants increases the risks of "adiposity rebound" and risk of subsequent cardiovascular and metabolic diseases.

Selected References

Agostoni C, Buonocore G, Carnielli VP, et al. Enteral nutrient supply for preterm infants: commentary from the European Society for Pediatric Gastroenterology, Hepatology, and Nutrition Committee on Nutrition. *J Pediatr Gastroenterol Nutr.* 2010;50: 85–91.

Bombell S, Mcguire W. Early trophic feeding for very low birth weight infants. *Cochrane Database Syst Rev.* 2009;CD000504.

Chacko SK, Ordonez J, Sauer PJ, Sunehag AL. Gluconeogenesis is not regulated by either glucose or insulin in extremely low birth weight infants receiving total parenteral nutrition. *J Pediatr.* 2011;158:891–896.

Deshpande G, Rao S, Patole S, Bulsara M. Updated meta-analysis of probiotics for preventing necrotizing enterocolitis in preterm neonates. *Pediatrics.* 2010;125:921–930.

Deshpande G, Simmer K. Lipids for parenteral nutrition in neonates. *Curr Opin Clin Nutr Metabol Care.* 2011;14:145–150.

Dyer JS, Rosenfeld CR. Metabolic imprinting by prenatal, perinatal and postnatal overnutrition: a review. *Semin Reprod Med.* 2011;29:266–276.

Ehrenkranz RA, Das A, Wrage LA, et al. Early nutrition mediates the influence of severity of illness in extremely low birth weight infants. *Pediatr Res.* 2011;69:522–529.

Grand A, Jalabert A, Mercier G, et al. Influence of vitamins, trace elements, and iron on lipid peroxidation reactions in all-in-one admixtures for neonatal parenteral nutrition. *JPEN J Parenter Enteral Nutr.* 2011;35:505–510.

Groh-Wargo S, Sapsford A. Enteral nutrition support of the preterm infant in the neonatal intensive care unit. *Nutr Clin Pract.* 2009;24:363–376.

Hay WW, Thureen P. Protein for preterm infants: how much is needed? How much is enough? How much is too much? *Pediatr Neonatol.* 2010;51:198–207.

Jansson LM. AMB clinical protocol # 21: Guidelines for breast feeding and the drug dependent woman. *Breastfeed Med.* 2009;4:225–228.

Kaempf JW, Kaempf AJ, Wu Y, Stawarz M, Niemeyer J, Grunkemeier G. Hyperglycemia, insulin and slower growth velocity may increase the risk of retinopathy of prematurity. *J Perinatol.* 2011;31:251–257.

Morgan J, Young L, McGuire W. Slow advancement of enteral feed volumes to prevent necrotising enterocolitis in very low birth weight infants. *Cochrane Database Syst Rev.* 2011;CD001241.

Moyer-Mileur LJ. Anthropometric and laboratory assessment of very low birth weight infants: the most helpful measurements and why. *Semin Perinatol.* 2007;31:96–103.

Rao R, Georgieff MK. Iron therapy for preterm infants. *Clin Perinatol.* 2009;36:27–42.

Schanler RJ. Outcomes of human milk-fed premature infants. *Semin Perinatol.* 2010;35:29–33.

Sinclair JC, Bottino M, Cowett RM. Interventions for prevention of neonatal hyperglycemia in very low birth weight infants. *Cochrane Database Syst Rev.* 2011;CD007615.

Sullivan S, Schanler RJ, Kim JH, et al. An exclusively human milk-based diet is associated with a lower rate of necrotizing enterocolitis than a diet of human milk and bovine based products. *J Peds.* 2010:156;562–567.

Tsang RC, Uauy R, Koletzko B, Zlotkin SH, eds. *Nutrition of the Preterm Infant: Scientific Basis and Practical Guidelines.* Cincinnati, OH: Digital Education Publishing; 2005.

Vlaardingerbroek H, van Goudoever JB, van den Akker CH. Initial nutritional management of the preterm infant. *Early Hum Dev.* 2009:85;691–195.

Wessel JJ, Kocoshis SA. Nutritional management of short bowel syndrome. *Semin Perinatol.* 2007;31:104–111.

Wong S, Ordean A, Kahan M, et al. Substance use in pregnancy. *J Obstet Gynaecol Can.* 2011;33:367–384.

11 Imaging Studies

COMMON RADIOLOGIC TECHNIQUES

I. **Radiographic examinations.** The need for radiographs must always be weighed against the risks of exposure of the neonate to radiation (eg, 3–5 mrem per chest radiographic view). The infant's gonads should be shielded as much as possible, and any person holding the infant during the x-ray procedure should also wear a protective shield. For the usual vertically oriented radiographic exposure, personnel need to be only 1 ft outside the zone of exposure.

A. Chest radiographs

1. **Anteroposterior (AP) view.** The single best view for identification of heart or lung disease, verification of endotracheal tube and other line positions, and identification of air leak complications of mechanical ventilation, such as pneumothorax.

2. **Cross-table lateral view.** Of limited diagnostic value except to determine whether a pleural chest tube is positioned anteriorly (best for drainage of a pneumothorax) or posteriorly (best for drainage of a pleural fluid collection).

3. **Lateral decubitus view.** Best at evaluating for a small pneumothorax or a small pleural fluid collection, as either can be difficult to identify on the AP view. For example, if a pneumothorax is suspected, a contralateral decubitus view of the chest should be obtained. An air collection between lung and chest wall will be visible on the side on which the pneumothorax is present. By contrast, for pleural fluid identification, the same side should be placed down (ipsilateral decubitus). The lateral decubitus view may not be safely obtainable in unstable infants.

4. **Upright view.** Rarely used in the neonatal intensive care unit (NICU), but can identify abdominal perforation by showing free air under the diaphragm.

B. Abdominal radiographs

1. **AP view.** The single best view for diagnosing abdominal disorders such as intestinal obstruction or mass lesions and checking placement of support lines such as umbilical arterial and venous catheters and intestinal tubes.

2. **Cross-table lateral view.** Helps diagnose abdominal perforation, but the left lateral decubitus view is better for this purpose. Abdominal perforations may be missed on the AP and cross-table lateral views if the amount of intraperitoneal air is limited or if the segment of perforated bowel contains only fluid.

3. **Left lateral decubitus view.** (With the infant placed left side down.) Best for diagnosis of intestinal perforation. Free intra-abdominal air resulting from bowel perforation will be visible as an air collection between the liver and right lateral abdominal wall.

C. **Babygram.** A radiograph that includes the whole body or just the chest and abdomen (thoracoabdominal babygram) on a single image. It is most commonly ordered for line placement.

D. **Barium contrast studies (barium swallow or barium enema).** Barium sulfate, an inert compound, is not absorbed from the gastrointestinal (GI) tract and results in little or no fluid shift.

1. **Indications.** The use of barium as a contrast agent is recommended for the following:

a. **GI tract imaging.** Barium enema is used to rule out lower intestinal tract obstruction from a variety of causes.

133

b. **Suspected H-type tracheoesophageal fistula (TEF) without esophageal atresia (type E).** Most esophageal atresias can be diagnosed by inserting a radiopaque nasogastric tube; the tube curls up in the blind-ending proximal esophageal pouch. If additional confirmation is required, air can be injected under fluoroscopy to distend the pouch. Barium or other contrast agent injection is rarely required. However, evaluation for the rare H-type TEF requires contrast injection, such as barium, into the esophagus.

c. **Suspected esophageal perforation.** Barium swallow is used only if previous studies using low-osmolality water-soluble contrast agents were negative.

d. **Suspected gastroesophageal reflux (GER).** The pH probe examination and the reflux nuclear scan more reliably identify and quantitate GER than does the upper GI (UGI) series.

2. **Contraindications.** Barium contrast studies are not recommended in infants with suspected abdominal perforation or if the destination of the administered contrast is unknown because barium is irritating to the peritoneum and can result in "barium peritonitis."

E. **High-osmolality water-soluble (HOWS) contrast studies.** Formerly widely employed in imaging, HOWS contrast agents have been replaced by low-osmolality contrast agents (LOWS).

F. **Low-osmolality water-soluble (LOWS) contrast agents.** These agents have many advantages over barium and have replaced high-osmolality contrast agents in neonatal imaging.

1. **Advantages**
   a. These agents do not cause fluid shifts.
   b. If bowel perforation is present, these substances are nontoxic to the peritoneal cavity. In addition, they do not damage the bowel mucosa.
   c. If aspirated, there is limited irritation (if any) to the lungs.
   d. They have very limited absorption from the normal intestinal tract and thus maintain good opacification throughout the intestinal tract on delayed imaging.

2. **Disadvantages.** None other than a higher cost than barium.

3. **Indications**
   a. Suspected H-type TEF.
   b. Suspected esophageal perforation.
   c. Evaluation of the bowel if perforation is suspected.
   d. Unexplained pneumoperitoneum.
   e. Evaluation of "gasless abdomen" in a neonate >12 hours of age.

G. **Radionuclide studies.** Radionuclide studies provide more physiologic than anatomic information and usually involve a lower radiation dose to the patient compared with radiographic examinations.

1. **Reflux scintiscan.** Used for documenting and quantitating gastroesophageal reflux and is comparable to the pH probe examination and superior to the upper GI series. Technetium-99m–labeled pertechnetate in a water-based solution is instilled into the stomach. The patient is then scanned in the supine position for 1–2 hours with a gamma camera.

2. **Radionuclide cystogram.** Used for documenting and quantitating vesicoureteral reflux. Advantages over the radiographic voiding cystourethrogram (VCUG) is a much lower radiation dose (by 50–100 times) and a longer monitoring period (1–2 hours). Disadvantages include much poorer anatomic detail; bladder diverticula, posterior urethral valves, or mild reflux cannot be reliably identified. This technique should not be the initial examination for evaluation of the lower urinary tract, especially in boys.

3. **Radionuclide bone scan.** Used for evaluation of possible osteomyelitis. This procedure involves a 3-phase study (blood flow, blood pool, and bone uptake) after intravenous injection of technetium-99m–labeled methylene diphosphonate.
   a. **Advantages.** Sensitivity to bony changes earlier than with the radiograph.

b. **Disadvantages.** Several. A bone scan may not identify the acute phase of osteo-myelitis (ie, the first 24–48 hours), and it requires absence of patient motion, gives poorer anatomic detail than radiographs, and has resultant areas of positive uptake ("hot spots") that are nonspecific.

4. **HIDA (hepatobiliary) scan.** Used in certain types of neonatal jaundice to assist in differentiating biliary atresia (surgical disorder) from neonatal hepatitis (medical disorder).

II. **Ultrasonography**

A. **Ultrasonography of the brain.** Performed primarily to rule out intraventricular hemorrhage, ischemic change (periventricular leukomalacia [PVL]), hydrocephalus, and developmental anomalies. It can be performed in any NICU with a portable ultrasound unit. No special preparation is needed. However, open anterior and posterior fontanelles must be present, and no intravenous catheters should be placed in the scalp. The **AAP recommends that routine cranial ultrasound be performed** on all infants <30 weeks' gestation once between 7 and 14 days of age and be repeated between 36 and 40 weeks postmenstrual age. The classification of intraventricular hemorrhage (IVH) based on ultrasonographic findings is demonstrated in Figures 11–1 through 11–4. Figure 11–5 shows a posterior fossa hemorrhage, and Figure 11–6 demonstrates ischemic changes of PVL. Grading of IVH in the neonate by sonography is as follows (based on Papile, 1978):

1. **Grade I.** Subependymal, germinal matrix hemorrhage.
2. **Grade II.** Intraventricular extension without ventricular dilatation.
3. **Grade III.** Intraventricular extension with ventricular dilatation.
4. **Grade IV.** Intraventricular and intraparenchymal hemorrhage.

B. **Abdominal ultrasonography.** Useful in the evaluation of abdominal distention, gall bladder disease, biliary obstruction, intraperitoneal fluid, abdominal masses, abscesses, and possible causes of renal failure. Abdominal sonography can be performed portably. The addition of duplex and color Doppler evaluation of regional vessels is a supplementary procedure that can identify portal hypertension and vascular occlusion resulting from thrombosis.

C. **Power Doppler sonography.** Better demonstrates amplitude of blood flow compared with color Doppler but does not define direction of blood flow and is very motion sensitive.

III. **Computed tomographic (CT) scanning**

A. **CT scanning of the head.** More complicated than ultrasonography because the patient must be moved to the CT unit and may require sedation. However, as CT scanning times progressively decrease due to technical improvements, the need for sedation is decreasing. CT scanning provides more global information than ultrasonography of the head, particularly at the periphery of the brain.

B. **This technique can be used to diagnose intraventricular, subdural, or subarachnoid bleeding and cerebral edema or infarction.** To diagnose cerebral infarction, infusion of contrast medium is necessary. If contrast is used, blood urea nitrogen and creatinine levels must be obtained before the CT test to rule out renal impairment, which may be a contraindication to the use of intravenous contrast media. An intravenous catheter must be placed, preferably not in the head.

C. **Imaging for the encephalopathic term infant.** Noncontrast CT should be done in an encephalopathic term infant with birth trauma, low hematocrit (Hct), or coagulopathy. This should be done early to rule out hemorrhage.

IV. **Magnetic resonance imaging (MRI).** Now an acceptable mode of imaging in the neonate, and its use is expanding. MRI is superior to CT for imaging the brainstem, spinal cord, soft tissues, and areas of high bony CT artifact. Supplemental magnetic resonance arteriography and magnetic resonance venography are now available to improve vascular anatomy and flow. In **encephalopathic term infants**, do an MRI if CT findings are inconclusive. MRI is recommended in the first postnatal week to document pattern of injury and predict neurologic outcome.

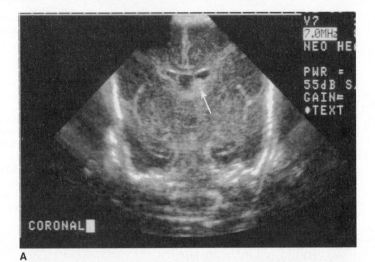

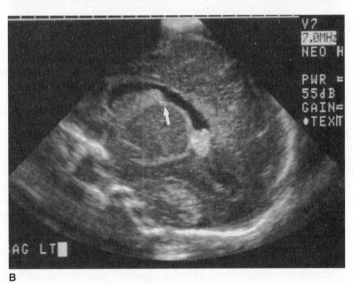

FIGURE 11–1. Ultrasonogram of the brain. Coronal (A) and left sagittal (B) views show a left germinal matrix hemorrhage (grade I or subependymal) at arrow.

  A. **Advantages.** The absence of ionizing radiation and visualization of vascular anatomy without contrast agents.
  B. **Disadvantages.** It cannot always be performed on critically ill infants requiring ventilator support, the scanning time is longer, and sedation is usually required.

COMMON RADIOLOGIC PREPARATIONS

See Table 11–1 for guidelines for common radiographic studies. Institutional guidelines may vary slightly from these.

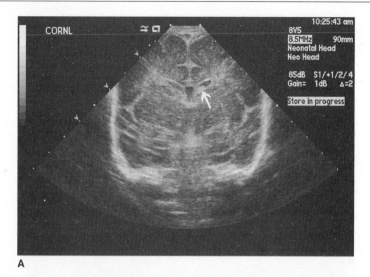

A

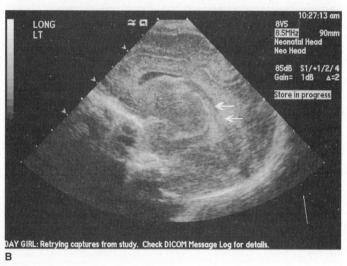

B

FIGURE 11–2. Ultrasonogram of the brain. Coronal (A) and left sagittal (B) views show a limited intraventricular hemorrhage (IVH) with minimal ventricular enlargement at arrows (grade II IVH).

RADIOGRAPHIC EXAMPLES

Invasive life support and monitoring techniques depend on proper positioning of the device being used. **Caution is necessary when identifying ribs** and correlating vertebrae in the newborn as a means for determining the proper position of a catheter or tube. Infants often have a noncalcified 12th rib; thus the 11th rib is mistaken for the 12th rib, and an incorrect vertebral count may occur.

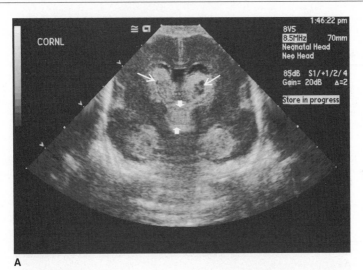

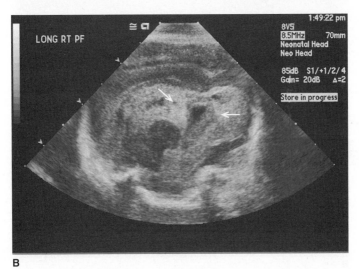

FIGURE 11–3. Ultrasonogram of the brain. Coronal (A) and right parasagittal (B) views demonstrate severe dilatation of both lateral (small arrows) as well as the third (large arrows) ventricles, which are filled with clots (grade III intraventricular hemorrhage).

  I. **Endotracheal intubation**
   A. **The preferred location of the endotracheal tube (ETT) tip** is halfway between the thoracic inlet (the medial ends of the clavicles) and the carina. Correct tube placement is shown in Figure 11–7.
   B. **If the ETT is placed too low,** the tip usually enters the right main bronchus, a straighter line than with the left main bronchus. The chest film may show asymmetric aeration with both hyperinflation and atelectasis. If the tube extends below the carina or does not match the tracheal air column in position, suspect esophageal intubation. Increased proximal intestinal air may also reflect esophageal intubation.

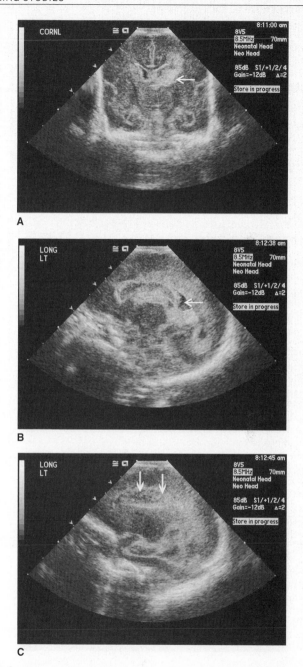

FIGURE 11–4. Ultrasonogram of the brain. Coronal (A) and left sagittal (B and C) demonstrate left intraventricular hemorrhage (IVH) with ventricular dilatation and localized left intraparenchymal hemorrhage (grade IV IVH) (arrows). (See next page for follow-up sonography.)

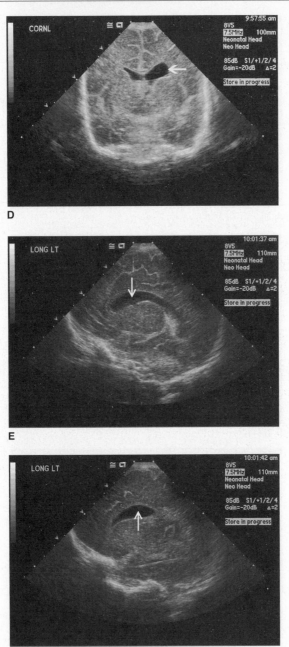

FIGURE 11–4. Ultrasonogram of the brain. Follow-up sonogram 3 months later (coronal view [D] and left sagittal [E and F] views) shows resolution of clot, residual mild ventriculomegaly, and focal porencephaly (arrow) at the site of previous parenchymal hemorrhage.

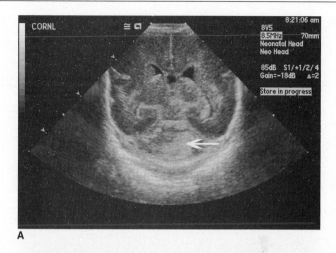

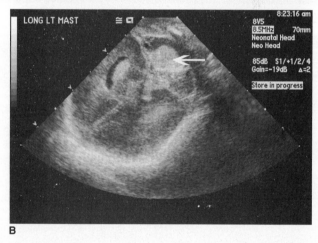

FIGURE 11–5. Ultrasonogram of the brain. Coronal (A) and mastoid (B) views demonstrate focal hemorrhage into the left cerebellar hemisphere (posterior fossa hemorrhage, arrow).

An ETT placed too high has the tip above the clavicle, and the x-ray film may show diffuse atelectasis.

II. **Naso/orogastric tube.** The naso/orogastric tube tip should be in the mid-stomach. Correct placement is shown in Figure 11–8.

III. **Transpyloric tube.** The weighted feeding tube is in the mid to distal duodenum. Correct placement is shown in Figure 11–9.

IV. **Umbilical vein catheterization (UVC).** The catheter tip should be at the junction of the inferior vena cava and right atrium, projecting just above the diaphragm on the AP chest radiograph. Degree and direction of patient rotation affect how the UVC appears positioned on the radiograph. **Due to its more anterior location, the UVC deviates more from the midline with patient rotation than will the umbilical artery catheterization (UAC).** Figure 11–10 shows correct UVC tip placement.

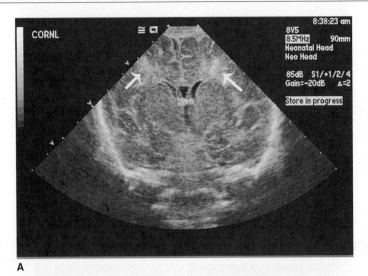

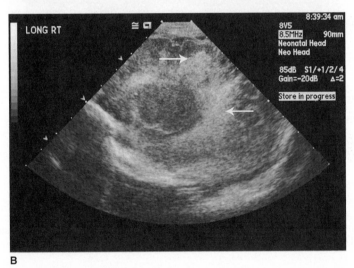

FIGURE 11–6. Ultrasonogram of the brain. Periventricular leukomalacia (PVL). Coronal (A) and right sagittal (B) views demonstrate increased periventricular echogenicity (PVE) suggesting ischemic white matter disease (arrows).

V. Umbilical artery catheterization (UAC). Cochrane review states that **high catheters should be used exclusively.** In certain instances, a catheter may have to be placed in the low position. The use of high versus low UAC placement used to depend on institutional preference. High catheters were once thought to be associated with a higher risk of vascular complications, but a recent analysis showed a decreased risk of vascular complications and no increased risk of hypertension, necrotizing enterocolitis (NEC), IVH, or hematuria. Low catheters are associated with an increased risk of vasospasms.

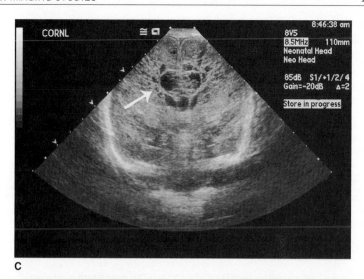

FIGURE 11–6. Ultrasonogram of the brain. Follow-up sonography of the brain 1 month later (coronal [C] and sagittal [D] views) shows extensive periventricular cystic change reflecting PVL.

A. **If high UAC placement is desired,** the tip should be between thoracic vertebrae 6 and 9 (above the diaphragm, which is above the celiac axis at T12, the superior mesenteric artery at T12–L1, and the renal arteries [L1]). (Figure 11–11).

B. **For low UAC placement,** the tip should be below the third lumbar vertebra, optimally between L3 and L4 (above the aortic bifurcation which is at L4–L5) (Figure 11–12). A catheter placed below L5 usually does not function well and carries a risk of severe vasospasm in small arteries. Note that the catheter turns downward

Table 11–1. **PREPARATORY PROCEDURES FOR PREMATURE AND NEWBORN INFANT RADIOLOGIC STUDIES**[a]

Neonatal Study	Preparation
Upper GI series	NPO for 1–2 hours for neonates and infants up to 2 years of age
Contrast enema	No preparation needed for evaluation of bowel obstruction or to rule out Hirschsprung disease
Renal sonography	No preparation
Abdominal sonography	NPO for 1 hour for filling of gall bladder
HIDA (hepatobiliary) scan	Oral phenobarbital (5 mg/kg/d) for 5 days prior to the examination
CT of abdomen/pelvis	Oral contrast beginning 2 hours prior to scanning
Voiding cystourethrogram (VCUG)	No preparation required

CT, computed tomography; GI, gastrointestinal; HIDA, hepatoiminodiacetic acid; NPO, nothing by mouth; VCUG, voiding cystourethrogram.
[a]Review your institution-specific recommendations before ordering.

and then upward on an abdominal x-ray film. The upward turn is the point at which the catheter passes through the internal iliac artery (hypogastric artery).

Note: If both a UAC and a UVC are positioned and an x-ray study is performed, it is necessary to differentiate the two so that line placement can be properly assessed. **The UAC turns downward and then upward on the x-ray film, whereas the UVC takes only an upward or cephalad direction.**

VI. **Extracorporeal membrane oxygenation/extracorporeal life support (ECMO/ ECLS).** ECLS is a type of external life support using a membrane oxygenator that can be applied to a neonate in severe but reversible respiratory or cardiac failure (see Chapter 18). See VA ECLS cannulae placement and VV ECLS cannulae placement radiographs (see Figures 18–2 and 18–3, respectively).

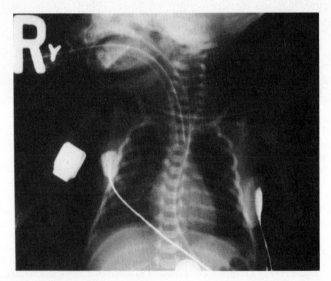

FIGURE 11–7. Chest radiograph showing proper placement of an endotracheal tube.

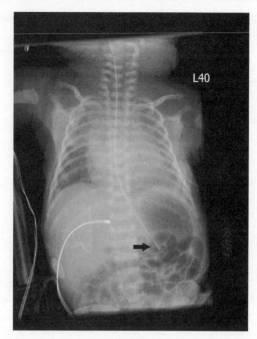

FIGURE 11–8. Chest abdomen film showing the nasogastric tube tip in the mid-stomach (arrow at distal tube).

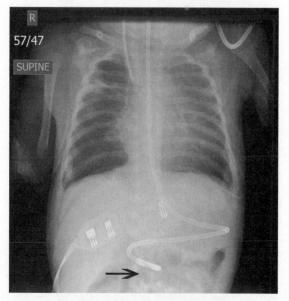

FIGURE 11–9. Chest abdomen film showing the transpyloric tube (weighted feeding tube tip) in the mid-to-distal duodenum (arrow at distal tube).

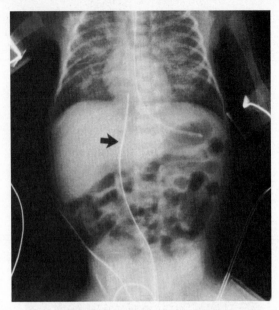

FIGURE 11–10. Radiograph showing correct placement of an umbilical venous catheter with tip at arrow. The tip of the nasogastric tube is properly positioned in the stomach.

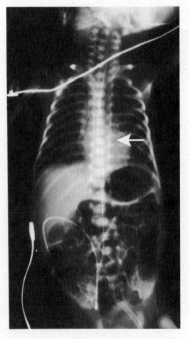

FIGURE 11–11. Radiograph showing correct positioning of a high umbilical artery catheter.

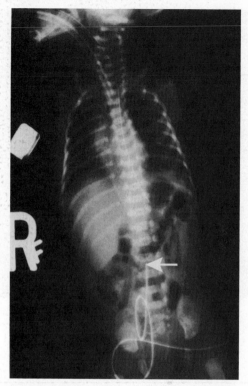

FIGURE 11–12. Radiograph showing correct positioning of a low umbilical artery catheter.

RADIOGRAPHIC PEARLS

I. **Pulmonary diseases**
   A. **Respiratory distress syndrome (RDS).** A fine, diffuse reticulogranular pattern is seen secondary to microatelectasis of the alveoli. The chest radiograph reveals radiolucent areas known as air bronchograms, produced by air in the major airways and contrasted with the opacified, collapsed alveoli (Figure 11–13).
   B. **Meconium aspiration syndrome (MAS).** Bilateral, patchy, coarse infiltrates and hyperinflation of the lungs are present (Figure 11–14). There is also an increased incidence of pneumothorax.
   C. **Pneumonia.** Diffuse alveolar or interstitial disease that is usually asymmetric and localized. Group B streptococcal pneumonia can appear similar to respiratory distress syndrome (RDS). Pneumatoceles (air-filled lung cysts) can occur with staphylococcal pneumonia. Pleural effusions or empyema may occur with any bacterial pneumonia (Figure 11–15).
   D. **Transient tachypnea of the newborn (TTN).** Hyperaeration with symmetric perihilar and interstitial streaky infiltrates are typical. Pleural fluid may occur as well, appearing as widening of the pleural space or as prominence of the minor fissure (Figure 11–16).
   E. **Bronchopulmonary dysplasia (BPD).** Now more commonly referred to as **chronic lung disease (CLD)**, the radiographic appearance is highly variable, from a fine, hazy

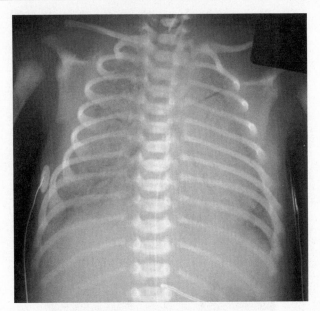

FIGURE 11–13. Chest radiograph showing diffuse granular opacification of the lungs with air bronchograms. In the premature neonate, this would almost always represent respiratory distress syndrome (RDS).

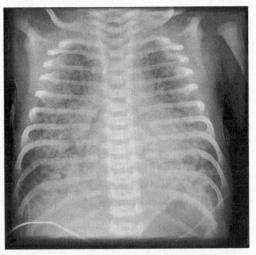

FIGURE 11–14. Chest radiograph showing diffuse coarse increase in lung markings accompanied by hyperinflation, typical for meconium aspiration syndrome (MAS).

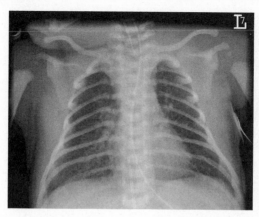

FIGURE 11–15. Diffuse increase in interstitial lung markings is typical with neonatal pneumonia but could also be produced by transient tachypnea of newborn.

appearance of the lungs to mildly coarsened lung markings to a coarse, cystic lung pattern (Figure 11–17). Typically occurring in ventilated premature neonates, CLD usually requires a minimum of 7–10 days to develop. Many centers no longer rely on the following grading system for this condition, but it is included for historical purposes.

1. **Grade I.** X-ray findings are similar to those of severe RDS.
2. **Grade II.** Dense parenchymal opacification is seen.
3. **Grade III.** A bubbly, fibrocystic pattern is evident.
4. **Grade IV.** Hyperinflation is present with multiple fine, lacy densities spreading to the periphery and with areas of lucency similar to bullae of the lung.

F. **Air leak syndromes**
1. **Pneumopericardium.** Air surrounds the heart, including the inferior border (Figure 11–18). Cardiac tamponade may result.
2. **Pneumomediastinum**
   a. **AP view.** A hyperlucent rim of air is present lateral to the cardiac border and beneath the thymus, displacing the thymus superiorly away from the cardiac silhouette ("angel wing sign") (Figure 11–19, left panel).
   b. **Lateral view.** An air collection is seen either substernally (anterior pneumomediastinum) or in the retrocardiac area (posterior pneumomediastinum) (Figure 11–19, right panel).
3. **Pneumothorax.** The lung is typically displaced away from the lateral chest wall by a radiolucent zone of air. The adjacent lung may be collapsed with larger pneumothoraces (as in Figure 11–20). The small pneumothorax may be very difficult to identify, with only a subtle zone of air peripherally, a diffusely hyperlucent hemithorax, unusually sharply defined cardiothymic margins, or a combination of these.
4. **Tension pneumothorax.** The diaphragm on the affected side is depressed, the mediastinum is shifted to the contralateral hemithorax, and collapse of the ipsilateral lobes is evident (Figure 11–20).
5. **Pulmonary interstitial emphysema (PIE).** Single or multiple circular radiolucencies with well-demarcated walls are seen in a localized or diffuse pattern. The volume of the involved portion of the lung is usually increased, often markedly so (Figure 11–21). PIE usually occurs in ventilated preemies with RDS within the initial few days of life.

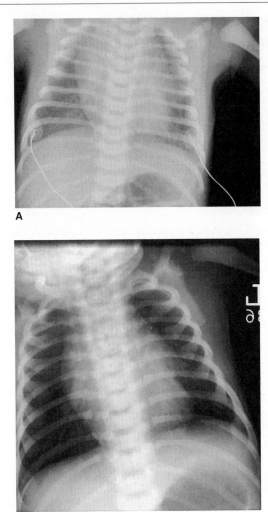

FIGURE 11–16. Chest radiograph (A) showing diffuse, mild increase in interstitial lung markings, consistent with transient tachypnea of newborn. The findings had typically resolved by the following day (B).

    G. **Atelectasis.** A decrease in lung volume or collapse of part or all of a lung is apparent, appearing as areas of increased opacity. The mediastinum may be shifted toward the side of collapse. Compensatory hyperinflation of the opposite lung may be present.

        1. **Microatelectasis.** Nonobstructive atelectasis associated with RDS.

        2. **Generalized atelectasis.** Diffuse increase in opacity ("whiteout") of the lungs is visible on the chest film. It may be seen in severe RDS, airway obstruction, if the endotracheal tube is not in the trachea, and hypoventilation.

        3. **Lobar atelectasis.** Lobar atelectasis is atelectasis of one lobe. The most common site is the right upper lobe, which appears as an area of dense opacity ("whiteout")

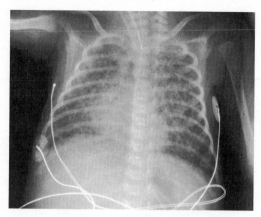

FIGURE 11–17. Chest radiograph showing a diffuse, moderately coarse increase in lung density, which in a 2-month-old ventilated ex-preemie is most consistent with bronchopulmonary dysplasia/chronic lung disease (BPD/CLD).

on the chest film. In addition, the right minor fissure is usually elevated. This pattern of atelectasis commonly occurs after extubation.

  H. **Pulmonary hypoplasia.** Small lung volumes and a bell-shaped thorax are seen. The lungs usually appear radiolucent.

  I. **Pulmonary edema.** The lungs appear diffusely hazy with an area of greatest density around the hilum of each lung. Heart size is usually increased.

II. **Cardiac diseases.** The cardiothoracic ratio, which normally should be <0.6, is the width of the base of the heart divided by the width of the lower thorax. An index >0.6 suggests cardiomegaly. The pulmonary vascularity is increased if the diameter of the descending branch of the right pulmonary artery exceeds that of the trachea.

  A. **Cardiac dextroversion.** The cardiac apex is on the right, and the aortic arch and stomach bubble are on the left. The incidence of congenital heart disease associated with this finding is high (>90%).

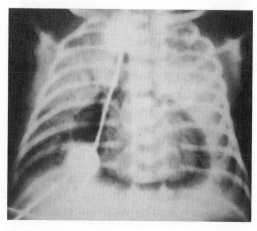

FIGURE 11–18. Chest radiograph showing pneumopericardium in a 2-day-old infant.

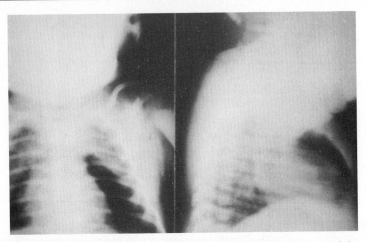

FIGURE 11–19. Pneumomediastinum on anteroposterior (left panel) and cross-table lateral (right panel) radiographs, demonstrating central chest air and elevation of the lobes of the thymus.

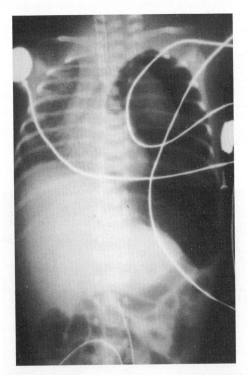

FIGURE 11–20. Left tension pneumothorax as shown on an anteroposterior chest radiograph in a ventilated infant on day 2 of life. Note the accompanying collapse of the left lung, depression of the left diaphragm, and contralateral shift of mediastinal structures, all signs of increased pressure within a pneumothorax.

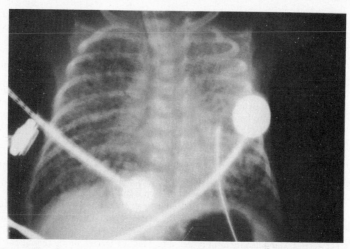

FIGURE 11–21. Chest radiograph showing bilateral pulmonary interstitial emphysema in a 7-day-old ventilated infant.

B. **Congestive heart failure.** Cardiomegaly, pulmonary venous congestion (engorgement and increased diameter of the pulmonary veins), diffuse opacification in the perihilar regions, and pleural effusions (sometimes) are seen.

C. **Patent ductus arteriosus.** Cardiomegaly, pulmonary edema, ductal haze (pulmonary edema with a patent ductus arteriosus), and increased pulmonary vascular markings are evident.

D. **Ventricular septal defect.** Findings include cardiomegaly, an increase in pulmonary vascular density, enlargement of the left ventricle and left atrium, and enlargement of the main pulmonary artery.

E. **Coarctation of the aorta**
   1. **Preductal coarctation.** Generalized cardiomegaly, with normal pulmonary vascularity, is seen.
   2. **Postductal coarctation.** An enlarged left ventricle and left atrium and a dilated ascending aorta are present.

F. **Tetralogy of Fallot.** The heart is boot shaped. A normal left atrium and left ventricle is associated with an enlarged, hypertrophied right ventricle and small or absent main pulmonary artery. There is decreased pulmonary vascularity. A right aortic arch occurs in 25% of patients.

G. **Transposition of the great arteries.** The chest film may show cardiomegaly, with an enlarged right atrium and right ventricle, narrow mediastinum, and increased pulmonary vascular markings, but in most cases the chest film appears normal.

H. **Total anomalous pulmonary venous return (TAPVR).** Pulmonary venous markings are increased. Cardiomegaly is minimal or absent. Congestive heart failure and pulmonary edema may be present, especially with type 3 (subdiaphragmatic) TAPVR.

I. **Hypoplastic left heart syndrome.** The chest film can be normal at first but then may show cardiomegaly and pulmonary vascular congestion, with an enlarged right atrium and ventricle.

J. **Tricuspid atresia.** Heart size is usually normal or small, the main pulmonary artery is concave, and pulmonary vascularity is decreased.

K. **Truncus arteriosus.** Characteristic findings include cardiomegaly, increased pulmonary vascularity, and enlargement of the left atrium. A right aortic arch occurs in 30% of patients.

L. **Atrial septal defect.** Varying degrees of enlargement of the right atrium and ventricle are seen. The aorta and the left ventricle are small, and the pulmonary artery is large. Increased pulmonary vascularity is also evident.

M. **Ebstein anomaly.** Gross cardiomegaly and decreased pulmonary vascularity are apparent. The right heart border is prominent as a result of right atrial enlargement.

N. **Valvular pulmonic stenosis.** Heart size and pulmonary blood flow are usually normal unless the stenosis is severe. Dilatation of the main pulmonary artery is the typical chest film finding.

III. **Abdominal disorders**

A. **Changes in the following normal patterns** should raise suspicion of GI tract disease.
1. **Air in the stomach.** Should occur within 30 minutes after delivery.
2. **Air in the small bowel.** Should be seen by 3–4 hours of age.
3. **Air in the colon and rectum.** Should be seen by 6–8 hours of age.

B. **Intestinal obstruction.** Gaseous intestinal distention is present. Gas may be decreased or absent distal to the obstruction. Air-fluid levels are seen proximal to the obstruction.

C. **Ascites.** Gas-filled loops of bowel, if present, are located in the central portion of the abdomen. The abdomen may be distended, with relatively small amounts of gas (**"ground-glass" appearance**). A uniform increase in the density of the abdomen, particularly in the flank areas, may be evident.

D. **Calcification** in the abdomen is most often seen secondary to meconium peritonitis, which may also cause calcifications in the scrotum in male infants. Calcifications in the abdomen may also be seen in infants with neuroblastoma or teratoma, or may signify calcification of the adrenals after adrenal hemorrhage.

E. **Pneumoperitoneum**
1. **Supine view.** Free air is seen as a central lucency, usually in the upper abdomen (Figure 11–22).

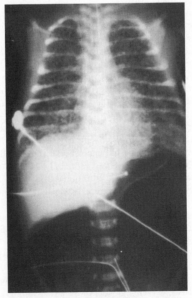

FIGURE 11–22. Radiograph showing pneumoperitoneum in a 3-day-old infant.

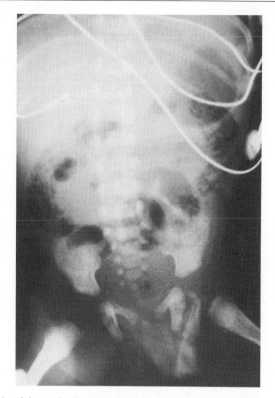

FIGURE 11-23. Abdominal radiograph showing pneumatosis intestinalis.

    2. Upright view. Free air is present in a subdiaphragmatic location.

    3. Left lateral decubitus view. Air collects over the lateral border of the liver, separating it from the adjacent abdominal wall.

  F. Pneumatosis intestinalis. Intraluminal gas in the bowel wall (produced by bacteria that have invaded the bowel wall) may appear as a string or cluster of bubbles (submucosal) or a curvilinear lucency (subserosal). It is most frequently seen in infants with NEC (Figure 11-23).

  G. Situs inversus (complete). The stomach, aortic arch, and cardiac apex all are right sided. There is only a limited increased incidence of congenital heart disease.

  H. Ileus. Distended loops of bowel are present. Air-fluid levels may be seen on the upright or cross-table lateral abdominal film.

  I. Absence of gas in the abdomen. Absence of gas in the abdomen may be seen in patients on muscle-paralyzing medications (eg, pancuronium) because they do not swallow air. It may also be evident in infants with esophageal atresia without tracheoesophageal fistula and in cases of severe cerebral anoxia resulting in central nervous system depression and absence of swallowing.

  J. Portal venous air. (Figure 11-24) Air is demonstrated in the portal veins (often best seen on a lateral view). This finding may indicate bowel necrosis, which can occur in an advanced degree of NEC; intestinal infarction secondary to mesenteric vessel occlusion; and iatrogenically introduced gas into the portal vein, which can occur during umbilical vein catheterization or exchange transfusion.

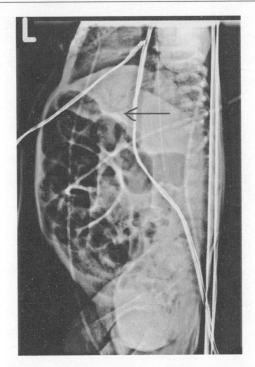

FIGURE 11–24. Cross-table lateral radiograph of abdomen showing portal venous gas.

Selected References

ACR Manual on Contrast Media, Version 7, 2012. American College of Radiology, Philadelphia, PA. http://www.acr.org/SecondaryMainMenuCategories/quality_safety/contrast_manual/FullManual.aspx. Accessed March 2012.

Agrons GA, Courtney SE, Stocker JT, Markowitz RI. Lung disease in premature neonates: radiologic-pathologic correlation. *Radiographics.* 2005;25:1047–1073.

Barrington KJ Editorial Group: Cochrane Neonatal Group. Umbilical artery catheters in the newborn: effects of position of the catheter tip. *Cochrane Database Syst Rev.* 2010. DOI:10.1002/14651858.CD000505.

Breysem L, Smet MH, Van Lierde S, Devlieger H, De Boeck K. Bronchopulmonary dysplasia: correlation of radiographic and clinical findings. *Pediatr Radiol.* 1997;27: 642–646.

Dinger J, Schwarze R, Rupprecht E. Radiologic changes after therapeutic use of surfactant in infants with respiratory distress syndrome. *Pediatr Radiol.* 1997;27:26–31.

Donnelly LF, Frush DP. Localized radiolucent chest lesions in neonates: causes and differentiation. *AJR.* 1999;172:1651–1658.

Donoghue V. *Radiological Imaging of the Neonatal Chest.* Berlin, Germany: Springer; 2002.

Ferguson EC, Krishnamurthy R, Oldham SA. Classical imaging signs of congenital cardiovascular abnormalities. *Radiographics.* 2007;27:1323–1324.

Greenspan JS, Fox WW, Rubenstein SD, Wolfson MR, Spinner SS, Shaffer TH. Partial liquid ventilation in critically ill infants receiving extracorporeal life support. *Pediatrics.* 1997;99(1):E2.

Gross GW, Cullen J, Kornhauser MS, Wolfson PJ. Thoracic complications of extracorporeal membrane oxygenation: findings on chest radiographs and sonograms. *AJR Am J Roentgenol.* 1992;158:353.

Gross GW, McElwee DL, Baumgart S, Wolfson PJ. Bypass cannulas utilized in extracorporeal membrane oxygenation in neonates: radiographic findings. *Pediatr Radiol.* 1995;25:337.

Papile LA, Burstein J, Burstein R, Koffler H. Incidence and evolution of subependymal and intraventricular hemorrhage: a study of infants with birthweights less than 1500 g. *J Pediatr.*1978;92:529– 534.

Veyrac C, Couture A, Saguintaah M, Baud C. Brain ultrasonography in the premature infant [symposium]. *Pediatr Radiol.* 2006;36:626–635.

12 Management of the Extremely Low Birthweight Infant During the First Week of Life

This chapter addresses the initial care of premature infants of <1000 g birthweight. Many aspects of the care of extremely low birthweight (ELBW) infants are ***controversial***, and each institution must develop its own philosophy and techniques for management. It is of utmost importance to follow the practices of your own institution. This chapter offers guidelines that the authors have found useful for stabilizing and caring for extremely small infants.

I. **Delivery room management**

    A. **Ethics.** The neonatologist and other health care team members should make every effort to meet with the family before delivery to discuss the treatment options for the ELBW infant. Counseling should include discussions with the parents regarding survival rate and both short- and long-term complications based on institutional statistics and the National Institute of Child Health and Human Development (NICHD) Neonatal Research Network calculator. Communication regarding treatment options for the 22–24 week gestation infant is crucial. Neonatal bioethics are discussed in detail in Chapter 21.

    B. **Resuscitation**

        1. **Thermoregulation.** A polyethylene wrap or bag used immediately after birth prevents heat loss at delivery in very preterm infants. The wrap is removed and infant is dried after being placed in a thermal-neutral environment in the neonatal intensive care unit (NICU).

        2. **Respiratory support.** Oxygen (O_2) use in resuscitation has been challenged in recent years. It takes 7–10 minutes for oxyhemoglobin saturations to rise to 90% after delivery. The Neonatal Resuscitation Program recommends availability of pulse oximetry and blended O_2 for resuscitation and low saturation protocol. For infants who require intubation,

surfactant is recommended; however, for infants breathing spontaneously it remains *controversial*. If the infant is breathing spontaneously and has a heart rate >100, continuous positive airway pressure (CPAP) of 4–6 cm of H_2O should be initiated to prevent atelectasis. CPAP cannot be delivered with a self-inflating bag.

3. **Transport.** As soon as possible, the infant should be transported to the NICU. Transport must be in a prewarmed portable incubator equipped with blended O_2 and CPAP availability. Occlusive wrap should remain in place, and the infant should be placed under warmed blankets with a knit hat. Infants transported from referring hospitals should be handled in a similar manner with the addition of an underlying thermal mattress.

II. **Temperature and humidity control.** Because the tiny infant has a relatively large skin surface area and minimal energy reserves, a constant **neutral thermal environment** (environmental temperature that minimizes heat loss without increasing O_2 consumption or incurring metabolic stress) is essential. To maintain minimal evaporative heat loss, it is best if the environmental humidity is 80%. Lower ambient humidity requires higher ambient temperatures to maintain infant skin temperature.

A. **Incubators and hybrid incubators.** ELBW infants should be admitted into prewarmed **double-walled incubators.** Until recently, only **radiant warmers** allowed accessibility to the infant; however, they caused large evaporative heat with water losses and somewhat higher basal metabolic rates. As a result, the development and exclusive use of hybrid humidified incubators has been on the rise, with many facilities converting to these multiuse incubators.

B. **Humidification.** ELBW infants have increased insensible water loss secondary to large body surface area and a greater proportion of body water to body mass. Transcutaneous water loss is enhanced by their thin epidermis and underdeveloped stratum corneum. Increased environmental humidity can minimize these losses. **Warm humidification within the incubator is recommended.** Double-walled incubators provide the best control for monitoring humidity levels.

1. **Use a respiratory care humidification unit.** Humidification and warming of administered ventilator gases are important to minimize insensible fluid losses and hypothermia. Infants receiving mechanical ventilation as well as noninvasive respiratory assistance require humidification. In-line warming of ventilator gas circuits minimizes "rainout" of the humidified air and O_2 and maintains airway temperature as close as possible to 35° C. The fluids used for humidification in these systems should be changed every 24 hours.

2. **Minimize nosocomial infection in humidified environments.** Minimize by not allowing nonmedical items inside the incubator and by changing linens regularly if the infant's condition is stable. Change bed every 7–10 days per manufacturer's recommendation.

C. **Monitoring and maintenance of body temperature.** Infants weighing <1000 g have poor mechanisms for regulation of temperature and depend on environmental support.

1. **Maintain axillary skin temperature of 36.0–36.5°C.** If skin temperature is outside the range, you may need to change from servo control to manual control for warming the smallest infants. Use extreme caution while in the manual temperature mode because the danger of hyperthermia does exist. Rectal thermometers are not to be used for tiny infants. Electronic thermometers have become standard in obtaining infant temperatures.

2. **Record skin temperature.** Using a servo-control skin probe, record skin temperature and environmental temperature every hour until the skin

temperature is stable (36.0–36.5°C) and thereafter with recordings at 2-hour intervals.

3. **Record the incubator humidity.** Record every hour until it is stable and then every 2 hours for maintenance.

4. **Weigh low birthweight infants at least once daily for management of fluids and electrolytes.** The incubator should be equipped with an in-bed scale for continuous weighing of the infant to minimize handling and loss of the thermal-controlled environment.

5. **Other heat-conserving practices.** These include the use of knit hats, fetal positioning, and air boost curtains on incubators.

6. **Accessory items for infant care must be prewarmed.** These items include intravenous (IV) fluids, stethoscope, saline lavages, and any other items that come in direct contact with the infant. Placement of these items in the infant's incubator 30 minutes before use warms them to avoid heat loss by conduction from the infant.

D. **Slow warming or cooling of infants.** Infants who become hypothermic must be gradually rewarmed.

1. **Warming.** If the infant's temperature is <36.0°C, set the warmer temperature 0.4°C higher than the infant's temperature. Continue this procedure until the desired temperature is achieved. Frequent observations of environmental and skin temperatures are essential to evaluate warming efforts. **Do not rewarm faster than 1°C/h.** When skin temperature of 36.5°C is achieved, rewarming efforts should be gradually discontinued and temperature maintenance by servo-control should be monitored. Rapid rewarming of ELBW infants must be avoided because core body temperatures >37.5°C cause increased insensible water losses, increased O_2 consumption, apneic episodes, increased incidence of intraventricular hemorrhage, deviations in vital signs, and a detrimental effect on neurodevelopment.

2. **Hyperthermia (skin temperature >37.0°C).** In case of hyperthermia, set the warmer temperature control to 0.4°C lower than the infant's skin temperature. Continue to reduce the warmer temperature until desired temperature is achieved. If increased temperature persists, consider evaluation for pathologic conditions such as sepsis, intraventricular hemorrhage, or mechanical overheating by exterior lamps. Do not turn off the warmer, as this may cause a sudden decrease in the infant's temperature.

III. **Fluids and electrolytes.** Because of increased insensible water loss and immature renal function, these infants have greater fluid requirements, necessitating IV fluid therapy (see Chapter 9).

A. **Intravenous fluid therapy**

1. **Insensible water loss.** Insensible water loss increases with the use of radiant warmers and low ambient humidity. Under these circumstances in which increased insensible fluid loss can occur, additional fluid supplementation is required. However, excessive fluid intake may contribute to the development of a hemodynamically significant patent ductus arteriosus (PDA).

2. **First day of life.** Table 12–1 gives suggested guidelines for total fluids per kilogram of body weight for the first day of life for infants in humidified incubators/omnibeds and on radiant warmers.

3. **Second and subsequent days of life.** Fluid management on the second and subsequent days depends on changes in body weight, renal function (blood urea nitrogen, creatinine, urine output), and serum electrolyte concentrations (see Chapter 9).

4. **Additional fluid may be required if phototherapy is used.** The fluid volume should be increased by 10–20 mL/kg/d.

Table 12–1. **ADMINISTRATION RATES FOR THE FIRST DAY OF LIFE FOR INFANTS IN HUMIDIFED INCUBATORS/OMNIBEDS AND RADIANT WARMERS**

Birthweight (g)	Gestational Age (wk)	Fluid Rate (mL/kg/d)	
		Incubators[a]	Radiant warmers[b]
500–600	23	60–80	140–200
601–800	24	60–80	120–150
801–1000	25–27	50–70	100–120

[a]Fluid rates based on 80% or higher humidity; fluids should be increased incrementally with decreasing environmental humidity.
[b]Fluid rates may be decreased with the addition of a humidity tent.

   a. **Incubators/omnibeds.** Fluid rates based on 80% or higher humidity; fluids should be increased incrementally with decreasing environmental humidity.
   b. **Radiant warmers.** Fluid rates may be decreased with the addition of a humidity tent.
  B. **Infusion of fluids.** Confirm appropriate line placement and document before infusion (see specific procedure chapter).
   1. **Umbilical artery catheter.** Use only for laboratory and hemodynamic monitoring if other IV access is available. Infuse 0.5 normal saline (NS) + 0.5 U heparin/mL or 0.5 sodium acetate + 0.5 U heparin/mL (sodium acetate aids in acid-base balance).
   2. **Umbilical venous catheter.** Fluids containing glucose and amino acids add 0.5 U heparin/mL to maintenance fluids.
   3. **Broviac or percutaneous central venous catheters.** Add 0.5 U heparin/mL to maintenance fluids.
   4. **Radial arterial line/posterior tibial arterial line.** Add 2 U heparin/mL to 0.5 NS.
  C. **For catheter flushes,** use the same fluids as those infused as IV fluids. Avoid NS as a flush solution because of excessive sodium. In addition, avoid hypotonic solutions (<0.45 NS or <5% dextrose); these solutions may cause red blood cell hemolysis.
  D. **Monitoring of fluid therapy.** The infant's fluid status should be evaluated at least twice daily during the first few days of life and the fluid intake adjusted accordingly. Fluid status is monitored via measurement of body weight, urine output, blood pressure measurements, serum sodium, hematocrit, and physical examination.
   1. **Body weight.** This is the most important method of monitoring fluid therapy. If an in-bed scale is used, weigh the infant daily. If unavailable, weighing may be delayed to every 48 hours, depending on the stability of the tiny infant, to prevent excessive handling and cold stress. A weight loss of up to 15% of birthweight may be experienced by the end of the first week of life. If weight loss is excessive, environmental controls for insensible fluid losses and fluid management must be carefully reviewed.
   2. **Urine output.** This is the second most important method of monitoring fluid therapy. For greatest accuracy, diapers should be weighed before use and immediately after urination.
    a. **First 12 hours.** Any amount of urine output is acceptable.
    b. **12–24 hours.** The minimum acceptable urine output is 0.5 mL/kg/h.

c. **Day 2 and beyond.** Normal urine output for the second day is 1–2 mL/ kg/h. After the second day of life, and during a diuretic phase, urine output may increase to 3.0–5.0 mL/kg/h; values outside this range warrant reevaluation of fluid management.

3. **Hemodynamic monitoring.** This is a valuable tool in assessing fluid status in the infant.

    a. **Heart rate.** The accelerated heart rate of the tiny infant averages 140–160 beats/min and is generally considered within normal limits. Tachycardia, with a heart rate >160 beats/min, may be a sign of hypovolemia, pain, inadequate ventilation, anemia, sepsis, or hyperthermia. Low heart rate (<100 beats/min) may be related to hypoxia or medication.

    b. **Arterial blood pressure.** This is most accurately measured via an indwelling arterial catheter and transducer. Cuff pressures are difficult to obtain because of the infant's small size and lower systemic pressures. A recognized standard is to maintain the infant's mean arterial pressure at or equal to the gestational age during the first 48 hours. Thereafter, mean blood pressure increases with chronological age. It is important to evaluate the infant's perfusion, urine output, and acid-base balance in conjunction with blood pressure monitoring.

4. **Electrolyte values.** Serum electrolyte levels should be monitored at least twice daily or every 8 hours for the most immature infants. Sodium and potassium are added as diuresis begins.

    a. **Sodium.** Initially tiny infants have a sufficient sodium level (132–138 mEq/L), and if there are no ongoing fluid losses, they will not require additional sodium. Serum sodium level may begin to decrease in the postdiuretic phase (usually third to fifth days of life). Subsequently, sodium chloride should be added to the IV fluids (3–8 mEq/kg/d of sodium). **Hyponatremia in the prediuretic phase usually indicates fluid overload, and hypernatremia during the same period usually indicates dehydration.** *Note:* Hypernatremia in the prediuretic phase is due to excessive insensible water loss. This can be effectively treated with sterile water intragastric drip. This avoids use of hyposmolar IV fluids. For subsequent monitoring of the serum sodium levels:

        i. **Hypernatremia Na$^+$ > 150 mEq/L.** Differential diagnosis is (**a**) premature addition of sodium in the prediuretic phase, or (**b**) dehydration, or (**c**) excessive Na$^+$ intake.

        ii. **Hyponatremia Na$^+$ <130 mEq/L.** Differential diagnosis is (**a**) fluid overload, or (**b**) inadequate Na$^+$ intake, or (**c**) excessive Na$^+$ loss.

    b. **Potassium**

        i. **During the first 48 hours after birth.** During this time, tiny infants are prone to increased serum potassium levels of ≥5 mEq/L (range, 4.0–8.0 mEq/L). Most clinicians recommend that no potassium be given during the prediuretic phase. The increase is mostly a result of the following:

            (a) Relative hypoaldosteronism

            (b) Shift of intracellular potassium to the extracellular space due to an immature Na+, K+-ATPase pump

            (c) Immature renal tubular function

            (d) Lack of arginine, a precursor to insulin

        ii. **K$^+$ >6 mEq/L mandates close ECG monitoring T-wave changes and rhythm disturbances along with electrolyte trends, acid-base status, and urine output.** Acidosis should be aggressively treated because this tends to cause intracellular potassium to leak out. Use of Kayexalate enemas is *controversial* in this age group and best avoided if possible. Albuterol metered-dose inhaler (MDI) (4 puffs every 2 hours;

1 puff = 90 mcg) can reduce high levels. Serum K^+ >7 mEq/L can also be treated with insulin, $NaHCO_3$, and calcium gluconate (see Chapter 60).

iii. **3–6 days after birth.** Usually by this time, the initially elevated K^+ level begins to decrease. When K^+ levels approach 4 mEq/L, add supplemental K^+ to IV fluids. Begin with 1–2 mEq/kg/d. Measure serum K^+ every 6–12 hours until the level is stabilized.

IV. **Blood glucose.** ELBW infants should be supported with 4–6 mg/kg/min glucose infusion; start with a 5–10% dextrose solution, depending on glucose needs. Amino acid used immediately after birth along with glucose solutions achieves better glucose homeostasis. Bedside glucose levels should be monitored frequently until a blood glucose level of 50–90 mg/dL has been established. Abnormal values should be confirmed with serum glucose.

A. **Hypoglycemia is <40 mg/dL for first 48 hours, thereafter < 50 mg/dL.** It may occur because of an inadequate glucose infusion rate or a physiologic lack of glycogen stores. Additionally, pathologic states such as sepsis, cold stress, or hyperinsulinemia need to be considered.

B. **Hyperglycemia >150 mg/dL.** This can cause osmotic glycosuria, resulting in excessive fluid loss. Hyperglycemia may be secondary to increased glucose infusion rate or pathologic causes such as sepsis, necrotizing enterocolitis (NEC), intraventricular hemorrhage (IVH), or a stress response. Determine the underlying etiology and recalculate glucose administration. Treatment with insulin infusion is *controversial*. An alternative is to decrease the glucose infusion rate (GIR); maintaining glucose infusion as low as 1.5 mg/kg/min has been demonstrated to provide adequate glucose for cerebral metabolism while not affecting proteolysis and protein turnover.

V. **Calcium.** Serum calcium should be monitored daily. Hypocalcemia in preterm infants is a serum calcium <6 mg/dL. Some institutions also evaluate ionized calcium. In our institution, we provide daily maintenance calcium along with total parenteral nutrition soon after birth (eg, 2 mg of calcium gluconate/mL IV solution). Asymptomatic hypocalcemia is not treated with additional calcium because it resolves with time. Symptomatic hypocalcemia is treated with calcium salts (for dosage, see Chapter 148). This decrease usually happens on the second day of life.

VI. **Nutrition for the metabolically stable infant**

A. **Parenteral nutrition** can be started on admission and continued until the infant is receiving sufficient enteral feeding to promote growth. Along with an adequate GIR of 4–6 mg/kg/min, amino acids are started at 2.5 g/kg/d and increased by 0.5 g/kg/d to a maximum of 3.5–4 g/kg/d.

B. **Intravenous lipids (20%)** should be started by 24 hours of age; start with 0.5 to 1 g/kg/d and increase by 0.5 g/kg/d every 24–48 hours up to 3 g/kg/d while monitoring triglyceride levels. Septic and thrombocytopenic infants require caution before advancing lipids. A generally acceptable safe triglyceride level is <200 mg/dL.

C. **Early feeds of small amounts of breast milk or premature formulas (10–20 mL/kg/d)** can promote gut development, characterized by increased gut growth, villous hypertrophy, digestive enzyme secretion, and enhanced motility. This approach is called **trophic feedings.** The decision to either advance or maintain trophic feedings at a constant level should take into account the clinical status of the infant. Trophic feeds should be started with maternal or donor breast milk. The incidence of infection, NEC, and retinopathy of prematurity is decreased when breast milk is used. Mothers should be provided information regarding the benefits of breast milk and should be encouraged to pump their breasts regularly. Once feedings are established, the breast milk can be fortified with supplements. If breast milk is not available, premature formulas can be used.

D. **Controversy** exists with regard to feeding infants while undergoing pharmacologic treatment for PDA closure and during blood transfusions.

VII. Respiratory support. ELBW infants have underdeveloped muscles of ventilation. Many of these infants initially require support by mechanical ventilation; however, others, if vigorous, may be supported with CPAP or high-flow nasal cannula (HFNC).

   A. Endotracheal intubation
   1. **Type of endotracheal tube (ETT).** When possible, use an ETT with 1-cm markings on the side. The internal diameter (ID) of the tube should routinely be 2.5 or 3.0 mm, according to body weight:
       a. <500–1000 g. 2.5 mm ID.
       b. 1000–1250 g. 3.0-mm ID.
   2. **ETT placement.** Described in detail in Chapter 29. Confirm proper placement by a chest radiograph study, performed with the infant's head in the midline position, noting the marking at the gum. *Note:* In ELBW infants, the carina tends to be slightly higher than T_4. As a means of subsequently checking proper tube position, on every shift the nurse responsible for the infant should check and record the numbers or letters at the gum line.

   B. Mechanical ventilation. With the advancement of ventilation technology, various modes are available, including volume ventilation, pressure support, and high-frequency ventilation. Ventilation applied appropriately assists the clinician in avoiding overexpansion of the lung or atelectasis.
   1. **Conventional ventilation.** Tiny infants respond to a wide range of ventilator settings. Some do relatively well on 20–30 cycles/min; others require 50–60 cycles/min with inspiratory times ranging from 0.25–0.35 seconds. The goal is to use minimal pressure and tidal volume for optimal expansion of the lung, avoiding volu-trauma and atelectasis. Seek to maintain mechanical breath tidal volumes of 4–6 mL/kg; this often may be achieved with as little as 8–12 cm inspiratory pressure and 3–5 cm positive end-expiratory pressure. Pressures can be kept to a minimum by allowing permissive hypercapnea (pH 7.25–7.32, Pco_2 45–60 mm Hg). The following conventional ventilator support guidelines are offered for the initiation of respiratory care. Each tiny infant requires frequent reassessment and revision of settings and parameters. Recommended initial settings for pressure-limited time-cycled ventilators in tiny infants are as follows (see also Chapter 8):
       a. **Rate.** 20–60 (usually 30) breaths/min.
       b. **Inspiratory time.** 0.25–0.35 seconds.
       c. **Peak inspiratory pressure (PIP).** Select PIP allowing optimal expansion of lungs.
       d. **Fio₂.** As required to maintain O_2 saturation 88–92%.
       e. **Flow rate.** 6–8 L/min.
       f. **Synchronized intermittent mandatory ventilation (SIMV) and volume/pressure control ventilators.** These have internal controls that adjust flow delivery. Current ventilators have incorporated enhancements for pressure support, resulting in increased triggering sensitivity, shortened response times, reduced flow acceleration, and improved breath termination parameters.
   2. **High-frequency ventilation.** Uses small (less than dead space) tidal volumes and extremely rapid rates. The advantage of delivering small tidal volumes is that it can be done at relatively low pressures, reducing the risk of barotrauma. A slight disadvantage is that infant positioning is restricted.
   3. **Nasal CPAP (nCPAP).** Some ELBW infants may not require mechanical ventilation, whereas others may require ventilation for a short period of time for surfactant replacement. nCPAP has become a mainstay of respiratory management in these infants, initiating soon after birth. Infants requiring intubation and mechanical ventilation should be transitioned to nCPAP as clinical condition allows. nCPAP helps maintain lung expansion and improves oxygenation without significant barotrauma. Care should be taken to use nasal prongs appropriately to prevent nasal injuries and septal breakdown. A gel form of normal saline can help keep nasal passages moist and prevent such injuries.

4. **High-flow nasal cannula (HFNC).** Nasal flows >1 L using blended gases are used as an alternative to NCPAP in the management of respiratory distress and apnea of prematurity. There are insufficient data to establish its safety and efficacy; thus caution should be used for this population, and it should be reserved for stable infants.

C. **Monitoring respiratory status**
   1. **Oxygenation**
      a. **Blood gas sampling.** Arterial catheterization (see Chapter 23 for percutaneous arterial catheterization or Chapter 24 for umbilical arterial catheterization) should be performed for frequent blood gas sampling. As the infant becomes clinically stable, frequency of laboratory testing should be decreased to minimize blood loss and the need for blood transfusions.
         i. **Desirable arterial blood gas values**
            (a) **Pao_2.** 45–60 mm Hg.
            (b) **$Paco_2$.** 45–60 mm Hg.
            (c) **pH.** 7.25–7.32 is acceptable.
         ii. **Abnormal blood gas values.** Indicate the need for assessment including ETT placement, chest wall movement, effectiveness of ventilation, ventilator malfunction, assessment for pneumothorax, and need for suction. Actions may include immediate chest radiographs, chest wall transillumination (see Chapters 11 and 40), and repeat blood gas determinations.
      b. **Continuous O_2 monitoring.** Should also be performed, preferably by pulse oximetry. To prevent skin breakdown, pulse oximetry sites should be changed every 8 hours and a protective barrier placed under the probe site. The O_2 mixture should be adjusted to maintain the pulse oximeter reading between 88% and 92% hemoglobin O_2 saturation. Excess oxygenation must be avoided in this group of infants. Failure to closely regulate the administration of O_2 can contribute to the development of retinopathy of prematurity and bronchopulmonary dysplasia.
   2. **Chest radiograph**
      a. **Indications**
         i. Abnormal change in blood gas values
         ii. Adjustment of the ETT (to confirm proper positioning)
         iii. Sudden change in the infant's status
         iv. Significant increase in O_2 requirement or frequent desaturations
      b. **Technique.** A chest radiograph should be taken with the infant's head in the midline position to check for ETT placement.
      c. **Radiograph evaluation.** Check the chest radiograph for expansion of the lung, chest wall, and diaphragm. Overexpansion (exhibited by hyperlucent lungs and diaphragm below the ninth rib) and underventilation (exhibited by hazy, white lung field—atelectasis) must be avoided. If overexpansion is present, differentiate between volu-trauma and air trapping based on the age of the infant and underlying disease process. Consider decreasing the peak airway pressure if volu-trauma is suspected. Under-expansion can be treated with the use of CPAP or increasing pressures (peak airway pressure or positive end expiratory pressure) via the ventilator.

D. **Suctioning.** Should be done on an as-needed basis. The need for suctioning can be determined with the use of flow-volume loop monitoring, which can illustrate restricted airflow caused by secretions.
   1. **Assessment of the need for suctioning.** The nurse or physician should consider the following:
      a. **Breath sounds.** Wet or diminished breath sounds may indicate secretions obstructing the airways and the need for suctioning.
      b. **Blood gas values.** If significant increase in $Paco_2$, consider ETT malposition, secretions blocking the airway passages, inadequate ventilation, prior bicarbonate/acetate

administration, or pain. Suctioning should be considered to clear the airways and avoid the "ball-valve" effect of thick secretions.

    c. **Airway monitoring.** By using airflow sensors and continuous computer graphic screen displays, abnormal waveforms indicative of accumulating secretions or airway blockage can be easily seen, and immediate steps can be taken to clear the airway.

    d. **Visible secretions in the ETT.**

    e. **Loss of chest wall movement.**

  2. **Suctioning technique**

    a. **In-line suctioning is recommended to minimize airway contamination.** Suctioning should be done only to the depth of the ETT. Use a suctioning guide or a marked (1-cm increments) suction catheter.

    b. **Suctioning without lavage solution is recommended.** An exception is the use of warm sterile normal saline lavage for thick secretions.

    c. **Suction should be regulated.** 80–100 mm Hg for in-line suction (closed system) and 60–80 mm Hg (open system).

E. **Extubation**

  1. **Preextubation.** Consider use of caffeine citrate loading as it improves respiratory drive and reduced length of time on mechanical ventilation. Recent reports also indicate caffeine to have neuroprotective effects when started at birth.

  2. **Indications.** When an ELBW infant has been weaned to a mean airway pressure of 6 cm H_2O and a low (30%) FIO_2, extubation should be considered. Most infants >26 weeks and 700 g birthweight can be extubated in the first 72 hours. These are the other indications for extubation:

    a. **Ventilator rate ≤10 breaths/min**

    b. **Regular spontaneous respiratory rate**

  3. **Postextubation care.** Frequent observation of breathing patterns, respiratory effort, auscultation of the chest, monitoring of vital signs, and blood gas analysis are necessary. After extubation, the infant is placed on CPAP or HFNC with blended O_2. Some neonatologists suggest that extubation to nasal prong or mask CPAP has beneficial effects on respiratory function and the prevention of atelectasis.

F. **Vitamin A.** Vitamin A as a mode of therapy for decreasing chronic lung disease in ELBW infants is well established in clinical trials. Dosing should begin the first week of life, 5000 IU intramuscularly (IM) 3 times per week for 4 weeks. Some institutions are reluctant in using this therapy because of the frequency of IM injections. Vitamin A delivery via IV fluids is not effective because it binds to the tubing.

VIII. **Surfactant.** Some literature supports early administration of surfactant during the first 4 hours of life to decrease chronic lung disease. Recent research supports early CPAP in the delivery room over prophylactic surfactant. Several preparations of surfactant are available; some have the advantage of smaller volume and dosing intervals. It should be administered according to the manufacturer's recommendations. Administration criteria for surfactant include absence of antenatal steroids, increased oxygen demand >30%, and a radiograph consistent with surfactant deficiency (see also Chapter 8).

IX. **PDA.** Incidence of persistent PDA is inversely proportional to gestational age. Infants should be monitored clinically for signs and symptoms of PDA. An echocardiogram is recommended to rule out other structural heart defects and confirmation of PDA when concerned. Efforts should be made to minimize the risk of PDA. **Overhydration must be avoided.** Up to 30% of PDAs spontaneously close. Currently it is unclear whether a conservative, pharmacologic or surgical approach is advantageous. If the decision is made to treat a hemodynamically significant PDA, indomethacin or ibuprofen is generally accepted (see Chapter 118). Renal and GI adverse effects are less common with administration of ibuprofen or with slower infusion rates of indomethacin. Indomethacin can also be considered for IVH prophylaxis, although its safety and benefit remain **controversial**. Concurrent administration of indomethacin and steroids should be avoided because of the associated risk for spontaneous intestinal perforation.

X. Transfusion. ELBW infants usually have low red blood cell volume, with a hematocrit <40%, and they are subjected to frequent phlebotomies. Most centers keep the hematocrit between 35% and 40%. Lower values may be acceptable if the infant is asymptomatic. Each institution should have transfusion guidelines established to minimize donor exposure and the number of transfusions.

XI. Skin care. Maintenance of intact skin is the tiny infant's most effective barrier against infection, insensible fluid loss, protein loss, and blood loss and provides for more effective body temperature control. Minimal use of tape is recommended because the infant's skin is fragile, and tears often result with removal. **Zinc-based tape** can be used. Alternatives to tape include the use of a **hydrogel adhesive**, which removes easily with water. Hydrogel adhesive products also include electrodes, temperature probe covers, and masks. In addition, the very thin skin of the tiny infant allows absorption of many substances. Skin care must focus on maintaining skin integrity and minimizing exposure to topical agents. Transparent adhesive dressings can be used over areas of bone prominence, such as the knees or elbows, to prevent skin friction breakdown and under adhesive monitoring devices that are frequently moved. Use of humidity helps maintain skin integrity until skin is mature (2–3 weeks). Humidity can be weaned as tolerated after 2 weeks. *Note:* **When the skin appears dry, thickened, and no longer shiny or translucent (usually in 10–14 days), these skin care recommendations and procedures may be modified or discontinued.**

A. Use a hydrogel skin probe or cut servo-control skin probe covers to the smallest size possible (try a 2-cm diameter circle). This will help to reduce skin damage resulting from the adhesive.

B. Monitoring of O_2 therapy is best accomplished by use of a pulse oximeter. The probe must be placed carefully to prevent pressure sores. The site should be rotated a minimum of every 8 hours. Alternative means of O_2 monitoring include umbilical catheter blood sampling.

C. Urine bags and blood pressure cuffs. These **should not be used routinely** because of adhesives and sharp plastic edge cuts. Bladder aspirations should be avoided.

D. Eye ointment for gonococcal prophylaxis. Should be applied per routine admission plan. If the eyelids are fused, apply along the lash line.

E. Cleansing for required procedures (eg, umbilical artery or chest tube). Use minimal povidone-iodine solution to cleanse the area. After the procedure is completed, the solution should be sponged off immediately with warm sterile water. The use of chlorhexidine in the ELBW infant is **controversial** and should be used per institution guidelines.

F. Attach ECG electrodes using as little adhesive as possible. Options include the following:
    1. Consider using limb electrodes.
    2. Consider water-activated gel electrodes.
    3. Use electrodes that have been trimmed down and secured with a flexible dressing material.

G. An initial bath. Not necessary, but if HIV is a consideration, those infants should receive a mild soap bath when the infant's temperature has stabilized. Warm sterile water baths are given only when needed during the next 2 weeks of life.

H. Avoid the use of anything that dries out the skin (eg, soaps and alcohol). Bonding agents should be avoided.

I. Sterile water-soaked cotton balls. Helpful for removing adhesive tape, probe covers, and electrode covers.

H. **Readmission.** Late preterms were almost twice as likely to require readmission to the hospital. Jaundice and infection were the most common diagnoses. The strongest risk factor for readmission was breast-feeding at discharge. Recent studies demonstrated that early follow-up visits or home nursing visits were effective at reducing rates of readmission.

I. **Respiratory syncytial virus (RSV) infection.** Late preterm infants have an increased susceptibility to RSV infection due to incomplete lung development and impaired immunity from immaturity and the relative lack of passively acquired maternal antibodies. **The risk of RSV bronchiolitis in infants born between 32 and 36 weeks is similar to those born before 32 weeks.** The risk of hospitalization due to RSV infection is twice as high in late preterm compared to term infants. Late preterms span from 34 0/7 to 36 6/7 weeks, and the AAP recommendations for palivizumab prophylaxis only goes up to 35 weeks only. Late preterm infants from 34 to 35 weeks with risk factors or those with chronic lung disease or congenital heart disease potentially qualify for treatment. The uncomplicated baby born at 34–35 weeks must also have either a sibling <5 years old or be attending day care, according to the AAP guidelines. Since few late preterm infants qualify for palivizumab, precautions such as decreasing contact with sick individuals and good hand washing by those handling these infants are of great importance. See Chapter 125.

J. **Long-term outcomes.** By comparison, moderately low birthweight infants (1500–2500 g) are more likely than infants >2500 g to have a special health care need, a chronic condition, a learning disability, or attention deficit hyperactivity disorder (ADHD). Moderately low birthweight infants are at increased risk for poor health outcomes.

IV. **Recommendations for management.** Iatrogenic prematurity should be prevented by prolonging pregnancy whenever feasible. To that end, the American College of Obstetrics and Gynecology have come out with recommendations that prohibit induction or scheduled repeat cesarean delivery before 39 weeks, to which most hospitals now adhere. Because late preterm infants are at risk for certain medical problems, previously outlined, specific management strategies should be developed for both their initial hospitalization as well as their care after discharge. Early monitoring of respiratory status, temperature, feeding ability, bilirubin, and glucose levels are critical. The AAP has issued specific recommendations for minimum discharge criteria for late preterm infants. In addition to those things performed for term infants, the late preterm infant requires:

A. **Accurate gestational age assessment.**

B. **Individualizing the time of discharge** based on the baby's condition with regard to temperature stability and adequacy of feeding.

C. **Identification of a medical home** following discharge.

D. **Normal vital signs for 12 hours before discharge.**

E. **Passing of one stool spontaneously.**

F. **The absence of excessive weight loss.**

G. **Screening for hyperbilirubinemia.**

H. **A car seat study** for apnea, bradycardia, or oxygen desaturation.

I. **Formal breast-feeding education** when applicable.

J. **Discharge follow-up.** Strategies should include closer follow-up of issues such as weight gain and development, as well as good family support.

Selected References

Adamkin DH. Feeding problems in the late preterm infant. *Clin Perinatol.* 2006;33:831–837.

Coffman S. Late preterm infants and risk for RSV. *MCN.* 2009;34(6):378–384.

Colin AA, McEvoy C, Castile RG. Respiratory morbidity and lung function in preterm infants of 32 to 36 weeks' gestational age. *Pediatrics.* 2010;126(1):115–128.

Engle WA, Tomashek KM, Wallman C, et al. "Late preterm" infants: a population at risk. *Pediatrics.* 2007;120(6):1390–1401.

Lee YM, Cleary-Goldman J, D'Alton ME. Multiple gestation and late preterm (near-term) deliveries. *Semin Perinatol.* 2006;30:103–112.

Medoff-Cooper B, Bakewell-Sach S, Buos-Frank ME, et al. The AWHONN Near Term Initiative: a conceptual framework for optimizing health for near-term infants. *JOGNN.* 2005;34(6):666–671.

Meier PP, Furman LM, Degenhardt M. Increased lactation risk for late preterm infants and mothers: evidence and management strategies to protect breastfeeding. *J Midwifery Women's Health.* 2007;52(6):579–587.

Morse SB, Zheng H, Tang Y, et al. Early school-age outcomes of late preterm infants. *Pediatrics.* 2009;123(4):e622–e629.

Petrini JR, Dias T, McCormick MC, et al. Increased risk of averse neurologic development for late preterm infants. *J Pediatr.* 2009;154:169–176.

Raju TN, Higgins RD, Stark AR, et al. Optimizing care and outcome for late-preterm (near-term) infants: a summary of the workshop sponsored by the NICHD. *Pediatrics.* 2006;118(3):1207–1214.

Tomashek KM, Shapiro-Mendoza CK, Weiss J, et al. Early discharge among late preterm and term newborns and risk of neonatal morbidity. *Semin Perinatol.* 2006;30:61–68.

14 Pain in the Neonate

Before the 1980s, it was a common belief that preterm infants lacked the neurodevelopmental capacity to feel pain. This resulted in severe undertreatment of pain in the neonate during their hospitalization. Although neonatology has made strides in the past 20 years to understand pain, it remains challenged to effectively assess and treat the various types of pain experienced in the neonatal intensive care unit (NICU).

I. **Physiology of pain in the neonate**
   A. **Definition.** Pain has been defined by the International Association for the Study of Pain as "an unpleasant sensory and emotional experience associated with actual or potential tissue damage or described in such terms of such damage." When an infant responds to pain, it involves a collection of biochemical, physiologic, and behavioral reactions. There are many different layers of an infant's response that can be understood by gestational age and development. Noxious stimuli lead to tissue damage, causing the release of sensitizing substances such as prostaglandins, bradykinin, serotonin, substance P, and histamine. These chemicals produce an impulse that is then transmitted to the nociceptive pathways. Nociception refers to the reflex movement occurring with exposure to noxious stimuli that does not require cortical involvement or the ability to perceive pain.
   B. **Development.** Development of sensory nerve endings begins very early in the process of nociception and follows as:
      1. **7.5–15 weeks' gestation.** Peripheral cutaneous sensory receptors develop in the perioral, facial, palmar, and abdominal areas and proximal extremities.
      2. **8–19 weeks' gestation.** Spinal reflexes are able to respond to noxious stimuli, and neurons populate the dorsal root ganglion.
      3. **20 weeks' gestation.** Mucous membranes and remaining cutaneous areas are populated with sensory nerve endings.
      4. **20–24 weeks' gestation.** Thalamic afferents involved in conscious perception of pain reach the subplate zone and the cortical plate.
      5. **23–27 weeks' gestation.** Thalamic afferents reach the visual cortex.
      6. **26–28 weeks' gestation.** Thalamic afferents reach the auditory cortical plate.

C. **Repeated exposure to noxious stimuli.** This can cause physiologic and behavioral disorganization, leading to changes in the neurodevelopmental system of the infant. This may cause the infant to develop an inability to respond to pain or an exaggerated physiologic response to painful stimuli in the future.

II. **Types of pain in the neonate**

A. **Birth trauma.** Neonatal pain associated with birth trauma is typically a result of vacuum-assisted births. Some babies may show signs of bruising on the face or head simply as a result of the trauma of passing through the birth canal. Forceps deliveries can leave temporary marks or bruises on the baby's face and head. Cephalohematomas are more common with forceps delivery or vacuum extraction. Tylenol may be used for the treatment of associated pain. Collarbone fractures are the most common birth-related fracture. If the fracture is painful, limiting movement of the arm and shoulder may be helpful.

B. **Acute procedural pain.** The frequency of painful procedures in the NICU can range from 5–15 per day. **The most optimal method of pain control is to minimize the amount of painful procedures. Painful procedures performed in the NICU** include endotracheal tube (ETT) suctioning, intubation, mechanical ventilation, chest tube insertion, retinopathy of prematurity (ROP) examinations, central line placement, intravenous (IV) placement, heelsticks, lumbar puncture, circumcision, patent ductus arteriosus (PDA) ligation, and peritoneal drain placement.

C. **Acute postoperative pain.** Postsurgical pain remains an issue in the NICU. The largest risk with postsurgical pain is undertreating. Postoperative pain protocols help standardize practice between health care professionals. Routine pain assessment should be performed using scales specific to postoperative or prolonged pain. **It is important to alternate pain medications for maximum pain control with minimal toxicity. Opioids are the medications of choice and can be given by continuous infusion or bolus.**

D. **Chronic pain.** Chronic pain remains to be well-defined within neonatology. Some view chronic pain as the extension of uncontrolled acute pain. Pain assessment tools should include validated measurement for chronic pain. Research needs to continue to develop in this critical area of pain.

III. **Assessment of pain in the neonate.** One of the most challenging aspects of neonatal pain is recognition of the symptoms. Careful assessment is critical when evaluating preterm infants for signs of pain. **Assessment must include physiologic as well as behavioral symptoms.**

A. **Common symptoms of pain in the neonate.** Commonly assessed symptoms of pain include **increased heart rate, changes in respiratory rate, and fluctuations in blood pressure, as well as changes in facial expression such as brow bulge, eyes squeezed shut, nasolabial furrow, crying, and increased movement.**

B. **Continued pain symptoms.** Infants experiencing prolonged pain may exhibit decreased heart rate, decreased respiratory rate, decreased oxygen consumption, lethargy, decreased perfusion, and cool extremities.

C. **Pain versus discomfort.** Differentiating between infant pain and discomfort can be challenging for health care professionals. Premature infants can exhibit minimal response to pain, especially if they are septic or physiologically stressed. Older infants who have experienced multiple incidents or prolonged pain may over or under react to pain. Lack of pain response can also be observed in infants with neurologic impairment or those who have been chemically paralyzed.

D. **Pain assessment scales.** Listed below are the four most commonly used pain scales and are compared in Table 14–1.

1. **Premature Infant Pain Profile (PIPP).** This scale addresses procedural and postoperative pain. It contains 2 physiologic indicators: heart rate and oxygen saturation. It includes 3 facial indicators (brow bulge, eye squeeze, and nasolabial furrow). Total scores of **7–12 indicate mild to moderate pain** requiring nonpharmacologic pain measures. **Scores >12 indicate moderate to severe pain** and require pharmacologic pain intervention in addition to comfort measures.

Table 14–1. COMPARISON OF COMMONLY USED PAIN SCALES

	PIPP	CRIES	NIPS	N-PASS
Facial expression	X	X	X	X
Cry	X	X	X	X
Extremities	X	X	X	X
Consolability			X	
Oxygen saturation		X	X	X
Vital signs				X
Activity state				X
Term infants	X	X	X	X
Premature infants	X	If >32 weeks	X	X

CRIES, crying, requires O_2 for SaO_2 <95%, increased vital signs, expression, sleepless; NIPS, Neonatal Infant Pain Scale; N-PASS, Neonatal Pain, Agitation, and Sedation Scale; PIPP, Premature Infant Pain Profile.

2. CRIES Neonatal Pain Assessment Tool (Crying; Requires O_2 for SaO_2 <95%; Increased vital signs; Expression; Sleepless). This scale addresses postoperative pain in 32–37 weeks' gestation infants as well as procedural pain in preterm and term neonates. It measures 5 parameters, including crying, increase in oxygen requirement, increase in vital signs, expression, and sleeplessness. Total scores range from 0–10. Scores <4 indicate mild pain requiring nonpharmacologic intervention. Scores ≥5 indicate moderate to severe pain requiring pharmacologic intervention as well as comfort measures.

3. Neonatal Infant Pain Scale (NIPS). This scale addresses procedural pain in preterm and newborn infants as well as postoperative pain. Total scores range from 0 to 7. No parameters for level of pain are included for this tool. Midlevel scoring indicates moderate to severe pain requiring pharmacologic management. It includes the assessment of 5 behaviors and 1 physiologic parameter: facial expression, crying, relaxation or tension in the arms and legs, state of arousal, and breathing pattern.

4. Neonatal Pain, Agitation, and Sedation Scale (N-PASS). This scale considers pain/agitation and sedation. It is used for both preterm and term neonates with the following types of pain: prolonged, postoperative, and mechanical ventilation. It contains 4 behavioral symptoms and 4 physiologic indicators: crying, irritability, behavioral state, extremities tone, heart rate, respiratory rate, blood pressure, and oxygen saturation. Points are added based on gestational age for a total score. Scores >3 indicate the need for nonpharmacologic or pharmacologic measures. Sedation scores between 5 and 10 are considered deep sedation.

IV. Pain intervention
   A. Nonpharmacologic. Preferable for mild procedural pain due to the short-term efficacy and absence of side effects. Most effective when combined with a reduction in lighting and sound. Not to be used in place of pharmacologic therapy with severe and chronic pain.
      1. Nonnutritive suck. The type of suck associated with a pacifier without breast milk or formula. When used in combination with oral sucrose (24%), it is effective in reducing the pain associated with heelsticks, peripheral IV catheter (PIV) placement, and ROP examinations.
      2. Positioning. A prone position can cause an improvement in breathing effort and decrease the infant's oxygen requirement.
      3. Swaddling. Wrapping an infant securely in a blanket can cause a decrease in heart rate, an increase in oxygen saturation, and an increase in ability to organize behaviors. Good to use with PIV starts, ROP examinations, and ETT suctioning.

4. **Facilitated tuck.** Holding the infant's arms and legs gently in a flexed position. Effective with PIV starts, ROP examinations, and ETT suctioning in decreasing heart rate and recovery time.

5. **Music.** Effective in infants >31 weeks' gestation. It assists with the regulation and reduction of heart rate as well as increase in oxygen saturation.

6. **Kangaroo care.** Research supports its use to decrease the pain response. It is effective for use in decreasing pain with heelsticks.

7. **Sucrose.** When combined with nonnutritive suck, shown to be very efficacious with heelsticks. Facilities should adopt a specific protocol to standardize the use of oral sucrose, which is most effective when combined with nonnutritive suck. **Dosage range is 0.012–0.12 g or 0.05–0.5 mL of a 24% solution.** Optimal pain relief is noted if given ~2 minutes before the heelstick followed by 1–2 minutes after completion. Sucrose is effective in infants >27 weeks' gestation; however, it is not approved by the US Food and Drug Administration. **Safety regarding repeated dosages of sucrose has been investigated and has been shown to demonstrate ongoing effectiveness.** Nonetheless, caution should be taken in administering multiple doses, and administration should be limited to the management of acute procedural pain.

B. **Pharmacologic.** Most often light pain and moderate pain of short duration are best dealt with by nonpharmacologic pain measures. Pain assessment scores >12 indicate moderate to severe pain and strongly suggest pharmacologic pain intervention along with comfort measures. **Procedures that require the use of pharmacologic pain intervention** include intubation, mechanical ventilation, chest tube insertion, central line placement, lumbar puncture, circumcision, PDA ligation, and placement of peritoneal drains. Commonly used pain relief drugs in neonates are (see Chapter 148 for specific drug dosing information) as follows: **topical:** EMLA (eutectic mixture of lidocaine and prilocaine) cream; **infiltration:** 0.5–1% lidocaine; **systemic:** morphine, fentanyl, diazepam, midazolam.

V. **Potentially better pain management practices.** As identified by the Neonatal Intensive Care Quality Improvement Collaborative include the following:

A. Reduce the frequency of avoidable painful procedures such as ETT suctioning and heelsticks.

B. Develop protocol for standardization of sucrose administration.

C. Perform frequent pain assessment.

D. Implement strategies to manage pain during the following: heelsticks, peripheral vascular procedures, circumcision, nonemergent intubation, mechanical ventilation.

E. Implement strategies to manage pain during the postoperative period.

F. Implement strategies to wean neonates effectively and safely from opiates.

VI. **Conclusion.** Pain continues to be an emerging field of study within the discipline of neonatology. Much research is needed regarding the ongoing assessment and treatment of neonatal pain. Heath care professionals need to diligently document pain assessment and follow-up scores postintervention to insure proper pain management. Clinical practice guidelines need to be developed for the neonatal community at large for standardization of practice. Research continues to evolve to support accurate assessment of pain in the neonate. Monitoring skin conduction scores during painful procedures is an area of current investigation. Research is also focused on measuring the impact of pain on the infant's brain. Measurements would include values during the experience of noxious stimuli and the long-term impact on the neurodevelopment of the infant. It is through continuous research and commitment to reducing the experience of pain for the neonate that we will fully understand and effectively treat the neonate while supporting their viability.

Selected References

American Academy of Pediatrics, Committee on Fetus and Newborn and Section on Surgery, Section on Anesthesiology and Pain Medicine, Canadian Pediatric Society and Fetus and Newborn Committee. Prevention and management of pain in the neonate: an update. *Pediatrics*. 2006;118:2231–2241. Reaffirmed May 2010.

Bouza H. The impact of pain in the immature brain. *J Matern Fetal Neonatal Med*. 2009;22: 722–732.

Epstein EG. Moral obligations of nurses and physicians in neonatal end-of-life care. *Nurs Ethics*. 2010;17:577–589.

Harrison D, Loughnan P, Manias E, Johnston L. Utilization of analgesics, sedatives, and pain scores in infants with a prolonged hospitalization: a prospective descriptive cohort study. *Int J Nurs Stud*. 2009;46:624–632.

Sharek PJ, Powers R, Koehn A, Anand KJ. Evaluation and development of potentially better practices to improve pain management of neonates. *Pediatrics*. 2006;118(suppl 2): S78–S86.

Walden M, Carrier C. The ten commandments of pain assessment and management in preterm neonates. *Crit Care Nurs Clin North Am*. 2009;21:235–252.

Yamada J, Stinson J, Lamba J, Dickson A, McGrath PJ, Stevens B. A review of systematic reviews on pain interventions in hospitalized infants. *Pain Res Manage*. 2008;13:413–420.

15 Newborn Screening

I. **Newborn screening (NBS).** This is a population-based system for the identification and early treatment of potentially devastating medical conditions. In the United States, this screening is mandated in every state, but the disorders included in the screening panels vary. A list of the screening tests provided by each state can be found on the National Newborn Screening and Genetics Resource Center website at http://genes-r-us.uthscsa.edu. An expert panel commissioned by the American College of Medical Genetics (ACMG) has recommended 29 conditions on newborn screening panels (Table 15–1). This chapter addresses selected disorders included in most state newborn screen panels, as well as special considerations related to discharge planning and follow-up. The American Academy of Pediatrics (AAP) has published newborn screening FACT sheets that address appropriate testing methods, follow-up, and diagnostic testing for all 29 disorders recommended by the ACMG.

II. **Timing and special considerations**
   A. **An initial specimen.** It is typically drawn between 24 and 72 hours of life.
   B. **Obtain the specimen prior to blood transfusion.** It is recommended practice to obtain a specimen prior to blood transfusion if a specimen has not already been sent.
   C. **Invalid results.** Any results judged to be invalid by the performing laboratory or any results that are reported as positive must have a repeat specimen.
      1. **Antibiotics.** It is important to note that antibiotic administration will increase the chance of a false-positive NBS, which will require a repeat NBS to ensure that the patient does not have the underlying disorder.
      2. **Preterm infants.** These infants are much more likely to have an abnormal newborn screen due to hepatic immaturity, parenteral nutrition, blood transfusions, and delayed enteral nutrition, which will frequently require these patients to have multiple NBS sent during their NICU course.

Table 15–1. **ESTIMATED INCIDENCE OF 29 DISORDERS (28 GENETIC/METABOLIC CONDITIONS AND HEARING SCREENING) RECOMMENDED BY ACMG FOR INCLUSION ON NEWBORN SCREENING PANELS**

	Estimated Incidence
Amino acid metabolism disorders	
Phenylketonuria (PKU)	1:10,000
Argininosuccinic acidemia (ASA)	1:70,000
Tyrosinemia type 1 (TYR 1)	<1:100,000
Citrullinemia (CIT)	1:100,000
Maple syrup urine disease (MSUD)	1:185,000
Homocystinuria (HCY)	1:300,000
Organic acid metabolism disorders	
Glutaric acidemia type I (GA I)	1:40,000
Methylmalonic acidemia due to mutase deficiency (MMA)	1:48,000
3-Methylcrotonyl-CoA carboxylase deficiency (3MCC)	1:50,000
Propionic acidemia (PROP)	1:75,000
Beta-ketothiolase deficiency (BKT)	<1:100,000
Hydroxymethylglutaric aciduria (HMG)	<1:100,000
Isovaleric acidemia (IVA)	<1:100,000
Methylmalonic acidemia cblA and cblB (Cbl A, B)	<1:100,000
Multiple carboxylase deficiency (MCD)	<1:100,000
Fatty acid oxidation disorders	
Medium-chain acyl-CoA dehydrogenase deficiency (MCAD)	1:10,000–20,000
Long-chain 3-OH acyl-CoA dehydrogenase deficiency (LCHAD)	1:100,000
Very long-chain acyl-CoA dehydrogenase deficiency (VLCAD)	1:100,000
Trifunctional protein deficiency (TFP)	Unknown
Carnitine uptake defect (CUD)	1:40,000
Hemoglobinopathies	
Sickle cell anemia (Hb SS)	1:2,500
Hb S/C disease (Hb S/C)	>1:25,000
Hb S/beta-thalassemia (Hbs/βTh)	>1:50,000
Others	
Hearing loss (HEAR)	2–3:1,000
Congenital hypothyroidism (CH)	1:3,000–4,000
Cystic fibrosis (CF)	1:3,500
Congenital adrenal hyperplasia (CAH)	1:15,000
Classical galactosemia (GALT)	1:47,000
Biotinidase deficiency (BIOT)	1:110,000

ACMG, American College of Medical Genetics.

III. Selected disorders included in newborn screening panels
   A. Amino acid metabolism disorders
      1. Phenylketonuria (PKU)
         a. **Screening process.** Increased concentrations of phenylalanine in the blood can be detected using fluorometric analysis and tandem mass spectrometry (sometimes referred to as MS/MS).
         b. **Follow-up.** Children diagnosed with PKU should receive diets with reduced phenylalanine. Subspecialty follow-up should be arranged with a nutritionist as well as with a pediatrician who specializes in metabolic disorders.

B. **Organic acid metabolism disorders**
   1. **Methylmalonic acidemia (MMA)**
      a. **Screening.** Elevated levels of propionylcarnitine are detected by tandem mass spectrometry.
      b. **Follow-up.** Abnormal screening results should be followed with plasma and/or urine organic acid analysis, which can establish the presence or absence of methylmalonic acid. A high level of methylmalonic acid is diagnostic. Treatment includes the institution of a low-protein diet. Follow-up care should be arranged with a pediatrician who specializes in metabolic disorders, as well as with a nutritionist. MMA has an autosomal recessive inheritance pattern. Genetic counseling should be provided.
C. **Fatty acid oxidation disorders**
   1. **Medium-chain acyl-CoA dehydrogenase deficiency (MCAD)**
      a. **Screening.** Tandem mass spectrometry is the screening tool of choice for MCAD. Levels of octanoylcarnitine are higher during the first 3 days of life, so screening is best performed in the newborn period. Prematurity, immaturity of hepatic function, and total parenteral nutrition can result in abnormal amino acid results, necessitating a repeat specimen.
      b. **Follow-up.** Diagnostic testing is done though plasma acylcarnitine analysis and urinary organic acid analysis. Molecular analysis to determine the particular gene involved provides prognostic information.
D. **Hemoglobinopathies**
   1. **Sickle cell anemia/disease**
      a. **Screening.** Hemoglobin variants are detected using isoelectric focusing, high-performance liquid chromatography (HPLC), or cellulose acetate electrophoresis. Retesting of abnormal screen samples is usually done by electrophoretic technique, HPLC, immunologic testing, or DNA assays. Blood transfusions that include red cell components can invalidate the screen results, so initial screening should be done prior to transfusion. (Plasma, platelets, and albumin transfusions do not affect screening results.)
      b. **Follow-up.** The majority of states require follow-up screening on normal screens 90 days after the last transfusion. Confirmatory testing should be done on abnormal screens before 2 months of age. A pediatric hematologist should be involved in follow-up care.
E. **Other**
   1. **Congenital hypothyroidism (CH).** See also Chapter 140.
      a. **Screening.** The primary measurement for most screens is thyrotropin/thyroid stimulating hormone (TSH) and T_4. Optimal timing is between 48 hours and 4 days of age. False-positive elevations in TSH may occur in infants screened at <48 hours of age due to a thyrotropin surge after birth. This surge may be delayed in preterm infants. Likewise, preterm infants with hypothyroidism have delayed elevation of TSH levels, presumably due to immaturity of the hypothalamic-pituitary-thyroid axis. Therefore, it may be prudent to consider a second routine screening on preterm infants between 2 and 6 weeks of age. Preterm infants also typically have lower T_4 levels, resulting in more false-positive results. Screening for hypothyroidism is unaffected by diet or transfusion, except in the case of total exchange transfusion.
      b. **Follow-up.** Abnormal screening results should be immediately followed up with TSH testing and free T_4. Etiology of hypothyroidism can be determined using thyroid ultrasound, thyroid uptake and scan, and/or thyrotropin-binding inhibitor immunoglobulin (in cases of suspected transient hypothyroidism related to maternal autoimmune thyroid disease). Diagnostic testing to determine etiology is optional but does not alter treatment, and it should never delay treatment. Prompt consultation with a pediatric endocrinologist and early initiation of adequate thyroid replacement therapy is paramount to improving lifelong outcome.

2. **Cystic fibrosis (CF)**
   a. **Screening.** It is estimated that ~15% of patients with CF have had a neonatal presentation, making CF an ideal disorder to be evaluated through NBS. Determination of sweat chloride concentrations is the hallmark diagnostic test for CF; however, it is impractical for most newborn infants, especially preterm infants of <36 weeks' gestation or a birthweight of <2000 g, and is not recommended. Alternative screening tests include immunoreactive serum trypsinogen (IRT) and fecal elastase-1. More specifically, genotyping can identify the more common mutations involving the CF transmembrane regulator, of which the ΔF508 mutation is the most frequently identified. Neonates diagnosed with meconium ileus (MI) should eventually have a sweat chloride test performed, due to the possibility of a false-negative IRT; 80–90% of patients with MI will have CF.
   b. **Follow-up.** Neonates who have a positive screen will require DNA testing to evaluate for their particular gene mutation. Additional follow-up should include referral to a pediatric pulmonologist for all infants who have a positive CF screening test or who have equivocal results on their sweat chloride test.
3. **Biotinidase deficiency (BIOT)**
   a. **Screening.** Filter paper spotted with whole blood is assessed for biotinidase activity by a semiquantitative colorimetric method. Up to 20% of patients with symptomatic biotinidase can be missed if screened with tandem mass spectrometry, so this methodology should not be used.
   b. **Follow-up.** Some states require a repeat specimen between 1 week and 4 months after the last red blood cell transfusion. A serum specimen for quantitative measurement of biotinidase activity should be obtained if the screening results were positive. Children with BIOT should be followed by someone who specializes in metabolic disorders for biotin therapy.
4. **Galactosemia (GALT)**
   a. **Screening.** Three different enzyme deficiencies may result in GALT. **Classic galactosemia**, which is the most common form, results from the deficiency of galactose 1-phosphate (GALT). **Galactokinase (GALK) deficiency** and **galactose-4-epimerase (GALE) deficiency** also result in galactosemia but are very rare. Screening tests vary by state and measure galactose, galactose 1-phosphate plus galactose, and/or GALT enzyme deficiency, which can be done using MS/MS. The GALT enzyme test is performed using red blood cells and is diagnostic only for classic galactosemia. It is not affected by the infant's diet but rather by red blood cell transfusions. Test results of galactose and galactose 1-phosphate are influenced by the infant's diet, so the infant should receive a galactose-containing formula or breast milk prior to screening.
   b. **Follow-up.** A false-negative result may persist for 3 months after a red blood cell transfusion, so a repeat test is needed 90 days after the last transfusion. All infants with positive screening results should receive a nutrition consultation and be placed on a galactose-restricted diet pending definitive diagnostic testing. Breast-milk feedings are contraindicated for infants with galactosemia, and soy-based formulas are commonly used. Quantitative analysis of galactokinase (GALK) and galactose-4-epimerase (GALE) identifies these less common types of galactosemia.
5. **Congenital adrenal hyperplasia (CAH)**
   a. **Screening.** Measurement of 17-hydroxyprogesterone (17-OHP) is performed through a variety of reagents/immunoassays or tandem mass spectrometry. A high rate of false-positive results occurs in samples taken at <1 day of age. Normal 17-OHP levels are affected by birthweight and gestational age; thus, prematurity and illness can result in false-positive screen results. Preterm infants tend to have higher levels. Levels are not affected by transfusions if they are drawn several hours after the transfusion. However, some states require

a repeat specimen with the timing of the repeat screen varying from 72 hours to 4 months after transfusion.

b. **Follow-up.** Abnormal screening results should be followed with a serum 17-OHP level. Serum electrolytes and serum 17-OHP levels should be obtained in neonates with a disorder of sex development. An adrenocorticotropic hormone stimulation test is useful for ruling out nonclassic CAH in infants with mild elevations of 17-OHP levels. Infants with CAH should be followed by a pediatric endocrinologist.

6. **Hearing loss (HEAR)**

a. **Screening.** Universal screening should be done before 1 month of age and/or prior to initial hospital discharge. Although automated auditory brainstem response (ABR) and otoacoustic emission are the primary methods used, ABR is the recommended screening tool for infants with neonatal intensive care unit (NICU) stays >5 days because of the high risk of neural hearing loss.

b. **Follow-up**

i. **Audiologic testing and medical follow-up** should be performed prior to 3 months of age for all infants who do not pass the initial screen. Rescreening of both ears is recommended.

ii. **Infants who have one or more risk factors** should be reassessed by an audiologist no later than 24–30 months of age regardless of initial screening results. **Risk factors include the following:** family history of sensorineural hearing loss, perinatal infections, craniofacial anomalies, hyperbilirubinemia necessitating exchange transfusion, ototoxic medications including chemotherapy, treatment with extracorporeal membrane oxygenation, bacterial meningitis, mechanical ventilation, neurodegenerative disorders, syndromes known to include hearing loss, or trauma.

iii. **Infants with confirmed hearing loss** should be evaluated by a pediatric otolaryngologist, a pediatric ophthalmologist for assessment of visual acuity, and early intervention services no later than 6 months of age. A genetic consultation should also be considered.

Selected References

American College of Medical Genetics Newborn Screening Expert Group Genetics Home Reference. Genetic conditions. Lister Hill National Center for Biomedical Communications, U.S. National Library of Medicine National Institutes of Health Department of Health & Human Services: Bethesda, MD; 2007. http://ghr.nlm.nih.gov. Accessed October 24, 2012.

Joint Committee on Infant Hearing. Year 2007 position statement: principles and guidelines for early hearing detection and intervention programs. *Pediatrics.* 2007;120(4):898–921.

Levy PA. An overview of newborn screening. *J Dev Behav Pediatr.* 2010;31:622–631.

Lockwood C, Lemons J, eds. *Guidelines for Perinatal Care.* 6th ed. Elk Grove, IL: American Academy of Pediatrics & The American College of Obstetricians and Gynecologists; 2007:223–224.

Lu KD, Engmann C, Moya F, Muhlebach M. Cystic fibrosis in premature infants. *J Perinatol.* 2011;31:504–508.

Newborn Screening Authoring Committee. Newborn screening expands: recommendations for pediatricians and medical homes—implications for the system. *Pediatrics.* 2008;121:192–217.

Watson MS, Mann MY, Lloyd-Puryear MY, Rinaldo P, Howell RR, American College of Medical Genetics Newborn Screening Expert Group. Newborn screening: toward a uniform screening panel and system—executive summary. *Pediatrics.* 2006;117:S296–S307.

16 Studies for Neurologic Evaluation

Continued improvements in neuroimaging and neuromonitoring have added insight into the developing brain and helped the clinician to identify infants at risk for poor neurologic outcome. However, available techniques continue to be limited in their ability to predict neurodevelopmental outcomes accurately. Moreover, given the enormous plasticity of the neonate's brain, even significant detectable defects may result in "normal" neurodevelopmental outcomes. Nevertheless, imaging and monitoring modalities hold future promise in assisting clinicians to better identify patients at risk for neurodevelopmental sequelae.

I. Neuroimaging

A. Ultrasonography

1. Definition. Using the bone window of a fontanelle, sound waves are directed into the brain and reflected according to the echodensity of the underlying structures. The reflected waves are used to create 2- and 3-dimensional images.

2. Indication. Ultrasonography is preferred for identification and observation of germinal matrix/intraventricular hemorrhage and hydrocephalus and is valuable in detecting midline structural abnormalities, hypoxic-ischemic injury, subdural and posterior fossa hemorrhage, ventriculitis, tumors, cysts, and vascular abnormalities. Ultrasonography of the developing cingulate sulcus has been suggested to reflect gestational age (see sample studies in Chapter 11).

3. Method. A transducer is placed over the anterior fontanelle, and images are obtained in coronal and parasagittal planes. The posterior fontanelle is the preferred acoustic window for the imaging of the infratentorium, including brainstem and cerebellum. Advantages include high resolution, convenience (performed at the bedside), safety (no sedation, contrast material, or radiation), noninvasiveness, and low cost. Disadvantages include the lack of visualization of nonmidline structures, especially in the parietal regions, and the lack of differentiation between gray and white matter.

4. Results. The integrity of the following structures may be evaluated with ultrasonography: all 4 ventricles, the choroid plexus, caudate nuclei, thalamus, septum pellucidum, and corpus callosum.

B. Doppler ultrasonography

1. Definition. Doppler ultrasonography also uses a bone window to direct sound waves into the brain. Moving objects (eg, red blood cells) reflect sound waves with a shift in frequency (Doppler shift) that is proportional to their speed. These changes are measured and expressed as the pulsatility index and resistance index (RI). The angle of the probe in relation to the flow affects the Doppler shift and requires exact standards for serial measurements.

2. Indication. Knowing the cross-section of the vessel (area), Doppler ultrasonography can provide information on cerebral blood flow (CBF) and resistance. CBF (cm^3/time) = CBF velocity (cm/time) $\times$ Area (cm^2) Doppler ultrasonography is of clinical value in states of cessation of CBF (eg, brain death or cerebrovascular occlusion), states of altered vascular resistance (eg, hypoxic-ischemic encephalopathy, hydrocephalus, or arteriovenous [AV] malformation), and ductal steal syndrome.

3. Method. Combined with conventional ultrasonography to identify the blood vessel, Doppler ultrasonography produces a color image indicating flow (red, toward the transducer; blue, away from the transducer). CBF velocity is measured as the area under the curve of velocity waveforms. Small body weight and low gestational ages negatively influence the success rate in visualizing intracranial vasculature. Contrast-enhanced ultrasonography with injection of gas-filled microbubbles (size of red cells) may offer improved cerebral perfusion measurement in the future.

   4. **Results.** Doppler ultrasonography measurements can be compared with age-adjusted norm values for systolic, end-diastolic, and mean flow velocity. Serial measurement of CBF and RI may be helpful in following lesions associated with increased cerebral pressure such as determining the need for a ventriculoperitoneal shunt in progressive hydrocephalus.
C. **Computed tomography (CT)**
   1. **Definition.** Using computerized image reconstruction, CT produces 2- and 3-dimensional images of patients exposed to ionizing radiation.
   2. **Indication.** CT is the preferred tool for evaluation of the posterior fossa and non-midline disorders (eg, blood or fluid collection in the subdural or subarachnoid space) as well as parenchymal disorders. It is also helpful in the diagnosis of skull fractures.
   3. **Method.** The patient is advanced in small increments in a scanner, and images (cuts) are obtained. Cerebral white matter (more fatty tissue in myelin sheaths around the nerves) and inflammation appear less dense (blacker) than gray matter. Calcifications and hemorrhages appear white. If a patient receives contrast material, blood vessels and vascular structures (eg, falx cerebri and choroid plexus) appear white. Spaces containing cerebrospinal fluid are clearly shown in black, making it easy to identify diseases that alter their size and shape. Bones also appear white but are poorly defined, and details are better evaluated in a "bone window." Disadvantages include the need for transportation and sedation, the potential for hypothermia, and radiation exposure.
   4. **Results.** CT provides detailed information on brain structures not accessible by ultrasonography and is superior to magnetic resonance imaging (MRI) in the diagnosis of intracranial calcifications. Caution should be exerted when considering the use of multiple diagnostic CT studies given the high exposure to ionizing radiation in infancy, which can play a role in future development of malignancies.
D. **Magnetic resonance imaging (MRI)**
   1. **Definition.** Inside a strong magnetic field, atomic nuclei with magnetic properties (hydrogen protons being most common) align themselves and emit an electromagnetic signal when the field is terminated and the nuclei return to their natural state. Computers reconstruct the signal into 2-dimensional image cuts. A variety of contrasts can be obtained in MRI and include T1- and T2-weighted imaging (reflecting 2 relaxation time constraints, longitudinal and transverse, respectively), diffusion-weighted imaging (DWI), blood-oxygen-level-dependent (BOLD) imaging, and proton-density weighted imaging. In functional MRIs (fMRI), such as BOLD and DWI, underlying brain physiology is reflected in the created images.
   2. **Indication.** MRI is the preferred tool for a number of brain disorders in the neonate that are difficult to visualize by CT, such as disorders of myelination or neural migration, ischemic or hemorrhagic lesions, agenesis of the corpus callosum, AV malformations, and lesions in the posterior fossa and the spinal cord. Diffusion-based MRI is the most sensitive to acute brain injury in the first week after injury. Conventional T1- and T2-weighted MRI is preferred after 1 week following the injury. Conventional MRI has been used at term equivalent or at the time of discharge from the hospital to predict neurologic outcome.
   3. **Method.** The patient is advanced in small increments in a scanner, and images (cuts) are obtained. Gray matter appears gray, and white matter, white. Cerebrospinal fluid and bones appear black; however, the fat content in the bone marrow and the scalp appear white. In T1 and T2 MRI, fluid may appear dark or bright, depending on the type of weighted image. Advantages of MRI include the ability to identify normal and pathologic anatomy without ionizing radiation and insight into neurologic prognosis. Disadvantages include the need for transportation, sedation, a ferro-magnetic free environment, the potential for hypothermia, and difficulties in monitoring during the procedure. Ventilated infants pose a special problem, and ferro-magnetic free MRI incubators have been developed and used

to help prevent motion artifact, provide improved cardiorespiratory monitoring, maintain temperature and fluid status, and improve image quality by using built-in head coils.

4. **Results.** MRI provides high-resolution images of the brain with exquisite anatomic detail and allows diagnosis of a number of illnesses easily missed by CT. The temporal development of the prenatal brain, including the emergence of sulci and gyri and the myelination process, has been described, allowing for a more meaningful interpretation of MRI in premature infants. Quantitative volumetric MRI has been used to demonstrate the effects of postnatal dexamethasone on cortical gray matter volume and to help provide long-term prognosis for neurologic outcome. Diffusion-weighted MRI can be used in the early diagnosis of perinatal hypoxic ischemic encephalopathy at *any* stage of development. fMRI promises new insights into the functional reorganization of the brain after injury. Diffusion tensor imaging (DTI) may demonstrate direction and integrity of neural fiber tracks through 3-dimensional diffusion of water molecules along the longitudinal axis of myelinated axons. Newer magnetic resonance spectroscopy allows the study of metabolic mechanisms through quantitative measurements of certain metabolites.

E. **Near-infrared spectroscopy (NIRS)**
   1. **Definition.** Light in the near-infrared range can easily pass through skin, thin bone, and other tissues of the neonate. At selected wavelengths, light absorption depends on oxygenated and deoxygenated hemoglobin as well as oxidized cytochrome *aa* 3, allowing for qualitative measurements of oxygen delivery, cerebral blood volume, and brain oxygen availability and consumption.
   2. **Indication.** Although NIRS is not widely used, it has potential as a bedside tool to follow cerebral oxygen delivery or CBF. It is a useful technique to assess the effects of new treatments and common interventions (eg, endotracheal suction, continuous positive airway pressure) on cerebral perfusion and oxygenation.
   3. **Method.** A fiberoptic bundle applied to the scalp transmits laser light. Another fiberoptic bundle collects light and transmits it to a photon counter.
   4. **Results.** NIRS allows qualitative determination of oxygen delivery, cerebral blood volume, and oxygen consumption. In intubated infants, NIRS has been used to identify pressure-passive cerebral circulation, a condition associated with a 4-fold increase in periventricular leukomalacia and severe intraventricular hemorrhage.

II. **Electrographic studies**
   A. **Electroencephalogram (EEG)**
      1. **Definition.** An EEG continuously captures the electrical activity between reference electrodes on the scalp. In the neonatal period, cerebral maturation and development result in significant EEG changes during different gestational ages that must be considered when interpreting results.
      2. **Indication.** Indications include documented or suspected seizure activity, events with potential for cerebral injury (eg, hypoxic-ischemic, hemorrhagic, traumatic, or infectious), central nervous system (CNS) malformations, metabolic disorders, developmental abnormalities, and chromosomal abnormalities.
      3. **Method.** Several electrodes are attached to the infant's scalp, and the electrical activity is amplified and measured. Recordings can be traced on paper or can be saved electronically. EEG waves are classified into different frequencies: delta (1–3/s), theta (4–7/s), alpha (8–12/s), and beta (13–20/s).
      4. **Results.** EEGs are sensitive to a number of external factors, including acute and ongoing illness, medications or drugs, position of the electrodes, and state of arousal. A number of abnormal findings can be documented on the EEG of the term and preterm infant, including the following:
         a. Abnormal pattern of development.
         b. Depression or lack of differentiation.

    c. Electrocerebral silence ("flat" EEG).

    d. Burst suppression pattern (depressed background activity alternating with short periods of paroxysmal bursts). Burst suppression patterns are associated with especially high morbidity and mortality and poor prognosis.

    e. Persistent voltage asymmetry.

    f. Sharp waves (multifocal or central).

    g. Periodic discharges.

    h. Rhythmic alpha-frequency activity.

B. Cerebral function monitor (CFM)/amplitude-integrated EEG (aEEG)

    1. **Definition.** CFM or an aEEG records a single EEG channel for each hemisphere. The range of the signal amplitude is displayed in microvolts. Discontinuity in the EEG results in a wider trace amplitude and a decreased lower margin.

    2. **Indication.** The cerebral function monitor allows for the fast identification of infants at risk for hypoxic-ischemic encephalopathy (HIE) and for assistance in the identification of clinical and subclinical seizure activity. In addition, it has been used to select patients for neuroprotective measures such as head or total-body cooling and has been useful in providing information on neurodevelopmental outcome in cases of HIE and intraventricular hemorrhages. Not available in all institutions, the aEEG has also been used in other conditions including metabolic disorders, congenital anomalies, extracorporeal membrane oxygenation, and postoperative monitoring.

    3. **Method.** Electrodes are attached to the scalp, and the aEEG channel is recorded at a speed of 6 cm/h. CFM cannot provide information on aEEG frequency or focal lesions. Unlike standard EEG, this technique requires fewer operating and interpreting skills, making it more readily available. The aEEG should be used in conjunction with the standard EEG to provide clinical information.

    4. **Results.** The aEEG provides information on the background pattern of electrical activity of the brain (Table 16–1), the presence or absence of the sleep-wake cycle (SWC), and/or the presence of epileptiform activity and other examples of neonatal aEEG patterns (Figure 16–1). After asphyxia, the occurrence of a moderately or severely abnormal aEEG trace has a positive predictive value >70% for abnormal neurologic outcome. For instance, burst suppression, low voltage, and flat trace in the first 12–24 hours after injury is associated with a poor prognosis. SWC returning before 36 hours is associated with good outcome and after 36 hours is associated with bad outcome.

Table 16–1. **SUMMARY OF NORMAL SINGLE-CHANNEL aEEG FEATURES IN NEWBORNS AT DIFFERENT GESTATIONAL/POSTCONCEPTIONAL AGES**

Gestational or Postconceptional Age (wk)	Dominating Background Pattern	SWC	Minimum Amplitude (mcV)	Maximum Amplitude (mcV)	Burst/h
24–25	DC	(+)	2–5	25–50 (to 100)	>100
26–27	DC	(+)	2–5	25–50 (to 100)	>100
28–29	DC/(C)	(+)/+	2–5	25–30	>100
30–31	C/(DC)	+	2–6	20–30	>100
32–33	C/DC in QS	+	2–6	20–30	>100
34–35	C/DC in QS	+	3–7	15–25	>100
36–37	C/DC in QS	+	4–8	17–35	>100
38 +	C/DC in QS	+	7–8	15–25	>100

(C), continuous; DC, discontinuous background pattern; QS, quiet/deep sleep; SWC, sleep-wake cycling; SWC (+), imminent/immature; SWC +, developed SWC.

Reproduced from Hellström-Westas L, Rosén I, de Vries LS, Greisen G. Amplitude-integrated EEG classification and interpretation in preterm and term infants. *NeoReviews.* 2006;7:e76.

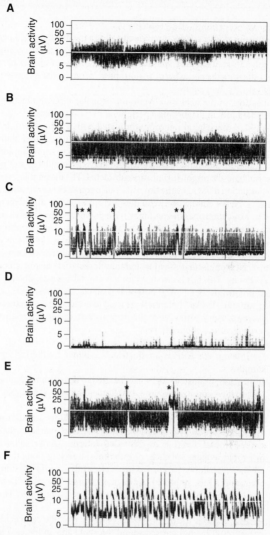

FIGURE 16–1. Sample aEEG patterns. The patterns are classified as follows: (A) **Continuous normal voltage** (normal background pattern for term infants characterized by continuous activity with lower amplitude at [5]–7–10 μV and maximum amplitudes at 10–25–[50] μV). (B) **Discontinuous normal voltage** (mildly abnormal in term infants, can be normal in some preterm infants depending on the postmenstrual age at the time of monitoring; characterized by discontinuous activity with some variability in the minimum amplitude, but mainly <5 μV and maximum amplitude >10 μV). (C) **Burst suppression** (abnormal background pattern characterized by minimum amplitude without variability at 0–2 μV intermixed with bursts of high-voltage activity >25 μV) with seven short seizures (asterisks). (D) **Isoelectric or flat trace** (severely abnormal background pattern with inactive background corresponding with electrocerebral inactivity. (E) **Two seizures** (asterisks) can be identified by a rise in the upper and lower margins against a discontinuous normal voltage background. (F) **Saw-tooth pattern** of status epilepticus. (*Modified from Bonifacio SL, Glass HC, Peloquin S, Ferriero D. A new neurological focus in neonatal intensive care. Nat Rev Neurol. 2011;7:485–494.*)

C. **Peripheral nerve conduction velocity**
   1. **Definition.** Nerve conduction velocity allows the diagnosis of a peripheral nerve disorder by measuring the transmission speed of an electrical stimulus along a peripheral (median, ulnar, peroneal) nerve. Because of smaller nerve fiber diameters affecting the nerve transmission speed, neonates have a lower nerve conduction velocity than adults.
   2. **Indication.** In the weak and hypotonic neonate, nerve conduction velocity is an important tool in diagnosing a peripheral nerve disorder.
   3. **Method.** A peripheral nerve is stimulated with a skin electrode, and the corresponding muscle action potential is recorded with another skin electrode. To determine the nerve conduction alone (as opposed to nerve conduction, synaptic transmission, and muscle reaction), the nerve is stimulated at 2 points, and the resulting muscle response times are subtracted. The distance between the 2 points of stimulation divided by the time difference equals the nerve conduction velocity.
   4. **Results.** Nerve conduction velocities are prolonged in disorders of myelination and in axon abnormalities and may have potential clinical value in combination with other tests (eg, muscle biopsy or electromyogram) in these disorders. Initially, infants with anterior horn cell disorders (eg, Werdnig-Hoffmann paralysis) have normal nerve conduction but may demonstrate decreased velocity later in the course. Neuromuscular junction and muscle disorders do not alter nerve conduction velocity. This test is also used for gestational age assessment.

D. **Evoked potentials.** An evoked potential is an electrical response by the CNS to a specific stimulus. Evoked potentials are used to evaluate the intactness and maturity of *ascending* sensory pathways of the nervous system and are relatively unaffected by state, drug, or metabolic effects.
   1. **Auditory evoked potential (AEP)**
      a. **Definition.** An AEP is an electrical response by the CNS to an auditory stimulus.
      b. **Indication.** Brainstem AEPs may be used to detect abnormalities in threshold sensitivities, conduction time, amplitudes, and shape and may be useful as a hearing screen in high-risk infants.
      c. **Method.** Although neonates respond to an auditory stimulus with brainstem as well as cortical evoked responses, the latter are variable, depending on the state of arousal, and thus are difficult to interpret. As a result, AEPs (generated by a rapid sequence of clicks or puretones) traveling along the eighth nerve to the diencephalon are recorded by an electrode over the mastoid and vertex as brainstem AEPs, amplified and digitally stored. The shape (a series of waves) and latency of brainstem AEPs depend on gestational age. This technique is sensitive to movement and ambient noise.
      d. **Results.** Injuries in the peripheral pathway (middle ear, cochlea, and eighth nerve) result in an increased sound threshold and an increase in latency of all waves, whereas central lesions cause only increased latency of waves originating from distal (in relation to the lesion) structures. Brainstem AEPs are used to demonstrate disorders of the auditory pathways caused by hypoxia-ischemia, hyperbilirubinemia, infections (eg, cytomegalovirus or bacterial meningitis), intracranial hemorrhage, trauma, systemic illnesses, drugs (eg, aminoglycoside or furosemide), or a combination of these. In low birthweight infants, brainstem AEPs have a high false-positive rate secondary to known gestational differences (longer latency, decreased amplitude, and increased threshold in preterm infants). Up to 20–25% of infants in the neonatal intensive care unit have abnormal (failed) tests, and most have normal tests at 2–4 months. In asphyxiated infants, abnormal brainstem AEPs are associated with neuromotor impairments. Because infants with congenital infection and persistent pulmonary hypertension may experience progressive hearing loss, they require serial hearing evaluations even if results are normal.

2. **Visual evoked potential (VEP)**
   a. **Definition.** A VEP is an electrical response by the CNS to a visual stimulus.
   b. **Indication.** A VEP may provide information on disorders of the visual pathway and has been used as an indicator for cerebral malfunctioning (eg, hypoxia).
   c. **Method.** An electrical response to a visual stimulus (eg, light flash in neonates or checkerboard pattern reversal in older children) is measured via a surface electrode. The electrical response is complex and undergoes significant developmental changes in the preterm infant.
   d. **Results.** When corrected for conceptional age, visual evoked responses allow the detection of various visual pathway abnormalities. Although generalized insults such as severe hypoxemia may result in temporary loss of visual evoked responses, local abnormalities may have similar results (eg, compression of the pathway in hydrocephalus). Persistent visual evoked response abnormalities in postasphyxiated infants have been strongly correlated with poor neurologic outcomes. Although VEPs may aid in the prognosis of long-term neurodevelopmental outcomes, they may not be helpful in predicting blindness or loss of vision. Improvements in visual evoked responses have also been applied to determine the success of interventions such as a ventricular-peritoneal shunt. The prognostic value in preterm infants is *controversial*.

3. **Somatosensory evoked potential (SEP)**
   a. **Definition.** An SEP is an electrical response by the CNS to a peripheral sensory stimulus.
   b. **Indication.** SEPs allow insight into disorders of the sensory pathway (peripheral nerve, plexus, dorsal root, posterior column, contralateral nucleus, medial lemniscus, thalamus, and parietal cortex).
   c. **Method.** SEPs have been recorded over the contralateral parietal scalp after providing an electric stimulus to the median or the posterior tibial nerve. SEPs are technically more difficult to obtain than auditory brainstem evoked potentials and are age dependent, with significant changes occurring in the first months of life.
   d. **Results.** SEPs may allow evaluation of peripheral lesions such as spinal cord trauma and myelodysplasia as well as cerebral abnormalities such as hypoxia, ischemia, hemorrhage, hydrocephalus, hypoglycemia, and hypothyroidism. SEP abnormalities in term infants have a high positive predictive value for neurologic sequelae and abnormal neurodevelopmental outcome. The significance of SEP remains *controversial* in the preterm infant.

III. **Clinical neurodevelopmental examination**
   A. **Definition.** The clinical neurodevelopmental examination combines the assessment of posture, movement, extremity and axial muscle tone, deep tendon reflexes, pathologic reflexes (eg, Babinski sign), primitive (or primary) reflexes, cranial nerve and oromotor function, sensory responses, and behavior by an experienced clinician.
   B. **Indication.** All infants should undergo a brief neurologic examination, including tone and reflex assessment, as part of their initial physical examination. A more detailed neurodevelopmental examination should be performed on high-risk infants. Important risk factors include prematurity, hypoxic-ischemic encephalopathy, congenital infection, meningitis, significant abnormalities on neuroimaging studies (eg, intraventricular hemorrhage, ventricular dilatation, intraparenchymal hemorrhage, infarct, or cysts), and feeding difficulties.
   C. **Method.** The experienced clinician should examine the infant when stable, preferably during the recovery phase. However, the examination may also be quite useful when performed serially, as with hypoxic-ischemic encephalopathy. The infant's state of alertness may affect many responses, including sensory response, behavior, tone, and reflexes. Normal findings change according to age (actual and postconceptional).
   1. **The full-term neonate.** The normal full-term neonate has flexor hypertonia, hip adductor tone, hyperreflexia (may have unsustained clonus), symmetric tone and

reflexes, good trunk tone on ventral suspension, some degree of head lag on pulling to a sitting from a supine position with modulation of forward head movement, presence of pathologic (eg, Babinski sign) and primitive reflexes (eg, Moro, grasp, and asymmetric tonic neck reflexes), alerting to sound, visual fixation, and a fixed focal length of 8 in.

2. **The preterm neonate.** Before 30 weeks' postconceptional age, the infant is markedly hypotonic. Extremity flexor and axial tone and the reflexes emerge in a caudocephalad (ie, lower to upper extremity) and centripetal (ie, distal to proximal) manner. Visual attention and acuity improve with postconceptional age. The extremely preterm infant can suck and swallow, but coordination of suck with swallow occurs at ~32–34 weeks' postconceptional age. Flexor tone peaks at term and then becomes decreased in a caudocephalad manner. In comparison with full-term neonates, preterm infants at term have less flexor hypertonia, more extensor tone, more asymmetries, and mild differences in behavior.

D. **Results.** Abnormalities on neurodevelopmental examination include asymmetries of posture or reflexes (especially significant if marked or persistent), decreased flexor or extremity tone or axial tone for postconceptional age, cranial nerve or oromotor dysfunction, abnormal sensory responses, abnormal behavior (eg, lethargy, irritability, or jitteriness), and extensor neck, trunk, or extremity tone. A normal neonatal neurodevelopmental examination is reassuring, but an abnormal examination cannot be used to diagnose disability in the neonatal period. The more abnormalities that are found on examination and the greater the degree of abnormality (eg, marked neck extensor hypertonia), the higher the incidence of later disability, including cerebral palsy and mental retardation.

Selected References

Allen MC, Capute AJ. Neonatal neurodevelopmental examination as a predictor of neuromotor outcome in premature infants. *Pediatrics.* 1989;83:498.

Bonifacio SL, Glass HC, Peloquin S, Ferriero D. A new neurological focus in neonatal intensive care. *Nat Rev Neurol.* 2011;7:485–494.

Di Salvo DN. A new view of the neonatal brain: clinical utility of supplemental neurologic US imaging windows. *Radiographics.* 2001;21:943.

Hellström-Westas L, Rosén I, de Vries LS, Greisen G. Amplitude-integrated EEG classification and interpretation in preterm and term infants. *NeoReviews.* 2006;7:e76.

Huppi PS, Inder TE. Magnetic resonance techniques in the evaluation of the perinatal brain: recent advances and future directions. *Semin Neonatol.* 2001;6:195.

Majnemer A, Rosenblatt B, Riley PS. Prognostic significance of multimodality response testing in high-risk newborns. *Pediatr Neurol.* 1990;6:367.

McCarville MB. Contrast-enhanced sonography in pediatrics. *Pediatr Radiol.* 2011;41:238–242.

Stapells DR, Kurtzberg D. Evoked potential assessment of auditory system integrity in infants. *Clin Perinatol.* 1991;18:497.

Van Bel F, Lemmers P, Naulaers G. Monitoring neonatal regional cerebral oxygen saturation in clinical practice: value and pitfalls. *Neonatology.* 2008;94:237–244.

Volpe JJ. *Neurology of the Newborn.* 5th ed. Philadelphia, PA: WB Saunders; 2008.

17 BLOOD COMPONENT THERAPY

I. Blood banking procedures
   A. Type and screen. Whenever possible, samples from both mother and infant should be obtained for initial ABO group and Rh(D) type determinations.
      1. Investigations of the maternal sample should include:
         a. ABO group and Rh(D) type.
         b. Screen for unexpected red cell antibodies by an indirect antiglobulin technique (IAT).
      2. Investigations of the infant (or umbilical cord) sample should include:
         a. ABO group and Rh(D) type.
         b. Direct antiglobulin test (DAT) performed on neonatal red cells.
         c. In the absence of maternal serum or plasma, the infant's serum or plasma is screened for unexpected antibodies by an IAT.
         d. If a non–group-O neonate is to be transfused with non–group-O erythrocytes, which are incompatible with the maternal ABO group, then the neonate's serum or plasma must be tested for anti-A and anti-B using an IAT. If either antibody is detected, then donor erythrocytes that lack the corresponding antigen must be chosen for transfusion.
         e. Unexpected (or atypical) red cell antibodies are clinically significant antibodies other than anti-A and/or anti-B whose presence may be expected depending on the ABO group. Repeat ABO group and Rh(D) type determinations may be omitted throughout the remainder of the neonate's hospital admission or until age 4 months is attained, whichever occurs sooner.
   B. Type and cross-match red blood cells (RBCs). Mix donor RBCs with maternal or infant serum or plasma (or both) and inspect for agglutination and/or hemolysis after incubation at 37°C (98.6°F). Infants very rarely make alloantibodies in the first 4 months of life. If the initial screen for red cell antibodies is negative, then there is no need to perform cross-matching during that period (or throughout the remainder of the neonate's hospital admission, whichever occurs sooner). **If the initial screen for red cell antibodies is positive, then additional testing should be done.**
      1. Perform testing to determine the specificity of any antibodies identified (involves reaction of maternal serum or plasma and/or umbilical cord serum or plasma against a panel of reagent erythrocytes of known antigen phenotype).
      2. Transfused red cells used must lack the corresponding antigen(s) or be compatible by antiglobulin cross-match until such antibodies are no longer demonstrable in the neonate's serum or plasma. The presence of multiple antibodies increases the difficulty of identifying compatible donors and delays blood availability.
II. Routine blood donation
   A. Voluntary blood donations. These are from screened donors with a negative history for potentially blood transmissible diseases. All blood donors are tested using serological enzyme immunoassays (EIAs) and nucleic acid amplification testing (NAT) for viral risks that include HIV (1 and 2), hepatitis viruses B and C (HBV and HCV), human T-cell lymphotrophic viruses (HTLV [I and II]), and West Nile virus (WNV). The only screening assay for parasites currently is an EIA for antibodies to *Trypanosoma cruzi* (cause of Chagas disease). In addition, EIA or microhemagglutination testing for *Treponema pallidum* (syphilis) is still required. Testing obviously is not performed for all blood-borne threats; testing for the following viruses is *not* routinely done: cytomegalovirus (CMV), parvovirus B19, hepatitis A virus (HAV), hepatitis G virus (HGV, also known as

GB virus-C [GBV-C]; no proven disease association), Torque teno virus (TTV or transfusion-transmitted virus; no proven disease association), Epstein-Barr virus (EBV), and human herpes virus-8 (HHV-8 or KSHV; associated with Kaposi's sarcoma and with multicentric Castleman's disease and primary effusion lymphoma in HIV-infected patients).

B. **The residual risks of transfusion per unit transfused are estimated to be:**
1. **HIV types 1 and 2.** 1 per 1,467,000.
2. **HCV.** 1 per 1,149,000.
3. **HBV.** 1 per 280,000.
4. **HTLV types I and II.** 1 per 2,993,000.
5. **West Nile virus.** Risk for WNV varies with location, date, and test method (mini pool NAT vs individual NAT) and has been decreasing in recent years, so a single risk estimate applicable to the Unites States is not possible. Risk for transfusion-transmitted *T. cruzi* is unknown.
6. **For perspective, selected comparative mortality odds ratios are: anesthesia**—1:7000–1:340,000; **flood**—1:455,000; and **lightning strike**—1:10,000,000.

III. **Donor-directed blood products.** Blood provided by a relative or friend of the family for a specified infant. This technique cannot be used in the emergency setting as it takes up to 48 hours to process the blood for use. There is no evidence that donor-directed transfusion is safer than blood provided by routine donation. Mothers are not ideal donors because maternal plasma frequently contains a variety of antibodies (against leukocyte and platelet antigens) that could interact with antigens expressed on neonatal cells. Similarly, transfusions from paternal donors present a risk because the neonate may have been passively immunized against paternal blood cellular antigens (by transplacental transfer of maternal antibodies against paternal antigens).

IV. **Autologous blood donation.** In adults, safety of transfusion is markedly enhanced with the use of autologous blood collected preoperatively.
A. **The fetoplacental blood reservoir** contains a blood volume of ~110 mL/kg and 30–50% of this volume is contained in the placenta. Thus, placental blood is autologous blood. Approximately 20 mL/kg can be harvested at birth and used for future transfusion. The potential for bacterial contamination coupled with the additional expense of collection have limited the widespread adoption of placental autologous blood transfusion.
B. **As an alternative, delayed cord clamping** for 30–45 seconds after birth allows the transfer of a significant amount of blood from the placenta to the infant. The blood volume of a newborn subjected to delayed cord clamping is 15–30 mL/kg larger than that of neonates with early cord clamping. **Beneficial effects** from this procedure are a reduction in transfusions needed, decreased iron deficiency at a later age, and possibly decreased risk of intraventricular hemorrhage in preterm infants.

V. **Irradiated/filtered blood components**
A. **The following adverse reactions to blood transfusion** are caused by passenger or contaminant leukocytes (white blood cells [WBCs])—whose numbers are maximal when fresh blood is used).
1. Sensitization to human leukocyte antigens (HLAs)
2. Febrile transfusion reactions
3. Immunomodulation, which may increase the risk of postoperative infection
4. CMV transmission
5. Transfusion-associated graft-versus-host disease (TA-GVHD) from engraftment of donor T lymphocytes
B. **HLA sensitization and febrile transfusion reactions** are unusual in infants, while transfusion-transmitted CMV and TA-GVHD can be life threatening.
1. **At greatest risk of severe CMV infection** are preterm infants (<1200 g) born to CMV-seronegative mothers.

2. Patients at risk for TA-GVHD include recipients of donor-directed units from first- and second-degree blood relatives, HLA-matched platelets, intrauterine transfusions, and massive fresh blood transfusions or exchange transfusions, as well as patients with suspected or proven severe T-lymphocyte immunodeficiency states (eg, DiGeorge syndrome).

3. For these high-risk patients, transfused blood components must be processed to remove passenger WBC.

    a. **Leukoreduction (removal of passenger WBC)**

        i. Such so-called leukoreduction is almost always performed by filtration of the blood component through proprietary hollow-fiber filters to which intact WBC adhere. (Centrifugation-based techniques are outdated.) Leukocyte counts can be reduced from 10^9 to 4–6×10^5 per RBC unit (4 log unit reduction) with third-generation filters.

        ii. Leukoreduction is effective in reducing HLA alloimmunization and transmission of cell-associated viruses (especially herpes viruses [such as CMV and HHV-8] and EBV)—as well as preventing some febrile transfusion reactions.

    b. **Gamma-irradiation** of cellular blood components delivers a dose of 25 Gy and prevents subsequent WBC mitoses, and thereby TA-GVHD.

VI. **Emergency transfusions.** For patients >4 months, uncross-matched (or "emergency release") blood is rarely transfused, because most blood banks can complete an IAT cross-match within 1 hour. In cases of massive, exsanguinating hemorrhage, "type-specific" blood (ABO and Rh[D]-matched only), usually available in 10 minutes, can be used. If this delay is too long (as in severe fetomaternal hemorrhage), type O Rh(D)-negative RBCs should be used.

VII. **Blood bank products**

  A. **Red blood cells**

    1. **Packed red blood cells (PRBCs)**

      a. **Indications.** PRBC transfusions are given to maintain the hematocrit (Hct) at a level judged best for the clinical condition of the baby. The selected target Hct is quite *controversial* and may vary greatly among neonatal units. In general the goal is to maintain the Hct:

        i. >35–40% in the presence of severe cardiopulmonary disease. The severity of cardiopulmonary disease is assessed based on the level of respiratory support (intermittent positive pressure ventilation [IPPV], continuous positive airway pressure [CPAP], Fio_2) required, symptoms of unexplained apnea and/or tachycardia, and/or poor growth.

        ii. 30–35% for moderate cardiopulmonary disease or major surgery.

        iii. 20–25% for infants with stable, so-called asymptomatic anemia.

      b. **Administration**

        i. **Type.** PRBC transfused throughout infancy should be screened in order to exclude donations from blood donors containing hemoglobin S.

        ii. **Dosage.** 10–20 mL/kg given over 1–3 hours (4 hours maximum). **Use the following formula as a guide:**

$$\text{Volume PRBC to transfuse (mL)} = 1.6 \times \text{weight (kg)} \times \text{desired rise in Hct (\%)}$$

    2. **"Adsol" PRBCs.** The traditional use of relatively fresh RBCs (<7 days storage) has been largely replaced by the practice of transfusing aliquots of RBCs from a dedicated unit of PRBCs stored for up to 42 days. This requires a sterile connecting device and is done to diminish the number of donor exposures among infants expected to require numerous transfusions during their stay in the neonatal intensive care unit (NICU) (infants whose birthweight is

<1500 g). PRBCs are suspended in a citrate-anticoagulated storage solution at an Hct of 55–60% stored at 1–6°C. The storage or additive solutions (AS or Adsol-1, -3, or -5) contain various combinations of preservatives (dextrose, sodium chloride, phosphate, adenine, and mannitol).

3. **Citrate phosphate dextrose PRBCs.** Because of concern about potential hepatorenal toxicity of adenine and mannitol, units of RBCs without extended storage medium are used for large-volume transfusions such as exchange transfusion and transfusions for major surgical procedures. PRBC units with only small amounts of adenine and devoid of mannitol have a hematocrit of 65–80% and a shelf life of 35 days. PRBC units with CPD formulations (citrate-phosphate-dextrose) lacking both adenine and mannitol also have a hematocrit of 65–80% but a shelf life of only 21 days. Washed Adsol PRBC units are an alternative if these other PRBC units are unavailable.

4. **Washed PRBCs.** During storage, potassium is progressively released from RBCs so that, by the end of the storage period, extracellular (plasma) potassium levels approximate 50 and 80 mEq/L for Adsol and CPD units, respectively. This leakage is increased in irradiated blood. For small-volume transfusions the amount of infused K is, in general, of little clinical significance (0.3–0.4 mEq/kg per 15 mL/kg RBC transfusion). But it may become hazardous for larger transfusion volumes such as in exchange transfusion. In such an event and in the absence of fresh whole blood (<2–3 days old), RBCs (typically O Rh[D] negative) washed free of their potentially hyperkalemic supernatant using normal saline and then reconstituted to a hematocrit of 50–55% with fresh frozen plasma (typically AB, termed "reconstituted whole blood") can be used. Irradiated reconstituted whole blood should be used for total exchange transfusion.

B. **Plasma—fresh-frozen plasma (FFP), thawed plasma.** Donated whole blood is centrifuged to separate the cells (RBCs) and the liquid (plasma). If the separation is done within 18 hours of the blood being donated and is frozen, it is called fresh-frozen plasma. FFP contains albumin, immune globulins, and clotting factors (some retain much of their activity after thawing, eg, von Willebrand factor [vWF]) and factors V, VII, and VIII (their activity may be reduced during processing before freezing).

1. **Indications**
   a. Correction of coagulopathy due to inherited deficiencies of some clotting factors, vitamin K deficiency (hemorrhagic disease of the newborn), or disseminated intravascular coagulation (DIC). When available, clotting factor concentrates are preferred to plasma in case of inherited clotting factor deficiency. There are no single factor concentrates available for factors II, V, and X. Prothrombin complex concentrates containing factors II, IX, and X are used for factor II and X deficiencies.
   b. Prophylaxis for dilutional coagulopathy that may ensue during massive blood transfusion administered for replacement of blood loss in excess of half of the blood volume.
   c. Preparation of reconstituted whole blood from washed PRBCs for total exchange transfusion.
   d. Although FFP provides excellent colloid volume support, it is not recommended for volume expansion or antibody replacement because safer components are available for these purposes.

2. **Administration**
   a. Transfused plasma should be ABO compatible with the patient's blood group. Incompatible antibodies in the donor plasma (such as anti-A or -B antibodies in group O plasma) may rarely, if given in sufficient volume, result in an acute hemolytic reaction in the transfused patient.
   b. Dosage: 10–20 mL/kg over 1–2 hours (4 hours maximum).

    c. Rapid transfusion may result in transient hypocalcemia due to the sodium citrate that is added to the original donated blood. If rapid infusion of FFP is needed, a small bolus of calcium chloride (3–5 mg/kg) may be considered.

C. **Cryoprecipitate.** Prepared from FFP by thawing it at 1–6°C. In this temperature range, a cryoprecipitate forms and is separated from so-called cryo-poor supernatant plasma by centrifugation. The pellet is then frozen as cryoprecipitate. Prior to use, it must again be thawed and dissolved off the interior surface of its plastic bag with normal saline (with a total volume of 10–15 mL). Cryoprecipitate is a concentrated source of the following blood clotting proteins: factor VIII, vWF, fibrinogen, and factor XIII (with some other proteins, eg, fibronectin).

    1. Indications

      a. To restore fibrinogen levels in patients with acquired hypofibrinogenemia (as occurs in DIC and massive transfusion)

      b. Factor XIII in deficient patients

    2. Administration

      a. Like plasma, it should be ABO compatible with the recipient's blood group.

      b. Dosage: 10 mL/kg (0.1–0.2 U/kg raises fibrinogen by 60–100 mg/dL).

      c. Infusion should be completed within 6 hours of thawing.

D. **Platelets.** Prepared from whole blood donations by centrifugation (termed "random donor") or by automated apheresis (termed "single donor" or "platelets pheresis"). Each random donor unit contains 5.5×10^{10} platelets in 50–70 mL of anticoagulated plasma. Each single-donor unit contains 3×10^{11} platelets, typically in 200–300 mL of anticoagulated plasma. Both are stored at room temperature (20–24°C) with agitation for a maximum of 5 days.

    1. Indications. There are no absolute guidelines regarding platelet counts that necessitate transfusion.

      a. In general, platelet transfusion is indicated for platelet counts below 50,000/μL.

      b. In the presence of active bleeding or prior to surgery, this "transfusion trigger" may be raised to 100,000, while in a nonbleeding, stable neonate platelet counts as low as 20,000–30,000 may be tolerated.

      c. In septic patients, platelet increments after transfusion may only be transient.

      d. Because of room temperature storage, bacterial contamination of platelet units is actively sought, typically by culture or direct testing of each component.

      e. Increased mortality and morbidity have been described among preterm infants receiving multiple platelet transfusions.

    2. Administration

      a. Infant and donor should be ABO identical if possible. When ABO-identical platelets are unavailable, group AB platelets are the most suitable substitute. However, the frequent unavailability of group AB platelets causes the use of group A platelets for group B recipients and vice versa. Group O platelets are the least suitable for non–group-O infants, as passively transfused anti-A or -B antibodies may lead to hemolysis.

      b. Rh(D)-negative platelets should be given whenever possible to Rh(D)-negative patients—especially female infants.

      c. For infants with alloimmune thrombocytopenia (AIT), platelets lacking platelet-specific antigens (HPAs) to which antibodies are directed are required. If such platelets are unavailable, then HPA 1a, 5b–negative platelets may be given since these will be compatible in 95% of AIT cases among Caucasians. If anti-HPA antibodies are not demonstrated, then anti-HLA antibodies may be present requiring HLA-matched platelets.

      d. **Dosage:** 10–20 mL/kg IV should raise neonatal platelet counts by 60,000–100,000/μL.

VIII. **Transfusion reactions**
   A. **Acute intravascular hemolysis.** Occurs due to incompatibility of donor RBCs with antibodies in the patient plasma. The most common antibodies responsible for complement-mediated acute hemolysis are isohemagglutinins (anti-A, anti-B). Newborns do not all make isohemagglutinins in high titer until 4–6 months of age.
      1. However, transfusion of ABO-incompatible donor RBCs (most commonly due to clerical error) may result in hemolysis if isoagglutinin titers are high enough. Accordingly, some neonatal units may transfuse all neonates with O Rh(D)-negative PRBCs (if the blood supplier can support this policy).
      2. Incompatible isoagglutinins are more often found in the neonatal circulation due to transfusion of the ABO-incompatible plasma in platelet units.
      3. Transplacental passage of group O maternal isohemagglutinins to a non–group-O fetus may also cause hemolysis of the neonate's own RBCs in the absence of transfusion (typically mild; "ABO HDFN"). Note that passively acquired anti-A and anti-B, whether of blood donor or maternal origin, are not detected by antibody screens but do cause incompatible cross-matches. Accordingly, cross-matches using an IAT are always necessary when clinically significant red cell antibodies, including isohemagglutinins, are present in neonatal plasma.
      4. Red cell T-antigen is present on all human erythrocytes but expressed only after exposure to neuramidinase produced by a variety of infectious organisms—in particular *Streptococcus*, *Clostridium*, and influenzae viruses. Anti-T antibodies are present in almost all adults but are not present in the plasma of infants until 6 months of age. Anti-T may be associated with hemolysis in patients whose red cells are "activated," eg, infants with necrotizing enterocolitis (NEC) or sepsis. When intravascular hemolysis occurs and T activation of neonatal RBCs is identified through peanut lectin testing, donor RBCs and platelets should be washed prior to use.
      5. Possible symptoms of intravascular hemolysis include hypotension, fever, tachycardia, hematuria, and hemoglobinuria. Diagnosis may be confirmed by an elevated free serum hemoglobin, absent haptoglobin (if it is not congenitally absent, as in about 10% of African-American infants), as well as the presence of schistocytes on a peripheral blood smear.
   B. **Nonhemolytic febrile reactions.** Usually mild, due to transfusion of cytokines released from donor WBCs during storage or of fragmented donor WBCs.
   C. **Allergic transfusion reactions.** Unusual in neonatal transfusion recipients. Due to antibodies in the patient's plasma reacting to epitopes on donor plasma proteins.
   D. **Transfusion-associated acute lung injury (TRALI).** Typically due to antibodies in donor plasma that react with the patient's HLA antigens. More likely to occur with blood components containing large amounts of plasma such as FFP or platelets.
   E. **Bacterial contamination.** There is a small but potentially fatal risk of bacterial infection on the order of 1 per 8–13 million for PRBCs but of 1 per 300,000 for platelets (because of room temperature storage). *Escherichia coli*, *Pseudomonas*, *Serratia*, *Salmonella*, and *Yersinia* are the most commonly implicated bacteria.
   F. **Hypothermia.** Large-volume transfusions of either reconstituted whole blood (exchange transfusion) or PRBCs (major surgery, large fetomaternal hemorrhages), which are stored at 1–6°C, will result in hypothermia unless a blood warmer is used.
   G. **Hyperkalemia.** At risk are infants receiving a large transfusion of RBCs such as in exchange transfusion, major surgery, or ECMO/ECLS. Reconstituted whole blood (washed PRBCs [<14 days old] with Hct adjusted using FFP) is recommended. In some neonatal units, fresh whole blood (<2–3 days) may be available.

Selected References

Baer VL, Lambert DK, Henry E, Snow GL, Sola-Visner MC, Christensen RD. Do platelet transfusions in the NICU adversely affect survival? Analysis of 16000 thrombocytopenic neonates in a multihospital healthcare system. *J Perinatol.* 2007;27:790–796.

Carson TH, Banbury MK, Beaton MA, et al. Standards for blood banks and transfusion services. *AABB.* 2011;27:32–38.

Nordmeyer D, Forestner J, Wall M. Advances in transfusion medicine. *Adv Anesth.* 2007;25:11–58.

Nunes dos Santos AM, Petean Trindade CE. Red blood cell transfusions in the neonate. *NeoReviews.* 2011;12:e13–e19.

O'Riordan JM, Fitzgerald J, Smith OP, Bonnar J, Gorman WA. Transfusion of blood components to infants under four months: review and guidelines. *Irish Medical J.* 2007;100(6):1–21.

Galel SA. Infectious disease screening. In: Roback JD, Grossman BJ, Harris T, Hillyer CD, eds. *AABB Technical Manual.* 17th ed. Bethesda, MD: American Association of Blood Banks. 2011;17:241–282.

Strauss RG. How I transfuse red blood cells and platelets to infants with anemia and thrombocytopenia of prematurity. *Transfusion.* 2008;48:209–217.

18 Extracorporeal Life Support in the Neonate

I. **Introduction. Extracorporeal life support (ECLS)** provides oxygen (O_2) delivery, carbon dioxide (CO_2) removal, and cardiac support in patients who have cardiac and/or respiratory failure by draining blood from the right atrium through a cannula with the aid of a pump and then propelling blood through an oxygenator, where gas exchange occurs. From there, it is returned to the patient into the aorta (venoarterial [VA]) or right atrium (venovenous [VV]) (Figures 18–1, 18–2, and 18–3). Uniform guidelines have been established to describe essential equipment, procedures, personnel, and training required for ECLS and can be found in the *ECMO Specialist Training Manual* published by the Extracorporeal Life Support Organization. (**Note: The term extracorporeal membrane oxygenation [ECMO] has generally been replaced by ECLS, reflecting an expanded role beyond oxygenation for this technology.**)

II. **Indications.** ECLS is used primarily for critically ill term and late preterm newborns with reversible respiratory and/or cardiac failure who have failed appropriate maximal medical management with ventilator support (conventional or high frequency), inhaled nitric oxide, volume expansion, or inotropic/vasopressor support. **Neonatal conditions treated with ECLS support include meconium aspiration syndrome, congenital diaphragmatic hernia, persistent pulmonary hypertension of the newborn, respiratory distress syndrome, sepsis, and pneumonia. ECLS can be used to support patients with cardiac failure owing to congenital heart disease, postcardiotomy heart failure, cardiomyopathy, or severe rhythm disturbances and may be used as a bridge to cardiac transplantation.**

III. **Appropriate patients for ECLS**
   A. **Weight ≥1.6–1.8 kg; gestational age ≥32–34 weeks.** The cannula size is determined by the infant's weight; the lower limit in weight is based on the limitation of cannula sizes available.
   B. **Respiratory criteria**
      1. **Oxygenation index (OI).** Historically, an OI >30–40 for 0.5–4 hours was routinely used to determine the severity of illness and establish when a neonate was felt to be at high risk for death if not treated with ECLS. Although OI levels can be helpful in establishing a trend, most centers rely on additional parameters to guide their decisions to initiate ECLS, including the inability to

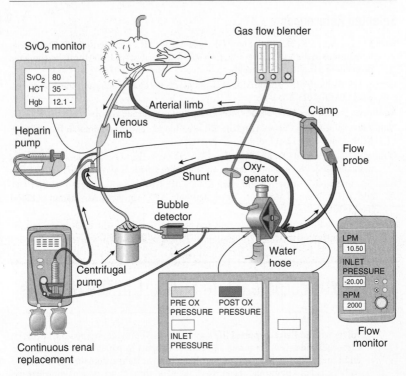

FIGURE 18–1. ECLS circuit. (*Reprinted, with permission, from Michaele Miller at Michaele Miller Projects LLC.*)

wean from 100% oxygen within a period of time and/or ongoing hypotension or metabolic acidosis.

$$OI = \frac{F_{IO_2} \times MAP \times 100}{Pa_{O_2}}$$

(F$_{IO_2}$, fraction of inspired O$_2$; MAP, mean airway pressure; Pa$_{O_2}$, partial pressure of oxygen, arterial)

2. **Acute deterioration with intractable hypoxemia.** Patients who have a Pa$_{O_2}$ <30–40 mm Hg or a preductal Sa$_{O_2}$ <80% for greater than an hour and are not responding to conventional therapies should be considered for ECLS support.

3. **Barotrauma.** Severe air leak from pneumothoraces that are not responsive to low tidal volume conventional ventilation or high-frequency oscillatory or jet ventilation may benefit from lung rest on ECLS.

C. **Cardiovascular/oxygen delivery criteria**

1. **Plasma lactate levels >5 mmol/L (45 mg/dL).** Patients with a metabolic acidosis not improving, or escalating, despite volume expansion and inotropic/vasopressor support can be supported with ECLS.

2. **Mixed venous oxygen saturations (Sv$_{O_2}$) <55–60% for 0.5–1 hour.** Low Sv$_{O_2}$ levels indicate a critical level of O$_2$ extraction and suggest an increased metabolic stress. With further decreases in Sv$_{O_2}$ levels, there is impending risk of cellular death if not reversed.

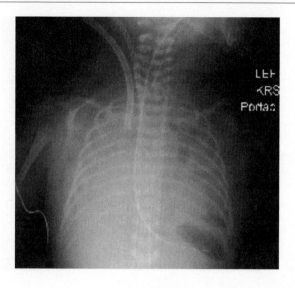

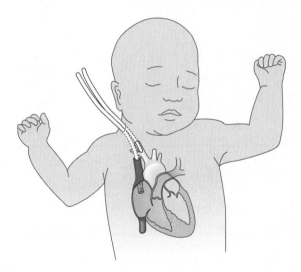

FIGURE 18–2. VA ECLS cannulae placement. The echogenic dot denoting the end of the venous cannula at T9 is hard to visualize.

   3. **Cardiac arrest.** ECLS during cardiopulmonary resuscitation (extracorporeal cardiopulmonary resuscitation [ECPR]) is available in many centers for patients with or without primary heart disease in situations in which the cardiac arrest is witnessed.
IV. **Relative contraindications to ECLS.** Decisions for determining contraindications to ECLS are institution based.

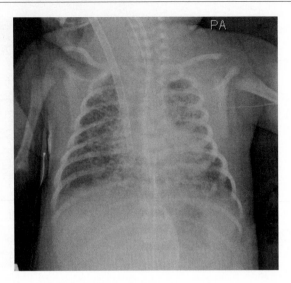

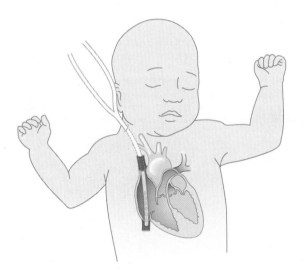

FIGURE 18–3. VV ECLS cannulae placement.

    A. Gestational age <32–34 weeks and/or a birthweight <1600–1800 g due to the risk of intracranial hemorrhage and surgical difficulties with vessel cannulation. Lower birthweight and gestational age infants are at risk for increased mortality and morbidity. With current technology requiring the use of systemic heparinization during ECLS, there is concern for a higher risk of intracranial hemorrhage in patients <32 weeks. Despite size limitations in preterm infants, newer technologies and smaller cannulae sizes are being developed, which may allow ECLS support at younger gestational ages and in smaller weight categories.

B. Mechanical ventilation >14 days due to the likelihood of irreversible lung disease.

C. Intracranial hemorrhage >grade II due to a higher risk of extending the hemorrhage. Those with an intracranial hemorrhage >grade II may be considered candidates for ECLS on an individual basis.

D. Severe congenital anomalies incompatible with long-term survival.

E. Cardiac lesions that cannot be corrected or palliated.

F. Congenital diaphragmatic hernia patients with best OI >45 or who have never had a preductal saturation >85% or $Paco_2$ <70. See references that follow.

G. Marked perinatal asphyxia

   1. Severe neurologic syndrome persisting after respiratory and metabolic resuscitation (stuporous, flaccid, and absent primitive reflexes).

   2. High plasma lactate levels

      a. Lactate levels >25 mmol/L (225 mg/dL) are highly predictive of death.

      b. Lactate levels >15 mmol/L (135 mg/dL) are highly predictive of adverse neurologic outcome.

   3. Base deficit >30 on 2 ABGs.

H. Multiple organ dysfunction syndrome in neonates can develop when there has been an acute sepsis, hypoperfusion, or hypoxia and may be preceded by a systemic inflammatory response. Neonates can often have respiratory failure, metabolic acidosis, a coagulopathy that doesn't resolve with transfusion therapy, and cardiac, renal, and gastrointestinal dysfunction. If a neonate has such significant multiple organ dysfunction that they are not likely to survive, ECLS may not provide any benefit.

V. Transfer of patients possibly needing ECLS. Patients should optimally be transferred early in their course. An OI of >25 suggests significant hypoxic respiratory failure, equating to a patient with a mean airway pressure of 15 with an Fio_2 of 1.0 who achieves a Pao_2 of only 60 mm Hg. Any patient requiring 100% oxygen without signs of improvement on high-frequency and/or inhaled nitric oxide within 2–3 hours or those who have persistent hypotension, acidosis, and/or lactic acidosis despite vasopressor/inotropic therapy should be considered a candidate for transport on their current therapy to an ECLS center.

VI. Parental consent. Before ECLS initiation, parents should be made aware of the potential complications. It is important to emphasize that ECLS is a supportive therapy rather than curative and that there are some circumstances where neonates may not survive. **Potential complications**:

A. Difficulties may arise during cannulation, including the inability to achieve adequate venous drainage or infusion secondary to a venous web, valve, or vessel spasm. Perforation of the right atrium leading to pericardial tamponade can occur suddenly and be life-threatening, requiring immediate surgical evacuation.

B. Hemorrhage may develop in any organ, most significantly the brain. Blood accumulation in the pericardium, abdomen, retroperitoneum, or chest can result in decreased pulse pressure, low SvO_2 levels, hypotension, and inability to maintain ECLS flows.

C. Thrombosis or emboli in the circuit may lead to an infarction in the brain, and is usually associated more commonly with VA ECLS.

D. Infections, hemolysis, renal failure, accidental decannulation, **arrhythmias** (due to the venous catheter being positioned in the atrium), and mechanical problems (ie, oxygenator failure, fracture of the tubing or connector sites) are other possible ECLS complications.

E. ECLS survivors are at risk for significant neurologic sequelae resulting from the underlying disease process and/or their treatment (see Section XXI). Decreased tone and poor feeding may lengthen hospital stay and necessitate ongoing rehabilitative services. Chronic lung disease may lead to future hospitalizations. Other long-term complications, including blindness, hearing loss, and cognitive problems requiring special support in school, can also occur. Despite these stated complications, most infants have excellent morbidity-free outcomes.

VII. **Pre-ECLS studies and preparation**

    A. **Before initiating ECLS,** patients require evaluation for structural heart disease and intracranial hemorrhage with an **echocardiogram and head ultrasound.**

    B. **Screening labs** should include electrolytes, ionized calcium, blood urea nitrogen, creatinine, glucose, complete blood count, differential, platelet count, coagulation studies including international normalized ratio (INR), fibrin breakdown products, total and direct bilirubin, arterial blood gas (ABG), lactate, activating clotting time (ACT), antithrombin III level, blood culture, and a blood type and screen. Labs should be followed daily to twice daily.

    C. **Bladder catheter, enteral feeding tube** or tube for low intermittent suction, and a rectal temperature probe should be inserted as needed. It is extremely important to place these tubes before the initiation of anticoagulation and ECLS given the risks of bleeding.

    D. **For VV ECLS,** a percutaneously placed internal jugular central line can serve as a guide for placement of the VV cannula. Other access for IV infusions, blood draws and arterial blood gases, and central blood pressure monitoring via percutaneously inserted central lines, umbilical arterial, and/or venous catheters or femoral arterial and/or venous catheters should preferably be placed before the initiation of ECLS as well.

VIII. **Pretreatment with glucocorticoids.** During ECLS, the patient's blood is exposed to plastic, silicone, polymethylpentene, and other circuit compounds, which can cause activation of the immune system with the release of inflammatory mediators (complement, leukotrienes, cytokines, and leukocytes). The coagulation cascade and fibrinolytic system are also activated. Consumption of platelets by the hollow fiber or membrane oxygenator or filter used for continuous renal replacement can exacerbate the coagulopathy and the additive responses can result in massive capillary leak. This process may be mitigated somewhat by pretreating neonates with a glucocorticoid, but the evidence for this has not been established.

IX. **Gas exchange.** Gas exchange through the **oxygenator** mimics pulmonary respiration (see Figure 18–1). Some oxygenators house hollow fibers. Blood flows around the fibers, in constant contact with the fiber surface. Oxygen flow, however, occurs through the fibers. The microporous nature of the fibers allows gas exchange by diffusion across the membrane based on concentration gradients, allowing O_2 delivery and CO_2 removal. The FIO_2 delivered to the oxygenator influences the oxygen delivered to the blood.

    Membrane oxygenators are designed to allow blood to flow on one side of the membrane, whereas gas flows on the other side. Again, concentration gradients are the driving force for diffusion. Membrane oxygenators are more likely to have complications with plasma leaks, air emboli, water vapor condensation, and thrombus formation.

    To provide varying oxygen concentrations for both types of oxygenators, the **gas blender** is used to dial in an appropriate O_2 concentration. To remove CO_2, the **flow meter** is adjusted, which provides gas flow or "sweep gas" through the oxygenator and serves to wash out CO_2 from the oxygenator system.

    A. **In patients on ECLS, O_2 delivery** is influenced by the following:

        1. O_2 **content** of the blood after it passes through the oxygenator

        2. **Rate of blood flow** through the ECLS circuit, particularly in membrane oxygenators

        3. O_2 **uptake** through the patient's lung

        4. **Native cardiac output**

        5. **Patient's hemoglobin**

B. Oxygenation through the circuit depends on the following:
1. The amount of O_2 in the gas phase (the driving concentration gradient).
2. The ease with which O_2 crosses the hollow fiber or membrane (permeability).
3. The ability of O_2 to diffuse through the blood layer (its solubility in plasma). Because there is more O_2 in the sweep gas than in the blood, there is always a large concentration gradient that never achieves equilibrium throughout the oxygenator. Sweep gas flow has little influence on oxygen exchange. Blood flow, however, may influence oxygenation. If the blood flows faster than the time it takes to achieve complete saturation of the hemoglobin with oxygen, blood will leave the oxygenator incompletely saturated. The "**rated flow**" is the pump blood flow rate at which maximal O_2 delivery is achieved. Oxygenation decreases at flows that exceed that rate. Additionally, the likelihood of hemolysis increases. Devices have a flow rated graph on their web site.
C. For patients on ECLS, CO_2 exchange is affected by 3 main factors:
1. The relative concentration of CO_2 on either side of the oxygenator hollow fibers or membrane (which is usually at least 45–50 mm Hg in the venous blood and zero in the sweep gas of the oxygenator, allowing very efficient transfer of CO_2).
2. The movement of gas through the oxygenator or sweep gas flow-rate (which constantly refreshes the concentration gradient by moving air through the oxygenator).
3. The surface area of the hollow fibers or membrane. Because the diffusion of CO_2 through blood and the hollow fibers or membrane occurs rapidly (6 times faster than O_2), it remains independent of blood flow rate through the oxygenator. Factors that decrease the functional surface area, however, will limit CO_2 transfer before affecting oxygenation.
X. Comparison of VA and VV ECLS
A. Advantages and disadvantages of VA and VV ECLS
1. VA ECLS. Provides cardiopulmonary bypass that runs in parallel to the native cardiac output. Blood from the right atrium serves as the source for ECLS pump preload, which is oxygenated and then infused into the brachiocephalic artery/aortic circulation.
a. VA ECLS advantages
i. May provide full cardiac and respiratory support for the nonfunctioning heart and lungs.
ii. May decrease the load on the heart, allowing for recovery. However, if left ventricular (LV) failure is severe, the flow through the arterial cannula may exceed the ability of the LV to eject. Under such conditions, acute pulmonary edema may occur, leading to dire outcomes if the left atrium (LA) is not decompressed.
b. VA ECLS disadvantages
i. Results in ligation of the carotid artery; reconstruction may or may not be possible. VA ECLS also causes temporary interruption of isohemispheric cerebral blood flow when carotid cannulation is used.
ii. Causes a higher incidence of central nervous system (CNS) hemorrhage.
iii. Potentially may allow emboli to enter the arterial circulation, which could cause a stroke.
iv. May compromise organ tolerance to hypoxia (especially in the brain and kidneys) because of the lack of pulsatility in the blood flow.
2. VV ECLS. Provides respiratory support (and indirectly circulatory support) that runs in series with the native cardiac output.
a. VV ECLS advantages
i. Maintains function of the carotid artery because it is not used for cannulation
ii. Preserves pulsatile flow, which may better preserve organ function

iii. Allows the lungs to serve as filters for emboli so embolic strokes are less likely

iv. Increases the availability of oxygen to the coronary circulation as blood is ejected from the left ventricle due to the arterial admixture of the mixed venous blood

b. **VV ECLS disadvantages**

i. Provides only indirect circulatory support by improving myocardial oxygenation; patients may continue to require inotrope/vasopressor support, but many patients experience improvement in cardiac function after cannulation for VV ECLS.

ii. May not provide full oxygen delivery. In this case, some native lung function may be necessary to sustain appropriate gas exchange.

iii. More prone to difficulties with cannula position. Provides less support due to recirculation. (See Section XVIII.B.4).

XI. **Cannulation guidelines and preparation**

A. **Circuit preparation.** Occurs once a patient is felt to need ECLS. The circuit tubing is connected and then primed with packed red blood cells, fresh-frozen plasma (FFP), sodium bicarbonate, calcium gluconate, and heparin. Some institutional preferences may include albumin or tris-hydroxymethyl amino-methane.

B. **Neonatal vascular access.** Usually through the right internal jugular vein and right common carotid artery for VA ECLS, each using a single lumen cannula for access, and the right internal jugular vein for VV ECLS with a dual lumen cannula for access.

C. **Patient positioning.** Patients should be positioned with the head turned to the left and the neck extended using a neck roll.

D. **Medications.** To provide analgesia/anesthesia and surgical preparedness, patients should receive a narcotic and neuromuscular blocking agent before the procedure. Sedatives and narcotics are usually provided throughout the ECLS course; however, most patients do not require ongoing therapy with neuromuscular blocking agents. For patients receiving muscle relaxants, the ventilator settings should be adjusted and the end tidal CO_2 followed.

E. **X-ray placement.** An x-ray cassette should be placed under the patient before initiation of surgical placement of the cannula(e).

F. **Heparin for anticoagulation.** Patients not already receiving anticoagulation should have an ACT drawn and be given a heparin bolus of 50–100 U/kg immediately before the insertion of the cannula(e) to prevent clot formation. After the ACT level falls to 250–300 seconds, a continuous heparin infusion is started. The typical starting dose is 10–20 U/kg/h, and the typical steady-state infusion rate is 20–40 U/kg/h. If ongoing bleeding and coagulopathy are a concern or the patient has recently had surgery, the heparin drip may be held until an appropriate coagulation status is achieved.

G. **Appropriate cannula positions/sizes.** See Figures 18–2 and 18–3. Cannula size choices should be determined based on the patient size. The size of the venous cannula is critical because restricted flow due to high resistance may cause blood-shearing resulting in hemolysis.

1. **For VA cannulation.** The arterial cannula tip should be in the brachiocephalic artery, at or just above the junction of the aortic arch. Optimal positioning is achieved when the cannula tip is at T3–4 (just above the carina) after the neck roll is removed. The tip of the venous cannula should be in the right atrium near the junction of the inferior vena cava. If the arterial cannula is positioned high in the right common carotid artery, streaming of blood can occur into the right subclavian artery, causing the right arm to appear more oxygenated than the rest of the body, invalidating any arterial blood gas sampling from a right radial artery. The catheter generally needs to be adjusted in these situations.

2. **For VV cannulation.** The cannula chosen should have the largest internal diameter to minimize resistance to blood flow. The cannula tip should be well into the right atrium at T7–8 or about 1–2 cm above the diaphragm for most cannulae. Removal of the neck roll may advance the catheter as much as 1 cm. Proper cannula position helps maintain appropriate flows, a critical feature of VV ECLS. Flows of 120 mL/kg/min should be achievable after intravascular volume expansion and removal of the neck roll. It is imperative to assess for signs of significant recirculation after VV cannulation. In this situation, venous saturations may be >85–90% and arterial saturations lower than their baseline levels. (See recirculation in Section XVIII.B.4.)

H. **Intravascular volume.** Before connecting the ECLS cannula(e) to the circuit, surgeons may allow backflow of the patient's blood in the cannula(e) to assure that there is no air in the circuit. During these times, blood pressures may drift downward momentarily, and intravascular volume may be needed.

I. **Ongoing heparin therapy.** The ACT range depends on the type of monitoring equipment and institution-specific standards. ACT levels are monitored regularly and **kept in a range between 200 to 220 seconds.** When disseminated intravascular coagulation (DIC) or bleeding occurs, clinicians may target a lower ACT goal, typically between 180 to 200 seconds. A heparin bolus may be necessary if the ACT falls below 180 seconds and the ECLS flow is interrupted for a circuit change or modification. Because the circuit flow rate also has an impact on thrombus formation, an attempt should be made to maintain ECLS flows >80 mL/kg/min whenever the ACT levels drop to <180 seconds.

The ACT assays whole blood clotting. As such, factors that affect ACT include heparin dosing, coagulation and anticoagulation factor levels, and antithrombin III (ATIII) levels, as well as the platelet count and function. If the ACT is at the lower end of the target range, a bolus of heparin (5–10 U/kg) may be needed when platelets are transfused. ACT levels may overestimate heparin effect and therefore lead to inadequate anticoagulation.

Furosemide often prompts a brisk diuresis. Diuresis increases heparin clearance, often necessitating an increase in the heparin infusion rate. Likewise, a spontaneous increase in urine output, continuous renal replacement therapy, or platelet transfusions often require an increase in the heparin rate to maintain the target ACT level.

J. **Management of coagulopathy and anemia.** Coagulopathies should be corrected at the earliest possible opportunity.

1. **Fibrinogen levels.** Should be kept >150 mg/dL using cryoprecipitate.
2. **INR levels.** Should be kept ≤1.4 by treating with FFP and/or cryoprecipitate.
3. **Platelet counts.** Generally maintained >80,000 μL or >100,000 if there is bleeding.
4. **Antithrombin III antigen levels.** Normally kept >60–100%, especially with excessive clot buildup in the circuit and/or a high heparin infusion rate (eg, >40 U/kg/h). Infants demonstrate physiologically low ATIII levels until 6–9 months of age depending on their gestational age and other illnesses. Furthermore, low ATIII levels may result from DIC, endothelial injury, ongoing protein losses from a chylothorax or nephrotic syndrome, dilutional effects of cardiac bypass, liver disease with synthetic failure, or from congenital deficiencies (rare).

ATIII, a serine protease inhibitor produced by the liver, is essential to endogenous anticoagulation by inhibiting the activity of thrombin and Xa. It also inactivates plasmin, IXa, XIa, and XIIa. ATIII is necessary for an adequate response to heparin. Heparin, a glycosaminoglycan produced by basophils and mast cells, works by binding to ATIII and upregulating the catalytic activity of ATIII a 1000-fold.

FFP has approximately 1 U of antithrombin/mL. ATIII concentrate, however, increases the serum level with a much smaller administration volume and so may be appropriate to use if a goal ATIII level is preferred. Larger protein losses, with the loss of other coagulation factors, may be more efficiently treated with FFP.

5. **Unfractionated heparin levels (anti-Xa).** Help to determine whether a prolonged ACT level is due to a heparin effect or coagulopathy. Normal goals are 0.25–0.5 IU/mL.
6. **Hematocrit levels.** Maintained at >35% for VA ECLS and >40% for VV ECLS.
7. **Thromboelastography.** Assays whole blood to provide information about intrinsic factor, platelet function, anticoagulation, and fibrinolytic function. As such, it may be used for further assessment in particularly challenging cases.

XII. **Monitoring during ECLS**

A. **Thrombus in the oxygenator.** Suspected when an increase in the preoxygenator pressure and a fall in the postoxygenator pressure occurs (see Figure 18–1). Trends in the change in pressures (Δ pressure) should be followed. If the Δ pressure is increasing to above acceptable parameters, the oxygenator or circuit should be changed. In addition, consumption of clotting factors and platelets suggests the presence of thrombi in the circuit, so called "circuit DIC." This often requires a change of the entire circuit.

B. **Gas pressure.** Monitored and controlled in the sweep gas line.

C. **SvO_2 levels.** During ECLS, SvO_2 levels reflect the degree of O_2 extraction and should normally be in the 75–80% range. SvO_2 levels <50% indicate a critical level of O_2 extraction and suggest that the rate of tissue metabolism dangerously exceeds the rate of O_2 delivery. Once this occurs, cells use the markedly less efficient anaerobic metabolism producing lactic acid. SvO_2 levels present a useful parameter to follow in VA ECLS, but due to the recirculation phenomenon in VV ECLS, they may sometimes be more difficult to interpret. (See Tables 18–1 and 18–2.)

XIII. **Lung rest during ECLS.** Neonates who receive ECLS already have substantial ventilator-associated lung inflammation and injury. An extremely important benefit of ECLS is to provide "resting" ventilator settings. Although centers vary in the level of rest ventilator settings, for VA ECLS patients, a low rate of 10 breaths/min (10–20), a modest to high positive end-expiratory pressure (PEEP) of 5–14 cm H_2O, a low peak inspiratory pressure (PIP) in the 12–20 cm H_2O range, with a low FIO_2 of ~40% is used. **In VA ECLS, the ventilator FIO_2 of ~ 40% may improve oxygenation of coronary blood.**

Higher ventilator settings may be necessary if appropriate gas exchange cannot be achieved on VV ECLS (ie, a rate of 20–30 breaths/min, PIP of 15–25 cm H_2O, PEEP of 5–10 cm H_2O, and FIO_2 from 30 to 50%). Some centers use high-frequency oscillatory ventilation for lung rest, usually with a mean airway pressure of 10–14 cm H_2O and low amplitudes.

Table 18–1. DECREASED SvO_2 LEVELS DURING EXTRACORPOREAL LIFE SUPPORT

O_2	Causes	Etiologies
↓ O_2 supply	↓ CO	Heart failure, cardiac depressants, arrhythmias, ↑ PEEP, ↓ preload
	↓ Sao_2	↓ Respiratory function, oxygenator failure, suctioning, insufficient ECLS flow, ↓ ECLS blender FIO_2
	↓ Hb	Anemia, methemoglobinemia
↑ O_2 demand	↑ VO_2	Fever, shivering, agitation, pain, seizures, infection
	↑ CO	↑ Work of breathing

CO, cardiac output; ECLS, extracorporeal life support; PEEP, positive end-expiratory pressure; VO_2, oxygen consumption.

Table 18–2. **INCREASED SvO$_2$ LEVELS DURING EXTRACORPOREAL LIFE SUPPORT**

O$_2$	Causes	Etiologies
↑ O$_2$ supply	↑ CO	Improved cardiac function
	↑ Sao$_2$	Improved lung function, excess ECLS flow, ↑ Fio$_2$
	↑ Hb	Blood transfusion
	↑ Flow	Recirculation
↓ O$_2$ demand	↓ VO$_2$	Hypothermia, anesthesia, muscle relaxation
	↓ Utilization	Sepsis, cyanide toxicity (from sodium nitroprusside), severe neurological injury

CO, cardiac output; ECLS, extracorporeal life support; PEEP, positive end-expiratory pressure; VO$_2$, oxygen consumption.

XIV. **Renal function during ECLS.** ECLS patients frequently need their urine output augmented with a diuretic. Particularly with VA ECLS, the kidneys may be sensitive to the nonpulsatile nature of the flow, resulting in a decrease in renal function. For patients with preexisting or developing renal failure and/or those with anasarca, hemofiltration may be added in parallel to the ECLS circuit via a small shunt. This system allows for removal of excess fluid and stabilizes electrolyte abnormalities. (See Figure 18–1.)

XV. **Medications and nutrition.** Antibiotics, sedatives, antianxiety medications, proton pump inhibitors, and total parenteral nutrition should be delivered to the patient if possible, but with limited access can be delivered into the ECLS circuit at patient venous access locations. Because the volume of distribution is higher due to the ECLS circuit volume, higher doses may be needed. If renal failure is present, doses may need to be decreased. Discussion with the pharmacist will help with correct dosing.

XVI. **Myocardial stun.** Myocardial stun may occur after an ischemic insult to the heart and after the initiation of VA or VV ECLS. In patients on VA ECLS, left ventricular (LV) stun can occur when the LV is not properly ejecting blood, becomes overdistended, and impedes cardiac ejection, potentially resulting in cardiac damage and pulmonary edema. Cardiac stun should be suspected any time there is a loss in pressure on ECLS that is not secondary to the recent initiation of VA ECLS, hypovolemia, pneumothorax, pneumopericardium, hemothorax, or hemopericardium. An echo showing minimal LV wall motion can confirm the diagnosis.

Management of cardiac stun is challenging. Increasing ECLS flow in an attempt to try to improve oxygenation may cause further LV dilation, increasing the LV afterload and increasing myocardial oxygen consumption. Additional volume to improve right heart filling, inotropic agents to improve left heart ejection, maximizing postmembrane oxygen content and total oxygen delivery, and reducing afterload with vasodilators may allow for recovery of the stunned ventricle.

Cardiac stun failing to improve within 4–5 days represents an ominous sign and suggests myocarditis or myocardial infarction. Decompression may be necessary by balloon septostomy with or without a stent in place. Alternatively, a transthoracic LV catheter may be connected to the venous drainage side of the ECLS circuit.

Right ventricular (RV) dysfunction can occur, particularly in neonates with severe pulmonary hypertension before the initiation of ECLS. In some cases, even while on VV ECLS, the RV becomes further dilated and dysfunctional, causing it to bow into the LV, compromising LV filling and cardiac output. Cardiac echo assessment is necessary, and the use of agents to reduce RV afterload, such as inhaled nitric oxide, milrinone, and/or sildenafil, are warranted. If medical management is not effective, patients may need to be converted to VA ECLS.

XVII. **Circuit changes/thrombosis.** Thrombosis in the circuitry may necessitate the need for a circuit change. During circuit changes, a large percentage of blood volume is exchanged, and there can be electrolyte imbalances and arrhythmias. Blood drug levels may need to be adjusted as well. Clots in the cannula(e) can be challenging to manage because removal of these thrombi requires temporary discontinuation of ECLS.

XVIII. **Practical considerations for ECLS management**
   A. **VA ECLS**
      1. **VA ECLS blood flows.** After cannulation, bypass flow is slowly increased. Typically, VA ECLS flow is maintained at ~60–80% of total blood flow (100–150 mL/kg/min), and the pulse pressure is generally around 10–20 mm Hg if the heart has effective contractility.

      The goal of VA ECLS is to provide adequate oxygen delivery to all tissues. As more blood is routed through the circuit with a high flow rate, the systemic arterial pulse contour may become dampened and then flatten if total bypass is achieved. In this situation, more blood drains into the circuit, decreasing both right and left heart preload and resulting in a decrease in the left ventricular stroke volume. Despite the lack of pulsatility, the mean blood pressure remains fairly constant and is the best gauge of blood pressure dynamics.

      2. **SvO_2 levels.** SvO_2 levels of 75–80% usually reflect adequate tissue oxygen supply.
      3. **Oxygen delivery/CO_2 removal.** In VA ECLS, part of the blood from the right atrium also circulates through the native lung into the left heart and out the aorta, returning again to the right heart. This blood will be exposed to variable ventilation, depending on lung function and status of the disease process. With improvement in native lung function and cardiac output, the oxygen content of the blood returning will be higher.

      A major strategy to improve oxygen delivery includes maintaining a higher hemoglobin level. Increasing the ECLS blender O_2 or ventilator FiO_2 will also improve the arterial saturations if they are low. A failing oxygenator (because of reduced functional surface area) may decrease oxygen delivery as well.

      Increasing the sweep gas flow rate will lower the CO_2. An increasing CO_2 level may be the first sign that the oxygenator is developing excessive clot formation.

      4. **Trialing off VA ECLS.** After the initial disease processes and inflammatory responses have subsided and pulmonary function has improved (demonstrated by improvement in chest radiographs and lung compliance), patients are ready to be weaned off VA ECLS. Before the trial, all infusions should be moved from the ECLS circuit to the patient if not done previously. Heparin may continue to run through the circuit or be split so that one-half is transfused to the patient and one-half to the circuit. The surgical team should be notified of the estimated time of possible decannulation.
         a. **Starting 12 hours before the anticipated trial off, the ECLS blood flows are decreased slowly** and ventilator settings adjusted as needed based on blood gases. The pump flow can be weaned hourly by 10–20 mL/min while gradually increasing ventilatory support. ECLS blood flows are weaned to a target "idling" flow of 50–100 mL/kg/min. Once this is accomplished, the cannulae are clamped and the bridge clamp is removed. To maintain integrity of the cannulae and circuit while trialing off, the cannulae are flushed every 5 minutes by opening the venous cannula, clamping the bridge or shunt, then opening the arterial cannula for 5–10 seconds, followed by reversing the sequence. Patient blood gases should be obtained with a frequency that assures adequate lung function throughout the trial. The low flow state of the trial increases the possibility of thrombosis formation in the circuit; the length of time for the trial may depend on cannulae and circuit integrity. If the patient does not appear ready for decannulation, infusions

may continue in the patient's vascular catheters or moved to the circuit. All heparin infusions will be moved back to the circuit. If parameters remain within the acceptable ranges, patients may be decannulated.

B. **VV ECLS**

1. **VV ECLS blood flows.** As with VA ECLS, flow is gradually increased to 100–120 mL/kg/min. With the use of a double-lumen VV ECLS catheter, blood is withdrawn simultaneously from the right atrium via one side of the cannula, oxygenated in the extracorporeal lung or oxygenator, then reinfused continuously back into the right atrium via the other side of the cannula; consequently, there is no net effect on the right atrial volume, intracardiac flow, or aortic blood flow. Ideally the output from the return port is directed toward the tricuspid valve. The native cardiac output propels oxygenated blood forward to the systemic arterial system and tissues. O_2 delivery can be augmented by increasing the O_2 content of the venous blood in the right atrium or by maneuvers that decrease recirculation (eg, increasing native cardiac output, repositioning the cannula). Because oxygenator blood mixes continuously with desaturated venous blood entering the right atrium, the final O_2 content of the blood reaching the aorta and tissues is limited by the amount of blood that can be drained into the ECLS circuit, oxygenated, and returned to the venous system. The optimal pump flow rate is one that provides the highest effective pump flow at the lowest revolutions per minute of the pump, resulting in the highest O_2 delivery and causing the least degree of tubing wear and/or hemolysis.

2. **Pao_2 levels.** Patients usually have arterial saturation levels of 80–95%, with Pao_2 levels of 50–80 mm Hg. During VV ECLS, only indirect circulatory support is achieved, and lower oxygen saturations often need to be tolerated. Pao_2 levels may rise as native pulmonary function improves.

3. **Ventilator strategies.** When the size of the venous cannula limits ECLS flow, maintenance of some native pulmonary gas exchange may be necessary to achieve adequate patient oxygenation. In this situation, using higher PEEP levels may facilitate O_2 delivery.

4. **Recirculation.** Occurs when oxygenated blood from the ECLS circuit delivered to the reinfusion lumen is siphoned back to the venous drainage lumen instead of flowing across the tricuspid valve. The recirculation fraction depends on the type of cannula, native cardiac output, and right atrial volume. When pump flow rises above optimal flow, recirculation increases and effective flow decreases. **Clinically significant recirculation is recognized by a decrease in patient arterial saturations and a rise in SvO_2 levels with increasing pump flow.** Higher degrees of recirculation decrease the effective O_2 delivery from the circuit, possibly contributing to increased hemolysis as well. Other factors that increase recirculation include the following:

   a. **Decreased right atrial volume** causes a higher percentage of returned oxygenated blood to be drained back to the pump.

   b. **A catheter malpositioned too high in the superior vena cava or too low in the inferior vena cava increases recirculation.** Furthermore, inappropriate positioning of the outflow ports may result in blood being directed away from the tricuspid valve, thus increasing the recirculation fraction. Catheters may migrate with changes in lung volume, increasing edema of the neck, a change in the patient's position or with the patient's movements, necessitating adjustment of the cannula to maintain adequate flows and minimize recirculation. Maintaining the catheter position is critical in VV ECLS.

   c. **Poor cardiac output** leads to greater recirculation because a smaller fraction of the oxygenated pump blood is propelled forward out of the right atrium.

5. **Oxygen delivery/CO_2 removal.** Major strategies to improve oxygen delivery in VV ECLS include increasing the hemoglobin, increasing ECLS flow, and improving the native cardiac output. Recirculation issues may not be amenable to changes in ECLS flow, forcing acceptance of suboptimal gas exchange. Increasing the sweep gas flow rate will lower the CO_2.

6. **Trialing off VV ECLS.** Given the dynamics of VV ECLS, circuit flow rates do not require weaning. Blood flow may remain constant (usually 60–100 mL/kg/min) followed by weaning the FIO_2 sweep gas flow rate to room air. During this time, the ventilator settings are increased to levels expected to achieve normal gas exchange. Then the sweep gas tubing is disconnected from the blender source, which functionally removes the patient from ECLS. ACT levels, blood gases, and SvO_2 levels are followed, and once assured of success after 1–2 hours, the patient may be decannulated and the heparin drip discontinued. If a percutaneous technique was used for VV cannula insertion, simply cutting the sutures and removing them and then the cannula is all that is required. Pressure at the site for 15–20 minutes should achieve adequate hemostasis.

XIX. **Complications of ECLS**

A. **Patient complications of ECLS.** Patient complications per the Extracorporeal Life Support Organization (ELSO) International Summary data as of July 2011 for neonatal respiratory patients are as follows: acute renal failure (continuous renal replacement required, 16.5%; dialysis required, 3.2%); hypertension requiring vasodilators, 12.3%; hypotension requiring inotropics, 20.1%; CNS infarction, 7.5%; intracranial hemorrhage, 7.0%; culture-proven infection, 6.0%; surgical bleeding, 6.3%; pulmonary hemorrhage, 4.5%; pneumothorax requiring treatment 6.1%; DIC, 2.5%; hemolysis,10.9%; seizures, 10.5%; brain death, 0.9%.

B. **Mechanical problems.** Include oxygenator clots, 17.2%; cannula problems, 11.7%; oxygenator failure, 6%; air in the circuit, 5.9%; pump failure, 1.7%; raceway rupture, 0.3%.

XX. **Prognosis.** The **Neonatal ECLS Registry** (established in 1985), as of July 2011, lists 29,839 neonatal patients. Currently, the overall cumulative neonatal survival rate is 75% for respiratory, 39% for cardiac, and 39% for extracorporeal cardiopulmonary resuscitation use of ECLS for patients with refractory cardiopulmonary arrest. The cumulative drop in survival over the years reflects a larger proportion of patients treated with high-mortality diagnoses. The registry also tracks cumulative survival rates for specific diseases: meconium aspiration syndrome, 94%; pulmonary hypertension, 78%; hyaline membrane disease, 84%; sepsis, 75%; pneumonia, 57%; airleak syndrome 74%; congenital diaphragmatic hernia, 51%; congenital heart defect 38%; cardiac arrest, 22%; cardiogenic shock, 39%; cardiomyopathy, 63%; myocarditis, 49%; cardiac transplant, 30%. Congenital diaphragmatic hernia and lower birthweight status in those patients treated for respiratory failure are variables associated with increased mortality and morbidity.

XXI. **Neurodevelopmental outcomes.** Results of a randomized study comparing patients treated with ECLS versus conventional support suggest that the underlying disease processes appear to be the major influence on morbidity at 7 years of age in former newborns with severe respiratory failure. When comparing the ECLS group with the conventionally treated group, a higher respiratory morbidity and increased risk of behavioral problems was noted in the group of children treated conventionally. There were no cognitive differences between the 2 trial groups (76% of the children available for follow-up testing in both groups were within the normal range, although they fell below population norms). Overall, 40% of the children had normal neuromotor development (43% of the children in the ECLS group and 35% in the conventionally treated group). Behavioral problems, particularly hyperactivity, were more common in the conventionally treated children. Progressive sensorineural hearing loss was found in both groups and could be late in onset and progressive. Inciting causes for certain neurologic sequelae were difficult to discern. However, it was felt that cannulation itself, causing disruption of the cerebral circulation, was not responsible for subsequent neurologic or behavioral consequences. The increased survival among children randomized to ECLS (67% compared with conventional survival at 41%) was not offset by disability among survivors.

Selected References

Extracorporeal Life Support Organization. *Registry Report, International Summary.* Ann Arbor, MI: Extracorporeal Life Support Organization; January 2011.

Extracorporeal Life Support Organization. Organization web site. www.elsonet.org.

Hansell DR. ECLS equipment and devices. In: Van Meurs K, Lally KP, Peek G, Zwischenberger JB, eds. *ECMO Extracorporeal Cardiopulmonary Support in Critical Care.* 3rd ed. Ann Arbor, MI: Extracorporeal Life Support Organization; 2005:108.

Hoffman SB, Massaro AN, Gingalewski C, Short BL. Survival in congenital diaphragmatic hernia: use of predictive equations in ECLS population. *Neonatology.* 2011;99:258–265.

McNally H, Bennett CC, Elbourne D, Field DJ; UK Collaborative ECMO Trial Group. United Kingdom collaborative randomized trial of neonatal extracorporeal membrane oxygenation; follow-up to age 7 years. *Pediatrics.* 2006;117:e845–e854.

Short BL, Williams L. *ECMO Specialist Training Manual.* 3rd ed. Ann Arbor, MI: Extracorporeal Life Support Organization; 2010.

19 Follow-Up of High-Risk Infants

Whenever an infant requires neonatal intensive care, concerns about survival are followed by concerns about the infant's quality of life. Follow-up clinics are a necessary adjunct to neonatal intensive care because they provide feedback regarding the child's ongoing health and development to families, pediatricians, neonatologists, and obstetricians. For families, neonatal intensive care unit (NICU) follow-up clinics provide the support and advice they need following NICU discharge.

I. Goals of a neonatal follow-up clinic

    A. **Early identification of neurodevelopmental disability.** These infants need comprehensive neurodevelopmental evaluations and appropriate community services.

    B. **Assessment of a child's need for early interventions.** Although NICUs refer many infants directly to community early intervention programs, children's needs change with neuromaturation, requiring periodic review.

    C. **Parent counseling.** Reassurance that their child is making good neurodevelopmental progress is always welcome, as this is a time of high anxiety for parents. Parents of children with developmental delay need realistic information about its significance, and advice about needed evaluations and interventions. Parents need to know as soon as possible if their child is demonstrating signs of neurodevelopmental impairment. A comprehensive evaluation can provide them with essential information. Physical and occupational therapists provide valuable suggestions regarding positioning, handling, and feeding infants. Even if their infant does well, parents of high-risk infants should be warned about early signs of school or behavior problems.

    D. **Identification and treatment of medical complications** that were not recognized or anticipated at the time of discharge from the NICU.

    E. **Referral for comprehensive evaluations and community services** as indicated.

    F. **Feedback for neonatologists, pediatricians, obstetricians, pediatric surgeons, and others** regarding neurodevelopmental outcomes, ongoing medical problems, and unusual or unforeseen complications in these infants is essential.

II. **Staff of the neonatal follow-up clinic.** Pediatricians, neurodevelopmental pediatricians, and neonatologists make up the regular staff of the clinic, and many clinics include neuropsychologists and physical, occupational, and/or speech and language therapists. In addition, some infants may need referrals to audiologists, ophthalmologists, neuropsychologists, social workers, respiratory therapists, nutritionists, gastroenterologists, orthopedic surgeons, or other subspecialists.

III. **Risk factors for developmental disability.** It is virtually impossible to diagnose developmental disability with certainty in the neonatal period, but a number of perinatal risk factors have been identified for selecting high-risk infants for close follow-up.

A. **Preterm birth.** The risks of cerebral palsy and intellectual disability increase with decreasing gestational age. Risk of disability, especially cognitive impairments, is highest in survivors born at the limit of viability (at or before 25 weeks' gestation). Children born preterm have higher rates of language disorders, visual perception problems, minor neuromotor dysfunction, attention deficits, executive dysfunction, and learning disabilities than full-term controls. Although most do well, children born at 33–36 weeks' gestation have higher rates of cognitive impairments, cerebral palsy, and school problems than children born full term. Besides gestational age, predictors of neurodevelopmental disability include poor growth (especially head growth), asphyxia, sepsis (especially meningitis), chronic lung disease, and retinopathy of prematurity. Risk is highest in infants with signs of brain injury on neonatal neurodevelopmental examination and neuroimaging studies (see Chapter 16).

B. **Intrauterine growth restriction (IUGR).** Full-term infants who are small for gestational age (SGA) have a higher risk of motor or cognitive impairments, attention deficits, specific learning disability, and school and behavior problems than appropriate for gestational age (AGA) infants. The etiology and severity of their IUGR, timing of the insult, and subsequent perinatal complications (eg, asphyxia, hypoglycemia, or polycythemia) influence their degree of risk (see Chapter 105). After 30 weeks' gestation, compensatory mechanisms for adverse intrauterine circumstances include accelerated maturation to improve survival if born preterm. Adverse intrauterine circumstances, preterm birth, and accelerated neuromaturation can adversely influence neurodevelopmental, especially cognitive, outcomes in preterm SGA infants.

C. **Neonatal encephalopathy (NE).** Neonatal encephalopathy is a clinical syndrome characterized by a constellation of findings, including seizures and abnormalities of consciousness, muscle tone, reflexes, respiratory control, and feeding. Etiologies include infection, inflammation, metabolic errors, drug exposures, brain malformations, stroke, hypoxia, ischemia, or any combination of these conditions. Etiology, severity of clinical symptoms, abnormal electroencephalogram (EEG) pattern (especially low voltage or burst-suppression patterns), and patterns of brain injury (eg, injury to the basal ganglia and thalamus) are much stronger predictors of neurodevelopmental disability than signs of fetal distress, cord pH, or Apgar scores. Infants with mild or moderate NE who do not develop major disability are at risk for more subtle disorders, including attention deficit, learning disability, and other school problems. Infants with severe NE have a high mortality rate; many of the survivors have severe, multiple disabilities, including intellectual disability, spastic quadriplegia, microcephaly, seizures, and sensory impairment. Treatment of infants with moderate to severe NE with hypothermia improves neurodevelopmental outcomes.

D. **Respiratory failure.** Some late preterm and full-term infants develop respiratory failure that can be due to pulmonary hypoplasia, pneumonia, meconium aspiration, or persistent pulmonary hypertension. Outcome studies for randomized controlled trials of treatments for severe respiratory failure (eg, inhaled nitric oxide, ECMO/ECLS) report cognitive impairment in up to one-quarter of survivors, cerebral palsy in up to 15%, and hearing impairment in up to 30%. When followed to school age, many have problems with attention deficit, specific learning disability, minor neuromotor dysfunction, and behavior problems. Health sequelae include poor growth

and reactive airway disease. Some survivors have demonstrated progressive hearing loss, so these children need serial hearing assessments.
  E. **Infection and/or inflammation.** Maternal, fetal, and neonatal infection or inflammation has been implicated as etiologies of preterm birth, brain injury (eg, white matter injury), cerebral palsy, and cognitive impairments.
  F. **Other risk factors**
    1. **Congenital infections (TORCH—*t*oxoplasmosis, *o*ther, *r*ubella, *c*ytomegalovirus, and *h*erpes simplex virus).** Infants with congenital cytomegalovirus infection, toxoplasmosis, or rubella who are symptomatic at birth have a high incidence (60–90%) of neurodevelopmental disability. Asymptomatic infants are at risk for sensory impairment and learning disability.
    2. **In utero exposures.** Maternal drugs reported to influence fetal development include narcotics, cocaine, alcohol, phenytoin, trimethadione, valproate, warfarin, aminopterin, and retinoic acid. There are concerns that environmental toxicants influence preterm birth and fetal development.
IV. **Terminology.** Communicating about preterm outcomes entails consistent definitions.
  A. **Gestational age.** Time between mother's first day of the last menstrual cycle to birth.
  B. **Postmenstrual age (PMA).** Infant's gestational age (GA) plus chronological age (from birth).
  C. **Corrected age.** Calculated from the infant's due date, the infant's age corrected for degree of prematurity (ie, chronological age minus number of weeks born preterm).
  D. Use PMA for preterm infants in an NICU and **corrected age** for preterm follow-up.
V. **Parameters requiring follow-up**
  A. **Growth (height, weight, head circumference, weight for height).** Should be assessed at each follow-up visit. Poor head growth is associated with lower cognitive scores. Most preterm infants "catch up" in growth, but some infants with IUGR, extremely preterm birth, chronic lung disease, or short gut syndrome remain smaller than their peers.
  B. **Blood pressure.** High blood pressure (BP) is a serious NICU sequelae; monitor BP.
  C. **Breathing disorders**
    1. **Apnea.** For infants discharged home on monitors, there is often uncertainty as to when to discontinue the monitor.
    2. **Chronic lung disease.** Infants with chronic lung disease have higher rates of respiratory infections, reactive airway disease, rehospitalization, and neurodevelopmental disability. Those on supplemental oxygen, monitors, diuretics, and other medications need subspecialty follow-up and protection from secondhand smoke. Anticipatory guidance against ever smoking themselves is essential.
  D. **Hearing.** Hearing is essential for language acquisition, so it should be identified as early as possible. Before hospital discharge, all neonates should have their hearing screened (eg, **brainstem auditory evoked potentials, transient evoked otoacoustic emissions**) and referred for a comprehensive audiologic evaluation if there are concerns. Hearing aids, cochlear implants, and other treatment strategies have had a profound effect on language acquisition. Infants who had congenital perinatal (eg, TORCH) infection, congenital malformations of the head or neck, persistent pulmonary hypertension, chronic otitis, a family history of hearing impairment, or a language delay warrant serial hearing assessments.
  E. **Vision. Retinopathy of prematurity (ROP)** is a disease of the developing retina in preterm infants (see Chapter 126). Infants at risk for ROP need serial eye examinations until their retinas are fully vascularized. Ophthalmological examinations are also indicated in infants with congenital infection, congenital anomalies, and neonatal encephalopathy. All high-risk infants should have their visual acuity when 1–5 years old.
  F. **Neuromaturation (the functional development of the central nervous system [CNS]).** A dynamic process; what is typical at one age is often abnormal at another age. Extremely preterm infants are hypotonic at birth and typically develop flexor tone, first in the legs then in the arms (eg, caudocephalad direction) as they approach term. Typical preterm infants at term and full-term infants have strong flexor tone

(ie, flexor hypertonia), as well as a number of primitive (eg, Moro) and pathological (eg, Babinski) reflexes. In the months following term, emergence of higher cortical control suppresses flexor tone and pathological and primitive reflexes. Examiners must know typical infant development and the significance of deviations from the norm.

G. **Neurodevelopmental examination.** Includes an assessment of posture, extremity and axial (neck and trunk) muscle tone, deep tendon reflexes, primitive reflexes, pathologic reflexes, postural reactions (eg, automatic movements needed to keep the body upright), and motor function.

H. **Neuromotor abnormalities.** Common in many high-risk infants during the first year, but they often resolve or become less prominent by 1–2 years. They persist and are accompanied by motor delay in infants who develop cerebral palsy. These infants should have a comprehensive multidisciplinary evaluation, as infants with cerebral palsy may have debilitating associated deficits. Infants with neuromotor abnormalities and mild or no motor delay have minor neuromotor dysfunction, which signifies increased risks of balance and coordination difficulties, learning disability, attention deficit, and behavior problems.

   1. **Hypotonia** (generalized or axial hypotonia) is common in preterm infants and infants with chronic lung disease.
   2. **Hypertonia** is most common at the ankles and hips. Persistent hypertonia (especially extensor) and hyperreflexia indicate spasticity. In preterm children, spastic diplegia (ie, of both lower extremities) is the most common type of cerebral palsy. Avoid standing activities until infants can pull up on furniture themselves.
   3. **Asymmetry** of function, tone, posture, or reflexes. Encourage parents to position infants in their crib so they will turn their head to each side. Some NICU infants develop such a strong head preference that they develop torticollis and plagiocephaly. Spastic hemiplegia is spasticity of an arm and ipsilateral leg.
   4. **Neck, trunk, and lower extremity extensor hypertonia and shoulder retraction** (ie, excessive arching, shoulders back) can interfere with head control, hand use, rolling, sitting, and getting in and out of a sitting position. Encourage families to hold and position infants with their head and shoulders in line with their body and to avoid standing activities until their children pull themselves up to stand against furniture.
   5. **Fine motor dysfunction** is difficulty using the hands for manipulating objects.
   6. **Feeding problems.** Tube-fed infants need oromotor stimulation programs to prevent oral aversion (eg, not tolerating anything in their mouth).

I. **Cognitive development.** Language and visual attention are early signs of cognitive development. Refer infants with language delay for a follow-up audiologic evaluation. Encourage families to talk and read to their infant, reinforce vocalizations, and, by 9–10 months, identify objects by name. Accuracy of cognitive assessments improves with age.

J. **Developmental assessment.** A number of standardized tests are available for developmental screening or assessment. Many of them are easy to learn and administer.

   1. **Infant developmental milestones.** History and observation of language, motor, and adaptive milestone attainment provides a quick overview of developmental progress.
   2. **Standardized screening and assessment tests.** A number of standardized tests are available, some for developmental screening, as well as comprehensive tests for developmental assessment.

VI. **Correction for degree of prematurity.** Most agree that one should correct for degree of prematurity in preterm infants, but correcting beyond 2–3 years is ***controversial***. The older a child, the less important correction is: by 5 years, arithmetically 3 months' difference (eg, 60 vs 57 months) matters little. Motor milestone attainment up to independent walking proceeds according to age corrected for degree of prematurity, but some data suggest correction influences cognitive scores in children born extremely preterm well beyond age 3.

VII. **Comprehensive evaluations.** Recognizing delay or disability is an indication for comprehensive evaluation of all areas of function. Brain damage is seldom focal and often diffuse. A comprehensive multidisciplinary evaluation recognizes areas of strength and helps develop strategies for intervention, provide realistic data for parent counseling, and identify community programs and resources.

Selected References

Accardo PJ. *Caputo & Accardo's Neurodevelopmental Disabilities in Infancy and Childhood.* Baltimore, MD: Paul H. Brookes Publishing Co.; 2008.

Allen MC. Assessment of gestational age and neuromaturation. *Ment Retard Dev Disabil Res Rev.* 2005;11:21–33.

Allen MC, Cristofalo EA, Kim C. Outcomes of preterm infants: morbidity replaces mortality. *Clin Perinatol.* 2011;38:441–454.

Behrman RE, Butler AS, Institute of Medicine (U.S.). Committee on Understanding Premature Birth and Assuring Healthy Outcomes. Preterm birth: causes, consequences, and prevention. Washington, D.C.: National Academies Press; 2007.

Council on Children With Disabilities; Section on Developmental Behavioral Pediatrics; Bright Futures Steering Committee; Medical Home Initiatives for Children With Special Needs Project Advisory Committee. Identifying infants and young children with developmental disorders in the medical home: an algorithm for developmental surveillance and screening. *Pediatrics.* 2006;118:405–420.

Dong Y, Yu JL. An overview of morbidity, mortality and long-term outcome of late preterm birth. *World J Pediatr.* 2011;7:199–204.

Engle WA. Age terminology during the perinatal period. *Pediatrics.* 2004;114:1362–1364.

Leppert M, Allen MC. Risk assessment and neurodevelopmental outcomes. In: Gleason CA Devaskar SU, eds. *Avery's Diseases of the Newborn.* Philadelphia, PA: Saunders Elsevier; 2012:920–935.

Shah PS. Hypothermia: a systematic review and meta-analysis of clinical trials. *Semin Fetal Neonatal Med.* 2010;15:238–246.

20 Complementary and Alternative Medical Therapies in Neonatology

I. **Introduction.** The wave of complementary/alternative care sweeping the country has virtually bypassed neonatal intensive care units (NICUs). However, if we listen, we find families asking for complements to traditional care in many aspects of medicine. The consciousness that patients wanted around their deathbeds wasn't even on the radar screen of most hospitals when the hospice movement began. Today, a new sense of nurturant care is struggling to take shape in our NICUs. **Complementary and alternative medical (CAM)** therapies may be one adjunct to help soften the high-tech environment of an NICU by imbuing the nurturing elements one would expect to find around newborns.

Early exposure to the ex utero environment, long before development is capable of handling it, has myriad sequelae. We can't escape the evolving realization of environmental and epigenetic influences on the development of the immature brain. These infants require developmental care equal to their acute and chronic medical care. CAM therapies give us some options that might help ameliorate some of the routinely expected morbidities.

This chapter briefly describes some of the most popular and promising CAM therapies, explores how these options are used in the NICU, provides some evidence-based support, and presents ideas on potential future CAM expansions. **The following standard categorizations of CAM modalities come from the National Center of Complementary Medicine:**

A. **Lifestyle therapies (called "developmental care" in neonatology).** Examples included are light and color therapies, sound and music therapies, aromatherapy, kangaroo care and positioning, as well as avoidance of negative factors such as loud noises and bright lights.

B. **Biomechanical therapies.** Massage, reflexology, osteopathy/craniosacral, and chiropractic care.

C. **Bioenergetic therapies.** Acupuncture, healing touch, Reiki, and energy workers.

D. **Biochemical therapies.** Homeopathy and herbal medicine.

II. **Lifestyle therapies.** Many CAM practices currently implemented in neonatal units are categorized under lifestyle therapies, but they are more commonly referred to in the NICU as developmental care intervention. Research shows that the environment of a newborn is an important influence on sensory, neural, and behavioral development. CAM therapies attempt to create an environment in the NICU that is reflective of the intrauterine environment.

A. **Developmental care.** Includes many interventions, both on the macro- and microenvironmental level. Many neonatal units have made tremendous efforts to modify existing nurseries or have designed new units with environmental modifications that include particular attention to noise levels, light exposure, organization of care, and family-centered care.

1. **Noise.** Adverse environmental auditory stimuli are a common concern. Most who work in the NICU have difficulty with the constant and confusing barrage of alarms. Imagine trying to sleep in that environment. Many NICUs incorporate a system of noise assessment and regulation. We also know one of the drawbacks of incubators is the approximate 77-decibel noise level and minimal vestibular stimulation, which differs markedly from the in utero environment. Ex utero, the auditory system is not shielded by the maternal tissues that significantly attenuate frequencies. Ambient noise in the NICU may cause distress, and attempts have been made to minimize the noise using ear plugs or using sound to negate other sounds, called sonic acoustic masking.

2. **Light.** Regulation of ambient light in the NICU is also an important concern. Constant exposure to light can result in disorganization of an infant's state. Unit lighting is now designed or modified to regulate light and to include developmentally supportive circadian dark/light cycling. Focused lighting for procedures and the use of eye covers or incubator drapes are all great adjuncts.

3. **Care organization.** Infant-specific care plans help better regulate the myriad intrusions of intensive care. Positioning, handling, and interactions should be coordinated when possible with cues of readiness from the infant. This is felt to help the infant minimize energy losses and allow for more optimal conditions for neurodevelopment maturation. Infants need more conscious developmental care when the situation allows.

4. **Family involvement.** For years parents have expressed a feeling of helplessness when given little opportunity to be involved in the care of their sick child. Many complementary therapies have the benefit of encouraging early participation by family members, encouraging parent–neonate interactions, and enhancing bonding. Many professionals, who wouldn't otherwise even consider some of the complementary therapies that follow, now look at these for no other reason than having something that allows more parental participation and connection. Parents

can create a loving environment, instill a sense of security, and foster a trusting responsiveness; however, when they are met with an authoritarian, "You can't touch your baby," they can feel pushed aside and confused.

We are just beginning to see how parents can be included in our expanded focus on the developmental aspects of care. What parents need is a context for their interactions—for someone to teach them how to titrate interactions while becoming aware of their infant's cues. The **Newborn Individualized Developmental Care and Assessment Program (NIDCAP)** has been especially influential in encouraging awareness of the use of an infants' communications as a basis for individualized care delivery. These can be detected by reading the infant's sign language or state-related behaviors such as finger splaying, frequent fisting, trunk arching, gaze aversion, or more typical behaviors such as cooing, babbling, or fussing with a frowning face. Awareness of these states has changed our understanding from thinking of an infant as a passive organism to an active partner in a feedback system of rich human interactions.

Maternal administration of physical activity such as passive limb movements has been shown to enhance bone mineral acquisition in VLBW infants. This could be a great way for a father to also feel included in the care of his baby. These care practices can also provide an opportunity for the infant to hear their parents' voices, as speech and language development is believed to be influenced by prenatal maternal speech. The long-term effects of missed exposure to maternal speech in late fetal life are not known.

5. **Kangaroo care (KC).** Usually used to promote bonding and attachment between the infant and the parent (the infant is usually wearing nothing more than a diaper while held on the parent's bare chest). KC was originally developed for a different purpose. Preterm infants in Bogota, Colombia, were dying of infection caused by cross-contamination from shared bedding space and equipment in the nursery. Colombian physicians decided to try having mothers stay in the hospital and incubate their infants next to their bodies until the babies were stable and discharged home.

   KC has many cogent justifications. It supports the growing consumer interest in participation in the care of hospitalized infants while giving a significant feeling of autonomy to the parents. When a parent holds their infant against his or her skin, the infant's breathing, oxygen saturation, heart rate, and tone improve. It has also been shown that skin-to-skin care results in fewer episodes of apnea, less disorganized sleep states, and a doubling in the periods of quiet regular sleep. Also, varying body position seems to affect gastric emptying and reflux. Mounting evidence for KC promoting physiologic stability has encouraged expanded studies with very immature and ventilated infants.

6. **Aromatherapy.** Several recent articles address the role of olfaction as a tool in preterm infants. The most illustrative was a French study (Marlier) that appeared in *Pediatrics* in 2005, demonstrating a 36% reduction in apnea with the introduction of the aroma vanillin (used because of its weak trigeminal nerve activation) when used in the treatment of apnea unresponsive to caffeine.

   Researchers have reported that newborns have an acute sense of smell. Odor forms part of the complex bonding process. The soothing effects of a mother's odor are in stark contrast to the noxious odors of alcohol, skin cleansers, and adhesives normally found in an NICU. In some cultures, familiar odors are often left in a newborn's crib to calm an infant in the mother's absence. One article assessed the effects of familiar odors (eg, maternal breast milk, amniotic fluid) used on healthy preterm infants during routine blood draws, noting a decrease in crying and grimacing compared with baseline.

   Through the use of aromas, neurotransmitters are released that calm, sedate, and decrease painful sensations or can be used for stimulation. Lavender has been the most studied; for example, when lavender is placed on pillows of adults, it is known to alleviate insomnia and stress.

Could we use lavender rather than sedatives for sleep or calming infants during procedures such as computed tomography or magnetic resonance imaging? As in the French study, could other aromatic stimulants like peppermint be used in incubators as "olfactory caffeine" to minimize apnea and bradycardia? Is it possible to use scents as anxiolytics or to enhance attachment? Can olfaction be used to minimize the deleterious effects of neonatal pain?

Aromatherapy could be helpful for NICU staff as well. In a study from Japan, keypunch operators were monitored 8 hours per day for 1 month. When the office air was scented with jasmine, error rates decreased 33%, and the scent was found to increase efficiency and relieve stress among employees.

A variety of aromatherapy oils are also used for diaper rashes, such as lavender sitz baths, almond oils, and beeswax. Brazilian guava oil has been found to have analgesic effects and is being investigated for use in infants.

7. Sound and music therapy. Lullabies have been linked with infants throughout history; music therapy carries this tradition over into the NICU. In the first meta-analysis of music therapy in premature infants, Standley reported heart and respiratory rates, oxygen saturations, weight gain, length of stay, feeding rate, and rates of nonnutritive sucking as all being positively influenced. Recently it has been shown that playing Mozart reduces the resting energy expenditure in preterm infants and might be an explanation for the improved weight gain. Music therapy has also been shown to calm distress after painful stimuli, resulting in faster return to more organized states and improves hypersensitivity that is associated with stimulation. Others document improvements in feedings, weight gain, and decreased salivary cortisol levels, as well as enhanced development and parental bonding.

A few studies seek to mimic in utero noises and movements by using waterbeds and vibroacoustic stimulation. Some music therapies are used for stimulation, whereas others are used to mask over stimulation—a sonic camouflage, all attempting to enhance a neonate's neurodevelopment environment. Recent literature on the pacifier-activated lullaby (a pacifier fitted with a pressure transducer that activates music) coordinates the infants sucking with music. Sucking rates during the periods of contingent music were 2.43 times greater than baseline (silence) sucking rates. Music reinforcement for nonnutritive sucking may aid in the development of nipple feeding.

There are still many unanswered questions about the potential for sound therapy in our nurseries. Should we use it? Which types of music are best in particular situations? Is the therapeutic benefit of live music greater than recorded? Is Shostakovich better, Vivaldi, or the nurses' favorite radio station? Can music affect the caregivers' mood and behavior? Is there a "sonic caffeine"— a music or sound pattern that could ameliorate apnea and bradycardia in preterm infants?

8. Color and light therapy. Health care workers tend to dismiss color and light therapy as something from the distant annals of medicine, but certainly neonatologists could expand awareness in this area due to the near omnipresent use of phototherapy in neonatal units. Research on phototherapy has shown the biologic significance of light exposure. Aside from the classically recognized effects of diminishing bilirubin and activation of vitamin D, numerous studies have shown other metabolic alterations with phototherapy to effect thyroid stimulation, alterations in renal and vascular parameters, and increased gut-transit times. Could it be that other wavelengths of light might have other physiologic effects? This has become the basis for the field of study for color and light therapy.

The current interest for light therapy in the NICU has less emphasis on the effect of different wavelengths (colors) on an infant's metabolic milieu; rather, it focuses on generalized lighting in the unit. Establishing circadian rhythmicity by varying light cycles in the infant's environment seems to minimize endocrine fluctuations, as well as the states of disorganization that come from constant light stimulation. We can only postulate the potential for long-term neurologic dysfunction that might come from constant light stimulation. Before 28 weeks, when not using incubator covers or eye patches, it has been suggested that overexposure to light may also interfere with the development of the other senses.

III. **Biomechanical therapies**

A. **Massage therapy.** Massage therapy has been used in the care of premature infants for many years, and a significant body of research has already shown its effectiveness. Tiffany Fields has conducted infant massage research since the 1970s, much of which has focused on the premature infant. Fields reported that massaged infants have improved weight gain and better organized sleep states; they become more responsive to social stimulation, have more organized motor development, and are commonly discharged 6–10 days earlier from the hospital. Fields' studies suggest that massage increases vagal activity, which in turn releases gastrin and insulin, and also increases levels of insulin-like growth factor-1. These findings may explain the weight gain in massaged premature infants. Recent studies have shown that massaged infants are found to be calmer on discharge with improved neurodevelopmental outcome at 2 years of corrected age.

The amount of massage or stimulation applied should be altered according to the infant's maturation, acuity, engagement cues, and response to touch. The various types of massage may include stroking, gentle touch without stroking, therapeutic touch, kinesthetic (bicycling) stimulation, or even confinement holds mimicking the womb. Being aware of the infant and his or her receptivity and alertness is important in determining the best time for a massage rather than relying on a predetermined time.

A significant emphasis has been placed on fathers performing massage as a bonding tool similar to what breast-feeding would be for the mother. It can also be a great way to get other family members, such as grandparents, involved. One day we may find that, just as important as the technologies of intensive care medicine, so will be the supportive touch of a parent in helping activate an optimal neurodevelopmental milieu. Data suggest that the mother, as the masseuse, benefits from lower stress hormone levels and decreased postnatal depression and anxiety.

Although there are numerous replicated studies, infant massage is not yet a mainstay of neonatal care. Concerns regarding whether infant massage can produce overstimulation and therefore adverse effects have been raised. Further research is needed through controlled trials to determine the benefits as well as the risks of this therapy; however, many CAM therapists feel this is a classic example of the difficulties of integrating CAM therapies in an NICU. If the extensive research in massage doesn't translate into a change in practice, many wonder what hope is there for other therapies? They believe that in the current medical milieu, if a drug were developed that had the same effects, it would surely be used.

B. **Osteopathy/craniosacral therapy.** Osteopaths believe that many problems begin at birth. Labor is seen as quite traumatic, and an infant may be altered both physically and psychologically by the experience. Craniosacral therapists feel that misalignment of structure that is not corrected can lead to potential alterations in function. Problems such as sucking/swallowing difficulties, suboptimal breast-feeding, and recurrent reflux after birth are so common that many mothers and doctors consider them to be normal; however, in osteopathy, they are believed to be based in craniosacral abnormalities. Recognition and treatment of these dysfunctions in the immediate postpartum period is considered an essential preventive measure. According to craniosacral theory, these can be easily rectified.

The occipital area is thought to sustain most of the trauma at delivery. A complex study by osteopath Viola Frymann explored the relationship between symptomatology in the newborn and anatomic disturbances. The study suggested that strains within the unfused fragments of the occipital bones produce problems in the nervous system, such as vomiting, reflux, hyperactive peristalsis, tremor, hypertonicity, and irritability. Frymann notes that compression at the point of the hypoglossal nerve egress can cause an infant to suck ineffectively. Symptoms left untreated may result in tongue thrust, deviant swallowing, speech problems, and, in later life, malocclusion. Decompress the condylar parts of the occiput, and the vomiting stops. In temporal bone development, misalignment may cause recurrent otitis media. If the sphenoid sinuses are involved, the child may have headaches. When the vagus nerve is compressed, recurrent vomiting or reflux can occur.

Osteopaths believe that every child should be structurally evaluated after any type of trauma, especially birth. Until the structural cause of a problem is recognized and addressed, the underlying pathophysiology will not change. A practitioner of this discipline gently realigns cranial bones, bringing them into proper relationship.

C. **Chiropractic therapy.** Chiropractic adjustments have been used on pregnant women, newborns, and infants for more than a century. The specialization of chiropractic pediatrics has emerged in the past decade. The need for spinal care immediately after birth is a focus of the chiropractic profession, particularly if there is any history of birth trauma.

A neonatal chiropractic examination consisting of observation, static and range of motion palpation, and spinal percussion is used to detect fixation or aberrant movement in the vertebral column. Gentle chiropractic adjustment is used to correct any detected abnormalities.

IV. **Bioenergetic therapies**

A. **Acupuncture.** Acupuncture is part of the traditional system of Chinese medicine. The main concept behind this system is that of chi (body energy not currently measurable by current instrumentation), which underlies and supports all aspects of the physical body. This chi/energy circulates throughout the body along specific pathways called meridians. Obstructions in the flow of chi may cause disease. By gently placing thin, solid, disposable, metallic needles into the skin along the meridians where chi is blocked, acupuncturists rebalance the flow of energy.

Acupuncture has shown promising results in use for anesthesia, postoperative pain, and addiction recovery. Auricular acupuncture has been used since the early 1970s for various forms of maternal addiction and withdrawal prenatally. It is also used to help reduce the effects of neonatal drug withdrawal.

Currently in China, acupuncture is used to treat infants with jaundice (augmenting "hepatic chi"), skin problems, teething, ear infections, constipation, conjunctivitis, and peripheral nerve injury. Researchers are currently considering whether acupuncture can help treat colic, constipation, diminished postoperative urine output, apnea, and bradycardia. It is used also in intraoperative and postoperative pain control.

B. **Healing touch.** Healing touch (HT) is an energy-based therapy based on clearing, aligning, and balancing the human energy system through touch. HT is an energy therapy that uses gentle hand techniques purported to help reconfigure a patient's energy field and accelerate healing.

One example of an HT technique that can empower parents to feel like they are actively participating in care of their infant is called comfort infusion and is used to relieve pain. Parents are taught to place their left palm over the infant, encouraging any pain the infant may be having to move up from the infant to the parent's palm and then through their body to drain out of their right hand. When parents no longer sense pain, the right hand is placed over the infant and the left one turned upward to infuse healing energy. When the parents are at a point of feeling totally helpless in their infant's plight, this can restore a feeling of energetic connection with no touch involved, so they can do this no matter how ill their infant may be.

C. **Reiki.** Reiki is a form of noninvasive energy healing, similar to HT, in which energy is transferred from the hands of a Reiki master to a patient using a sequence of hand positions above the body. Reiki relaxes and heals by clearing energy meridians and chakras (vortices of energy along the spine). Energy blockages are dissolved, allowing the vibration frequency of the body to increase, thus restoring balance. As a calming balance occurs, respirations slow, blood pressure normalizes, and pain is relieved—all of which are felt to accelerate the healing process.

D. **Reflexology.** Reflexology is an ancient form of healing, somewhat similar to traditional acupuncture. In this modality, chi is restored by manipulation of reflex points in the hands and feet that have specific correlates to organs, glands, and body parts. Reflexology may benefit infants by increasing blood flow to specific organs, such as increasing perfusion to the kidneys or increasing cardiac output.

Imagine the distress to a newborn brought about by a heelstick; the affects of reflexology are just the opposite. Instead of a painful stick, this modality is thought to provide a grounding for a patient—a balancing and soothing of their bioenergies.

E. **Energy workers.** Energy-based healing is growing in popularity. Energy workers are a contemporary twist on some of the ancient traditions working with chi. Their ability to "read" energy patterns can provide some novel ideas in caring for infants. There are numerous energetic observations made around birthing and bonding. One is known as "psychic umbilica," a persistent energetic connection between the mother and infant after delivery. This connection is felt to diminish over the course of time, such that if breast-feeding duration is left to the infant's natural instincts, a child stops breast-feeding exactly when this energetic connection can no longer be seen or felt by a practitioner. Energy workers mention the striking alterations they feel in this energetic connection depending on the birth method (ie, medicated vs. nonmedicated vaginal deliveries or cesarean section deliveries).

Another interesting concept is one from India, where it is felt that along with the standard corporeal nutrition of breast milk, there are small energetic openings (or chakras—as in Reiki healing) in the mother's nipples that supply the infant with energetic nourishment.

V. **Biochemical interventions**

A. **Homeopathy.** The basic idea behind homeopathy is that the body's internal wisdom will defend and heal itself by choosing the most beneficial response. Homeopathy is based on the "like cures, like principle": a symptom in a patient is treated with a remedy that causes this same symptom, thus further stimulating the body's natural responses (similar in philosophy to a vaccine). Homeopathy can be considered a catalyst to jump-start the body's healing process. Homeopathic remedies are an enigma to those unaware of the concept of the memory of water and the potentiating successions that are believed to enhance that memory.

Homeopaths prescribe medicine that is very patient specific, and they base these prescriptions on past health history, past medical treatments, genetic inheritance, and a constellation of physical, emotional, mental, and spiritual symptomatology. Apparently, titrating individualized medicine(s) for newborns is not always easy. Chubby infants require different constitutional remedies than small or low-birthweight infants, as do infants who sleep through the night compared with those who do not.

Some examples of homeopathic therapies are for infants who endure traumatic labors with bruising or other injuries (ie, postnatal intravenous infiltrates). They are considered to benefit from a remedy called **arnica** and **hypericum perforatum,** which are thought to optimize the body's attempts to heal wounds, both physical and psychological. It is hypothesized that homeopathic remedies such as these, as well as **staphysagria** and **calendula,** can help circumcised newborns heal from the physical and psychological trauma of the procedure.

In Europe, where homeopathic remedies are much more commonly used, **carbovege** is used for apnea and bradycardia. **Aethusa** is used for milk intolerance as well as for reflux. **Nux vomica** and **chamomilla** are used for colic. **Magnesium phosphorica** is used to relieve symptoms of gas, bloating, and burping. **Topical calendula** is used for diaper dermatitis.

B. **Herbal medicine.** The World Health Organization estimates that ~75% of the world population relies on botanical medicines; indeed, 30% of Americans also use botanical remedies, and the practice is growing in popularity. It behooves health care professionals to be familiar with the expanding field of herbal medicine. Many mothers use herbal remedies during pregnancy. They are especially popular among breast-feeding women. Knowing what, if any, herbal remedies nursing mothers use is essential because the substances can be passed through breast milk to children. **Galactogogue herbs** have gained a reputation for increasing breast milk. (See Section VI.D.) **Sage** and **parsley** can dry up milk supply. **St. John's wort** is commonly used for postpartum depression. It has been speculated that the increased incidence of neonatal unconjugated hyperbilirubinemia in Asians may result from maternal ingestion of certain ethnically characteristic herbal medications or foods. Some of these herbal remedies can cause hemolysis in infants with glucose-6-phosphate dehydrogenase deficiency.

Caffeine is probably the herbal medicine most used in neonatal care. Many credit the use of **probiotics,** a hot topic in neonatology for prevention of necrotizing enterocolitis, as originating from the field of herbal medicine. Many others are herbal folk remedies. **Aloe vera** is used as a skin protectant or for burns and skin irritations. Creams made from **comfrey, plantain,** or **marigolds** are used for treatment of rashes and cradle cap. **Calendula** is used in Russia for conjunctivitis. **Tree tea oil** is used as an antifungal. Dandelion is used as a diuretic. **Peppermint** stimulates bile flow and decreases lower esophageal sphincter pressure. **Tripola** increases intestinal peristalsis. **Milk thistle** increases enterohepatic circulation. In China, **artemisia, Scutellaria, rheum officinale, glycyrrhiza,** and **coptis chinensis** are prescribed to jaundiced infants often in combination with phototherapy. **Kava** can be used to induce oral numbness, which would be helpful with endotracheal tube discomfort.

VI. **Supportive care**

A. **Hospice care.** Another CAM focus, increasingly prevalent in the NICU setting, is hospice care. Many NICUs are developing stronger links with hospice care teams to address the process of dying and the stages of grief for parents and family members.

Hospice has even extended its philosophical trajectory to the prenatal arena, so that families not opting to abort infants with known lethal anomalies receive support services while the child is in utero.

B. **Palliative care.** Multiple lines of evidence suggest that early repeated and prolonged pain exposure (eg, IV and heelsticks, x-rays, ventilation, peripherally inserted central catheter lines, ultrasounds) may contribute to altered development of pain systems, behavior, cognition, and learning in former preterm infants later in childhood. Early recurrent pain and thereby stress may reset arousal and thereby affect interactions with the environment. We have a lot to learn about integrating sensory stimulation and the use of CAM therapies in alleviating pain and stress.

C. **Emotional care.** Another complementary area of focus is the myriad of options that address the emotional and spiritual needs of parents. Support groups can help parents gain perspective on their situation. These groups may help to obviate the emotional trauma parents may feel about having such a vulnerable infant, or they may address the extreme disruption families experience in the usual stages of pregnancy, which may influence their preparation for nurturing their child. The same idea can be used to meet the often overlooked needs of siblings.

D. **Galactagogues.** Therapies in the management of inadequate breast milk supply are of special concern to neonatologists. Prescription galactagogues and increased fluid intake are traditional mainstays, but many mothers prefer more natural therapies when breast-feeding. CAM therapies that have been used for centuries include herbal galactagogues, such as Fenugreek, chaste tree, blessed thistle, fennel, trobangun leaves (thought to antagonize the dopamine receptors, and thereby increasing prolactin release), and biomechanical galactagogues, which vary from massage, kangaroo care, and relaxation therapies, to auricular acupuncture, which is used in China for the treatment of hypogalactia.

VII. **Conclusion.** As neurodevelopmental care emerges as neonatology's new frontier, CAM therapies challenge us to think of the many options for supporting and nurturing the complexities of health and healing in infants. Many of these provide the possibility of using structured stimuli to help reduce stress and other noxious environmental factors. For example, recent neuroscience research has shown that environmental enrichment can accelerate the maturation of EEG activity and visual function in neonates.

Because mainstream medicine has traditionally viewed CAM therapies with suspicion, research will be needed to demonstrate the efficacy of many of these therapies, as well as to assess the short- and long-term benefits and burdens.

Selected References

Als H, Duffy FH, McAnulty GB, et al. Early experience alters brain function and structure. *Pediatrics.* 2004;113:846–857.

Fields TM. *Touch in Early Development.* Mahwah, NJ: Erlbaum; 1995.

Frymann VM. *The Collected Papers of Viola M. Frymann, DO: Legacy of Osteopathy to Children.* Ann Arbor, MI: Edward Brothers; 1998.

Guzzetta A, Baldini S, Bancale A, et al. Massage accelerates brain development and the maturation of visual function. *J Neurosci.* 2009;29:6042–6051.

Kramer LI, Pierpont ME. Rocking waterbeds and auditory stimuli to enhance growth of preterm infants. *J Pediatr.* 1976;88:297–299.

Lubetzky R, Mimouni FB, Dollberg S, Reifen R, Ashbel G, Mandel D. Effect of music by Mozart on energy expenditure in growing preterm infants. *Pediatrics.* 2010;125:e24–e28.

Marlier L, Gaugler C, Messer J. Olfactory stimulation prevents apnea in premature newborns. *Pediatrics.* 2005;115:83–88.

Moyer-Mileur LJ, Ball SD, Brunstetter VL, Chan GM. Maternal-administered physical activity enhances bone mineral acquisition in premature very low birth weight infants. *J Perinatol.* 2008;28:432–437.

Procianoy R, Mendes EW, Silveira RC. Massage therapy improves neurodevelopment outcome at two years corrected age for very low birth weight infants. *Early Hum Dev.* 2010;86:7–11.

Standley JM. A meta-analysis of the efficacy of music therapy for premature infants. *J Pediatric Nurs.* 2002;17:107–113.

21 Neonatal Bioethics

I. **Introduction. Ethics** is a term that describes "doing good." The study of bioethics as a field separate from medicine itself is a recent phenomenon. Physicians have historically set and maintained policies concerning ethical behavior in medical practice. During the last 30 years, the distinct study of bioethics has come into being. The obligation to act in an ethical manner in medical practice requires that we know something about how we should act and what internal and external guidelines should be followed to accomplish that end. Bioethical issues should be examined from the perspectives of the patient and family, the physician, and society as a whole.

II. **Bioethics perspectives**

    A. **The patient.** Patient-centered bioethics deals with basic principles in which every interaction should be filtered. This protects patients in their more vulnerable position and allows equal treatment. The principles that govern physician–patient interaction are respect of **autonomy, nonmaleficence, beneficence, and justice.**

    B. **The physician.** Despite an increasing public distrust of physicians' motives, the practice of medicine requires physicians to perform in an exceptionally professional manner. Indeed, the very idea of "professional" is closely linked to good conduct and virtuous behavior. Several important virtues make the practice of medicine a profession as opposed to everyday work.

        1. **Fidelity to trust.** Trust is an important virtue in any human relationship. This involves not only truth telling but also aspects of consistency, integrity, and confidence. The medical relationship between physician and patient extends even further into this idea of trust. The relationship between professionals such as physicians, lawyers, and ministers is termed a fiduciary relationship. In such a relationship, the patient trusts the physician to help the patient, and the physician is expected to provide this help to the best of his or her ability. In other words, as physicians, we should always be found trustworthy.

        2. **Compassion.** If there is one aspect of a physician's character most scrutinized by patients, it is compassion. Compassion, although difficult to define precisely, is the quality most associated with ethical behavior. The word compassion (*com* meaning "with" and *passion* meaning "suffering") literally means to "suffer with" your patient.

        3. **Phronesis.** The term phronesis was used by Aristotle for the virtue of practical wisdom, the capacity for moral insight, the capacity, in a given set of circumstances, to discern what moral choice or course of action is most conducive to the good of the agent or the activity in which the agent is engaged. In short, phronesis can be defined as "common sense."

        4. **Justice.** It is defined as "the rendering to one what is due." As physicians, we have a specific obligation to render to our patients what is due: the patient's healing. The virtue of justice also indicates an unfailing quality. This quality is linked to the rule of nonmaleficence or the avoidance of doing harm to the patient.

        5. **Fortitude.** Describes not only physical but also mental and emotional courage. We tend to think of courage in terms of a soldier in battle, but physicians display courage in a variety of ways: caring for patients with HIV infection, continuing in our care long past any hour that reasonable jobs would require, and facing the emotional wear and tear of dealing with families in crisis situations.

        6. **Temperance or prudence.** Usually thought of in terms of social activities or moral life. The physician, too, would be wise to consider this; however, temperance in medicine deals with our use of technology.

        7. **Integrity.** To integrate is to "bring all parts together." In the same sense, physicians need to have all the parts together. Our outward presentation to patients and families should be that of consistency and predictability. This virtue is important in developing trust in our physician–patient relationships. True integrity, as opposed to a facade of self-confidence, requires ongoing self-examination and reflection.

        8. **Self-effacement.** To avoid the elevation of oneself above another. Although physicians are highly trained and skilled in the art of medicine, it is important to remember our place; we are to help the parents (or guardians) in caring for the patient. Self-effacement also involves attitudes toward patients in research studies and protocols.

        9. **Society.** In some instances, the good of society outweighs individual rights. In cases of quarantine for infectious diseases or mandatory treatment to prevent epidemics, we must understand that the temporary loss of rights is for the greater good of all people. This perspective should always be thought of in health care decisions but should not have primacy in that unjust loss of rights might result.

III. **Pediatric issues**

A. **The best-interest standard.** When physicians work with patients who cannot talk, either because of age or because of mental incapacity, we cannot obtain direct consent for treatment and procedures. In these cases, we must decide which treatment options the patient would choose. This is called the "best interest standard," which describes what we should do as physicians: provide care that is in the patient's best interest. In the case of young children, we normally assume that the parents have the best idea of what constitutes the child's best interest. In other cases, the patient's best interests are decided by a guardian, or legal appointee. Physicians sometimes assume this role in emergencies when there is not enough time to contact other responsible family members.

B. **Parents as patient advocates**

1. **Parental rights.** In the care of infants and children, the parents are uniformly thought to represent the patient's best interests. They are intimately involved in the child's situation and will be long after the physician is out of the picture. Unless imminent harm will come to the child, the parents should be permitted to make all decisions concerning the welfare of their child.

2. **Exception cases.** There are a few cases in which parental rights are not maintained. The widest known of these concerns blood transfusions in children of families who belong to the Jehovah's Witness sect. The parent's right to refuse potentially lifesaving therapy, however, commonly does not extend to the children. The reasoning is that this particular request is outside of what is "normal and usual" in American society, and thus the parental right to refuse this therapy is challenged. Normally, a physician can seek a court order that will place the child in the custody of the state, which then consents to blood transfusion. This same standard has been applied to other parental requests that are outside what would be reasonably expected. Refusal of surgery for a correctable anomaly or demand for treatments that have no effectiveness are cases in which parental rights may be refused.

C. **Minors as parents.** Increasingly, we see teenagers—minors themselves—giving birth to children. In most circumstances, the minor parent is treated with adult status. In many cases, there may be an overseer figure, such as a grandparent, who helps in this decision process. Note, however, that the parent does have final say in issues of consent and treatment unless that minor parent is otherwise incapacitated.

D. **Child abuse.** Normally, we think of child abuse as occurring after birth when we see a number of injuries and problems associated with this, such as physical and emotional abuse, neglect, or sexual abuse. Several states, however, have made proposals to prosecute prenatal child abuse by mothers who act in a harmful or neglectful manner toward their unborn infants. Continued intravenous or cocaine drug abuse is considered directly harmful to the fetus and, in some instances, has been prosecuted. In these cases, the child becomes a ward of the state after birth.

IV. **Specific ethical issues in neonatology**

A. **Informed consent is a recent term.** It implies the two components required for proper treatment of patients. First, they must be informed completely of the disease and its short- and long-term ramifications. Additionally, the treatment or procedures should be performed in a like manner. Potential major complications, long-term side effects, and indications and benefits of the treatment or procedure must be explained to the understanding of the parents. Possible alternative treatment should also be presented. As physicians, we also need to evaluate the consent that is given. Do the parents have a good understanding of the child's disease, prognosis, and therapeutic options? Are the parents capable of acting in the child's best interest and thus capable of giving consent? Obviously, it is impossible to discuss every complication or ramification of the operation; however, some mention should be made that other complications exist, and the major complications should be listed. These should be explained more fully if the parent desires. The consent obtained should always be durable and written, not assumed merely because the parent voices no dissenting opinion. Emergency and life-threatening situations complicate our ability to obtain informed consent. It is prudent, therefore, to try to discuss potential problems before they develop.

B. **Withholding care.** There is sometimes a feeling among physicians that, to provide optimal care, patients should be offered every technological treatment or procedure possible. In many cases, however, the application of highly technical procedures is not in the best interest of the patient. Frequently, critically ill infants who are not responding to present therapy should have further or more advanced therapy withheld. The decision in these cases rests on whether further therapy will

1. Have its intended effect
2. Reverse the process
3. Restore the quality of life that is acceptable to the patient or the caregivers

    With these goals in mind, one can see that it is as important to obtain informed consent for withholding care as it is for the application of procedures. The physician should not withhold care without discussing this course of action with the parents. Likewise, the decision to withhold care should be discussed with the other physicians and nursing staff involved. The indications for and benefits of withholding care should be clearly defined.

C. **Withdrawing care.** In some cases, care can and should be withdrawn for a number of reasons.

1. **The care or treatment** rendered no longer accomplishes its intended purpose (ie, futility of care).
2. **Ongoing evaluations or tests** reveal information changing the diagnosis or prognosis of the patient. In these cases, reevaluation and discussion with the patient's parents are required to provide for the patient's best interest with this new information.
3. **Care given in an emergency** should be withdrawn if it is contrary to the parents' wishes when they are informed. As noted, there are a few legal exceptions to this rule. Overall, the withdrawal of care hinges on the idea of futility. Does the patient benefit from such care? Can we expect the therapy to accomplish both short- and long-term goals? As an example, the use of pressor agents in a moribund infant may reach the point of futility. If the short-term goal (ie, raising the blood pressure) is not accomplished and neither is the long-term goal (ie, restoring health), then therapy is no longer useful and should be withdrawn. The difficulty with withdrawing care rests on the definition of futility. This may depend on the health care worker's perspective. The ability of a physician to use the virtues of compassion, phronesis, and temperance comes into play when discussing these issues. At every step, the patient's parents should be clearly informed of the decisions and possible outcomes.

D. **Nutrition and patient comfort. Nutrition** has been classified as a therapy, that is, as a medicine that could potentially be withdrawn or, in other instances, as one of the patient's basic rights for comfort. In any discussion of ethics and patient care, there is consensus that the patient should be provided some basic comforts despite what other circumstance may be in question. The comfort of nursing care, cleanliness, pain relief, and mere presence are factors considered to be basic to human life and not subject to diminution or withdrawal, secondary to end-of-life issues. In most cases, nutrition (ie, food and water) is classified as one of these basic comfort cares. This has been contested in the legal system in a variety of cases, with a broad spectrum of varying opinions. With this in mind, it is probably wise to assume nutrition and feeding to be basic rights for patient care and to challenge this position only in extreme circumstances. The parents' understanding of nutrition as therapy or as a basic right is important. Agreement among the parents, caregivers, administration, and legal authorities must be obtained if the withdrawal of nutrition is contemplated. The activation and opinion of the institution's bioethics committee may be very helpful in resolving these issues.

E. **Delivery room issues.** Neonatal care in the delivery room requires rapid assessment and quick decision making. In infants with severe congenital anomalies or extreme prematurity, these first few moments of life are critical. In these instances, the pediatrician is called on to make critical decisions within seconds concerning viability, quality of life, and prognosis. Care during this period should be guided by the following general principles.

1. **Discuss as fully as possible** with the parents their wishes and expectations before actual delivery of the child. Coordination between the pediatricians and obstetricians can facilitate this dialogue (counseling parents before high-risk delivery is discussed in Chapter 50).

2. **Err on the side of life.** If the mother is unable to express her wishes, then emergency therapy must be performed. It is much better to err on the side of life-sustaining therapy than to withhold such therapy. If in the aftermath of this crisis it is discovered that the parents wish no such therapy, then it is appropriate to withdraw therapy. This, however, gives the parents the opportunity to form their own opinion and exercise their right in protecting the child's best interest.

3. **Noninitiation of resuscitation** in the extremely immature infant or in cases of severe congenital anomaly is a challenging problem in neonatology. According to guidelines from the American Heart Association and American Academy of Pediatrics, noninitiation of resuscitation appears appropriate in confirmed gestation of <23 weeks or birthweight <400 g, anencephaly, or confirmed trisomy 13 or 18. In these cases, all data suggest that resuscitation of these infants is highly unlikely to result in survival or survival without severe disability. In cases in which the antenatal information may be unreliable or with uncertain prognosis, options include a period of resuscitation with the option of discontinuation of the resuscitation if assessment of the infant after delivery does not support the continued efforts. Initial resuscitation and subsequent withdrawal of support may allow time to gather key clinical information and to counsel the family appropriately.

4. **Discontinuation of resuscitation** may be appropriate if the infant fails to have return of spontaneous circulation within 15 minutes. This is based on strong data suggesting that after a period of 10 minutes of asystole, survival or survival without severe disability is highly unlikely. The Guideline Committee of the American Academy of Pediatrics and American Heart Association recommends that each institution develop local discussions of these issues based on the availability of resources and outcome data.

V. **Conflict resolution**

A. **Identifying conflict. Conflict** is any dispute or disagreement of opinion. This may occur between the physician and the patient or the patient's guardian. Alternatively, conflicts can arise between the physician and the nursing staff, health care workers, and administrative staff or any combination of these. Most ethical issues arise as conflict between differing values or moral ideals. Therefore, the identification of conflict is a key or essential ingredient in bioethical decisions. Conflict is best identified by ongoing communication. Normally, we think of this as communication between physician and patient. However, this is just the first step. Continued communication among members of the health care team, parents, family members, and others involved in the case will uncover unvoiced concerns and opinions. These should be dealt with in an open and honest fashion to obtain consensus about ethical issues.

B. **Putting virtue into practice.** Section II of this chapter describes various virtues or attributes that will assist a physician in making ethical decisions. Many of these virtues are common for all humans. Others, however, apply specifically to the obligations and responsibilities of a physician. If used, many of these virtues will help the physician defuse or avoid completely many ethical issues. Careful attention to the physician's responsibility and behavior creates an environment in which open dialogue and an exchange of ideas and values can occur between the patient and the physician. This ongoing dialogue automatically corrects many of the miscommunications or conflicts that lead to ethical crises.

C. **The bioethics consult: obtaining an outside perspective.** Many institutions have standing bioethics committees or departments that can aid in resolving bioethical conflicts. Despite our best intentions, we are sometimes unable to resolve conflict with patients or cannot fully explain the necessity of action to patients, causing confusion. In these instances, an outside perspective may be of value. A consultation from the bioethics committee is simply an outside review of the facts and values associated with a particular crisis. This outside observer may be a physician, another health care worker, or a member of the clergy. The purpose of the consult is not to render a "more expert" opinion but to uncover differing moral values and miscommunication that lead to conflict. In many instances, this is all that is needed to resolve these problems. If consensus cannot be obtained in this manner, further interventions are warranted.

D. **The bioethics committee is usually multidisciplinary in membership.** Composed of administrators, lawyers, physicians, nursing staff, and clergy, the committee reviews ethical dilemmas put before it. Many bioethics committees also have a standing role in monitoring the ethical behavior of physicians and health care workers at their institution. Activation of the bioethics committee, as opposed to a consult, is a more involved process. The committee's purpose is to not only resolve conflict in particular instances but also to provide policy and general guidelines for ethical behavior at that institution. Because of the potential legal ramifications, this group may routinely consult the judiciary system for further advice. It is the usual policy of most committees that physicians or other health care workers, family members, clergy, or other interested parties may query the group. These queries can be put forth without fear of retribution or chastisement from other staff members. The procedure for activating the bioethics committee should be posted in the residents' or physicians' handbook or nursing manual for that patient unit.

E. **The legal system.** On occasion, conflict arises that cannot be resolved by the physician, bioethics consult, or committee opinion. In these instances, outside judiciary opinions should be sought. The bioethics committee can usually be helpful in obtaining this legal opinion. Not only does the committee have familiarity with accessing the judiciary system, but they should also be able to frame the question in such a way to provide the most concise legal response. Activation of the legal system in this way also protects the physician from direct consequence from legal action.

Selected References

Barber B. *The Logic and Limits of Trust.* New Brunswick, NJ: Rutgers University Press; 1983.

Beauchamp TL. *Principles of Biomedical Ethics.* 4th ed. New York, NY: Oxford University Press; 1994.

Kattwinkel J. *Textbook of Neonatal Resuscitation.* 6th ed. Elk Grove, IL: American Heart Association/American Academy of Pediatrics; 2011.

Pellegrino ED. Socrates at the bedside. *Pharos Alpha Omega Alpha Honor Medical Society* 1983;46(1):38.

Pellegrino ED, Thomasma DC. *The Virtues in Medical Practice.* New York, NY: Oxford University Press; 1993.

Purdy IB. Embracing bioethics in neonatal intensive care, part I: evolving toward neonatal evidence-based ethics. *Neonatal Netw.* 2006;25(1):33–42.

Purdy IB, Wadhwani RT. Embracing bioethics in neonatal intensive care, part II: case histories in neonatal ethics. *Neonatal Netw.* 2006;25(1):43–53.

Winyard A. The Nuffiend Council on Bioethics report—critical care decisions in fetal and neonatal medicine: ethical issues. *Clin. Risk.* 2007;13(2):70–73.

Principles of Neonatal Procedures

INFORMED CONSENT

Upon admission to the neonatal intensive care unit (NICU), most facilities provide a parental blanket or general informed consent for routine procedures performed on newborns (eg, phlebotomy, intravenous placement) and emergency procedures for life-threatening situations. For nonemergent invasive bedside procedures that may carry significant risk, parental or guardian permission should be obtained. Risks, benefits, and alternative procedures, if appropriate, should be discussed. Major surgical procedures require informed consent. Refer to your local unit policy manual for detailed guidance.

STANDARD PRECAUTIONS

Standard precautions integrate and expand the elements of the previously adopted **universal precautions** and are designed to protect both health care workers and patients. **Standard precautions** apply to contact with blood, all body fluids, secretions, and excretions except sweat, nonintact skin, and mucous membranes. **Standard precautions** must be used in the care of all patients, regardless of their infection status.

In the case of a known transmissible infection, additional precautions known as **expanded or transmission-based precautions** are recommended. These are used to interrupt the spread of diseases that are transmitted by airborne, droplet, or contact transmission. Most bedside procedures incorporate principles of **standard precautions**.

Standard Precautions Key Components

- **Hand hygiene** before and after patient contact.
- **Gloves** for contact with blood, body fluids, secretion, contaminated items, mucous membranes, and nonintact skin.
- **Personal protection equipment (masks, goggles, face masks)** when contact with blood and body fluids is likely.
- **Gowns** for blood or body fluid contact and to prevent soiling of clothing.
- **Sharps precautions.** Avoid recapping used needles; avoid bending, breaking, or manipulating used needles by hand; and place used sharps in puncture-resistant containers. Use self-shielding needle devices whenever possible.

Time Out

JCAHO (Joint Commission on Accreditation of Health Care Organizations) has produced a universal protocol for "The Prevention of Wrong Site, Wrong Procedure and Wrong Person Surgery." The 3 principal components of the Universal Protocol include a preprocedure verification, site marking, and a time out. Originally developed for the operating room, many facilities use this before bedside invasive procedures. All activity ceases, a moment will be taken ("time out"), and the following will be verified verbally by each member of the team:

- Correct patient identity
- Correct side and site
- Agreement on the procedure to be done
- Correct patient position
- Availability of correct equipment and/or special requirements

227

NICU PROCEDURE CONSIDERATIONS
Latex Allergy

There is a growing concern over latex exposure in the hospital. Certain pediatric populations are at higher risk for latex allergies such as in spina bifida. Many hospitals are converting to a latex-free environment. Latex-free equipment is recommended when available in the NICU.

Hand Hygiene

Hand hygiene is the most effective method of decreasing health care–related infections. It is best to follow your hospital-based infection prevention protocols.
1. A 3- to 5-minute scrub (surgical, washing up to the elbows) or rub is usually required before entering the NICU. This is also necessary for certain major procedures (eg, lumbar puncture, chest tube, central line placement or cut down).
2. A 2- to 3-minute scrub (up to elbows) or rub is recommended for a minor procedure (bladder aspiration, blood drawing, intravenous lines).
3. A 30-second hand wash or shorter alcohol-based hand rub is indicated before and after each patient contact.

Antiseptic Solutions

1. General rules
   a. Always allow antiseptics to dry on the site (at least 30 seconds recommended).
   b. Remove iodophor solutions off the wider area at the end of the procedure except right at the insertion procedure site.
2. Commonly used antiseptics
   a. Alcohol (60–90% ethyl or isopropyl) is commonly used for skin prep of minor procedures (eg, phlebotomy); not for mucous membranes. Apply 3 times in a circle starting at the center of the site and going outward. Not for major procedures and may cause burns in premature infants.
   b. Iodine preparations have broad spectrum antimicrobial activity (bacteria, viruses, fungi, spores).
      i. Topical iodine (1%) is not recommended as it can cause skin hypersensitivity, iodine overload, and transient hypothyroidism.
      ii. Iodophor solutions (iodine plus a solubilizing agent such as surfactant or povidone). One example is Povidone iodine (polyvinylpyrrolidone plus elemental iodine) which releases iodine slowly. It is not recommended for premature newborns, but can be used in term newborns (small risk of transient hypothyroidism with large area of the body or >5 days use). Typically 10% solutions of povidone iodine (Betadine, Wescodyne) are recommended for major procedures.
   c. Chlorhexidine solutions
      i. Hibiclens (chlorhexidine gluconate 4% solution) is good for hand washing and used in the following procedures in preparation or maintenance: central venous catheter insertion, umbilical venous catheter prep, others. Use with care in premature infants or infants < 2 months old. May cause irritation or chemical burns.
      ii. Chloraprep (2% chlorhexidine in 70% isopropyl alcohol) is used for PIV, PICC, umbilical line art puncture, chest tube insertion. Do not use on nonintact skin, below neck, infants <26 weeks, infants <1000 g, lumbar punctures, urethral catheter. Approved for infants >2 months of age.
   d. Hexachlorophene (Phisohex) is used for hand washing and only recommended for term infants during outbreak of *Staphylococcus aureus*.

PAIN MANAGEMENT IN THE NEONATE

The American Academy of Pediatrics (AAP) has recommended that every health care facility caring for neonates have an effective pain prevention program and use pharmacologic and nonpharmacologic therapies to prevent pain with procedures. Each procedure in this section has a designated section on pain. This information is based on the AAP recommendations plus a review of international guidelines (see references). Chapters 14 and 76 provide additional details.

1. Pharmacologic pain management. Topical and systemic agents are reviewed in Chapters 14 and 76. EMLA (eutectic mixture of lidocaine and prilocaine) should be used with caution in very premature infants and with repeated use for multiple procedures.

2. Nonpharmacologic pain prevention and relief techniques. Refers to breast-feeding, nonnutritive sucking (pacifier), kangaroo care, facilitated tuck (arms and legs are held in a flexed position), swaddling, and developmental care (lateral positioning, supportive bedding, attention to behavioral clues [brow bulge, eye squeeze] and limiting environmental stimuli). Sucking on a pacifier releases endorphin possibly through a pressure point in the roof of the mouth.

   a. Oral sucrose/glucose

      i. Sucrose. Eliminates electroencephalogram changes associated with a painful procedure (mechanism unknown). Intra-oral (not intra-gastric) administration of sucrose without suckling is effective. Doses 0.012–0.12 g (0.05–0.5 mL of 24% solution) given 2 minutes before and 1–2 minutes after are more effective than single dose. Sucrose does not totally eliminate pain; use with other nonpharmacologic therapies.

      ii. Glucose. Diminishes pain from venipuncture; does not decrease oxygen consumption or energy expenditure.

   b. Breast-feeding or breast milk. This can alleviate procedural pain in neonates undergoing a single painful procedure. Administration of glucose/sucrose seems to be similar in effectiveness.

Selected References

American Academy of Pediatrics Committee on Fetus and Newborn; American Academy of Pediatrics Section on Surgery; Canadian Paediatric Society Fetus and Newborn Committee; Batton DG, Barrington KJ, Wallman C. Prevention and management of pain in the Neonate: an update. *Pediatrics.* 2006;118:2231–2241. Policy statement reaffirmation, August 1, 2010.

Guideline Statement: management of procedure related pain in neonates. Royal Australasian College of Physicians, 2005. http://www.racp.edu.au/. Accessed September, 2012.

Joint Commission. Standards. http://www.jointcommission.org/standards_information/up.aspx. Accessed July 2012.

Lago P, Garetti E, Merazzi D, Tavares EC, Yerkes Silva YP Guidelines for procedural pain in the newborn. *Acta Pediatrica.* 2009;98:932–939.

Marcatto Jd'O, Tavares EC, Yerkes Silva YP. Topical anesthesia in preterm neonate: a reflection on the underutilization in clinical practice. *Revista Brasileira de Terapia Intensiva.* 2010;22.

22 Arterial Access: Arterial Puncture (Radial Artery Puncture)

I. **Indications**
   A. **To obtain arterial blood for blood gas measurements.**
   B. **When blood is needed and venous or capillary blood samples cannot be obtained.** Not preferred.
   C. **To obtain ammonia levels.** Venous blood can be used if it is collected, transported appropriately, and done quickly.
   D. **To obtain lactate and pyruvate levels.** Free-flowing arterial blood; stasis of blood increases lactate.

II. **Equipment.** A 23–25-gauge scalp vein (butterfly) needle or a 23–25-gauge venipuncture needle (safety-engineered self-shielding), 1- or 3-mL syringe, povidone-iodine and alcohol swabs, 4 × 4 gauze pad, gloves, 1:1000 heparin or self-contained blood gas kit, high-intensity fiber optic light for transillumination, or a Doppler ultrasound (optional, can be useful to locate the artery). Smaller needles preferred (25 gauge for preterm infants, 23 gauge for term infants).

III. **Procedure**
   A. **For a blood gas, most hospitals have kits with 1-mL syringes coated with heparin.** If this is not available, draw a small amount of heparin (1:1000) into the blood gas syringe (coat the surfaces and discard excess heparin from the syringe). The small amount of heparin coating the syringe is sufficient to prevent coagulation. Excessive heparin may interfere with laboratory results (see later). If any other laboratory test is to be performed, do not use heparin.
   B. **The radial artery is the most frequently used site and is described in detail here.** One of the advantages of the radial artery site is that the radial nerve does not lie close to the artery so there is no concern of nerve damage. Alternative sites are the posterior tibial (preferred second site) or the dorsalis pedis artery. Femoral arteries should be reserved for emergency situations. Brachial arteries should not be used (unless absolutely necessary) because there is minimal collateral circulation and a risk of median nerve damage. Temporal arteries should not be used because of the high risk of neurologic complications.
   C. **Check for collateral circulation and patency of the ulnar artery by means of the Modified Allen's test.** Elevate the arm and simultaneously occlude the radial and ulnar arteries at the wrist; rub the palm to cause blanching. Release pressure on the ulnar artery. If normal color returns in the palm in <10 seconds, adequate collateral circulation from the ulnar artery is present. If normal color does not return for >15 seconds or does not return at all, the collateral circulation is poor, and it is best not to use the radial artery in this arm. The radial and ulnar arteries in the other arm should then be tested for collateral circulation. Because of concern on the reliability of the modified Allen test, other methods such as the modified Allen test with Doppler ultrasound evaluation of collateral flow are being used (***controversial***). One study found that the best way to perform the Allen test was using the laser Doppler flowmetry method. Some are combining the use of pulse oximetry with the modified Allen test.
   D. **Pain. Use of topical local anesthetic agents (EMLA)** may diminish pain from arterial puncture. Evidence of distress responses exist even before and after a radial arterial puncture. The literature is conflicting concerning the utility of EMLA for arterial puncture, but there may be some benefit. Oral sucrose, breast milk, and/or pacifier are preferred. Other nonpharmacologic techniques are also recommended.
   E. **To obtain the sample.** Take the patient's hand in your left hand (for a right-handed operator) and slightly extend the wrist. Hyperextension can occlude the vessel.

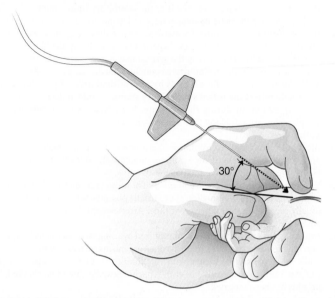

FIGURE 22-1. Technique of radial arterial puncture in the neonate.

Palpate the radial artery with the index finger of your left hand (Figure 22-1). **Transillumination** with a high-intensity fiber optic light and marking the puncture site with a fingernail imprint may be helpful (see Chapter 40). A **Doppler ultrasound** by noting characteristic sounds or **real-time 2-dimensional ultrasonography** can also help locate the vessel. **Real-time ultrasound** can result in fewer attempts and less chance of a hematoma as compared with palpation.

F. **Clean the puncture site.** Clean with a povidone-iodine swab and then with an alcohol swab.

G. **Puncture the skin at about a 30-degree angle.** Then slowly advance the needle and penetrate the artery with the bevel up until blood appears in the tubing (see Figure 22-1). If the entire artery is perforated (anterior and posterior wall) and no blood is obtained, slowly withdraw the needle until blood is obtained. Because the artery can spasm, you may need to wait for blood return. **For a more superficial artery or in a premature or extremely low birthweight infant,** puncture the skin at 15-25 degrees with the bevel down. With arterial blood samples, little aspiration is usually needed to fill the syringe. If there is no return of blood, withdraw the needle slowly because the artery may have been punctured through and through. (Best to limit to 2 attempts.)

H. **Collect the least amount of blood needed.** The volume of blood taken at one time should not exceed 3–5% of the total blood volume (the total blood volume in a neonate is ~80 mL/kg). As an example, if 4 mL of blood is drawn from an infant weighing 1 kg, this represents 5% of the total blood volume.

I. **Withdraw the needle and apply firm, but not occlusive, pressure to the site for ≥5 minutes with a 4 × 4 gauze pad to ensure adequate hemostasis.** Shield and dispose the needle in appropriate container. Check fingers for adequate circulation.

J. **Before submitting an arterial blood gas sample, expel air bubbles from the sample and tightly cap the syringe.** Failure to do this can lead to errors in testing. (See the following discussion of inaccuracy of blood gas results.)

K. Place the syringe in ice, and take it to the laboratory immediately. Note the collection time and the patient's temperature and hemoglobin on the laboratory slip.

L. Inaccurate blood gas results. Excessive heparin in the syringe may result in a falsely low pH and $Paco_2$. Remove excess heparin before obtaining the blood sample. Air bubbles caused by failure to cap the syringe may falsely elevate the Pao_2 and falsely lower the $Paco_2$. Crying during arterial puncture can decrease $Paco_2$, decrease HCO_3, and oxygen saturation. **Blood gases by intermittent arterial punctures may not accurately reflect the infant's respiratory status.** A sudden decrease in the $Paco_2$ and Pao_2 can occur during the puncture. *Note:* **Neutrophil counts** are lower in samples from arterial blood than venous samples.

IV. Complications
  A. Bleeding/hematoma. To minimize hematoma risk, use the smallest gauge needle possible and hold pressure for 5 minutes immediately after withdrawing the needle. Hematomas usually resolve spontaneously.
  B. Vasospasm, thrombosis, and embolism. These can cause distal ischemia and can be minimized by using the smallest gauge needle possible. With thrombosis, the vessel usually recanalizes over a period of time. Arteriospasm usually resolves spontaneously (see Chapter 79).
  C. Infection. Risk is rare and can be minimized by using strict sterile technique. Infection is commonly caused by gram-positive organisms such as *Staphylococcus epidermidis*, which should be treated with nafcillin or vancomycin and gentamicin (see Chapter 148). Drug sensitivities at the specific hospital should be checked. Osteomyelitis has been reported.
  D. Arteriovenous fistula. May occur after multiple arterial punctures and is treated surgically. Because the brachial artery and median cubital vein are anatomically very close, a single puncture can cause a fistula. Diagnosis is by Doppler flow of the brachial vessels.
  E. Nerve damage. Median nerve damage has been reported after brachial artery puncture. Posterior tibial and femoral nerve damage have also been reported.
  F. Rare complications. **Forearm compartment syndrome** with brachial artery puncture. **Extensor tendon sheath injury** from repeated radial artery punctures. **Pseudoaneurysm of the brachial artery** can occur from trauma to the wall of an artery and may require surgical treatment.

23 Arterial Access: Percutaneous Arterial Catheterization (Radial Arterial Line)

I. Indications
  A. When frequent arterial blood samples are required and an umbilical arterial catheter cannot be placed or has been removed because of complications.
  B. Intra-arterial blood pressure monitoring.
  C. To measure preductal Pao_2 (usually done with pulse oximeter of the right hand or finger if catheterization not necessary). Right upper extremity catheterization must be done for preductal measurement.
  D. Exchange transfusions (for removal of blood only). Used in peripheral vessel exchange transfusion (PVET) when drawing blood from a peripheral artery and infusing through a peripheral vein.
  E. Not for infusion of hyperalimentation, medications, hypertonic or hypotonic solutions, glucose solutions, or blood product administration.

II. **Equipment.** Safety-engineered catheter over needle access device based on local practices (22 or 24 gauge; 24 gauge preferred for infants <1500 g), arm board (or two tongue blades taped together), adhesive tape, sterile drapes, gloves, povidone-iodine or skin disinfectant, gloves, antiseptic ointment, suture material optional (needle holder, suture scissors, 4–0 or 5–0 silk sutures), 0.5 or 0.25% normal saline flush solution (latter preferred in premature infants, decreases hypernatremia risk) with heparin (0.25–0.50 unit of heparin/1 mL saline), pressure bag (to prevent backflow and keep the line free of clots), connecting tubing, pressure transducer for continuous blood pressure monitoring, optional: fiber optic light for transillumination or a Doppler/real-time ultrasound to locate the artery.

III. **Procedure.** Two methods are described here using the **radial artery**, the most common site because of low complication rates. Methods can be adapted to other arteries. Another common site is the **posterior tibial artery**, as both the radial and posterior tibial arteries have good collateral circulation. **Ulnar** (to be used only in the absence of previous radial artery puncture attempt) and **dorsalis pedis** arteries are alternative sites. The temporal, brachial, and femoral arteries are not recommended. Axillary artery cannulation is very difficult and also not recommended. Temporal artery catheterization may have adverse neurologic sequelae. The brachial artery does not have good collateral flow and can have a lot of complications. **Lateral or posterior wrist transillumination or Doppler/real-time ultrasound may be helpful in locating the artery in premature infants.** Arterial catheterization requires patience.

A. **Locate the artery by palpation, transillumination, or Doppler/real-time ultrasound.** Palpation of the artery can be done at the following sites: radial artery (lateral wrist), ulnar artery (medial wrist), posterior tibial artery (posterior to the medial malleolus), and dorsalis pedis artery (on top of the foot). For technique on transillumination, see Chapter 40. Use of real-time ultrasound and color Doppler imaging can identify the artery and help one guide the catheter in the vessel. It can lead to a shorter time required, a higher first attempt success rate, and a decrease in complications.

B. **Verify adequate collateral circulation in the hand using the modified Allen test.** (See Chapter 22.) Some recommend doing a Doppler evaluation to verify collateral flow since there can be false positives with the modified Allen test.

C. **Pain management.** Oral sucrose or breast milk and/or pacifier is recommended with other nonpharmacologic pain prevention and relief techniques. Use of topical local anesthetic agents (EMLA, eutectic mixture of lidocaine and prilocaine) or subcutaneous infiltration of lidocaine can also be considered. Consider dose of opioid if IV access available. (See Chapters 14 and 76.).

D. **Place the infant's wrist on an arm board** (some prefer IV bag) and slightly hyperextend the wrist by placing gauze underneath it. Tape the arm and hand securely to the board (Figure 23–1).

E. **Scrub or rub and put on gloves. Cleanse the site** with antiseptic solution and place sterile drapes around the puncture site.

F. **Methods of insertion**
  1. **Standard method** (preferred for any newborn infant that is not premature)
     a. **Puncture (with bevel up) both the anterior and posterior walls of the artery** at a 30- to 45-degree angle. Remove the stylet. There should be little or no backflow of blood.
     b. **Pull the catheter back slowly until blood is seen;** this signifies that the arterial lumen has been entered.
     c. **Advance the catheter** after attaching the syringe and flush the catheter. Never use hypertonic solutions to flush an arterial catheter.
     d. **Securely tape the catheter** with Steri-strips™ and Tegaderm™ (preferred) or secure the catheter with 4–0 or 5–0 silk sutures in 2 places (may promote skin infection and is not recommended).
     e. **Connect the tubing** from the heparinized saline pressure bag to the catheter.
     f. **Iodophor ointment** on the area is no longer recommended because it can obscure the site and may promote infection. Secure the cannula with a transparent dressing to allow visualization of the site.

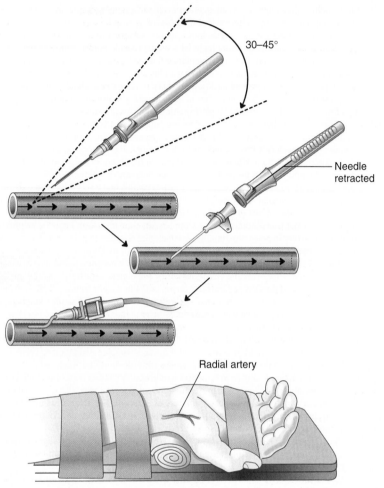

FIGURE 23–1. When placing an indwelling arterial catheter, the wrist should be secured as shown. The catheter assembly is introduced at a 30- to 45-degree angle.

2. **Premature infant method**
   a. **With the bevel down, at an angle of 10 to 15 degrees, puncture the anterior wall of the artery until blood return is seen.** At this point, the catheter should be in the lumen of the artery. Vasospasm is common, and the procedure should be performed slowly.
   b. **Advance the catheter into the artery while simultaneously withdrawing the needle.** The blood should be flowing freely from the catheter if the catheter is properly positioned.
   c. **Attach the syringe and flush the catheter.** Secure the line as in the standard method.

IV. **Additives**
   A. **Heparin is recommended in the flushes and the pressure line.** Dosage range: 0.5 to 2 U/mL, per Pediatric Advanced Life support text. Doses as low as 0.25 U/mL

have been used with success in umbilical artery catheters and peripheral intravenous catheters. Use the lowest amount recommended. Follow institution guidelines. American College of Chest Physicians Evidence-Based Clinical Practice Guidelines (2012) recommends UFH continuous infusion at 0.5 U/mL at 1 mL/h for neonates with peripheral arterial catheters.

B. Papaverine. Added to the arterial line (30 mg/250 mL) may prolong patency of peripheral arterial lines *(controversial)*.

C. Lidocaine. Sometimes given intra-arterially if there is a problem with a vasospasm *(controversial)*.

V. Radial artery catheter removal

A. Remove the dressing and sutures if present.

B. Slowly remove the catheter. Have sterile gauze available.

C. Apply pressure to the site for 5 to 10 minutes and dress site.

VI. Complications

A. Vasospasm/embolism/thrombosis. (See Chapter 79.) Vascular endothelium, injured from catheters, reacts by eliciting an inflammatory response with hemostasis and thrombus formation resulting in tissue ischemia and release of potent vasoconstrictors. Use the smallest gauge catheter possible, minimize the infusion rate, and avoid large or rapid infusions and withdrawals. Avoid hypertonic solutions and blood products. Remove catheter at the earliest signs of ischemia. These events can cause a wide spectrum of complications:

1. Temporary blanching of the extremity.

2. Skin ulcers with sloughing of skin.

3. Tissue ischemia, skin necrosis, gangrene, and partial loss of digits. Transient ischemia of the forearm and hand has been reported with radial artery cannulation.

4. Cerebral embolization from a clot from a catheter in the radial or temporal artery and retrograde thrombosis of the posterior auricular artery have been reported from a temporal artery catheterization. Retrograde emboli to the central nervous system (CNS) can occur if the catheter is flushed too vigorously.

5. Temporary occlusion. Reversible total occlusion of the artery has been reported after a radial arterial catheterization.

B. Air embolism. Can be prevented by making certain that air is not introduced into the catheter and the catheter is flushed with heparinized saline.

C. Hemorrhage/hematoma at puncture site. If the catheter becomes dislodged, bleeding can occur. Tightly secure connections.

D. Infection. Low infection risk, rarely associated with bloodstream infection. Local infection, sepsis, cellulitis, and abscess have been reported. Prophylactic antibiotics are not recommended.

E. Extravasation/infiltration of solution. See Chapter 31.

F. Nerve damage. Median, ulnar, posterior tibial, and peroneal nerve damage based on the catheter site.

G. Hypernatremia. Use 0.25% normal saline (NS) in low birthweight infants.

H. Pseudoaneurysm. Rare.

Selected Reference

Monagle P, Chan AK, Goldenberg NA, et al. Antithrombotic therapy in neonates and children: Antithrombotic Therapy and Prevention of Thrombosis. 9th ed. American College of Chest Physicians Evidence-Based Clinical Practice Guidelines. *Chest.* 2012;141(suppl 2):e737S.

24 Arterial Access: Umbilical Artery Catheterization

I. **Indications**
   A. Frequent or continuous measurements of arterial blood gases.
   B. Continuous arterial blood pressure monitoring.
   C. Access for exchange transfusion (to withdraw blood).
   D. Angiography.
   E. Administration of emergency resuscitation medications and fluids. *Note:* Umbilical vein preferred.
   F. Infusion of maintenance solutions.
   G. Short-term infusion/emergency infusion of volume expanders, parenteral nutrition, and/or medications (*controversial*). Parenteral nutrition can be given through a UAC, a route that has been used in some centers, especially in very low birthweight (VLBW) infants; however, the umbilical artery is not preferred and should be used with caution. The maximum dextrose concentration that can be administered using this method is 15%. If necessary, antibiotics can be given via UAC, but this also is not a preferred method. Indomethacin, vasopressor medications (epinephrine, dopamine, dobutamine), calcium boluses, and anticonvulsants **should not** be given via the UAC (umbilical venous catheter [UVC], central venous line preferred).
   H. Blood products (*controversial,* emergency only). Blood products can be given via a UAC, but UVC or peripheral/central access preferred. UAC is less preferred, as this may enhance the risk of thrombosis.
II. **Equipment**
   A. **Basic.** Prepackaged umbilical artery catheterization trays (usually include sterile drapes, tape measure, a needle holder, suture scissors, hemostat, forceps, scalpel, 3-way stopcock), umbilical tape, silk tape (eg, Dermicel), 3–0 silk suture, gauze pads, antiseptic solution, sterile gown, gloves, mask, hat, 10-mL syringe, 0.5% normal saline (NS) flush solution (0.25% NS for very small infants to decrease hypernatremia risk), NS with heparin (0.25–1.0 U/mL) in continuous infusion calibrated pressure transducer for pressure monitoring. Ultrasound equipment is optional to guide catheter insertion.
   B. **Umbilical artery catheter (sizes 2.5F, 3.5F, 5F, 12–15 inch).** Size recommendations vary based on institutional guidelines. Some general guidelines:
      1. **UAC recommendation 1.** 2.5F if <800–1000 g, 3.5F >1000 g, 5F in a term infant.
      2. **UAC recommendation 2.** 3.5F if <1.2 kg or 1.5 kg, 5F for an infant weighing >1.2 or 1.5 kg.
      3. **If using catheter without a hub.** Cut off wide part of catheter and insert blunt needle: No. 18 for 5F, No. 20 for 3.5F.
      4. **Single-lumen UAC recommended.** Multiple-lumen catheters are not recommended (recommended for UVC use only). End-hole catheters are associated with a decreased risk of aortic thrombosis when compared with side-hole catheters. Avoid side-hole catheters.
      5. **Feeding tubes used as catheters.** Associated with increase in thrombosis; avoid use.
      6. **Cochrane review notes that there is no benefit of using a heparin bonded polyurethane catheter versus the standard polyvinyl chloride (PVC) catheter.** A catheter made of Silastic (silicone) is more difficult to use because it is softer but may reduce aortic thrombosis compared with PVC tubing. Teflon or polyurethane catheters have been associated with fewer infections and thrombogenicity than PVC or polyethylene catheters.

III. Procedure
   A. Important UAC tips
      1. The 2 umbilical arteries (1 umbilical artery in ~1% of births) are muscular walled vessels (2–3 mm) that carry deoxygenated blood from the fetus to the placenta. The umbilical arteries are the direct continuation of the internal iliac arteries. The catheter enters the umbilical artery at the umbilicus; it courses downward into the internal iliac artery and then into the common iliac and then the aorta.
      2. The umbilical arteries usually constrict within seconds after birth and close a few minutes later. They can be dilated and used for the first 3–4 days of life. It is easiest to put the UAC in on the first day of life. After the first day, it helps to place a saline gauze on the umbilical stump for 45–60 minutes before attempting the procedure.
      3. Unless it is an emergency (where you put the UVC first), put the UAC in first if putting in both a UAC and UVC. The UAC is the more difficult one to put in, and often a second cut of the umbilical stump needs to be done when inserting a UAC.
      4. Blood cultures. Blood cultures can be drawn from the UAC for up to 6 hours after insertion (right after insertion preferred, venipuncture preferred).
      5. Heparin use. Cochrane reviews note the use of heparin (as low as 0.25 U/mL) is recommended to prolong the life of the catheter by decreasing the incidence of catheter occlusion. It does not decrease the incidence of aortic thrombosis. Heparinization of intermittent flushes alone is ineffective in preventing catheter occlusion. American Academy of Pediatrics (AAP) recommends low doses of heparin (0.25–1.0 U/L) through the umbilical arterial catheter. The American College of Chest Physicians Evidence-Based Clinical Practice Guidelines (2012) recommends prophylaxis with a low-dose UFH infusion via the UAC (heparin concentration of 0.25–1.0 U/mL, total heparin dose of 25–200 U/kg/d) to maintain patency.
      6. Prophylactic antibiotic use (controversial). Cochrane review found that there was not enough evidence to support or refute the use of prophylactic antibiotics in infants with UACs.
      7. Ultrasound guidance. Faster and results in fewer manipulations and x-rays as compared with conventional placement.
   B. "High" versus "low" catheter. Catheter position used to be determined by institutional guidelines. High catheters were once thought to be associated with a higher risk of vascular complications, but a recent analysis showed a decreased risk of vascular complications and no increased risk of hypertension, necrotizing enterocolitis (NEC), IVH, or hematuria. Low catheters are associated with an increased risk of vasospasms. Cochrane review now recommends high catheters exclusively. They found that high catheters have fewer complications and lesser need for replacement and reinsertion. The American College of Chest Physicians Evidence-Based Clinical Practice Guidelines (2012) suggests high UAC placement rather than low position. A low position may only be needed if there is a problem placing a high catheter. Be certain you know whether you will insert a high or low catheter and the correct length of catheter to be inserted. See Figure 24–1 for vascular landmarks.
      1. High catheter/line. UAC tip lies above the diaphragm at the level of T6–T9. This position is above the celiac artery (T12), the renal arteries (L1), and the superior mesenteric artery (T12–L1). High positioning is associated with decreased vascular complications, lower incidence of blanching and cyanosis of the extremities with longer duration of catheter use, and no statistically significant increase in hypertension, intraventricular hemorrhage, necrotizing enterocolitis (NEC), or hematuria. However, high positioning is associated with hypoglycemia and hyperglycemia.
      2. Low catheter/line. UAC tip lies between the level of L3 and L4 (above the L4–L5 aortic bifurcation) and is associated with more episodes of lower extremity vasospasm.

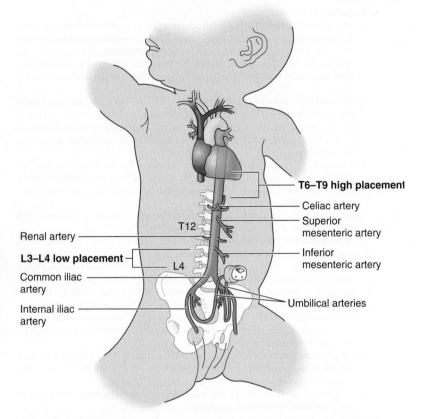

Renal artery

L3–L4 low placement

Common iliac artery

Internal iliac artery

T12

L4

T6–T9 high placement

Celiac artery

Superior mesenteric artery

Inferior mesenteric artery

Umbilical arteries

FIGURE 24–1. Important landmarks, related vessels, and the path of the umbilical artery. The internal iliac artery is also called the hypogastric artery.

C. **Length of UAC necessary.** This can be obtained from several methods, with not one universally accepted. **Remember to add the umbilical stump length.**
   1. **Dunn method.** Uses the shoulder-to-umbilicus length (SUL) and a nomogram to determine the insertion length. It can be used for **high or low UAC** placement (Figure 24–2).
   2. **Shukla and Ferrara method.** Uses the birthweight (BW) and the following formula for a **high UAC.** Shukla method was more accurate than the Dunn method for determining UAC insertion length.
      a. **Modified BW equation.** UAC length (cm) = (birthweight in kg × 3) + 9 cm.
      b. **Exact BW equation.** 2.5 × BW in kg + 9.7.
   3. **Wright formula.** For low birthweight infants (<1500 kg) and is only for **high position of the catheter.**

   UAC length (cm) = (birthweight in kg × 4) + 7 cm

D. **Pain management.** Because the umbilical cord is denervated, pain will be minimal. Avoid the placement of the hemostat or any sutures on the skin around the umbilicus as this will cause pain. Consider any nonpharmacologic methods of pain relief (see Chapter 14).

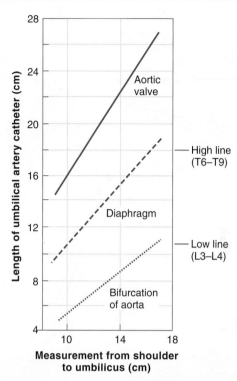

FIGURE 24–2. The umbilical artery catheter can be placed in 1 of 2 positions. The **low catheter** is placed below the level of L3 to avoid the renal and mesenteric vessels. The **high catheter** is placed between the thoracic vertebrae from T6 to T9. The graph is used as a guide to help determine the catheter length for each position. The **low line** corresponds to the aortic bifurcation in the graph, whereas a **high line** corresponds to the diaphragm. To determine catheter length, measure (in centimeters) a perpendicular line from the top of the shoulder to the umbilicus. This determines the shoulder-umbilical length. Plot this number on the graph to determine the proper catheter length for the umbilical artery catheter. Add the length of the umbilical stump to the catheter length. (*Data from Dunn PM. Localization of the umbilical catheter by postmortem measurement.* Arch Dis Child. *1966;41:69.*)

E. **Technique**
1. **Place the patient supine.** Wrap a diaper around both legs and tape the diaper to the bed. This stabilizes the patient for the procedure and allows observation of the feet for vasospasm.
2. **Put on sterile gloves, a mask, a hat, and a sterile gown.**
3. **Prepare the UAC tray.** Attach the stopcock to the blunt needle and then attach the catheter to the blunt needle. Fill the 10-mL syringe with flush solution, and inject it through the catheter.
4. **Clean the umbilical cord area with antiseptic solution (povidone-iodine).** Place sterile drapes around the umbilicus, leaving the feet and head exposed.
5. **Tie a piece of umbilical tape around the base of the umbilical cord** tight enough to minimize blood loss but loose enough so that the catheter can be passed easily through the vessel (ie, snug but not tight). Cut off the excess umbilical cord with scissors or a scalpel, leaving a 1-cm stump (Figure 24–3A). A scalpel usually makes a cleaner cut so that the vessels are more easily seen. There are *usually*

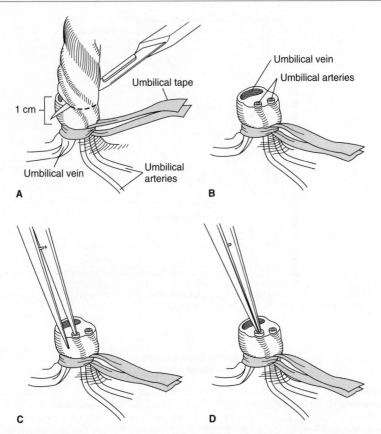

FIGURE 24–3. (A) The umbilical cord should be amputated, leaving a 1-cm stump. (B) Identification of the umbilical cord vessels. (C and D) A forceps is used to gently dilate the umbilical artery.

2 umbilical arteries (1 and 7 o' clock positions). The vein usually has a large floppy thin wall at the 12 o'clock position (Figure 24–3B).

6. Using the curved hemostat, grasp the end of the umbilicus to hold it upright and steady.

7. Use the iris forceps to open and dilate the umbilical artery. Remember, the diameter is only 2–3 mm. First, place one arm of the forceps in the artery, and then use both arms to gently dilate the vessel (Figure 24–3C and D).

8. Once the artery is sufficiently dilated, insert the catheter caudally or towards the feet. It is common to have some resistance at either the abdominal wall or at the level of the bladder. If resistance is met, apply gentle pressure for about 30–60 seconds. Avoid repeated probing. Approximately 5–10% will have difficulty passing the catheter. If there is difficulty passing the catheter:

   a. The most common cause of failure to catheterize an umbilical artery is inadequate dilation of the artery.

   b. Use 0.5 mL of lidocaine and drip into the vessel until it dilates (*controversial*).

   c. Use of the "double catheter technique" (as for UVC). **Not recommended** due to greater risk of perforation.

  d. If in a false channel (no blood return). Remove and use other artery.

  e. Incorrect path. Rarely the UAC will go from the umbilical artery to the femoral artery (by way of the internal iliac artery, common iliac artery, and external iliac artery) or to the gluteal artery (by way of the internal iliac artery). Using a small catheter in a large infant increases the risk of the catheter going into the gluteal artery. This line is not usable and will have to be removed.

 9. Once the catheter is in position, aspirate to verify blood return. Never advance the catheter once sterile technique is broken. It is better to advance it too high and withdraw it. Once sterile field has been compromised, one can only reposition it by pulling it out, not pushing it in.

 10. Secure the catheter. Several methods are described.

  a. Method 1. See Figure 24–4A. The silk tape is folded over part way, the catheter is placed, and the remaining portion of the tape is folded over. Suture the silk tape to the base of the umbilical cord (through the Wharton jelly, not the skin or vessels) using 3–0 silk sutures. Connect the tubing to the monitor and flush it. No special dressing is needed. The umbilical stump with the catheter in place is left open to the air. Once the catheter is secure, loosen the umbilical tape.

  b. Method 2. Place a purse string around the base of the cord, and then wrap the ends of the suture around the catheter and tie.

  c. Method 3. Secure the catheter with a tape bridge. (See Figure 24–4B, "goal post" method.) Make 2 tabs from tape and place on either side of the umbilicus. Then take another piece of tape and wrap it around the 2 tabs.

  d. Method 4. A commercially available NeoBridge (NEOTECH, Valencia, CA) can also be used.

 11. Do not use topical antibiotic ointment on the umbilical catheter insertion site. This can promote fungal infections.

 12. Obtain an abdominal radiograph. To verify the position of a low catheter or a chest radiograph to check the position of a high catheter. Figure 24–1 shows landmarks and the relationship of umbilical arteries to the other major abdominal arteries. Radiographs showing positioning can be found in Chapter 11 (for high UAC, see Figure 11–11 and for low UAC, see Figure 11–12). An **ultrasound** can also be used to assess catheter tip position.

 13. Centers for Disease Control and Prevention recommends that UACs only stay in no more than 5 days. Other sources state 5–7 days. The duration of UACs was a risk factor for aortic thrombosis. One study of UACs in for up to 28 days had no increased risk of thrombus.

IV. UAC removal. Make sure the tie is lightly tied around the stump.

 A. Withdraw the catheter slowly until about 5 cm remains in the vessel.

 B. Tighten the umbilical tie.

 C. Discontinue the infusion and pull the catheter slowly (1 cm/min).

 D. If bleeding, apply pressure to the cord.

V. Complications have been reported in the range of 5–32%.

 A. Infection (septic emboli, cellulitis, omphalitis, sepsis). The catheter disrupts the integrity of the skin, introducing bacteria or fungi and causing an infection; minimize by using strict sterile technique. No attempt should be made to advance a catheter once it has been placed in position; instead, the catheter should be replaced. Prophylactic antibiotics are not recommended. VLBW infants who received antibiotics for >10 days were at increased risk for catheter-related bloodstream infections in one study. AAP recommends the catheter to be removed and not replaced if there are any signs of central line–associated bloodstream infection.

 B. Vascular accidents. **Vasospasm, thrombosis, embolism, and infarction can occur.** Heparin use in UACs did not decrease the rate of aortic thrombi. Air embolism has also been reported. Doppler ultrasound is useful to examine the aorta and renal vessels. AAP recommends removing the UAC if thrombosis is present. See Chapter 79 for treatment plans.

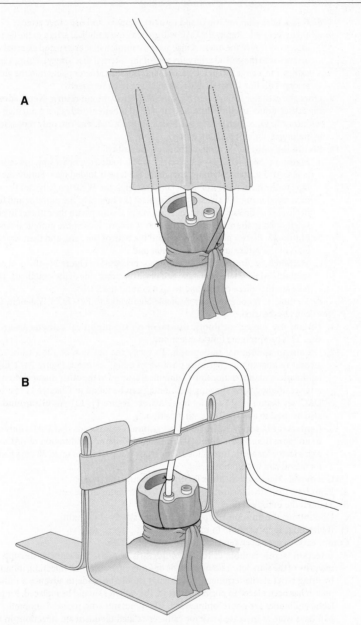

FIGURE 24–4. (A) The umbilical artery catheter is secured with silk tape, which is attached to the base of the cord (through the Wharton jelly, not the skin or vessels). (B) The umbilical catheter is secured with a tape bridge ("goal post" method). (*From The Johns Hopkins Hospital. Tshudy MM, Arcara KM, eds. The Harriet Lane Handbook. 19th ed. Philadelphia, PA: Elsevier; 2012.*)

1. Arterial vasospasm. This can cause blanching and cyanosis of the buttocks, legs, feet, and toes. It is increased in low-lying catheters. Loss of extremity is rare but can occur. If the leg blanches, warm the other leg (reflex vasodilatation).
2. Thrombosis. This can cause dampening of the arterial tracing and is classified as follows:
   a. Femoral artery thrombosis. Limb ischemia, gangrene.
   b. Renal artery thrombosis. Hematuria, hypertension, renal failure.
   c. Mesenteric artery thrombosis. Ischemia of the gut, necrotizing enterocolitis.
   d. Aortic thrombosis. Congestive heart failure, hematuria, paraplegia, renovascular hypertension, leg-growth discrepancy.

C. Hemorrhage. This can be secondary to perforation of the vessel, umbilical cord site bleeding around the catheter, disconnection of the catheter at any point in the system, and accidental line dislodgment. The tubing stopcocks must be securely fastened.

D. Vessel perforation. The catheter should never be forced into position. If the catheter cannot be easily advanced, use of another vessel should be attempted. If perforation occurs, surgical intervention may be necessary.

E. Gastrointestinal complications. UACs may lead to gastrointestinal ischemia, intestinal necrosis (embolization to the gut), or localized perforation. Data do not support that UACs alter the incidence of NEC whether they are high or low or regardless of enteral feeding status.

F. Improperly placed catheter. This can cause perforation of a vessel, false aneurysm, perforation of the peritoneum, sciatic nerve palsy, and refractory hypoglycemia (catheter tip opposite celiac axis). Necrosis of the left buttock has been reported.

G. Hematuria. Injury to the bladder has been reported.

H. Hypertension secondary to renal artery embolus. This can occur as a long-term complication caused by stenosis of the renal artery as a result of improper catheter placement near the renal arteries.

I. Patent urachus. If the urachal tract is not obliterated during embryonic development, a patent urachus can result. If urine is obtained from a UAC and not blood, there may be a patent urachus. Urology or pediatric surgery consult is needed.

J. Other complications. Injury and rupture of the bladder, urinary ascites, Wharton jelly or cotton fiber emboluts, hypernatremia, peroneal nerve palsy, factitious hypernatremia or hyperkalemia, and hypoglycemia.

Selected References

Barrington KJ. Umbilical artery catheters in the newborn: effects of position of the catheter tip. *Cochrane Database Syst Rev.* 2000;CD000505.

College of Respiratory Therapists of Ontario. Central Access: Umbilical Artery and Vein Cannulation. http://www.crto.on.ca/pdf/PPG/Umbilical_CBPG.pdf. Assessed September, 2012.

Monagle P, Chan AK, Goldenberg NA, et al. Antithrombotic therapy in neonates and children: Antithrombotic Therapy and Prevention of Thrombosis. 9th ed. American College of Chest Physicians Evidence-Based Clinical Practice Guidelines. *Chest.* 2012;141 (suppl 2):e737S.

25 Bladder Aspiration (Suprapubic Urine Collection)

I. **Indication.** To obtain urine for culture when a less invasive technique is not possible. It is the **most accurate and preferred culture source** for infants and children <2 years of age when compared with urethral catheterization and bag urine specimens. Any bacteria or growth on a suprapubic culture is considered abnormal and requires treatment. **Other common terms** include suprapubic bladder aspiration (SBA), suprapubic aspiration (SPA), and bladder tap.

II. **Equipment.** Safety-engineered needle: 23- or 25-gauge 1-inch needle or 21- to 22-gauge 1.5-inch needle (large infant) or 23-gauge butterfly (for preemie) attached to a 3-mL syringe, sterile gloves, povidone-iodine solution, 4 × 4 gauze pads, gloves, and sterile container; transillumination light source or portable ultrasound recommended.

III. **Procedure**

   A. **Contraindications.** Empty bladder, thrombocytopenia, presence of abdominal distension, bleeding disorders, genitourinary anomalies, cellulitis at the site, after recent lower abdominal or urologic surgery.

   B. Note that before the age of 2 years, the bladder is an abdominal organ and this makes the procedure easier. After 2 years of age, the bladder moves into the pelvis.

   C. Verify that voiding has not occurred within the previous hour so there will be enough urine in the bladder for the procedure. Has there been a recent wet diaper? Is the diaper wet now?

      1. **Palpate or percuss the bladder.** Dullness to percussion 2 fingers above the pubic symphysis suggests urine in the bladder. The neonatal bladder extends above the pubic symphysis as it fills.

      2. **Transillumination** can determine bladder height and verify the presence of urine. With the lights dim, the transillumination source is pointed at the bladder. The area will glow red if urine is present. (See Chapter 40.)

      3. **Ultrasound of the bladder** can help determine the size and location of the bladder and the volume of urine in the bladder. Portable ultrasound can significantly improve the diagnostic yield; a minimum volume on ultrasound of 10 mL is associated with a 90% successful bladder aspiration. If the cephalocaudal diameter of the bladder (sagittal view) is >20 mm and the anteroposterior diameter is >15 mm, the success rate approaches 100%.

   D. **Pain management.** This procedure is significantly more painful than transurethral catheterization (as evidenced by brow bulging in one study). Nonpharmacologic pain procedures can be used. **EMLA** (eutectic mixture of lidocaine and prilocaine) alone or **EMLA plus local injection of lidocaine** can be used. In one study EMLA use 1 hour before the suprapubic aspiration was found to reduce pain scores more than without EMLA. Local injection of lidocaine often turns this from a "one stick" to a "two stick" procedure.

   E. **Bedside ultrasonography** if available can be used to **help guide needle insertion** and **puncture of the bladder wall.** When used, fewer needle insertions are necessary.

   F. An assistant should hold the infant in a supine position with the legs in the frog-leg position.

   G. Locate the site of bladder puncture, which is ~1–2 cm above the pubic symphysis in the midline of the lower abdomen (look for the transverse lower abdominal skin crease just above the pubic symphysis). See Figure 25–1A.

   H. To avoid the bladder from emptying (reflex urination) when the needle is inserted, have an assistant hold pressure at the base of the penis in a male infant, or in a female infant apply anterior rectal pressure after inserting the fingertip in the anus.

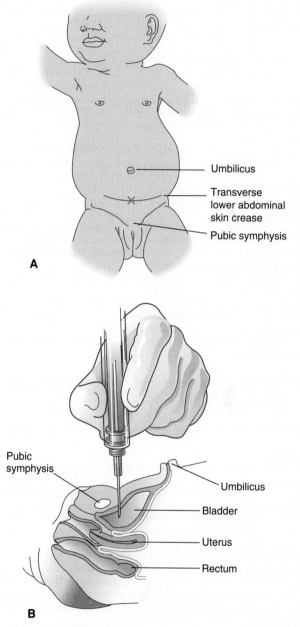

FIGURE 25–1. Technique of suprapubic bladder aspiration. (A) Landmarks and recommended site for suprapubic bladder aspiration. (B) Technique of suprapubic aspiration.

I. Put on sterile gloves, and clean the entire suprapubic area of skin (from pubic symphysis to the umbilicus) with antiseptic solution three times. Place sterile drapes around the insertion site.

J. Palpate the pubic symphysis. Insert the needle with syringe attached 1–2 cm above the pubic symphysis (at the transverse lower abdominal skin crease in the midline) at a 90-degree angle (Figure 25–1B).

K. Advance the needle while aspirating ~2–3 cm. Do not advance the needle once urine is seen in the syringe, to reduce risk of posterior wall bladder perforation. Use only gentle aspiration to prevent the needle from suctioning the bladder wall.

L. If no urine appears, do not advance or redirect the needle. Withdraw the needle and reattempt the procedure in a minimum of 1 hour; consider ultrasound to evaluate bladder filling.

M. Collect sample, withdraw the needle, maintain pressure over the site of puncture, and apply a bandage (optional). Place a sterile cap on the syringe or transfer the specimen to a sterile urine cup, and submit the specimen to the laboratory.

IV. Complications. Serious complications are very rare.

A. Bleeding and hematomas. Hematuria is the most common complication; it is usually microscopic, rarely causes concern, and resolves. Gross hemorrhage is more likely if there is a bleeding disorder; transient gross hematuria is reported in up to 3.4% of cases. Thrombocytopenia is a contraindication. Hematomas (abdominal wall, pelvic, supravesical, and bladder wall), massive hemoperitoneum, and vaginal bleeding are rare.

B. Infection. Rare and not likely to occur if strict sterile technique is used. Sepsis, bacteremia, abdominal wall abscess, suprapubic abscess formation, and osteomyelitis of the pubic bone have all been reported.

C. Perforation of the bowel or other pelvic organs. With careful identification of the landmarks and not advancing the needle too far, this complication is rare. If the bowel is perforated (aspiration of bowel contents), close observation is recommended, and intravenous antibiotics should be considered. Surgical consultation may be obtained.

D. Needle breakage.

26 Bladder Catheterization

I. Indications

A. To collect a urine specimen when a clean-catch specimen cannot be obtained or is unsatisfactory or a suprapubic aspiration cannot be performed. Bladder catheterization is an alternative to suprapubic aspiration but is not the method of first choice. It has a higher false-positive rate than suprapubic aspiration and it can also introduce bacteria and cause a urinary tract infection (UTI).

B. To monitor urinary output, relieve urinary retention, or to instill contrast to obtain a cystogram or voiding cystourethrogram.

C. To determine a bladder residual urine volume.

II. Equipment. Sterile gloves, cotton balls, povidone-iodine solution, sterile drapes, lubricant, a sterile collection bottle (often packaged together as a commercial set), and choice of catheter (balloon retention [Foley] catheters are not used in newborns).

A. Use the smallest catheter possible. Recommendations vary widely; it is best to follow your institution's guidelines if available.

B. Urethral catheters. Commercially available sizes: 3.5, 5.0, 6.5, and 8F.
1. 3.5F for weight <1000 g.
2. 5F for weight 1000–1800 g.
3. 6.5F for weight 1800–4000 g.
4. 8F for weight >4000 g.

C. **National Association of Neonatal Nurses (NANN) recommendations.** 3.5F for weight <1000 g; 5F for weight 1000–1800 g; 8F for weight >1800 g.

D. **Feeding tubes.** When used as an alternative, they may increase the risk of trauma or knotting (tubes are softer). 5F feeding tube is sometimes used (not preferred).

E. **3.5F or 5F umbilical catheter.** May be used as an alternative: 3.5F for weight <1000 g; 5F for weight >1000 g.

III. **Procedure**

A. **When performing catheterization to obtain a specimen, it is best to wait until 1–2 hours after voiding.** Ultrasound the bladder to determine the **urinary bladder index measurement** (product of anteroposterior and transverse diameters, expressed in centimeters squared), which will identify whether there is sufficient urine in the bladder. A urinary bladder index <2.4 cm² means there is lack of urine volume and the catheterization may be unsuccessful. A urinary bladder index >2.4 cm² suggests an adequate urine volume.

B. **Pain management.** Consider the use of topical and intraurethral lidocaine-enhanced lubricant. Nonpharmacologic pain-reducing methods are also recommended.

C. **Male catheterization.** See Figure 26–1.

1. **Place the infant supine, with the thighs abducted (frog-leg position).**

2. **The newborn male infant has a physiologic phimosis, and the penis cannot be retracted fully.** Gently retract the foreskin just enough to expose the meatus; do not force retraction of the foreskin. The meatus can usually be aligned with the opening in the prepuce.

3. **Put on sterile gloves, and drape the area with sterile towels.**

4. **Cleanse the penis with povidone-iodine solution.** Begin with the meatus and move in a proximal direction. Infant smegma (white discharge from cell shedding) can be gently wiped away.

5. **Place the tip of the catheter in sterile lubricant.**

6. **Hold the penis approximately perpendicular to the body to straighten the penile urethra and help prevent false passage.** Use a small amount of pressure at the base of the penis to avoid reflex urination.

7. **Advance the catheter until urine appears. Length of insertion in males** is generally as follows: weight <750 g, >5 cm; weight >750 g, ~6 cm. A slight resistance may be felt as the catheter passes the external sphincter; therefore, hold the catheter in place with minimal pressure. Gentle continuous pressure enables the catheter to pass when the sphincter relaxes. Never force the catheter because urethral trauma or false passage can occur.

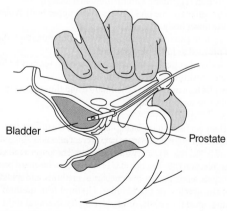

FIGURE 26–1. Bladder catheterization in the newborn male.

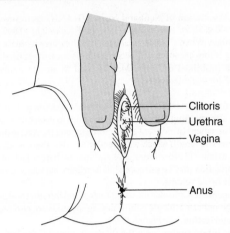

FIGURE 26–2. Landmarks used in catheterization of the bladder in newborn females in supine position.

8. **Collect the urine specimen.** If the catheter is to be removed, gently withdraw it. If the catheter is to remain in place, connect it to a closed urinary collection system. It should be taped to the lower abdomen rather than to the leg in males to help decrease stricture formation caused by pressure on the posterior urethra. Contrast can be injected at this point if the catheter has been placed for a radiographic study.

D. **Female catheterization.** See Figure 26–2.

1. **Supine position technique**

   a. Place the infant supine, with the thighs abducted (frog-leg position).

   b. Put on sterile gloves, and drape sterile towels around the labia.

   c. Separate the labia, and cleanse the area around the meatus with povidone-iodine solution. Use anterior-to-posterior strokes to prevent fecal contamination.

   d. Spread the labia with 2 fingers. See Figure 26–2 for landmarks. Lubricate the catheter, and advance it in the urethra until urine appears. **General length of insertion:** weight <750 g, generally <2.5 cm; weight >750 g, up to 5 cm.

   e. Tape the catheter to the leg if it is to remain in position.

2. **Prone position technique.** Used for a female infant who cannot be placed in the supine position (eg, infant with meningomyelocele).

   a. Place the infant prone on blankets so the upper body is elevated as compared with the lower body.

   b. Tape a gauze pad over the anus to avoid contamination. Place sterile drapes.

   c. Then proceed as for supine position.

3. If urine does not appear in the catheter, the catheter may be in the vagina. Check the catheter position and replace if necessary.

IV. **Catheter removal.** Once urine has been obtained and flow has stopped, gently withdraw the catheter. Observe for urine output.

V. **Complications**

A. **Infection.** There is a risk of introducing bacteria into the urinary tract and then the bloodstream. Sterile technique is necessary to help prevent infection. "In-and out" catheterization carries a small (<5%) risk of urinary tract infection. The longer a catheter is left in place, the greater is the infection risk. The risk of UTI is high in catheterized patients. Infections that can occur include sepsis, cystitis, pyelonephritis, urethritis, and epididymitis.

B. **Trauma to the urethra or the bladder.** Urethral tear, urethral false passage, erosion, stricture, meatal stenosis, or bladder injury (perforation) is more common in males. Minimize by adequately lubricating the catheter and stretching the penis to straighten the male urethra. Never force the catheter if resistance is felt. Use the smallest catheter possible, and advance only until urine is obtained.

C. **Hematuria.** Hematuria is usually transient but may require irrigation with normal saline solution. Gross hematuria on insertion may indicate a false passage.

D. **Urethral stricture.** More common in males. It is usually caused by a catheter that is too large or by prolonged or traumatic catheterization. In males, taping the catheter to the anterior abdominal wall helps decrease the pressure on the posterior urethra.

E. **Urinary retention.** Secondary to urethral edema.

F. **Catheter knot.** Rare but can happen if the catheter advances too far and is more common if feeding tubes are used. Insert only enough to obtain urine and never force a catheter. Using appropriate lengths based on age and sex may help prevent this complication. If this occurs, a urology consultation may be necessary.

G. **Malpositioned catheter.** The catheter can be accidently placed in the vagina. If this happens during cystography, the vagina can mimic the bladder. The clue to this is that fluid is in the peritoneal cavity (contrast material flowed through the uterus and fallopian tubes into the peritoneal cavity).

H. **Obstructive bilateral hydroureteronephrosis.** Rare.

Selected Reference

Milling TJ Jr, Van Amerongen R, Melville L, et al. Use of ultrasonography to identify infants for whom urinary catheterization will be unsuccessful because of insufficient urine volume: validation of the urinary bladder index. *Ann Emerg Med.* 2005;45:510–513.

27 Chest Tube Placement

I. **Indications**

A. **Evacuation of pneumothorax** compromising ventilation and causing increased work of breathing, hypoxia, and increased $Paco_2$.

B. **Relieve tension pneumothorax** causing respiratory compromise and decreased venous return to the heart, resulting in decreased cardiac output and hypotension. **This is an emergency that should be handled by immediate needle aspiration before chest tube placement.** (See Chapter 70.)

C. **Drainage of significant pleural fluid** (pleural effusion, empyema, chylothorax, hemothorax, extravasation from a central venous line). Studies have shown that placement of a drainage catheter rather than aspiration alone is more effective and just as safe.

D. **Postsurgical drainage** after repair of a tracheoesophageal fistula, bronchopleural fistula, esophageal atresia, or other thoracic procedure.

II. **Equipment.** Prepackaged chest tube tray (sterile towels, 4 × 4 gauze pads, 3-0 silk suture, curved hemostats, a no. 11 or 15 scalpel, scissors, a needle holder, antiseptic solution, antibiotic ointment, 1% lidocaine, 3-mL syringe, 25-gauge needle); sterile gloves, mask, eye protection, hat, gown, suction-drainage system (eg, the Pleur-Evac system). A high-intensity fiber optic light for transillumination is helpful (see Chapter 40). Chest tube types and sizes are as follows:

A. **Standard (traditional) chest tube insertion.** Requires a skin incision with blunt chest wall dissection and sutures. Use polyvinyl chloride (PVC) chest tubes 8, 10, or 12F. **Recommended size for weight:** 8 or 10F <2000 g, 12F >2000 g.

B. **Percutaneous chest tube with pigtail catheter.** Does not require a skin incision. The pigtail catheter is inserted through a needle. This is an easier and less invasive technique requiring less anesthesia. Disadvantages are that the catheter may kink and become obstructed since they are softer. It may not drain a pneumothorax with an ongoing air leak. **Pigtail catheter sizes** range from 5F to 12F with 8 and 10F most commonly used.

III. Procedure

A. The site of skin insertion for the elective chest tube insertion is the same for both air and fluid, but the direction of the tube is determined by examining the anteroposterior and cross-table lateral or lateral decubitus chest films for air or fluid. Air collects in the uppermost areas of the chest, and fluid in the most dependent areas. For air collections, place the tube anteriorly. For fluid collections, place the tube posteriorly and laterally.

B. Transillumination of the chest may help detect pneumothorax but not a small pneumothorax (see Chapter 40). With the room lights turned down, a strong light source is placed on the anterior chest wall above the nipple and in the axilla. The affected side usually appears hyperlucent ("lights up") and radiates across the chest as compared with the unaffected side. Unless the infant's status is rapidly deteriorating, a chest radiograph should be obtained to confirm pneumothorax before the chest tube is inserted. A lateral decubitus or cross-table lateral x-ray film should be done. If air is suspected, the infant should be lying on his or her side with the suspect side up; if fluid is suspected, the infant should be placed with the suspect side down. See Figure 11–20 for a radiograph showing a left tension pneumothorax.

1. **False-positive transillumination.** Subcutaneous air, severe pulmonary interstitial emphysema, lobar emphysema, pneumomediastinum, large air bubble in the stomach, and too dim of a light source.

2. **False-negative transillumination.** Weak light source, bright room lights, small pneumothorax, thick chest wall with edema, thick skin folds on a large baby, and dark pigmented skin.

C. Position the patient so the site of insertion is accessible. The most common position is supine, with the arm at a 90-degree angle on the affected side. Some say position the infant with a rolled up towel to 60-75 degrees off bed to evacuate air, and 15-30 degrees for fluid, chyle, blood, or pus.

D. Select the appropriate site

1. **Emergency needle aspiration (tension pneumothorax).** Needle aspiration is done at the **second intercostal space at the midclavicular line** on the suspected side of the pneumothorax. The needle is inserted above the third rib. See Chapter 70 and Figure 70–1. The **fourth intercostal space at the anterior axillary line** can also be used (needle would be inserted above the fifth rib).

2. **For air or fluid.** Placement is the same except the tube is directed differently. The chest tube should be at the **fourth or fifth intercostal space between the anterior axillary line and midaxillary line (modified Buelau position).** This site is safe for both thoracic sides, for both preterm and term infants, as only lung parenchyma and no organ structures are found. See Figure 27–1.

   a. **Air.** Skin incision is at fifth or sixth rib. If skin incision is at the fifth rib, the pleura is punctured above the fifth rib in the fourth intercostal space. If the skin incision is at the sixth rib, the pleura is punctured above the sixth rib in the fifth intercostal space. **Insert the tube anteriorly and toward the apex.**

   b. **Fluid.** Skin incision at the fifth or sixth intercostal space. If skin incision is at the fifth rib, the pleura is punctured above the fifth rib in the fourth intercostal space. If the skin incision is at the sixth rib, the pleura is punctured above the sixth rib in the fifth intercostal space. **Insert the tube posteriorly and inferiorly.**

3. **The nipple is a landmark for the fourth intercostal space.** Do not place the tube in the nipple area of a female, as this can cause future asymmetrical breast tissue development.

E. Put on a sterile gown, mask, hat, and gloves. Cleanse the area of insertion with povidone-iodine solution, and drape.

F. Prophylactic antibiotics. **Cochrane review** states there is no evidence to recommend or refute the use of prophylactic antibiotics in infants when a chest tube is placed.

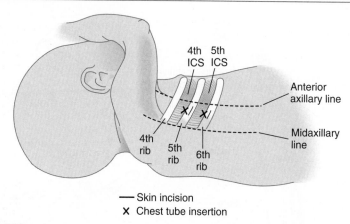

FIGURE 27–1. Recommended site for skin incision and chest tube insertion in the neonate: fourth and fifth intercostal space between the anterior and midaxillary line. ICS, intercostal space.

   G. **Pain management.** There are no prospective studies on pain management for chest tube insertion.

      1. **The American Academy of Pediatrics (AAP) recommends slow infiltration** of the area with a local anesthetic before incision (unless life-threatening instability) and the use of systemic analgesia with a rapidly acting opiate (fentanyl). If there is not enough time to infiltrate before the chest tube is inserted, infiltration should be done after the chest tube is in (may decrease later pain responses).

      2. **Local anesthetic.** Slowly infiltrate the area superficially with 0.5–1% lidocaine and then down to the rib. Infiltrate into the intercostal muscles and along the parietal pleura.

      3. **Systemic analgesia** with a rapidly acting opiate (fentanyl).

      4. **General nonpharmacologic measures** should also be used.

   H. **Standard (traditional) chest tube insertion**

      1. **Make a small incision** (approximately the width of the tube, usually ≤0.5–75 cm) in the skin over the rib just below the intercostal space where the tube is to be inserted (see Figure 27–1).

      2. **Insert a closed curved hemostat into the incision,** and spread the tissues down to the rib. Using the tip of the hemostat, **puncture the pleura just above the rib** (avoids the subcostal blood vessels, minimizes vascular injury) and spread gently. The intercostal vein, artery, and nerve lie below the ribs (Figure 27–2A). This creates a subcutaneous tunnel that aids in closing the tract when the tube is removed. This tunnel can be carried superiorly over the next rib, anteriorly (for air) or posteriorly (for effusion) parallel to the ribs, or obliquely.

      3. **When the pleura has been penetrated, a rush of air is often heard or fluid appears.** Insert the chest tube through the opened hemostat (Figure 27–2B). Be certain that the side holes of the tube are within the pleural cavity. The presence of moisture in the tube usually confirms proper placement in the intrapleural cavity in a pneumothorax. Use of a trocar guide is usually unnecessary and may increase the risk of complications such as lung perforation. **The chest tube should be inserted 2–3 cm for a small, preterm infant and 3–4 cm for a term infant.** (These are guidelines only; the length of tube to be inserted varies based on the size of the infant.) An alternative approach to tube insertion is to measure the length from the insertion site to the apex of the lung (approximately the midclavicle) and tie a silk suture around the tube the same distance from the tip. Position the tube until the silk suture is just outside the skin.

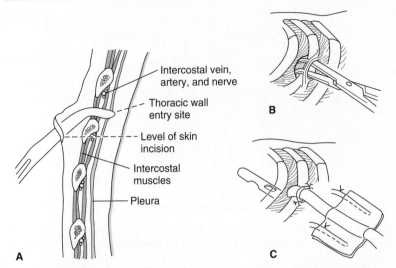

FIGURE 27–2. Procedures of standard chest tube insertion. (A) Level of skin incision and thoracic wall entry site in relation to the rib and the neurovascular bundle. (B) Opened hemostat, through which the chest tube is inserted. (C) The chest tube is then secured to the skin with silk sutures.

4. Hold the tube steady first and then allow an assistant to connect the tube to a water seal vacuum drainage system (eg, Pleur-Evac system). Five to ten centimeters of suction is usually used. Start at the lower level of suction and increase as needed if the pneumothorax or effusion does not resolve. Some recommend starting at 10 cm increasing 20 cm, if necessary. Excessive suction can draw tissue into the side holes of the tube. Systems such as the Pleur-Evac provide both continuous suction and water seal. A water seal prevents air from being drawn back into the pleural space.

5. Secure the chest tube with 3–0 silk sutures and silk tape (Figure 27–2C). Close the skin opening with sutures, if necessary. Use a purse-string suture around the tube or a single interrupted suture on either side of the tube.

6. Obtain an immediate chest radiograph (AP and lateral) to verify placement and check for residual fluid or pneumothorax. Look for tachypnea, dyspnea, increasing oxygen requirement, hypotension, or worsening arterial blood gas. Positioning of the tube must always be verified by a chest radiograph. Place a sterile clear occlusive dressing at the site. Figure 27–3 shows a standard chest tube in position.

I. Modified Seldinger technique using a pigtail (Fuhrman) catheter. Advantages include speed, safety (fewer complications), improved discomfort, and easily learned. This is the preferred chest tube placement in tiny preemies. The catheter is a coiled, single-lumen polyurethane catheter (5–12F) with 8 or 10F being commonly used.

1. Follow the site and anesthetic selections as noted above.

2. Insert an 18-gauge needle with the syringe attached (or an 18-gauge IV catheter) into the skin over the top of the rib at the designated site into the pleural space. Pull back on the syringe while inserting the needle. Do not advance more than 2 cm in depth. Verify placement by aspirating for fluid or air. When air or fluid is obtained, stop insertion.

3. Secure the needle and remove the syringe, keep lumen occluded. If an 18-gauge IV catheter is used, the IV catheter will act as the introducing needle.

4. Straighten the J tip of the guide wire and insert into the hub of the needle or the IV catheter. Advance the guide wire into the needle about 2 to 3 cm past the tip of the needle or until the coloured line on the wire is at the level of the hub.

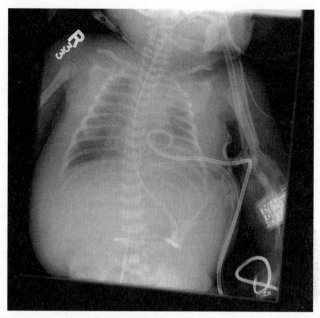

FIGURE 27–3. Unusual chest radiograph showing both a standard chest tube and pigtail catheter in the same patient.

5. Withdraw the needle or IV catheter while holding the guide wire.
6. Thread the dilator down over the guide wire. Twist the dilator to dilate the skin, muscles, and pleura. The site has to be well dilated so the catheter will fit. Once dilated, remove the dilator while securing the guide wire.
7. Straighten the pigtail catheter and insert over the guide wire. Advance until all holes are inside the skin and pleural cavity and then 1 to 2 cm further.
8. Slowly remove the guide wire while holding the tube in place. The pigtail catheter will curl up inside the pleural cavity. Immediately connect the tube to the underwater sealed drainage (see Section III.H.4).
9. For a pigtail catheter, one does not have to usually suture, since the skin often closes around the catheter. Place a sterile clear occlusive dressing at the site.
10. Obtain an immediate chest radiograph (AP and lateral). To verify placement and check for residual fluid or pneumothorax (see Section III.H.6). Figure 27–3 shows a pigtail catheter in position.

IV. **Chest tube removal**

A. **Pain management.** Removing a chest tube is known to be painful. **AAP recommends** general nonpharmacologic measures and a short-acting rapid-onset systemic analgesic. Methohexital has been used with good pain control and without major respiratory compromise. Some recommend EMLA (eutectic mixture of lidocaine and prilocaine) at the site of insertion and a slow IV opiate bolus.

B. **For pneumothorax.** If there is no more bubbling in the underwater seal or presence of air for 24 to 48 hours, discontinue the suction and leave the underwater seal for 4 to 12 hours (some units will leave it for 24 hours). Transilluminate, or preferably check an x-ray. If there is no air on x-ray or transillumination, it is okay to remove the chest tube. *Never* clamp a chest tube (tension pneumothorax risk).

C. **Clean the skin area around the chest tube with an antiseptic solution.** Remove any tape or sutures but leave the wound suture. Cover entry site with gauze and your fingertips to prevent air from entering chest as the tube is withdrawn, then cover with petroleum gauze. Keep pressure on it. Cover with gauze and remove sutures when healed.

D. **Clinical signs and symptoms of respiratory distress** will identify almost all patients with significant pneumothoraces following chest tube removal. Monitor for tachypnea, dyspnea, increasing oxygen requirement, hypotension, or worsening arterial blood gas. Transillumination and chest x-ray may be necessary.

V. **Complications**

A. **Infection.** Strict sterile technique minimizes infections. Cellulitis is common. Intrapleural inoculation of *Candida* has been reported after chest tube placement. Many institutions recommend prophylactic antibiotics (eg, Nafcillin) when a chest tube is placed (*controversial*). Empyema requires antibiotics and drainage.

B. **Bleeding.** May occur if one of the major vessels (intercostal, axillary, pulmonary, or internal mammary) or the myocardium is perforated, or if the lung is damaged during the procedure. It can cause a hematoma or hemothorax. This complication can be avoided if landmarks are properly identified. Bleeding is less likely if a trocar is not used. Bleeding may stop during suctioning; however, if significant bleeding continues, immediate surgical consultation is necessary. Tears of subclavian vessels and thymic trauma can occur with hemorrhage. Bleeding can be more significant with a coagulopathy.

C. **Nerve damage.** Passing the tube over the top of the rib helps avoid injury to the intercostal nerve running under the rib. Horner syndrome, diaphragmatic paralysis, or eventration from phrenic nerve injury has been reported. The medial end of the chest tube should be no less than 1 cm from the spine on frontal chest radiograph (phrenic nerve paralysis is related to the abnormal location of the medial end of the chest tube). The main nerve tract lies outside the pericardium in the middle mediastinum. The tip should not be against the mediastinum.

D. **Trauma.** The premature lung is at greater risk of trauma because the chest wall is thin and the lung tissue is fragile. Lung trauma (perforation or laceration) can be minimized by never forcing the tube into position. Trauma can also occur to the breast tissue. Iatrogenic tracheobronchial perforation (tube through esophagus, carina, right main bronchus) and tracheoesophageal fistula have been reported. Liver trauma with hemoperitoneum can occur. Damage to the heart, great vessels, diaphragm, thymus, and liver and spleen can all occur but are rare.

E. **Subcutaneous emphysema.** Secondary to a leak through the pleural opening.

F. **Chylothorax.** Results if the catheter causes trauma to the thoracic duct. It is best to avoid penetration into the posterior superior mediastinum.

G. **Cardiac tamponade.** See Chapter 38.

H. **Fluid and electrolyte imbalance/hypoproteinemia.**

I. **Rare complications.** Myocardial perforation, severing the phrenic nerve, subclavian vessel tear with blood loss, thymic trauma with blood loss, trauma to the liver with hemoperitoneum, traumatic arteriovenous fistula, aortic obstruction, compression of the aorta, and displacement of the trachea can all occur.

Selected Reference

Eifinger F, Lenze M, Brisken K, Welzing L, Roth B, Koebke J . The anterior to midaxillary line between the 4th or 5th intercostal space (Buelau position) is safe for the use of thoracostomy tubes in preterm and term infants. *Paediatr Anaesth.* 2009;19(6):612–617.

28 Defibrillation and Cardioversion

Defibrillation and cardioversion are used for rapid termination of a tachyarrhythmia (a fast abnormal rhythm originating either in the atrium or ventricle) that is unresponsive to baseline treatment or is causing the patient to have cardiovascular compromise (inadequate systemic perfusion). Baseline treatment consists of correcting metabolic problems, use of vagal maneuvers (bag of ice water over the eyes and face of the infant without obstructing the airway, pressure on closed eyelids), use of medications (adenosine, digoxin, propranolol, verapamil, amiodarone, procainamide, lidocaine, or magnesium sulfate), or transesophageal pacing. It is best to try these maneuvers or medical therapy if intravenous access is available. **Neonatal arrhythmias are rare, and the majority of them can be treated with these initial measures.**

Current defibrillators are capable of delivering 2 modes of shock: synchronized and unsynchronized. Synchronized shocks are lower dose and used for cardioversion. Unsynchronized shocks are higher dose and used for defibrillation. **Pediatric cardiology consultation is recommended for all infants with a tachyarrhythmia.**

I. Indications
   A. Cardioversion (synchronized cardioversion)
      1. Unstable patients with tachyarrhythmias who have a perfusing rhythm but evidence of poor perfusion, heart failure, or hypotension (signs of cardiovascular compromise). Examples of tachyarrhythmias are:
         a. Tachycardia (supraventricular tachycardia [SVT] or ventricular tachycardia [VT]) with a pulse and poor perfusion
         b. Supraventricular tachycardia with shock and no vascular access
         c. Atrial flutter with shock
         d. Atrial fibrillation with shock (very rare in infants)
      2. Elective cardioversion in infants with **stable** SVT, VT, or atrial flutter (good tissue perfusion and pulses) unresponsive to other treatments. This is always done under the close supervision of a pediatric cardiologist. Sedation and a 12-lead electrocardiogram are recommended before cardioversion.
   B. Defibrillation (asynchronized). Used in pulseless arrest with a shockable rhythm (VT and ventricular fibrillation). It is used in between cardiopulmonary resuscitation (CPR) and **not used in asystole or pulseless electrical activity (PEA).** The most common cause of a ventricular arrhythmia in a neonate is electrolyte imbalance. Defibrillation will not stop the arrhythmia in these patients. **Defibrillation is the most effective treatment for ventricular fibrillation and pulseless ventricular tachycardia.**
II. Equipment
   A. External standard defibrillator (manual or semiautomated) and 2 paddles of the correct sizes with conductive pads. For infants, use the smallest size (usually measuring 4.5 cm). It is important to be familiar with your institution's equipment because there are many different types and models of machines. Pediatric-capable automatic external defibrillators (adult-automated external defibrillators with energy reducer pads) can be used for infants.
   B. Other equipment. Heart rate monitor, airway equipment, resuscitation medications, antiarrhythmic medications, and equipment used in basic and advanced life support.
III. Procedure
   A. Adequate sedation (may not be possible in emergency situations), preoxygenation, and continuous heart monitoring are essential. Emergency airway equipment should be readily available.

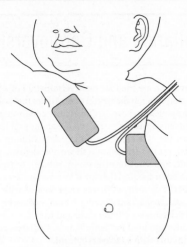

FIGURE 28–1. Anterolateral pad and paddle placement.

    B. **Pain management.** During a code, pain relief is not focused on. Depending on the type of procedure, sedation may be considered.
       1. **Planned cardioversion.** Use propofol (short-acting, side effects are rare). Induction dosing: 2.5–3.5 mg/kg over 20–30 seconds, then 200–300 mcg/kg/min.
       2. **Emergent cardioversion.** These patients are usually too unstable to wait for appropriate sedation. It is best to proceed with cardioversion without sedation.
       3. **Defibrillation.** These patients are unconscious, so do not require sedation.
    C. **Wipe any cream or soap off the chest.**
    D. **Place the pads firmly on the chest wall.** To prevent skin burns, be sure the conductive pad totally covers the paddle and that the skin is not in contact with any noninsulated part of the paddle. If the pads are in contact with each other, this can cause the electric current to arch across the chest instead of toward the heart. There are 2 different positions for pad placement (see Figures 28–1 and 28–2).

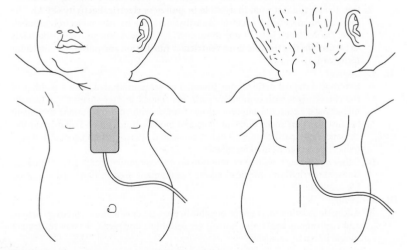

FIGURE 28–2. Anteroposterior pad and paddle placement.

1. Anterolateral positioning. (Figure 28–1)The anterior pad is placed to the right of the upper sternum, and the posterior pad is placed below the left nipple toward the axilla.
2. Anteroposterior positioning. (Figure 28–2) This may be preferred in atrial tachycardia. The anterior pad is placed on the midsternal border, and the posterior pad is placed between the scapulae. The paddles or pads should not be in contact with one another. **With dextrocardia, the pads need to be placed across the right chest.**

E. Charge the defibrillator
1. Cardioversion uses lower energy. Charge the defibrillator to **0.5 J/kg** and synchronize. **The SYNC button must be activated each time because the default setting on a defibrillator is on the asynchronized setting.**
2. Defibrillation uses higher energy. Charge the defibrillator to **2 J/kg.**
3. Once charged, make sure everybody is clear of the patient, including the person holding the oxygen. Ask if everyone is clear, and visually check while they answer. Use the accepted phrase **"I'm clear, you're clear, oxygen clear."** Verify that oxygen is not flowing across the area. It is best to disconnect the bag and verify that no one is touching the endotracheal tube or any part of the ventilation circuit. The machine will indicate that it is charged and ready for discharge with an audible signal and/or a flashing red light either on the machine or the end of the paddle based on the model.

F. Deliver the shock by pressing both buttons together
1. Cardioversion. If the first attempt does not work, additional attempts should be made. **Repeat steps C–E using 1 J/kg, then up to a max of 2 J/kg.**
2. Defibrillation. In pulseless infants, continue CPR with appropriate compressions, ventilation, and medications between attempts. Additional attempts should be made by repeating steps C–E. **The second and any subsequent shock should have a dose of 4 J/kg.** Acidosis and hypoxia decrease the success of defibrillation, and correction increases the likelihood of success.

IV. Complications. Risk of complications are increased when there is an increased energy dose, multiple shocks, increased impedance, or decreased interval between shocks.
A. Altered skin integrity. Soft tissue injury, chest wall lesions, skin burns, bruising, and pain can occur. Burns can be moderate to severe in 20–25% of patients. They are usually due to improper pad placement.
B. Pulmonary edema. A rare complication. It is most likely due to left ventricular dysfunction, but true mechanism is unknown.
C. Neurologic impairment. This can occur from a stroke from a thromboembolic event after cardioversion and most often occurs when cardioverting atrial flutter or atrial fibrillation. A preelective cardioversion echocardiogram to evaluate for atrial clots could aid in determining whether the patient is at risk for an embolic event.
D. Cardiac arrhythmias. Dysrhythmias due to enhanced automaticity such as digitalis toxicity or catecholamine-induced arrhythmias have increased risk of VT/VFib with shock. Premature beats can also occur. Vfib can also occur with poor synchronization of the shock administration.
E. Myocardial necrosis. When excessive energy is delivered, heart tissue can be damaged. This can cause necrosis with elevated ST segments seen on electrocardiogram. If myocardial damage is severe enough, this can cause shock.
F. Cardiogenic shock. Patients can develop transient decreased cardiac output with left ventricular diastolic dysfunction and damage of the myocardium after cardioversion or defibrillation.
G. Fire (rare). Fire has resulted from sparks in the presence of oxygen and cotton. The infant's stocking cap and part of the sheet caught on fire. Use of oxygen can increase the risk of fire. To avoid this, place the oxygen at least 1 meter away from the patient before defibrillation.

H. **Electrical shock to health care providers.** This can result in tingling, minor burns, or transient lethargy.

Selected References

Minczak BB. Cardioversion and defibrillation. In: Roberts JR, ed. *Roberts: Clinical Procedures in Emergency Medicine.* 5th ed. Philadelphia, PA: Saunders; 2009.

Sutton RM, Berg RA, Nadkarni V. Performance of cardiopulmonary resuscitation in infants and children. In: Fuhrman BP, ed. *Fuhrman: Pediatric Critical Care.* 4th ed. Philadelphia, PA: Saunders; 2011.

29 Endotracheal Intubation and Extubation

I. **Indications**
   A. Provide mechanical respiratory support.
   B. Obtain aspirates for culture.
   C. Assist in bronchopulmonary hygiene ("pulmonary toilet").
   D. Alleviate upper airway obstruction (subglottic stenosis).
   E. Clear the trachea of meconium.
   F. Perform selective bronchial ventilation.
   G. Assist in the management of congenital diaphragmatic hernia (to avoid bowel distention).
   H. Administer medications ("NEAL" or "LANE" see Section III.O) in the emergency setting while intravenous access is established.
   I. Administration of surfactant.
   J. Management of apnea.

II. **Equipment.** Correct endotracheal tube (ETT) and suction catheter (Table 29–1), a pediatric laryngoscope handle with a Miller blade ("00" blade for extremely preterm infants, "0" blade for preterm infants, "1" blade for full-term infants; straight blades [Miller blades] are preferred over curved blades [Macintosh blade] because of better visualization), an ETT adapter, a suction apparatus, suction catheters, tape, scissors, tincture of benzoin, a malleable stylet (*optional*), personal protection equipment,

Table 29–1. **GUIDELINES FOR ENDOTRACHEAL TUBE SIZE, DEPTH OF INSERTION, AND SUCTION CATHETER SIZE BASED ON WEIGHT AND GESTATIONAL AGE**

Weight (g)	Gestational Age (wk)	Endotracheal Tube Size, Inside Diameter (mm)	Depth of Insertion (tip of tube to upper lip[a] in cm)
<1000	<28	2.5	6 (if <750 g)–7
1000–2000	28–34	3.0	7–8
2000–3000	34–38	3.5	8–9
>3000	>38	3.5–4.0	9 (3000 g) –10 (4000 g)

[a]"Tip to lip."
Data from guidelines from Kattwinkel J. *Textbook of Neonatal Resuscitation.* 6th ed. Elk Grove, IL: American Heart Association/American Academy of Pediatrics; 2011.

bag-and-mask apparatus with 100% oxygen, and pressure manometer should be available at the bedside. The mechanical ventilator should be checked and ready. Monitoring with electrocardiogram and pulse oximetry is essential if time permits. A colorimetric device or capnograph to confirm the position of the tube. Suctioning equipment and catheters.

III. Procedure

    A. Orotracheal versus nasotracheal intubation

        1. **Orotracheal intubation.** More commonly performed emergently and is described here. It is easier and quicker than nasotracheal intubation. The orotracheal tube should be precut to eliminate dead space (cut to 15 cm).

        2. **Nasotracheal intubation.** More commonly performed in the elective setting or if anatomy precludes the oral route. Nasotracheal intubation can be used in overly active infants or in those infants who have copious secretions. It offers tube stability but can be associated with an increase in postextubation atelectasis and a risk of nasal damage. In nasotracheal intubation the procedure is the same except the lubricated nasotracheal tube is passed into the nostril, then pharynx and into cords following to the back of the throat. Small doses of 2% lidocaine gel can be used.

        3. **Cochrane review.** Did not find any differences in the effect of nasal versus oral intubation.

    B. Pain/premedication

        1. Premedication is not necessary in the case of an emergency intubation in the delivery room or after an acute deterioration in a neonatal intensive care unit (NICU). It is also not necessary in some cases of infants with upper airway anomalies (such as Pierre Robin sequence).

        2. If IV access is not available, the IM route should be considered.

        3. **Premedication.** Many intubations require more than one attempt and take longer than the recommended time frame; therefore, premedication can improve intubation and also alleviate the pain associated with it. **Premedication for nonemergency intubation in the neonate is safer and more effective** than when awake, but the ideal combination of premedication has not been established. Preferred medications are with a rapid onset and short duration of action. One preferred sequence is as follows:

           a. Administer oxygen.

           b. Vagolytic agent to prevent bradycardia. Atropine preferred.

           c. Analgesic (fentanyl preferred) and/or sedative/hypnotic. None preferred.

           d. Muscle relaxant. Vecuronium or rocuronium preferred.

        4. Because optimal protocols and medications have not been established, each unit should adopt its own pain and premedication protocols. See Table 29–2 for a listing of elective intubation medications reviewed by the American Academy of Pediatrics (AAP). Key premedication points:

           a. Do not use a sedative without an analgesic agent.

           b. Do not use a muscle relaxant without an analgesic agent.

           c. Analgesic or anesthetic dose of a hypnotic drug should be given.

           d. Vagolytic and muscle relaxants (rapid onset) should also be considered.

        5. **Rapid sequence intubation (RSI).** Involves premedication prior to intubation with atropine, a sedative, and a neuromuscular blocker. It is commonly used in the emergency department for rapid intubation. When RSI is used in neonates, there is better visualization of the airway, no movement from the infant, and intubation is quicker with lesser attempts. One recommendation: atropine IV push (0.01–0.03 mg/kg, minimum dose 0.1 mg), fentanyl (2–3 mcg/kg per dose), and lastly vercuronium (0.1 mg/kg per dose). Further research is needed before definite recommendations can be made on using RSI in the neonate.

    C. **Confirm that the laryngoscope light source is working** before beginning the procedure. Place the stylet (if used) in the endotracheal tube (ETT). Malleable stylets

Table 29–2. **MEDICATIONS FOR PREMEDICATION FOR NONEMERGENCY INTUBATION**

Drug	Route/ Dose	Onset of Action	Duration of Action	Common Adverse Effects	Comments[a]
Analgesic					
Fentanyl	IV or IM:[b] 1–4 mcg/kg	IV, almost immediate; IM, 7–15 minutes	IV, 30–60 minutes; IM,1–2 hours	Apnea, hypotension, CNS depression, chest wall rigidity	Preferred analgesic Effects reversible with naloxone Give slowly (preferably over 3–5 minutes, at least over 1–2 minutes) to avoid chest wall rigidity Chest wall rigidity can be treated with naloxone and muscle relaxants
Remifentanil	IV:1–3 mcg/kg; may repeat in 2–3 minutes if needed	IV, almost immediate	IV, 3–10 minutes	Apnea, hypotension, CNS depression, chest wall rigidity	Acceptable analgesic Short duration of action and limited experience in neonates Effects reversible with naloxone Give slowly over 1–2 minutes to avoid chest wall rigidity Chest wall rigidity can be treated with naloxone and muscle relaxants
Morphine	IV or IM: 0.05–0.1 mg/kg	IV, 5–15 minutes; IM, 10–30 minutes	IV, 3–5 hours; IM, 3–5 hours	Apnea, hypotension, CNS depression	Acceptable analgesic agent Use only if other opioids are not available; if selected, must wait at least 5 minutes for onset of action Effects reversible with naloxone

Hypnotic/sedative

Midazolam	IV or IM: 0.05–0.1 mg/kg	IV, 1–5 minutes; IM, within 5–15 minutes	IV, 20–30 minutes; IM, 1–6 hours	Apnea, hypotension, CNS depression	Acceptable sedative for use in term infants in combination with analgesic agents Hypotension more likely when used in combination with fentanyl Not recommended in premature infants Effects reversible with flumazenil
Thiopental	IV: 3–4 mg/kg	IV, 30–60 seconds	IV, 5–30 minutes	Histamine release, apnea, hypotension, bronchospasm	Acceptable hypnotic agent Hypotension more likely when used in combination with fentanyl and/or midazolam
Propofol	IV: 2.5 mg/kg	Within 30 seconds	3–10 minutes	Histamine release, apnea, hypotension, bronchospasm, bradycardia; often causes pain at injection site	Acceptable hypnotic agent Limited experience in newborns Neonatal dosing has not been well established
Muscle relaxant					
Pancuronium	IV: 0.05–0.10 mg/kg	1–3 minutes	40–60 minutes	Mild histamine release, hypotension, tachycardia, bronchospasm, excessive salivation	Acceptable muscle relaxant Relatively longer duration of action Effects reversible with atropine and neostigmine
Vecuronium	IV: 0.1 mg/kg	2–3 minutes	30–40 minutes	Mild histamine release, hypertension/ hypotension, tachycardia, arrhythmias, bronchospasm	Preferred muscle relaxant Effects reversible with atropine and neostigmine

(*Continued*)

Table 29-2. **MEDICATIONS FOR PREMEDICATION FOR NONEMERGENCY INTUBATION** (*CONTINUED*)

Drug	Route/ Dose	Onset of Action	Duration of Action	Common Adverse Effects	Comments[a]
Rocuronium	IV: 0.6–1.2 mg/kg	1–2 minutes	20–30 minutes	Mild histamine release, hypertension/ hypotension, tachycardia, arrhythmias, bronchospasm	Preferred muscle relaxant Effects reversible with atropine and neostigmine
Succinylcholine	IV: 1–2 mg/kg; IM:[b] 2 mg/ kg	IV, 30–60 seconds; IM, 2–3 minutes	IV, 4–6 minutes; IM, 10–30 minutes	Hypertension/ hypotension, tachycardia, arrhythmias, bronchospasm, hyperkalemia, myoglobinemia, malignant hyperthermia	Acceptable muscle relaxant Contraindicated in presence of hyperkalemia and family history of malignant hyperthermia
Vagolytic					
Atropine	IV or IM: 0.02 mg/kg	1–2 minutes	0.5–2 hours	Tachycardia, dry hot skin	Preferred vagolytic agent
Glycopyrrolate	IV: 4–10 mcg/kg	1–10 minutes	~6 hours	Tachycardia, arrhythmias, bronchospasm	Acceptable vagolytic agent Limited experience in newborns Contains benzyl alcohol as preservative

Note: Most of these drugs have limited pharmacokinetics data from newborns and are not approved for use in the newborn, but they have been used in newborns.

CNS, central nervous system; IM, intramuscularly; IV, intravenously.

[a]Preferred and acceptable designation of medications is based on consensus opinion after review of available evidence.

[b]Consider only if no intravenous access.

Reproduced, with permission, from Kumar P, Denson SE, Mancuso TJ; Committee on Fetus and Newborn, Section on Anesthesiology and Pain Medicine. Clinical report—premedication for nonemergency endotracheal intubation in the neonate. *Pediatrics.* 2010;125:608–615.

are optional but may help guide the tube into position more efficiently. Be sure the tip of the stylet does not protrude out of the end of the ETT. The stylet should be 1–2 cm proximal to the distal end of the ETT.

D. Place the infant in the "sniffing position" (with the neck slightly extended); a small roll behind the neck may help with positioning. Hyperextension of the neck in infants may cause the trachea to collapse. It displaces the cords anteriorly and makes it difficult to pass the ETT. The infant's head should be at the same level as the operator.

E. Cautiously suction the oropharynx as needed to make the landmarks clearly visible.

F. Preoxygenate the infant with a bag-and-mask device, and monitor the heart rate, color, and pulse oximeter. **To limit hypoxia, limit each intubation attempt to**

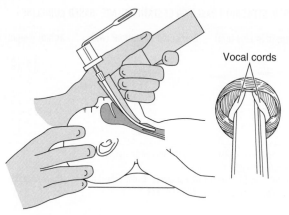

Vocal cords

FIGURE 29–1. Endotracheal intubation in the neonate.

<20 seconds before reoxygenation. Infants frequently deteriorate during an intubation attempt.

G. **Hold the laryngoscope with your left hand.** Insert the scope into the right side of the mouth, and sweep the tongue to the left side. Some practitioners move the tongue to the left by using the index finger of the right hand placed alongside the head. To perform this maneuver, stabilize the head and hold the mouth open.

H. **Advance the blade a few millimetres**, passing it beneath the epiglottis.

I. **Lift the blade vertically to elevate the epiglottis** and visualize the glottis (Figure 29–1). *Note:* The purpose of the laryngoscope is to lift the epiglottis vertically, not to pry it open. To better visualize the vocal cords, an assistant may place gentle external pressure on the thyroid cartilage. If the cords are together, wait for them to open (never force a tube between closed cords). Do not touch the closed cords as this may cause spasm.

J. **Pass the ETT along the right side of the mouth** and down past the vocal cords during inspiration. Advance the tube *only* 2–2.5 cm into the trachea to avoid placement in the right main stem bronchus (no more than 1–2 cm below the vocal cords). If a stylet was used it should be removed gently while the tube is held in position. **If the tube is needed for suction (as in meconium aspiration), connect to a meconium aspirator.**

K. **Multiple ETT depths of insertion methods are described:**

1. **7-8-9 rule (Tochen rule).** The depth of ETT insertion in centimeters ("tip to lip") is estimated as 6 plus the weight in kilograms. Tape the ETT at the lip when the tube has been advanced 7 cm in a 1-kg infant, 8 cm in a 2-kg infant, 9 cm in a 3-kg infant, or 10 cm in a 4-kg infant ("**1, 2, 3, 4, 7, 8, 9, 10**"). Do not use this in infants <750 g (overestimates the depth of insertion) or in infants with severe neck or orofacial deformities. Infants weighing <750 g may only require a 6-cm insertion (see Table 29–1).

2. **ETT length based on gestation-based guidelines.** ETT length is more related to gestation in a linear manner than to birthweight. Using gestation-based guidelines are associated with a decrease in uneven lung expansion and a decrease in the number of tubes that need to be repositioned. See Table 29–3.

3. **Nasal tragus length (NTL) and sternal length (STL).** One method that allows length assessment in ~10 seconds and does not require weight is the NTL (base of the nasal septum to the tragus of the ear); the other method is the STL (suprasternal notch to the tip of the xiphoid process).
   a. **Orotracheal route.** NTL or STL plus 1.
   b. **Nasotracheal route.** NTL or STL plus 2.

Table 29–3. ETT LENGTH BASED ON GESTATIONAL AGE–BASED GUIDELINES

ETT Length at Lips (cm)	Corrected Gestation[a] (wk)	Actual Weight[b] (kg)
5.5	23–24	0.5–0.6
6.0	25–26	0.7–0.8
6.5	27–29	0.9–1.0
7.0	30–32	1.1–1.4
7.5	33–34	1.5–1.8
8.0	35–37	1.9–2.4
8.5	38–40	2.5–3.1
9.0	41–43	3.2–4.2

[a]Corrected gestation is gestation at birth plus postnatal age.
[b]Actual weight is weight at intubation.
Data from Kempley ST, Moreiras JW, Petrone FL. Endotracheal tube length for neonatal intubation. *Resuscitation.* 2008;77(3):369–373.

L. **Confirm the position of the tube immediately after insertion.** Detection of exhaled carbon dioxide plus clinical assessment are the most reliable initial methods to confirm placement of a tracheal tube in a neonate.
   1. **Auscultation.** The resuscitation bag is attached to the tube using the adapter, and an assistant provides mechanical breaths while the operator listens for equal breath sounds on both sides of the chest. Some recommend the stethoscope laterally and high on the axilla of the chest. Auscultate the stomach to be certain that the esophagus was not intubated. **Caution is necessary** as breath sounds heard over the anterior part of the chest can come from the stomach or esophagus. If correctly intubated there should be an increase in heart rate and color. Breath sounds are audible over lung fields and are absent in the stomach. There should be no gastric distension and vapor condensing on the inside of the tube during exhalation.
   2. **CO_2 detectors.** To confirm ETT position.
      a. **Colorimetric device.** Changes color in the presence of CO_2 and is the most commonly used device. End tidal carbon dioxide detectors connected to the ETT are commercially available that rapidly confirm proper endotracheal placement. One such device (Pedi-Cap CO_2 detector, Nellcor) displays violet in the absence of CO_2 and yellow means presence of CO_2 (tube in trachea).
      b. **Capnographs.** These have a special electrode at the ETT connector, and a waveform shows oscillation with each breath if the tube is in the correct place.
      c. **Limitations of ETT CO_2 detectors.** With some cyanotic congenital heart disease, they may underestimate the true arterial CO_2 level. If the cardiac output is low or absent and there is no heartbeat, the CO_2 monitor may not change color because not enough CO_2 is exhaled to detect. Any acidic substance (gastric acid, endotracheal epinephrine) can contaminate the colorimetric device and cause a false-positive result.
M. **Paint the skin with tincture of benzoin and tape the tube securely in place.** A Neofit tube grip (Ackrad Laboratories, Cranford, NJ) eliminates the need for tape use and provides stabilization. It fits tube sizes 2.5–4.0 mm. A Neobar (Valencia, CA) can also be used.
N. **After the ETT is secured, obtain a chest radiograph to confirm proper placement** of the tube. Figure 11–7 shows proper placement of a neonatal ETT. Some sources indicate that the ETT tip should be placed at the level of the body of the first thoracic vertebra, and to not use the medial end of the clavicles (most common reference point) as their position may be variable. Others state that the ETT tip should be placed 2 cm above carina.
O. **Certain emergency medications can be given through the ETT.** These medications are *l*idocaine, *a*tropine, *n*aloxone, and *e*pinephrine. These can be remembered by

the mnemonic **"LANE" or "NEAL." Epinephrine given by intravascular route is recommended as the most effective route, since absorption by the lungs is slow and unpredictable**; however, it can be given by the ETT route while the IV is being started. A higher dose of epinephrine (0.5–1 mL/kg of 1:10,000) is necessary even though studies do not validate the safety of this. There are no studies confirming that endotracheal naloxone is effective.

IV. Endotracheal extubation

A. The decision to remove an endotracheal tube is a complex clinical decision. Issues surrounding ventilatory support are discussed in Chapter 8. When adequate ventilation is maintained with minimal settings, extubation is attempted. Manage postextubation atelectasis intensively with chest physiotherapy.

B. Use of medications prior to extubation

1. Dexamethasone use is *controversial*

a. Stridor. Some advocate systemic dexamethasone given before and after extubation to reduce the incidence of stridor. A Cochrane review states that using corticosteroids in neonates to prevent or treat stridor after extubation is not effective.

b. Reintubation risk. Dexamethasone IV given prior to extubation reduces the need for reintubation in high-risk neonates. A Cochrane review states that it is best to use in infants at risk (repeated and prolonged intubations) for airway edema and obstruction.

c. Systemic corticosteroids. Early corticosteroid therapy (first 2 weeks after birth) reduced the risk of BPD/CLD and shortened the time to extubation. Steroid therapy after 3 weeks promoted earlier extubation. Because of long-term studies showing poor neurodevelopment, use is not recommended routinely. Cochrane review states steroid therapy should be limited until further studies are done.

2. Methylxanthines used prophylactically (eg, caffeine) increases the chance of successful extubation of preterm infants within 1 week of life. The caffeine group had lower rates of patent ductus arteriosus ligation, cerebral palsy, death, bronchopulmonary dysplasia/chronic lung disease (BPD/CLD), or major disability at 18–21 months. The majority of preterm infants are given caffeine before extubation and are maintained on this medication while on nasal continuous positive airway pressure (NCPAP) or nasal ventilation.

3. Other medications. Cochrane review states there is not enough evidence to support the routine use of prophylactic **doxapram** and there is no evidence for or against the use of nebulized **racemic epinephrine**.

C. Extubation procedure

1. Perform chest physiotherapy and suction.

2. Remove tape and any devices that are holding the ETT in place.

3. Remove the tube. Best to use your own unit's recommendation on how and when to remove the tube. **Recommendations vary**:

a. Give positive pressure inspiration while slowly removing the tube.

b. Suction, give positive pressure breaths, remove the ETT.

c. Using manual ventilation, give the infant a sigh breath, and withdraw the tube during exhalation.

4. Chest physiotherapy. Cochrane review found that fewer babies had to go back on ventilator support when chest physiotherapy postextubation was used.

D. Other postextubation procedures. Level of respiratory support varies and depends on the clinical status of the patient. (See also Chapter 8.) Possibilities include:

1. Supplemental oxygen by hood or high-flow nasal cannula (HFNC) >3–6 L/min. Limit flows in extremely low birthweight (ELBW) infants to less than 6 L/min (*controversial*). High-flow nasal cannula may be associated with a higher rate of reintubation than NCPAP in preterm infants. Cochrane review states that there is not enough evidence to use HFNC as a form of respiratory support in preterm infants.

2. **Nasal continuous positive airway pressure (NCPAP).** Cochrane review found that NCPAP reduced the incidence of apnea, respiratory acidosis, and increased oxygen requirements after extubation in preterm infants. Cochrane review states that binasal prongs are more effective than single prongs after weaning in reducing reintubation. NCPAP is used with a nasal interface such as nasal prongs (eg, Hudson type). Other forms of postextubation support are **bubble CPAP**, and **N-BiPAP (nasal biphasic positive airway pressure).**

3. **Nasal ventilation. Nasal intermittent positive pressure (NIPPV) is better than NCPAP** in preventing reintubation on extubated infants. Both NIPPV and synchronized nasal intermittent positive pressure ventilation (SNIPPV) seem to be equally effective.

E. **Observe for atelectasis.** If the infant has an increasing oxygen requirement and signs of respiratory distress a chest radiograph should be obtained.

V. **Complications**

A. **Hypoxia, apnea, hypoventilation, and bradycardia can all occur during the intubation process.** This can be secondary to a prolonged attempt or vagal reflex.

B. **Hypopharyngeal or tracheal perforation/rupture and trauma.** Tracheal perforation is a rare complication requiring surgical intervention and is prevented by careful use of the laryngoscope and the ETT. Hemorrhage, edema of the larynx, and injury to the vocal cord can all occur. Tracheal injury usually presents with rapid occurrence of subcutaneous emphysema, pneumomediastinum, and respiratory failure. Contusions of the gums, tongue, and airway can occur.

C. **Esophageal perforation.** Usually caused by traumatic intubation, and treatment depends on the degree of perforation. Most injuries can be managed conservatively by use of parenteral nutrition until the leak seals, use of broad-spectrum antibiotics, and observation for signs of infection. A barium swallow contrast study may be necessary after several weeks to evaluate healing or rule out stricture formation.

D. **Laryngeal edema.** Usually seen after extubation and may cause respiratory distress. A short course of steroids (eg, dexamethasone) can be given intravenously before and just after extubation. However, systemic dexamethasone has no effect in reducing acute postextubation stridor in neonates.

E. **Improper tube positioning (esophageal intubation, right main stem bronchus).** Signs of esophageal intubation include poor chest movement, no breath sounds heard, zero mist in the tube, continued cyanosis, gastric distension, and air heard over the stomach. Signs of right main stem bronchus intubation include breath sounds heard over the right chest and none heard over the left, and no improvement in color. ETT in right main stem bronchus causes overventilation of the right lung and hypoventilation or atelectasis of the left lung. If the tube is in the right main stem bronchus, it needs to be pulled back to the position where the breath sounds on both sides of the chest become equal.

F. **Tube obstruction or kinking.** Try suctioning or possibly reintubation.

G. **Infection.** Pneumonia and trachea-bronchitis can occur.

H. **Palatal/alveolar grooves.** Palatal and alveolar grooves are usually seen in cases of long-term intubation and typically resolve with time.

I. **Subglottic stenosis.** Subglottic stenosis is most often associated with long-term (>3–4 weeks') endotracheal intubation. It is the most serious long-term complication and is secondary to posttraumatic fibrosis of the infant larynx. Surgical correction is usually necessary. With prolonged intubation, consideration may be given to surgical tracheostomy to help prevent stenosis.

J. **Other complications.** Aspiration, atelectasis, pneumothorax, increased intracranial pressure, and hypertension can all occur.

Selected References

Davis PG, Henderson-Smart DJ. Intravenous dexamethasone for extubation of newborn infants. *Cochrane Database Syst Rev.* 2001;(4). DOI:10.1002/14651858.CD000308.

Davis PG, Henderson-Smart DJ. Prophylactic doxapram for the prevention of morbidity and mortality in preterm infants undergoing endotracheal extubation. *Cochrane Database Syst Rev.* 2000;(3). DOI:10.1002/14651858.CD001966.

Davies MW, Davis PG. Nebulized racemic epinephrine for extubation of newborn infants. *Cochrane Database Syst Rev.* 2010. DOI:10.1002/14651858.CD000506.

Kaye S, Peter B. Nasal versus oral intubation for mechanical ventilation of newborn infants. *Cochrane Database Syst Rev.* 1999;(2). DOI:10.1002/14651858.CD000948.

Kempley ST, Moreiras JW, Petrone FL. Endotracheal tube length for neonatal intubation. *Resuscitation.* 2008;77(3):369–373.

Peterson J, Johnson N, Deakins K, Wilson-Costello D, Jelovsek JE, Chatburn R. Accuracy of the 7-8-9 rule for endotracheal tube placement in the neonate. *J Perinatol.* 2006;26:333–336.

Whyte KL, Levin R, Powls A. Optimal positioning of endotracheal tubes in neonates. *Scott Med J.* 2007;52(2):25–27.

Wilkinson D, Andersen C, O'Donnell CP, De Paoli AG. High flow nasal cannula for respiratory support in preterm infants. *Cochrane Database Syst Rev.* 2011;11(5). DOI:10.1002/14651858.CD006405.

30 Exchange Transfusion

I. **Indications**
   A. **Hyperbilirubinemia. Exchange transfusion (ET)** is most commonly done for infants with hyperbilirubinemia of any origin when the serum bilirubin level reaches or exceeds a level that puts the infant at risk for central nervous system toxicity (see Chapters 58 and 100). Serum levels of bilirubin for which to begin an ET are under considerable debate. **Double-volume ETs** taking 50–70 minutes are used for removal and reduction of serum bilirubin. Efficiency of bilirubin removal is increased in slower paced exchanges to allow for time of extravascular and intravascular bilirubin equilibration.
   B. **Hemolytic disease of the newborn.** Results from destruction of fetal red blood cells (RBCs) by passively acquired maternal antibodies. ET aids in removing antibody-coated RBCs and replaces them with uncoated donor RBCs that lack sensitizing antigen, thereby prolonging intravascular RBC survival. It also reduces a potentially toxic bilirubin concentration, the result of the antibody destruction of RBCs. Intravenous immunoglobulin (IVIG) is now used to reduce the need for ET in hemolytic disease of the newborn. American Academy of Pediatrics guidelines recommend IVIG if the total serum bilirubin (TSB) is rising despite intensive phototherapy or the TSB level is within 2–3 mg/dL of the exchange level.
   C. **Sepsis.** May be associated with shock caused by bacterial endotoxins. ET may help remove bacteria, toxins, fibrin split products, and accumulated lactic acid. It may also provide immunoglobulins, complement, and coagulating factors.
   D. **Disseminated intravascular coagulation (DIC).** ET may provide necessary coagulation factors and help reduce the underlying cause of the abnormal coagulation. Repletion of clotting factors by transfusion of fresh-frozen plasma (10–15 mL/kg) may be all that is necessary in less severe cases of DIC.

E. **Metabolic disorders causing severe acidosis.** Partial exchanges are usually acceptable and beneficial; however, peritoneal dialysis may also be needed to treat severely acidotic disorders of metabolism.

F. **Severe fluid or electrolyte imbalance.** Isovolumetric partial exchanges can be used to modulate electrolyte fluctuations with each aliquot of blood exchanged. The process allows for a gradual correction of electrolyte imbalances.

G. **Polycythemia.** This can be managed by partial ET using normal saline. Normal saline is preferred because it reduces both the polycythemia and the hyperviscosity of the infant's circulating blood volume. (See also Chapter 71 and 122.)

H. **Severe anemia.** Normovolemic or hypervolemic anemia causing cardiac failure, as in hydrops fetalis, is best treated with a partial ET using packed RBCs.

I. **Any disorder requiring complement, opsonins, or gamma globulin.** Infants with these conditions may require frequent exchanges, and their fluid status must be carefully managed. Partial exchanges are recommended.

II. **Types of exchange transfusions**

A. **Single-volume exchange blood transfusion.** Refers to 1 times the estimated blood volume at ~60% of infant's blood volume.

B. **Double-volume exchange blood transfusion.** Refers to 2 times the estimated blood volume at ~85% of infant's blood volume. This is indicated for severe hyperbilirubinemia (to remove bilirubin), for alloimmune hemolytic disease of newborns, to remove antibodies and abnormal proteins, and for idiopathic severe hypermagnesemia, DIC, congenital leukemia, neonatal sepsis, malaria, malignant pertussis, drug overdose, and metabolic toxin removal (hyperammonemia, organic academia, lead poisoning). **Cochrane review** states that there are insufficient data to support or refute the use of single-volume ET as opposed to double-volume ET in newborns with jaundice. Double-volume ET is still recommended for infants with severe jaundice and Rh hemolytic disease.

C. **Isovolumetric double-volume exchange blood transfusion.** Exchange is done simultaneously pulling blood out of the umbilical artery and pushing blood into the umbilical vein. Indicated in sick and unstable neonates because of less fluctuation of blood pressure and cerebral hemodynamics (eg, hydrops fetalis).

D. **Partial-volume exchange (<2 volumes) transfusion.** This type of exchange is indicated in neonates with polycythemia (to decrease the hematocrit and whole blood viscosity) or to correct severe anemia (usually associated with congestive cardiac failure or hypervolemia).

III. **Equipment.** An assistant needed to help maintain a sterile field, monitor and assess the infant, and record the procedure and exchanged volumes. Also needed are radiant warming bed or hybrid incubator, equipment for cardiorespiratory monitoring, support and resuscitation, immediate access to blood gas determinations, equipment for umbilical artery and umbilical vein catheterization (see Chapters 24 and 44), disposable ET tray, and nasogastric tube for evacuating the stomach before beginning the transfusion. Temperature-controlled device must be used for warming of the blood before and during the transfusion (should have an internal disposable coil and connectors to the donor blood bag and the ET circuit. The blood should be warmed to 37°C. Use of makeshift water baths or heaters is not advised because blood that is too warm may hemolyze).

IV. **Choice of blood**

A. **Blood collection**

1. **Homologous blood.** Blood donated by an anonymous donor with a compatible blood type is most commonly used. Donor-directed blood (blood donated by a selected blood type–compatible person) is another option.

2. **Cytomegalovirus (CMV).** Seronegative donor blood is preferred. White blood cells harboring CMV can be removed using leukodepletion filters during blood preparation. The use of frozen deglycerolized RBCs, reconstituted with fresh-frozen plasma, is another means of using seropositive blood free of viable CMV.

3. Hemoglobin S (sickle cell trait). Precautions should be taken to avoid ET with donor blood from a carrier. If the donor blood with sickle trait becomes acidic, sickling can occur, with expected complications to the patient.

4. Graft-versus-host disease. Consideration should be given for using irradiated donor blood to avoid graft-versus-host disease in known immune-compromised infants and low birthweight infants. Preterm infants who have been transfused in utero or who have received >50 mL of transfused blood are candidates for irradiated blood.

B. Blood typing and cross-matching

1. Infants with Rh incompatibility. The blood must be type O, Rh-negative, low titer anti-A, anti-B blood. It must be cross-matched with the mother's plasma and RBCs.

2. Infants with ABO incompatibility. The blood must be type O, Rh-compatible (with the mother and the infant) or Rh-negative, low-titer anti-A, anti-B blood. It must be cross-matched with both the infant's and mother's blood.

3. Other blood group incompatibilities. For other hemolytic diseases (eg, anti-Rhc, anti-Kell, anti-Duffy), blood must be cross-matched to the mother's blood to avoid offending antigens.

4. Hyperbilirubinemia, metabolic imbalance, or hemolysis not caused by isoimmune disorders. The blood must be cross-matched against the infant's plasma and RBCs.

C. Freshness and preservation of blood. In newborn infants, it is preferable to use blood or plasma that has been collected in citrate phosphate dextrose (CPD). The blood should be <72 hours old. These 2 factors ensure that the blood pH is >7.0. For disorders associated with hydrops fetalis or fetal asphyxia, it is best to use blood that is <24 hours old. **Use of irradiated blood** less than 24 hours before the ET is recommended for all ETs to decrease the potassium in the blood and to decrease graft-versus-host disease.

D. Hematocrit (Hct). Most blood banks can reconstitute a unit of blood to a desired Hct of 50–70%. The blood should be agitated periodically during the transfusion to maintain a constant Hct.

E. Potassium levels in donor blood. Should be determined if the infant is asphyxiated or in shock, and renal impairment is suspected. If potassium levels are >7 mEq/L, consider using a unit of blood that has been collected more recently or a unit of washed RBCs.

F. Temperature of the blood. Warming of blood is especially important in low birthweight and sick newborn infants.

V. Procedure

A. Simple 2-volume exchange transfusion is used for uncomplicated hyperbilirubinemia

1. The normal blood volume in a full-term newborn infant is 80 mL/kg. In an infant weighing 2 kg, the volume would be 160 mL, and twice the volume of blood is exchanged in a 2-volume transfusion. Therefore, the amount of blood needed for a 2-kg infant would be 320 mL. Blood volume of low birthweight and extremely low birthweight newborns, which may be up to 95 mL/kg, should be taken into account when calculating exchange volumes.

2. Allow adequate time for blood typing and cross-matching at the blood bank. The infant's bilirubin level increases during this time, and this increase must be taken into account when ordering the blood.

3. Perform the transfusion in an intensive care setting. Place the infant in the supine position. Restraints must be snug but not tight. A nasogastric tube should be passed to evacuate the stomach and should be left in place to maintain gastric decompression and prevent regurgitation and aspiration of gastric juices.

4. Scrub and put on a sterile gown and gloves.

5. Perform umbilical vein catheterization and confirm the position by radiograph. (See Figure 11–10.) If an isovolumetric exchange is to be performed, then an umbilical artery catheter (high position preferred) must also be placed and

Table 30–1. ALIQUOTS USUALLY USED IN NEONATAL EXCHANGE TRANSFUSION

Infant Weight	Aliquot (mL)
3 kg	20
2–3 kg	15
1–2 kg	10
850 g–1 kg	5
<850 g	1–3

confirmed by radiograph (see Figure 11–11 for correct positioning of a high umbilical artery catheter and Figure 11–12 for correct positioning of a low umbilical artery catheter).
6. Have the unit of blood prepared
   a. Check the blood types of the donor and the infant.
   b. Check the temperature of the blood and warming procedures.
   c. Check the Hct. The blood should be agitated regularly to maintain a constant Hct.
7. Attach the bag of blood to the tubing and stopcocks according to the directions on the transfusion tray. The orientation of the stopcocks for infusion and withdrawal must also be checked by the assistant (ie, a procedure "time out").
8. Establish the volume of each aliquot. (Table 30–1)
B. Isovolumetric double-volume exchange transfusion. Performed using a double setup, with infusion via the umbilical vein and withdrawal via the umbilical artery. This method is preferred when volume shifts during simple exchange might cause or aggravate myocardial insufficiency (eg, hydrops fetalis). Two operators are needed; one to perform the infusion and the other to handle the withdrawal.
   1. Perform steps 1–6 as in double-volume ET. In addition, perform umbilical artery catheterization.
   2. Attach the unit of blood to the tubing and stopcocks attached to the umbilical vein catheter. The catheter may be left in place after the ET to monitor central venous pressure. It should be placed above the diaphragm with placement confirmed by chest radiograph.
   3. The tubing and the stopcocks of the second setup are attached to the umbilical artery catheter and to a sterile plastic bag for discarding the exchanged blood.
   4. If isovolumetric exchange is being performed because of cardiac failure, the central venous pressure can be determined via the umbilical vein catheter. It should be placed above the diaphragm in the inferior vena cava.
C. Partial exchange transfusion (PET). Performed in the same manner as double-volume ET. If a partial exchange is for polycythemia (using normal saline) or for anemia (using packed RBCs), the following formula can be used to determine the volume of the transfusion.
   1. To calculate volume to exchange for polycythemia:

$$\text{Volume of exchange (mL)} = \frac{\text{Estimated blood volume (mL)} \times \text{Weight (kg)} \times (\text{Observed Hct} - \text{Desired Hct})}{\text{Observed Hct}}$$

   2. To calculate volume to exchange for anemia:

$$\text{Volume of exchange (mL)} = \frac{\text{Estimated blood volume (mL)} \times \text{Weight (kg)} \times (\text{Desired Hct} - \text{Observed Hct})}{\text{PRBC Hct} - \text{Observed Hct}}$$

D. **Isovolumetric partial exchange transfusion with packed RBCs.** Best procedure if the diagnosis is severe hydrops fetalis.

E. **Ancillary procedures**

1. **Laboratory studies.** Blood should be obtained for laboratory studies before and after ET.

   a. **Blood chemistry.** Total calcium, sodium, potassium, chloride, pH, $Paco_2$, acid-base status, bicarbonate, and serum glucose.

   b. **Hematologic studies.** Hemoglobin Hct, platelet count, white blood cell count, and differential count. Blood for retyping and cross-matching after exchange is often requested by the blood bank to verify typing and re–cross-matching and for study of transfusion reaction, if needed.

   c. **Blood culture.** Recommended after ET (*controversial*).

2. **Administration of calcium gluconate.** The CPD buffer in stored blood binds calcium and transiently lowers ionized calcium levels. Treatment of suspected hypocalcemia in patients receiving transfusions is *controversial*. Some physicians routinely administer 1–2 mL of 10% calcium gluconate by slow infusion after 100–200 mL of exchange donor blood. Others maintain that this treatment has no therapeutic effect unless hypocalcemia is documented by electrocardiogram showing a change in the QT interval.

3. **Phototherapy.** Begin or resume phototherapy after ET for disorders involving a high bilirubin level (for phototherapy guidance, see Chapters 58 and 100).

4. **Monitor serum bilirubin levels after transfusion at 2, 4, and 6 hours and then at 6-hour intervals.** A rebound of bilirubin levels is to be expected 2–4 hours after the transfusion.

5. **Remediation.** Patients receiving antibiotics or anticonvulsants need to be remedicated. Patients receiving digoxin should not be remedicated, unless the cardiac status is deteriorating or serum digoxin levels are known to be low. The percentage of lost medications is extremely variable. As little as 2.4% of digoxin is lost, but up to 32.4% of theophylline may be lost during a 2-volume ET. Determination of drug levels after ET is advisable

6. **Antibiotic prophylaxis after the transfusion should be considered on an individual basis.** Infection is uncommon but is the most frequent complication.

VI. **Complications.** See also complications related to umbilical vein catheterization, Chapter 44.

A. **Infection.** Bacteremia (usually a *Staphylococcus* organism), hepatitis, CMV, malaria, and HIV have been reported.

B. **Vascular complications.** Clot or air embolism, vasospasm of the lower limbs, thrombosis, and infarction of major organs may occur. Perforation of vessels can occur.

C. **Cardiac.** Arrhythmias, cardiac arrest, and volume overload can occur.

D. **Bleeding/coagulopathies.** Coagulopathies may result from thrombocytopenia or diminished coagulation factors. Platelets may decrease by >50% after a 2-volume ET.

E. **Electrolyte abnormalities.** Hyperkalemia, hypernatremia, hyperglycemia, hypercalcemia, hypomagnesemia, and hypocalcemia can occur.

F. **Hypoglycemia.** Especially likely in infants of diabetic mothers and in those with erythroblastosis fetalis because of islet cell hyperplasia and hyperinsulinism. Rebound hypoglycemia may result in these infants in response to the concentrated glucose (300 mg/dL) contained in CPD donor blood.

G. **Metabolic acidosis.** Metabolic acidosis from stored donor blood (secondary to the acid load) occurs less often in CPD blood.

H. **Metabolic alkalosis.** Metabolic alkalosis may occur as a result of delayed clearing of citrate preservative from the donated blood by the liver.

I. **Necrotizing enterocolitis.** An increased incidence of NEC after ET has been suggested. For this reason, the umbilical vein catheter should be removed after the procedure unless central venous pressure monitoring is required. Also, it is recommended that feedings be delayed for at least 24 hours to observe the infant for the possibility of a post-ET ileus.

J. **Miscellaneous.** Feeding intolerance, hypothermia, hyperthermia, graft-versus-host disease, apnea, bradycardia.

31 Peripheral IV Extravasation and Infiltration: Initial Management

I. **Indication.** To minimize initial injury resulting from infiltration of IV fluids into the tissue. **Infiltration** refers to the inadvertent leakage of **nonvesicant** (nonirritating) fluid from the vein into the surrounding tissues. Infiltration is usually considered benign unless a very large amount of fluid causes compression of nerves or compartment syndrome. **Extravasation** refers to the inadvertent leakage of **vesicant fluid** (highly caustic fluid or medication that is capable of causing tissue necrosis) from the vein into the surrounding tissues. This can cause a mild skin reaction or severe tissue necrosis or an injury so severe it leads to amputation.

II. **Procedures**

A. Initial treatment is determined by the stage of the infiltration, the type of infiltrating solution, and the availability of specific antidotes. There is a lack of conclusive evidence regarding optimal care after IV extravasation in the newborn. Available information in the literature is primarily anecdotal or from descriptive case reports. A staging system has been proposed that provides guidance concerning the appropriate initial treatment options (Table 31–1). This chapter refers only to the initial management and not to the management of long-term complications (scarring, contractures, tissue loss, vascular compromise).

Table 31–1. **STAGING OF IV INFILTRATES[a]**

Stage	Description	Treatment Options[a]
I	Painful IV site No redness or swelling	1. Remove IV cannula. 2. Elevate extremity.
II	Painful IV site Slight swelling (0–20%)	1. Remove IV cannula. 2. Elevate extremity.
III	Painful IV site Marked swelling (30–50%) Blanching Skin cool to touch, but with good pulse and brisk capillary refill below infiltration site	1. Leave IV cannula in place. Using 1-mL syringe, aspirate as much fluid as possible. 2. Remove cannula unless it is needed for administration of an antidote. 3. Elevate extremity. 4. Consider antidote (eg, hyaluronidase, phentolamine).
IV	Painful site Very marked swelling (>50%) Blanching Skin cool to touch Decreased or absent pulse Delayed capillary refill <4 seconds Skin breakdown, blistering, or necrosis	1. Leave cannula in place. Using 1-mL syringe, aspirate as much fluid as possible. 2. Remove cannula unless needed for administration of antidote. 3. Elevate extremity. 4. Consider antidote. 5. If site is tense with swelling and skin is blanched, use multiple needle puncture technique (see Section II.C).

[a]Data from Millam D. Managing complications of IV therapy. *Nursing.* 1988;18:34–43; and Thigpen JL. Peripheral intravenous extravasation: nursing procedure for initial treatment. *Neonatal Netw.* 2007;26(6):379–384.

B. Specific antidotes
 1. Hyaluronidase
  a. Appropriate for stage III extravasation of IV fluids except vasoconstrictors.
  b. Administer within 1 hour after insult if possible, and not after 3 hours.
  c. Clean area with antimicrobial agent.
  d. Inject 1 mL (150 U) as 5 separate 0.2-mL subcutaneous injections around the periphery of the extravasation site. Use aseptic technique and change the needle after each injection.
  e. Cover with hydrogel dressing (Intrasite, Smith and Nephew, London) for 48 hours.
 2. Phentolamine (Regitine)
  a. The drug of choice for extravasation of dopamine and other vasoconstrictors.
  b. Clean area with antimicrobial agent.
  c. Inject a 0.5-mg/mL solution subcutaneously into the affected area. Usual amount needed is 1–5 mL, depending on size of infiltrate. May repeat if necessary.
C. Multiple needle puncture technique
 1. May be used to create an avenue for fluid to escape and help to minimize tissue damage.
 2. Clean with antimicrobial agent.
 3. Using a 20-gauge needle, puncture the skin subcutaneously in multiple areas of the edematous tissue. Change the needle after each injection.
 4. Cover with saline-soaked gauze to absorb the fluid, and elevate the extremity.
 5. Evaluate every 1–2 hours for 48 hours.
III. Complications. Initial management may cause the following:
A. Infection. Use strict aseptic technique during injections.
B. Trauma to site. Handle skin gently; remove skin disinfectant with sterile saline pad.
C. Hypotension. Could potentially occur with a large dose of phentolamine or with absorption of topical nitroglycerin.

Selected References

Chandavasu O, Garrow E, Valda V, Alsheikh S, Dela Vega S. A new method for the prevention of skin sloughs and necrosis secondary to intravenous infiltration. *Am J Perinatol.* 1986;3(1):4–5.

Lawson EE, Lehmann CU, Nogee LM, Terhaar M, McCullen KL, Pieper B. Neonatal extravasation injuries associated with intravenous infusions. *eNeonatal Rev.* 2008;5(11).

Ramasethu J. Pharmacology review: prevention and management of extravasation injuries in neonates. *NeoReviews.* 2004;5:E491–E497.

Thompson Reuters Clinical Editorial Staff. *Neofax 2011, A Manual of Drugs Used in Neonatal Care.* New York, NY:PDR Network; 2011:205, 324–325.

32 Gastric and Transpyloric Intubation

In gastric intubation, a gastric tube is inserted through the nose (NG) or mouth (OG) to the stomach. In **transpyloric intubation**, a transpyloric tube is inserted through the nose or mouth through the pylorus into the duodenum or jejunum.

Gastric Intubation

I. Indications
A. Enteric feeding in the following situations:
 1. High respiratory rate. Enteric feedings are used at some centers if the respiratory rate is >60 breaths/min to decrease the risk of aspiration pneumonia (*controversial*).

2. **Neurologic disease.** If it impairs the sucking reflex or the infant's ability to feed. An abnormal gag reflex is an indication for a gastric tube.
3. **Premature infants.** May have immature sucking and swallow mechanisms that normally develop after 32 weeks. Preemies have immaturity of motor function and tire before they can take in enough calories to maintain growth.
4. **Insufficient oral intake.**

B. **Gastric decompression.** In infants with necrotizing enterocolitis (NEC), bowel obstruction, or ileus.
C. **Administration of medications.**
D. When a transpyloric tube is placed, a gastric tube is needed to empty gastric contents and administer medications.
E. **Analysis of gastric contents.**

II. **Equipment.** Infant feeding tube (3.5 or 5F if <1000 g or 5–8F if ≥1000 g), for decompression dual-lumen vented Replogle tube (6, 8, 10F) (*Note:* tubes come with and without stylets), stethoscope, sterile water (to lubricate the tube), syringes (10–20 mL), 1/2-inch adhesive tape, benzoin, gloves, suctioning equipment, cardiac monitor, stethoscope, pH paper, and bag-and-mask ventilation with 100% oxygen (in case of emergency). Recommended: colorimetric device (eg, CO2nfirm Now CO_2 detector [Covidian, Mansfield, MA] or capnograph) to help confirm the position of the tube by absence of CO_2 within the tube.

III. **Procedure**
A. **Monitor heart rate and respiratory function throughout the procedure.** Place the infant in the supine position, with the head of the bed elevated. The infant can be swaddled to provide comfort.
B. There are 4 methods of estimating gastric tube insertion length:
1. **OG tube insertion.** Table 32–1 provides OG guidelines for very low birthweight infants <1500 g.
2. **Age-related/height-based (ARHB) method**
    a. **Less than 1 month of age: NG only**
        i. NG tube insertion length (cm) = 1.950 cm + 0.372 × (infant's length in centimeters)
    b. **Greater than 1 month of age (if greater than 44.5 cm in length)**
        i. OG tube insertion distance = 13.3 cm + 0.19 × (infant's length in centimeters)
        ii. NG tube insertion distance = 14.8 cm + 0.19 × (infant's length in centimeters)
3. **NEMU (nose/ear/mid-umbilicus) for NG/OG tubes.** Measure the distance from the tip of the nose to the bottom of the ear (earlobe) to the midpoint between the xiphoid and the umbilicus. This measurement proved to be the **most accurate** in one study.

Table 32–1. GUIDELINES FOR MINIMUM OROGASTRIC TUBE INSERTION LENGTH TO PROVIDE ADEQUATE INTRA-GASTRIC POSITIONING IN VERY LOW BIRTHWEIGHT INFANTS

Weight (g)	Insertion Length (cm)
<750	13
750–999	15
1000–1249	16
1250–1500	17

Data from Gallaher KJ, Cashwell S, Hall V, Lowe W, Ciszek T. Orogastric tube insertion length in very low birth weight infants. *J Perinatol.* 1993;13:128.

4. NEX (nose/ear/xiphoid). Distance from the tip of the nose to the bottom of the ear to the xiphoid (*controversial*). This technique gave an insertion distance that was too short in infants with a high error rate and is considered inaccurate by some.

C. Mark the length on the tube. Measure based on choice of the preceding calculations and lubricate the tube by moistening the end of the tube with sterile water. (Note that smaller tubes such as 3.5F clog easily).

D. Pain management. Consider nonpharmacologic methods such as oral sucrose, swaddling, or containment by flexing and holding the infant. Make sure appropriate tube lubrication is used.

E. The tube can be placed in 1 of 2 insertion points, oral or nasal. Most units use indwelling technique as opposed to the intermittent intubation.

   1. Many centers preferentially use NG tubes as they do not limit breast or bottle feeds. **Do not use nasal insertion** with nasal trauma, recent esophageal surgery, choanal atresia, nasal prong continuous positive airway pressure (CPAP), respiratory distress, grunting, with oxygen requirement (CPAP, nasal ventilation, or nasal supplemental oxygen). In these cases, the oral route is preferred.

   2. Oral insertion. Less traumatic and does not impact respiration. It is easier for the infant to dislodge and may limit breast and bottle feeding.

   3. Nasal insertion. Avoid NG in very low birthweight infants <2 kg because of increased incidence of respiratory compromise.

      a. Check nostrils for patency.

      b. Flex the neck, push the nose up, and insert the tube, directing it straight back (toward the occiput).

      c. Tilt head slightly forward. Advance the tube to the desired distance.

   4. Oral insertion. Push the tongue down with a tongue depressor and pass the tube into the oropharynx. Slowly advance the tube the desired distance.

F. Do not push against any resistance (perforation potential). Remove stylet if present.

G. Continue to observe the infant for respiratory distress and/or bradycardia. Stop procedure immediately until the patient is stabilized.

H. Determine the location of the tube and never instill materials into the tube until the position is verified. **Radiologic verification** can be done and is considered the gold standard and is recommended at the time of initial tube placement or tube change. The radiograph should be read before feeding or medication instillation by an appropriate trained health care provider. **Nonradiologic verification** can be done by the following methods:

   1. Auscultation is done but is not reliable as the only method to verify placement. Injecting air into the tube with a 10–20 mL syringe and listen for a rush of air (a gurgle in the stomach commonly referred to as the "whoosh test"). This may be unreliable because a rush of air can occur when the tip is in the distal esophagus and respiratory tract air can be heard by auscultation.

   2. Visual inspection of the aspirate has not been reliable when used alone as gastric contents can vary in color. Normal gastric contents can be blood tinged, yellow, pale green, off white, clear, milky, or tannish in color. Small bowel aspirates are usually golden yellow or greenish brown. Respiratory secretions can be yellow, straw colored, clear, or white. Respiratory and gastric aspirates may be similar in color therefore the result may be misinterpreted. If used with pH it may be more beneficial. Grossly bloody aspirate may indicate a perforation.

   3. CO_2 at the proximal end of the tube. **Absence of CO_2** suggests placement in the alimentary tract and CO_2 with a normal capnograph tracing suggests placement in the trachea and distal airways. Inadvertent insertion in the trachea and distal airway occurs from 0.3% to 15%.

   4. Gastric aspirate pH testing using pH paper or a pH meter (pH paper is preferred over litmus paper). A pH aspirate <5 suggests gastric placement. If the pH

is >6, then the placement should be questioned. The mean values of pH are not usually affected by feeding status or use of acid suppression medications. *Note:* Swallowed amniotic fluid may transiently raise gastric pH, and some preterm infants have a decreased ability to produce gastric HCl. Gastric pH at birth is high (pH 6–8) because of alkaline amniotic fluid. Gastric fluid has a much lower pH than respiratory or intestinal fluid. To differentiate intestinal and respiratory fluid, pH is less effective because both have a high pH.

5. Testing aspirate for bilirubin, pepsin, and trypsin can help identify site of tube placement. Usually not practical for routine procedures. **Gastric aspirate testing:** bilirubin <5, high pepsin, low trypsin. **Intestinal aspirate testing:** bilirubin >5, low pepsin, high trypsin. **Respiratory aspirate:** little or no trypsin or pepsin. A bilirubin <5 mg/dL, pepsin ≥100 mcg/mL, and trypsin ≤30 mcg/mL indicates gastric placement.

6. If the location is still in question, obtain a radiograph. **However, this only verifies the location at the exact time of the radiograph. The tube tip should be below T12.** See Figure 11–8, which demonstrates a nasogastric tube properly positioned in the stomach.

7. It is best to verify placement after insertion, once per shift, before each feeding, and with medication administration. Some recommend radiography to verify placement if planning to initiate enteral feeding or administering medication.

   I. Aspirate the gastric contents and secure the tube to the cheek with benzoin and 1/2-inch tape. For NG tubes, make certain the tube does not press on the nasal ala. For feeding, attach the tube to a syringe. For decompression, connect the tube (preferably a dual-lumen **Replogle tube**) to low continuous suction.

   J. When not in use, the tube should be left open in a dependent drainage position below the level of the stomach.

IV. Removal of tube. Disconnect suction (if attached) and pinch gastric tube closed when pulling it out so contents will not go into the pharynx.

V. Complications

   A. Apnea and bradycardia. Usually mediated by a vagal response and resolve without specific treatment.

   B. Hypoxia. Always have bag-and-mask ventilation with 100% oxygen available to treat this problem.

   C. Misplaced tube. Incorrect placement in trachea, esophagus, Eustachian tube, trachea, or oropharynx. Twisting, coiling, or knotting of the tube.

   D. Perforation of the esophagus, posterior pharynx, stomach, or duodenum. The tube should never be forced during insertion

   E. Aspiration. If feeding has been initiated in a tube that is accidentally inserted into the lung or if the gastrointestinal tract is not passing the feedings out of the stomach. Periodically check the residual volumes in the stomach to prevent over distention and aspiration. (See Chapter 54.) Any NG or OG tube may increase gastroesophageal reflux and risk of aspiration pneumonia.

   F. Nasopharyngeal complications. Irritation, bleeding, infections. Grooved palate with prolonged OG placement.

Transpyloric Intubation

Transpyloric intubation requires a gastric tube for aspiration, drainage, and medication administration. Cochrane review found that transpyloric tubes are not recommended in premature infants because there was no evidence of any beneficial effect of transpyloric feeding in preterm infants, with increased adverse effects. Feedings with human milk via transpyloric tubes may reduce apnea and bradycardia in preterm infants with suspected gastroesophageal reflux.

I. Indications
   A. Enteric feeding in the following conditions:
      1. Not tolerating gastric feeding (eg, severe gastroesophageal reflux)
      2. Infants at risk for aspiration (the transpyloric tube is below the pyloric sphincter)
      3. Delayed gastric emptying
      4. Motility disorders
      5. Severe gastric distension
      6. Plain intolerance of gastric feeds (persistent gastric residuals)
   B. To test duodenal and jejunal contents
   C. Postoperative duodenal atresia
II. **Equipment.** Weighted infant feeding tube (silastic tubes preferred with or without stylet) 6F <1500 g, 8F >1500 g, stethoscope, sterile water (to lubricate the tube), a syringe (20 mL), 1/2-inch adhesive tape, pH paper, continuous infusion pump and tubing, gloves, suctioning equipment, and bag-and-mask ventilation with 100% oxygen.
III. Procedure
   A. **Determine insertion length.** Measure from using the ARHB, NEMU, or NEX method. Add the distance from the designated point to the right lateral costal margin. Mark the point on the tube with tape.
   B. **Follow initial steps for gastric intubation** as noted on page 275. Confirm the initial gastric position as previously described.
   C. **Place infant into a right lateral position.** With the patient on his right side, elevate the head of the bed 30–45 degrees.
   D. **To distend the stomach.** Inject 10 mL/kg of air through the tube and then close the tube.
   E. **Insert the tube to the desired length.** Keep the infant in the right side down position for 1–2 hours to allow the weighted tube to migrate into the duodenum.
   F. **Periodically, inject 2–3 mL air and aspirate the tube.** No air ("snap test," high-pitch crackles and inability to aspirate air) suggests the tube is in position in the duodenum. An alkaline (pH >6) and a bilious (gold to green) aspirate suggests proper placement. (See also Section III.E.5.)
   G. **Place an OG/NG tube** as described on page 275 for aspiration and medication delivery. *Note:* Consult PharmD specialist for medications that are administered into the stomach or duodenum.
   H. **Check placement by checking the pH and color of the aspirate.** If pH >6 and the color of the aspirate is golden yellow, the tube is probably in the transpyloric position. To further confirm, **check bilirubin** level in the aspirate (a value >5 is seen if tube is in transpyloric position).
   I. **Confirm placement with a radiograph.** The tip of the tube should be just beyond the second portion of the duodenum. See Figure 11–9. **Aspirate contents** or initiate tube feeding.
   J. **Flushing the tube with 3 mL of water** after each use will limit tube obstruction. Avoid flushing tubes with small caliber syringes (1–5 mL) as they generate high pressure and may rupture tubing.
   K. **If long-term use anticipated,** consider changing the tube very 2–4 weeks.
IV. **Removal of tube.** Discontinue the infusion, pinch off the tube, and withdraw slowly. Gastric tube can be left in place or removed as described on page 276.
V. **Complications.** These are similar to the NG/OG tube placement (page 276). Other complications may include:
   A. **Inability to pass tube beyond pylorus.** Fluoroscopic guidance may be necessary.
   B. **Aspiration.** Transpyloric feeding tubes do not have a decreased risk of aspiration as compared with gastric feeding tubes.
   C. **Infection.** Local infection or sepsis can occur. Enterocolitis can occur secondary to *Staphylococcus* or NEC.
   D. **Malabsorption.** Enteral feeds bypass the stomach: fat malabsorption, increased frequency of bowel movements, some medications may not be absorbed.

E. **Rare complications.** Intussusception, pyloric stenosis, enterocutaneous fistula, methemoglobinemia in very premature from intestinal obstruction and inflammation induced by the transpyloric tube, pyloric stenosis, bronchopleural fistula, and pneumothorax.

Reference

Cirgin Ellett ML, Cohen MD, Perkins SM, Smith CE, Lane KA, Austin JK. Predicting the insertion length for gastric tube placement in neonates. *AWHONN.* 2011;40(4):412–421. DOI:10.1111/j.1552-6909.2011.01255.x.

33 Heelstick (Capillary Blood Sampling)

I. **Indications**
   A. **Collect blood samples** when only a small amount of blood is needed or when there is difficulty obtaining samples by venipuncture or other source. Common studies include complete blood count (CBC), chemistries, liver function tests, sickle cell anemia, thyroid, bilirubin levels, toxicology/drug levels, bedside glucose monitoring, and newborn metabolic screening. Coagulation studies, chromosomal analyses, immunoglobulin titers, and some other, more sophisticated tests cannot be done on capillary sampling.
   B. **Capillary blood gas determination** gives satisfactory pH and Pco_2, but not Po_2.
   C. **Blood cultures** when venous access or other access is not possible. Sterile technique is required but heelstick is not the preferred method.
   D. **Newborn metabolic screen** is ideally performed in the first 48–72 hours of life (however, can be done after 24 hours). It should be done before a transfusion and antibiotic therapy and ideally after receiving breast milk or formula to ensure accurate testing. See Chapter 15.
II. **Equipment.** Automated self-shielding lancets are preferred in neonates (Table 33–1); sterile manual lancets are not recommended but may be used in some units if automated lancets are not available (sizes: 2 mm for <1500 g and 4 mm for >1500 g). Capillary tube (for rapid hematocrit and bilirubin tests) or larger BD Microtainer™ collection tubes (if more blood is needed [eg, for chemistry determinations]), filter paper card for newborn screening (if appropriate), clay to seal the capillary tube, a warm washcloth or heel warming device (eg, a chemical activated packet), antiseptic solution, gloves, and a diaper.
III. **Procedure**
   A. **Automated self-shielding lancets are preferred in neonates because they are associated with fewer complications and decreased pain.** Automated devices cause less hemolysis and less lab value error, and provide an exact width and depth of incision. **Manual unshielded lancets** are no longer recommended (unless automated lancets are not available) because they cause more pain, may penetrate too deeply, and can injure health care providers. Studies have shown that using the Tenderfoot Preemie™ (ITC, Edison, NJ) automated lancet versus a manual lancet resulted in fewer heel punctures, less collection time, and a lower recollection rate. There are two types of devices: puncture and incision (see Table 33–1).
      1. **Puncture devices.** (eg, BD Microtainer Contact-Activated Lancet.) Activate only when positioned and pressed against the skin. These puncture the skin by inserting a blade or needle vertically into the tissue. Puncture-style devices typically deliver a single drop of blood and are better for sites that are repeatedly punctured (eg, for glucose testing).
      2. **Incision devices.** (eg, BD Microtainer Quickheel Lancets, Tenderfoot, BD, babyLance.) These devices slice through the capillary beds. These are less painful and

Table 33–1. COMMONLY USED AUTOMATED SELF-SHIELDING LANCETS FOR SAMPLE COLLECTION IN NEWBORNS

Device	Infant	Characteristics
Tenderfoot MicroPreemie[a]	<1000 g	Blue: depth 0.65 mm, length 1.40 mm Incision type
Tenderfoot Preemie[a]	Low birthweight, 1000–2500 g	White: depth 0.85 mm, length 1.75 mm Incision type
Tenderfoot Newborn[a]	Birth to 3–6 months, >2500 g	Pink/blue: depth 1.0 mm, length 2.5 mm Incision type
BD Microtainer Quikheel Preemie Lancet[b]	Low birthweight (>1.0 kg and <1.5 kg) premature infants or full term for lower blood volume	Pink: depth 0.85 mm, length 1.75 mm Incision type
BD Microtainer Genie Lancet[b,c]	Infant heelsticks for glucose testing	Purple: 1.25 mm × 28 g Puncture type
BD Microtainer Quikheel Infant Lancet[b]	Infants who need high flow, full term with high blood volume needed	Teal: depth 1.00 mm, length 2.50 mm Incision type
babyLance Preemie: BLP[d]	Preemie	Green: depth 0.85 mm Incision type
babyLance Newborn[d]	Newborn	Blue: depth 1.00 mm Incision type

[a]ITC Edison, NJ.
[b]BD, Franklin Lakes, NJ.
[c]BD Microtainer Genie Lancet (pink/green/blue) are for finger sticks and not for heelsticks in infants.
[d]MediPurpose, Duluth, GA.

require fewer repeat incisions and shorter collection times, and are recommended for infant heelsticks. Incision devices deliver a small flow of blood as opposed to a drop and are better to fill Microtainer tubes.

B. **Capillary blood sampling is considered the most common painful procedure but the least invasive and safest of all the blood drawing methods done in the neonatal intensive care unit (NICU).** Sampling is done by puncturing the dermis layer of the skin to access capillaries running through the subcutaneous layer of the skin. The sample is a mixture of arterial and venous blood (from arterioles, venules, and capillaries) plus interstitial and intracellular fluids. The proportion of arterial blood is greater than that of venous blood due to increased pressure in the arterioles leading into the capillaries. Warming of the puncture site further arterializes the blood. The areas on the bottom surface of the heel contain the best capillary bed. *Note:* **Cochrane review states that venipuncture, not capillary blood sampling, by a skilled operator is the method of choice for blood sampling in term neonates. Lower pain scores are seen with venipuncture.**

C. **Heelsticks are contraindicated.** If there is local infection, poor perfusion, significant edema, any injury of the foot, or any congenital anomaly of the foot.

D. **Infant should be supine.** Some advocate for infant to be on stomach with the limb lower than the level of the heart to increase blood flow.

E. **Wrap the foot in a warm washcloth and then in a diaper for 3–5 minutes (moist heat helps to increase blood flow).** Commercial packs are available to heat the heel and should be applied for 5 minutes. A warming pad may be used, but its temperature should not exceed 40°C (104°F). This prewarming of the blood (arterialization of capillary blood) increases the local blood flow and reduces the difference between the arterial and venous gas pressures. Although not mandatory, it will produce hyperemia, which increases vascularity, making blood collection easier. It is mandatory when collecting a sample for a blood gas or pH determination. One study suggests that heel warming is an unnecessary step. Topical nitroglycerine did not facilitate blood collection in a heelstick study.

F. **Pain management.** Factors that contribute to pain responses from a heelstick are size of needle, gestational age, repeated exposure, squeezing of the heel, severity of illness, and behavioral state of the infant.

    1. **The American Academy of Pediatrics (AAP) recommends nonpharmacologic pain prevention** such as oral sucrose/glucose, breast milk, kangaroo care, swaddling, pacifier, or other methods.

    2. **EMLA (eutectic mixture of lidocaine and prilocaine). Not found to be effective** in heelsticks.

    3. **Automated devices.** Cause less pain than manual devices.

    4. **Other methods found to help.** Sugar-coated pacifier, pacifier-activated lullaby, Yakson therapy (Korean touching method of laying a hand on the back and caressing the abdomen for 5 minutes), and mechanical vibration.

G. **Choose the area of puncture.** (Figure 33–1) Blue area on the picture is preferred. An alternative site is the area between the sides of the heel (plantar area), but it should

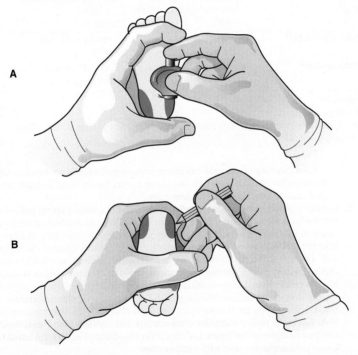

FIGURE 33–1. Preferred sites and technique for heelstick in an infant. Use the shaded area when performing a heelstick in an infant. (A) Use of an automated self-retracting lancet (BD Quikheel) for heelstick in an infant is illustrated. The automated lancet is held at 90 degrees to the axis of the foot and activated. (B) Standard lancet technique is shown. The automated lancet is held at 90 degrees to the axis of the foot and activated. (*Reproduced with permission from Gomella LG, Haist SA, eds. Clinician's Pocket Reference. 11th ed. New York: McGraw-Hill; 2007.*)

only be used if the other areas are used extensively. Avoid the end (crown) of the heel (the posterior curvature of the heel where the calcaneus bone is close to the skin), as this area is associated with an increased incidence of osteomyelitis. Fingertips and toes are not recommended in infants and are only recommended in children >1 year. Vary the sites to prevent bruising. **One recommendation to prevent osteomyelitis** is to use the most medial or lateral portions of the plantar surface of the heel, at a depth no more than 2.4 mm; never on the posterior curvature and not through a previous heelstick site.

H. Wipe the area with povidone-iodine, followed by a saline wipe. Some advocate only a 70% alcohol prep pad and let dry. Do not use cotton balls. (*Note*: Povidone-iodine can interfere with potassium, bilirubin, phosphorus, and uric acid. If the area is wet with alcohol, hemolysis may occur, altering the results.)

I. Two general devices are available: automated and manual
   1. Using an automated lancet (preferred method). Common devices are noted in Table 33–1. Prepare the unit and hold the device 90 degrees to the surface. The device can be oriented perpendicularly or at 90 degrees to the long axis of the foot (see Figure 33–1A). Depress the trigger with your index finger to activate the device and automatically make the puncture. Immediately discard the device.
   2. Using a standard manual heel lancet. Encircle the heel with the palm of your hand and index finger (Figure 33–1B). Make a quick, deep (<2.0 mm) puncture. Never puncture more than 2 mm to avoid complications.

J. Wipe off the first drop of blood with gauze as the first drop of blood is often contaminated with tissue fluid and may have a high potassium level, causing specimen dilution, hemolysis, and clotting. Wiping off the first drop also permits the sample to flow better as platelets aggregate at the site and may stop bleeding. Gently apply pressure to the heel ("tennis racket grip"), and place the collection tube at the site of the puncture. The capillary tubes will automatically fill by capillary action; gently "pump" the heel to continue the blood flow to collect drops of blood in a larger tube. Allow enough time for capillary refill of the heel, and apply pressure so the incision is opened with each pumping maneuver. Do not squeeze, milk, scoop, scrape, or massage the area as these may affect the test results.

K. Seal the end of the capillary tube with clay. Collect the larger samples in the BD Microtainer or similar tubes.

L. Collect the blood gas sample first. The blood becomes more venous if the collection is delayed. Send it to the lab promptly, making sure there are no air bubbles. Hematology studies should be done next, then chemistry. Also, if the CBC is delayed there is an increased chance of erroneous cell counts due to platelet clumping. Use the following **"Order of Draw"**: blood gases, ethylenediaminetetraacetic acid (EDTA) tubes, other additive tubes, serum tubes.

M. For filter paper newborn screening. (See Chapter 15.) The paper can be directly applied to the heel or the blood can be transferred to a capillary tube (without anticoagulants) and then applied to the filter paper. This testing is usually done at least 24 to 48 hours after birth.

N. Maintain pressure on the puncture site with a dry sterile gauze pad until the bleeding stops and elevate the foot. A 4 × 4 gauze pad can be wrapped around the heel and left on to provide hemostasis; adhesive bandages are not recommended.

O. Inaccurate laboratory results. Falsely elevated glucose/dextrostix, potassium, hematocrit, and inaccurate blood gas values (slightly lower pH, slightly higher Pco_2, and markedly lower Pco_2) can occur with heelstick sampling. Milking or squeezing causes hemolysis and inaccurate values.

IV. Complications
   A. Infection
      1. Cellulitis. Risk can be minimized with the proper use of sterile technique. A culture from the affected area should be obtained and the use of broad-spectrum antibiotics considered.

2. **Osteomyelitis.** Usually occurs in the calcaneus bone. Avoid the center area of the heel, and do not make the puncture opening too deep. If osteomyelitis occurs, tissue should be obtained for culture, and broad-spectrum antibiotics should be started until a specific organism is identified. Infectious disease and orthopedic consultation is usually obtained.

3. **Other infections.** Abscess and perichondritis have been reported.

B. **Scarring of the heel.** Occurs when there have been multiple punctures in the same area. If extensive scarring is present, consider another technique of blood collection, such as central venous sampling.

C. **Pain.** Caused by heelsticks in premature infants can cause declines in hemoglobin oxygen saturation as measured by pulse oximetry.

D. **Calcified nodules.** These can occur but usually disappear by 30 months of age.

E. **Other complications.** Include nerve damage, tibial artery laceration (medial aspect of heel), burns, bleeding, bruising, hematoma, and bone calcification.

34 Laryngeal Mask Airway

The laryngeal mask airway (LMA) consists of a soft elliptical mask with an inflatable cuff that is attached to a flexible airway tube. The mask covers the laryngeal opening with an inflatable cuff that occludes the esophagus. It can provide positive pressure ventilation. To quote the 2011 American Academy of Pediatrics/American Heart Association *Textbook of Neonatal Resuscitation*, when you "can't ventilate and can't intubate," the device may provide a successful rescue airway.

I. **Indications**
   A. **Ineffective face mask ventilation in neonates with the following:**
      1. Abnormal facial anatomy (eg, cleft lip, cleft palate)
      2. Unstable cervical spine (eg, osteogenesis imperfecta, arthrogryposis, trisomy 21)
      3. Upper airway obstruction (eg, Pierre-Robin sequence, micrognathia, large tongue, reductant tissues, and oral, pharyngeal, or neck tumors)
   B. **Rescue procedure after failed intubation or intubation not feasible.**
   C. **For short-term positive pressure ventilation in neonatal intensive care unit.**
   D. **Resuscitation** (delivery room or other) when face mask and endotracheal intubation fail. If necessary, chest compressions can be attempted with LMA in place.

II. **Equipment.** Appropriate LMA (size 1 for neonate; see Figure 34–1; reusable and disposable types), lubricant (water-soluble), 5-mL syringe, gloves.

III. **Procedure**
   A. **LMA limitations.** To suction meconium, to give intratracheal medications (may leak), prolonged ventilator support (not enough evidence, high ventilation pressures are needed, and air may leak), extremely small infants (<1500 g), when chest compressions are performed (ETT preferred, but if not possible chest compressions can be attempted with LMA).
   B. **With significant gastric distension.** Consider a temporary orogastric tube to decompress the stomach and remove.
   C. **The LMA covers the laryngeal opening.** The inflated cuff conforms to the hypopharynx and occludes the esophagus. See Figure 34–2.
   D. **Use size 1 LMA.** Commercially available masks are designed for infants >2000 g, but can be used in smaller infants (>1500 g) if needed.
   E. **Follow standard precautions.** Gloves, eye protection, etc.
   F. **Check cuff for leakage by inflating with 2–3 mL of air.** Fully deflate the cuff before insertion.

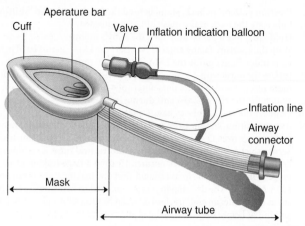

FIGURE 34–1. Basic laryngeal mask airway design. (*Reproduced, with permission, from Trevisanuto D, Micaglio M, Ferrarese P, Zanardo V. The laryngeal mask airway: potential applications in neonates.* Arch Dis Child Fetal Neonatal Ed. *2004;89:F485–F489. Review.*)

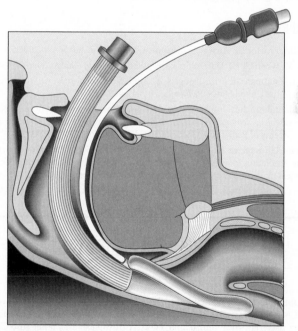

FIGURE 34–2. Demonstration of correct anatomical positioning of the laryngeal mask airway cuff around laryngeal inlet. (*Reproduced, with permission, from Trevisanuto D, Micaglio M, Ferrarese P, Zanardo V. The laryngeal mask airway: potential applications in neonates.* Arch Dis Child Fetal Neonatal Ed. *2004;89:F485–F489. Review.*)

G. Position patient on back, stand behind the head, put in the "sniffing position."
H. Lubricate the back of the mask of LMA if needed.
I. Hold LMA like a pencil and open the baby's mouth.
J. With the aperture facing anteriorly, insert the LMA against hard palate and using your index finger guide the LMA. Insert until resistance felt.
K. Inflate the mask with 2–4 mL of air to provide adequate seal. Do not exceed maximum recommended by manufacturers of 4 mL of air in a size 1 mask.
L. Watch for the rise of LMA cuff during inflation.
M. Connect the end of tube to bag, T-piece, or ventilator.
N. Assess position, similar to endotracheal tube. Check chest movement, equal breath sounds, improved O_2 saturation, increased heart rate, and colorimetric CO_2 monitor.
O. Secure the LMA with tape similar to endotracheal tube. Remember, grunting and crying through the device is normal. Hearing a large leak of air or presence of a bulge in the neck of the infant should alert one that the LMA is not properly placed.
P. LMA removal. The decision to remove the mask is based on the infant's respiratory status or whether an endotracheal tube can be successfully placed. Suction the mouth and throat before the cuff is deflated and remove the LMA.

IV. Complications
A. Air leak around LMA may result in ineffective ventilation.
B. Abdominal distention and aspiration.
C. Malposition.
D. Laryngospasm and bronchospasm.
E. Soft tissue trauma.
F. Prolonged use in adults (incidence in infants not available) can cause lingual edema and oropharyngeal nerve damage.

Selected References

Bingham RM, Proctor LT. Airway management. *Pediatr Clin North Am.* 2008;55:873–886.

El-Orbany M, Woehlck HJ. Difficult mask ventilation. *Anesth Analg.* 2009;109:1870–1880.

Karlsen KA, Trautman M, Price-Douglas W, Smith S. National survey of neonatal transport teams in the United States. *Pediatrics.* 2011;128:685–691.

Kattwinkel J. Endotracheal intubation and laryngeal mask airway insertion. In: Kattwinkel J, ed. *Textbook of Neonatal Resuscitation.* 6th ed. Elk Grove Village, IL/Dallas, TX: American Academy of Pediatrics/American Heart Association; 2011:189–195.

Keidan I, Fine GF, Kagawa T, Schneck FX, Motoyama EK. Work of breathing during spontaneous ventilation in anesthetized children: a comparative study among the face mask, laryngeal mask airway and endotracheal tube. *Anesth Analg.* 2009;91:1381–1388.

35 Lumbar Puncture (Spinal Tap)

I. Indications
A. Obtaining cerebrospinal fluid (CSF) for the diagnosis of central nervous system (CNS) disorders such as meningitis/encephalitis. Infections that can be diagnosed are bacterial, viral, fungal, and **TORCH** (*t*oxoplasmosis, *o*ther [usually syphilis], *r*ubella, *c*ytomegalovirus, and *h*erpes simplex virus). Meningitis can be present in as many as 15–25% of cases of neonatal sepsis.
B. Aid in the diagnosis of intracranial hemorrhage. CSF studies are indicative but not diagnostic for intracranial hemorrhage: large number of red blood cells (RBCs),

xanthochromia, increased protein content, and hypoglycorrhachia (abnormally low CSF glucose content).

C. **Diagnose an inborn error of metabolism.** CSF amino acid analysis can be obtained to rule out nonketotic hyperglycinemia. Postmortem CSF (1- to 2-mL specimen, frozen) is recommended: suspected inborn error of metabolism.

D. **Draining CSF in communicating hydrocephalus associated with intraventricular hemorrhage.** (Serial lumbar punctures for this are *controversial*.) Cochrane review states that early repeated CSF tapping cannot be recommended for neonates at risk of developing posthemorrhagic hydrocephalus.

E. **Administration of intrathecal medications.** Chemotherapy, antibiotics, or anesthetic agents or contrast material.

F. **Monitoring efficacy of antibiotics used to treat CNS infections** by examining CSF fluid.

G. **Diagnose CNS involvement with leukemia.**

H. **For the initial sepsis workup** (*controversial*). If CNS involvement is suspected or blood cultures are positive, some recommend a lumbar puncture (LP). Because signs and symptoms of neonatal meningitis are so vague and unspecific, some clinicians advise that all infants with proven or suspected sepsis undergo LP.

II. **Equipment.** Lumbar puncture kit (usually contains three sterile specimen tubes; four sterile tubes are often necessary); sterile drapes; sterile gauze; 20-, 22-, or 24-gauge 1.5-inch spinal needle with stylet (**do not use a butterfly needle,** as it may introduce skin into the subarachnoid space and form a dermoid cyst); 1% lidocaine; 25- to 27-gauge needle, 1-mL syringe; sterile gloves; mask; gown; hat; and skin disinfectant (10% povidone-iodine solution).

III. **Procedure**

A. **Contraindications** include increased intracranial pressure (risk of CNS herniation), uncorrected bleeding abnormality, severe bleeding diathesis, infection near puncture site, severe cardiorespiratory instability, and lumbosacral abnormalities that may interfere with identification of key structures.

B. **If significant increased intracranial pressure is suspected** obtain a computed tomography (CT) or magnetic resonance imaging (MRI) of the head. Herniation rarely occurs in the neonate with open cranial sutures, but is reported.

C. **Pain management**

1. **AAP recommends** that topical anesthetics (**EMLA** [eutectic mixture of lidocaine and prilocaine] or other topical agents) be applied 30 minutes before the procedure. Nonpharmacologic pain management, if appropriate, can be used.

2. **Lidocaine 0.5–1%** (in a 1-mL syringe with a 25- or 27-gauge needle) can be injected subcutaneously. *Note:* Physiologic instability is not reduced with lidocaine use and is not recommended by some sources.

3. **Systemic therapy.** Other recommendations include sedation with a slow IV opiate bolus if the infant is intubated; if not intubated, a bolus of midazolam in a term infant can be used (see Chapter 76).

D. **An assistant should restrain the infant in either a sitting or a lateral decubitus position,** with the spine flexed as in Figure 35–1, depending on personal preference. An intubated, critically ill infant must be treated in the lateral decubitus position. Some advocate that if CSF cannot be obtained in the lateral decubitus position, the sitting position should be used. In the lateral decubitus position, the spine should be flexed (knee-chest position). The neck should not be flexed because of an increased incidence of airway compromise; maintain airway patency. Supplemental oxygen can prevent hypoxemia. Monitor vital signs and pulse oximetry during the procedure.

E. **Once the infant is in position, check for landmarks.** (See Figure 35–1.) Palpate the iliac crest and slide your finger down to the L4 vertebral body. Then use the L4-L5 interspace (preferred LP site to avoid cord penetration) as the site of the lumbar puncture. Make a nail imprint at the exact location to mark the site.

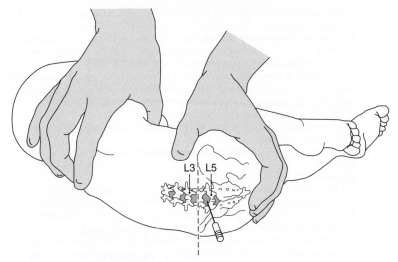

FIGURE 35–1. Positioning and landmarks used for lumbar puncture. The iliac crest (dotted line) marks the approximate level of L4.

F. **Prepare the materials.** Open sterile containers, pour antiseptic solution into the plastic well located in the lumbar puncture kit.

G. **Put gloves on and clean the lumbar area with antiseptic solution, starting at the interspace selected.** Prep in a widening circle from that interspace up and over the iliac crest.

H. **Drape the area with one towel under the infant and one towel covering everything but the selected interspace.** Keep the infant's face exposed. Palpate again to find the selected interspace.

I. **Insert the needle in the midline** with steady pressure aimed toward the umbilicus.
   1. **Guidelines for spinal needle depth.** 1–1.5 cm in term infant, <1 cm in a preterm, or calculate depth of needle insertion: 0.03 × body length (in centimeters). Advance the needle slowly and then remove the stylet to check for appearance of fluid. The fluid should be clear but may be slightly xanthochromic (common and associated with maternal labor preceding delivery).
   2. **Remove the stylet frequently to keep from going too far and getting a bloody specimen.** Early stylet removal improves the success rate. A "pop" as the ligamentum flavum and dura are penetrated is not usually found, as is the case with older children and adults. Rotate the needle if no fluid is seen, and never aspirate with a syringe.

J. Collect 0.5–1 mL of CSF in each of the 4 sterile specimen tubes by allowing the fluid to drip into the tubes. **CSF white blood cell (WBC) and glucose values can decrease over time (>2 hours)**; therefore, these need to be sent immediately. For routine CSF examination, send 4 tubes of CSF to the laboratory in the following recommended order:
   1. **Tube 1.** Gram stain, bacterial culture, and sensitivity testing.
   2. **Tube 2.** Glucose and protein levels. Others if metabolic disease suspected.
   3. **Tube 3.** Cell count and differential.
   4. **Tube 4.** Optional and can be sent for rapid antigen tests for specific pathogens (eg, group B *Streptococcus*) or PCR (polymerase chain reaction; eg, herpes).

K. **For the treatment of communicating hydrocephalus with intraventricular hemorrhage.** Remove 10–15 mL/kg of CSF.

L. If a bloody specimen is obtained in the first tube:
 1. **Observe for clearing in the second and third tubes.** An RBC count on the first and last tubes determines if there is a difference in the number of RBCs/mm³. If the last tube has fewer RBCs than the first, the tap was likely traumatic (usually puncture of the epidural venous plexus on the post surface of the vertebral body). *Note:* Adjustment of WBC counts in a traumatic lumbar puncture does not aid in the diagnosis of meningitis in neonates.
 2. **If blood does not clear but forms clots.** A blood vessel has probably been punctured. Because CSF has not been obtained, a repeat tap must be done.
 3. **If blood does not clear and does not clot and there are equal numbers of RBCs in the first and last tubes.** The infant probably has intracranial bleeding.
M. **Replace the stylet before removing the needle to prevent trapping the spinal nerve roots.** Withdraw the needle. Maintain temporary pressure and clean and bandage on the site.
N. **A repeat tap in 24 to 48 hours is recommended.** If the first tap is not diagnostic and the clinical picture is concerning.
IV. **Complications.** There is no evidence that LP-related headache occurs in infants.
 A. **Contamination of CSF specimen with blood.** (See Section III.L, above.) Correction of WBCs for RBCs is not useful. Repeat LP in 12–24 hours.
 B. **Infection.** Sterile technique reduces risk. Bacteremia may result if a blood vessel is punctured after the needle has passed through contaminated CSF. Meningitis can occur if LP is performed during bacteremia. Abscess (spinal and epidural) and vertebral osteomyelitis are rare.
 C. **Intraspinal epidermoid tumor.** Results from performing LP with a needle that does not have a stylet. The cause is the displacement of a "plug" of epithelial tissue into the dura. The incidence of traumatic lumbar puncture is not reduced by the use of a needle without a stylet. Do not use a butterfly or any needle without a stylet.
 D. **Herniation of cerebral tissue through the foramen magnum.** Uncommon in neonates because of the open fontanelle.
 E. **Spinal cord and nerve damage.** To avoid this complication, use the L4-L5 interspace. Between 25 and 40 weeks' gestation the spinal cord terminates between the second and fourth lumbar vertebrae. After 2 months post term, the cord is in the normal adult position.
 F. **Intramedullary hemorrhage resulting in paraplegia.** It is important to consider the location of the conus medullaris in a preterm infant.
 G. **Bleeding/hematoma.** Spinal epidural hematoma, intracranial or spinal subdural hematoma, and intracranial or spinal subarachnoid hematomas have all been reported.
 H. **Cerebrospinal fluid leakage.** Frequent complications are seen on sonograms.
 I. **Apnea and bradycardia.** Sometimes occur from respiratory compromise caused by the infant being held too tightly during the procedure.
 J. **Hypoxia.** Commonly seen; increasing the oxygen during the procedure may help. Preoxygenation may also help.
 K. **Cardiopulmonary arrest.**
V. **Interpretation of CSF fluid findings.** Normal CSF values are listed in Table 35–1. Remember that neonatal meningitis can occur with normal CSF values. No single CSF value can exclude CSF meningitis. CSF values in the neonate that indicate meningitis are ***controversial*. Use caution** when interpreting results in the premature infant. Data suggests that results in premature infants cannot be reliably used to exclude meningitis.
 A. **Bloody CSF fluid.** See Section III.L.
 B. **CSF protein and WBC count.** Decrease with increasing postnatal age. CSF protein decreases by about 6.8% with each week of age.
 C. **Elevated CSF protein without increased CSF WBC counts.** Seen in congenital infections, intracranial hemorrhage, and para-meningeal infections (eg, brain abscess).

Table 35–1. **NORMAL CEREBROSPINAL FLUID VALUES IN NEONATOLOGY**

	WBC (mm³)	Protein (mg/dL)	Glucose (mg/dL)
Term	0–32 (mean 61% PMN)	20–170	34–119
Preterm (970–2500 g)	0–29 (mean 57% PMN)	65–170	24–63
VLBW (550–1500 g)	0–44 (range 0–66% PMN)	45–370	29–217

PMN, polymorphonuclear neutrophils; VLBW, very low birthweight.
Data from Rodriguez AF, Kaplan SL, Mason EO Jr. Cerebrospinal fluid values in the very low birth weight infant. *J Pediatr.* 1990;116(6):971–974; Sarff LD, Platt LH, McCracken GH Jr. Cerebrospinal fluid evaluation in neonates: comparison of high-risk infants with and without meningitis. *J Pediatr.* 1976;88(3): 473–477; and Martín-Ancel A, García-Alix A, Salas S, Del Castillo F, Cabañas F, Quero J. Cerebrospinal fluid leucocyte counts in healthy neonates. *Arch Dis Child Fetal Neonatal Ed.* 2006;91(5):F357–F358.

D. **CSF WBC counts.** Higher in gram-negative meningitis than gram-positive meningitis.

E. **Number of bands in a CSF specimen.** Does not predict meningitis.

F. **CSF glucose.** This is 80% of term blood glucose, 75% of preterm blood glucose. **A low CSF glucose** has the greatest specificity for meningitis.

G. **CSF glucose and protein.** Cannot accurately diagnose meningitis.

H. Generally CSF protein is higher in preterm infants when compared to term infants. For CSF glucose, values tend to be higher or similar in preterm infants compared to term infants.

I. Other values suggestive of meningitis
   1. CSF WBC count >20–30 cells with predominance of polymorphonuclear (PMN) leukocytes (with bacterial meningitis: infants >34 weeks, median WBC 477/mm³; infants <34 weeks, median WBC 110/mm³).
   2. CSF protein >150 mg/dL in preterm infants, >100 mg/dL in term infants (96% of infants with meningitis have a CSF protein >90 mg/dL).
   3. CSF glucose <20 mg/dL in preterm infants, <30 mg/dL in term infants.
   4. Meningitis can occur with normal CSF values.

J. Values suggesting meningitis is not present
   1. CSF mean WBC count in preterm and term <10 cells/m³.
   2. CSF protein in term infants <100 mg/dL. With preterm infants it varies with gestational age.
   3. Age-specific protein values, mean 0–14 days, 79 mg/dL; 15–28 days, 69 mg/dL; 29–42 days, 58 mg/dL.

Selected References

Polin RA; Committee on Fetus and Newborn. Management of neonates with suspected or proven early onset bacterial sepsis. *Pediatrics.* 2012;129(5):1006–1015.

Shah S, Ebberson J, Kestenbaum LA, Hodinka RL, Zorc JJ. Age-specific reference values for cerebrospinal fluid protein concentration in neonates and young infants. *J Hosp Med.* 2011;6(1): 22–27.

Whitelaw A. Repeated lumbar or ventricular punctures in newborns with intraventricular hemorrhage. *Cochrane Database Syst Rev.* 2001. DOI:10.1002/14651858.CD000216.

36 Ostomy Care

I. **Indications.** A variety of surgical procedures may require an **ostomy**, a **temporary or permanent intestinal diversion.** The majority of these ostomies in the neonatal intensive care unit are for the management of **necrotizing enterocolitis (NEC).** Other indications are anorectal malformations, meconium ileus (related to cystic fibrosis or due to very low birthweight), Hirschsprung disease, volvulus, and intestinal atresias and these are discussed elsewhere in this book. A **gastrostomy (surgical opening in the stomach)** may be necessary for feeding or decompression in a variety of conditions, such as the inability to swallow (neurologic or congenital anomalies such as Pierre Robin sequence), or esophageal abnormalities.

II. Ostomy classification
   A. Ileostomy. Stoma opening from the ileum, used for NEC, intestinal malrotation or volvulus, and small bowel atresia or stenosis.
   B. Colostomy. Stoma opening from the colon, used for NEC, Hirschsprung disease, malrotation or volvulus, imperforate anus, and colonic atresia.
   C. Mucous fistula. Distal nonfunctioning limb of intestine secured flush to skin with a mucocutaneous anastomosis.
   D. Hartman pouch. Distal intestine is left in the abdominal cavity rather than removed or secured as mucous fistula, allowing reconnection to stoma at later date.
   E. Double-barrel stoma. Loop of bowel is completely divided and 2 ends brought out as stomas to abdominal surface. Skin and fascia are closed between ends to provide separation of stomas.
   F. End ostomy. Intestine is completely divided. The functioning proximal end is everted, elevated above skin, and secured circumferentially.
   G. Loop ostomy. The intestine is incompletely divided with an opening at the antimesenteric side, while leaving the mesenteric side intact. This is used when temporary diversion or minimal surgical procedure is needed. It is not performed as often as end ostomy.
   H. Gastrostomy. Surgical opening into the stomach, where a gastrostomy tube (GT "or g-tube") is inserted into the opening for nutritional support, medications, or gastrointestinal decompression.

III. Equipment
   A. Ostomy. Ostomy bag or pouch (1-piece or 2-piece system), skin barrier wafer, skin preparation agents, sterile water, gauze pads, petroleum gauze, and gloves. **Products that improve security of pouch** include plasticizing skin sealants, skin barrier paste (protect exposed skin), adhesive agents (improve adherence), and skin barrier powder (dusted onto denuded skin to form protective crust).
   B. Gastrostomy tube. 12–14F balloon or mushroom gastrostomy tube; similar-sized Foley catheters are sometimes used. Silicone is preferred over latex, skin barrier as for ostomies.

IV. Procedures
   A. Ileostomy and colostomy
      1. Postoperative ileostomy and colostomy care
         a. No bag is applied first 24–48 hours postop due to minimal stool production.
         b. Apply petrolatum gauze to stoma until first stool output appears.
         c. Measure effluent output. Volume >2 mL/kg/h should be replaced with 1/2 normal saline (NS). Some institutions add 10–20 mEq KCl/L.
      2. Changing ostomy bags. Not a sterile procedure, but regular hand washing and gloves are important. Goals are containment of stool/odor and protection of the peristomal skin. Minimize skin sealants, adhesives, and adhesive removers in premature infants due to more permeable skin.

      a. Empty bag and carefully remove from skin.

      b. Clean skin and stoma with warm water and dry thoroughly. Inspect stoma and peristomal skin.

      c. Measure stoma at base using stoma-measuring guide or template. Cut appropriate size hole in soft silicone bordered dressing or wafer for bag; do not constrict stoma but ensure that the skin is covered by the appliance.

      d. Prepare skin for wafer application. If there is no skin compromise, apply skin sealant to surface area. Apply stoma adhesive paste around stoma for better adherence. Apply skin barrier powder to denuded skin to form protective crust.

      e. Position wafer on skin around stoma and mold to contour of skin.

      f. Adhere closed-ended ostomy bag or pouch to wafer.

      g. Position bag in lateral position to allow for easy drainage.

      h. Empty bag regularly when one-third to one-half full. Change bag with any evidence of leaking.

  B. **Gastrostomy tubes (GT)**

    1. Types of gastrostomy tubes

      a. **Balloon tip.** Initial placement requires abdominal surgery. Tube has balloon on distal end, similar to indwelling urinary catheter.

      b. **Mushroom tip.** Mushroom tip portion secures tube to stomach wall.

      c. **Percutaneous endoscopic gastrostomy (PEG).** Placed by endoscopy. Tube has internal bumper secured against abdominal mucosa and external bumper stabilizes tube.

      d. **Low profile gastrostomy ("button").** Replaces original tube once the stoma tract has matured, about 6–8 weeks. Access device is flush to the skin.

    2. Care of all gastrostomy tubes

      a. Flush tubing every 4 hours during continuous feedings or before and after intermittent feedings with at least 3 mL of warm water.

      b. Give only one medication at a time and flush between mediations.

      c. Assess site daily for breakdown, warmth, redness, edema, purulent drainage, leakage, foul odor or pain.

      d. Clean GT site with warm water and mild soap to remove drainage or crusting. Dry skin thoroughly; the site should be kept clean and dry.

      e. Do not use hydrogen peroxide to clean site.

V. Complications

  A. **Ileostomy and colostomy.** Consider consultation with an ostomy nurse specialist for persistent ostomy issues.

    1. **Peristomal skin breakdown.** Common problem as small bowel effluent contains a high concentration of digestive enzymes.

      a. Careful cleansing of the stoma and surrounding skin requires gentle technique to avoid abrasions.

      b. To minimize contact dermatitis from digestive fluids, fecal material, or adhesives, select a bagging system that is correctly sized to minimize skin exposure.

      c. Use protective skin products (see earlier) that will further prevent contact between skin and ostomy output.

    2. **Excessive output may cause dehydration and/or electrolyte imbalance.** Daily liquid output is normally 10–15 mL/kg; ileostomy output is usually greater than colostomy.

      a. Replace excessive output with appropriate fluids (1/2 NS). Some institutions add 10–20 mEq KCl/L to the replacement fluids; others supplement potassium in the daily fluids. Consider consultation with gastroenterology.

      b. **Malabsorption.** A risk in situations involving surgical loss of overall small intestine length. Also, dehydration may occur if usual stoma output is abnormal.

      c. **Diarrhea.** Diarrhea secondary to infectious agents or osmotic enteral loads is a constant threat. Replace fluid losses intravenously and evaluate electrolyte balance.

d. Management. May involve changes in enteral feeds such as continuous feeds or elemental formulas to improve absorption or tolerance. Probiotics may improve gut flora. Cholestyramine may reduce diarrhea related to short gut and excessive bile acids.

3. If dermatitis is suspected (contact, fungal, or otherwise), change bag and barrier every 24–48 hours to reassess for further treatment. Fungal skin infections may appear in the form of pustules or papules. Apply antifungal (eg, nystatin) powder to area before applying skin barrier wafer and bag. Consider consultation with an ostomy nurse specialist or a dermatologist for persistent signs of dermatitis.

4. Bleeding a small amount from the stoma tissue itself after cleaning is normal. A pediatric surgeon should be notified about excessive bleeding or blood coming from lumen of the stoma.

5. Peristomal hernia. A defect in abdominal fascia that allows intestine to bulge into peristomal area. Surgical intervention will be necessary if hernia is incarcerated.

6. Stomal stenosis. An impairment of drainage due to narrowing or contraction of stoma tissue at the skin or subcutaneous fascial level; may require revision.

7. Retraction of a stoma. Stoma tissue being pulled below skin level. Surgical reevaluation is suggested. Adequate bag adherence can be challenging if the stoma cannot be revised.

8. Necrosis of stoma tissue can occur from impaired blood flow. Stomas are usually moist and pink-red in color. Color changes can occur when infant cries, but should return to normal when calm. A dark maroon or black stoma may indicate necrosis.

9. Prolapse is a telescoping of intestine through the stoma beyond skin level. This requires surgical assessment for perfusion, length, and stoma function. If ischemia or obstruction is suspected, then surgical intervention will be required.

B. Gastrostomy

1. Leaking around tube. This can result from tube displacement, improper balloon inflation, inadequate tube stabilization, or increased abdominal pressure.

2. Skin irritation. Possible causes include leakage, sutures, and infection. Topical treatments include antifungal powder or ointment, zinc oxide, and skin barrier wafer. Cover site with dry gauze or foam dressing under stabilizer to pull drainage off skin until irritation resolves.

3. Infection. Most likely occurs within first 2 weeks after tube placement. Risk factors include skin breakdown, immunosuppressed patient, chronic corticosteroids, and excessive handling/manipulation of tube.

4. Granulation tissue formation. A proliferation of capillaries that present as red, raw, beefy, painful or bleeding tissue protruding from stoma. Possible causes include moisture, infection, tube not stabilized, and use of hydrogen peroxide.

5. Tube occlusion. May be caused by inadequate tube flushing, kink in tube, formula, or medication precipitation in tube.

6. Accidental removal. Site can close within 1–4 hours. Immediately place Foley catheter in stoma if tube is removed to maintain patency.

Selected References

Celegato M, Gancia P. Medical and nursing care in post-operative period to the newborn with surgical problems and intestinal ostomy. *Early Hum Dev.* 2011;87S:S83.

Colwell JC, Beitz, J. Survey of wound, ostomy, and continence (WOC) nurse clinicians on stomal and peristomal complications: a content validation study. *J Wound Ostomy Continence Nurs.* 2007;34:57–69.

Goldberg E, Barton S, Xanthopoulos MS, Stettler N, Liacouras CA. A descriptive study of complications of gastrostomy tubes in children. *J Pediatr Nurs.* 2010;25:72–80.

Hansen A, Puder M. Part 11: Ostomy diversions and management. In: *Manual of Neonatal Surgical Intensive Care*. 2nd ed. Shelton, CT: People's Medical Publishing House; 2009:353–370.

Wound, Ostomy, and Continence Nurse Society. Management of gastrostomy tube complications for the pediatric and adult patient. http://www.health.state.nm.us/ddsd/ClinicalSvcsBur/Initiatives/documents/WOCNguidelines.pdf.

---

37 Paracentesis (Abdominal)

I. Indications

A. **To obtain peritoneal fluid for diagnostic tests** to determine the cause of ascites. **Ascites** is an excessive amount of fluid in the peritoneal cavity and in the neonate it is usually urinary, biliary, or chylous. Other causes can occur but are less common.

1. **Urinary ascites.** Due to perforation of the ureter, intrarenal collecting system, or bladder (intraperitoneal) often caused by a distal obstruction. The most common cause is posterior urethral valves. Other causes: ureterocele, ureteral stenosis, urethral stenosis/atresia, neurogenic bladder, urogenital sinus, congenital nephrotic syndrome, bladder neck obstruction, and renal vein thrombosis.

2. **Biliary ascites.** Due to perforation of bile duct (more common), injury to the bile ducts, or a choledochal cyst.

3. **Chylous ascites.** Slightly more common in males and usually idiopathic. Other causes include a congenital lymphatic abnormality (more common), or disruption of the lymphatic ducts from trauma or surgery.

4. **Hepatocellular ascites.** Can be caused by neonatal hepatitis, viral hepatitis, congenital hepatic fibrosis, Budd-Chiari syndrome, or hepatic/portal vein thrombosis.

5. **Pancreatic ascites.** Usually caused by trauma or pseudocysts.

6. **Gastrointestinal causes of ascites.** Any perforation of the gastrointestinal tract (gastric, others), necrotizing enterocolitis (NEC) with perforation/peritonitis, meconium peritonitis, perforation of the Meckel diverticulum, atresia, malrotation, volvulus, gastroschisis, omphalocele, postabdominal surgery, or intussusception. **Peritonitis** in neonates is most commonly associated with gastrointestinal tract perforations.

7. **Infections.** Most common is congenital (CMV, toxoplasmosis, syphilis, and others) but can also be from fungal, viral (parvovirus, enterovirus), or bacterial infections.

8. **Inborn errors of metabolism.** Glycogen storage disorders, lysosomal storage disorders, and galactosemia can all cause ascites. Examples include infantile free sialic acid storage disorder (ISSD), Salla disease, GM1 gangliosidosis and Gaucher disease, α_1-antitrypsin deficiency.

9. **Cardiac abnormalities.** Congestive heart failure and right-sided heart obstruction can cause ascites.

10. **Chromosomal causes.** Turner syndrome and trisomy 21.

11. **Iatrogenic.** Can occur from fluid from central venous catheters or intraperitoneal extravasation of total parenteral nutrition (TPN) from a umbilical vein catheterization-related vessel perforation. See Chapter 44.

12. **Hemoperitoneum (bloody ascites).** Uncommon but can be nontraumatic (hepatoblastoma) or secondary to birth trauma (hepatic, splenic, or adrenal) or secondary to a ruptured internal organ. Splenic trauma can be associated with consumptive coagulopathy.

B. As a therapeutic procedure, such as removal of **peritoneal fluid from massive ascites or air from a pneumoperitoneum** to aid in ventilation in a patient with cardiorespiratory compromise.

II. Equipment. Sterile drapes, sterile gloves, topical disinfectant such as povidone-iodine solution, sterile gauze pads, tuberculin syringe, 1% lidocaine, sterile tubes for fluid, a 10- to 20-mL syringe on a 3-way stopcock, safety engineered 22- or 24-gauge catheter-over-needle assembly (24 gauge for <2000 g, 22–24 gauge for >2000 g). Consider the use of ultrasound to guide needle placement.

III. Procedure

A. Contraindications and precautions. Paracentesis can be done with thrombocytopenia or coagulopathy if corrected before the procedure. With massive bowel distension, attempt to reduce distension with a nasogastric (NG) or rectal tube. Avoid surgical scar sites.

B. Diagnosis of ascites. Ascites is usually diagnosed by clinical examination and ultrasound (prenatal or postnatal). Ascites is usually obvious by clinical examination (abdominal distention, increasing abdominal girth, increased weight gain, bulging flanks dullness to percussion, and dilated superficial veins). The majority of these infants are also very edematous. Ascites obvious by clinical examination usually indicates a fluid volume of 200 cc or greater. Ascites not obvious by physical examination usually means that the volume of ascitic fluid is under 100 cc.

C. Position the infant supine with both legs restrained. To restrict all movements of the legs, a diaper can be wrapped around the legs and secured in place. Slightly elevate the flank side you are not using so the intestines float up and the fluid becomes more dependent.

D. Choose the site for paracentesis. The area between the umbilicus and the pubic bone is not generally used in neonates because of the risk of perforating the bladder or intestines. The sites most frequently used are the right and left flanks. A good rule is to draw a line from the umbilicus to the anterior superior iliac spine, and plan to use the area two-thirds of the way from the umbilicus to the anterior superior iliac spine (Figure 37–1). **Ultrasound guidance can be used and is recommended.**

E. Prepare the area with povidone-iodine in a circular fashion, starting at the puncture site. Put on sterile gloves, and drape the area. Perform "time out" per unit protocol.

F. Pain management. Topical anesthetic (eutectic mixture of lidocaine and prilocaine [EMLA]) can be used if the procedure is not emergent, or infiltrate the area with a tuberculin needle (skin to peritoneum) with lidocaine 0.5–1%. Use other nonpharmacologic pain prevention such as oral sucrose, breast milk, and others.

G. Connect the 10- to 20-mL syringe to the catheter and needle assembly.

H. Insert the needle at the selected site. (See Section D, above.) The needle is positioned toward the back at a 45-degree angle. A "Z-track" technique is usually used to minimize persistent leakage of fluid after the tap. Insert the needle perpendicular to the skin. When the needle is just under the skin, move it 0.5 cm before puncturing the abdominal wall.

I. Advance the needle, aspirating until fluid appears in the barrel of the syringe. Hold the assembly steady and remove the needle. Aspirate the contents slowly with the syringe and stopcock connected to the catheter. It may be necessary to reposition the catheter to obtain an adequate amount of fluid. Once the necessary amount of fluid is taken (usually 5–10 mL for specific tests and at least 10–15 mL, enough to aid ventilation), remove the catheter. If too much fluid is removed or it is removed too rapidly, hypotension may result. If there is no fluid, the catheter could be attached to the intestine or in the retroperitoneum; withdraw or remove the catheter and retry.

J. Cover the site with a sterile gauze pad until leakage has stopped.

K. Distribute the fluid in containers as appropriate for the clinical setting. Cell count and differential, Gram stain, culture and sensitivity, protein, albumin, triglycerides,

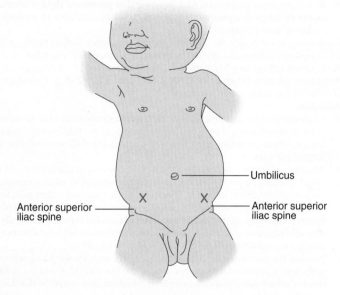

FIGURE 37-1. Recommended sites for abdominal paracentesis noted by the Xs.

cholesterol, bilirubin, glucose, electrolytes, creatinine, inclusion bodies and treponemes, sialic acid, and amylase.

L. **Ascitic fluid analysis. Brown with debris** suggests fecal matter secondary to intestinal perforation or gangrene such as NEC; **Gram stain positive for bacteria**—perforation or peritonitis; **ascites creatinine > serum creatinine**—urinary leak; **elevated bilirubin**—biliary or intestinal leak; **milky fluid, elevated triglycerides** with predominant lymphocytes and elevated cholesterol—chylous ascites; **elevated amylase and lipase**—pancreatic ascites; **high serum-to-ascites albumin gradient >1.1 g/dL**—hepatocellular disease (hepatitis, α_1-antitrypsin deficiency); **iatrogenic fluid or TPN ascites**—values consistent with infusate; **inclusion bodies** (congenital infections) and **treponemes** (syphilis); and **sialic acid** (infantile free sialic acid storage disease), **bloody (hemorrhagic) fluid**—birth trauma involving liver, spleen, or adrenal glands, or a ruptured internal organ.

IV. Complications
   A. **Cardiovascular effects.** Hypotension, tachycardia, and decreased cardiac output can occur. **Hypotension** can be caused by removing too much fluid or removing fluid too rapidly. To minimize this possibility, take only the amount needed for studies or what is needed to improve ventilation and always remove fluid slowly.
   B. **Infection.** The risk of peritonitis is minimized by using strict sterile technique.
   C. **Perforation of a viscus.** To help prevent perforation, use the shortest needle possible and take careful note of landmarks (see Section III.D). If perforation occurs, broad-spectrum antibiotics may be indicated with close observation for signs of infection. Usually the puncture site heals spontaneously. **Perforation of the bladder** is normally self-limited and requires no specific treatment.
   D. **Persistent peritoneal fluid leak.** The Z-track technique (see Section III.H) usually prevents the problem of persistent leakage of fluid. Persistent fluid leaks may have to be bagged to quantify the volume. Applying pressure over the site for a few minutes, or applying a pressure dressing and monitoring the site can be done.

E. **Pneumoperitoneum.** Observation is usually required (see Figure 11–22 for radiograph of a pneumoperitoneum).

F. **Bleeding.** Bleeding from the liver or intra-abdominal vessels, if severe, may require emergency surgery consultation. An **abdominal wall hematoma** can occur but is usually self-limiting. Correct abnormal clotting factors if necessary.

G. **Scrotal swelling.** Occurs in males for extravasation of ascitic fluid between body wall layers and is usually self-limiting.

38 Pericardiocentesis

I. **Indications**

A. **Emergency evacuation of air or fluid in the treatment of cardiac tamponade** (inability of the heart to expand with decreased stroke volume and cardiac output) caused by **pericardial effusion (accumulation of excess fluid)** or **pneumopericardium (accumulation of air)** in the pericardial space. Early recognition and intervention are paramount.

1. **Cardiac tamponade secondary to a pericardial effusion. A rare but life-threatening complication of central venous catheters, including percutaneous central venous catheters (CVP) and umbilical venous catheters (UVC).** Etiology is unclear but proposed causes include a direct puncture of a vessel or myocardium by the tip of the catheter during insertion or delayed perforation secondary to erosion of the cardiac or vascular wall. **Keep a high index of clinical suspicion in a neonate who has a central line and suddenly has cardiovascular collapse** that does not respond to resuscitation or resistance to external cardiac compressions and has no air leak by thoracic transillumination. It is more common with lines in the right atrium, and the median time to occurrence is 3 days after a central venous catheter insertion. A chest radiograph may not be diagnostic; an echocardiogram is but may delay treatment. Mortality is high.

2. **Cardiac tamponade secondary to a pneumopericardium. Rare** but is very dangerous and usually occurs with other air leak syndromes, with severe lung pathology, with a history of vigorous resuscitation, and/or a history of assisted ventilation. (See Figure 11–18 for a radiograph of pneumopericardium.)

B. **To obtain pericardial fluid for diagnostic studies** in infants with a pericardial effusion. Pericardial effusion is rare in neonates and most commonly occurs in a **hydropic** or **septic** infant. Other causes include thyroid dysfunction, cardiac and pericardial tumors, congenital anomalies (diaphragmatic hernia/eventration, ruptured ventricular diverticulum), infections, surgically related (postoperative), autoimmune, idiopathic, and other causes.

II. **Equipment.** Povidone-iodine solution, sterile gloves, gown, sterile drapes, a safety-engineered 22- or 24-gauge 1-inch catheter-over-needle assembly, extension tubing, 10-mL syringe, 3-way stopcock, lidocaine, and underwater seal if the catheter is to be left indwelling, transillumination device for pneumopericardium, transthoracic echocardiogram/ultrasound device.

III. **Procedure.** *Note:* If a central venous catheter is in place and a pericardial effusion is suspected, stop infusion of fluids into the catheter immediately.

A. **Ideally, pericardiocentesis is performed with the help of echocardiography/ ultrasound.** Besides diagnosing the pericardial effusion, it helps guide needle insertion to reduce complications. With a pneumopericardium, thoracic transillumination may be helpful. **With sudden cardiovascular collapse, time does not allow these** tests, and an immediate aspiration is necessary. **Emergency pericardiocentesis should not be delayed, as it is life-saving.** In certain cases, a quick betadine prep, followed by a "blind" needle insertion with aspiration, is necessary. **If time permits, it is best to follow these steps.**

B. **Perform an echocardiogram to diagnose and show the pericardial effusion.** It will also help to determine the site and angle of entry and allow an estimation of the distance the needle should go in. Imaging can also help in monitoring the effusion while the procedure is done.

C. **If a pneumopericardium is suspected.** Thoracic transillumination can be done to help diagnose and also to help monitor the air evacuation while the procedure is done (see Chapter 40).

D. **Monitor electrocardiogram and vital signs.**

E. **Prep the area (xiphoid and precordium) with antiseptic solution.** Put on the sterile gloves and gown and drape the area, leaving the xiphoid and a 2-cm circular area around it exposed.

F. **Pain management.** If time permits, local anesthesia can be administered (0.25–1.0 mL of 1% lidocaine subcutaneously).

G. **Prepare the needle assembly.** Attach the catheter over needle to a short piece of extension tubing that is attached to a 3-way stopcock. A syringe is attached to the stopcock. Alternative method is to just use a 22- to 24-gauge needle attached to a syringe (no cannula is placed when fluid or air can no longer be aspirated the needle is removed).

H. **Identify the site where the needle is to be inserted.** Most commonly is ~0.5 cm to the left of and just below the infant's xiphoid (Figure 38–1).

I. **Insert the needle at about a 30-degree angle, aiming toward the midclavicular line on the left.** (See Figure 38–1.) Have an assistant apply constant suction on the syringe while advancing the needle.

J. **Once air or fluid is obtained (depending on which is to be evacuated).** Stop advancing the needle, advance the cannula over the needle, remove the needle from the catheter, and reconnect the cannula to the extension tubing.

K. **Withdraw as much air or fluid as possible.** The goal is to relieve the symptoms or obtain sufficient fluid for laboratory studies.

L. **If an indwelling catheter is to be left in place.** Secure it with tape and attach the tubing to continuous suction (10–15 cm H_2O is used).

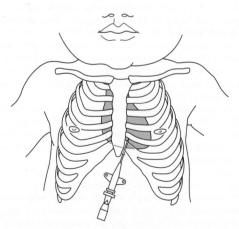

FIGURE 38–1. Recommended sites for pericardiocentesis.

M. Obtain a chest radiograph or ultrasound. To confirm the position of the catheter and the effectiveness of drainage. Transillumination can also be done.
IV. Complications
  A. Puncturing the heart. **Grossly bloody fluid may indicate that the needle punctured the heart.** Perforation of the right ventricle can be avoided by advancing the needle only far enough to obtain fluid or air. **Ultrasound guidance** is recommended if time permits. **Another technique** to avoid puncturing the heart (if ultrasound is not available) is to attach the electrocardiogram (ECG) anterior chest lead to the needle with an alligator clip. If changes are seen on the ECG (eg, ectopic beats, changes in the ST segment, increase in the QRS voltage), the needle has contacted the myocardium and should be withdrawn. Avoid leaving a metal needle indwelling for continuous drainage. Most needle perforations heal spontaneously. If cardiac perforation occurs, emergency intervention and cardiac surgeon consultation needed.
  B. Pneumothorax or hemothorax. This can occur if landmarks are not used and "blind" punctures are done. If this complication has occurred, a chest tube on the affected side is usually needed.
  C. Infection. Strict sterile technique minimizes the risk of infection.
  D. Arrhythmias. Usually transient. Repositioning the needle is usually effective, but with persistent arrhythmia, treatment may be necessary.
  E. Bleeding. Bleeding is usually superficial and controlled with pressure. Hepatic puncture can occur.
  F. Hypotension. May occur if a significant amount of fluid is drained. A fluid bolus may be necessary.
  G. Pneumomediastinum. Observation is only required.
  H. Pneumopericardium. Treat as above.

39 Therapeutic Hypothermia

I. Indication. To reduce mortality in infants with perinatal hypoxia ischemia when initiated before 6 hours of age. It is indicated in the treatment of infants (36 0/7 weeks' gestation or greater, younger than 6 hours) who fulfill the criteria for the diagnosis of moderate to severe hypoxic ischemic encephalopathy (HIE). Cooling can be done by **selective head** (Olympic Cool-Cap System, Olympic Medical Corporation, Seattle, WA) or **total-body cooling**. This chapter discusses total body cooling.
II. Eligibility for hypothermia. Infants should be evaluated for eligibility by **(step A) clinical and physiological criteria followed by (step B) complete neurological examination. Infants have to meet both physiologic and neurologic criteria.** Eligibility criteria are for either whole-body cooling by blanket or mattress or head cooling by a fitted cap. **For head cooling** a step C is required, which includes an amplitude-integrated electroencephalogram (aEEG) (recording at least 20 minutes duration) that shows either moderately or severely abnormal aEEG background activity or seizures.
  A. Step A: clinical and physiological criteria. All infants should be evaluated as follows:
    1. Blood gas (a cord blood gas or an arterial [preferred] or venous/capillary blood gas within the first hour of life): pH <7 or base deficit >16, proceed to step B.
    2. No blood gas or arterial/venous/capillary blood gas pH 7–7.15 or base deficit of 10–15.9 with an acute perinatal event (cord prolapse, abruption placenta, severe fetal heart rate [FHR] abnormality, variable or late decelerations; maternal trauma, hemorrhage, or cardiac arrest) plus either a or b (below), then proceed to step B.
      a. 10-minute Apgar ≤5.
      b. Continued need for ventilation initiated at birth and continued for at least 10 minutes.

B. **Step B: complete neurologic examination.** Once infant meets step A clinical and physiological criteria, perform a complete standardized neurologic examination. **Moderate to severe encephalopathy is defined as seizures or the presence of one or more signs in 3 of the 6 categories in staging of HIE** (level of consciousness, spontaneous activity, posture, tone, primitive reflexes, and autonomic system). The number of moderate or severe signs will determine the extent of encephalopathy; if signs were equally distributed, the designation is based on the level of consciousness.

   1. **If seizures are documented or are occuring, the infant is automatically eligible for cooling.**
   2. **No seizures are reported, the infant has to have at least 3 out of the 6 neurologic signs in moderate or severe encephalopathy** (Table 39–1) to be eligible for cooling.

C. Infant is eligible for cooling once criteria in step A and B are met.

III. **Equipment. Hyper-hypothermia machine** used to raise or lower a patient's temperature to a target level through conductive heat transfer; **infant-sized hyper-hypothermia blanket**, single-patient use, able to provide both heating and cooling to maintain patient's target temperature; **infant esophageal probe and cable** for continuous monitoring of patient's core temperature; 2–3 gallons of distilled water for initial setup; **drainage hose**; **open infant critical care bed** with warming capability at the **conclusion of the therapeutic hypothermia.** Cooling device unit (eg, Blanketrol III with cooling blankets, Kool-Kit Neonate, Cincinnati Sub-Zero, Cincinnati, OH).

IV. **Procedure**

A. **Confirm the eligibility for cooling as noted in Section II.**

B. **Gather equipment for cooling.** Follow preparation instructions of the hyper-hypothermia machine per operation manual. The author's institution uses the Blanketrol III Model 233 hyper-hypothermia cooling device unit.

C. **Pain management.** No specific analgesics or anesthetics are recommended. Sedation throughout the procedure is based on needs for mechanical ventilation and/or seizure control. Most commonly used sedation is morphine.

D. **Precool the blanket to 5°C for whole-body cooling to maintain an esophageal temperature of 33.5°C ± 0.5°C for neuroprotection.** Lay infant supine on the precooled blanket with occiput resting on the blanket. A single-layer thin blanket may be placed between the infant and the cooling blanket to prevent soiling of equipment (Figure 39–1).

Table 39–1. STAGING AND EVALUATION OF HYPOXIC ISCHEMIC ENCEPHALOPATHY

Category	Moderate Encephalopathy	Severe Encephalopathy
1. Level of consciousness	Lethargic	Stupor/coma
2. Spontaneous activity	Decreased activity	No activity
3. Posture	Distal flexion, full extension	Decerebrate
4. Tone	Hypotonia (focal, general)	Flaccid
5. Primitive reflexes		
Suck	Weak	Absent
Moro	Incomplete	Absent
6. Autonomic system		
Pupils	Constricted	Skew deviation/dilated/nonreactive
Heart rate	Bradycardia	Variable heart rate
Respirations	Periodic breathing	Apnea

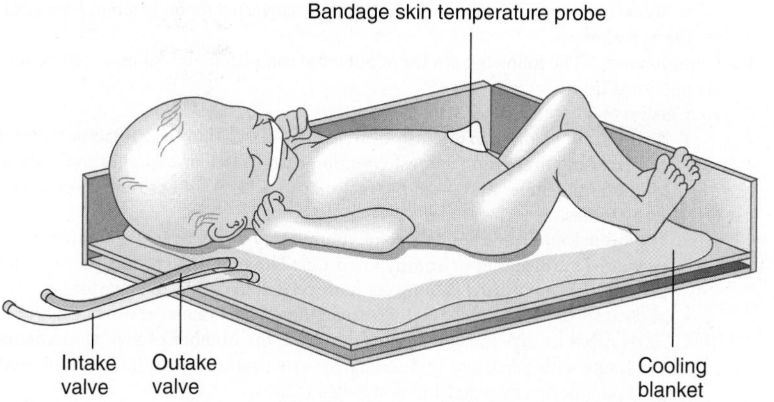

Bandage skin temperature probe

Intake valve · Outake valve · Cooling blanket

FIGURE 39–1. Hypothermia procedure; infant positioning on cooling blanket. (*Reproduced, with permission, from Cincinnati Subzero.*)

E. **Insert the esophageal temperature probe into an external naris.** Probe may be softened by placing in warm water for a few minutes. The probe should be positioned in the lower third of the esophagus (desired length = distance from nares to ear to the mid-sternum minus 2 cm). Secure the probe by taping with adhesive to the side of the infant's nose. Connect the probe to the cooling unit and begin temperature monitoring straight away. Confirm probe placement with a radiograph but do not wait for a radiograph to initiate cooling.

F. **Use an open critical care bed for optimal monitoring.** Skin temperature will be monitored by skin temperature probe on the lower abdomen attached to the radiant warmer. The radiant warmer is set to "manual mode" with the heat turned off (allow continuous skin temperature monitoring without any heat output). Do not use any other source of exogenous heat.

G. **Operate the cooling unit in automatic mode** with a core temperature goal of 33.5°C ± 0.5°C. Follow your neonatal intensive care unit [NICU]-specific cooling device instruction manual.

H. **The infant's esophageal temperature will begin to decrease soon after the initiation of the cooling therapy.** The cooling blanket system adjusts automatically to achieve 33.5°C in ~90–120 minutes. Once stable at 33.5°C, some esophageal temperature fluctuation around the setpoint is to be expected, but should not be greater than ±0.5°C. Monitor and record esophageal, skin, and water temperatures, as well as all vital signs at 15-minute intervals during cooling (or follow unit-specific policy). **Total period of cooling is 72 hours.**

I. **Gradual rewarming is done over 6 hours after completion of 72-hour cooling period.** The automatic cooling unit setpoint temperature is increased by 0.5°C every hour to a maximum setpoint of 36.5°C. The goal is to slowly increase the temperature 0.5°C per hour to reach normothermia by the end of 6 hours. Monitor vital signs (especially temperature) throughout the rewarming period. Hyperthermia must be avoided at all cost.

J. **At the end of 6-hour rewarming period, turn off hyper-hypothermia unit and remove cooling blanket and esophageal probe.** Follow cooling unit maintenance per local NICU protocol.

K. **During the cooling and rewarming process, the infant should receive routine clinical care appropriate for the level of acuity, including laboratory blood studies for surveillance of respiratory, cardiovascular, hematologic, and renal** dysfunction. Blood gas measurements must be corrected for body temperature during hypothermia.

V. **Complications.** The following is a list of potential complications and may include others not noted here.

A. **Cardiovascular and respiratory**

1. **Arrhythmia.** Hypothermia can decrease depolarization of cardiac pacemaker cells, causing bradycardia (most common cardiovascular complication). Maintain infant's temperature within target of $33.5°C \pm 5°C$ to prevent more severe arrhythmias.

2. **Hypotension.** Decreases in stroke volume and heart rate may contribute to decreased cardiac output and hypotension. The requirement for inotropes for pressure support during cooling are more related to physician behavior.

a. **Pulmonary hypertension.** Increased pulmonary vascular resistance has been reported in hypothermic infants; however, the number of hypoxic-ischemic infants with persistent pulmonary hypertension in large clinical trials were similar between cooled and noncooled infants.

b. **Blood gases.** Hypothermia decreases O_2 consumption and CO_2 production; therefore, ventilator settings need to be monitored and adjusted to avoid hyperventilation that can cause cerebral vasoconstriction. Blood gas values are temperature dependent, and if blood samples are warmed to 37°C before analysis (as is common in most laboratories), Po_2 and Pco_2 will be overestimated and pH underestimated in hypothermic patients. For accurate interpretation, samples should be analyzed at the patient's real temperature. If this is not possible, Polderman suggests blood gas values assayed at 37°C can be estimated as follows:

i. Subtract 5 mm Hg Po_2 per 1°C that the patient's temperature is <37°C;

ii. Subtract 2 mm Hg Pco_2 per 1°C that the patient's temperature is <37°C;

iii. Add 0.012 pH units per 1°C that the patient's temperature is <37°C.

B. **Dermatologic**

1. **Skin breakdown.** Vasoconstriction during extreme cold can lead to decreased blood flow, and localized damage is caused to skin and other tissues. Regular inspection of the infant's skin is part of routine care during cooling.

2. **Subcutaneous fat necrosis.** Cause is unknown and is associated with perinatal asphyxia. Hypothermia causes vasocontriction that worsens skin perfusion that has already been compromised by asphyxia, thereby leading to fat necrosis. Most of the reported cases occurred after completion of cooling. Serum calcium levels should be monitored in affected infants due to risk of hypercalcemia (Plate 9).

C. **Hematologic.** Serial follow-up of hematologic parameters is an important part of surveillance during cooling.

1. **Hypothermia-induced thrombocytopenia** is due to **increased platelet destruction** (platelet sequestration in the liver and spleen) and **disseminated intravascular coagulation (DIC)**, resulting in early thrombocytopenia and bone marrow suppression with reduced platelet production.

2. **Coagulopathy** induced by mild hypothermia with the risk for severe bleeding associated with therapeutic cooling is relatively small.

D. **Metabolic**

1. **Metabolic acidosis.** Decreased cardiac output leading to reduced clearance of lactic acid.

2. **Altered glucose metabolism.** Hypothermia decreases insulin sensitivity and secretion, leading to hyperglycemia; higher doses of insulin may be needed. During rewarming process, infants treated with insulin may be at risk for hypoglycemia as sensitivity to insulin is restored.

3. **Drug metabolism** and excretion of drugs and metabolites might be modified by cooling, as well as the presence of hepatocellular and renal impairment complicating HIE. Metabolism of drugs such as phenobarbital, morphine, and vecuronium

are slowed by effects of the temperature-dependent hepatic cytochrome P450 system. **Potentially toxic levels of drugs can accumulate in the system if metabolism and excretion are impaired.**

E. Infections. Cooling has immunosuppressive and anti-inflammatory effects. Meta-analysis of large trials did not show any increased incidence of infection in cooled infants.

Selected References

Blanketrol® III, Operation Manual, Model 233 Hyper-Hypothermia Units. Cincinnati Sub-Zero Products, Inc.

Polderman KH. Mechanism of action, physiological effects and complications of hypothermia. *Crit Care Med.* 2009;37:S186–S202.

Sarkar S, Barks JD. Systemic complications of hypothermia. *Semin Fetal Neonatal Med.* 2010;15:270–275.

Shah PS. Hypothermia: a systematic review and meta-analysis of clinical trials. *Semin Fetal Neonatal Med.* 2010;15(5):238–246.

Shankaran S, Laptook AR, Ehrenkranz RA, et al. Whole-body hypothermia for neonates with hypoxic-ischemic encephalopathy. *N Engl J Med.* 2005;353(15):1574–1584.

Strohm B, Hobson A, Brocklehurst P, Edwards AD, Azzopardi D; UK TOBY Cooling Register. Subcutaneous fat necrosis after moderate therapeutic hypothermia in neonates. *Pediatrics.* 2011;128:e450–e452.

Zanelli S, Buck M, Fairchild K. Physiologic and pharmacologic considerations for hypothermia therapy in neonates. *J Perinatol.* 2011;31:377–386.

40 Transillumination

I. Indications. Transillumination is the use of a strong light as a noninvasive tool for bedside diagnosis and aiding in procedures. By shining a bright light through an area of the body or an organ, one can diagnose abnormal air, fluid, or a nonsolid mass. One can also localize vessels, verify urine in the bladder, and aid in insertion in many procedures.
A. Procedures
1. Localize an artery or vein for vessel cannulation or blood sampling.
2. Bladder aspiration. Transillumination verifies the presence of urine in the bladder and shows the size and location of the bladder.
3. Cannulation of umbilical vessels. Transillumination identifies path of the vessels and can identify a false passage of an umbilical catheter.
4. Aid in oro/nasoduodenal feeding tube insertion (by gauging distension of stomach with air).
5. Chest tube thoracostomy/pericardiocentesis. Transillumination can document the success of air removal in a pneumothorax or in a pneumopericardium.
6. Serial transillumination for infants at high risk for pneumothorax.
B. Diagnostic. Air or fluid or nonsolid masses will light up brightly when transilluminated. Solid masses will appear dark. Normally there is a 2-cm area of lucency around the probe. If there is more than 2-cm lucency, the test is abnormal and further testing may have to be done.
1. Chest abnormalities. Air leaks in infants (such as pneumothorax, pneumomediastinum, and pneumopericardium) can be suspected and some diagnosed at the

bedside with transillumination. The thin wall of the infant's chest makes it easy to transilluminate, and as little as 10 mL of free air can be detected. Obtain a baseline transillumination on any infant at a high risk for an air leak.

2. **Abnormalities in the head.** Such as hydrocephaly, intracranial hemorrhage, subdural effusion, subdural hematoma, skull fractures, hydrocephalus, hydranencephaly, anencephaly, porencephaly, encephalocele, and large cerebral cysts. Transillumination of the skull is known as **skull diaphanoscopy.** It can be used as a screening tool for macrocephaly.

3. **Differentiate cystic from solid masses.** Such as cystic hygroma, a congenital macrocystic lymphatic malformation commonly found in the left base of the neck, that reveals complete transillumination.

4. **Abdominal abnormalities.** Such as ascites, distended bowel, pneumoperitoneum, cysts, perforated bowel in male infants with a patent processus vaginalis.

5. **Genitourinary abnormalities.** Such as distended bladder, hydrocele, hydronephrosis, cystic kidneys.

II. **Equipment.** Light source such as mini–light-emitting diode light, high-intensity fiber optic light source, commercially available transilluminators (eg, Veinlite, TransLite LLC, Sugarland, TX; Pediascan, Sylvan Fiberoptics, Irwin, PA), simple otoscope with light, disposable plastic cover or sterile glove to cover light source for aseptic technique, alcohol swab.

III. **Procedure.** Clinical examination is always necessary with transillumination. It is best to transilluminate the contralateral side of the body to compare changes.

A. **Clean end of light source with an alcohol swab** and cover with either a disposable plastic cover or sterile glove.

B. **Turn the lights in the room down and set light on the lowest intensity and increase as needed.** Limit skin contact time with light source.

C. **Head exam.** The light source is placed on the anterior fontanel and if transillumination of more than 2 cm around the edge of the beam or asymmetry is noted, this may be abnormal, and further studies are needed. The light source should be moved around all over the skull. Examples: subdural effusion (increased transillumination superior to the tentorium), subdural hematoma (decreased transillumination), hydrocephalus (increased lucency in supratentorial region), hydranencephaly (increased lucency in areas superior to the posterior fossa).

D. **Vessel location.** Place light source opposite the puncture site (ventral side, such as on the palm for hand cannulation) so the light goes through to show the vessel. Vessels are seen as dark lines against a transilluminated background; arteries are fixed, veins move with the skin.

E. **Genitourinary system/abdomen**

1. **Scrotum.** Place the light underneath the scrotum. If the entire scrotum lights up, a collection of fluid (hydrocele or patent processus vaginalis) is the likely cause. The testicles will appear as marble-sized shadows. With particulate matter or gas bubbles in the scrotum, suspect intestinal perforation.

2. **Kidneys/bladder. For kidney:** the infant is placed on its side, and the transilluminator is placed anteriorly over the kidney area. The kidney needs to be manipulated against the abdominal wall. Normal kidneys do not transilluminate. **For Bladder:** the transilluminator is pointed at the bladder area above the pubic symphysis. The area will glow red if urine is present. The size of the bladder on transillumination correlates with the actual size on excretory urography.

3. **Abdomen.** Place the transilluminator in the left paramedian position and direct the probe toward the midline. If the peritoneal cavity glows brightly, suspect a pneumoperitoneum. The falciform ligament can usually be seen as a dark band. In differentiating air from fluid in the abdomen, place the infant in a lateral decubitus position, ascites will light up inferiorly and free air will light up superiorly.

F. Chest
   1. Pneumothorax. Place transilluminator on the anterior chest wall above the nipple and in the axilla or along the posterior axillary line on the side of chest where air is suspected. Normally there is a 2- to 3-cm lucent area around the probe tip. In a pneumothorax, the area of lucency is huge (sometimes the entire side of the chest). Compare the other side of the chest. The affected side will appear hyperlucent and radiates across the chest as compared with the unaffected side. Note that a small pneumothorax may not be seen. Compare the other side of the chest, especially if concerned about a small accumulation of air.
   2. Pneumopericardium. Place the transilluminator in the third or fourth intercostal space on the left midclavicular line and angle toward the xiphoid process. The pericardium will light up. It will appear as a crown in the lower left chest.
   3. Pneumomediastinum. Differentiating between a pneumomediastinum and a pneumothorax is difficult. Cardiac pulsations within the area of lucency suggest air in the mediastinum.
   4. Hydrothorax and chylothorax. Abnormal accumulation of fluid in the pleural space will light up.
IV. Complications
   A. Burns and thermal blisters from the light source. Limit light source contact time.
   B. False-positive and false-negative results. Limit these by using a sufficiently bright light source and dimming the room lights. **Individuals with deutan color vision** (red-green blindness) may have difficulty with this technique.
      1. False positive. Pneumothorax example: subcutaneous air or edema, severe pulmonary interstitial emphysema, lobar emphysema, pneumomediastinum, large stomach air bubble.
      2. False negative. Pneumothorax example: small air leak, thick chest wall with edema, thick skin folds on a large baby, darkly pigmented skin, room not dark enough.

Selected References

Buck JR, Weintraub WH, Coran AG, Wyman M, Kuhns LR. Fiberoptic transillumination: a new tool for the pediatric surgeon. *J Pediatr Surg.* 1977;12(3):451–463.

Donn SM, Faix RG. Transillumination in neonatal diagnosis. *Clin Perinatol.* 1985;12(1):3–20.

41 Venous Access: Intraosseous Infusion

I. Indications. **Intraosseous (IO) infusion** is used for emergency vascular access (fluids and medications) when other access methods have been attempted and cannot be quickly established or have failed. The **umbilical vein is the preferred route** in a hospital setting, but IO access can be considered if rapid intravenous access is essential and the operator is not experienced in umbilical vein catheter (UVC) placement.
II. Equipment. Povidone-iodine solution, 4 × 4 sterile gauze pads, sterile towels, gloves, IO device (devices approved for newborns are available; Table 41–1), syringe with saline flush, IV fluid, and infusion setup.
III. Procedure
   A. Contraindications include bone diseases (eg, osteogenesis imperfecta, osteopetrosis), infection of the overlying skin, presence of a fracture, and thermal injury to the overlying skin. There is limited data but IO seems safe in preterm infants.

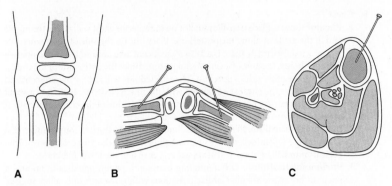

FIGURE 41–1. Technique of intraosseous infusion. (A) Anterior view of sites on the tibia and the fibula. (B) Sagittal view. (C) Cross-section through the tibia. (*Reproduced with permission from Hodge D. Intraosseous infusion: a review.* Pediatr Emerg Care. *1985;1:215.*)

    B. **The proximal tibia (anteromedial surface) is the preferred site in the infant** (vs the sternum in adults) and is described here (Figure 41–1). The intramedullary vessel in the tibial marrow empties into the popliteal vein and into the femoral vein. The other 2 most common sites used in newborns are the **distal femur** and **distal tibia**.

    C. **Select the area in the midline on the flat surface of the anterior tibia, 1–2 cm below the tibial tuberosity.** Some recommend inserting a minimum of 10 mm (1 cm) distal to the tibial tuberosity: this avoids epiphyseal growth plate injury, and the thinner cortex here ensures an easier insertion.

    D. **Restrain the patient's lower leg** and place a small sandbag or IV bag behind the knee for support.

    E. **Clean the area** with povidone-iodine solution. Sterile drapes can be placed around the area.

    F. **Pain management.** Lidocaine (0.5–1%) can be injected into the skin, soft tissue, and periosteum, but this is optional as this is usually an emergency procedure.

    G. **IO needle insertion.** (See specific devices in Table 41–1.) Insertion site should be at least 10 mm distal to tibial tuberosity to avoid epiphyseal growth plate.

Table 41–1. COMPARISON OF INTRAOSSEOUS DEVICES USED IN NEONATOLOGY

IO Device	Features
Butterfly needle or standard IV catheter over needle	Simple needle, 18 to 20 gauge (***Note:*** not recommended; absence of stylet increases incidence of obstruction by bony spicules)
Spinal needle[a]	Straight needle with stylet, 18–20 gauge
Bone marrow biopsy needle[a]	Hollow needle with handle and stylet, 18 gauge
Intraosseous needle	Specialized handles and stylets with short needle shafts, 18 gauge
EZ-IO Pediatric (Vidacare, San Antonio, TX)	Reusable lithium-powered drill; 15-gauge needle; length 15 mm for infants 3–39 kg
Bone Injection Gun, Pediatric (B.I.G., WaisMed, Houston Texas)	Automatic (spring-loaded) device; uses the "position and press" mechanism; 18 gauge <12 years; dial in age for needle depth

[a]Best for emergency use where specifically designed IO device is not available.
Data form Tobias JA, Ross AK. Intraosseous infusions: a review for the anesthesiologist with a focus on pediatric use. *Anesth Analg.* 2010;110:391–401. www.vidacare.com. Accessed July 2012.

1. Spinal, bone marrow biopsy, or intraosseous needle. Insert the needle at a 10-to 15-degree angle toward the foot to avoid the growth plate. Advance the needle until a lack of resistance is felt (usually no more than 1 cm is necessary), at which point entry into the marrow space should have occurred. *Note:* It is best not to place the other hand under the tibia for stabilization, as excessive force may cause the needle to pass through the bone and exit on the other side.

2. B.I.G. Pediatric device. Dial the age to get the appropriate needle depth. Position device at 90 degrees to the skin and hold firmly with one hand while the other hand pulls out the safety latch. It uses a "position and press" mechanism with a spring-loaded device that penetrates the cortex when the button is pushed. No additional force is needed other than holding the device firmly against the skin. Manufacturer-recommended site for infants is 0.5 inches medial and distal to the tibial tuberosity.

3. EZ-IO Pediatric. (Only recommended for infants >3 kg.) Device operates like a drill. It has a tip that rotates into the IO space at a preset depth. Once the needle enters the space, the stylet is withdrawn and a metal catheter remains with a Luer lock attachment. Manufacturer recommends removal within 24 hours.

H. Once the device is in place, remove the stylet and tape needle in place. Bone marrow aspiration for laboratory studies can be done, if needed. Bone marrow aspirates can be sent for chemistry, pH, Pco_2, hemoglobin, culture and sensitivity (C&S), blood type, and cross match. Even if marrow can't be aspirated, the IO needle can be used if it flushes without extravasation. If appropriate, secure the needle to the skin with tape to prevent it from dislodging.

I. Attach the needle to IV fluids and infuse at same rate used for IV route. Hypertonic and alkaline solutions should be diluted 1:2 with normal saline. Administer at the same rate as that for an IV infusion. Any fluid or medication that can be used via a peripheral IV can be used via the IO route (Table 41–2).

Table 41–2. **FLUIDS AND MEDICATIONS THAT HAVE BEEN ADMINISTERED BY THE INTRAOSSEOUS ROUTE**

IV Fluids

Blood and blood products (fresh frozen plasma, whole blood)	Crystalloids (lactated Ringer's, sodium chloride solutions)	Dextrose solutions (D50 should be diluted)	Colloids

Medications

Adenosine	Aminophylline	Amiodarone	Anesthetic agents
Antibiotics (various)	Atracurium	Atropine	Calcium chloride and
Contrast media (dilute if possible)	Dobutamine	Diazepam	gluconate
	Heparin	Dopamine	Diazoxide
Digoxin	Lidocaine	Fentanyl	Furosemide
Epinephrine	Methylprednisolone	Insulin	Labetalol
Levarterenol	Pancuronium	Lorazepam	Magnesium sulfate
Naloxone	Succinylcholine	Midazolam	Morphine
Potassium chloride	Vecuronium	Phenobarbital	Phenytoin
Sodium bicarbonate (should be diluted)		Propranolol	Rocuronium
Vasopressin		Thiamine	Thiopental

Data from www.vidacare.com. Accessed July 2012.

J. **Confirm appropriate IO needle placement** by aspiration of blood or bone marrow and also by the free gravity flow of crystalloid without extravasation. Ultrasound confirmation can be obtained, but a plain radiograph confirms position and is usually obtained to rule out fracture. Because of the risk of a fracture, a follow-up radiograph should be obtained in all infants in whom IO was attempted.

K. **IO vascular access should optimally be used for <2 hours** to minimize the risk of infectious complications, with some devices U.S. Food and Drug Administration (FDA) approved for longer use. When completed, withdraw the needle, apply pressure, and dress the site.

L. **With unsuccessful IO placement** do not repeat attempts at the same site or use the same site for 1–2 days.

IV. Complications

A. **Most common is extravasation.** If giving caustic/vasoconstrictive medications, such as dopamine, and extravasation occurs, tissue damage is possible. Subperiosteal infiltration of fluid can also occur.

B. **Infections.** Localized cellulitis, subcutaneous abscess, periostitis, and sepsis have all been reported. Osteomyelitis is rare (<0.6%). To prevent osteomyelitis, hypertonic and alkaline solutions and all medications should be diluted. Sterile technique is important and if compromised consider antibiotic coverage.

C. **Clotting of bone marrow.** Results in loss of vascular access.

D. **Iatrogenic bone fracture.** Radiograph confirmation of the needle should be done to confirm position and rule out fracture (tibial fracture is most common).

E. **Compartment syndrome.** Due to prolonged infusion and extravasation. The leaking fluid collects in the spaces between the muscles of the leg.

F. **Blasts in the peripheral blood.** These have been noted after IO infusions.

G. **Fat embolism.** Much less likely in infants than adults. Before the age of 5 years, the intramedullary space consists mainly of red marrow, which is more vascular and has a lower fat component.

H. **Bone growth concerns have been ruled out.** Studies have shown there is no long-term effect on tibial growth after IO infusion with a properly placed IO needle trocar. At the tibia, IO blood transfusions may result in transient radiologic changes but do not impact bone growth.

I. **Needle dislodgement.**

Selected Reference

Tobias JA, Ross AK. Intraosseous infusions: a review for the anesthesiologist with a focus on pediatric use. *Anesth Analg.* 2010;110:391–401.

42 Venous Access: Percutaneous Central Venous Catheterization

I. **Indications.** Percutaneous central venous catheterization (also called **peripherally inserted central catheter [PICC]**) involves inserting a long small-gauge catheter into a peripheral vein and threading it into a central venous location. The catheter is placed peripherally but is longer than the usual intravenous (IV) device, and hence its tip lies in a more central location. The catheter can be placed in large vessels such as the cephalic and basilic veins in the arm or the saphenous vein in the leg.

A. When IV access is anticipated for an extended period of time.

B. In low birthweight infants when it is anticipated that full enteral feedings will not be achieved within a short period.

C. For the delivery of fluids, nutritional solutions, and medications when other venous access is not acceptable (eg, hypertonic IV solutions).

II. **Equipment**

A. **Basic supplies.** Cap, mask, sterile gloves, a sterile gown, transparent dressing, and sterile tape strips (for stabilization of the catheter), a sterile tray (multipurpose tray or umbilical artery catheter tray), povidone-iodine solution or locally approved bactericidal skin prep, a sterile tourniquet (or a rubber band), saline flush solution, and a T-connector.

B. **Percutaneous catheter device.** Two types of insertion devices are available: silastic (silicone) catheters (usually without introducer wire) and polyurethane catheters (usually with an introducer wire). Several sizes and double-lumen catheters are also available. National Association of Neonatal Nurses (NANN) guidelines recommend the following catheter sizes: infants <2500 g, 1.1–2F (28- to 23-gauge catheter); infants ≥2500 g, 1.9–3F (26- to 20-gauge catheter).

III. **Procedure.** There are 2 commonly used types of catheters, and some of the smaller ones come with guide wires. The procedure varies if a guide wire is or is not present because the guide wire needs to be removed before blood is withdrawn or the catheter is flushed. **It is suggested that the person placing the catheter should be familiar with the specific manufacturer's guidelines for placement of the catheters used. Special training is suggested before the placement of these devices.** A review of the NANN *Guideline for Peripherally Inserted Central Catheters* (see Selected Reference) is also suggested and is helpful.

A. **Obtain informed consent and perform a time out.** Gather the equipment and assemble the tray with the catheter using sterile technique.

B. **Select a suitable vein in the arm, such as the cephalic or basilic vein, or use the saphenous vein in the leg.** (See Figure 43–1.) Position the infant so that the selected vessel is accessible. Restrain the infant to prevent contamination of the sterile field with the other extremities. It is helpful to have a second person available to help stabilize the infant's position, to help maintain sterility, and to offer a pacifier and comfort measures.

C. **Determine the length of the catheter.** Measure the distance between the insertion site and the desired catheter tip location. (For catheters placed in the upper extremities, measure to the level of the superior vena cava or the right atrium; for catheters placed in the lower extremities, measure to the inferior vena cava.) Catheters are typically marked at 5-cm increments.

D. **Put on the cap and mask, wash your hands, and then put on the sterile gown and gloves.** If others are helping or observing at the bedside, anyone within about 3 ft of the bedside should don a cap and mask and observe maximal sterile barrier precautions. Anyone assisting and scrubbed in should have full cap, mask, gown, and gloves.

E. **Prepare the area of insertion.** This should be done with a triple prep of povidone-iodine solution or unit-approved bactericidal agent, and allow the solution to dry. Some catheters warn against using alcohol due to degradation of the catheters. (Consult your manufacturer's guidelines.) *Note:* Catheters that do not contain a guide wire require flushing with saline before being inserted into the vessel (see specific product package insert).

F. **Pain. The American Academy of Pediatrics recommends topical anesthetics** for IV catheter insertion (topical anesthetics proved not to be effective in one study for PICC placement). Other nonpharmacologic pain prevention and relief techniques can be used. Other recommendations include systemic opiate-based analgesia.

G. **Have an assistant apply the tourniquet if using a nonsterile tourniquet.**

H. **Place sterile drapes over most of the patient.** Allow for maximal sterile barrier precaution, a large sterile field around the area of insertion, and cover most of the infant.

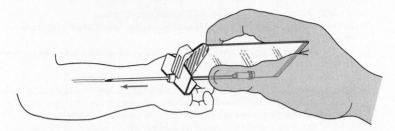

FIGURE 42–1. Technique for insertion of the introducer needle into the vein.

I. Remove the plastic protector from the introducer needle.

J. Insert the introducer needle into the vein. Confirm entry into the vein by observing for a flashback of blood in the needle. Do not advance the introducer needle once the flashback (or the blood) has been noted, or you may puncture through the other side of the vessel (Figure 42–1).

K. Release the tourniquet.

L. Hold the introducer needle to maintain the position in the vein. Slowly advance the catheter through the introducer needle with a pair of smooth forceps or fingers into the vein. **Do not use a hemostat or ridged forceps because it may damage the catheter** (Figure 42–2).

M. Once the catheter has been advanced to the premeasured location, stabilize the catheter by placing a finger over the vessel where the catheter has been introduced (~1–2 cm above the tip of the introducer needle). Then carefully withdraw the introducer needle completely out of the skin. The area may bleed around the catheter. Hold sterile gauze to the area until the bleeding resolves (Figure 42–3).

N. Separate the introducer needle from the catheter by using the technique specified by the manufacturer of the needle. Grasp the opposite halves of the introducer needle, and carefully peel each half apart until the needle splits completely (Figure 42–4).

O. While removing the needle, occasionally the catheter also partially pulls out of the vein and has to be readvanced to the desired location.

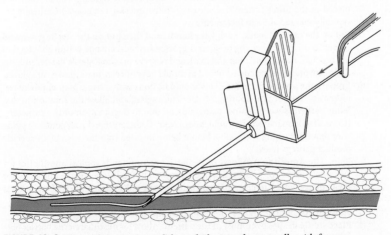

FIGURE 42–2. The catheter is inserted through the introducer needle with forceps.

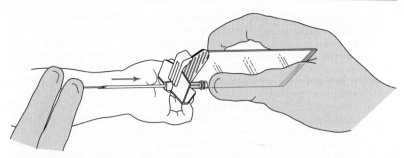

FIGURE 42–3. The catheter is stabilized while withdrawing the needle.

P. If a guide wire is present, remove the wire slowly and steadily from the catheter. Do not attempt to reintroduce the wire once it has been removed from the catheter.

Q. As the introducer wire is withdrawn, a blood return may or may not be observed in the catheter, depending on the size of catheter. Smaller catheters are less likely to have blood return. Using a 3-mL syringe, aspirate the blood through the catheter until the blood reaches the hub. (Slightly more pressure is necessary to withdraw blood through the very small diameter of the catheter; however, if blood is returning, the catheter is patent and in the intravascular system.) Once the blood has been aspirated back to the catheter hub, place a T-connector and flush the catheter with normal saline. (Because of the small diameter of the catheter, it will take slightly more pressure on the syringe to aspirate the blood and to flush solution through the catheter; however, do not use excessive pressure when flushing the catheter because it can cause catheter rupture or fragmentation with possible embolization.) *Note:* Practice the flushing technique on another catheter before attempting insertion and flushing of a catheter in a patient if you are unfamiliar with this type of catheter.

R. Secure the catheter to the extremity by placing a sterile tape strip over the catheter at the insertion site to anchor the catheter. Curl the remaining external catheter, making sure there are no kinks, and cover with a sterile transparent dressing. **Do not suture the catheter in place.**

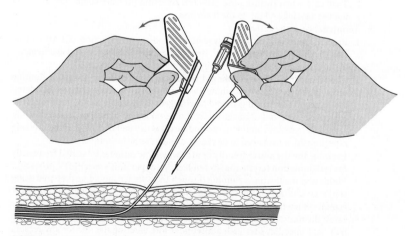

FIGURE 42–4. Technique for removing the needle wing assembly of most catheters.

S. **Connect the IV fluid.** New fresh sterile IV fluids should be connected to the new catheter. **Heparin** should be used. Cochrane review recommends prophylactic use of **heparin** in peripherally placed central venous lines because it allows a higher number of infants to complete their therapy, and reduces the risk of catheter occlusion. The American College of Chest Physicians Evidence-Based Clinical Guidelines (2012) recommends UFH continuous infusion 0.5 U/kg/h to maintain patency in neonates with central venous access devices.

T. **Obtain a radiograph to verify the central catheter tip location.** Most catheters are radiopaque and therefore can be seen on radiograph; however, because of its small size, it may be difficult to assess the location of the tip. Some manufacturers suggest injecting contrast medium (~0.3–1 mL) through the catheter just before the radiograph to assess catheter tip placement. *Note:* Ideally, the position of the catheter tip should be in a central location in the superior vena cava for upper body insertions and the thoracic inferior vena cava for lower extremity insertions. However, if the catheter has a blood return and is patent but could not be advanced to a central location, it may be pulled back in the proximal portion of the extremity and used as a midline catheter. Hypertonic solutions should not be infused through a midline catheter.

U. **When placing the PICC in the lower extremity.** A cross-table lateral x-ray should be done to assess the proper placement of the catheter in the inferior vena cava.

V. **Chart the size and the length of catheter that has been inserted** and the position of the catheter on radiograph.

W. **Precautions**
  1. **Do not measure the infant's blood pressure on the extremity containing the percutaneous catheter.** Occlusion or damage to the catheter may occur.
  2. **Do not trim the catheter before placement unless specified by the manufacturer.** A rough cut end may increase thrombus formation.
  3. **Do not use a hemostat or ribbed forceps to advance the catheter** because it could damage the catheter.
  4. **When inserting the catheter through the introducer needle, do not pull the catheter back through the introducer needle.** Doing so could sever the catheter.
  5. **Do not suture the catheter itself.** The catheter is very small, and a suture would occlude it.
  6. **Do not attempt to infuse blood products or viscous solutions through the catheter.** This could cause the catheter to become occluded.
  7. **Take care when flushing the catheter.** Excessive pressure could rupture it. Do not use a syringe <3 mL to the flush line.

X. **Maintenance of the catheter**
  1. **Prevention of central line–associated bloodstream infection (CLABSI)** (see later) begins before insertion with strict guidelines for placement and maintenance of the catheters. Strict hand washing technique is also necessary.
  2. **The transparent dressing should remain in place over the catheter.** Routine dressing changes are not recommended because of the risk of tearing or dislodging the catheter. The dressing should be changed, using sterile technique, only if the current dressing has drainage under it or is no longer occlusive. Assess dressing each shift to assess condition, making sure it is dry and occlusive. If the dressing is peeling up, it may need to be changed using sterile technique.
  3. **Examine the site and extremity or area where the catheter is located frequently** for inflammation (erythema) or tenderness (as per unit's specific IV protocol).
  4. **Fluids and medications running through the catheter should be prepared using sterile conditions and heparinized** according to hospital or unit protocol for central catheters.
  5. **Limit the number of times the catheter is accessed to decrease infection.** Clean hubs and injection sites with antiseptic before entering the line for any reason. Research suggests that the hub is a common site of contamination and subsequent

infection. The number of times the hub is opened and the duration of catheter use are both related to the presence of catheter associated infections.

Y. **Removal of the catheter.** The catheter can remain in place for several weeks. Several studies have shown an increase in the infection rate after ~2–3 weeks.

1. Gently remove the occlusive dressing from the extremity and the catheter, being careful not to tear the dressing from the catheter.

2. Grasp the catheter tubing near the insertion site, and gently pull the catheter in a continuous movement. If resistance is met, do not apply force and do not stretch the catheter. Doing so could cause the catheter to rupture.

3. Apply a moist, warm compress to the area above the catheter tract for several minutes, and then reattempt removal of the catheter. If catheter is still resistant, consult NANN Practice Guidelines (see Selected Reference). It may take several hours to days to remove some catheters.

4. Once the catheter is removed, inspect and measure it to make sure the entire catheter was removed from the vein. Compare this length with the initial measurement at the time of placement. Cover the area with a sterile dressing.

IV. **Complications.** Only the most common complications are listed. Refer to the manufacturer's enclosures for a list of further complications. Special training is needed for the placement of these devices.

A. **Infiltration.** As with any intravascular device, infiltration is a risk and the area will swell. Because the catheters are longer than peripheral IV catheters, it is necessary to assess for swelling in the area where the tip of the catheter is located, not just at the insertion site.

B. **Catheter occlusion.** This catheter is extremely small, fragile, and easily occluded during taping or if the infant bends the extremity containing the catheter. When securing the catheter with the dressing and tape, avoid kinking the catheter; doing so could create an occlusion. If resistance is met when flushing the catheter, do not attempt to flush it any further. Doing so could result in catheter rupture with possible embolization.

C. **Infection or sepsis. A catheter-associated bloodstream infection is the most common health care–associated infection in the NICU. The prevention of CLABSI is extremely important.** Each unit should develop a strategy to track CLABSI and develop strategies for prevention, including during placement, and maintenance of the line. Refer to NANN guidelines (see Selected Reference) and Centers for Disease Control and Prevention guidelines for risk reduction strategies. Infants requiring a PICC are at an increased risk for nosocomial infections (poor skin integrity, immature immune system, multiple invasive procedures, exposure to multiple pieces of equipment). PICC infection appears to be related to the length of time the catheter remains in place; catheters indwelling for >3 weeks appear to be at greater risk for catheter-related sepsis. The catheter should only be accessed when necessary to change fluids and limit the breaks in the line. Coagulase-negative Staphylococci account for more than 50% of infections. Other pathogens include gram negatives (20%), *Staphylococcus aureus* (4–9%), *Enterococcus* (3–5%), and *Candida* (10%). Paired samples should be drawn (catheter and a peripheral vein) from neonates with suspected sepsis to isolate a potentially infected catheter. Treatment of neonates with suspected CLABSI should be treated with broad-spectrum antibiotics to cover both gram-positive and gram-negative organisms.

D. **Air embolism.** Because these catheters are in a central location, air embolism is a risk. The catheter should be cared for like any central catheter. Special precautions should be taken to avoid air in the line.

E. **Catheter embolus.** Do not pull the catheter back through the introducer needle, which could cause the catheter to sever.

F. **Catheter migration/malposition.** Catheters can move after initial placement. Assess the catheter position with an x-ray 2–3 days after insertion and periodically each week (some twice a week) thereafter to assess position after initial placement. (Coordinate with other needed x-rays patient may need, if possible).

G. Pericardial effusions are a rare but life-threatening complication of percutaneous central venous catheters. Keep a high index of clinical suspicion in a neonate who has a central line and suddenly has cardiovascular collapse that does not respond to resuscitation, resistance to external cardiac compressions, and has no air leak by thoracic transillumination. It is more common with lines in the right atrium, and the median time to occurrence is 3 days after percutaneous central catheter insertion. Chest radiograph may not be diagnostic; echocardiography is diagnostic but may delay treatment. Mortality is high. See Chapter 38.

Selected References

Monagle P, Chan AK, Goldenberg NA, et al. Antithrombotic therapy in neonates and children: Antithrombotic Therapy and Prevention of Thrombosis. 9th ed. American College of Chest Physicians Evidence-Based Clinical Practice Guidelines. *Chest.* 2012;141 (suppl 2):e737S.

Pettit J, Wyckoff MM. *Peripherally Inserted Central Catheters: Guideline for Practice.* 2nd ed. Glenview, IL: National Association of Neonatal Nurses (NANN); 2007.

Shah PS, Shah VS. Continuous heparin infusion to prevent thrombosis and catheter occlusion in neonates with peripherally placed percutaneous central venous catheters. *Cochrane Database Syst Rev.* 2008;(2). DOI:10.1002/14651858.CD002772.

43 Venous Access: Peripheral Intravenous Catheterization

I. Indications
  A. Vascular access in nonemergent and emergent situations for the administration of intravenous (IV) fluids and medications
  B. Administration of parenteral nutrition
  C. Administration of blood and blood products
  D. Blood sampling (only after initial IV placement)
II. Equipment
  A. Basic. Armboard, adhesive tape, tourniquet, alcohol swabs, normal saline for flush (0.5% normal saline if hypernatremia is a concern), povidone-iodine solution/swabs, transparent dressing material; appropriate IV fluid and connecting tubing, transillumination equipment (optional). In-line filters are sometimes used.
  B. Intravenous catheter. Safety-engineered (shielded) devices preferred: 23- to 25-gauge scalp vein ("butterfly") needle or a 22- to 24-gauge catheter-over-needle. Use at least 24-gauge for blood transfusion.
III. Procedure
  A. Scalp vein ("butterfly") needle
    1. Select the vein. Neonatal IV sites are shown in Figure 43–1. It is useful to select the "Y" or crotch region of the vein, where 2 veins join together for the insertion. To help identify the vein, use palpation, visualization, and transillumination. The dorsum of the hand is the best choice to preserve the sites for potential central venous catheters (cephalic, brachial, greater saphenous veins) if needed. Avoid areas of flexion.
       a. Scalp. Supratrochlear, superficial temporal, or posterior auricular vein (last resort).

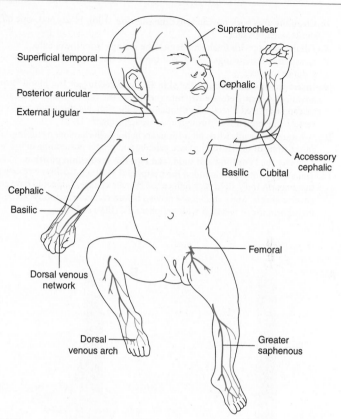

FIGURE 43–1. Frequently used sites for venous access in the neonate.

    b. **Back of the hand.** Preferred site using the dorsal venous network. This includes the dorsal metacarpal veins.

    c. **Forearm.** At the wrist area is the cephalic and basilic vein. Median antebrachial or accessory cephalic vein are higher up on the forearm.

    d. **Foot.** Dorsal venous arch.

    e. **Antecubital fossa.** Basilic or cubital veins.

    f. **Ankle.** Greater and small saphenous veins.

2. **Shave the area if a scalp vein is to be used.** Try to place needle behind the hair line in the event of cosmetic scarring.

3. **Restrain the extremity on an armboard.** Or have an assistant help hold the extremity or the head.

4. **Pain management. The American Academy of Pediatrics (AAP) recommends** topical anesthetics (eg, eutectic mixture of lidocaine and prilocaine [EMLA]) applied 30 minutes before the procedure. Oral sucrose/glucose, pacifier, swaddling, and other nonpharmacologic methods can be used for pain reduction.

5. **Apply a tourniquet proximal to the puncture site.** If a scalp vein is to be used, a rubber band can be placed around the head, just above the eyebrows.

6. Clean the area with povidone-iodine solution. Allow to dry and wipe off with sterile water or saline.
7. Fill the tubing with flush and detach the syringe from the needle.
8. Grasp the plastic wings. Using your free index finger, **pull the skin taut** to help stabilize the vein.
9. Insert the needle through the skin in the direction of the blood flow and advance ~0.5 cm before entry into the side of the vessel. Alternatively, the vessel can be entered directly after puncture of the skin, but this often results in the vessel being punctured "through and through" (Figure 43–2).
10. Advance the needle when blood appears in the flash chamber or tubing. **Gently inject some of the flush** to ensure patency and proper positioning of the needle.
11. Connect the IV tubing and fluid, and tape the needle into position.
12. Heparin is not recommended for peripheral IV lines. Cochrane review states that heparin in IV fluid may reduce the IV tube changes but could have serious adverse effects. More studies are needed before recommendations can be made on heparin use in neonates with peripheral IV (PIV) catheters.

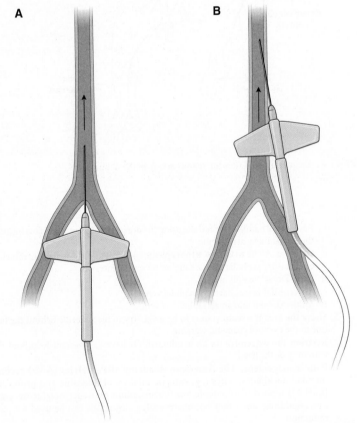

FIGURE 43–2. Two techniques for entering the vein for IV access in the neonate. (A) Direct puncture. (B) Side entry.

B. Catheter-over-needle assembly
   1. Follow steps 1–6 for the scalp vein needle.
   2. Fill the needle and the hub with flush via syringe, then remove the syringe.
   3. Pull the skin taut to stabilize the vein.
   4. Puncture the skin then enter the side of the vein in a separate motion. Alternately, the skin and the vein can be entered in one motion.
   5. Carefully advance the needle until a flash of blood appears in the hub.
   6. Activate the shield to sheathe the needle and advance the catheter. Injecting a small amount of flush solution into the vein before advancing the catheter may help.
   7. Remove the tourniquet and gently inject some normal saline into the catheter to verify patency and position.
   8. Connect the IV tubing and fluid and tape securely in place using transparent dressing.

IV. Complications
   A. Hematoma (most common complication) at the site can often be managed effectively by gentle pressure.
   B. Phlebitis (inflammation of the vein) risk increases the longer a catheter is left in place, especially if >72–96 hours. Sites are rotated at 72- to 96-hour intervals to decrease phlebitis and infection.
   C. Vasospasm rarely occurs when veins are accessed and usually resolves spontaneously.
   D. Infection risk can be minimized by using sterile technique, including antiseptic preparation. The risk of infection rises after 72 hours. Rarely associated with bloodstream infection.
   E. Embolus (air or clot). Never allow the end of the catheter to be open to the air, and make sure that the IV catheter is flushed free of air bubbles before it is connected. Don't use excessive force when flushing.
   F. Infiltration/extravasation injury results from the leakage of fluid from a vein into the surrounding tissue, usually due to improper catheter placement or damage to the vessel. **Infiltration** of nonvesicant fluid does not cause necrosis, but a large volume can cause compression of the neurovascular structures, leading to compartment syndrome. **Extravasation** can cause a mild injury or severe necrosis (blisters, tissue injury, and necrosis) and may result in the need for skin grafting. To limit this, confirm intravascular placement of the catheter with the flush solution before the catheter is connected to the IV tubing. Infiltration often means that the catheter needs to be removed. Avoid hyperosmolar solutions for peripheral infusion, and use caution with dopamine, which can cause constriction. Vialon catheter material was found to reduce the risk of infiltration (35% in infants <1500 g) as compared to Teflon. See Chapter 31 for details on management of infiltration and extravasation.
   G. Calcification of subcutaneous tissue secondary to infusion of a calcium-containing solution.
   H. Fluid overload, electrolyte problems (hypernatremia).

Selected Reference

Shah PS, Ng E, Sinha AK. Heparin for prolonging peripheral intravenous catheter use in neonates. *Cochrane Database Syst Rev.* 2005;(4). DOI:10.1002/14651858.CD002774.pub2.

44 Venous Access: Umbilical Vein Catheterization

I. **Indications**

   A. **Immediate, primarily postnatal access** for intravenous (IV) fluids or emergency medications.

   B. **Central venous pressure monitoring** (if UVC passed through the ductus venosus).

   C. **Exchange or partial exchange transfusion** (catheter tip should not be in the intrahepatic venous system or the portal system).

   D. **Long-term central venous access** in extremely low birthweight infants or sick infants for administration of IV fluids, total parenteral nutrition, medications.

   E. **Delivery of blood and blood products.**

   F. **Other reported indications** include general venous access in difficult peripheral IV access, administration of fluids and total parenteral nutrition, infusion of hypertonic solutions (>12.5% only if catheter tip in inferior vena cava), infusion of vasoactive drugs, antibiotics, and medications.

   G. **Secondary aid in the diagnosis** of cardiovascular or other anomalies by an unusual course of the umbilical venous catheter or the blood gas samples are suspicious.

   1. **Congenital diaphragmatic hernia.** Umbilical venous catheter (UVC) is left of the midline because of the anomalous positioning of the liver in the chest.

   2. **Persistent left superior vena cava.** Diagnosed by the path of a UVC. UVC catheter extended beyond the lung (it had entered the persistent left superior vena cava and entered the left jugular vein).

   3. **Congenital absence of the ductus venosus.** This can cause an abnormal path of UVC. (Caudal loop is seen on radiograph in a UVC.)

   4. **Infracardiac total anomalous pulmonary venous return.** Diagnosed by high partial pressure of oxygen in a UVC below the diaphragm.

II. **Equipment**

   A. **Basic.** Identical to umbilical artery catheterization (see Chapter 24, page 236).

   B. **UV catheters**

   1. **Types. Single lumen:** 2.5F, 3.5F, 5.0F; **dual lumen:** 3.5F, 5.0F; **triple lumen:** 5.0F, 8.0F.

   2. **Size guideline. Preterm:** 3.5F; term and late preterm: 5F. Other guidelines: 3.5F or 5F catheter <3.5 kg, 5F or 8F >3.5 kg. An 8F catheter is recommended for exchange transfusion or a large volume replacement. **Dual-lumen catheters** are sometimes recommended in infants <28 weeks and <1000 g, in infants that need inotropes or insulin, and any critically ill neonates such as persistent pulmonary hypertension or meconium aspiration syndrome.

III. **Procedure**

   A. **Important UVC tips**

   1. **There is only 1 umbilical vein, and it remains open and viable for cannulation for up to 1 week after birth.** The umbilical vein carries oxygenated blood from the placenta to the fetus. The UVC passes into the umbilical vein through the umbilicus and follows this path: junction of the right and left portal vein in the liver, the ductus venosus, crosses at the level of the right and left hepatic vein, and enters the inferior vena cava up to the junction of the inferior vena cava and right atrium.

   2. **In an emergency postnatal situation (delivery room).** The UVC can be rapidly inserted only until adequate blood return is obtained (usually 2–4 cm in a term infant, less in preterm) as an emergency venous access. Resuscitation medications, volume, and blood can be given.

3. Cochrane review does not make any recommendations on using **single- versus multiple-lumen catheters.** Double-lumen catheters decreased the number of additional venous lines during the first week of life, but double-lumen catheters broke, leaked, and clogged more (smaller diameter). No difference in catheter placement difficulty, misplacement, catheter-related infections or blood clots, or rate of infant mortality was noted. More studies are needed; consider using the least amount of lumens required.

4. Suspect cardiac tamponade in a neonate with a UVC (even if properly placed) who develops a sudden unexplained clinical deterioration in cardiopulmonary status. Urgent echocardiography or pericardiocentesis should be considered. Routine radiography to verify tip placement is recommended by some to check for tip migration.

5. Catheter duration recommendations. Centers for Disease Control and Prevention, 14 days; others sources: 7 days, up to 28 days if absolutely necessary. The American Academy of Pediatrics (AAP) states catheters can be used up to 14 days if used aseptically.

6. Heparin use in UVCs is *controversial*. The literature is conflicting since there are recommendations for and against its use. The majority of NICUS use heparin in UVCs. Our recommendation: heparin (lowest dose at least 0.25 U/mL) in all fluids via the UVC. Use of heparin flushes only are not effective in maintaining patency. The American College of Chest Physicians Evidence-Based Clinical Practice Guidelines study does recommend heparin in central venous access devices. They recommend UFH continuous infusion at 0.5 U/kg/h to maintain CVAD patency.

7. Blood cultures can be obtained from the UVC right after placement (venipuncture preferred).

8. Ultrasound guidance. Faster and results in fewer manipulations and x-rays as compared with conventional placement.

B. Determine the length of UVC needed. There are multiple methods reported; refer to institutional guidelines if possible.

1. Dunn method. Measures the shoulder-umbilicus length and uses a nomogram to determine the insertion length. This method was more accurate than the Shukla method in one study. The catheter tip should be placed between the level of the diaphragm and the left atrium on the graph (Figure 44–1).

2. Shukla method. Based on birthweight (BW):
   a. Modified BW equation. UAC line calculation divided by 2 + 1 cm (**UAC**: BW in kilograms × 3 + 9).
   b. Exact BW equation. 1.5 × BW in kilograms + 5.6.

3. Measure from the xiphoid to the umbilicus and add 0.5–1.0 cm. This number indicates how far the venous catheter should be inserted.

4. UVC length (in centimeters) = shoulder (distal end of clavicle) to umbilicus length × 0.66

C. Pain management. Since the umbilical cord is denervated, pain may be minimal. No formal anesthesia is usually needed if you avoid using a hemostat to grab the skin or avoid putting sutures through the skin around the umbilicus. Use any nonpharmacologic pain prevention and relief techniques if possible.

D. Technique

1. Place the infant supine with a diaper wrapped around both legs for stabilization.

2. Prepare the area around the umbilicus with povidone-iodine solution. Use a gown, gloves, and mask.

3. Prepare the tray as you would for the umbilical artery catheterization. (See Chapter 24, page 239.) Fill the lumen with infusion solution so it is air free.

4. Place sterile drapes, leaving the umbilical area exposed. Use gown, mask, and gloves.

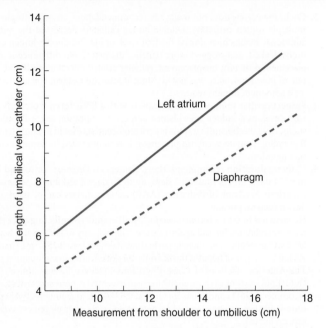

FIGURE 44–1. The umbilical venous catheter is placed above the level of the diaphragm and below the left atrium. Determine the shoulder-umbilical length as for the umbilical artery catheter. Use this number and determine the catheter length using the graph. Add the length of the umbilical stump to the length of the catheter. The catheter length should be between the diaphragm and left atrium on the graph. *(Data from Dunn PM: Localization of the umbilical catheter by post-mortem measurement.* Arch Dis Child. *1966;41:69.)*

5. Tie a piece of umbilical tape or a purse string suture around the base of the umbilicus.
6. Cut the excess umbilical cord with a scalpel or scissors, leaving a stump of ~0.5–1.0 cm. Identify the umbilical vein. The umbilical vein is thin-walled, larger than the 2 arteries, and close to the periphery of the stump (see Figure 24–3B, page 240.)
7. Grasp the end of the umbilicus with the curved hemostat to hold it upright and steady. (Figure 44–2A).
8. Open and dilate the umbilical vein with the forceps. If a later insertion, remove any visible clots in the lumen with the forceps. Once the vein is sufficiently dilated, **insert the catheter** (Figure 44–2B) the desired length. Direct the catheter toward the head/cephalad with a hand providing liver immobilization, as this improves the rate of insertion of the UVC into the inferior vena cava. Some units use **ultrasound to help guide the catheter**, and this has been found to reduce complications during UVC insertion.
9. Occasionally, a catheter enters the portal vein. (Figure 44–3) Suspect portal vein entry if you meet resistance and cannot advance the catheter the desired distance or if you detect a "bobbing" motion of the catheter. Several options are available to correct this.
   a. Withdraw the catheter 2–3 cm, rotate it, and try to reinsert it.
   b. Try injecting flush as you advance the catheter. Sometimes this makes it easier to pass the catheter through the ductus venosus.

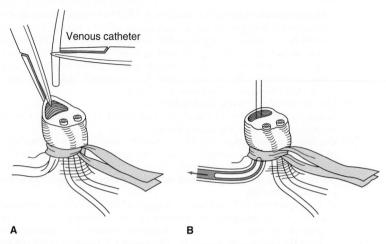

FIGURE 44–2. Umbilical vein catheterization. (A) The umbilical stump is held upright before the catheter is inserted. (B) The catheter is passed into the umbilical vein.

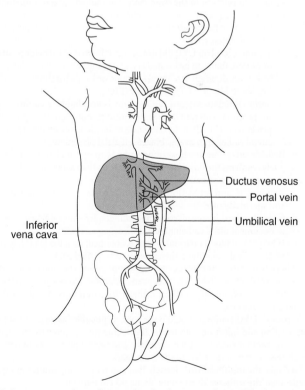

FIGURE 44–3. Anatomic relationships used in the placement of an umbilical venous catheter.

   c. **Double-catheter technique** is based on the fact that once the first catheter occupies the wrong vessel, the second catheter will have to enter the correct vessel because the wrong one is blocked. Leave the misplaced catheter in and pass another catheter through the same opening. Sometimes this allows one catheter to go through the ductus venosus while the other enters the portal system. The one in the portal system can then be removed (reported 50% success rate).This technique increases the risk of perforation.
10. **Connect the catheter to the fluid and tubing.**
11. **Secure the catheter just like the UAC.** (See Figure 24–4, page 242.) Never advance a catheter once it is secured in place.
12. **Confirm placement.** Incorrect UVC placement is associated with a higher complication rate. The UVC should be placed in the inferior vena cava below the level of the right atrium and above the level of the ductus venosus. Recently, some centers have used **ultrasound combined with radiography** for catheter placement and to verify position.
    a. **Anteroposterior (AP) and lateral "babygram"** (includes the abdomen and chest) are the radiographs of choice for catheter placement to confirm the position (see Figure 11–10). The UVC should be **above the diaphragm** but below the right atrium of the heart. The correct UVC position is catheter tip 0.5–1.0 cm (reported ranges 0–2 cm) above the right diaphragm (UVC tip at thoracic vertebrae 8–9 corresponding to the junction of the right atrium [RA] and inferior vena cava [IVC]). **The lateral image is necessary to show the exact location and will show the course of the umbilical vein and ductus venosus in relation to the liver.** *Note:* On the radiograph, sometimes air can be seen in the portal venous branches immediately after UVC insertion. As an isolated transient finding, it should not be confused with portal air due to necrotizing enterocolitis.
       i. Thoracic level on CXR did not accurately predict catheter position. UVC lines were found to be located at a wide range of vertebral bodies (T6–T11) by echocardiogram. Recommendations vary on what thoracic level the UVC line should be at T8-T9, T9, or T9-T10.
       ii. Some clinicians suggest radiography is unreliable in confirming catheter tip position. Lateral CXRs were found to not accurately predict catheter placement. The AP underestimates the incidence of left atrial placement and lateral radiograph overestimates left atrial placement.
    b. **Bedside ultrasound/echocardiography** is an option. Ultrasound more accurately confirms the position of the catheter tip than x-ray and reduces the exposure of ionizing radiation.
    c. **Venous Po$_2$ and saturation** can be obtained, but only has a sensitivity of 45% and specificity of 95%.
    d. **Gold standard** is considered echocardiography with saline contrast injection to document distal catheter location.
    e. If bright red blood (arterial blood) is obtained, then the UVC has crossed the foramen ovale, and the catheter needs to be pulled back.
13. There is insufficient evidence to support or refute the routine use of prophylactic antibiotics with UVC (Cochrane reviews). Do not use topical antibiotic ointment or creams at umbilical catheter insertion sites, as these will promote fungal infections.
IV. **UVC removal.** UVC removal should be as soon as possible because of the higher risk of colonization and infection with longer indwelling times. Compare the markings on the UVC to another catheter of the same size and review placement to determine the distance needed to pull the UVC to the 2-cm mark.
    A. Make sure the umbilical tie is loosely tied and remove any sutures or tape.
    B. Withdraw the catheter slowly until about 2-5 cm remains.
    C. Tighten the umbilical tie and stop the infusion.
    D. Pull the rest of the catheter out slowly (rate of 1 cm/min).

    E. Apply pressure and once bleeding has stopped, loosen the umbilical tie.

    F. Send tip for culture if suspect infection. **Observe stump** for excessive oozing or hemorrhage.

V. **Complications.** Risk of complications is high (10–50%). Keep the catheter tip in the ductus venosus or inferior vena cava and not at the foramen ovale, portal vein, or hepatic vein. Remember, you can have complications from appropriately placed UVC.

    A. **Infection.** The most commonly reported adverse effect. Minimize the risk by strict sterile technique, never advancing a catheter that has already been positioned, and limiting indwelling time. Sepsis is the most common, cellulitis, omphalitis, endocarditis, septic emboli, liver abscess, and lung abscess (with malposition of UVC into right pulmonary vein). AAP recommends to remove and not replace the line if any signs of central line–associated bloodstream infection are present.

    B. **Cardiac complications.** Pericardial effusion is the second most common complication. It can be asymptomatic and suspected in infants with catheters and progressive cardiomegaly. Right atrial arrhythmias can be caused by a UVC inserted too far and irritates the heart. Cardiac tamponade, cardiac perforation, pneumopericardium, and thrombotic endocarditis have also been reported.

    C. **Thrombotic or embolic phenomenon.** The most important risk factor is placement of central catheters. Never allow air to enter the end of the catheter. A nonfunctioning catheter should be removed. Never try to flush clots from the end of the catheter. Emboli can be in the lungs (if catheter passes through ductus venosus), liver, (catheter at portal system and ductus venous is closed), or anywhere in systemic circulation (catheter is through the ductus venosus, and there is right to left shunting through the ductus arteriosus or foramen ovale). Careful monitoring is indicated in very low birthweight infants who have a hematocrit >55% in the first week of life, as there is an increase in UVC-associated thrombosis in this group. AAP recommends removing the line if thrombosis is present.

    D. **Blood loss/hemorrhage.** Occurs if tubing becomes disconnected (use Luer lock connections).

    E. **Retroperitoneal fluid extravasation** (genital, buttocks, thigh, abdominal), total parenteral nutrition/IV fluid, ascites, hemoperitoneum.

    F. **Necrotizing enterocolitis.** Thought to be a complication of UVCs, especially if left in place for >24 hours.

    G. **Fungal infections of the right atrium.** Reported complication of 13%.

    H. **Pulmonary edema, hemorrhage, infarction** (with/without hydrothorax), hydrothorax can occur from a catheter lodged in or perforated pulmonary vein.

    I. **Portal vein hypertension.** Caused by a catheter positioned in the portal system.

    J. **Hepatic complications** include necrosis, calcification, laceration, abscess, biliary venous fistula formation, infusate ascites, subcapsular fluid collections, and portal venous air/hematoma/erosion. Do not allow a catheter to remain in the portal system. In case of emergency placement, the catheter should be advanced only 2–3 cm (just until blood returns) to avoid hepatic infusion. If the UVC perforates an intrahepatic vascular wall, a hematoma may result.

    K. **Other rare complications.** Creation of a false luminal tract, vessel perforation, hydrothorax, hepatic cyst, digital ischemia, perforation of the peritoneum, hemorrhagic infarction of the lungs, colon perforation, perforation of the Meckel diverticulum (UVC inserted through a narrow lumen in the umbilical cord mistaken for an umbilical vein), persistent neonatal hypoglycemia, ascites with peritoneal perforation), fluid in the peritoneal cavity from a perforated umbilical vein, Wharton jelly embolism, gangrene of the extremity (UVC placed in iliac artery branches).

Selected References

College of Respiratory Therapists of Ontario. Central Access: Umbilical Artery and Vein Cannulation: Clinical Best Practice Guideline. http://www.crto.on.ca/pdf/PPG/Umbilical_CBPG.pdf. Accessed September, 2012.

Kabra NS, Kumar M, Shah SS. Multiple versus single lumen umbilical venous catheters for newborn infants. *Cochrane Database Syst Rev.* 2005;CD004498.

Monagle P, Chan AK, Goldenberg NA, et al. Antithrombotic therapy in neonates and children: Antithrombotic Therapy and Prevention of Thrombosis. 9th ed. American College of Chest Physicians Evidence Based Clinical Practice Guidelines. *Chest.* 2012;141;e737S-e801S.

45 Venous Access: Venipuncture (Phlebotomy)

I. **Indications.** *Note:* Cochrane review states that **venipuncture**, by a skilled operator, is the **method of choice for blood sampling** in term infants. It was found to be less painful than heelstick sampling and a more effective sampling method.
   A. **To obtain a blood sample for routine analysis or blood culture.** Venipuncture typically allows a larger volume of blood (recommended if ≥1 mL needed) to be collected and is the method of choice for obtaining **blood cultures.** It is preferred over capillary blood sampling for certain tests (drug levels, hemoglobin/hematocrit, karyotype, coagulation studies, cross-matching blood, and ammonia, lactate, and pyruvate). Arterial blood is preferred for lactate, pyruvate, and ammonia.
   B. **To obtain a central hematocrit.** Venipuncture is more reliable than heelstick.
   C. **Administer medications.**
   D. **Venous blood gas.** This can be used in some diseases (neonatal sepsis/respiratory distress syndrome [RDS]) to diagnose acid-base imbalance if an arterial blood gas can't be obtained. Although arterial blood gas is preferred, venous samples show good validity in terms of pH, Pco_2, and HCO_3.
II. **Equipment.** Gloves, 23- or 25-gauge safety engineered scalp vein needle or needle (23 gauge preferred to reduce risk of hemolysis or clotting), alcohol swabs, 3 povidone-iodine swabs (for blood culture), appropriate specimen containers (eg, red-topped tube), a tourniquet or rubber band (for the scalp), 4 × 4 sterile gauze pads, syringe, transilluminator for vein imaging (optional) (see Chapter 40).
III. **Procedure**
   A. **Use distal venous sites first to preserve venous access.** Decide which vein to use. Use Figure 43–1 as a guide. Veins to use: antecubital fossa, dorsum of the hand or foot, wrist, greater saphenous vein at the ankle, scalp vein, external jugular. Avoid draws proximal to IV sites.
   B. **In cases of difficult vein localization.** Transillumination for vein imaging can be used and is described in Chapter 40.
   C. **Have an assistant restrain the infant.** If an assistant is not available, restrain the specific area selected for venipuncture by taping the extremity on an armboard.
   D. **Pain management**
      1. **The American Academy of Pediatrics (AAP) recommends** topical anesthesia (eg, eutectic mixture of lidocaine and prilocaine [ELMA], applied 30 minutes prior to procedure) and a combination of oral sucrose/glucose and nonpharmacologic pain prevention and relief techniques (combination is more effective).
      2. **Other recommendations** based on venipuncture studies (often with conflicting results): sucrose/human milk was comparable to EMLA in one study. Combination of sucrose and EMLA showed better results than sucrose alone in preterm

infants. Some recommend liposomal lidocaine 4% since it has a faster onset of action and it does not require occlusion dressing.

E. **"Tourniquet" the extremity to occlude the vein.** Use a rubber band (for the head), a tourniquet, or an assistant's hand to encircle the area proximal to the vein. Removing and reapplying may optimize the distension of the vein.

F. **Prepare the site with antiseptic solution.** For blood cultures, wipe at least 3 times in concentric circles starting at the puncture site.

G. **With the bevel up** (for optimal blood flow and less chance of occlusion by wall of vein), puncture the skin, and then direct the needle into the vein at a 25- to 45-degree angle. Use the vessel bifurcation if possible.

H. **Once blood enters the tubing.** Attach the syringe and collect the blood slowly (or administer the medication).

I. **Remove the tourniquet.** Then remove and press the button to shield the needle. Apply gentle pressure on the area until hemostasis has occurred (usually 2–3 minutes). Distribute blood samples to the appropriate containers; gently mix tubes with additives.

IV. **Complications**

A. **Infection** is a rare complication that can be minimized by using sterile technique. Septic arthritis of the hip has been reported from femoral venipuncture.

B. **Venous thrombosis/embolus** is often unavoidable, especially when multiple punctures are performed on the same vein and the vein is large.

C. **Hematoma or hemorrhage** is avoided by applying pressure to the site long enough after the needle is removed to ensure hemostasis. If a coagulation defect is present, hemorrhage can occur.

D. **Scarring of the dorsum of the hand** from multiple venipunctures in very low birthweight (VLBW) neonates.

E. **Cervical dural puncture** from internal jugular venipuncture in an infant. This is secondary to insertion of the needle at excessive depth.

F. **Laceration of artery** near the vein.

Selected References

Bilan N, Behbahan AG, Khosroshahi AJ. Validity of venous blood gas analysis for diagnosis of acid-base imbalance in children admitted to the pediatric intensive care unit. *World J Pediat.* 2008;4(2):114–117.

Shah VS, Ohlsson A. Venipuncture versus heel lance for blood sampling in term neonates. *Cochrane Database Syst Rev.* 2011;(10). DOI:10.1002/14651858.CD001452.pub4.

46 Abnormal Blood Gas

I. **Problem.** An abnormal blood gas value for a neonate is reported by the laboratory.

II. **Immediate questions**

   A. **What component of the blood gas is abnormal?** Accepted normal values for an arterial blood gas on room air are pH 7.35–7.45 (pH varies with age, a pH >7.30 is generally acceptable), $Paco_2$, 35–45 mm Hg (slightly higher accepted if the blood pH remains normal), and Pao_2 50–95 mm Hg (depends on gestational age). (See Table 8–1, page 72.) Blood gas measures pH, Pco_2, and oxygen (O_2), and all the other components (base excess, bicarbonate concentration, and oxygen saturation) are calculated based on the 3 levels measured. General blood gas concepts are as follows:

   1. pH is proportional to HCO_3 (base excess)
      a. **Metabolic acidosis.** Abnormal ↓ in HCO_3 with ↓ pH.
      b. **Metabolic alkalosis.** Abnormal ↑ HCO_3 with ↑ pH.
   2. pH is inversely proportional to Pco_2
      a. **Respiratory acidosis.** Abnormal ↑ Pco_2 with ↓ pH.
      b. **Respiratory alkalosis.** Abnormal ↓ Pco_2 with ↑ pH.

   B. **Is this blood gas value very different from the patient's previous blood gas determination?** If the patient has had metabolic acidosis on the last 5 blood gas measurements and now has metabolic alkalosis, it might be best to repeat the blood gas measurements before initiating treatment. **Do not treat the infant on the basis of one abnormal gas value,** especially if the infant's clinical status has not changed.

   C. **How was the sample collected?** Blood gas measurements can be reported on **arterial, venous,** or **capillary (heelstick)** blood samples.

   1. **Arterial blood samples.** Best indicator of pH, $Paco_2$, and Pao_2. The gold standard of obtaining a blood gas is to obtain one from an indwelling arterial catheter (peripheral or umbilical). Blood gases by intermittent arterial punctures may not accurately reflect the infant's respiratory status. A sudden decrease in the $Paco_2$ and Pao_2 can occur during the puncture. Crying can decrease the $Paco_2$, HCO_3 and oxygen saturation.
   2. **Venous blood samples.** Give a lower pH value, significantly lower Po_2, and a higher Pco_2 than arterial samples. It is good for HCO_3 estimation,
   3. **Capillary (heelstick) samples.** Give a satisfactory assessment of the infant's pH and Pco_2 but do not give an accurate Pao_2. Capillary samples give a similar or lower pH value (not as low as venous pH), similar or slightly higher Pco_2, and lower Po_2 than arterial samples; capillary blood gas measurements are not reliable in an infant who is hypotensive or in shock.

   D. **Is the infant on ventilatory support?** Management of abnormal blood gas levels is approached differently in an intubated infant than in a patient breathing room air.

III. **Differential diagnosis**

   A. **Metabolic acidosis (pH <7.30–7.35 with a normal to low CO_2).** After birth it is normal for an infant to have a mild metabolic acidosis. The 3 main causes of metabolic acidosis are loss of base (mainly bicarbonate) from renal or gastrointestinal (GI) cause, decreased renal excretion of acid, or an increased production of acid. Metabolic acidosis is classified as anion gap (increased, high) or non–anion (normal) gap acidosis. **Determining the anion gap will help decide the cause of the acidosis.**

3. **Ventilator malfunction or insufficient respiratory support.**
4. **Ventilator strategy that allows permissive hypercapnia** (controlled mechanical hypoventilation) is *controversial.* Use caution with permissive hypercapnia until further studies are done. Severe hypercapnia or hypocapnia should be avoided. In infants with BPD/CLD, higher CO_2 is sometimes tolerated to wean them from mechanical ventilation.
5. **Increasing respiratory failure; lung diseases** such as RDS, pneumonia, transient tachypnea (TTN), BPD/CLD, pleural effusion, pulmonary hypoplasia, atelectasis.
6. **Pneumothorax.**
7. **Hypoventilation or poor respiratory effort** from maternal anesthesia, medications, neuromuscular disorders, congenital central hypoventilation syndrome, sepsis, intracranial hemorrhage, or hypoglycemia.
8. **PDA with pulmonary edema.** Suspect a PDA if the infant has a systolic murmur, active precordium, bounding pulses, and increased pulse pressure. Other clinical signs and symptoms may include congestive heart failure, deteriorating blood gases with an increase in the ventilator settings, and cardiomegaly with increased pulmonary vascularity on chest radiograph.
9. **Others.** Congenital diaphragmatic hernia, phrenic nerve paralysis, and other causes.

E. **Low O_2 (hypoxia).** See also Chapter 51.
   1. **Agitation**
   2. **Improper ETT position or inadequate ventilatory support**
   3. **Congenital heart disease (cyanotic)**
   4. **Respiratory diseases**
      a. **Primary lung disease.** RDS, TTN, BPD/CLD, others.
      b. **Airway obstruction.** Mucus plug, choanal atresia, other congenital malformations (macroglossia, cystic hygroma, etc.).
      c. **External compression of the lungs.** Air leak syndrome (eg, pneumothorax) or congenital defects (eg, congenital diaphragmatic hernia).
   5. **Apnea of prematurity**
   6. **Pulmonary hypertension**
   7. **CNS/neuromuscular disorders**
   8. **Metabolic abnormalities**
   9. **Hematologic disorders**
   10. **Sepsis /hypotension**

IV. **Database**
   A. **Physical examination.** Evaluate for signs of sepsis (eg, hypotension or poor perfusion). Check for equal breath sounds; asymmetric breath sounds suggest pneumothorax or incorrect ETT placement. Observe for chest wall movement. Listen for breath sounds over the chest versus the epigastric region, which may help determine whether the ETT is malpositioned. Listen to the heart for any murmur, and palpate for cardiac displacement.
   B. **Laboratory studies**
      1. **Repeat blood gas measurement.** Repeat if the result is unexpected. Do not make a major clinical decision based on a venous or capillary blood gas values or on 1 arterial gas result.
      2. **Serum electrolytes.** To include blood urea nitrogen, creatinine, glucose, potassium (severe metabolic alkalosis can cause hypokalemia). Serum Na, K, Cl, and bicarbonate (from arterial blood gas) to determine anion gap.
      3. **Urine chloride.** To evaluate metabolic alkalosis. May not be valid in the setting of diuretic use.
      4. **Urinary ketones.** If absent or small, think lactic acidosis; if moderate or large, suspect organic acidemias (maple syrup urine disease, glycogen storage disease, disorders of pyruvate metabolism, others).

5. **Plasma ammonia level.** If normal, may be RTA; may be increased in urea cycle defects, may be increased in some organic acidemias (acidosis and hyperammonemia).
6. **Serum potassium level.** Severe metabolic alkalosis can cause hypokalemia.
7. **Measure the anion gap.** Correct for hypoalbuminemia by adding 2.5 mEq/L to the anion gap for every gram per deciliter that the concentration of serum albumin is reduced below the normal value of 3.5 g/dL.
8. **Plasma lactate.** Increased in lactic acidosis. It is important to do this in infants who have a normal anion gap but in whom lactic acidosis is suspected. Infants with lactic acidosis do not always have an increased anion gap. Normal and elevated lactate can be seen in organic acidemias.
9. **Complete blood count with differential.** If sepsis is being considered.
10. **Further sepsis workup if indicated.** Blood culture, urinalysis and culture, lumbar puncture if indicated.
11. **Metabolic screen if indicated.** Urine and plasma for amino acids and organic acids.

C. **Imaging and other studies**
1. **Pulmonary mechanics.** Check the tidal volume (VT) delivered on the ventilator. The normal VT is 5–6 mL/kg. If the VT is low, it could mean that not enough pressure is given or there is an obstruction in the ETT.
2. **Transillumination of the chest.** If pneumothorax is suspected (see Chapter 70).
3. **Chest radiograph.** Should be performed if an abnormal blood gas value is reported, unless there is an obvious cause. An anteroposterior view should be obtained to check ETT placement (see Figure 11–7), rule out air leak (eg, pneumothorax, see Figure 11–20), check heart size and pulmonary vascularity (increased or decreased) and determine whether the infant is being hypoventilated or hyperventilated.
4. **Abdominal radiograph.** If NEC is suspected in a patient with **severe metabolic acidosis.** See Figure 11–23.
5. **Ultrasonography of the head.** To diagnose IVH. See Figures 11–1 through 11–4 for examples of IVH.
6. **Echocardiography.** May detect PDA or other cardiac abnormality and can be used to diagnose low cardiac output.
7. **Ultrasonography of the abdomen with color Doppler studies.** To evaluate for NEC and bowel necrosis.

V. **Plan**
A. **Overall plan.** Verify the blood gas result, find the cause of the problem, and provide treatment for the specific cause. First, examine the infant. If the infant's clinical status has not changed, repeat blood gas measurements to verify the report. If the clinical status has changed, the abnormal report is probably correct; repeat blood gas measurements and begin further evaluation of the infant.
B. **Specific management**
1. **Metabolic acidosis.** The primary treatment is to **treat the underlying cause.** Correct hypoxia, hypovolemia, low cardiac output, and anemia. Treatment with bicarbonate is not recommended as a supportive therapy and its use is very *controversial*. It has been quoted as "basically useless therapy" and associated with adverse sequelae (hypernatremia, intracranial hemorrhage, fluctuations in cerebral blood flow, cardiac deterioration, and worsening acidosis).
a. **Important and *controversial* points in the treatment of metabolic acidosis**
i. **Sodium bicarbonate in the delivery room (*controversial*).** American Academy of Pediatrics and American Heart Association guidelines state that the use of sodium bicarbonate is *controversial* during resuscitation in the delivery room. It is not recommended early on, and if used later in resuscitation or during a prolonged resuscitation not responding to therapy, make sure the lungs are adequately ventilated. Sodium bicarbonate is

hyperosmolar and may cause IVH if given rapidly. **Cochrane review** states there are insufficient data to make a recommendation on using sodium bicarbonate during resuscitation.

ii. **Sodium bicarbonate in an asphyxiated newborn** (*controversial*). If metabolic acidosis is severe or persistent, some institutions may use sodium bicarbonate. Rapid infusion increases serum osmolality, and alkalinization may decrease cerebral blood flow. **Some institutions only do 24-hour corrections** in patients with profound postasphyxia acidosis.

iii. **Sodium bicarbonate in preterm infants** (*controversial*). **Cochrane review** states there is insufficient evidence to state that use of sodium bicarbonate in preterm infants with metabolic acidosis reduces mortality and morbidity.

iv. **Sodium bicarbonate in a cardiac arrest** (*controversial*). May cause harm and there is no evidence of benefit.

v. **If sodium bicarbonate is given and the infant does not respond,** think inborn error of metabolism.

vi. **Watch for hypokalemia** as metabolic acidosis is corrected.

vii. **Do not treat metabolic acidosis with hyperventilation.**

viii. **Replacement of base for ongoing GI and renal losses.** Not proven but is often accepted as reasonable therapy.

ix. **Fluid therapy for metabolic acidosis.** Volume expansion should not be used to treat acidosis unless there are signs of hypovolemia. Severe acidosis causes a decrease in myocardial contractility. **Cochrane review** states that there is insufficient evidence to state that a fluid bolus reduces morbidity and mortality in preterm infants with metabolic acidosis.

b. Medications for metabolic acidosis. **It is best to correct the underlying cause of the metabolic acidosis.** Some institutions treat acidosis if severe with an alkali infusion if the base excess is >−5 to − 10 or if the pH is ≤7.25 (*controversial*). The alkali can be given as IV push, 1 dose over 30 minutes, or can be given as an 8–24-hour correction. If the acidosis is mild, usually only 1 dose is given and repeat blood gas measurements are obtained. If the acidosis is severe, a dose is given and correction is started at the same time. One of 3 medications is used:

i. **Sodium bicarbonate** can be used if the infant's serum sodium and Pco_2 are not high. It is the most common medication used. If used, it is recommended to give a diluted formulation and a slow correction. If given to a premature infant, it is important to give it slower than recommended.

(a) **One-time dose.** 1–2 mEq/kg/dose, given as a 4.2% solution (0.5 mEq/mL); infuse at 1 mEq/kg/min max over at least 30 minutes.

(b) **IV push (for cardiac arrest, routine use not recommended,** *controversial*). 1 mEq/kg slow IV push, given as 0.5 mEq/mL (4.2% concentration). Maximum rate in neonates and infants is 10 mEq/min. May repeat with a 0.5-mEq/kg dose in 10 minutes one time as indicated by patient's unstable acid-base status.

(c) **Slow correction** should be given over 8–24 hours in IV fluids. Give half the correction at first, then reassess. The total dose required to correct the base deficit is as follows:

$$HCO_3^- \text{ dose (mEq)} = \text{Base deficit (mEq/L)} \times \text{weight (kg)} \times 0.3$$

ii. **Tromethamine (THAM)** can be used in infants who have a severe metabolic acidosis but have a high serum sodium (>150 mEq/L) or high Pco_2 (>65 mm Hg) despite aggressive assisted ventilation. It does not increase CO_2 or sodium as bicarbonate does. It is not indicated for metabolic acidosis caused by bicarbonate deficiency. **Use only in infants with good urine output (hyperkalemia risk) and monitor for hypoglycemia.** (*Controversial:* Many institutions do not use THAM because of side effects: higher osmolar load, risk of hypoglycemia, others). See dose in Chapter 148.

   iii. **Polycitrate (Polycitra) (oral solution).** This alkali can be helpful in patients with acidosis associated with chronic renal insufficiency, intrinsic renal disease, or renal wasting or on medications that promote acidosis such as acetazolamide (Diamox). It consists of 1 mEq Na$^+$, 1 mEq K$^+$, and 2 mEq citrate. Each 1 mEq citrate equals 1 mEq bicarbonate. The dose is 2–3 mEq/kg/d polycitrate in 3–4 divided doses; adjust to maintain a normal pH.

   iv. **Sodium or potassium acetate (IV preparations)** can be used to treat chronic metabolic acidosis through the conversion of acetate to bicarbonate. It is used in hyperalimentation for bicarbonate replacement as part of urinary losses in preterm infants and treatment of metabolic acidosis. See doses in Chapter 148.

  c. **Specific treatments for metabolic acidosis**

   i. **Sepsis.** Initiate a septic workup and consider broad-spectrum antibiotics. (See Chapter 130.)

   ii. **NEC.** See Chapter 113.

   iii. **Hypothermia or cold stress.** See Chapter 7.

   iv. **Periventricular-intraventricular hemorrhage.** Weekly ultrasonographic examinations of the head and daily head circumferences are indicated. Monitor the infant for signs of increased intracranial pressure (convulsions, vomiting, and/or hypotension). (See Chapter 104.)

   v. **PDA.** If hemodynamically significant, PDA should be treated. (See Chapter 118.)

   vi. **Shock/ low cardiac output.** Give volume expansion if hypovolemic or vasoactive medications based on cardiac function. (See Chapter 65.)

   vii. **Renal tubular acidosis.** Treated with alkaline therapy such as sodium bicarbonate or one of citrate and citric acid solutions.

   viii. **Inborn errors of metabolism.** Rare cause (see Chapter 101).

   ix. **Maternal use of salicylates.** Acidosis usually resolves without treatment.

   x. **Renal failure.** See Chapter 123.

   xi. **Congenital lactic acidosis.** Supportive care, correction of the metabolic acidosis with sodium bicarbonate.

   xii. **Parenteral hyperalimentation.** Preterm infants usually need acetate supplementation in hyperalimentation to correct for ongoing bicarbonate losses. It should be given to infants with a base deficit >–5. The use of acetate in total parenteral nutrition reduces the severity of the acidosis and the incidence of hyperchloremia.

2. **Metabolic alkalosis.** Mild or even moderate alkalosis may not require correction. First treat any underlying cause. Volume replacement can be used in cases of volume contraction and chloride depletion. If hypokalemia is present, that should be treated. Chloride replacement as KCl can be used, but infusion rate may have to be limited. HCL or ammonium chloride can be considered in severe persistent cases but must be given carefully. Acetazolamide has been used in some pediatric cardiac patients with chloride-resistant metabolic alkalosis.

  a. **Excess administered alkali.** Adjust or discontinue the dose of THAM, sodium bicarbonate, or polycitrate; reduce acetate in hyperalimentation.

  b. **Hypokalemia.** This can cause a shift of hydrogen ions into cells as potassium is lost. The infant's potassium level should be corrected (see Chapter 63).

  c. **Prolonged nasogastric suction.** Treated with IV fluid replacement, usually with 1/2 normal saline with 10–20 mEq KCl/L, replaced mL/mL each shift.

  d. **Vomiting and loss of chloride from diarrhea.** Give IV fluids and replace deficits.

  e. **Compensation for respiratory acidosis.** Correct ventilation.

  f. **Diuretics.** These can cause mild alkalosis; no specific treatment is usually necessary. Stop the dose temporarily, or decrease the diuretic dose if necessary, or add a potassium-sparing diuretic such as spironolactone.

  g. Bartter syndrome. Treated with indomethacin and potassium supplements. Replace electrolyte losses.

  h. Primary hyperaldosteronism. Treatment depends on the cause. Acute therapies include diuretics, angiotensin-converting enzyme inhibitors, and steroids.

 3. Other causes of abnormal blood gases

  a. ETT problems. Determine whether there are any changes on the pulmonary function test measurements on the ventilator that may indicate a problem with the ETT. Colorimetric CO_2 detectors can be used to determine airway patency, with a color change from purple to yellow if there is exhaled CO_2 gas. If no color change, there is airway obstruction and possible ETT problem. Mark position on the ETT when it is correctly placed to note whether the tube is out of position.

   i. Mucus plug. With decreased bilateral breath sounds and retractions, a plugged ETT is possible. Pulmonary function measurements on specific ventilators may also define this if the Vt is low. The infant can be suctioned, and, if clinically stable, repeat blood gas measurements can be obtained. If the infant is in extreme distress, replace the tube.

   ii. ETT placement problems. An infant with a tube placed down the right main stem bronchus has breath sounds on the right only. An infant with a tube that has dislodged has decreased or no breath sounds on chest auscultation.

  b. Ventilator issues. Changes in blood gas levels based on changes in routine ventilator settings can be found in Table 46–1. Advanced ventilator management for high-frequency devices can be found in Chapter 8, page 86.

   i. Overventilation. If the blood gas levels reveal overventilation, the ventilation parameters need to be adjusted. Deciding which parameter to adjust depends on the patient's lung disease and the disease course.

    (a) If the oxygen level is high. Decrease the FIO_2. Other options include decreasing the positive end-expiratory pressure (PEEP), peak inspiratory pressure (PIP), inspiratory time, rate and flow.

    (b) If the CO_2 level is low. Decrease the rate. Other options include decreasing the PIP, expiratory time, or flow.

   ii. Insufficient respiratory support. If the infant's chest is not moving, the PIP is not high enough; an adjustment of the ventilator setting is needed. Also check the Vt; if it is low, it could mean not enough pressure is given.

    (a) If the oxygen is low. One or more of the following can be increased: FIO_2, PIP, PEEP, inspiratory time, rate, and flow rate.

    (b) If the CO_2 is high. One or more of the following can be increased: rate, PIP, flow rate, or expiratory time. Decreasing PEEP will increase tidal volume and decrease CO_2.

Table 46–1. CHANGES IN BLOOD GAS LEVELS CAUSED BY CHANGES IN VENTILATOR SETTINGS

Variable	Rate	PIP	PEEP	IT	FIO_2
To increase Paco$_2$	↓	↓	NA	NA	NA
To decrease Paco$_2$	↑	↑	NA[a]	NA[b]	NA
To increase Pao$_2$	↑	↑	↑	↑	↑
To decrease Pao$_2$	NA	↓	↓	NA	↓

FIO_2, fraction of inspired oxygen; IT, inspiratory time; NA, not applicable; PEEP, positive end-expiratory pressure; PIP, peak inspiratory pressure.
[a]In severe pulmonary edema and pulmonary hemorrhage, increased PEEP can decrease Paco$_2$.
[b]Not applicable unless the inspiratory-to-expiratory ratio is excessive.

      iii. **Ventilator malfunction.** Notify respiratory therapy to check the ventilator and replace it if necessary.

   c. **Agitation.** May cause the infant to drop in oxygenation; sedation may be needed (*controversial*) or ventilator settings adjusted. See also Chapter 76.

      i. *Note:* Agitation can be a sign of hypoxia, so a blood gas level should be obtained before ordering sedation. If there is documented hypoxia, attempt to increase oxygenation.

      ii. **Sit by the bedside and try different ventilator rates.** To see whether the infant fights less.

      iii. **Routine sedation. Usually not recommended** because in very low birthweight infants and premature infants, it is associated with an increase in severe IVH, delay in diuresis, and ileus. **If sedation is used,** use the preferred agent at your institution (see Chapter 76 for agents used: diazepam, lorazepam, midazolam, fentanyl, chloral hydrate, morphine).

   d. Acute change in clinical pulmonary status

      i. **Pneumothorax.** See Chapter 70.

      ii. **Atelectasis.** Treatment consists of percussion and postural drainage and possibly increased PIP or PEEP. Avoid percussion in small preterm infants; a study showed a strong link between IVH and porencephaly with chest physiotherapy in extremely premature infants.

      iii. **Pulmonary edema.** Diuretics (eg, furosemide) are the primary treatment with mechanical ventilation as indicated.

      iv. **Persistent pulmonary hypertension.** See Chapter 120.

47 Apnea and Bradycardia ("A's and B's")

I. **Problem.** An infant has just had an apneic episode with bradycardia. **Apnea is the absence of breathing for >20 seconds or a shorter pause (>10 seconds) associated with oxygen desaturation or bradycardia (<100 beats/min).** Shorter apnea <10 seconds without hypoxemia or bradycardia is due to immaturity and is not clinically important. The incidence of apnea of prematurity (AOP) is inversely correlated with gestational age and birthweight. Apnea occurs in >50% of infants <1500 g and in 90% of infants <1000 g. **Types of apnea** with approximate incidence are:

A. **Central apnea.** Complete absence of the brainstem stimulus to breathe, resulting in no respiratory effort (40%).

B. **Obstructive apnea.** Infant breathes but no airflow is present because of an obstruction by mucus or airway collapse (10%).

C. **Mixed apnea.** Elements of both central and obstructive apnea. This is the type found in most preterm infants (>50%).

D. **Periodic breathing.** Three or more respiratory pauses lasting >3 seconds separated by normal respiratory intervals not >20 seconds and not associated with bradycardia. Periodic breathing can occur in 2–6% of healthy term neonates and in up to 25% of preterm infants.

E. **Apnea of infancy (AOI).** American Academy of Pediatrics (AAP) definition: "an unexplained episode of cessation of breathing for 20 seconds or longer or a shorter respiratory pause associated with bradycardia, cyanosis, pallor, and/or marked hypotonia" in an infant >37 weeks' gestational age.

F. **Apnea of prematurity (AOP).** Sudden absence of breathing that lasts at least 20 seconds or is associated with bradycardia or cyanosis (oxygen desaturation) in an infant <37 weeks' gestational age. It is most commonly central or mixed apnea. AOP is a developmental disorder usually of physiologic immaturity of respiratory control but other diseases may contribute. AOP may be hereditary. AOP usually presents on days 2–7. If apnea presents in the first 24 hours of life or after day 7, it is very unlikely to be AOP. **Note:** Apnea of prematurity is a diagnosis of exclusion.

   G. **Persistent apnea.** Apnea persists in a neonate ≥37 weeks postmenstrual age. It usually occurs in infants born at <28 weeks' gestation.

   H. **Secondary causes of apnea.** Apnea that has a specific cause (eg, sepsis, anemia, asphyxia, temperature instability, pneumonia, and others). Remember **immaturity** can worsen any apnea that is associated with a specific cause.

II. **Immediate questions**

   A. **Did you observe the apnea? What was going on when the apnea occurred? Do you know what type of apnea it is?** Try to distinguish the type; obstructive apnea is the easiest to detect visually while central and mixed are more difficult. A thorough history of the event may help differentiate the type of apnea. If it occurred during feeding with a naso- or orogastric tube, is the tube in proper position? (Stimulation of laryngeal receptors causes central apnea.) Did it occur with insertion of a naso-/orogastric tube? Think vagal response. (Stimulation of the vagal nerve resulting in central apnea.) Does it just occur with feeding? (Possible gastroesophageal reflux; mixed apnea.) If the infant has no respiratory effort on the monitor or on physical examination (absent breath sounds, chest wall not moving), think central apnea. What position was the infant in when it occurred? Neck flexion can obstruct the airway and cause obstructive apnea. Was the infant just suctioned when the apnea occurred? (Aggressive pharyngeal suctioning can cause central apnea.) Does the infant have excessive secretions? (Obstructive apnea.)

   B. **What is the gestational age of the infant?** A's and B's are common in premature infants (~70% experience apnea before 34 weeks' gestation) and uncommon in term infants In term infants apnea is usually associated with a serious disorder or related to a maternal condition (magnesium treatment or maternal exposure to narcotics). **Apnea in a term infant is never physiologic; it requires a full workup to determine the cause.**

   C. **Was significant stimulation needed to return the heart rate to normal?** An infant requiring significant stimulation (eg, oxygen by bag-and-mask ventilation) usually needs an immediate evaluation. An infant who has had one episode of apnea and bradycardia not requiring oxygen supplementation may not need a full evaluation unless the infant is term.

   D. **If the patient is already receiving medication (eg, methylxanthine) for apnea and bradycardia, is the dosage adequate?** Determine the serum drug level.

   E. **Did the episode occur during or after feeding?** It has been stated that gastroesophageal reflux (GER) causes apnea and bradycardia because it was observed when regurgitation of formula into the pharynx occurred after feeding. This has been a source of much debate, with recent studies showing no temporal relationship. Consider aspiration in an infant who has been doing well and feeding. Insertion of a nasogastric (NG) tube may cause a vagal reflex, resulting in apnea and bradycardia.

   F. **How old is the infant?** Apnea in the first 24 hours is usually pathologic. The peak incidence of apnea of prematurity occurs between 5 and 7 days postnatal age.

   G. **Is there a change in the frequency or increase in severity of episodes? Is this the first episode or has the pattern changed?** If the pattern changes or the amount and severity of each episode increases, then something new may be going on and a workup should be done.

III. **Differential diagnosis.** Causes of A's and B's can be classified according to diseases and disorders of various organ systems, gestationale age, or postnatal age. **Apnea of prematurity is a diagnosis of exclusion; therefore, it is important to diagnose and treat any secondary cause.**

   A. **Diseases and disorders of various organ systems**

     1. **Head and central nervous system**

       a. Perinatal asphyxia.

       b. Intraventricular/intracranial or subarachnoid hemorrhage.

    c. Meningitis.

    d. Hydrocephalus with increased intracranial pressure.

    e. Cerebral infarct with seizures.

    f. Seizures (apnea is an uncommon presentation of a subtle seizure). Consider a seizure if apnea occurs without bradycardia; tachycardia can be seen before or during the apneic attack.

    g. Birth trauma.

    h. Congenital myopathies or neuropathies.

    i. Congenital malformations.

    j. Congenital central hypoventilation syndrome.

    k. Encephalopathy.

2. Respiratory system

    a. Hypoxia

    b. Airway obstruction/malformation

    c. Lung disease/pneumonia/respiratory distress syndrome (RDS)/aspiration

    d. Inadequate ventilation or performing extubation too early

    e. Surfactant deficiency

    f. Pulmonary hemorrhage

    g. Pneumothorax

    h. Hypercarbia

3. Cardiovascular system

    a. Congestive heart failure.

    b. Patent ductus arteriosus.

    c. Cardiac disorders such as cyanotic congenital heart disease, congenital heart block, hypoplastic left heart syndrome, and transposition of the great vessels.

    d. Hypovolemia/hypotension/hypertension.

    e. Increased vagal tone. There is increased vagal tone in newborns especially in the postdelivery period. Vagal hyperreactivity has been described in sudden infant death syndrome (SIDS).

4. Gastrointestinal (GI) tract

    a. Necrotizing enterocolitis (NEC). Apnea has been associated with the onset of NEC.

    b. Gastroesophageal reflux (GER). Thought by some investigators to be related to AOP; however, to date, no research has shown a relationship between the two. Some studies suggest that antireflux surgery can reduce apnea in preterm infants at highest risk. It is a rare/infrequent cause of apnea in a full-term infant.

    c. Feeding intolerance.

    d. Oral feeding.

    e. Abdominal distension.

    f. Bowel movement.

    g. Non-rotavirus infection causes apnea in a premature infant.

    h. Esophageal hematoma. Rare.

5. Hematologic system

    a. Anemia. There is no specific hematocrit at which apnea and bradycardia occur and can be seen in infants with anemia of prematurity. These infants show improvement after transfusion; it has been shown that liberal blood transfusion may reduce apnea compared with more restrictive blood transfusion.

    b. Polycythemia. More common in term infants.

6. Other diseases and disorders

    a. Temperature instability. Especially hyperthermia, but also hypothermia, can cause apnea and bradycardia. Note the incubator temperature; the infant may have a normal body temperature but may have a rise in incubator temperature (the infant is hypothermic) or may require a lower incubator temperature (the infant is hyperthermic). Any rapid fluctuation of temperature can cause apnea.

Cold stress can occur after birth or during transport or a procedure, and it may produce apnea.

b. **Infection (sepsis).** Check for bacterial, fungal, and viral infections. Respiratory syncytial virus, *Ureaplasma urealyticum*, and botulism can all cause apnea in preterm infants.

c. **Metabolic/electrolyte imbalance and inborn errors of metabolism.** Hypoglycemia, hypo-/hypernatremia, hypermagnesemia (during parenteral nutrition), hyperkalemia, hyperammonemia, and hypo-/hypercalcemia can cause apnea and bradycardia. Hypothyroidism and inborn errors of metabolism can also cause apnea and bradycardia.

d. **Vagal reflex.** May occur secondary to nasogastric tube insertion, feeding, and suctioning.

e. **Acute/chronic pain.**

f. **Head/body position (neck flexion).**

g. **Drugs/drug withdrawal.** Oversedation from **maternal drugs** such as **magnesium sulfate**, narcotics such as opiates, and general anesthesia can cause apnea in the newborn. Apnea can be seen in drug withdrawal of infants born to drug-addicted mothers. **In the infant**, high levels of phenobarbital or other narcotics or sedatives, such as diazepam and chloral hydrate, may cause apnea and bradycardia. Topical eye drops for routine eye examinations can sometimes cause changes in apnea pattern. Prostaglandin E_1, γ-aminobutyric acid (GABA), and adenosine therapy can cause apnea.

h. **Immunization.** Apnea increases in preterm infants after immunization with the whole-cell pertussis component. New studies have shown an increase in apnea/bradycardia/desaturation after the DTaP-IPV-HIb and DTaP-IPV-HIb-HBV in premature infants with chronic disease. It is recommended to give these at 8 weeks if still hospitalized, with close observation. Infants with significant lung disease or sepsis can experience apnea after immunization. There is a risk of recurrence of apnea in premature infants who had apnea with their first immunization. Monitoring for a minimum of 24 hours after their next immunization is recommended.

i. **Kangaroo care.** Early studies showed a relationship, but recent studies have found no adverse effects. Observe head positioning during holding.

j. **Surgery.** This can cause postoperative apnea in premature infants.

k. **Retinopathy of prematurity (ROP).** ROP examination has been reported as a cause.

B. **Gestational age.** See Table 47–1.

1. **Full-term infants.** Usually do not have apnea and bradycardia from physiologic causes; the disease or disorder must be identified. The onset of apnea in a term infant at any time is a **critical event** that requires immediate investigation.

2. **Preterm infants.** The most common cause is AOP, usually presenting between days 2 and 7 of life (usually <34 weeks' gestation, <1800 g, and no other identifiable cause) and is a diagnosis of exclusion.

C. **Postnatal age can be a clue to the cause of apnea**

1. **Onset within hours after birth.** Oversedation from maternal drugs, asphyxia, seizures, hypermagnesemia.

2. **Apnea on day 1.** Usually pathologic; consider sepsis or respiratory failure.

3. **Apnea on days 1–2.** Sepsis, hypoglycemia, respiratory failure, polycythemia.

4. **Onset <1 week.** Patent ductus arteriosus, periventricular-intraventricular hemorrhage, sepsis, respiratory failure, or AOP.

5. **Onset >1 week of age.** Posthemorrhagic hydrocephalus with increased intracranial pressure or seizures, postextubation atelectasis, outgrown dose of caffeine or theophylline.

6. **Onset after 2 weeks in a previously well premature infant.** Something new is going on that needs an immediate evaluation, usually indicative of a serious illness such as sepsis, meningitis, or other causes.

Table 47–1. **MORE COMMON CAUSES OF APNEA AND BRADYCARDIA ACCORDING TO GESTATIONAL AGE**

Premature Infant	Full-Term Infant	All Ages
Apnea of prematurity	Cerebral infarction	Sepsis
PDA	Polycythemia	NEC
RDS		Meningitis
Respiratory insufficiency of prematurity		Aspiration
PV-IVH		GER
Anemia of prematurity		Pneumonia
Posthemorrhagic hydrocephalus		Cardiac disorder
		Postextubation atelectasis
		Seizures
		Cold stress
		Asphyxia

GER, gastroesophageal reflux; NEC, necrotizing enterocolitis; PDA, patent ductus arteriosus; PV-IVH, periventricular-intraventricular hemorrhage; RDS, respiratory distress syndrome.

7. Onset 4–6 weeks. Respiratory syncytial virus (RSV) infection.
8. Variable onset. Sepsis, NEC, meningitis, aspiration, GER, cardiac disorder, pneumonia, cold stress, or fluctuations in temperature.

IV. Database. Determine any prenatal risk of sepsis. A history of feeding intolerance increases the suspicion of NEC.

A. Complete physical examination with attention to the following signs:
1. Head. Signs of increased intracranial pressure, central nervous system (CNS) depression, or irritability.
2. Nares. Pass a small-diameter feeding tube through the nares to rule out choanal atresia.
3. Heart. Listen for a murmur or gallop.
4. Lungs. Check for adequate movement of the chest if mechanical ventilation is being used. Check for signs of respiratory distress.
5. Abdomen. Check for abdominal distention, which is one of the earliest signs of NEC. Other signs of NEC are decreased bowel sounds and visible bowel loops.
6. Skin. An infant with polycythemia has a ruddy appearance. Pallor is associated with anemia.
7. Neurologic examination. Do a complete neurologic examination and look for seizure activity. Is there hypotonia?

B. Laboratory studies
1. Immediate studies
   a. Arterial blood gas. To rule out hypoxia and acidosis.
   b. Complete blood count (CBC) with differential. May suggest infection, anemia, or polycythemia.
   c. Cultures of the blood, urine, and cerebrospinal (CSF) fluid. If infection is suspected and tests indicated. **C-reactive protein** at 36–48 hours after birth may be useful as an infection screen. Polymerase chain reaction (PCR) analyses and viral cultures are appropriate if a viral infection is suspected. **Lumbar puncture and CSF analysis** if meningitis is suspected or if increased intracranial pressure from hydrocephalus is causing apnea and bradycardia.
   d. Serum electrolyte, calcium, magnesium, and glucose levels. To rule out metabolic abnormality.
   e. Serum phenobarbital and methylxanthine levels. To check levels if indicated.

2. **Additional studies**
   a. **If an inborn error of metabolism is suspected.** Test for organic acid levels, amino acid profiles, ammonia, pyruvate, and lactate. Ketones in the urine may indicate an organic acidemia.
   b. **Stool analysis.** To rule out infant botulism or other organisms.
C. **Imaging and other studies**
   1. **Immediate studies**
      a. **Chest radiograph.** Should be performed immediately if there is any suspicion of heart or lung disease.
      b. **Electrocardiogram (ECG).** If cardiac disease is suspected.
      c. **Abdominal radiograph.** Should be performed immediately if indicated. It may detect signs of NEC (see Figure 11–23).
      d. **Ultrasonography of the head.** To rule out periventricular-intraventricular hemorrhage, hydrocephalus, or any congenital abnormalities.
   2. **Additional studies**
      a. **Echocardiography and cardiac consultation.** ECG can reveal changes in the R-wave amplitude and QRS duration, appearing at the onset and termination of apnea and bradycardia episodes. Also rules out prolonged QT syndrome.
      b. **Electroencephalography.** Apnea and bradycardia may be a manifestation of seizure activity.
      c. **Computed tomography (CT) of the head.** To detect cerebral infarction and subarachnoid hemorrhage. Use adjusted scanning protocol to limit radiation exposure. The **American Academy of Pediatrics (AAP) recommends** early non-contrast CT in term encephalopathic infants to rule out hemorrhage. **Magnetic resonance imaging (MRI)** may be indicated because of the concern for radiation exposure. Term infants may require an MRI for a more extensive workup.
      d. **Abdominal sonography or gastric emptying study.** Useful where GI motility disorder is suspected.
      e. **Barium swallow.** To rule out GER (only in cases of apnea and bradycardia associated with feeding). It is helpful if the infant has a swallowing dysfunction or you suspect tracheoesophageal (TE) fistula or esophageal web. A video-fluoroscopic swallow study (VFSS or VSS) is a modified barium swallow study.
      f. **Esophageal pH probe testing (acid reflux test of Tuttle and Grossman).** Useful in determining whether acidic GER is present. A small-caliber tube with a pH electrode is passed into the distal esophagus. Continuous monitoring can be carried out over 4–24 hours. If the pH is acidic, acidic GER is occurring. Most reflux in infants is not acidic. pH monitoring is of limited use in preemies because their gastric pH is >4 ~90% of the time.
      g. **Multichannel intraluminal impedance.** Measures reflux from retrograde flow of liquid from the stomach through the esophagus going up to the oropharynx. It can detect as small as 0.1 mL of volume by changes in impedance. This technique allows for detection of pH-neutral reflux, which may be as much as 75% of reflux in an infant.
      h. **Reflux scintiscan (termed "milk scan" if used with milk or formula).** This test is used to document GER. It is comparable to the pH probe and superior to the barium swallow. Technetium-99m–labeled pertechnetate is put in a water-based solution or milk (milk scan) and is instilled into the stomach. The patient is scanned in the supine position for 2 hours with the gamma camera. Positive scintigraphy has no correlation with symptoms.
      i. **Lateral neck radiography, head and neck tomography (3 dimensional), and otolaryngology evaluation.** May help to evaluate the upper airway in obstructive apnea.
      j. **Polygraphic recording.** (Usually multichannel, which can include many physiologic parameters.) Continuous recordings for up to 24 hours may help in the differential diagnosis of apnea. There are many different types of devices used.

      i. **Polysomnography.** This is the collective process of monitoring and recording physiologic data during sleep. It includes respiration, perioral electromyography, oxygen saturation, heart rate, electroencephalography, electrocardiography, and electrooculography.

      ii. **Thermistor pneumocardiogram.** This incorporates a thermistor, which detects the changes in nasal and mouth airflow. It incorporates a pH probe to study the acidity in the esophagus.

      iii. **Impedance pneumography.** This measures chest wall movements, oronasal flow, heart rate, and O_2 saturation by a multichannel recorder to help identify different types of apnea.

V. **Plan.** See also Chapter 83.

  A. **Prophylactic therapy and recommended monitoring**

    1. **At-risk infants.** Cochrane review does not support prophylactic caffeine for premature infants at risk of apnea, bradycardia, or hypoxemic episodes.

    2. **Postoperative apnea/bradycardia.** Caffeine can be used to prevent postoperative apnea/bradycardia and oxygen desaturation in preterm infants. Infants <46 weeks postconceptional age should be monitored a minimum of 12 hours postoperatively.

    3. **Postimmunization of preemies.** Infants who had apnea after their first immunization should receive cardiorespiratory monitoring for a minimum of 24 hours after immunization.

    4. **Cobedding of preterm twins.** A decrease in central apnea occurs with cobedding of preterm twins.

  B. **General plan**

    1. **Emergency treatment.** Tactile stimulation, oxygen if the infant is hypoxic, bag-and-mask ventilation, and intubation may be necessary if the infant is not responding. Once the infant is stabilized, evaluation should begin. Send stat labs, get a chest x-ray (CXR) and possible abdominal radiograph. Rule out simple causes: Is temperature okay in isolette? Is the NG tube, endotracheal tube (ETT) in the correct position? Is the position of the infant okay?

    2. **Determine the cause of apnea and bradycardia and treat if possible. Sepsis is a cause that cannot be overlooked** because antibiotics need to be started. Rule out sepsis/infection and other treatable causes (such as intraventricular hemorrhage [IVH], seizures, PDA, anemia, NEC, and others) before diagnosing and treating the infant with apnea of prematurity.

    3. **Apnea of prematurity (AOP)**

      a. **Nonpharmacologic treatments**

        i. **Environmental temperature.** Overheating may play a role in apnea. Keep the environmental thermoneutral or at the lower end of the range; a specific environmental temperature cannot be recommended. Some recommend humidification of warm gas.

        ii. **Infant positioning.** In infants receiving other treatments, these positions did not result in a further decrease of AOP. **Remember that the infant needs to be transitioned to be on the back before discharge.**

          (a) **Prone position.** Avoid neck flexion or extension, which can decrease the patency of the airway. **Prone position reduces apnea,** improves oxygenation and ventilation, decreases GER, and reduces energy expenditure in respiration. Only recommended for infants with apnea in the neonatal intensive care unit (NICU). Nursing in the prone position is also done.

          (b) **Head elevated tilt position ("HETP").** The bed is tilted in an inclined position of 15 degrees so the head and neck are elevated 15 degrees from the prone position; this position reduces episodes of hypoxia.

          (c) **Three stair position ("TSP").** The head and abdomen are maintained at horizontal position. The head is on 3 blankets, the thorax is on

2 blankets, and the pelvis is on one. Airway obstruction and neck inclination do not occur. This position was shown to improve apnea, bradycardia, and desaturation.

   iii. Stimulation

      (a) Tactile stimulation. Provides excitatory activity in the brainstem to stimulate respiratory activity. This is the most common intervention. Provide tactile stimulation (eg, rubbing the skin, stroking the back, patting the infant, tapping or tickling the feet).

      (b) Olfactory stimulation. Introducing a pleasant odor (vanillin) into the incubator decreased apnea (study only 24 hours) in infants who were unresponsive to caffeine or doxapram (see Chapter 20).

      (c) Kangaroo care. Conflicting results: effect is similar to prone positioning.

      (d) Kinesthetic stimulation (oscillating mattress). Not effective in clinically significant apnea. **Stochastic mechanosensory stimulation** has been shown to decrease the duration of oxygen desaturation and potentially decrease apnea.

   iv. Maintain nasal patency. Because nasogastric tubes increase nasal airway resistance and an increase in upper airway resistance may increase apnea of prematurity, **orogastric tubes** have been preferred in premature infants with apnea. Recent studies show that there is no difference in the two for feeding infants with AOP. The placement of the oral versus nasal feeding tubes also had no effect on hypoxia and bradycardia. **Transpyloric feedings (especially when only human milk is used)** may reduce apnea and bradycardia in preemies with suspected GER.

C. Management. **Deciding on which infants to treat usually depends on how many episodes of apnea are occurring, the severity of each episode, and the required intervention to stop the episode of apnea.** If there are multiple or severe apneic episodes, medical treatment may be necessary. Different institutions have different guidelines on when to start treatment. **Some recommendations** are: >6 apneic episodes every 12 hours requiring only minimal stimulation, or >2 apneic episodes per hour requiring minimal stimulation over a couple of hours, or >1–2 apneic episodes in 24 hours requiring vigorous stimulation, or any episode that the infant does not respond to tactile stimulation, or when the infant requires bag-and-mask ventilation with oxygen.

  1. Respiratory support. Maintain adequate oxygen saturation with supplemental oxygen (indicated if there is desaturation or bradycardia). Avoid vigorous suctioning.

    a. Low-flow oxygen. This **may** decrease the rate of intermittent hypoxia and apnea. Avoid hyperoxia.

    b. Nasal cannula oxygen This is a small, tapered cannula that is used to deliver oxygen or blended oxygen. It can cause nasal irritation, causing arousal, and may help to prevent apnea.

      i. Low-flow nasal cannula (<1 L/min) can be used as an adjunct for apnea. Low-flow oxygen does decrease the rate of intermittent hypoxia and apnea.

      ii. High-flow nasal cannula (HFNC) can provide high concentrations of oxygen and also deliver a positive end-expiratory pressure and can be used as an alternative to nasal continuous positive airway pressure (NCPAP). The rates are 1–6 L/min. One study showed that nasal cannula oxygen was just as effective as nasal CPAP (NCPAP). HHHFNC (heated humidified high-flow nasal cannula) is preferred over HFNC.

    c. Continuous positive airway pressure (CPAP). **CPAP via nasal prongs** reduces apneic spells. (**Note:** Different sources cite different CPAP parameters. Ranges reported: 2–4, 3–6, 4–6, and 5–8 cm H_2O.) **A range of 4–6 cm H_2O seems to be cited frequently and is safe.** Use the settings recommended by your institution. It can be used in conjunction with medication (after a therapeutic level has been obtained). Side effects of CPAP include bowel distension, nasal trauma, barotrauma, and pneumothorax.

d. **Noninvasive ventilation (NIV). NIV** is a method of ventilation without tracheal intubation that uses constant or variable pressure to provide ventilatory support. It is often used with CPAP. **Nasal intermittent positive pressure ventilation (NIPPV)** is a type of noninvasive ventilation that combines nCPAP with superimposed positive pressure breaths. Cochrane review states that NIPPV reduced the frequency of apneas more effectively than NCPAP. NIPPV via nasal prongs is more effective than NCPAP alone in apnea of prematurity. NIPPV also reduces the incidence of extubation failure more effectively when compared with NCPAP. More research is recommended.

e. Mechanical ventilation. Should only be used if apnea and bradycardia cannot be controlled by other interventions (drug therapy or nasal CPAP or NIPPV). Low pressures (minimal peak inspiratory pressure) are used at the rate necessary to prevent apnea.

2. Pharmacotherapy. See doses in Chapter 148.

a. Caffeine is the drug of choice for apnea. Theophylline and caffeine seem to have equal efficacy (both reduce apnea within 2–7 days of beginning treatment), but caffeine offers benefits (fewer side effects, once-daily dosing, and increased CSF penetration). Caffeine therapy is associated with improved neurodevelopmental outcome and survival at 18–21 months in infants 500–1250 g and a reduction in death, incidence of cerebral palsy, cognitive delay, and severe ROP. Therapy can usually be discontinued by postconceptional age, usually 35–37 weeks, depending on the weight of the infant (usually 1800–2000 g) or if the infant has been free of apnea for 5–7 days.

b. If apnea persists, begin doxapram. (**Controversial, not recommended as routine therapy.**) Doxapram appears to be efficacious when theophylline, caffeine, and CPAP have failed; it can reduce apnea within 48 hours after other methods have failed. There are concerns with side effects: risk of reduced cerebral blood flow with mental delay later; increased QTc interval, second-degree heart block, lower mental developmental index at 18 months; irritability, gastric retention, hypertension, seizures, and GI disturbance; metabolic acidosis (has benzyl alcohol preservative). If acidosis occurs, consider stopping the medication.

D. Specific treatment

1. Anemia. Transfusion is not routinely recommended as data are conflicting and evidence is insufficient. Most institutions do not treat anemia if the infant is asymptomatic, the infant is feeding and growing, and the reticulocyte count is >5–6%. If the hematocrit (Hct) is low (<21–25% based on institutional guidelines), transfusion may be indicated. If the infant is symptomatic (significant apnea and bradycardia, defined as >9 episodes in 12 hours or >2 episodes in 24 hours requiring bag-and-mask ventilation), on therapeutic doses of methylxanthines, not feeding well, or on oxygen or respiratory support and the reticulocyte count is not appropriate for the low hematocrit (ie, reticulocyte count <2–3%), transfusion may be indicated to a Hct level of ≥30% or higher (**controversial**). Some data suggest that blood transfusion in extremely low birthweight infants is associated with an increase risk in bronchopulmonary dysplasia/chronic lung disease (BPD/CLD) and NEC. The use of recombinant human erythropoietin (rHuEPO) with iron for anemia of prematurity, decreasing the need for transfusions, is **controversial** and may increase the incidence of progression of ROP.

2. Gastroesophageal reflux (GER). Common in premature infants. Apnea is unrelated to GER in most studies. The impression that apnea and bradycardia are more prevalent after feeding is not supported by the literature. Most institutions treat GER because of the possible association. Non-acid GER is responsible for a variable number of AOPs after GER. If clinical assessment (significant reflux or emesis with feeds) warrants intervention, then treatment options include:

a. **Feedings.** Consider a change in feeding volume, method of feeding, or type of feeding. Overfeeding can aggravate reflux, so small volumes more frequently are recommended. Continuous tube feedings may help. Thickened feedings are recommended but *controversial* because randomized trials are inconclusive (starch thickening may be associated with an increase in human milk osmolality, which may make GER worse). Small-volume, thickened milk is preferred. A change in formula may be necessary if a food allergy is suspected. A diet change for the mother with a breast-feeding infant may be necessary. **Transpyloric feedings with human milk** may reduce apnea and bradycardia in preterm infants with GER.

b. **Position.** Hold the infant upright in your arms at least 30 minutes after feeding. Prone head-elevated positioning showed a reduction in apnea and bradycardia and is preferred in infants with GER, but it has become *controversial* because of its association with SIDS. Infants with GER should sleep on their backs. Prone or left lateral position in the postprandial period limits GER.

c. Medications for reflux have limitations based on inconclusive effectiveness and concern for side effects. If needed, the following can be used. Some clinicians advocate a prokinetic agent (eg, metoclopramide). If there is true acid reflux (documented by esophageal pH probe studies), then an H_2 blocker or proton pump inhibitor is used. Acid suppression therapy has been associated with an increase in lower respiratory infections and an increase in gram-negative infections due to the potential for GI colonization. See doses in Chapter 148.

   i. **Prokinetic agents** increase the muscle tone of the digestive tract.

      (a) **Metoclopramide (Reglan).** Improves GI motility and reduces feeding intolerance. In GER of prematurity it is commonly used but *controversial.* (See Chapter 148 for dosing and other information.) Effectiveness is inconclusive and side effects are a concern: drowsiness, restlessness, extrapyramidal symptoms.

      (b) **Erythromycin.** A prokinetic agent; it increases gastric motility and has been used in GER. Cochrane review states that there is insufficient evidence to recommend low or high doses of erythromycin for feeding intolerance in preterm infants. Studies in infants >32 weeks using high-dose erythromycin did show improvement in feeding intolerance.

   ii. **Antacids (Maalox and Mylanta).** Neutralize acid but their use increases the risk of infection and feeding intolerance in infants receiving gavage feedings, and there is a risk of concretion formation. Side effects include diarrhea or constipation. If used, the dosage is 0.5–1 mL/kg by mouth every 4 hours by nasogastric tube. **Alginate-based formulations** (sodium alginate, Gaviscon dose 0.25 mL/kg per dose QID) was shown to decrease the degree and acidity of GER but had no effect on non-acid GER. It doesn't reduce the total number of apneas or gastroesophageal apneas. Side effects have included bezoar formation and adverse effects from the aluminum content. Further studies need to be done.

   iii. **H_2 blockers.** Inhibit gastric acid production in neonates and are usually recommended. Of the 4 H_2 blockers available, ranitidine and famotidine are most commonly used in infants. They are preferred because of fewer side effects. H_2-blocker therapy is associated with higher rates of NEC in very low birthweight (VLBW) infants and an increased risk of Candida infections with H_2 blockers (predisposes to gastric colonization and increases the risk of bacteremia). They may also increase the risk of gram-negative sepsis. Ranitidine is associated with increased infections, increased NEC, and an increase in fatal outcome in VLBW infants and should be used with caution in newborns <1500 g.

   iv. **Proton pump inhibitors (PPIs).** Found not to be effective in reducing GER symptoms in infants. Physicians should use caution when prescribing

PPIs in infants and only use them if there is documented disease with strict monitoring. The studies show that evidence is lacking supporting the safety of PPIs in infants. Lansoprazole (Prevacid) and omeprazole (Prilosec) have been used the most in infants (only U.S. Food and Drug Administration [FDA] approved for infants >1 year). Like the H_2 blockers, they also increase the risk of Candida infections. There is also an increase in the risk of gram-negative sepsis.

E. **Persistent apnea.** Apnea of prematurity usually resolves by 36 weeks. Persistent apnea is apnea that persists ≥37 weeks postmenstrual age. It usually occurs in infants born <28 weeks' gestation. These infants are usually ready to go home except they continue to have apnea. These infants can be at risk for serious episodes of apnea, bradycardia, and cyanosis for several months. How to manage these infants at home is not well studied and recommendations are lacking.

  1. **A comprehensive polygraphic recording is sometimes done before discharge.** This does not predict the risk of SIDS or a severe cardiopulmonary event. It may give a more detailed explanation of the apnea and help in the decision process.
  2. **Medication is continued.** Decision when to stop depends on institutional guidelines.
  3. **Apnea home monitoring.** Cardiorespiratory monitoring at home with an event recorder can be recommended. Parents need to be instructed in the use of the monitor and be trained in cardiopulmonary resuscitation (CPR). Home monitoring does not prevent SIDS. **AAP recommendations on home monitoring:** may be justified in premature infants who are at high risk for recurrent apnea, bradycardia, and hypoxemia; infants with symptomatic BPD/CLD; infants who are respiratory technology dependent; and infants with medical conditions affecting their breathing. Use is limited after episodes stop or ~43 weeks postmenstrual age.

References

Committee on Fetus and Newborn. Apnea, sudden infant death syndrome, and home monitoring. *Pediatrics*. 2003;111:914.

Davis PG, Lemyre B, de Paoli AG. Nasal intermittent positive pressure ventilation (NIPPV) versus nasal continuous positive airway pressure (NCPAP) for preterm neonates after extubation. *Cochrane Database Syst Rev*. 2001;(3):CD003212.

Lemyre B, Davis PG, De Paoli AG. Nasal intermittent positive pressure ventilation (NIPPV) versus nasal continuous positive airway pressure (NCPAP) for apnea of prematurity. *Cochrane Database Syst Rev*. 2002;(1):CD002272.

Zhao J, Gonzalez F, Mu D. Apnea of prematurity: from cause to treatment. *Eur J Pediatr*. 2011;170:1097–1105.

48 Arrhythmia

I. **Problem.** An infant has an abnormal tracing on the heart rate monitor.
II. **Immediate questions**
  A. **What is the heart rate?** The heart rate in newborns varies from 70–190 beats/min. It is normally 120–140 beats/min but may decrease to 70–90 beats/min during sleep and increase to 170–190 beats/min with increased activity such as crying. See Table 48–1 for normal heart rate values.
  B. **Is the abnormality continuous or transient?** Transient episodes of sinus bradycardia, tachycardia, or arrhythmias (usually lasting <15 seconds) are benign and

Table 48–1. **HEART RATES IN NEWBORNS**

Age	Term Infants		Preterm Infants	
	Mean HR	**Range HR**	**Mean HR**	**Range HR**
1 minute	80	20–140	100	50–145
2 minutes	140	80–200	120	80–160
3 minutes	150	100–200	140	105–175
4 minutes	160	120–195	155	120–183
5 minutes	160	120–190	160	120–180
10 minutes	160	110–185	160	129–195
Normal Newborns				
Up to 24 hours	119	84–145		
1–7 days	133	100–175		
8–30 days	163	115–190		

HR, heart rate.
Data from Hastreiter AR, Abella JE. The electrocardiogram in the newborn period: I. The normal infant. *J Pediatr.* 1971;78:146. Dawson JA, Kamlin CO, Wong C, et al. Changes in heart rate in the first minutes after birth. *Arch Dis Child Fetal Neonat Ed.* 2010;95:F177–F181, 2010. Brady JP, James LS. Heart rate changes in the fetus and newborn infant during labor, delivery and immediate neonatal period. *Am J Obstet Gynecol.* 1962;84:1–12. Davidson S, Reina N, Shefi O, Hai-Tov U, Akselrod S. Spectral analysis of heart rate fluctuations and optimal thermal management for low birth weight infants. *Med Biol Eng Comput.* 1997;35:619–625.

do not require further workup. Episodes lasting >15 seconds usually require full electrocardiogram (ECG) assessment.

C. **Is the infant symptomatic?** A symptomatic infant may need immediate treatment. Signs and symptoms of some pathologic arrhythmias include tachypnea, poor skin perfusion, lethargy, hepatomegaly, and rales on pulmonary examination. All of these signs and symptoms may signify congestive heart failure (CHF), which may accompany arrhythmias. CHF resulting from rapid cardiac rhythms is unusual with heart rates <240 beats/min.

III. **Differential diagnosis**

A. **Heart rate abnormalities.** Heart rates in the normal newborn vary dramatically. Some evidence, using computer programs to assess heart rate variability in the neonatal period, suggests that the lower heart rates early on are due to the inability of the infant's sympathetic system to inhibit the parasympathetic (or vagal) response.

1. **Tachycardia.** Heart rate >2 standard deviations (SD) above the mean for age (see Table 48–1).

a. **Benign causes.** Postdelivery, heat or cold stress, painful stimuli, medications (eg, atropine, caffeine, epinephrine, intravenous glucagon, pancuronium bromide, tolazoline, and isoproterenol).

b. **Pathologic causes**

i. **Common.** Fever, shock, hypoxia, anemia, sepsis, patent ductus arteriosus, and CHF.

ii. **Uncommon.** Hyperthyroidism, metabolic disorders, cardiac arrhythmias, and hyperammonemia.

2. **Bradycardia.** Bradycardia is a heart rate >2 SD below the mean for age (see Table 48–1). Transient bradycardia is fairly common in newborns; rates range from 60–70 beats/min.

a. **Benign causes.** During defecation, vomiting or micturition, gavage feedings, suctioning, medications (eg, propranolol, digitalis, atropine, and infusion of

calcium, maternal long-acting β-blockers to treat hypertension given within 24 hours of delivery).
  b. Pathologic causes
    i. Common. Hypoxia, apnea, convulsions, airway obstruction, air leak (eg, pneumothorax), CHF, intracranial bleeding, severe acidosis, and severe hypothermia.
    ii. Uncommon. Hyperkalemia, cardiac arrhythmias, pulmonary hemorrhage, diaphragmatic hernia, hypothyroidism, and hydrocephalus.
B. Arrhythmias
  1. Benign arrhythmias. Include any transient episode (<15 seconds) of sinus bradycardia and tachycardia and any of the benign causes of sinus tachycardia and bradycardia noted in Section III.A.1 and III.A.2. Sinus arrhythmia, a phasic variation in the heart rate often associated with respiration, is also benign.
    a. Premature atrial beats. These can occur in the newborn and are usually benign. The QRS is narrow, and the T waves are often discordant. (See the example in Figure 48–1C.) They tend to decrease in number or go away entirely in the first few months of life. A workup is usually not indicated unless the infant has the premature atrial beats in association with structural cardiac disease.
    b. Unifocal premature ventricular beats. Fairly frequent in the newborn. The QRS is wide, and the T wave is discordant with the sinus T wave. (See Figure 48–1D.) If seen in a newborn, obtain a 12-lead ECG. Do not treat unless the infant is symptomatic. Sometimes premature ventricular contractions (PVCs) become less frequent when the sinus rate increases. PVCs tend to decrease in number or go away entirely in the first few months of life.
    c. Benign bradycardia. Unusual.
  2. Pathologic arrhythmias
    a. Supraventricular tachycardia (SVT). The most common type of cardiac arrhythmia seen in the neonate (Figure 48–1A).
    b. Atrial flutter. Difficult to distinguish from other SVTs, unless the block is >2:1. Administration of adenosine may increase the block to 3:1 or 4:1, allowing the flutter waves to become more visible on the ECG tracing.
    c. Atrial fibrillation. Less common than SVT or atrial flutter.
    d. Wolff-Parkinson-White syndrome (WPW). (A short PR interval and delta wave and slow upstroke of the QRS complex.) Difficult to identify when the rate is fast (Figure 48–1B).
    e. Ectopic beats.
    f. Ventricular tachycardia.
    g. Atrioventricular (AV) block with symptoms. Occurs in newborns with complete block and ventricular rates <55 beats/min. Premature infants may even require a higher rate. Because cardiac output in premature and young term babies can increase only by rate increase (their stroke volume is fixed by the small size of the ventricles), fevers, sepsis, and other stressors are tolerated poorly by babies with complete heart block.
  3. Secondary to extracardiac disease
    a. Sepsis (usually tachycardia).
    b. Diseases of the central nervous system (usually bradycardia).
    c. Hypoglycemia.
    d. Drug toxicity. Digoxin (potentiated by hypokalemia, alkalosis, hypercalcemia, and hypomagnesemia); theophylline (less frequently used in neonatal intensive care units).
    e. Electrolyte abnormalities such as potassium, sodium, magnesium, or calcium abnormalities.
    f. Other. Metabolic acidosis or alkalosis, adrenal insufficiency.

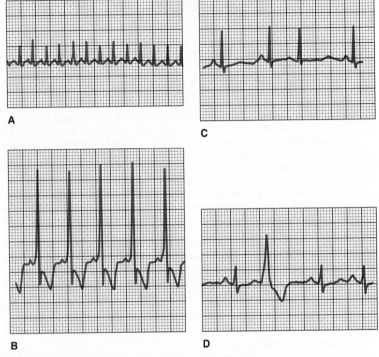

FIGURE 48–1. (A) Supraventricular, narrow QRS tachycardia with a rate of 300 beats/min. The PR interval is long for this rate. (B) Wolff-Parkinson-White syndrome with a short PR interval and a delta upstroke on the QRS complex. The T waves are often discordant. (C) A premature atrial beat. The QRS is narrow, and the T wave is concordant with sinus T waves. (D) A premature ventricular beat. The QRS is wide, and the T wave is discordant with the sinus T wave.

IV. Database

   A. **Physical examination.** Check for signs of CHF (ie, tachypnea, rales on pulmonary examination, enlarged liver, and cardiomegaly). Vomiting and lethargy may be seen in patients with digoxin toxicity. Hypokalemia can cause ileus.

   B. **Laboratory studies**

   1. **Electrolyte, calcium, and magnesium levels**
   2. **Blood gas may reveal acidosis or hypoxia**
   3. **Drug levels to evaluate for toxicity**
      a. **Digoxin.** Normal 0.5–2.0 mcg/mL (sometimes up to 4 mcg/mL). Elevated levels of digoxin alone are not diagnostic of toxicity; clinical and ECG findings consistent with toxicity are also needed, and many neonates have naturally occurring substances that interfere with the radioimmunoassay test for digoxin.
      b. **Caffeine.** Toxicity is manifested by tachycardia and feeding intolerance. Reduce dose or skip dose.

   C. **Imaging and other studies**

   1. **ECG.** Should be performed in all infants who have an abnormal rhythm that lasts >15 seconds or is not related to a benign condition. Diagnostic features of the common arrhythmias are listed next. Although PR interval varies with heart rate, a **PR interval of >160 milliseconds** is abnormal in any newborn.

a. **Supraventricular tachycardia** (see Figure 48–1A)
   i. Ventricular rate of 180–300 beats/min
   ii. No change in heart rate with activity or crying
   iii. An abnormal P wave or PR interval
   iv. A fixed R-R interval
b. **Atrial flutter**
   i. Atrial rate is 220–400 beats/min.
   ii. A sawtooth configuration seen best in leads V_1–V_3 but often difficult to identify when a 2:1 block or rapid ventricular rate is present.
   iii. The QRS complex is usually normal.
c. **Atrial fibrillation**
   i. Irregular atrial waves that vary in size and shape from beat to beat.
   ii. The atrial rate is 350–600 beats/min.
   iii. The QRS complex is normal, but ventricular response is irregular.
d. **Wolff-Parkinson-White syndrome** (see Figure 48–1B)
   i. A short PR interval
   ii. A widened QRS complex
   iii. Presence of a delta wave
e. **Ventricular tachycardia**
   i. Ventricular premature beats at a rate of 120–200 beats/min and a widened QRS complex
f. **Ectopic beats**
   i. Abnormal P wave and widened QRS complex
g. **Atrioventricular block**
   i. **First-degree block** (Figure 48–2A)
      (a) A prolonged PR interval (normal range, 0.08–0.12 second)
      (b) Normal sinus rhythm
      (c) A normal QRS complex
   ii. **Second-degree block**
      (a) **Mobitz type I.** (Figure 48–2B)
         • A progressively prolonged PR interval until a ventricular beat is dropped (Wenckebach)
         • A normal QRS complex
      (b) **Mobitz type II.** (Figure 48–2C) A constant PR interval with dropped ventricular beats or nonconducted P waves
   iii. **Third-degree block** (Figure 48–2D)
      (a) Regular atrial beat.
      (b) Slower ventricular rate.
      (c) Independent atrial and ventricular beats.
      (d) Atrial rate increases with crying and level of activity. The ventricular rate usually stays the same.
h. **Hyperkalemia**
   i. Tall, tented T waves
   ii. A widened QRS complex
   iii. A flat and wide P wave
   iv. Ventricular fibrillation and late asystole
i. **Hypokalemia**
   i. Prolonged QT and PR intervals
   ii. Depressed ST segment
   iii. Flat T wave
j. **Hypocalcemia.** A prolonged QT interval. QT interval prolongation may also be due to myocardial stress at the time of delivery and may resolve. Persistent prolongation of the PR interval with normocalcemia mandates questions about family history of arrhythmia or sudden death. ECG on the parents may be indicated.

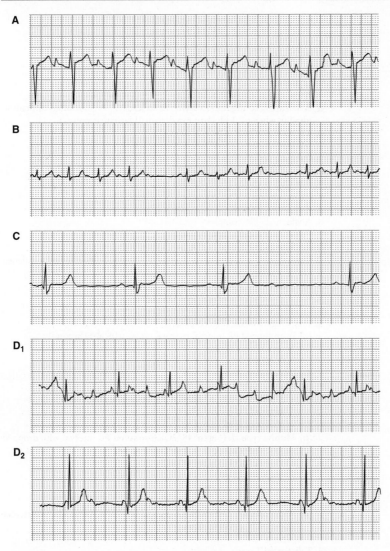

FIGURE 48–2. Types of AV block. (A) First-degree AV block: PR interval is long. (B) Mobitz type I second-degree block (Wenckebach): progressive lengthening of PR interval until ventricular beat is blocked. (C) Mobitz type II second-degree block: PR interval is constant; ventricular beat is blocked. (D_1) Infant with complete or third-degree heart block: atrial rate is 175 beats/min, ventricular rate is 62 beats/min; no relationship between P waves and QRS complexes. (D_2) same infant at 2 months of age: atrial rate is 119 beats/min, ventricular rate is 54 beats/min; still no relationship between P waves and QRS complexes.

   k. Hypercalcemia. Shortened QT interval.
   l. Hypomagnesemia. Same as for hyperkalemia.
   m. Hyponatremia
      i. Short QT interval
      ii. Increased duration of the QRS complex
   n. Hypernatremia
      i. Prolonged QT interval
      ii. Decreased duration of the QRS complex
   o. Metabolic acidosis
      i. Prolonged PR and QRS intervals
      ii. Increased amplitude of the P wave
      iii. Tall, peaked T waves
   p. Metabolic alkalosis. Inverted T wave.
   q. Digoxin
      i. Therapeutic levels. Prolonged PR interval and a short QT interval.
      ii. Toxic levels. Most common are sinoatrial block, second-degree AV block, and multiple ectopic beats; also seen are AV block and bradycardia.
   r. Caffeine
      i. Therapeutic levels. Desired effect is decreased frequency and duration of apneic spells; no significant changes on ECG.
      ii. Toxic levels. Tachycardia with feeding intolerance.
  2. Chest radiograph. Perform in all infants with suspected heart failure or air leak.
V. Plan
  A. General management. Decide whether the arrhythmia is benign or pathologic, as noted. If it is pathologic, full ECG evaluation must be performed. Any acid-base disorder, hypoxia, or electrolyte abnormality needs to be corrected.
  B. Specific management
   1. Heart rate abnormalities
    a. Tachycardia
      i. Benign. No treatment is necessary because the tachycardia is usually secondary to a self-limited event.
      ii. Medications. With certain medications, such as caffeine, observe infant for other signs of toxicity and decrease or skip the next dose.
      iii. Pathologic conditions. The underlying disease should be treated.
    b. Bradycardia. Confirm it is sinus bradycardia and not complete heart block.
      i. Benign. No treatment is usually necessary.
      ii. Drug related. Check the serum drug level if possible and then consider lowering the dosage or discontinuing the drug unless it is necessary.
      iii. Pathologic. Treat the underlying disease.
        (a) In severe hypotension or cardiac arrest, check the airway and initiate breathing and cardiac compressions.
        (b) Administer atropine, epinephrine, or isoproterenol to restore normal rhythm. (See Chapter 148 for dosing.)
   2. Arrhythmias. For dosages and other pharmacologic information, see Chapter 148; for details on cardioversion, see Chapter 28.
    a. Benign. Observation.
    b. Pathologic. Treat any underlying acid-base disorders, hypoxia, or electrolyte abnormalities.
      i. Supraventricular tachycardia
        (a) If the infant's condition is critical. Electrical cardioversion is indicated, with digoxin started for maintenance therapy, if sinus rhythm without preexcitation is present after cardioversion. Propranolol is drug of choice in babies with preexcitation (WPW).
        (b) If the infant's condition is stable. Vagal stimulation (ice or an ice-cold washcloth applied to the infant's face for a few seconds) can be tried.

Adenosine, 100 mcg/kg, IV push into a central vein, converts SVT to sinus rhythm. It may be necessary to double the dose to 200 mcg/kg (300 mcg/kg maximum). **Never use verapamil in infants.** Digoxin should be started as a maintenance drug, unless there is preexcitation. Another drug that may be used instead of or in addition to digoxin is propranolol. SVT refractory to digoxin and propranolol may be treated with flecainide or amiodarone.

   ii. **Atrial flutter**
     (a) **If the infant's condition is critical (severe CHF or unstable hemo-dynamic state).** Perform electrical cardioversion, with digoxin started for maintenance.
     (b) **If the infant is stable.** Start digoxin, which slows the ventricular rate. A combination of digoxin and propranolol may be used instead of digoxin alone.
     (c) **If rate is rapid and 2:1 block present.** Atrial flutter may be hard to identify on ECG. May give adenosine (see above) to increase block to 3 or 4:1.
   iii. **Recurrent atrial flutter management.** Same as that for atrial flutter.
   iv. **Atrial fibrillation (unusual in infants).** Management is the same as for atrial flutter.
   v. **Wolff-Parkinson-White syndrome.** Often accompanied by SVT. β-Blockers are preferred because digoxin may promote 1:1 conduction and demise.
   vi. **Ventricular tachycardia.** Perform electrical cardioversion (except in digitalis toxicity), with lidocaine started for maintenance therapy. Although lidocaine is the drug of choice, other drugs that may be used are procainamide or phenytoin.

3. **Ectopic beats**
   a. **Asymptomatic.** No treatment is necessary.
   b. **Symptomatic.** With underlying heart disease, in the unlikely event that ectopic beats compromise cardiac output, suppress with phenytoin, propranolol, or amiodarone.

4. **Atrioventricular block**
   a. **First degree.** No specific treatment necessary.
   b. **Second degree.** Treat the underlying cause.
   c. **Third degree (complete heart block)**
     i. **Rate >70 beats/min.** If the infant is asymptomatic, observe. Generally at this rate, no problems develop.
     ii. **Rate <50 beats/min.** The patient usually needs emergency transvenous pacing, with the need for subsequent permanent pacing.
     iii. **Rate between 50 and 70 beats/min.** Gray zone. Monitor urine output as an index of end-organ perfusion and measure serum lactate. Check the mother for SAA or SSA antinuclear antibodies (association with complete heart block and cardiomyopathy). Infants with nonimmune complete heart block generally fare better than those whose heart block is caused by maternal antibodies. Mothers who have given birth to an infant with complete heart block because of autoimmune-related SSA or SAA antibodies have a 50–69% chance of subsequent infants having complete heart block. Standard of care for these mothers' subsequent pregnancies include maternal treatment with Plaquenil and following PR interval of the fetus weekly starting at 12 weeks. In an effort to increase fetal heart rate, maternal terbutaline is sometimes used if the infant's heart rate is slow enough to worry about fetal demise.

5. **Arrhythmias secondary to an extracardiac cause**
   a. **Pathologic conditions.** Treat the underlying disease.
   b. **Digoxin toxicity.** Check the PR interval before each dose, obtain a stat serum digoxin level, and hold the dose. Consider digoxin immune Fab (Digibind).
   c. **Theophylline toxicity.** Reduce the dosage or discontinue medication.

6. Electrolyte abnormalities
   a. Check serum electrolyte levels with repeat determinations.
   b. Treat electrolyte abnormalities accordingly.
VI. **Technique of defibrillation/cardioversion.** Presented in Chapter 28.
VII. **Fetal considerations.** A multidisciplinary approach in any fetus with any arrhythmia serious enough to cause fetal hydrops is mandatory. Perinatologists, neonatologists, and cardiologists must be prepared to exert efforts in concert if such infants are to survive. Usually there is at least some warning that such an infant is being delivered, but in the event that specialists are not all in attendance, the physician assuming responsibility for care must be ready to intubate, do pleural and pericardial taps and a paracentesis if necessary, and treat the arrhythmia responsible for fetal CHF.

Selected References

Baruteau A, Fouchard S, Behaghel A, et al. Characteristics and long-term outcome of non-immune isolated atrioventricular block diagnosed in utero or early childhood: a multicentre study. *Eur Heart J.* 2012;33:622–629.

Costedoat-Chalumeau N, Georgin-Lavialle S, Amoura Z, Piette JC. Anti-SSA/Ro and anti-SSB/La antibody mediated congenital heart block. *Lupus.* 2005;14:660–664.

Friedman DM, Kim MY, Copel JA, et al. Utility of cardiac monitoring in fetuses at risk for congenital heart block: the PR Interval and Dexamethasone Evaluation (PRIDE) prospective study. *Circulation.* 2008;117:485–493.

Glickstein J, Buyon J, Kim M, Friedman D; PRIDE investigators. The fetal Doppler mechanical PR interval: a validation study. *Fetal Diagn Ther.* 2004;19:31–34.

Izmirly PM, Kim MY, Llanos C, et al. Evaluation of the risk of anti-SSA/Ro-SSB/La antibody-associated cardiac manifestations of neonatal lupus in fetuses of mothers with systemic lupus erythematosus exposed to hydroxychloroquine. *Ann Rheum Dis.* 2010;69:1827–1830.

Kleinman CS, Neghme RA. Cardiac arrhythmias in the human fetus. *Pediatr Cardiol.* 2004;25:234–251.

Orozco-Gregorio H, Mota-Rojas D, Villanueva H, et al. Caffeine therapy for apnoea of prematurity: pharmacological treatment. *African J Pharmacy Pharmacol.* 2011;5:564–571.

49 Bloody Stool

I. **Problem.** A newborn infant has passed a bloody stool. This is generally a benign and self-limiting disorder. In a large majority of patients, the cause is unknown, but it is important to detect the cases that have significant underlying pathology.
II. **Immediate questions**
   A. **Is the stool grossly bloody?** **Hematochezia (bright red or maroon colored stool)** is usually an ominous sign; **an exception is a bloody stool as a result of swallowed maternal blood, which is a benign condition.** A grossly bloody stool usually signifies **lower gastrointestinal (GI) bleeding** (typically below the ligament of Treitz, which is the anatomic landmark of the duodenojejunal junction): it includes the jejunum, ileum, cecum, colon, rectum, and anus. Hematochezia can occur rarely with massive upper gastrointestinal tract bleeding. **Necrotizing enterocolitis (NEC)** is the most common cause of bloody stool in premature infants and should be strongly suspected.

B. Is the stool otherwise normal in color but with streaks of blood? What is the consistency of the stool? This is more characteristic of a lesion in the anal canal, such as anal fissure. **Anal fissure** is the **most common cause of bleeding** in well infants. A hard stool usually signifies a fissure; a loose or diarrheal stool signifies colitis.

C. Is the stool black and tarry looking? **Melena (black or tarry stools)** suggests **blood in the stool** from the **upper gastrointestinal tract** (proximal to the ligament of Treitz: esophagus, stomach, or duodenum). It can also be from bleeding from the small bowel or proximal ascending colon if transit is slow enough to allow bacteria to denature the hemoglobin. Nasogastric trauma and swallowed maternal blood are common causes.

D. Is it occult blood (fecal occult blood testing/hemoccult) positive only? Microscopic blood as an isolated finding is usually not significant. Tests for occult blood are very sensitive and can be positive with repeated rectal temperatures or any perianal dermatitis.

E. Was the infant given vitamin K at birth? Hemorrhagic disease of the newborn or any coagulopathy may present with bloody stools.

F. What medications are the mother and infant on? Certain medications can cause bleeding. If the **mother** was on thiazides, phenobarbital, oral anticoagulants, or anticonvulsants, these can cross the placenta and cause coagulation abnormalities in the infant. If the **infant** has been given nonsteroidal anti-inflammatory drugs, heparin, tolazoline, indomethacin, or dexamethasone, these are all associated with bleeding.

G. Is the infant well or is the infant ill? Infants with NEC, Hirschsprung enterocolitis, or volvulus are ill; infants with an anal fissure, a milk protein allergy, or nodular lymphoid hyperplasia can appear well.

III. **Differential diagnosis.** The most common routine reasons are swallowed maternal blood and fissures. Significant hemorrhages are usually caused by a duodenal or gastric ulcer.

A. **Melena (black tarry stools).** Usually from the upper GI tract but can be from the small bowel or proximal colon, as noted previously.

1. Maternal blood. **Swallowing of maternal blood during delivery (melena neonatorum) accounts for 30% of infant "GI bleeding."** Infant has normal meconium, then swallowed blood usually appears in the stool on the second or third day of life (second or third stool has blood). **Swallowing of blood during breast-feeding** (secondary to cracked and bleeding nipples) can also cause this. **Swallowing of bloody amniotic fluid** from antepartum hemorrhage associated with bleeding into the amniotic fluid for several hours before birth is rare. This usually presents in the first stool.

2. Nasogastric tube trauma.

3. Coagulopathies. **Hemorrhagic disease of the newborn** occurs from a deficiency in vitamin K–dependent coagulation factors and can be prevented if vitamin K is administered at birth. Melena typically appears on the second or third day of life. Severe hemorrhage can occur in about 0.25–0.50% of neonates. **Other coagulopathies:** liver failure found in some metabolic disorders (iron storage disorder) or ischemic injuries, infections (sepsis).

4. Formula intolerance/dietary protein intolerance. Milk protein sensitivity is secondary to cow's milk or soybean formula, and symptoms of blood in the stool usually occur in the second or third week of life. Infants usually have a mucoid bloody diarrhea.

5. Other GI causes
   a. NEC. Usually presents with bloody stool but can also have melena.
   b. Gastritis/stress ulcer/esophagitis/erosions/gastritis. Occurs in up to 20% of infants in the neonatal intensive care unit (NICU). Prematurity, stress, and mechanical ventilation are associated with stress gastritis. **Hemorrhagic gastritis** can occur from tolazoline and theophylline therapy. Indomethacin is

associated with gastric mucosal injury. **Stress ulcer** is a common cause and can occur in the stomach or duodenum and is associated with prolonged severe illness or steroid therapy. Maternal stress in the third trimester may increase maternal gastrin secretion and contribute to a peptic ulcer in the newborn. **Esophagitis** can occur from trauma from pharyngeal, esophageal, or gastric suction at birth. A gastric and esophageal lesion together is unique to neonates. **Erosions** of the esophageal, duodenal, and gastric mucosa are a common cause of bloody stool. **Mallory-Weiss** or iatrogenic tear is a tear in the esophagus that is an unusual cause of upper gastrointestinal bleeding in an infant.

    c. Congenital GI tract malformations
       i. Anatomic. Intestinal malrotation, duplication cysts, anatomic duplications, Meckel diverticulum, Hirschsprung disease.
      ii. Vascular. Gastrointestinal hemangiomas can present with GI bleeding. **Associated syndromes with vascular malformations** of the GI tract are Down syndrome, Klippel-Trenaunay syndrome, Osler Weber Rendu disease, and blue rubber bleb nevus syndrome.
  6. Unknown cause. Many cases of bloody stool in an infant have no identifiable cause.
  7. Rare causes. Gastric teratoma, gastric Dieulafoy lesion, GI tract telangiectasia, heterotopic pancreatic tissue in the stomach, pyloroduodenal intestinal duplication, and dengue shock syndrome.
B. Grossly bloody stool (hematochezia). Usually from lower GI tract (jejunum, ileum, colon) but can be from the upper GI tract with rapid transit time (rare).
  1. Swallowing of maternal blood with rapid transit time.
  2. Necrotizing enterocolitis. Rare in the first couple of days of life. Emergency room (ER) presentation at 16 days of age with bloody stool in a term neonate.
  3. Coagulopathies. **Disseminated intravascular coagulation (DIC)**—there is usually bleeding from other sites and it may be secondary to an infection. **Hemorrhagic disease of the newborn** occurs from a deficiency in vitamin K–dependent coagulation factors and can be prevented if vitamin K is administered at birth. Bloody stools typically appear on the second or third day of life. Severe hemorrhage can occur in 0.25–0.50% of neonates. **Bleeding diathesis**—platelet abnormalities and clotting factor deficiencies can cause bloody stools. Hemophilia can present as GI hemorrhage. **Severe liver disease** can cause a coagulopathy.
  4. Surgical diseases
    a. Malrotation with midgut volvulus. Obstruction after birth and possible bleeding with ischemic damage or other causes of volvulus.
    b. Meckel diverticulum. **Painless rectal bleeding** (rule of 2's: 2% of population, length 2 inches, within 2 ft of ileocecal valve, 2 times as common in males, diagnosed in the first 2 years of life, 2 types of tissue present).
    c. Hirschsprung enterocolitis. Ten to thirty percent present with GI bleeding and abdominal distension; failure to pass meconium and feeding intolerance.
    d. Intussusception. Rare in the neonatal period; incidence is greatest in infants 3 months to 1 year of age. Most present with typical symptoms: bloody stool ("currant jelly" stool), abdominal mass, vomiting, and intermittent screaming. Intrauterine intussusception presents with a complete ileus.
    e. Gastrointestinal duplications. Colonic and tubular are least uncommon but do occur; presents with obstruction or abdominal mass and bleeding can occur due to presence of ectopic gastric mucosa or stasis.
    f. Incarcerated inguinal hernia. Infants are typically very irritable, refuse to eat, and on physical examination have a tender firm mass in the inguinal canal.
    g. Rare causes. Rectal polyp (more common in toddlers but can occur in newborns); acute appendicitis; duplication cyst induced by a congenital ileal polyp.

5. Colitis can be secondary to the following:
   a. **Intestinal infections (bacterial enteritis).** Rare in neonatal period and more common in older children and adults.
   b. **Food allergy (common cause in newborns).** Dietary/formula intolerance factors, including allergy and dietary protein-induced colitis. The top allergens are cow's milk products and soy. **There are multiple disorders: Allergic enterocolitis** can present with massive bloody stool, and lab data show no eosinophilia. Rectal mucosal biopsy shows eosinophilic infiltration. **Neonatal transient eosinophilic colitis**—there are cases of infants with this with no known allergic component involved (no prior feeding had occurred). **Eosinophilic gastrointestinal disorders (EGIDs)** are disorders where there is primary eosinophil inflammation in the gastrointestinal tract. **Food protein-induced proctocolitis (FPIPC)**—presents with bright red rectal bleeding with mucus in healthy neonate. Infant can occasionally have mild peripheral eosinophilia. Mainly in breast-fed infants but can be found in infants receiving cow's milk or soy. Nodular hyperplasia is found on endoscopy. **Food protein-induced enterocolitis syndrome (FPIES)/dietary protein-induced enterocolitis syndrome (DPIES):** non–IgE-mediated immune reaction in GI tract portions or entire GI tract involvement. Rare in breast-fed infants. **Hematochezia in exclusively breast-fed infants** presents at an average age of 7.4 weeks. Diarrhea is the most common symptom (also mild anemia, red and white cells in stool, negative culture, colitis on colonoscopy) and may represent sensitivity to protein eaten by the mother. The hematochezia disappears after the mother is on a protein-free diet.
C. **Streaks of bright red blood coating a normal or hard stool.** Most commonly associated with a perianal disorder.
   1. **Anal fissure** can be secondary to constipation and straining. This is the **most common cause of bleeding in infants**: spots of blood in the diaper or a strip of blood on the outside of one side of the stool. Etiology is a tear of the anal canal at the mucocutaneous line from a hard stool. Deeper rectal fissures can also occur.
   2. **Rectal trauma** may be secondary to temperature probes.
   3. **Perianal irritation and excoriations** can cause small amounts of blood. **This can be from a diaper rash.**
   4. **Rare causes. Rectal prolapse** is reported with chronic constipation, cow's milk allergy, *Shigella* diarrhea, rectal parasite infections, Hirschsprung disease, high anorectal malformations, and cystic fibrosis. **Perianal abscess/fistula in ano** is common in infants <1 year of age. It can originate from anal cryptitis, which then forms a perianal abscess. **Proctitis**—eosinophilic proctitis from cow's milk protein intolerance can present with rectal bleeding and proctitis.
D. **Bright red blood mixed in with a normal /loose stool.** This suggests bleeding from the lower GI tract. May occur from a proximal source with some degree of digestion of blood.
   1. **Eosinophilic proctocolitis. This is also called protein-induced proctitis or milk-induced enterocolitis.** Blood mixed with normal stools (sometimes with mucus) in a healthy infant that occurs most commonly in breast-fed infants, but can occur with cow's milk, soy protein–based, or hydrolysate formula.
   2. **Lymphonodular/nodular lymphoid hyperplasia (of the rectosigmoid area).** Characterized by multiple masses of lymphoid nodules that are usually present in the terminal ileum or colon. It disrupts the normal mucosa and leads to thinning of the mucosa and bleeding. Etiology is unknown. It can occur from cow's milk allergy or an immunologic response.
E. **Occult GI blood by fecal occult blood testing/hemoccult**
   1. **Positive fecal occult blood test/hemoccult test/stool guaiac.** As an isolated finding, is usually not significant. Tests for occult blood are very sensitive and can be positive with repeated rectal temperatures or any perianal dermatitis.

    2. **Can be positive earlier** in breast/cow's milk–fed infants and in more significant diseases such as esophagitis, gastritis, Meckel diverticulum, vascular malformations, eosinophilic gastroenteritis, polyps, colitis and others.

    3. **NEC.** Presence of occult blood does not correlate with the development of NEC.

  F. **Blood spots in a diaper (non-GI causes).** This can be from other **etiologies beside the gastrointestinal tract:** hematuria, severe diaper rash with excoriation, blood from a circumcision, vaginal bleeding in a female infant (**pseudomenses**—withdrawal of maternal hormones). Reddish-orange spots ("brick stain") in the diaper are from uric acid crystals in the urine and are usually benign but may indicate concentrated urine. A red stained diaper can also be from bile pigments or porphyrins.

IV. Database. The age of the infant is important. If the infant is <7 days old, swallowed maternal blood is a likely cause; in older infants, this is unlikely. Ask the mother about medications taken during pregnancy. Is the infant breast-feeding? Get a detailed description of the stool since type of stool and color of blood can all help to differentiate the bleeding source (see Section III above).

  A. **Physical examination**

    1. **Evaluate the infant's peripheral perfusion.** An infant with NEC can be poorly perfused and may appear to be in early or impending shock. Bruising may suggest a coagulopathy.

    2. **Examine naso-/oropharyngeal area for a source of bleeding.**

    3. **Abdominal examination.** Check for bowel sounds and tenderness. Hyperactive bowel sounds are more common in upper gastrointestinal bleeding. If the abdomen is soft and nontender and there is no erythema, a major intra-abdominal process is unlikely. If the abdomen is distended, rigid, or tender, an intra-abdominal pathologic process is likely. Abdominal distention is the most common sign of NEC. Abdominal distention may also suggest intussusception or midgut volvulus. If there are red streaks and erythema on the abdominal wall, suspect NEC with peritonitis. Malrotation with ischemic bowel can also present with peritonitis. If there is an abdominal mass, consider duplication. Consider Hirschsprung disease or malrotation if there is obstruction. Hepatomegaly, splenomegaly, or jaundice may indicate liver disease.

    4. **GU/anal examination.** Does the infant have a rash? If the infant's condition is stable, perform a visual examination of the anus to check for anal fissure or tear. Look for polyps, masses, or fistulas. Gentle digital rectal examination with a lubricated pinky finger may reveal fissures or polyps. Bedside "anoscopy" can be done by placing a lubricated blood collection tube into the anus.

  B. **Laboratory studies**

    1. **Initial studies**

      a. **Fecal occult blood testing (FOBT). Hemoccult or other test** for the presence of blood. This is not useful for screening for NEC. It is positive in more cow's milk–fed infants than formula-fed infants.

      b. **Apt test.** To differentiate maternal from fetal blood if swallowed maternal blood is suspected. A positive test indicates that the blood is due to either gastrointestinal or pulmonary bleeding from the neonate. A negative test would indicate that the blood is of maternal origin.

      c. **CBC with differential.** If a large amount of blood is lost acutely, it takes time for it to be evident on hemoglobin results; therefore, initial hemoglobin values may be unreliable. An increased white blood count suggests infection or thrombocytopenia (can be associated with NEC, sepsis).

      d. **Chemistry panel.** High BUN can be seen in upper GI bleeding (resorption of blood in GI tract).

      e. **Coagulation studies.** To rule out DIC or a bleeding disorder. The usual studies are partial thromboplastin time (PTT), prothrombin time (PT), fibrinogen level, and platelet count. Thrombocytopenia can also be seen with cow's milk–protein allergy. An elevated PT can indicate a coagulopathy. A prolonged PTT may indicate hemophilia.

    f. **Suspected NEC.** If NEC is suspected, the following studies should be performed:

      i. **CBC with differential.** To establish an inflammatory response and to check for thrombocytopenia and anemia.

      ii. **Serum potassium levels.** Hyperkalemia secondary to hemolysis may occur.

      iii. **Serum sodium levels.** Hyponatremia can be seen secondary to third spacing of fluids.

      iv. **Blood gas levels.** To rule out metabolic acidosis, which is often associated with sepsis or NEC.

  2. **Further studies**

    a. **Stool studies.** Certain pathogens cause bloody stools, but they are rare in the neonatal nursery. Obtain stool cultures for common pathogens, ova, and parasites. Stool smear for white blood cells (WBCs; elevated with colitis) and eosinophils (suggests allergic colitis).

    b. **Allergic enterocolitis diagnosis.** Difficult because there is no specific laboratory test. Eosinophilia may be present in the serum and can be present in the stool. A rectal mucosal punch biopsy can show eosinophilic infiltration suggestive of an allergic origin.

C. Imaging and other studies

  1. **Immediate study**

    a. **Abdominal radiograph.** A plain radiograph of the abdomen is useful if NEC or a surgical abdomen is suspected. Look for an abnormal gas pattern, a thickened bowel wall, pneumatosis intestinalis, or perforation. Pneumatosis can appear as a "soap bubble" area (see Figure 11–23). If a suspicious area appears on the abdominal radiograph in the right upper quadrant, it is usually not stool. A left lateral decubitus view of the abdomen may show free air if perforation has occurred and it cannot be seen on a routine anteroposterior (AP) film. Surgical conditions usually show signs of intestinal obstruction. Most common sign in intussusception in premature infants is dilated bowel loops.

  2. **Additional studies**

    a. **Abdominal ultrasound with color Doppler studies** to diagnose intussusception. A pseudo kidney (longitudinal appearance of the intussuscepted segment of bowel) is seen with intussusception and Meckel diverticulum.

    b. **Contrast studies** can be done for diagnosis of obstruction.

    c. **Endoscopy of upper gastrointestinal tract** allows visualization of the esophagus, stomach, and duodenum and helps to identify the site of bleeding in the upper tract.

    d. **Electronic gastroscopy** can be done in infants at 0–3 months. This can be used to assess upper gastrointestinal bleeding.

    e. **Meckel scan** (technetium-99m pertechnetate nuclear scan) can help diagnose Meckel diverticulum.

    f. **Radioactive tagged red blood cell (RBC) scan** can localize the site of lower GI bleeding if the source is unknown.

    g. **Colonoscopy** can be done to rule out colitis, polyps, or other masses.

    h. **Rectal mucosal biopsy** can show eosinophilia in the lamina propria in cases of allergic enterocolitis.

    i. **CT scan** to evaluate for obstruction or see gastrointestinal hemangiomatosis.

V. Plan. Based on the clinical status of the infant: Is the infant critically ill? Is the infant in shock? Is the infant who presents with blood in the stool well?

  A. Critically ill infant. Follow basic ABCs, and pass nasogastric/orogastric (NG/OG) tube. Aggressive volume replacement if hypotension/hypovolemia is present. Make NPO and consider broad-spectrum antibiotics. Correct acidosis and fluid disturbances if appropriate. Do immediate laboratory and radiograph studies. Consider surgical consultation and initiation of peripheral nutritional support.

B. **Noncritically ill infant.** Rule out non-GI causes of blood, especially if there was just blood on a diaper (see Section III.F). Rule out swallowed maternal blood, blood from breast-feeding, and an anal fissure. Then do the following:
   1. **Place the infant NPO.**
   2. **Start the workup.** Initial laboratory tests and abdominal radiograph.
   3. **Antibiotics.** Some institutions will start the infant on antibiotics while the workup is done depending on the clinical status of the infant.
   4. **For isolated rectal bleeding.** Placing the infant NPO for 1 day and antibiotics for 2 days was not associated with increased deterioration or recurrent episodes of isolated rectal bleeding.

C. **Individual plans as follows:**
   1. **Swallowed maternal blood.** Observation only.
   2. **Anal fissure and rectal trauma.** Observation is indicated. Petroleum jelly applied to the anus may promote healing.
   3. **Necrotizing enterocolitis.** See Chapter 113.
   4. **Nasogastric trauma.** In most cases of bloody stool involving nasogastric tubes, trauma is mild and requires only observation. If the tube is too large, replacing it with a smaller one may resolve the problem. If there has been significant bleeding, **gastric lavages** are helpful; it is ***controversial*** whether tepid water or normal saline is best. Then, if possible, removal of the nasogastric tube is recommended.
   5. **Formula intolerance.** Difficult to document acutely, and is usually diagnosed if the patient has remission of symptoms when the formula is eliminated. In breast-fed infants with rectal bleeding, the use of lactobacillus was not supported by the literature. Cow's milk allergy should be treated with a cow's milk–free diet and then those who become symptom-free should be rechallenged to reduce the number of false-positive diagnoses.
   6. **Gastritis or ulcers.** Treatment usually consists of ranitidine (preferred because of fewer side effects) or famotidine. Use of antacids in neonates is ***controversial***; some clinicians believe that concretions may result from the use of antacids. Use of antacids increases the risk of infection and feeding intolerance in infants receiving gavage feedings. (See Chapter 55.)
   7. **Unknown cause.** If no cause is found, the infant is usually closely monitored. In the majority of the cases, the bleeding subsides.
   8. **Nodular lymphoid hyperplasia.** Change the infant's formula to a hypoallergenic type.
   9. **Intestinal infections.** Antibiotic treatment and isolation are standard treatment.
   10. **Hemorrhagic disease of the newborn.** Intravenous vitamin K is usually adequate therapy (see Chapter 87). Fresh frozen plasma (FFP) and red cell transfusions are sometimes needed.
   11. **Surgical conditions (eg, NEC, perforation, volvulus).** All require immediate surgical evaluation. Intussusception can be reduced with an enema in most cases.

50 Counseling Parents Before High-Risk Delivery

I. **Problem.** The nurse calls to notify you of a pending high-risk delivery. You are on delivery room duty, and you are asked to counsel the parents before their infant is delivered.

II. **Immediate questions**

   A. **Are both parents and other important family members available? Is a translator needed?** Discuss the situation with the obstetric staff. A family member is often too emotionally involved to accurately translate.

B. **Is the mother too sick or uncomfortable to be able to adequately participate in the discussion?** In this situation, it is essential to include other family members.

C. **How well do the parents understand their current situation?** Discuss the circumstances with the obstetric staff, and ask the parents what they understand.

D. **What do they know about neonatal intensive care units (NICUs), pregnancy and neonatal complications, chronic health problems, and neurodevelopmental disability?** This helps you in beginning the discussion.

III. **Differential diagnosis.** Neonatologists are called to counsel expectant parents in a variety of circumstances. These include:

A. Preterm birth

B. Intrauterine growth restriction (IUGR)

C. Maternal drug use

D. Signs of fetal distress

E. Congenital anomalies

IV. **Database**

A. **Maternal/paternal data.** Obtain information regarding the age of both parents; mother's obstetric, past medical, and social history; history of the pregnancy, medications, and pertinent laboratory data; and family history.

B. **Fetal data.** Review fetal information with the obstetric staff, including accuracy of pregnancy dating, findings on prenatal ultrasounds, and signs of fetal distress.

V. **Plan**

A. **General approach to parent counseling.** Although circumstances are often less than ideal, it is important to communicate as effectively and empathetically as possible. Sit down, communicate at eye level, take time to introduce yourself and your role, and talk in a clear and unhurried manner. Explain all medical terms, avoid using abbreviations and percentages (many people cannot comprehend them), and acknowledge uncertainties. Ask if they understand, and summarize the most important points. Ask if they have any questions and offer to follow-up with them if they have more questions.

B. **Goal of counseling session.** Because a complete discussion is often unrealistic, your goal is to help parents anticipate and to provide a framework for understanding what happens during delivery and in the NICU.

C. **Content of discussion.** Discuss the infant's chances of survival, possible complications, and the range of long-term outcomes. Review appropriate references and other chapters in this book and textbooks for more information. Describe the anticipated activity during delivery. Giving them the opportunity to tour the NICU allows them to see the monitoring and life support equipment, so that they can better see their own baby underneath it all.

D. **Bedside manner.** For many, the shock and anxiety of facing difficult circumstances challenges their ability to process. Avoid overloading the family with information. Your communication is most effective if conveyed in a caring, empathetic, and unhurried manner. *Understand that hope helps people get through the most dire situations.*

VI. **Specific counseling issues.** Although medical terms are used in this section, avoid using medical terms as much as possible when counseling parents.

A. **Preterm delivery.** The more immature the infant, the greater are the risks of death, complications, health sequelae, and neurodevelopmental disability (Table 50–1). Gestational age serves as a proxy for maturity when counseling parents before delivery.

1. **Immediate questions.** Why is the mother delivering preterm? What is the gestational age of the fetus? Are there concerns about fetal growth, fetal distress, or infection?

2. **Specific issues to address with the parents**

a. **Mortality.** Even with aggressive intervention, the lower limit of viability is 23–24 weeks' gestation, with occasional survival reported at 22 weeks' gestation.

Table 50–1. **ESTIMATES OF MORBIDITY USEFUL IN COUNSELING PARENTS**

Risk Factor	Cerebral Palsy (%)	Intellectual Disability (%)	Sensory Impairment (%)
None	0.1–0.4	1–2	0.1–0.2
Prematurity			
GA 33–36 weeks	0.6–0.7	1–2	0.1–0.2
GA 29–32 weeks	4	2–3	0.4–2
GA ≤ 28 weeks	8–12	12–16	2–4
GA ≤ 25 weeks	17–40	27–47	4–9

GA, completed weeks of gestation at birth (birthweight data are difficult to accurately determine for prenatal counseling).

  b. **Complications of prematurity.** Complications of prematurity include respiratory distress syndrome; electrolyte and metabolic problems; infection; necrotizing enterocolitis; patent ductus arteriosus; apnea and bradycardia; anemia; and intraventricular hemorrhage and other signs of brain injury. Chronic complications include bronchopulmonary dysplasia/chronic lung disease (BPD/CLD); retinopathy of prematurity with subsequent visual problems; hearing impairment; and neurodevelopmental impairment. Complication rates increase with decreasing gestational age.

  c. **Long-term neurodevelopmental outcome.** Rates of neurodevelopmental disabilities increase with decreasing gestational age at birth, with the highest rates in those born before 25 weeks' gestation (see Table 50–1). Even late preterm children (born at 34–36 weeks' gestation) have higher rates of cerebral palsy and school problems than do infants born full term. Learning disability, language delays, visual perceptual deficits, minor neuromotor dysfunction, executive dysfunction, attention deficits, and behavior problems are more frequent in school-age children born preterm than in controls born full term. Nonetheless, the majority of preterm survivors have normal intelligence, graduate from high school, and become functioning adults in their communities.

B. **Intrauterine growth restriction (IUGR).** See also Chapter 105.

  1. **Immediate questions.** What is the cause of the IUGR and when was it detected? Are there signs of fetal decompensation?

  2. **Specific issues to address with parents**

   a. **Prediction of outcome.** The most important determinant of IUGR outcome is its cause. Infants with chromosomal disorders and congenital infections (eg, toxoplasmosis, cytomegalovirus) experience early IUGR, often do not tolerate labor and delivery well, and commonly have a disability. When there is fetal deprivation of uterine supply, the fetus initially compensates by reducing weight and length before head growth and, after 30 weeks' gestation, may accelerate fetal maturation. Although accelerated maturation improves fetal survival if delivered preterm, there is a cost in terms of cognitive development. Adverse intrauterine circumstances that overwhelm compensatory mechanisms lead to progressive damage to fetal organs, including the brain, and may result in fetal death.

   b. **Complications of IUGR.** IUGR infants are vulnerable to complications, including perinatal asphyxia, cold stress, polycythemia, and hypoglycemia.

   c. **Long-term outcome.** Full-term IUGR infants with fetal deprivation of supply have an increased risk of motor and cognitive impairments (cerebral palsy, minor neuromotor dysfunction, learning disability, attention deficits, behavior problems) and, as adults, cardiovascular disease, obesity, and diabetes. Preterm IUGR infants are vulnerable to the complications of both preterm delivery and IUGR.

C. **Maternal use of drugs**
1. **Immediate questions.** Which drugs did the mother use? When and how much?
2. **Specific issues to address with parents**
   a. **IUGR.** Infants with intrauterine exposure to opiates, cocaine, alcohol, cigarettes, and some prescription drugs can be diagnosed with IUGR (see preceding Section VI.B).
   b. **Specific syndromes and risks.** Fetal alcohol and fetal hydantoin syndromes are well defined but often difficult to diagnose in the neonatal period. Both carry an increased risk of intellectual disability. (See Chapter 88.)
   c. **Neonatal withdrawal syndrome.** Infants with intrauterine exposure to opiates, cocaine, alcohol, or some prescription medications may demonstrate neonatal withdrawal syndrome (see Chapter 103). These infants require close observation after delivery and may require medications to help them through the withdrawal period. Later, these infants have an increased incidence of school and behavior problems.
   d. **Cocaine exposure and risks.** Maternal cocaine use is associated with increased rates of miscarriage, stillbirth, abruption, preterm labor, and IUGR. Infants with central nervous system infarctions resulting from cocaine exposure are at risk for cerebral palsy, especially hemiplegia, as well as cognitive and sensory impairments.

D. **Signs of fetal distress**
1. **Immediate questions.** Which signs of fetal distress are evident and for how long?
2. **Specific issue to address.** The type of fetal distress and, after birth, evidence of neonatal encephalopathy and brain injury on neuroimaging, electroencephalogram, and neurodevelopmental examination (see Chapter 16) are prognostic indicators. Nonetheless, the majority of infants who demonstrate signs of fetal distress do not develop neonatal encephalopathy, persistent pulmonary hypertension, or neurodevelopmental disability.

E. **Congenital anomalies**
1. **Immediate questions.** What anomalies have been detected and how were they noted? Is the anomaly life-threatening? What workup has been done? Have any other anomalies been detected?
2. **Specific issues to address with the parents.** See Chapter 88.
   a. **Diagnosis.** The type of congenital anomaly, its severity, and whether further evaluation has identified other anomalies or etiology, to determine how you should counsel the parents.
   b. **Prognosis.** Clinical courses and outcomes have been well described for most chromosomal disorders (eg, trisomy 21, 22q11 deletion), many multiple congenital anomaly syndromes (eg, VATER/VACTERL [vertebral defects, anal atresia, tracheoesophageal fistula, and radial or renal dysplasia/vertebral defects, anal atresia, cardiac malformations, tracheoesophageal fistula, renal dysplasia and limb abnormalities] association, arthrogryposis), and some specific single anomalies (eg, meningomyelocele, congenital heart disease). The presence of a congenital anomaly increases an infant's risks of preterm birth, neurodevelopmental outcome.
   c. **Counseling parents.** Mothers who were counseled after prenatal diagnosis of a congenital anomaly reported in an interview a week after delivery that the consultation helped to prepare them. The study concluded that "parents want realistic medical information, specific to their situation, provided in an empathetic manner and want to be allowed to hope for the best possible outcome."

Selected References

Allen MC. Assessment of gestational age and neuromaturation. *Ment Retard Dev Disabil Res Rev*. 2005;11:21–33.

Allen MC. Risk assessment and neurodevelopmental outcomes. In: Gleason CA, Devaskar SU, eds. *Avery's Diseases of the Newborn*. Philadelphia: Saunders/Elsevier, 2012:920–935.

Allen MC, Cristofalo EA, Kim C. Outcomes of preterm infants: morbidity replaces mortality. *Clin Perinatol*. 2011;38:441–454.

Behrman RE, Butler AS, eds. *Preterm Birth: Causes, Consequences, and Prevention. Committee on Understanding Premature Birth and Assuring Healthy Outcomes*. Washington, DC: National Academies Press; 2007.

Donohue PK, Boss RD, Shepard J, Graham E, Allen MC. Intervention at the border of viability: perspective over a decade. *Arch Pediatr Adolesc Med*. 2009;163:902–906.

Graham EM, Ruis KA, Hartman AL, Northington FJ, Fox HE. A systematic review of the role of intrapartum hypoxia-ischemia in the causation of neonatal encephalopathy. *Am J Obstet Gynecol*. 2008;199:587–595.

Miquel-Verges F, Woods SL, Aucott SW, Boss RD, Sulpar LJ, Donohue PK. Prenatal consultation with a neonatologist for congenital anomalies: parental perceptions. *Pediatrics*. 2009;124:e573–e579.

Raz S, Debastos AK, Newman JB, Batton D. Intrauterine growth and neuropsychological performance in very low birth weight preschoolers. *J Int Neuropsychol Soc*. 2012;18:200–211.

Shankaran S, Lester BM, Das A, et al. Impact of maternal substance use during pregnancy on childhood outcome. *Semin Fetal Neonatal Med*. 2007;12:143–150.

51 Cyanosis

I. **Problem.** During a physical examination, an infant appears blue. Cyanosis can be caused by a rise in deoxygenated hemoglobin (more common) or an abnormal hemoglobin disorder.

II. **Immediate questions**

A. **Does the infant have respiratory distress?** If the infant has increased respiratory effort with increased rate, retractions, and nasal flaring, respiratory disease should be high on the list of differential diagnoses. **Cyanotic heart disease** usually presents without respiratory symptoms ("happy blue baby") but can have effortless tachypnea (rapid respiratory rate without retractions). **Blood disorders** usually present without respiratory or cardiac symptoms.

B. **Does the infant have a murmur?** A murmur usually implies heart disease, but in infants with congenital heart malformations, <50% have a murmur in the newborn period. Transposition of the great vessels can present without a murmur (~60%). Muffled heart sounds can indicate pericardial effusions or pneumopericardium.

C. **Was the infant cyanotic at birth?** Infants with **transposition of the great vessels** and **tricuspid atresia** can present almost immediately at birth with cyanosis. In the perinatal period, infants with truncus arteriosus, total anomalous pulmonary venous return, and tetralogy of Fallot can present with cyanosis.

D. **Is the cyanosis continuous, intermittent, cyclical, sudden in onset, or occurring only with feeding or crying?** **Intermittent cyanosis** is more common with neurologic disorders; these infants may have apneic spells alternating with periods of normal breathing. **Cyclical cyanosis** can occur with nasal obstruction. **Continuous**

cyanosis is more commonly associated with intrinsic lung disease or heart disease. **Cyanosis with feeding** can occur with esophageal atresia and severe gastroesophageal reflux. **Sudden onset of cyanosis** may occur with an air leak, such as pneumothorax. **Cyanosis that disappears with crying** may mean choanal atresia. **Cyanosis only with crying** can occur in infants with tetralogy of Fallot. **Cyanotic spells** with no or minimal coughing can occur with pertussis. **Crying** may improve cyanosis in respiratory disease and worsen it in cardiac disease.

E. **Is the pulse oximeter normal and the infant blue?** The pulse oximeter measures oxygen saturation of hemoglobin that is available to bind oxygen. If there is abnormal hemoglobin, it will not be measured. If you see a normal pulse oximeter in a cyanotic infant, think methemoglobinemia.

F. **Has the baby had the recommended pulse oximetry screening for congenital heart disease?** This has been recommended by the American Academy of Pediatrics (AAP) in all newborns (see page 43) as a useful method for screening for critical congenital cyanotic heart disease.

G. **Is there differential cyanosis (DC)?** Differential cyanosis is when there is cyanosis of the upper or lower part of the body only, and it usually signifies serious heart disease. **The prerequisite for this to happen is the presence of a right-to-left shunt through the patent ductus arteriosus (PDA).** To diagnose this, oxygen saturation should be measured in the preductal (right hand is preferred since it accurately reflects preductal value) and postductal (foot). There are 2 different types of differential cyanosis.

1. **Pink upper half of the body, cyanosis lower part of body (more common).** (Oxygen saturation is greater in the right hand than in the foot.) It occurs with severe coarctation of the aorta or interrupted aortic arch. It can also occur with persistent pulmonary hypertension (PPH) with right-to-left shunting through the ductus arteriosus.

2. **Cyanosis in the upper half of the body, pink lower part of the body. This type is very rare (reversed differential cyanosis [RDC]) and occurs when oxygen saturation is lower in the right hand than in the foot.** This is seen in complete transposition of the great arteries with shunt through the PDA with persistent pulmonary hypertension or aortic interruption/coarctation. It can also be seen in an infant with supracardiac total anomalous pulmonary venous connection (TAPVC) to the superior vena cava with a shunt through the PDA.

H. **What is the prenatal and delivery history?** Did the mother have a prenatal sonogram? It may show a cardiac anomaly. An infant of a diabetic mother has an increased risk of hypoglycemia, TTN, polycythemia, respiratory distress syndrome, and heart disease (TGA). Infection, such as that which can occur with premature rupture of membranes, may cause shock and hypotension with resultant cyanosis. Coxsackie B viral infections cause myocarditis in newborn infants. Amniotic fluid abnormalities, such as oligohydramnios (associated with pulmonary hypoplasia) or polyhydramnios (associated with esophageal atresia), may suggest a cause for the cyanosis. Cesarean section is associated with increased respiratory distress, transient tachypnea of the newborn (TTN), and persistent pulmonary hypertension of the newborn (PPHN). Pregnancy-induced hypertension can be associated with intrauterine growth restriction (IUGR), polycythemia, and hypoglycemia. Congenital infections can lead to cardiac abnormalities. Advanced maternal age can be associated with birth defects such as Down syndrome and Turner syndrome, which include heart defects. **Certain perinatal conditions increase the incidence of congenital heart disease.**

1. **Medications used by the mother can cause an increase in congenital heart disease.** Anticonvulsants, lithium, indomethacin, nonsteroidal anti-inflammatory drugs (NSAIDs), ibuprofen, sulfasalazine, thalidomide, trimethoprim, sulfonamide, vitamin A, selective serotonin reuptake inhibitors (SSRIs), marijuana, alcohol, cigarette smoking, cocaine, and exposure to organic solvents.

2. **Maternal illnesses that increase the risk of congenital heart disease.** Untreated phenylketonuria (PKU), maternal pregestational diabetes, febrile illness during the first trimester, influenza, maternal rubella, epilepsy, and maternal lupus/connective tissue disease.

3. **Maternal congenital heart disease and/or congenital heart disease in a first-degree relative.** Increased incidence of heart disease in the child.

III. **Differential diagnosis.** Cyanosis becomes visible when there is >3–5 g/dL of deoxygenated hemoglobin/dL. The degree of cyanosis depends on both oxygen saturation and hemoglobin concentration. Cyanosis can be a sign of severe cardiac, respiratory, or neurologic compromise. **The most common etiology of cyanosis in a newborn infant is respiratory.** Cyanosis can also be caused by a reduced blood oxygen–carrying capacity secondary to an abnormal form of hemoglobin, such as methemoglobinemia. Cyanosis may not be apparent in a severely anemic infant or may be difficult to see in a darkly pigmented newborn. The causes of cyanosis can be classified as arising from respiratory, cardiac, central nervous system (CNS), or other disorders.

A. **Respiratory diseases.** Include primary pulmonary diseases, airway obstruction, and extrinsic compression of the lungs and congenital defects. **Pulmonary diseases are the most common cause of cyanosis in the newborn.**

1. **Primary pulmonary diseases.** Respiratory distress syndrome (RDS), TTN, aspiration syndromes, pneumonia, bronchopulmonary dysplasia/chronic lung disease (BPD/CLD), pulmonary interstitial emphysema (PIE), pulmonary hemorrhage.

2. **Airway obstruction.** Mucous plug, Pierre Robin syndrome, choanal atresia, vocal cord paralysis, macroglossia, atelectasis, and others.

3. **External compression of the lungs.** Any air leak syndrome, pleural effusion, and others.

4. **Congenital defects.** Congenital diaphragmatic hernia, pulmonary hypoplasia, cystic adenomatoid malformation, lobar emphysema, and others.

B. **Infections. Sepsis is the second most common cause of cyanosis in infants.** Sepsis causes increased oxygen utilization, which results in cyanosis. Meningitis can also present with cyanosis.

C. **Hypotension and shock.** This can be secondary to sepsis, cardiogenic, neurogenic, or hypovolemic, and all can present with cyanosis. (See Chapter 65.)

D. **Cardiac diseases.** The majority of congenital heart diseases that present in the first couple of weeks of life are ductal-dependent cardiac lesions.

1. **All cyanotic heart diseases which include the 5 T's.** Transposition of the great arteries is the most common cyanotic congenital heart disease in newborns.
   a. *Transposition of the great arteries.*
   b. *Total anomalous pulmonary venous return.*
   c. *Tricuspid atresia.*
   d. *Tetralogy of Fallot.*
   e. *Truncus arteriosus.*
   f. Sixth T ("tons of others"/"terrible T's") includes all the others: severe pulmonic stenosis, double outlet right ventricle, pulmonary atresia with intact ventricular septum/or with ventricular septal defect (VSD), variations on single ventricle, Ebstein anomaly of the tricuspid valve, hypoplastic heart syndrome with intact foramen ovale (no mixing at the atrial level), and others.

2. **Persistent pulmonary hypertension of the newborn (PPHN).** In PPHN, infants do not transition from fetal to newborn circulation. Pulmonary hypertension causes right-to-left shunting of blood, a decrease in pulmonary blood flow, and cyanosis.

3. **Severe congestive heart failure.** This can occur from cardiomyopathies (infant of diabetic mother [IDM], inborn errors of metabolism, genetic or neuromuscular disease), myocarditis (bacterial or viral), congenital cardiac disease, sepsis, perinatal asphyxia, and sustained tachyarrhythmias.

4. **Pneumopericardium or pericardial effusion.**

5. **Other congenital anomalies** such as those associated with cardiac malformations: Turner syndrome, Noonan syndrome, etc. **Pulmonary arteriovenous malformation** is a rare cause of cyanosis in the newborn.

E. **Central nervous system diseases.** CNS disorders can cause apnea, seizures, and decreased respiratory effort.
  1. **Infectious.** Bacterial or viral CNS infection (meningitis, encephalitis).
  2. **Seizures.** Infection, metabolic, CNS injury, genetic syndrome, congenital disorder, primary seizure disorder.
  3. **Hypoxic ischemic encephalopathy (HIE).**
  4. **Hemorrhage.** Periventricular/intraventricular hemorrhage, subdural hemorrhage, subarachnoid hemorrhage, intracerebellar hemorrhage, infarction.
  5. **Congenital disorders.** Congenital hydrocephalus, spinal muscle atrophy, congenital central hypoventilation syndrome.
  6. **Drug toxicity (opioid toxicity).**

F. **Neuromuscular disorders.** Werdnig-Hoffman disease, Pompe disease, Barth syndrome, Duchenne or Becker muscular dystrophy, limb-girdle muscular dystrophy, congenital myopathy, neonatal myasthenia gravis, phrenic nerve injury, and congenital myotonic dystrophy.

G. **Hematologic disorders.** A hemoglobin disorder can interfere with the transport of oxygen and cause cyanosis.
  1. **Methemoglobinemia (normal arterial O_2).** Because the arterial blood is brown in color, it gives off a bluish hue in the skin of Caucasian people. It can be congenital (familial) or secondary to a toxin (medications such as eutectic mixture of lidocaine and prilocaine [EMLA], sulfonamides, others) or environmental substances.
  2. **Polycythemia/hyperviscosity syndrome (normal arterial O_2).** Infants with this can present with peripheral cyanosis, tachypnea, congestive heart failure (CHF), and cardiomegaly. Cyanosis is detectable at a higher value of Sao_2. Polycythemia can cause pulmonary hypertension.
  3. **Severe anemia** from hemorrhage or bleeding disorders.

H. **Metabolic abnormalities can present with apnea and cyanosis**
  1. **Drug withdrawal.**
  2. **Hypoglycemia, hypermagnesemia, severe metabolic acidosis.**
  3. **Inborn errors of metabolism.**
  4. **Rarely abnormalities** of calcium, potassium, and phosphorus can cause hypoxia and cyanosis. Calcium and potassium abnormalities can cause cardiac arrhythmias.

I. **Other disorders**
  1. **Apnea and bradycardia**
  2. **Hypothermia**
  3. **Hypoadrenalism/hypopituitarism**
  4. **Abdominal distension** with elevation of the diaphragm
  5. **Respiratory depression** secondary to maternal medications (eg, magnesium sulfate and narcotics) or sedation

J. **Pseudocyanosis.** Caused by fluorescent lighting.

IV. **Database.** Obtain a prenatal and delivery history (see Section II.H).
  A. **Physical examination**
    1. **Assess the infant for central, peripheral, acrocyanosis, versus differential cyanosis**
      a. **Central cyanosis.** Skin, lips, and tongue appear blue. This indicates generalized cyanosis. This is caused by reduced arterial oxygen saturation.
      b. **Peripheral cyanosis.** Skin is bluish but the oral mucous membranes are pink. Seen in methemoglobinemia, caused by a normal arterial oxygen saturation and increased oxygen extraction.
      c. **Acrocyanosis.** Hands and feet are blue but nothing else. This can be present in normal infants in the first 24–48 hours. It is caused by immature vascular tone

or vasoconstriction secondary to a cold environment. Less commonly it may indicate poor tissue perfusion or a decrease in cardiac output.

    d. Circumoral cyanosis. Blue appearance around the mouth. There is a venous plexus around the mouth that gets engorged during feeding. Usually a normal finding, it can be an expression of peripheral cyanosis.

    e. Poor peripheral perfusion with cyanosis. Seen in sepsis, hypoglycemia, dehydration, and hypoadrenalism.

    f. Differential cyanosis. Cyanosis of the upper or lower part of the body only (see Section II.G).

2. **Assess the heart.** Check for any murmurs and for heart rate and blood pressure. Increased second heart sound intensity can be seen in pulmonary hypertension. Single second heart sound can be seen with transposition of the great vessels, aortic atresia, truncus arteriosus, pulmonary atresia, and conditions with pulmonary hypertension. Remember not all infants with congenital heart disease have a murmur. (Transposition of the great vessels can have no detectable murmur.) Muffled heart sounds can signify pneumopericardium or pericardial effusion. A displaced cardiac impulse may mean dextrocardia or dextroposition. Not all infants with murmurs have congenital heart disease.

3. **Assess the respiratory system.** Is there retraction, nasal flaring, or grunting? Retractions are usually minimal in heart disease. Check the nasal passage for choanal atresia. Infants with pulmonary disease will have tachypnea and distressed breathing, whereas infants with cardiac disease do not.

4. **Assess the abdomen.** Check for an enlarged liver. The liver can be enlarged in CHF and hyperexpansion of the lungs. A scaphoid abdomen may suggest a diaphragmatic hernia. Hepatomegaly can indicate high venous pressure.

5. **Check the pulses.** In coarctation of the aorta, the femoral pulses are decreased. In patent ductus arteriosus, the pulses are bounding.

6. **Consider neurologic problems.** Check for apnea and periodic breathing, which may be associated with immaturity of the nervous system. Observe the infant for seizures, which can cause cyanosis if the infant is not breathing during seizures.

7. **Assess for multiple malformations on the examination.** These may suggest underlying heart or pulmonary defects ("CHARGE" or "VATER/VACTERL" anomalies).

B. **Laboratory studies**

1. **Arterial blood gas measurements on room air.** If the patient is not hypoxic, it suggests methemoglobinemia, polycythemia, or CNS disease. If the patient is hypoxic, perform the hyperoxia test, described later. Pulse oximetry can be used to check arterial saturation but is not a good indicator of central cyanosis. An **increased CO_2** can indicate pulmonary, PPHN, or CNS disorders. **Metabolic acidosis** can indicate sepsis, severe hypoxemia, or shock. A **low or normal CO_2** can indicate cardiac disease.

2. **Complete blood count (CBC) with differential.** This may reveal an infectious process. A central hematocrit of >65% confirms polycythemia.

3. **Sepsis workup.** Blood culture and C-reactive protein (CRP), urine culture, and lumbar puncture (LP) if indicated.

4. **Serum glucose level.** To detect hypoglycemia.

5. **Methemoglobin level.** If the infant has methemoglobinemia, the blood will not turn red when exposed to air. It will have a chocolate hue. To confirm the diagnosis, the laboratory should perform a spectrophotometric determination.

C. **Imaging and other studies**

1. **Transillumination of the chest.** (See Chapter 40.) Should be done on an emergent basis if pneumothorax is suspected.

2. **Chest radiograph.** If normal, it suggests a CNS disease or other cause for the cyanosis (see Section III). It can verify lung disease, air leak, or diaphragmatic hernia. It can also help diagnose heart disease by evaluating the heart size and pulmonary vascularity. The **heart size** may be normal or enlarged in hypoglycemia, polycythemia,

shock, and sepsis. In cardiac lesions with cyanosis and increased pulmonary blood flow there will be **cardiomegaly**. **Decreased pulmonary vascular markings** represent decreased blood flow through the pulmonary circulation and can be seen in tetralogy of Fallot, pulmonary atresia/stenosis, truncus arteriosus, and Ebstein anomaly. **Increased pulmonary arterial markings** can be seen in truncus arteriosus, single ventricle, and transposition of the great arteries. **Increased venous markings** can be seen in hypoplastic left heart syndrome and total anomalous pulmonary venous return. **Shape of the heart** can be important:
   a. **Boot-shaped heart.** Tetralogy of Fallot, tricuspid atresia
   b. **Egg-shaped heart ("egg on a string").** Transposition of the great arteries
   c. **Large globular heart.** Ebstein anomaly
   d. **Dextrocardia/mesocardia.** Congenital heart disease
   e. **"Snowman" or "figure 8."** Total anomalous pulmonary venous return
3. **Hyperoxia test.** Because of intracardiac right-to-left shunting, the infant with cyanotic congenital heart disease in contrast to the infant with pulmonary disease is unable to raise the arterial saturation. Measure arterial oxygen on room air. Then place the infant on 100% oxygen for 10–20 minutes. Then remeasure arterial oxygen. It is best not to use pulse oximetry since it may not give an accurate result. *Note:* A value of >150 mm Hg does not always rule out cyanotic heart disease. Diagnosis of cardiac disease can be delayed from a misleading hyperoxia test and has been reported (pulmonary disease with cardiac disease, infracardiac total anomalous pulmonary venous connection with Pao_2 >250 mm Hg). Echocardiogram should be done if unsure.
   a. **Normal infant.** Pao_2 >300.
   b. **Pulmonary disease.** Pao_2 >150 mm Hg. In an infant with severe pulmonary disease, the arterial oxygen saturation may not increase significantly.
   c. **Cardiac disease.** Pao_2 <50–70 mm Hg. In cyanotic heart disease the Pao_2 most likely will not increase significantly (usually <100 mm Hg and often <70 mm Hg). The hyperoxia test can also help in differentiating the different types of heart disease. Infants with transposition of the great arteries or severe pulmonary outflow obstruction will usually have a Pao_2 <50 mm Hg. Infants with disease with both right-to-left and left-to-right shunting (truncus arteriosus, TAPVC without obstruction, hypoplastic left heart syndrome, single ventricle with PDA) can have an increase in Pao_2 but rarely >150 mm Hg.
   d. **PPHN.** In infants with PPHN, it may or may not increase significantly. If the Pao_2 increases to <20–30 mm Hg, PPHN should be considered.
   e. **Neurologic disease.** Pao_2 >150 mm Hg.
   f. **Methemoglobinemia.** Pao_2 >200 mm Hg but pulse oximetry remains low.
4. **Right-to-left shunt test.** Done to rule out PPHN. Best way to do this is with pulse oximetry. Place 2 pulse oximeters on the infant (one preductal on the right hand, one postductal on either foot). If the simultaneous difference is >5% between preductal and postductal oxygen saturations, it is indicative of a right-to-left shunt. One can also draw a simultaneous sample of blood from the right radial artery (preductal) and the descending aorta or the left radial artery (postductal). If there is a difference of >10–15 mm Hg (preductal more than postductal), the shunt is significant.
5. **Hyperventilation test.** Hyperventilating the infant for 10 minutes (lowering $Paco_2$ and increasing the pH) will result in a marked improvement in oxygenation (>30 mm Hg increase in Pao_2) in PPHN. This may help differentiate the infant with PPHN from that with cyanotic congenital heart disease (little or no response in CHD).
6. **Electrocardiography (ECG).** Usually normal in patients with methemoglobinemia or hypoglycemia. With polycythemia, pulmonary hypertension, or primary lung disease, the ECG is normal but may show right ventricular hypertrophy. The ECG is usually nondiagnostic because of the normal neonatal right-axis deviation

and dominant right wave in the right chest leads. It is very helpful in identifying patients with tricuspid atresia; it will show left-axis deviation and left ventricular hypertrophy. ECG can be normal in transposition of the great vessels.
7. **Echocardiography.** Should be performed immediately if cardiac disease is suspected or if the diagnosis is unclear. It is the **gold standard** and definitive diagnostic test for congenital heart disease. It can confirm pulmonary hypertension.
8. **Computed tomography (CT) and CT angiography.** May help identify anomalies of the pulmonary venous return.
9. **Ultrasonography of the head.** Performed to rule out periventricular/intraventricular hemorrhage.
10. **Polysomnographic recording.** Helps diagnose apnea and its type.
11. **Electroencephalogram (EEG).** If seizure is suspected.

V. **Plan**
A. **General management.** Act quickly and accomplish many of the diagnostic tasks at once. Perform resuscitation (ABCs) if necessary and provide respiratory support, volume resuscitation if necessary, and antibiotics as indicated. Inotropic support and correcting metabolic acidosis are essential.
  1. **Perform a rapid physical examination.** What is the blood pressure? Other vital signs? Transilluminate the chest (see Chapter 40). If a tension pneumothorax is present, rapid needle decompression may be needed.
  2. **Order immediate studies.** For example, blood gas levels, CBC, and chest radiograph. Consider echocardiography.
  3. **Perform the hyperoxia test.** See Section IV.C.3.
B. **Specific management**
  1. **Lung disease.** (See the appropriate disease chapter.) Respiratory depression caused by narcotics can be treated with naloxone (Narcan) (see Chapter 148 for dosing).
  2. **Air leak (pneumothorax).** See Chapter 70.
  3. **Congenital defects.** Surgery is indicated for diaphragmatic hernia.
  4. **Cardiac disease.** Prostaglandin E_1 (PGE_1) is indicated for any clinical condition in which blood flow must be maintained through the ductus arteriosus to sustain pulmonary or systemic circulation until surgery can be performed.
    a. **Give PGE_1 to increase pulmonary blood flow** for pulmonary atresia/stenosis, tricuspid atresia, tetralogy of Fallot, and Ebstein anomaly of the tricuspid valve. Other ways of improving pulmonary blood flow are with supplemental oxygen, maintaining a respiratory alkalosis, sildenafil, and inhaled nitric oxide.
    b. **Give PGE_1 to increase systemic blood flow** for hypoplastic left heart syndrome, coarctation of the aorta, critical aortic stenosis, aortic arch interruption.
    c. **Give PGE_1 to improve mixing** in transposition of the great arteries.
    d. **PGE_1 is not recommended** in respiratory distress syndrome, PPHN, total anomalous venous return with obstruction (PGE_1 may minimize obstruction but does not help clinically), and dominant left-to-right shunt (patent ductus arteriosus, truncus arteriosus, or ventricular septal defect).
    e. **If the diagnosis is uncertain, a trial of PGE_1 can be given over 30 minutes in an effort to improve blood gas values.**
    f. **Other management.** D-transposition of the great arteries requires urgent balloon atrial septostomy under echocardiogram in the nursery if hypoxia or acidosis occurs. TAPVR, transposition of the great arteries with VSD, and truncus arteriosus require further cardiac evaluation and possible surgery.
  5. **PPHN.** See Chapter 120.
  6. **CNS disorders.** Treat the underlying disease.
  7. **Methemoglobinemia.** Treat the infant with methylene blue only if the methemoglobin level is markedly increased and the infant is in cardiopulmonary distress (tachypnea and tachycardia). Administer intravenously 1 mg/kg of a 1% solution of **methylene blue** in normal saline. The cyanosis should clear within 1–2 hours.
  8. **Shock.** See Chapter 65.

9. **Polycythemia.** See Chapters 71 and 122.
10. **Choanal atresia.** Usually requires surgery (see Chapter 135).
11. **Hypothermia.** Rewarming is necessary as described in Chapter 7.
12. **Hypoglycemia.** See Chapter 62.

52 Death of an Infant

I. **Problem.** A newborn infant is dying or has just died. The mortality rate in the United States for newborns is 4.56 per 1000 live births. Recent reviews have focused on the importance of bereavement support and the profound effect health care providers can have on parents who have lost an infant. Studies have shown that a health care provider's insensitivity to a parent can contribute to difficulties in coping and may increase the risk of a complicated grief reaction. Nurses who received training for bereavement care were more likely to have a positive attitude toward perinatal bereavement care. Studies show that more physicians than nurses never received any formal training in bereavement care. Hospitals should establish training and protocols for an infant death so they can potentially decrease the traumatic effects.

II. **Immediate questions**
   A. **Has the family been prepared for the death, or was it unexpected?** It is important to prepare the family in advance, if possible, for the death of an infant and to be ready to answer questions after the event.
   B. **Was this an early or late neonatal death?** Early neonatal death describes the death of a live-born infant during the first 7 completed days of life. Late neonatal death refers to the death of a live-born infant after 7 but before 28 completed days of life. After 28 days, it is considered an infant death.
   C. **Which family members are present?** Usually, several immediate family members in addition to the parents are present at the hospital, which is good for emotional support. Each of the family members may adopt a special role. The family should be allowed to go through the immediate process of grieving the way they feel most comfortable (eg, on their own, with the chaplain, with their favorite nurse, or with the physician they trust) and in the location they feel most comfortable (eg, the neonatal intensive care unit [NICU] or family conference room). Attention should focus on both parents.
   D. **If the family members are not present, is a telephone contact available?** It is standard practice to ensure there is a contact telephone number available for any sick infant. If the family members are not present, telephone contact must be made as soon as possible to alert the family that their infant is dying or has already passed away. In either case, urge the family to come in and be with their infant.
   E. **Are there any religious needs expressed by the family?** The religious needs must be respected and the necessary support provided (eg, priest, rabbi, chaplain, or pastoral care). Every hospital has pastoral services, and it is useful to inform the chaplain in advance because some parents may request that their child be baptized before death. Remember that a patient's culture or religion may influence the families' decision on how to handle the time of death, autopsy, and funeral.

III. **Differential diagnosis.** Not applicable.

IV. **Database.** Remember that the dying infant may continue with a gasp reflex for some time even without spontaneous respiration and movement. The heartbeat may be very faint; therefore, auscultation for 2–5 minutes is advisable. Legal definitions of "death" vary by state. It is essential to be familiar with the local legal requirements for declaring death.

Table 52–1. BEHAVIORS VIEWED MOST FAVORABLY BY PARENTS AFTER PERINATAL DEATH

Offering emotional support
Stay with the family and spend extra time with them as much as practical.
Talk about the baby by name.
Allow parents to grieve or cry.
Be sensitive to comments that could be perceived as trite or minimizing of grief.
Return to see family on multiple occasions, if possible.

Attending to physical needs of parents and baby
Continue routine postpartum nursing and medical care for mother.
Treat infant's body respectfully.
Consider dressing, bathing, or wrapping infant as for a live baby.
Be flexible about hospital policies that may not be appropriate for bereaved families.
Help parents create tangible memories of their infants.

Educating parents
Communicate loss to all staff to help avoid inappropriate comments or actions.
Help parents anticipate what normal grieving will be like.
Provide straightforward information about cause of death if known. Use lay language.
Take time to sit down with parents when discussing information.

Reproduced with permission from Gold KJ. Navigating care after a baby dies: a systematic review of parent experiences with health providers. *J Perinatol.* 2007:27:230–237.

V. **Plan**
   A. **Preparations.** A recent review has reported on the behaviors viewed most favorably by parents after their infant has died, outlined in Table 52–1.
      1. **The NICU environment.** The noise level should be kept to a minimum. The staff should be sensitive to the emotions of the parents and the family. The infant and family members should be provided privacy in an isolated quiet room or a screened-off area in the NICU. Examination of the infant by the physician to determine death may be done in that same private area, with the family.
      2. **The infant.** The equipment (eg, IVs and endotracheal tubes) may be removed from the infant unless an autopsy is anticipated. In that case, it is best to leave in place central catheters and possibly the endotracheal tube. The parents should be allowed to hold the infant for as long as they desire. This type of visual and physical contact is important to begin the grieving process in a healthy manner and try to relieve any future guilt. Treating the infant carelessly by staff members is not tolerated well by parents. The practice reported in the literature of placing the deceased infant on an uncovered metal table or placed into a bucket after delivery is unacceptable. Parents are acutely aware how nurses care for the deceased infant. Bathing and dressing the infant in a caring manner and treating the deceased infant with respect is appreciated by the family. Families also appreciate when nurses took special photos of the infant and gave the family special mementos so they could have some memories.
   B. **Discussion of death with the family**
      1. **Location.** Parents and immediate family members should be in a quiet, private consultation room, and the physician should calmly explain the cause and inevitability of death.
      2. **News of the death.** Studies show parents value clear communication. The physician needs to offer condolences to the family concerning their loss. News of the infant's death can be very difficult for the physician to convey and the family to accept. The physician must be sensitive to the emotional reactions of the family. Nurses, in one review, were perceived as the health care provider who was most likely to provide

emotional support. The nurse's ability to partner with the family is very important in helping the family take steps in their ability to grieve. It is important that nurses participate in this process because they can provide more ongoing support through this difficult time. They can also guide new mothers and fathers of caring tasks that they can perform for their baby and create memories that will provide them a sense of comfort later on. Communicate the news of the death to all staff members who will be taking care of the mother if she is hospitalized at the time of the infant death. This includes dietary staff and housekeepers so they know the appropriate way to act.

3. **Areas of dissatisfaction from parents.** Reviews have emphasized that parents are upset by lack of communication between staff members. Staff who did not know the infant had died and made comments, staff who avoided or were silent with the family, and staff who showed insensitivity or lack of emotional support all created great stress in the families of the deceased. Treating the mother and deceased infant with respect is important.

C. Effects on the family

1. **Emotional (grieving).** A brief outline of the normal grieving process may be discussed. The stages Kübler-Ross identified are **denial** ("This isn't happening to me!"); **anger** ("Why is this happening to me?"); **bargaining** ("I promise I'll be a better person if . . ."); **depression** ("I don't care anymore"); and **acceptance** ("I'm ready for whatever comes"). Temes has described 3 particular types of behavior exhibited by those suffering from grief and loss: numbness (mechanical functioning and social insulation), disorganization (intensely painful feelings of loss), and reorganization (reentry into a more "normal" social life). Physicians who offered specifics to the family in what to expect in the grieving process were rated as the most competent physicians.

2. **Physical.** Loss of appetite and disruption of sleep patterns.

3. **Siblings.** It is important to discuss the impact of death on a sibling. A study was done to assess the developmental impact of surviving a sibling who died in the NICU; it showed that siblings born both before and after a death of an infant are at risk and in need of psychological support. Photos and family rituals are important for parents and siblings. Clinicians should allow siblings to be active participants in the infant's life and death.

4. **Surviving twin or multiple.** Staff must be aware of the added stress on the parents looking in on a surviving twin or multiple birth.

D. Practical aspects

1. **Perinatal bereavement programs.** Because the neonatal staff plays a major role in helping families cope with the loss of their infant, it is important for each unit to set up a comprehensive program to help families deal with their grief. Some units have set up a bereavement support service that includes a bereavement suite, bereavement coordinators, bereavement support (funerals and blessings, 24-hour communication, financial advice and benefits, provision of mementoes and keepsakes, sibling involvement and counseling, and follow-up). It is important to not only focus on the neonate's physical needs but to address the family's spiritual, religious, and existential needs. Recent studies show that intergenerational services should be offered and provide benefit for the entire family. **Hospice care teams** are getting involved in the prenatal arena (mothers with infants with known lethal anomalies) and give support while the infant is in utero and also in the NICU to address the process of dying and stages of grief for parents.

2. **Education.** Recent reviews have reported that parents appreciated education from the health care providers. Parents want to have information regarding why the infant died and also specific information on the grieving process. Parents have indicated that staff members who kept them informed and provided honest answers with consistent information were valued the most. *Hello Means Good-Bye* by Paul Kirk and Pat Schwiebert (www.griefwatch.com) is an often recommended lay book that can help the family cope with the loss of an infant.

3. **Additional support.** Family members should be asked whether they need any support for transport or funeral arrangements and whether they need a note to the employer regarding time off from work and so on. Social workers or case workers are usually available to assist in the hospital setting. Questions regarding maternity leave benefits and returning to work can be answered. Some units offer a 24-hour dedicated telephone line for bereaved families to be able to contact as needed.

4. **Bereavement photography.** Gives consolation to parents after a perinatal loss. Includes pictures of the infant either alone or with family members done by staff, a professional photographer, or several organizations that help to ease the grief of NICU parents by taking professional photographs. These images can serve as a link to memories and feelings and help parents grieve and heal. Parents may wish to dress their baby in clothes or include mementoes in the pictures. It is important to respect the parents' wishes.

5. **Rituals.** Rituals provide an ordered way to say goodbye to a loved one. They can be beneficial to individuals and families who have experienced the death of a child. These can include funerals, memory boxes (with name bands, cord clamp, lock of baby's hair, etc.), naming the baby, religious practices, and specific cultural traditions.

6. **Written permission.** Should be obtained for the following: photography, mementos, autopsy, or biopsy.

7. **Organ donation.** Occasionally, parents and immediate family members may have discussed organ donation before the death of the infant. If not, it can be brought up gently with the family, who will be given adequate time to reflect on it, taking into consideration the requirements for organ donation. Sometimes the parents may want to donate an organ, but this may not be possible because of the presence of infection or inadequate function of the organ before death. This should be explained carefully to the parents. Follow your institution's procedure for requesting organ procurement.

8. **Autopsy.** Autopsy can be a vital part of determining the cause of death and may be important in counseling the parents for future pregnancies. It is always a very sensitive issue to discuss with the parents, especially after the loss of their loved one. Parents should always be allowed adequate time to discuss this themselves and with the family if they have not already made up their minds. A recent study on bereaved parents' perception on autopsy revealed that it is important to openly discuss the benefits of an autopsy; 90% of parents valued autopsy as a way to find out why their child died, and 77% knew it contributed to medical knowledge. Forty-two percent felt that the autopsy examination added to their grief, 30% found it a comfort, and 41% said it helped them with their loss.

9. **Documentation**
   a. **Neonatal death summary note.** The physician may include a brief synopsis of the infant's history or a problem list. The events leading up to the infant's death that day, whether it was sudden or gradual, and the treatment or interventions performed must be noted. It is also important to note conversations with family members while the infant was dying, if not written earlier in separate notes.
   b. **Death certificate.** The physician declaring the infant dead initiates the death certificate, following strict guidelines for each county/state.

E. **Follow-up arrangements**
1. **Family contact.** A telephone call from one of the medical team members should be arranged within the first week of death. A letter of sympathy can be sent. Another contact can be made at the end of the first month to comfort the family, share any further information, and answer questions. Some NICU teams may make contact again at the 1-year anniversary.

2. **Counseling.** It is extremely important to discuss the arrangements for future counseling and refer the parents to high-risk obstetrics if appropriate. Genetic counseling may also be appropriate based on the specific case. Parents should be

allowed to grieve for the death of their child and should be given the opportunity to contact the physician at a later date when they are more receptive emotionally. Siblings are at risk and may require psychological support.

3. **Autopsy follow-up.** If consent for autopsy has been obtained, an autopsy follow-up conference after ~6–8 weeks is essential. The presence of a geneticist at this follow-up may be appropriate. This autopsy conference not only provides the parents with concrete information but also assists in the process of grieving.

4. **The obstetrician, pediatrician, and family physician involved with the care of the mother or family should be notified of the death.**

5. **The needs of the caregivers also should be considered.** Dealing with grief, loss, and bereavement is one of the major stressors in the NICU setting. Several units have developed specific programs in this area, and resources should be made available to the staff as well. Some units have a palliative care team that receives specific training. They offer debriefing sessions for anyone in the NICU to attend.

53 Eye Discharge and Conjunctivitis

I. **Problem.** A purulent eye discharge is noted in a 3-day-old infant. Eye discharge in a neonate is usually caused by conjunctivitis or congenital lacrimal duct obstruction. **Neonatal conjunctivitis (ophthalmia neonatorum)** is an inflammation of the surface or covering of the eye that presents with eye discharge and hyperemia in the first 4 weeks of life. It is the most common ocular disease in neonates. Most infections are acquired during vaginal delivery. In the United States the incidence of infectious conjunctivitis is 1–2%; in the world it is 0.9–21%. **Congenital lacrimal duct obstruction (CLDO)** (dacryostenosis) is a condition where there is a blockage of the lacrimal drainage system. It occurs in ~5–6% of infants. The symptoms are persistent tearing and a mucoid discharge in the inner corner of the eye.

II. **Immediate questions**

A. **How old is the infant?** Age may be helpful in determining the cause of eye discharge. For conjunctivitis: in the first 6–24 hours of life, conjunctivitis is often due to ocular prophylaxis (usually silver nitrate drops; it may also be from tetracycline, erythromycin, or gentamicin). After 24–48 hours, a bacterial infection is most likely; the most common neonatal organisms are *Neisseria gonorrhoeae* (2–7 days but can present later) and *Staphylococcus aureus* (5–14 days). *Chlamydia trachomatis* conjunctivitis is usually seen after the first week of life (5–14 days) and often presents as late as the second or third week. Herpes conjunctivitis is seen 6–14 days after birth. *Pseudomonas aeruginosa* infections are typically seen between 5 and 18 days. *Note: Bacterial infections can occur anytime.* Lacrimal duct obstruction usually manifests at 2 weeks of age, but can be seen in the first few days to the first few weeks after birth.

B. **Is the discharge unilateral or bilateral? Unilateral** conjunctivitis is most often seen with S. *aureus*, P. *aeruginosa*, and herpes simplex (HSV) and adenovirus. **Bilateral** conjunctivitis is seen with infection caused by *N. gonorrhoeae* or by the use of ocular prophylaxis. Chlamydia usually develops in one eye but affects the other after 2–7 days. Lacrimal duct obstruction usually causes unilateral discharge, but up to 20 % of infants have bilateral obstruction.

C. **What are the characteristics of the discharge (purulent vs watery)?** Purulent discharge is more common with bacterial infection. A serous discharge is more common with a viral infection. Gonorrhea has a profuse purulent discharge. Greenish discharge is more characteristic of *P. aeruginosa*. Chlamydial infection can be watery early and purulent later, but a blood-stained discharge is typical. Herpes conjunctivitis usually has a nonpurulent and serosanguineous discharge. **Lacrimal duct obstruction** can cause watery tears in the corner of the eye or tears draining from the eyelid down the cheek. It can also cause a mucus or yellowish discharge in the eye.

D. **Did the infant receive eye prophylaxis?** Prophylaxis is used to decrease the risk of developing ocular gonorrheal infection (prevent blindness) and it also decreases the risk of nongonococcal and nonchlamydial conjunctivitis in the first 2 weeks of life. Remember, infants can still get gonococcal conjunctivitis with prophylaxis (risk drops from 50 to 2%). Prophylaxis is mandatory in the United States but may not be in other countries. Failure rates of eye prophylaxis and better screening and maternal therapy is causing a reevaluation of this process, especially in areas where maternal infection is low. **Proper technique is as follows:** give within 1 hour of birth; wipe each eyelid with sterile cotton; 2 drops of 1% silver nitrate solution or a 1-cm ribbon of either 1% tetracycline or 0.5% erythromycin are introduced into each lower conjunctival sac and not rinsed out. Ointment may be wiped away after 1 minute. Massage the eyelids to spread the ointment. Single-dose containers are recommended. For the very premature infant with fused eyes, apply the prophylactic agent without separating the eyelids. Prophylaxis can be with 1% tetracycline ophthalmic ointment or solution (evidence suggests better outcomes and more effectiveness), 2.5% povidone-iodine solution (not approved in United States but is used elsewhere), 1% silver nitrate solution (recommended over erythromycin if the patient population has a high number of penicillinase-producing *N. gonorrhoeae*), and 0.5% erythromycin ointment. Other alternatives are neomycin, chloramphenicol and azithromycin (used when there was a shortage of erythromycin), and gentamicin (used during a shortage but caused severe ocular reactions, so not recommended). A newer therapy is fusidic acid.

E. **Does the mother have a history of sexually transmitted infections?** Infants who pass through the birth canal of an infected mother with gonorrhea or chlamydia have an increased conjunctivitis risk. Neonatal conjunctivitis is frequently diagnosed in infants born to human immunodeficiency virus (HIV)-infected mothers.

F. **Is the infant at high risk?** Neonates are **at increased risk for conjunctivitis** and a more serious case of it because of decreased tear production, lack of immunoglobulin IgA in tears, decreased immune function, absence of lymphoid tissue of the conjunctiva, and decreased lysozyme activity. Risk factors may include mode of delivery, exposure of the infant to infectious organisms, no or inadequate prophylaxis after birth, ocular trauma/local eye injury during delivery, poor hygienic conditions, premature rupture of membranes (PROM), prolonged delivery, prematurity, mechanical ventilation, increased birthweight, history of midwife interference, HIV-infected mother, poor prenatal care, documented or suspected sexually transmitted infection, infection after delivery from direct contact from health care worker, or aerosolization. Neonates are at **an increased risk for congenital lacrimal duct obstruction** with Down syndrome, Goldenhar sequence, clefting syndromes, any midline facial anomaly, hemifacial microsomia, and craniosynostosis.

G. **Is the infant low birthweight and low gestational age?** An infant with conjunctivitis who has a low birthweight and low gestational age has a higher risk of having a conjunctivitis caused by a **gram-negative organism** (*Klebsiella* spp., *Escherichia coli, Serratia marcescens, P. aeruginosa,* and *Enterobacter* spp.). Premature infants have an increased risk of congenital lacrimal duct obstruction.

III. **Differential diagnosis. Eye discharge** can be **conjunctivitis** (ophthalmia neonatorum due to infectious, chemical/inflammatory cause) or due to an **obstruction** (congenital lacrimal duct obstruction). Other diagnoses that may cause an eye discharge in an infant are foreign body, orbital or preseptal cellulitis, entropion, trichiasis, eye trauma (corneal abrasion following delivery), dacryocystitis, keratitis, subconjunctival hemorrhage (breakage of vessels during delivery), congenital anomalies of the nasolacrimal system, corneal epithelial disease, neonatal abstinence (lacrimation), and congenital glaucoma.

A. **Chemical/inflammatory conjunctivitis.** Usually secondary to silver nitrate ocular drops and is the most common cause of conjunctivitis in underdeveloped countries. Chemical conjunctivitis can occur from other prophylactic ocular antibiotics used after birth, but it occurs less often. It is a nonpurulent inflammation of the eye that causes a watery discharge, conjunctival injection, and swelling within several hours of instilling the medication. The conjunctivitis shows a maximum inflammatory response around 48 hours and usually clears by the fourth day.

B. **Infectious conjunctivitis.** Bacterial, viral, or chlamydial infectious conjunctivitis in the newborn is caused by *C. trachomatis* (2–40%), *N. gonorrhoeae* (<1%), herpes simplex (<1%), and other bacterial microbes (30–50%). Other microbes include *Staphylococcus* spp., *Streptococcus pneumoniae, Haemophilus influenzae, Streptococcus mitis*, group A and B streptococci, *Enterobacter, Acinetobacter, Neisseria cinerea, Corynebacterium* spp., *Moraxella catarrhalis, S. marcescens, Stenotrophomonas maltophilia, E. coli*, viridans streptococci, *Klebsiella pneumoniae, Eikenella corrodens*, and *P. aeruginosa*. Epidemiology of gram-negative conjunctivitis: *Klebsiella* spp. (23%), *E. coli* (17%), *S. marcescens* (17%), *P. aeruginosa* (3%), and *Enterobacter* spp. (2%).

1. **Mechanisms of infection**
   a. **Infections acquired through vaginal birth.** Typically *N. gonorrhoeae, C. trachomatis*, group B streptococci, or HSV. They tend to reflect sexually transmitted infections in the community. Any bacteria that are normally present in the vagina (not sexually transmitted) can also cause neonatal conjunctivitis.
   b. **Cesarean section delivery can be associated with ascending infections.** Risk factors include amniotic fluid leak, vaginal examinations, and use of internal monitors.
   c. **Postnatally acquired infections.** Infection from organisms which are present in the environment (normal skin flora or nasopharyngeal flora). Examples are *S. aureus* (coagulase negative most common in one study), *Staphylococcus epidermidis, Streptococcus* spp., *Pseudomonas* spp., *Serratia* spp., *Klebsiella* spp., and *Enterococcus* spp. *Pseudomonas* infections are more typical in hospitalized preemies beyond 5 days of birth.

2. **Gonococcal conjunctivitis.** Most commonly transmitted from the mother during vaginal birth. The transmission rate from an infected mother to her newborn is 30–50%. It tends to occur 3–5 days after birth with abrupt onset. Usually bilateral, the eyes are very red (hyperacute conjunctivitis) with a thick, purulent drainage and swelling. The lid has chemosis (edema) and a conjunctival membrane may be present. This is an emergency because, left untreated, it can cause a corneal ulcer and perforation within hours. The incidence is low because of prophylactic ocular treatment immediately after birth. Infants can have systemic manifestations: sepsis, meningitis, rhinitis, stomatitis, arthritis, and anorectal infection.

3. **Chlamydial conjunctivitis.** Transmitted from the mother and develops in 30–40% of infants delivered vaginally to infected untreated mothers. **Topical prophylaxis with erythromycin does not prevent but reduces the incidence of chlamydial ophthalmia neonatorum.** Prophylaxis does not eradicate nasopharyngeal colonization or pneumonia. The eyes have a moderate drainage, redness, and conjunctival and eyelid swelling. It can be unilateral or bilateral and usually starts out as a watery discharge that becomes purulent and copious later. Corneal opacification, chemosis, and pseudomembranes may be present. Pneumonia is present in 10–20% of infants with chlamydial conjunctivitis. Otitis, pharyngeal, and rectal colonization can occur. Repeated and chronic infections of *C. trachomatis* can cause **trachoma** (rare in the United States), which is a **chronic follicular keratoconjunctivitis** that causes scarring and neovascularization of the cornea that can result in blindness.

4. **Pseudomonas conjunctivitis.** Usually a nosocomial infection and is becoming more common in nurseries. It can lead to a devastating corneal ulceration, perforation, endophthalmitis, and death. The organism thrives in moisture-filled environments such as respiratory equipment and occurs most often in hospitalized

premature infants or those with depressed immunity. It can be responsible for epidemic conjunctivitis in premature infants. Infants with pseudomonas conjunctivitis can have systemic complications.

5. **Herpes simplex keratoconjunctivitis.** Herpes simplex type 2 (HSV-2) can cause unilateral or bilateral conjunctivitis, optic neuritis, chorioretinitis, and encephalitis, and it is the most frequent viral cause of conjunctivitis. The conjunctivitis can be superficial or may involve the deeper layers of the cornea; vesicles may appear on the nearby skin. The infants can have lid edema, conjunctival injection, and a watery nonpurulent discharge. A conjunctival membrane may be present. Most of these infections are secondary to HSV-2 sexually transmitted infection (maternal genital tract ascending infection) or through the birth canal or by transplacental mechanisms; 15–20% are caused by HSV-1. Suspect herpes if the conjunctivitis is not responding to antibiotic therapy. Most neonatal HSV-1 infections are related to contact with someone with an active infection (fever blister or cold sore) in the perinatal period.

6. **Viral causes (other than herpes).** These are usually associated with other symptoms of respiratory tract disease due to adenovirus, enterovirus, and parechovirus. There is usually redness, and it is more commonly unilateral. The discharge is usually mild and watery and is rarely purulent. Preauricular adenopathy can be seen.

7. **Other bacterial infections.** (See Section III.B.) The conjunctivitis from other microbial agents usually presents **as a milder form of conjunctivitis**. It can cause conjunctival injection, chemosis, and a discharge. Infections caused by *Haemophilus* spp. and *S. pneumoniae* are associated with dacryocystitis (inflammation of the nasolacrimal sac). **Staphylococcal conjunctivitis** is usually a nosocomial infection. It is the most frequent isolate, but may not cause conjunctivitis in infants who are colonized. It can cause conjunctival hyperemia. Methicillin-resistant *S. aureus* (**MRSA**) **conjunctivitis** can also occur and has been associated with nurseries and neonatal intensive care units (NICUs).

C. **Congenital lacrimal duct obstruction (dacryostenosis) occurs in** ~5–6% of infants. The nasolacrimal duct may fail to canalize completely at birth. The obstruction is usually at the nasal end of the duct and is usually unilateral. The symptoms are persistent tearing and a mucoid discharge in the inner corner of the eye. One in 5 infants may have transient discharge (watery and sticky, particularly after sleep) due to a delay in the normal development and opening of the tear duct that resolves spontaneously. **Dacryocystitis** is a secondary infection in the lacrimal sac.

IV. **Database**

A. **Physical examination**

1. **Ophthalmic examination.** Examine both eyes/eyelids for swelling and edema and check the conjunctiva for injection (congestion of blood vessels) and chemosis (conjunctival swelling). A purulent discharge, edema, and erythema of the lids as well as injection of the conjunctiva are suggestive of bacterial conjunctivitis. Check for ulcerations and the presence of a red reflex.

2. **Perform a physical examination.** To rule out signs of respiratory or systemic infection. Evaluate for periorbital edema and adenopathy.

B. **Laboratory studies**

1. **Gram-stained smear of the discharge** to check for white blood cells (a sign of infection) and bacteria (to identify the organism). **A sample of the discharge should also be submitted for culture and sensitivity testing** (chocolate agar and/or Thayer martin media for N. gonorrhoeae and blood agar for other bacteria). **Findings on Gram stain:**

a. *N. gonorrhoeae* conjunctivitis. Gram-negative intracellular diplococci and white blood cells (WBCs).

b. *S. aureus* conjunctivitis. Gram-positive cocci in clusters and WBCs.

c. *P. aeruginosa* conjunctivitis. Gram-negative bacilli and WBCs.

d. Conjunctivitis caused by *Haemophilus* spp. Gram-negative coccoid rods.

D. **Chlamydial conjunctivitis.** Evaluate for systemic disease (pneumonia, otitis, pharyngeal and rectal colonization). Pneumonia has been reported in 20% of infants with chlamydial conjunctivitis.

1. **Recommended neonatal prophylaxis** does not prevent neonatal chlamydial conjunctivitis.
2. **Topical treatment with antibiotics** is ineffective and unnecessary.
3. **Oral erythromycin base** or ethylsuccinate, 50 mg/kg/d, in 4 divided doses for 14 days by mouth is recommended. Azithromycin therapy (20 mg/kg qd for 3 days) may be effective but data are limited. Oral sulfonamides may be used after the immediate neonatal period for infants who do not tolerate erythromycin. A second course of antibiotics is sometimes required because ~20% of cases recur after antibiotic therapy. **Infantile hypertrophic pyloric stenosis (IHPS) has been seen in infants <6 weeks treated with erythromycin.** Counsel patients about the risk and signs of IHPS. The American Academy of Pediatrics (AAP) still recommends erythromycin because other treatments have not been well studied.
4. **Macrolide antibiotics** such as azithromycin, clarithromycin, and roxithromycin may be more effective against chlamydia but have not been well studied in this group.
5. **Infants born to mothers with untreated chlamydia** are at a high risk for infection. Prophylactic antibiotic treatment is not indicated. Monitor for infection. If adequate follow-up is not possible, some clinicians advocate treatment. Mothers and sexual partners of infected infants should be treated for *C. trachomatis*.

E. **Pseudomonas conjunctivitis**

1. **Isolate the patient** and implement standard precautions unless infection is resistant where contact precautions are indicated.
2. **Evaluate for systemic disease if indicated** (sepsis, meningitis, pneumonia, brain abscess, and others). Infants with low birthweight and lower gestational age have an increased risk for systemic disease.
3. **Parenteral therapy is recommended** because *Pseudomonas* is a virulent organism. Use a β-lactam antibiotic or an appropriate cephalosporin plus an amino-glycoside (gentamicin) for a minimum of 10–14 days. For infections that include meningitis, ampicillin or cephalosporin plus an aminoglycoside is recommended for 21 days. Remember there is increasing antibiotic resistance; therefore, some are recommending third- and fourth-generation antibiotics.
4. **Treat with gentamicin ophthalmic ointment** 4 times per day for 2 weeks. Treat with fortified topical antibiotics.
5. **Ophthalmology consultation** is critical because the infection may be devastating. **Infectious disease consult** may also be helpful, especially with *Pseudomonas* meningitis.

F. **Herpes simplex conjunctivitis**

1. **Isolate the patient**; implement contact precautions.
2. **Obtain a complete set of viral cultures** (blood, cerebrospinal fluid, eyes, stool or rectum, urine, mouth or nasopharynx, and any lesions). Obtain a CSF PCR.
3. **Administer topical ophthalmic therapy** with 3% vidarabine ointment or 1% trifluridine ointment or 0.1% iododeoxyuridine (all are proven to be effective) 5 times per day for 10 days (every 2 hours for 14 days).
4. **Systemic acyclovir therapy** for a minimum of 14 days if SEM (skin, eye, mouth) disease. If central nervous system disease or disseminated disease is present, treat for a minimum of 21 days. (For dosage, see Chapter 148.) The dose is 60 mg/kg/d IV divided tid.
5. **Ophthalmologic evaluation** and follow-up are necessary because chorioretinitis, cataracts, and retinopathy may develop.

G. **Other bacterial infections**

1. Local saline irrigation.
2. **Topical antibiotics** only are usually required. For gram-positive organisms: erythromycin or bacitracin. For gram-negative organisms: gentamicin or tobramycin

or ciprofloxacin. Some authors recommend Neosporin ophthalmic for most bacterial infections. Ophthalmic ointment: 0.5- to 1-cm ribbon in each eye every 6 hours for 7 days. Ophthalmic solution: 1–2 drops into each eye every 4 hours for 7 days. Ointment preferred over eye drops for neonates because they have reduced washout effect.

3. *Haemophilus influenzae* infection may require further evaluation of the infant (rule out sepsis, meningitis, and other infections if indicated), and systemic antibiotics may be necessary.

4. MRSA conjunctivitis. Treatment depends on the clinical situation; some do not need to be treated. Topical chloramphenicol eye drops have been used but are not recommended. Tobramycin/Polytrim ophthalmic solutions are recommended. See Chapter 110.

5. For gram-negative conjunctivitis in premature low birthweight infants remember there is increasing antibiotic resistance, especially among the β-lactam antibiotics. Third- and fourth-generation antibiotics are recommended.

H. Lacrimal duct obstruction
1. Most clear spontaneously without treatment. Massaging the inside corner of the eye over the lacrimal sac, with expression toward the nose, may help to establish patency.
2. If the problem does not resolve and symptoms persist (usually after 6–7 months), the infant should be evaluated by an ophthalmologist. Probing of the duct is indicated with a success rate of >90%.
3. Dacryocystitis. Treated with probing of the duct and either topical or systemic antibiotics depending on the severity of the infection.

Selected Reference

Pickering LK, Baker CJ, Kimberlin DW, Long SS, eds. *Red Book: 2012 Report of the Committee on Infectious Diseases.* 29th ed. Elk Grove Village, IL: American Academy of Pediatrics, 2012.

54 Gastric Aspirate (Residuals)

I. Problem. The nurse alerts you that a gastric aspirate has been obtained in an infant. **Gastric aspiration before feeding** is a procedure by which the stomach is aspirated with an oral or nasogastric tube. The procedure is usually performed before each feeding to determine whether the feedings are being tolerated and digested. The amount of residual is measured and recorded (**gastric residual**). Gastric residuals indicate the rapidity of gastric emptying and can be an indicator of feeding intolerance, infection, or other diseases such as bowel obstruction/perforation if the gastric aspirate volume or color is abnormal. Isolated gastric aspirates in very low birthweight infants can reflect delayed gut maturation and motility and may not signify a gastrointestinal (GI) problem, especially if no other warning signs exist.

II. Immediate questions
A. What is the volume of the aspirate? A volume of >20–30% of the total formula given at the last feeding may be abnormal and usually requires evaluation. A gastric aspirate of >10–15 mL is considered excessive. A prefeed gastric aspirate of >20% may predict (with other factors) late-onset sepsis.
B. What is the color and characteristic of the aspirate (eg, bilious, nonbilious, nonyellow, bloody, yellow aspirate)? This is important in the differential diagnosis (see Section III.A–D). Some neonatal intensive care units (NICUs) are introducing color charts to help identify bilious aspirates.

    C. **Are the vital signs normal?** Abnormal vital signs may indicate a pathologic process, possibly an intra-abdominal process.

    D. **Is the abdomen soft, with good bowel sounds, or distended, with visible bowel loops? Has the abdominal girth increased >2 cm?** Absence of bowel sounds, distention, tenderness, and erythema are all abnormal signs and may indicate a pathologic process. Absence of bowel sounds suggests an ileus. An increase in abdominal girth >2 cm is considered abnormal. Palpation of the abdomen may reveal a pyloric "olive" (pyloric stenosis).

    E. **When was the last stool passed?** Constipation resulting in abdominal distention may cause feeding intolerance and increased gastric aspirates.

    F. **What medications is the infant on?** Theophylline delays gastric emptying in very low birthweight infants. Cisapride (not available in United States) use increases the daily total gastric aspirate volume. Doxapram can cause gastric residuals.

    G. **Is the infant premature?** Delayed gastric emptying and feeding intolerance is common in premature infants. They have decreased duodenal motor activity, gastrointestinal dysmotility, and slower intestinal transit time. Feeding intolerance is less common in term infants; therefore, if there is a bilious or bile-stained aspirate, a workup needs to be done.

III. **Differential diagnosis.** The characteristics of the aspirate can provide important clinical clues to the cause of the problem and are outlined next. It is important to be able to identify bilious aspirates. A bilious aspirate is an aspirate that is light to dark green but can be bright yellow in the initial phases. Colostrum may appear yellow in color. Remember, overidentification of bilious aspirates can lead to infants going NPO and getting unnecessary evaluations.

    A. **Bilious (light to dark green) aspirate.** Usually indicates an intestinal obstruction distal to the ampulla of Vater, usually in the proximal small bowel. Distal bowel obstruction can also result in bilious vomiting or aspirates. A bilious aspirate can be a surgical emergency (especially if it occurs in the first 72 hours of life) and usually means bowel obstruction until proven otherwise. Especially in the **term infant**, GI pathology needs to be investigated, and early surgical consultation should be obtained. In the **premature infant**, bilious aspirates can occur without serious bowel pathology and may indicate **immaturity of the bowel**. Not all cases of bilious aspirates are caused by intestinal obstruction. In one study of bilious vomiting, 62% of infants did not have intestinal obstruction and had resolution with conservative management.

        1. **Malpositioned nasogastric tube.** Passage of the feeding tube into the duodenum or the jejunum instead of the stomach can cause a bilious aspirate.

        2. **Necrotizing enterocolitis (NEC).** This occurs mainly in premature infants. Ten percent of the cases involve term infants. Usually presents 10–12 days after birth.

        3. **Bowel obstruction.** Studies show that 30–38% of infants with bilious vomiting in the first 72 hours of life had obstruction, of whom 20% required surgery. **Bowel perforation with pneumoperitoneum** can present with increased bilious gastric residuals.

            a. **Malrotation with midgut volvulus.** Most common and found in 22% of infants with bilious vomiting. Presents at 3–7 days of age. Bilious gastric aspirate may be the only early sign of small bowel volvulus.

            b. **Duodenal atresia.** (If obstruction distal to ampulla of Vater, which is seen in 80% of cases.) One can see bilious emesis without abdominal distension. Duodenal obstruction is seen with associated anomalies in more than 50% of cases (Down syndrome, imperforate anus, Cornelia del Lange, VATER/VACTERL [*v*ertebral defects, *a*nal atresia, *t*racheo*e*sophageal fistula, and *r*adial or *r*enal dysplasia/*v*ertebral defects, *a*nal atresia, *c*ardiac malformations, *t*racheo*e*sophageal fistula, *r*enal dysplasia and *l*imb abnormalities], and others).

            c. **Jejunoileal atresia. Small bowel atresia** including distal duodenum and jejunal and ileal atresia can cause bilious aspirates. Presents within 24 hours of birth.

     d. Meconium ileus/plug. Presents soon after birth with abdominal distention and bilious aspirates/vomiting.

     e. Hirschsprung disease. Usually presents with abdominal distension and no stool but can have bilious or yellow aspirate or vomiting.

   4. Ileus can be associated with sepsis, prematurity, hypokalemia, effects of maternal drugs (especially magnesium sulfate), pneumonia, hypothyroidism, and other etiologies.

   5. Prematurity and bilious aspirates. Some premature infants will have bilious aspirates from gastric dysmotility and immaturity. These infants do not have a bowel obstruction or pathologic process.

   6. Gastroesophageal and duodenogastric reflux can cause bilious aspirates/vomiting.

   7. Idiopathic. No cause is found.

B. Nonbilious, nonyellow aspirate (white, clear, cloudy, undigested or digested formula)

   1. Problems with the feeding regimen. Undigested or digested formula may be seen in the aspirate if the feeding regimen is too aggressive and is more likely in small premature infants who are given a small amount of formula initially and then are given larger volumes too rapidly, or after adding fortifier to breast milk.

     a. Aspirate containing undigested formula. May be seen if the interval between feedings is too short or if too much formula is being given.

     b. Aspirate containing digested formula. May be a sign of delayed gastric emptying or overfeeding. Also, if the osmolarity of the formula is increased by the addition of vitamins, retained digested formula may be seen.

   2. Other

     a. Formula intolerance. An uncommon cause of aspirate but should be considered. Some infants do not tolerate the carbohydrate source in some formulas. If the infant is receiving a lactose-containing formula (eg, Similac or Enfamil), perform a stool pH to rule out lactose intolerance. If the stool pH is acidic (>5.0), lactose intolerance may be present. There is usually a strong family history of milk intolerance. Diarrhea is more common than gastric aspirates with lactose intolerance.

     b. Constipation. This is a factor especially if the abdomen is full but soft and no stool has passed in 48–72 hours.

     c. NEC or post-NEC stricture.

     d. Pyloric stenosis. Pyloric stenosis typically presents at 3–4 weeks with nonbilious projectile vomiting.

     e. Incarcerated hernia.

     f. Infections. One study found a prefeed aspirate >20% (along with other factors) can help in predicting late-onset sepsis.

     g. Hypermagnesemia. This can present with increased gastric aspirates and delayed passage of meconium.

     h. Retinopathy of prematurity (ROP) examination. Gastric aspirates are associated with ROP eye examination. Feeding is recommended 1 hour before ROP examination.

     i. Other rare causes. Bowel obstruction can present with nonbilious aspirates or vomiting, inborn errors of metabolism, and adrenogenital syndrome.

C. Bloody aspirate. (See also Chapter 55.) Upper gastrointestinal bleeding is blood loss proximal to the ligament of Treitz in the distal duodenum. This is bleeding from the esophagus, stomach, or duodenum.

   1. Swallowed maternal blood. Must be ruled out to verify whether there is true fetal bleeding.

   2. Trauma from nasogastric intubation. A common reason.

   3. Coagulopathies. Vitamin K deficiency (hemorrhagic disease of the newborn; should be considered if they did not receive vitamin K prophylaxis at birth), disseminated intravascular coagulation from infection, coagulopathy from liver failure, and any congenital coagulation factor deficiency can cause a bloody aspirate.

4. **Stress gastritis/esophagitis/erosions** of the esophageal, gastric, or duodenal mucosa/gastroduodenal ulcers can all have a bloody aspirate.

5. **Allergic colitis.** Milk or soy enterocolitis or milk protein intolerance. Cow milk intolerance. Lower GI bleeding is the more common presentation.

6. **Severe fetal asphyxia.**

7. **Medications** that can cause a bloody aspirate are theophylline (rare), indomethacin, heparin, nonsteroidal anti-inflammatory drugs, and corticosteroids. Tolazoline, especially by continuous infusion, can cause massive gastric hemorrhage. Maternal use of aspirin, cephalothin, and phenobarbital can cause coagulation abnormalities in their infants.

8. **Rare causes.** NEC, GI perforations, gastric volvulus or duplication, intestinal duplications, duplication cyst, and vascular anomalies to include hemangiomas, telangiectasias, arteriovenous malformations, Hirschsprung enterocolitis, and Meckel diverticulitis.

D. **Yellow aspirates. Non–bile-stained yellow aspirates** can be associated with intestinal obstruction and should not be ignored. Some infants will have bilious aspirates that are initially bright yellow in color. Clinical evaluation may be warranted in this situation and further workup depending on the evaluation. Remember that colostrum may also be yellow in color.

IV. Database

A. **Physical examination.** Check for any temperature instability or any new subtle signs that could indicate a pathologic process. How is the infant's perfusion? Is there any apnea? Is there anything else going on besides gastric aspirates? Are the stools normal? Pay particular attention to the **abdominal examination.** Check for bowel sounds (absent bowel sounds may indicate ileus), abdominal distention, tenderness to palpation and erythema of the abdomen (may signify peritonitis), or visible bowel loops. Check for hernias (may cause obstruction). **Abdominal distension (an increase in abdominal circumference >2 cm)** is a serious sign and should not be ignored.

B. **Laboratory studies**

1. **Immediate studies**

a. **Complete blood count with differential.** To evaluate for sepsis, if suspected. The hematocrit and platelet count may be checked if bleeding has occurred.

b. **Blood culture.** If sepsis is suspected and before antibiotics are started.

c. **Serum potassium level** if ileus is present. To rule out hypokalemia.

d. **Arterial blood gas.** To rule out acidosis. If metabolic acidosis occurs, this is a red flag in this setting, and a further workup should be done.

2. **Additional studies**

a. **Stool pH.** (See Section III.B.2a.) If there is a family history of milk intolerance, a stool pH should be obtained to rule out lactose intolerance (stool pH is usually >5.0).

b. **Coagulation profile.** (Prothrombin time, partial thromboplastin time, fibrinogen, and platelets.) A bloody aspirate may signify the presence of a coagulopathy.

C. **Imaging and other studies**

1. **Immediate studies**

a. **Plain radiograph (flat plate) of the abdomen** should be obtained if the aspirate is bilious, if there is any abnormality on physical examination, or if aspirates continue. The radiograph will show whether the nasogastric tube is in the correct position and will define the bowel gas pattern. Look for an unusual gas pattern, pneumatosis intestinalis, ileus, or evidence of bowel obstruction. Dilated bowel loops and air fluid levels suggest a surgical abdomen. Duodenal atresia has a double bubble sign. (See Chapter 11 for radiographic examples.)

      b. **A left lateral decubitus film** is useful because a perforation can be easily missed on the anteroposterior film. A gasless abdomen can be seen with mid gut volvulus.

  2. **Additional studies**

    a. **Gastroesophageal reflux scintigraphy ("milk scan").** The infant is fed liquid (or milk) mixed with a technetium-99m–labeled pertechnetate. The infant is scanned in the supine position for 1–2 hours with a gamma camera to show whether there is delayed emptying of the stomach or reflux.

    b. **Endoscopy** should be considered for ulcer evaluation.

    c. **Abdominal ultrasound and contrast studies of the GI tract** if indicated.

V. **Plan.** The approach to management of the neonate with increased gastric aspirates is usually initially based on the nature of the aspirate (if the aspirate is increasing with each feed, if it is greater than the volume of the feed, or if the aspirate is persistent) and whether the physical examination is abnormal. **General rules when called to evaluate an infant with an aspirate include the following:**

  A. **Examine the infant thoroughly.** Careful examination of the abdomen is essential.

    1. **If the examination is abnormal.** Distended abdomen, palpable loop on examination, abnormal/no stool, vital signs abnormal, apnea and bradycardia, or any other abnormal signs: Place the infant NPO while starting the workup. Order abdominal radiographs as soon as possible and consider antibiotics once sepsis evaluation is done. Surgical consultation should be considered.

    2. **If the examination is normal.** No systemic signs or any other red flags, and if the infant is premature, can consider feeding with close observation. **If term,** consider baseline radiograph and close observation.

  B. **Treatment of specific types of aspirates**

    1. **Bilious aspirate**

      a. **Malpositioned nasogastric tube. Rule this out first.** An abdominal radiograph will confirm the position of the nasogastric tube distally in the duodenum. Replace or reposition the tube in the stomach.

      b. **GI pathology.** The majority are initially managed by making the **infant NPO** and placing a nasogastric tube to rest and decompress the gut while doing a workup. Order an abdominal radiograph.

        i. **NEC.** See Chapter 113.

        ii. **Ileus.** May be secondary to sepsis, hypokalemia, effects of maternal drugs (especially magnesium sulfate), pneumonia, and hypothyroidism. NPO status and nasogastric tube are indicated. Treat underlying cause.

        iii. **Other surgical problems (eg, bowel obstruction, malrotation, volvulus, meconium plug).** Abdominal series should be ordered in addition to ultrasound and contrast studies. Pediatric surgical consultation should be obtained immediately.

      c. **Prematurity and bilious aspirates.** Follow the infant closely. If the infant has a normal examination, it is acceptable to feed with close observation. If the bilious aspirates persist or anything changes on the vitals or examination, then the infant needs to be reevaluated, a baseline radiograph obtained, and a bowel obstruction (malrotation) needs to be ruled out.

      d. **Gastroesophageal and duodenogastric reflux.** See Chapter 47.

      e. **Idiopathic bilious aspirates.** Conservative management.

    2. **Nonbilious nonyellow aspirate.** Usually involves undigested or digested formula.

      a. **Aspirate containing undigested formula.** If the volume of undigested formula in the aspirate does not exceed 20–30% of the previous feeding or is >10–15 mL total and the physical examination and vital signs are normal, the gastric aspirate can be replaced. If gastric aspirates continue and the examination of the infant is normal, the following can be tried:

        i. **The time interval between feedings may not be long enough** for digestion to take place. If the infant is being fed every 2 hours and aspirates continue, the feeding interval may be increased to 3 hours.

      ii. **Decreasing the volume** of the feeds can be tried.

      iii. **Continuous gavage feedings** may be tried. The patient may also have to be fed intravenously to allow the gut to rest.

      iv. **If elevated aspirates still continue, or if the aspirate exceeds >20–30% of the previous feeding, or is >10–15 mL total, the patient must be reevaluated.** If the infant has physical findings, work up the infant and withhold feeds. An abdominal radiograph should be obtained.

  b. Aspirate containing digested formula. The aspirate is usually discarded, especially if it contains a large amount of mucus. If the physical examination and vital signs are normal, continue feedings. If elevated aspirates continue, the patient must be reassessed. If the examination is normal, consider **decreasing the amount of feeds**. The number of calories should be calculated to make certain that overfeeding (usually >130 kcal/kg/day) is not occurring. If the examination is not normal, further workup must be done.

  c. Other

      i. **Formula intolerance.** A trial of lactose-free formula (eg, ProSobee or Isomil) can be instituted if lactose intolerance is verified. (See formula components in Chapter 10.)

      ii. **NEC or post-NEC stricture.** See Chapter 113.

      iii. **Pyloric stenosis.**

      iv. **Constipation.** Anal stimulation can be attempted. If this fails, a glycerin suppository can be given. (See Chapter 67.)

      v. **Infections.** If sepsis is likely, broad-spectrum antibiotics are started after a laboratory workup is performed. A penicillin (usually ampicillin) and an aminoglycoside (usually gentamicin) are given initially until culture results are available. The patient is usually not fed orally if this diagnosis is entertained; an infant with sepsis usually does not tolerate oral feedings.

      vi. **Inborn errors of metabolism.** See Chapter 101.

      vii. **Adrenogenital syndrome.** Hormone/steroid replacement, fluid and electrolyte management, and surgery are indicated.

      viii. **Hypermagnesemia.** See Chapter 107.

 3. Bloody aspirate. See also Chapter 55.

  a. Swallowed maternal blood. Observation only.

  b. Nasogastric trauma. Nasogastric trauma may occur if the nasogastric tube is too large or insertion is traumatic. Use the smallest nasogastric tube possible. Observation is indicated. Because the bleeds are usually minimal, active management is not necessary.

  c. Coagulopathies. GI hemorrhage from disseminated intravascular coagulation, vitamin K deficiency, and others are discussed in detail in Chapter 87.

  d. Stress gastritis. See page 389.

  e. Allergic colitis. Change formula.

 4. Non–bile-stained yellow aspirate. Full clinical examination and possible abdominal radiograph. If anything abnormal is found, further studies are needed to rule out any intestinal obstruction. These infants need to be followed closely.

C. Medications. If there is **no obstruction or any other treatable cause** of the aspirates, some institutions will try prokinetic agents such as metoclopramide and erythromycin to stimulate gastric emptying and decrease gastric residual volume.

 1. Metoclopramide. Used to treat gastroesophageal reflux and decrease gastric residual volumes in infants. The concern is that it may have limitations based on inconclusive effectiveness and concern for side effects. Cochrane review states that metoclopramide may have some benefit in comparison with placebo, but this must be weighed against the side effects.

 2. Erythromycin. Infants can have GI motility immaturity that causes feeding problems. Erythromycin is a motilin agonist (the GI peptide that stimulates contractility) and produces a prokinetic effect on the gut that may help with feeding problems. Trials involving **erythromycin as a prokinetic agent** are conflicting. Infants on erythromycin had significantly fewer episodes of large residual gastric aspirates over 10 days. Erythromycin administration is given at some centers in high-risk premature infants with severe feeding intolerance or with documented delay in gastric emptying by decreased motility on the milk scan. **Cochrane review** states that there is not enough evidence to recommend the use of erythromycin to prevent or treat premature infants with feeding issues. Use within 2 weeks after birth; treatment duration more than 14 days increases the risk of hypertrophic pyloric stenosis.

3. **Gaviscon infant.** An antacid that is a reflux suppressant. Studies show its effect is only a marginal decrease in the height of the refluxate.

55 Gastrointestinal Bleeding from the Upper Tract

I. **Problem.** Vomiting of bright red blood or active bleeding from the nasogastric (NG) tube is seen. **Upper gastrointestinal (GI) bleeding** is bleeding that occurs proximal to the ligament of Treitz in the distal duodenum (esophagus, stomach, or duodenum). The majority of GI bleeds in neonates are benign, self-limiting, and require minimal workup and treatment, but it is important to detect the cases that have significant underlying pathology.

II. **Immediate questions**

A. **What are the vital signs?** If the blood pressure is dropping and there is active bleeding, urgent crystalloid volume replacement is necessary.

B. **What is the hematocrit?** A spun or STAT hematocrit should be done as soon as possible. The result is used as a baseline value and to determine whether blood replacement should be performed immediately. **With any acute episode of bleeding, the hematocrit may not reflect the blood loss for several hours.**

C. **Is blood available in the blood bank should transfusion be necessary?** Verify that the infant has been typed and cross-matched so that blood will be quickly available if necessary.

D. **Is there bleeding from other sites?** Bleeding from other sites suggests disseminated intravascular coagulation (DIC) or other coagulopathy. If bleeding is coming only from the NG tube, disorders such as stress ulcer, nasogastric trauma, and swallowing of maternal blood are likely causes to consider in the differential diagnosis.

E. **How old is the infant?** During the first day of life, vomiting of bright red blood or the presence of bright red blood in the NG tube is frequently secondary to swallowing of maternal blood during delivery. Infants with this problem are clinically stable with normal vital signs.

F. **What medications are being given?** Certain medications are associated with an increased incidence of GI bleeding. The most common of these medications are indomethacin (Indocin), tolazoline (Priscoline), nonsteroidal anti-inflammatory drugs (NSAIDs), theophylline (rare), heparin, and corticosteroids. Some maternal medications can cross the placenta (aspirin, cephalothin, and phenobarbital) and cause coagulation disorders in the infant. Thiazides in pregnancy can be associated with neonatal thrombocytopenia.

G. **Was vitamin K given at birth?** Failure to give vitamin K at birth may result in a bleeding disorder, usually at 3–4 days of life.

H. **Does the infant have a syndrome or condition that is associated with gastrointestinal bleeding? Down syndrome:** Meckel diverticulum, Hirschsprung disease, pyloric stenosis. **Turner syndrome:** venous ectasia, inflammatory bowel disease. **Klippel Trenaunay syndrome and blue rubber bleb nevus syndrome (BRBNS):** vascular malformations. **Osler Weber Rendu syndrome (hereditary hemorrhagic telangiectasia):** epistaxis and vascular malformations, acute and chronic digestive tract bleeding. **Epidermolysis bullosa:** anal fissures, esophageal lesions, and strictures of the colon. **Ehlers Danlos and pseudoxanthoma elasticum:** fragile blood vessel wall structure. **Hermansky-Pudlak syndrome:** platelet dysfunction, inflammatory bowel disease. **Glycogen storage disease type 1b:** inflammatory bowel disease. **Zellweger cerebrohepatorenal syndrome:** GI bleeding.

I. **Is there a history of melena?** Melena signifies significant upper gastrointestinal bleeding or possibly swallowed maternal blood (see also Chapter 49).

III. **Differential diagnosis**

A. **Benign conditions that are not a true gastrointestinal bleed. Swallowing of maternal blood accounts for ~10% of cases.** Typically, blood is swallowed during cesarean delivery, but can occur with a vaginal birth as well. Swallowed blood irritates the stomach and can cause vomiting. **Swallowing of blood from a cracked nipple** or fissure during breast-feeding can also cause it. **Swallowing of amniotic fluid** with an antepartum hemorrhage bleeding into the amniotic fluid normally presents with melena stools but can present with upper GI bleeding.

B. **True gastrointestinal bleed**

1. **Idiopathic.** More than 50% of cases have no clear diagnosis and usually resolve within several days.

2. **Stress-induced gastric bleeding/ulcers.** These can be caused by an increase in gastric acid secretion and laxity of gastric sphincters in infants. Prematurity, neonatal distress, and mechanical ventilation are associated with stress gastritis. Maternal stress in the third trimester with increased maternal gastrin may also play a part. Upper gastrointestinal bleeding in healthy full-term infants is often associated with clinically relevant mucosal lesions of the upper GI tract.

   a. **Esophagus.** Esophagitis (hemorrhage or ulcerative), Mallory Weiss tear.

   b. **Gastric.** Gastritis, ulcer.

   c. **Duodenum.** Duodenitis, duodenal mucosal lesions, ulcer, vascular malformation; single stress ulcers are more common in duodenum than in stomach in a neonate.

   d. **Gastroesophageal lesions.** Infants tend to have gastric and esophageal lesions together.

3. **Trauma.** Infants can swallow their own blood from trauma.

   a. **Nasogastric trauma.** Forceful insertion or too large a tube can cause trauma. Frequent aspiration to identify gastric residuals can cause trauma. The bleeding from this is usually minimal.

   b. **Endotracheal tube insertion.**

   c. **Vigorous suctioning.**

   d. **Traumatic esophagitis.** This has been reported in newborns possibly from pharyngeal, esophageal, or gastric suction at birth.

4. **Coagulopathy**

   a. **Hemorrhagic disease of the newborn (vitamin K–dependent coagulation factors deficiency) and DIC.** Account for ~20% of cases. This is rare due to vitamin K prophylaxis. Mothers who are on certain medications that interfere with vitamin K metabolism (eg, oral anticoagulant, isoniazid, rifampin, anticonvulsants) are at risk for hemorrhagic disease of the newborn.

   b. **Congenital coagulopathies.** Most commonly factor VIII deficiency (hemophilia A) and factor IX deficiency (hemophilia B) can cause GI bleeding from the upper tract.

    c. DIC. This can occur after infection, sepsis, shock, liver failure, and severe fetal asphyxia.

    d. Liver disease/failure in the newborn. Metabolic disorders that cause liver failure have associated coagulopathies that can present with GI bleeds. Ischemic injury to the liver can also present with GI bleeding. Portal vein thrombosis can cause bleeding.

    5. Allergic colitis is caused by allergy to cow's milk or soy after it has been introduced. Can present with upper GI or rectal bleeding. Rectal bleeding is a more common presentation.

    6. Sepsis can cause GI bleeding in a newborn.

    7. Necrotizing enterocolitis (NEC) is a rare cause of upper GI tract bleeding that indicates extensive disease.

    8. Medications (drug-induced bleeding). Indomethacin, corticosteroids, tolazoline, heparin, NSAIDs, sulindac, and other drugs may cause upper GI tract bleeding. Theophylline is a rare cause. High-dose dexamethasone is associated with stress and perforated ulcers and hemorrhage in the newborn. **Maternal use** of aspirin, cephalothin, and phenobarbital can cause coagulation abnormalities in neonates. Prenatal use of cocaine can predispose to GI bleeds.

    9. Congenital GI defects such as gastric volvulus, malrotation with volvulus, Hirschsprung disease with enterocolitis, intussusception, gastric/intestinal duplication, duplication cyst, and Meckel diverticulitis.

    10. Vascular anomalies such as arteriovenous malformations, extensive telangiectasias, gastrointestinal hemangiomas, etc with or without a related syndrome can present with GI hemorrhage.

    11. Pyloric stenosis presents at the third to fourth weeks of life with nonbilious projectile vomiting (occasionally bloody).

    12. Rare causes include gastric teratoma/gastric tumors, gastric Dieulafoy lesion, infection with *Serratia marcescens*, arteriovenous malformations, complication from intrapulmonary percussive ventilation (IPV) therapy, telangiectasia involving the entire GI tract, pyloroduodenal intestinal duplication, and heterotopic pancreatic tissue in the stomach.

IV. Database

    A. Physical examination should focus attention on other possible bleeding sites. Note bowel sounds, abdominal distension and if there is any abdominal wall erythema.

    B. Laboratory studies

        1. Initial tests

        a. Apt test. Should be performed if swallowed maternal blood is a possible cause. This test differentiates maternal from fetal blood. The test relies on the fact that hemoglobin F is not hydrolyzed by a strong base, whereas maternal hemoglobin A hydrolyzes to a yellow brown. However, a negative test does not completely rule out swallowed maternal blood.

        b. Hematocrit. Should be checked as a baseline and serially to gauge the extent of blood loss.

        c. Complete blood count (CBC) with differential. A change in the white blood cell (WBC) count may indicate infection. Thrombocytopenia is associated with NEC and sepsis.

        d. Coagulation studies (platelet count, prothrombin time [PT], partial thromboplastin time [PTT], fibrinogen, and international normalized ratio [INR]). To rule out DIC and other coagulopathies. An elevated PT and prolonged PTT may indicate a coagulopathy.

        e. Biochemistry panel. An elevated BUN (blood urea nitrogen) can be seen in a massive GI bleed.

        2. Additional tests

        a. Liver function. If cholestasis is a concern, total and direct bilirubin and liver function tests should be done.

      b. **Serum pepsinogen level.** Elevated levels can indicate severe atrophic gastritis and gastric atrophy and can be elevated in infants with gastric and duodenal lesions.

C. **Imaging and other studies**

1. **Immediate tests**

      a. **Abdominal radiograph.** Assesses the bowel gas pattern and rules out NEC. The film also shows the position of the NG tube and indicates a possible surgical problem. It can help identify a pneumoperitoneum, small bowel dilatation, and pneumatosis.

2. **Additional tests**

      a. **Upper GI series.** A barium contrast study can be done for nonemergent bleeding. It can evaluate for upper GI bleed or midgut volvulus. Not recommended when acute bleeding is occurring.

      b. **Fiber optic/flexible upper GI endoscopy (esophagogastroduodenoscopy [EGD]).** Should be considered and can reveal the source of bleeding in 90% of patients with upper GI bleeding. It is safe and should be considered in bleeding that is persistent or recurrent, or in cases of severe hemorrhage requiring blood transfusion. It can examine the esophagus, stomach, and duodenum, and biopsies can be taken. In one study the most common lesion identified by endoscopy was gastroesophagitis (unique to neonates).

      c. **Ultrasound.** If pyloric stenosis is suspected, ultrasound of the abdomen should be done. It can also show portal hypertension.

      d. **Hepatobiliary scan.** To rule out biliary atresia and neonatal hepatitis.

D. **Nasogastric lavage** can identify blood within the stomach and can help determine if the bleeding is ongoing. The presence of fresh blood in the stomach is diagnostic of upper GI bleeding, including duodenal hemorrhages. If the lavage is negative, then there is no active UGI bleeding.

V. **Plan**

A. **General measures.** The most important goal is to stop the bleeding in every case except those involving infants who have swallowed maternal blood. Infants with this problem are usually only a few hours old, are not sick, and usually have a positive Apt test result. Once stomach aspiration is performed, no more blood is obtained. Pediatric gastroenterologist/pediatric surgery consultation is recommended for significant upper GI bleeding.

B. **Significant upper GI bleed** with signs of decreased vascular volume.

1. **Volume replacement.** If the blood pressure is low or dropping, crystalloid (usually normal saline) can be given immediately. **Blood replacement** may be indicated, depending on the amount of blood loss and the result of hematocrit values obtained from the laboratory. Fresh frozen plasma (FFP) and platelet transfusions may be necessary.

2. **Supplemental oxygen therapy** should be started if needed.

3. **Stop the acute episode of GI bleeding**

      a. **Gastric lavage** (with tepid water, 1/2 normal saline [NS], or NS 5 mL/kg) by NG tube until the bleeding has subsided. (*Note:* There is *controversy* about which fluid to use. Some believe that hyponatremia may occur if water is used and hypernatremia if NS is used. Follow your institution's guidelines.) **Never use cold-water lavages** (lowers the infant's core temperature too rapidly). Gastric lavage is *controversial* and there is no definitive evidence to support that it controls hemorrhage. This should not be done beyond 10 minutes if the NG fluid does not clear.

      b. **Epinephrine lavage** (1:10,000 solution), 0.1 mL diluted in 10 mL of sterile water, can be used if tepid water lavages do not stop the bleeding (*controversial*).

      c. **Endoscopic hemostatic techniques** may be necessary in massive bleeds and includes electrocoagulation, laser photocoagulation, heater probe thermocoagulation, and the injection of sclerosing agents and epinephrine.

C. **Upper GI bleed that is benign and minimal** can be observed if there is no evidence of active bleeding and a normal hematocrit. Antisecretory medications (H_2 blockers and proton pump inhibitors) can be used if indicated (see next section).

D. **Disease-specific measures**

1. **Idiopathic.** When no cause is determined, the bleeding usually subsides and no other treatment is necessary.

2. **Swallowing of maternal blood.** Observation only.

3. **Stress ulcer/mucosal lesions.** Commonly diagnosed after an episode of GI bleeding by endoscopy. This disorder is difficult to confirm using radiologic studies; thus, they are not often requested. Remission usually occurs; recurrence is rare. Rarely surgery is necessary.

   a. **Antacids** may be used (eg, Maalox, 0.5–1 mL/kg or 0.25 mL/kg, 6 times per day, placed in the NG tube until bleeding has subsided). This is *controversial* because it may cause concretions in the GI tract. Antacids may increase the risk of infection and feeding intolerance in infants receiving gavage feedings. Calcium- and aluminum-containing antacids cause diarrhea; magnesium-containing antacids cause constipation.

   b. **H_2 blockers** inhibit gastric acid production in neonates and are usually recommended. **Start ranitidine or famotidine** (see Chapter 148 for dosing). Ranitidine and famotidine are preferred because they have fewer side effects. Follow your institution's guidelines. Cimetidine is rarely used because of adverse effects and clinically significant drug interactions. H_2-blocker therapy is associated with higher rates of NEC in very low birthweight infants and infections.

   c. **Proton pump inhibitors** are used if H_2 blockers do not work and are superior to H_2 blockers in the treatment of peptic ulcer after endoscopy. These include esomeprazole (Nexium), omeprazole (Prilosec), lansoprazole (Prevacid), rabeprazole (AcipHex), and pantoprazole (Protonix). Studies with these agents are promising but they are not approved in neonates (Prilosec and Prevacid are approved in children >1 year of age). As with the H_2 blockers, there is an increased risk of infections. See doses in Chapter 148.

4. **Diffuse ulcerative esophagitis, gastritis, and duodenal mucosa lesions.** Treatment is supportive (maintain adequate oxygenation; nasogastric suction plus the use of IV H_2 blockers is recommended). Acid-reducing agents are sometimes used prophylactically in high-risk patients to reduce the risk. Surgery is rarely needed.

5. **Allergic colitis.** Eliminate the formula and change to a hypoallergenic formula.

6. **Nasogastric trauma.** May occur if the NG tube is too large or insertion is traumatic. Use the smallest NG tube possible. Observation is indicated. Because the bleeds are usually minimal, active management is not necessary.

7. **Necrotizing enterocolitis.** Severe cases of NEC cause upper GI bleeding.

8. **Coagulation disorders.** See Chapter 87.

   a. **Hemorrhagic disease of the newborn.** When vitamin K deficiency is suspected, vitamin K should be administered IV or subcutaneously. Intramuscular injection can result in severe hematoma. One milligram of vitamin K IV stops the hemorrhage within 2 hours. There are 3 forms of **vitamin K deficiency:**

      i. **Early form** (first day of life) is related to maternal medications affecting production of vitamin K by the neonate (barbiturates, phenytoin, rifampin, isoniazid, warfarin).

      ii. **Classic form** between days 2 and 7 of life is more commonly seen in infants with inadequate intake of breast milk and when an infant has not received vitamin K at birth (eg, home delivery).

      iii. **Late form** occurs between 2 weeks and 6 months of age. This is secondary to inadequate vitamin K intake (breast-fed infants) or hepatobiliary disease.

   b. **DIC.** Associated with bleeding from other sites. Coagulation studies are abnormal (increased PT and PTT with decreased fibrinogen levels). Treat the underlying condition and support blood pressure with multiple transfusions of colloid as needed. Platelets may be required. The cause of DIC (eg, hypoxia, acidosis, bacterial or viral disease, toxoplasmosis, NEC, shock, or erythroblastosis fetalis) must be investigated. Several obstetric disorders, including abruptio placentae, chorioangioma, eclampsia, and fetal death associated with twin gestation, may give rise to DIC.

   c. **Congenital coagulopathies.** The most common that present with bleeding are secondary to factor VIII deficiency (hemophilia A) and factor IX deficiency (hemophilia B). Specific laboratory testing and appropriate consultation with a pediatric hematologist are appropriate.

  9. **Drug-induced bleeding.** The drug responsible for the bleeding should be stopped, if possible.

  10. **Congenital defects such as gastric volvulus, malrotation with volvulus, Hirschsprung disease with enterocolitis, gastric duplication.** Urgent surgical consultation is recommended.

  11. **Pyloric stenosis.** Hydration and surgical pyloromyotomy are necessary.

  12. **GI bleeding from liver disease**

   a. **Octreotide (Sandostatin).** Dosage recommended (safety and dosing not firmly established) is 1 mcg/kg IV bolus, followed by 1 mcg/kg/h IV infusion. If no bleeding occurs in 12 hours, decrease the dose by 50%. Then stop the medication when the dose is 25% of the initial dose.

   b. **Vasopressin (Pitressin).** Used in neonates but has many adverse effects, so it not recommended.

56 Hematuria

  I. **Problem.** A nurse reports that an infant has a red-stained diaper and states the infant may have hematuria. Hematuria is the presence of gross or microscopic blood in the urine. It is defined as ≥5 red blood cells per high power field (HPF) on a centrifuged urine sample. Some authors recommend that 2 of 3 urinalyses show microhematuria before an evaluation is undertaken. Hematuria is rare in newborns.

  II. **Immediate questions**

   A. **Does the infant have normal urine output?** Low urine output should raise concern for obstruction of the urinary tract. Beyond the first 24 hours of life, urine output should be 1–2 mL/kg/h. Spontaneous voiding may not occur until after 24 hours of life. If the newborn is not symptomatic and does not have a distended bladder, continuing observation for the wet diaper is appropriate.

   B. **Were prenatal ultrasounds normal?** Abnormalities including hydronephrosis, renal/abdominal masses, and renal cystic changes may lead to hematuria.

   C. **Has there been any instrumentation to the urinary tract?** Traumatic catheterization, bladder aspiration, or instrumentation of the urinary tract may lead to hematuria that is usually transient.

   D. **Was there a maternal history of diabetes?** Maternal diabetes should raise suspicion of renal vein thrombosis.

   E. **Has vitamin K been given?** Consider hemorrhagic diseases of the newborn.

   F. **Is there an umbilical artery catheter?** Presence of a catheter with hematuria should raise question of possible aortic or renal artery thrombosis.

  III. **Differential diagnosis.** Hematuria is not common in newborns, and most normal newborns do not have hematuria. Transient hematuria is common in critically ill infants. The most common cause is acute tubular necrosis (see Chapter 123).

A. **Rule out causes that are not hematuria.** A red-stained diaper usually signifies hematuria but may be due to bile pigments, porphyrins, or urate crystals. Rule out extraurinary sources of bleeding: vaginal bleeding (pseudomenses), rectal bleeding, post circumcision, or a severe diaper rash with excoriation. In myoglobinuria or hemoglobinuria, the urine looks red and the dipstick is positive for blood, but there are no red blood cells on microscopic examination.

B. **Causes of hematuria**

1. **Trauma.** Birth or iatrogenic, such as bladder aspiration or catheterization, nephrostomy tubes. Transient hematuria in asphyxiated newborns.

2. **Vascular.** Renal vein or artery thrombosis, hyperosmolar infusions into umbilical catheters, umbilical arterial catheters with or without thrombus. Consider renal venous thrombosis in an infant of diabetic mother (IDM), cyanotic congenital heart disease, or infants with an umbilical venous catheter.

3. **Renal.** Renal cortical or medullary necrosis, acute tubular necrosis, neonatal glomerulonephritis (most commonly caused by syphilis), interstitial nephritis (medications), autosomal recessive polycystic kidney disease, multicystic renal dysplasia, congenital nephrotic syndrome.

4. **Urologic.** Any cause of obstruction or anatomic anomaly: posterior urethral valves, ureteropelvic junction obstruction, reflux, ureterocele, etc. Obstruction, nephrocalcinosis, urolithiasis (after chronic Lasix administration).

5. **Infection.** Inflammation will lead to hematuria. Urinary tract infection.

6. **Neoplasms.** Uncommon in newborns: rhabdomyosarcoma, Wilms tumor, neuroblastoma, nephroblastoma, angiomas, congenital mesoblastic nephroma.

7. **Hematologic.** Coagulopathy, hemorrhagic disease of the newborn, disseminated intravascular coagulation (DIC), clotting factor deficiency, severe thrombocytopenia.

IV. **Database**

A. **Physical examination.** Note blood pressure, bruising, or edema. Abdominal mass (obstruction, neoplasm, renal vein thrombosis) may be noted. Note the presence of urinary or umbilical artery catheters.

B. **Laboratory studies**

1. **Urinalysis.** Microscopic examination and dipstick testing confirm presence of blood or other causes of "red" urine. Red blood cell casts are seen with intrinsic renal disease such as glomerulonephritis. Bacteria or white blood cells suggest infection.

2. **Urine culture.** Collection of urine by catheterization or suprapubic bladder aspiration.

3. **Serum blood urea nitrogen and creatinine levels.** Abnormal levels may indicate renal insufficiency; may also reflect maternal renal function during the first week of life.

4. **Serum cystatin C levels.** Estimates glomerular filtration rate (GFR), although not validated in patients <2 years.

5. **Coagulation studies.** Thrombocytopenia may indicate renal vein thrombosis. Abnormal prothrombin time and partial thromboplastin time may indicate DIC or hemorrhagic diseases of the newborn.

C. **Imaging and other studies**

1. **Ultrasonography** may show upper urinary tract dilation, congenital anomalies of the urinary tract, renal vein thrombosis, or neoplasms.

2. **Computed tomography/magnetic resonance imaging** may be used for evaluation of neoplasms.

3. **Nuclear renography** may be used to assess for functional renal parenchyma.

V. **Plan.** Most cases are transient and resolve without any specific therapy. Persistent hematuria requires urologic or nephrology consultation.

A. **Trauma.** Expectant management for minor birth trauma or instrumentation of the urinary tract.

B. **Urinary tract infection.** Treat with appropriate antibiotics. (See Chapter 148.)

C. **Renal vein thrombosis.** Intravenous hydration, may consider attempt at revascular-
ization/thrombolysis. (See Chapter 87.)
D. **Obstruction.** Indwelling urethral catheter for bladder outlet obstruction. May
require acute or nonurgent operative intervention for congenital anomalies of the
urinary tract. Consult urology.
E. **Neoplasms.** Operative intervention may be needed. Consultation with pediatric
oncologist.
F. **Hematologic.** Correct coagulopathies. (See Chapter 87.)
G. **Renal.** Supportive measures and treatment of the specific cause. Restrict fluid intake
and replace insensible losses. May require renal replacement therapy (dialysis or
transplantation). (See Chapter 123.)

Selected References

Ballard RA, Wernosky G. Clinical evaluation of renal and urinary tract disease. In: Gleason
CA, Devaskar SU, eds. *Avery's Diseases of the Newborn.* 8th ed. Philadelphia, PA: Elsevier
Saunders; 2005:1267–1271.

Meyers KE. Evaluation of hematuria in children. *Urol Clin North Am.* 2004;31:559–573.

Palmer LS, Trachtman H. Renal functional development and diseases in children. In:
Wein AJ, Kavoussi LR, et al., eds. *Campbell-Walsh Urology.* 10th ed. Philadelphia, PA:
Elsevier Saunders; 2012:3002–3027.

57 Hyperbilirubinemia, Conjugated

I. **Problem.** An infant's direct (conjugated) serum bilirubin level is 3 mg/dL. The guidelines from the North American Society for Pediatric Gastroenterology, Hepatology, and
Nutrition use the following definition for abnormal direct bilirubin: **direct bilirubin
is >1 mg/dL if total bilirubin is <5 mg/dL, or direct bilirubin is >20% of the total
if the total bilirubin is >5 mg/dL. Conjugated hyperbilirubinemia is never normal
or physiologic.** It occurs in 1 in every 2500 infants. A persistent or increasing elevated
direct bilirubin is always pathologic and must be evaluated promptly. **Early diagnosis is
urgent and treatment is essential** because it means a better outcome for the infant and
can be potentially lifesaving (eg, biliary atresia). The goal is to complete the evaluation by
45 to 60 days of age (surgery for biliary atresia has its best outcome if performed before
the age of 45–60 days).
II. **Immediate questions**
A. **Is the urine dark, and what color is the stool?** It is best to examine the stools because
history obtained by someone else may not be accurate. **Dark urine** is a nonspecific
indicator of increased conjugated bilirubin. **Persistent pale or clay-colored stools**
occur with cholestasis and obstruction needs to be ruled out. One or two pale stools
usually do not indicate disease, and infants with biliary atresia have presented with
normal stools. There is a high specificity of persistent pale stools.
B. **Is the infant receiving total parenteral nutrition (TPN)?** TPN may cause direct
hyperbilirubinemia by an unknown mechanism and usually does not occur until the
infant has been on TPN for >2 weeks. It is more common in sick premature infants.
C. **Is the infant gaining weight?** Failure to gain weight can be seen in neonatal hepatitis
and some metabolic diseases.
D. **Does the infant appear sick?** Infants with cholestatic jaundice caused by **bacterial**
sepsis appear acutely ill. Infection may cause hepatocellular damage, leading to

increased direct bilirubin levels. **Infants with urinary tract infection, galactosemia, tyrosinemia, hypopituitarism, fructosemia, hemochromatosis, any metabolic disorder, acute common duct obstruction, gallstones with cholestatic jaundice, or hemolysis** can also appear ill. These disorders require immediate diagnosis and treatment.

E. **Did direct hyperbilirubinemia occur only after feedings had been established?** This suggests that a metabolic disorder such as galactosemia may be present.

F. **Have any risk factors been identified?** The **most important risk factors** include low gestational age, early or prolonged exposure to parenteral nutrition, lack of enteral feeding, and sepsis. Episodes of sepsis can be associated with an increase of 30% in the bilirubin level. Other risk factors include neonatal hepatitis, congenital infections, ABO incompatibility, and trisomy 21. Anesthesia may be a risk factor with direct bilirubin levels being higher in the spinal and epidural group than the inhalation group at 24 hours.

G. **Is the infant being treated for jaundice for another condition and not improving?** Any infant who is being treated for jaundice and whose jaundice does not resolve or improve needs to be evaluated for cholestasis.

H. **How old is the infant? Conjugated hyperbilirubinemia in the first 24 hours of life is abnormal and can indicate an infection. If presentation with liver failure in the first couple of days occurs, consider the following:** infection (hepatitis, herpes simplex virus [HSV], cytomegalovirus [CMV], and others), hemochromatosis, α_1-antitrypsin deficiency, inborn error of metabolism (tyrosinemia, galactosemia, others), ABO incompatibility, congenital leukemia, neuroblastoma, ischemic event (hepatic vein thrombosis and shock), biliary atresia, and hemoglobinopathy. Onset of jaundice in an asymptomatic infant **after 8 days** may mean a urinary tract infection. **Jaundice at 2 weeks of age** is common (2.4–15%) of newborns. Most is unconjugated and caused by breast milk jaundice.

III. **Differential diagnosis.** See Table 99–1. **Bilirubin** is the main waste product of hemoglobin breakdown when the liver breaks down old red blood cells. There are 2 forms of circulating bilirubin: **indirect and direct. Direct bilirubin** can be measured directly in blood and is a product of bilirubin metabolism within the liver (**indirect bilirubin** is conjugated in the liver to become direct bilirubin). Direct bilirubin is excreted into bile, stool, and urine. Statistics vary on what are the most common causes of direct hyperbilirubinemia. The **North American Society for Pediatric Gastroenterology, Hepatology, and Nutrition Guidelines Committee** states that the most common causes are **biliary atresia and neonatal hepatitis.** The most common cause in the neonatal intensive care unit (NICU) is probably **TPN use** in premature infants.

A. **Common causes.** *Note:* The diagnosis of one disease does not exclude that another disease may also exist.

1. **Biliary atresia.** This is a progressive obliterative process involving the bile ducts and is fatal if untreated. It is the most common cause of end-stage liver disease in this age group. These infants usually have clay-colored stools and dark urine. It is the most common cause in term infants. The infants usually look well.

2. **Idiopathic neonatal hepatitis/neonatal giant cell hepatitis.** Diagnosed after all other known causes have been excluded. No known infectious or metabolic cause can be found. **Idiopathic neonatal hepatitis can occur in premature infants** due to an immature biliary tree. They can have feeding difficulties and hypoglycemia.

3. **Genetic intrahepatic cholestasis.** Includes many proposed subtypes of intrahepatic cholestasis. Some of these include progressive familial intrahepatic cholestasis (PFIC1 [formerly Byler disease], PFIC2, and PFIC3), Alagille syndrome, disorders of bile acid biosynthesis and conjugation, and others. Each one of these diseases is rare, but collectively as a group this is a common cause of conjugated hyperbilirubinemia. These are chronic diseases, and many can progress and require liver transplantation.

4. **Hyperalimentation.** (TPN-induced cholestasis or parenteral nutrition–associated conjugated hyperbilirubinemia). Common in premature or very low birthweight infants. Long duration of hyperalimentation is a risk factor along with prematurity/ low birthweight, necrotizing enterocolitis (NEC), and sepsis. Infants can present with hepatomegaly and acholic stools. TPN can also cause biliary sludge.

5. **Infections.** Cholestatic jaundice and liver enzyme abnormalities have been reported in sepsis in the neonate. **In infants with conjugated bilirubin levels >0.5 mg/dL and <2 mg/dL, an infection must be ruled out.**

   a. **Bacteria.** Most commonly sepsis or urinary tract infection (UTI). **Gram-negative infections are the most common.** Others are group B *Streptococcus*, syphilis (*Treponema pallidum*), *Listeria monocytogenes*, *Staphylococcus*, and tuberculosis. If the onset of jaundice occurs after 8 days of age in an asymptomatic infant, suspect a gram-negative UTI.

   b. **Viral. Most common appear to be human immunodeficiency virus (HIV) and CMV.** Others include Epstein-Barr virus, adenovirus, enterovirus, coxsackievirus, reovirus, herpes (simplex, HV-6, zoster) virus, hepatitis (A [rare], B, C, E), varicella zoster, and echovirus 14 and 19. **Intrauterine infections include TORCH (*t*oxoplasmosis, *o*ther infections, *r*ubella, *c*ytomegalovirus, and *h*erpes simplex virus), hepatitis B and C, and syphilis. These account for about 20% of neonatal hepatitis. CMV has been found to be the most common in some studies. Congenital parvovirus B19 and B6 infection can also be involved. Human papilloma virus has been linked to neonatal giant cell hepatitis.

   c. **Parasitic.** *Toxoplasma gondii*, malaria.

6. **Hemolytic disease. Inspissated bile syndrome** is excessive bilirubin that results from hemolytic disease. It can be from vitamin K deficiency, Rh or ABO incompatibility, extracorporeal support/extracorporeal membrane oxygenation (ECMO/ ECLS), and other causes. **Ceftriaxone pseudolithiasis** can cause inspissated bile syndrome.

7. **Choledochal cyst.** Infants present with jaundice at 1–3 weeks, acholic stools; some may have obvious hepatomegaly, palpable mass in right upper quadrant, rarely vomiting or fever.

8. α_1-**Antitrypsin deficiency.** This is the **most common genetic cause** of cholestasis (5–15% of cases). These infants can present with intrauterine growth restriction (IUGR) and hepatomegaly.

9. **Galactosemia.** This the **most well-known metabolic disorder** that presents with prolonged jaundice.

10. **Perinatal hypoxia-ischemia.** This has been identified as an important causal factor in transient neonatal cholestasis. **Shock** can cause hepatic insult. **Acute circulatory failure** from congenital heart disease, myocarditis, and severe asphyxia can cause fulminant liver failure and conjugated hyperbilirubinemia.

B. **Less common causes of direct hyperbilirubinemia**

1. **Cholelithiasis (gallstones), biliary sludge.**

2. **Paucity of intrahepatic bile ducts.**

3. **Cholecystitis (acute and chronic).**

4. **Bile duct stenosis/spontaneous perforation of the bile duct.**

5. **Neonatal sclerosing cholangitis.** Etiology is unknown; presents in early infancy and then resolves.

6. **Inborn errors of metabolism.** Wolman disease, Niemann-Pick diseases A and C, glycogen storage disease type IV, Gaucher disease, Zellweger syndrome (cerebrohepatorenal syndrome), neonatal hemochromatosis, tyrosinemia, fructosemia, mevalonic aciduria, and citrullinemia. Cystic fibrosis rarely presents with liver disease in the neonatal period. Bile acid synthetic defects, disorders of fatty acid oxidation, and citrin deficiency can all cause cholestasis. Mitochondrial respiratory chain defects can cause liver failure.

7. **Endocrine disorders.** Hypothyroidism, panhypopituitarism.
8. **Congenital. Rotor syndrome** exhibits high direct and indirect hyperbilirubinemia. **Dubin-Johnson syndrome** is a genetic defect in the canalicular transport system that exhibits high direct and indirect hyperbilirubinemia. **Caroli disease** is a congenital disease that has saccular dilatations of the intrahepatic bile ducts and is associated with polycystic kidney disease. Other rare diseases include **Aagenaes syndrome, North American Indian familial cirrhosis, and hair-like bile duct syndrome.**
9. **Genetic.** Trisomy 21, 18, 13; monosomy X; partial trisomy 11; cat-eye syndrome.
10. **Neoplasm (rare).** Includes mesenchymal hamartoma, rhabdomyosarcoma of the biliary tree, neuroblastoma, and neonatal leukemia.
11. **Medications.** Prolonged use of chloral hydrate. Drugs that can cause cholestasis: anticonvulsants, cephalosporins, trimethoprim-sulfamethoxazole, and fluconazole.

IV. **Database.** The clinical hallmarks of the disease include **icterus, acholic or pale stools, dark urine, hepatomegaly, and splenomegaly.** See Figure 57–1 for an approach to an infant with cholestasis.

A. **History.** Should include prenatal (evaluate for intrauterine infection or hemolytic disease) and postnatal (feeding history with questions about the composition of formula, as well as the presence of any acholic stools). Have other family members had this problem? This can imply genetic disease. Consanguinity increases the risk of autosomal recessive inheritance. Was a fetal ultrasound done, and what are the results? This may identify a choledochal cyst (cystic structure inferior to the liver or incomplete gastric obstruction by a large cyst) or other abnormalities such as bowel duplication. Is there excessive bleeding, which could signify a coagulopathy or vitamin K deficiency? Is the infant lethargic or irritable? Lethargy can mean hypothyroidism or panhypopituitarism. Irritability can signify a metabolic disorder. Does the formula contain galactose (galactosemia); does it contain fructose or sucrose (hereditary fructose intolerance)? Vomiting may indicate pyloric stenosis, metabolic disease, or bowel obstruction. Delayed stooling is associated with hypothyroidism or cystic fibrosis (CF). With failure to thrive, neonatal hepatitis and metabolic disease are to be ruled out.

B. **Physical examination.** Does the infant appear sick? Think of sepsis, hypopituitarism, galactosemia, or gallstone. Vital signs, weight assessment (small for gestational age [SGA] implies fetal involvement), and general assessment of nutrition and observation for any signs of sepsis. Is there macroglossia (hypothyroid)? Check for bruises or petechiae on the skin (coagulopathy). Is there evidence of pneumonia on the chest examination? Is there a murmur or evidence of heart failure (Alagille syndrome or biliary atresia)? Be familiar with the characteristics of the syndromes noted here in the differential. Attention should be given to examination of the abdomen. Is it distended? Palpate for an enlarged liver or spleen or for any masses. Check for a palpable mass in the right side of the abdomen (choledochal cyst). Splenomegaly is more common in neonatal hepatitis but can be a late sign in biliary atresia. Jaundice has a greenish hue compared with unconjugated jaundice, which is more yellow. **"Bronze baby syndrome"** (a bronze discoloration of the skin as a result of dermal accumulation of coproporphyrins) occurs in infants with direct hyperbilirubinemia who are exposed to phototherapy. Ask the nurses about the diaper examination. Is the urine dark (conjugated hyperbilirubinemia), and what color are the stools (light stools suggest cholestasis)?

C. **Laboratory studies. Check the newborn screen** for hypothyroidism (unconjugated and early-onset conjugated hyperbilirubinemia) and galactosemia as these conditions require urgent treatment to prevent or decrease serious sequelae. If it was not done, a repeat one can be sent, or urine for reducing substance and serum thyroxine and serum thyroid-stimulating hormone (TSH) can be obtained. Sepsis evaluation should also be done early in any ill infant with jaundice to improve outcome.

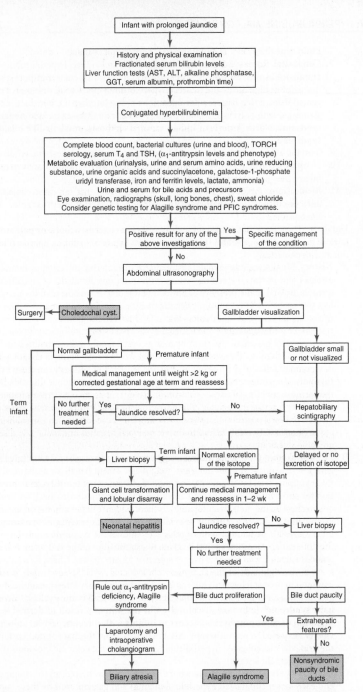

FIGURE 57–1. An approach to a full-term or premature infant with cholestasis. ALT, alanine transaminase; AST, aspartate transaminase; PFIC, progressive familial intrahepatic cholestasis; TORCH, *t*oxoplasmosis, *o*ther infections, *r*ubella, *c*ytomegalovirus, and *h*erpes simplex virus; TSH, thyroid-stimulating hormone. (*Reproduced, with permission, from Venigalla S, Gourley GR: Neonatal cholestasis. Semin Perinatol. 2004;28:348–355.*)

Perform tests based on results of history and physical examination first and rule out the most common etiologies.

1. **In infants with a conjugated bilirubin level >0.5 mg/dL and <2mg/dL infection must be ruled out (most are unexplained).** If the conjugated bilirubin continues to increase and is ≥2 mg/dL, assessment of the hepatobiliary system is needed.

2. **Testing guidelines from the North American Society for Pediatric Gastroenterology, Hepatology, and Nutrition.** Any infant with jaundice at 2 weeks of age should be evaluated for cholestasis by getting a total and direct bilirubin. Breast-fed infants should be evaluated at 3 weeks of age (if the history and physical examination is normal with no dark urine or light stools). **Retest any infant with** an acute illness or one whose jaundice does not improve with treatment.

3. **American Academy of Pediatrics (AAP) guidelines for jaundiced infants ≥35 weeks' gestation.** Total and direct bilirubin should be obtained in any sick infant, or if jaundice is present at or beyond 3 weeks of age. If the direct bilirubin is elevated, do a urinalysis and urine culture. Perform a sepsis evaluation if indicated by history and physical examination. Evaluate for causes of cholestasis including checking the results of the newborn thyroid and galactosemia screen. Look for signs and symptoms of hypothyroidism in the infant.

4. **Common causes.** The workup is as follows:

   a. **Bilirubin levels (total and direct) are the most important tests. A urine bilirubin** detects a substantial elevation of conjugated bilirubin. When serum levels exceed 3–4 mg/dL, bilirubin will be found in the urine.

   b. **Liver function tests.** Aspartate aminotransferase (AST/SGOT), alanine aminotransferase (ALT/SGPT), alkaline phosphatase, and gamma-glutamyltranspeptidase (GGTP). **Elevated levels of AST and ALT** signify hepatocellular damage. **Elevated alkaline phosphatase** levels may signify biliary obstruction (nonspecific because it is found in the liver, kidney, and bone). **Elevated GGTP** is a sensitive but nonspecific marker of biliary obstruction or inflammation. It was used in the past to differentiate biliary atresia from neonatal hepatitis, but wide variability in results makes interpretation difficult. **Elevated GGTP** suggests bile duct obstruction: biliary atresia or diseases that damage the bile ducts. **Low/normal GGTP** suggests progressive familial intrahepatic cholestasis type 1 or 2, bile acid synthesis defect, or neonatal hepatitis (giant cell hepatitis on histology). **A very low GGTP and high alkaline phosphatase** suggests metabolic and genetic causes of intracellular cholestasis. **Lipoprotein X is not routinely recommended.**

   c. **CBC with differential and platelet count.** May help determine whether infection is present. **Blood and urine cultures** if sepsis or urinary tract infection suspected. A **C-reactive protein (CRP)** as a screen for infection.

   d. **Urine analysis and culture.** Indicated for any infant with elevated direct bilirubin.

   e. **Serum glucose levels.** Hypoglycemia can be seen in metabolic liver disease, poor hepatic reserve, or hypopituitarism.

   f. **Direct Coombs test.** Used to test for hemolytic disease/inspissated bile syndrome.

   g. **Serum cholesterol, triglycerides, and albumin levels. Cholesterol and triglycerides** can be checked for assessment of liver failure and albumin for hepatic function.

   h. **Prothrombin time and partial thromboplastin time.** To evaluate hepatic function.

   i. **Reticulocyte count.** May be elevated (ie, >4–5%) if bleeding has occurred or hemolysis is present.

   j. **Testing for viral disease.** Determine the serum total immunoglobulin M (IgM) level. If high, test for TORCH infections (see Chapter 141). Urine is tested for cytomegalovirus, and a serum hepatitis profile is obtained (hepatitis surface antigen and IgM hepatitis A antibody). Hepatitis B markers should be tested in both the mother and the infant with **polymerase chain reaction (PCR) studies** being the most specific.

k. **Serum ammonia levels.** If elevated, can be caused by liver failure.

l. **Serum ferritin levels** are elevated, serum transferrin level is low but hypersaturated and lactate dehydrogenase (LDH) is elevated in neonatal hematochromatosis.

m. **Urine testing for reducing substances.** If galactosemia is suspected. Galactose in the urine results in a positive reducing substance in the urine on a Clinitest, but will have a negative urine test for glucose (glucose oxidase). Urine for succinylacetone should be done and if detected can be seen in hereditary tyrosinemia type 1.

n. **Serum thyroxine and thyroid-stimulating hormone levels.** If hypothyroidism is suspected.

5. **Less common causes.** Perform the following:

a. **Sweat chloride test/immunoreactive trypsin.** To rule out cystic fibrosis.

b. **Serum cortisol.**

c. **Plasma and urine amino acid screening.** Urine organic acid and plasma amino acid are screens for inborn errors that cause liver dysfunction.

d. **Karyotype.** To test for genetic disorders.

e. **Serum α_1-antitrypsin levels and phenotype.** To rule out deficiency.

D. **Imaging and other studies**

1. **Chest radiograph.** To check for cardiovascular or situs anomalies that may suggest biliary atresia. Infants with biliary atresia can have polysplenia syndrome. Alagille syndrome may have butterfly vertebrae on chest x-ray.

2. **Ultrasonography of the liver and the biliary tract (hepatic ultrasound).** Recommended for all infants with cholestasis per guidelines. It can rule out anatomic abnormalities such as choledochal cyst (cystic mass seen), stones, tumor, and masses and also provide information on the gallbladder. The absence of or finding a small gallbladder suggests, but cannot be used to rule out, biliary atresia. The procedure is operator dependent. **"Triangular cord"** (thickness of the echogenic anterior wall of the right portal vein of more than 4 mm on longitudinal scan) and an abnormal gallbladder length may be positive in the diagnosis of biliary atresia.

3. **Magnetic resonance imaging (MRI).** Best study for neonatal hemochromatosis to detect excess iron in the liver.

4. **Hepatobiliary scanning (scintigraphy).** Radionuclide scans such as **hepatobiliary iminodiacetic acid (HIDA), diisopropyl iminodiacetic acid (DISIDA),** or **paraisopropyl iminodiacetic acid (PIPIDA)** scans allow evaluation of the biliary anatomy. Injected radioactive material is normally excreted into the intestine. If there is no visualization after 24 hours, biliary obstruction or hepatocellular dysfunction may be present (high sensitivity for biliary atresia but low specificity). Tests are expensive, time-consuming, and have many false-positive and false-negative results and are not routinely recommended.

5. **Magnetic resonance cholangiopancreatography (MRCP) and endoscopic retrograde cholangiopancreatography (ERCP).** These can be done for diagnosis and therapy for bile duct stones. They are not routinely done, but ERCP may be useful if done by an experienced operator. MRCP requires deep sedation or general anesthesia and is not routinely recommended.

6. **Percutaneous liver biopsy.** Typically performed after extensive evaluation without definitive diagnosis and is guideline recommended. It is useful in infants with cholestasis of unknown etiology. Evidence indicates that this test can be performed safely in small infants. **Some studies have shown that this procedure had the greatest diagnostic accuracy and should be done before surgery to diagnose biliary atresia.** Results should be interpreted by a pathologist with pediatric liver disease expertise and experience.

7. **Duodenal aspirate.** May be useful in remote areas where other tests are not available. Fluid is obtained from the duodenum and then the aspirate is sent for bilirubin concentration. With obstruction the aspirate bilirubin concentration is less than or equal to the bilirubin concentration in the serum.

8. **Exploratory laparotomy and operative cholangiography.** These should be considered if all other tests have been done and are inconclusive, and biliary atresia needs to be diagnosed.

V. **Plan.** See Figure 57–1 for an approach to a full-term or premature infant with conjugated hyperbilirubinemia. The cause of direct hyperbilirubinemia is determined and specific treatment is directed at the cause. As few conditions are treatable, care is mostly supportive. Treatment involves dietary measures, medications, and surgery. This section also discusses some of the more common causes of conjugated hyperbilirubinemia, with more detailed management information in Chapter 99. **Consultation with a pediatric gastroenterologist is recommended for all infants.**

A. **Diagnose the infant who appears sick and requires urgent treatment**

1. **Sepsis.** If signs of sepsis are present, appropriate cultures should be performed and empirical antibiotic therapy initiated.

2. **Urinary tract infection.** Appropriate antibiotic therapy.

3. **Metabolic disorders.** (Galactosemia, tyrosinemia, fructosemia, hematochromatosis.) Immediate elimination of lactose- and galactose-containing products from the diet is required. **Hematochromatosis** requires supportive care (respiratory, ventilation, pressors) and treatment with chelation and other agents. Liver transplantation may be necessary.

4. **Hypothyroidism.** Treatment is ʟ-thyroxine. See Chapter 140.

5. **Hemolytic disease/hemolysis.** Treatment depends on etiology (vitamin K, etc.).

6. **Hypopituitarism.** Hormone replacement, fluid, and electrolyte therapy.

7. **Gallstones with acute common duct obstruction.** Surgery is indicated.

8. **Intrauterine infection.** Appropriate antiviral agents or other medications should be started, if indicated.

B. **Parenteral nutrition–associated cholestasis (PNAC).** If the infant has been on parenteral nutrition (PN) for 2 weeks and has not been fed, then the infant may have PN-associated cholestasis. Consider stopping TPN completely, cycling TPN, or using partial parenteral nutrition with some enteral feedings. Enteral feeding can reduce the incidence and severity of PNAC. Most infants recover with clearing of cholestasis in 1–3 months after normal feedings have begun. The use of phenobarbital therapy is ***controversial***. Ursodeoxycholic acid is being used investigationally in high-risk neonates with TPN cholestasis with good results. Cholecystokinin as a treatment or prophylactic agent has less conclusively shown benefit. Erythromycin by increasing motility may be helpful in preventing or treating PNAC. Fish oil–based lipid emulsions may be able to reverse TPN cholestasis and may be beneficial, but are not readily available. The only known effective treatment is to stop the parenteral nutrition and transition to full enteral feedings.

C. **Biliary atresia.** Biliary atresia must be differentiated from neonatal hepatitis. Earlier diagnosis of biliary atresia and surgical repair leads to a better outcome. Exploratory surgery with intraoperative cholangiography is often the initial step. Hepatic portoenterostomy (the **Kasai procedure**) is currently the initial procedure of choice in infancy. It has the greatest chance of reestablishment of bile flow and the longest-term survival of the infant's liver if performed before the age of 45–60 days. **Orthotopic liver transplantation** is selectively performed for those infants or children with progressive liver failure. Liver transplantation offers improved survival and quality of life to those for whom the Kasai operation is not successful.

D. **Other etiologies**

1. **Choledochal cyst.** The treatment is surgical removal of the cyst and biliary bypass.

2. **Idiopathic neonatal hepatitis.** Supportive care (medications, specific formulas, vitamins) with a fair prognosis exists. Those who develop cirrhosis may require a liver transplant.

3. **α₁-Antitrypsin deficiency.** Infants initially can be managed with nutritional support, vitamins, and treatment of cholestasis. The only curative therapy is liver transplantation.

4. **Inspissated bile.** Inspissated bile secondary to hemolytic disease is treated with supportive management. The use of phenobarbital is *controversial.*

E. **General recommendations**

1. **Dietary.** Most of these infants require special formulas (eg, Pregestimil, Enfaport, Portagen) that include medium-chain triglycerides (MCTs) that can be absorbed better with a bile salt deficiency. Supplemental MCTs can be given to breast-fed infants. Supplemental vitamins (A, D, E, K) are needed in many of these infants. Some infants may require other dietary restrictions.

2. **Medications.** Ursodeoxycholic acid, phenobarbital, and cholestyramine are used often and are discussed in detail in Chapter 99, page 671.

3. **Surgery.** Surgery includes the Kasai procedure and liver transplantation.

Selected References

American Academy of Pediatrics: Subcommittee on Hyperbilirubinemia. Management of hyperbilirubinemia in the newborn infant 35 or more weeks of gestation. *Pediatrics.* 2004;114:297–316.

Guideline for the evaluation of cholestatic jaundice in infants: recommendations of the North American Society for Pediatric Gastroenterology, Hepatology, and Nutrition. *J Pediatric Gastroenterol Nutr.* 2004;39:115–128.

Venigalla S, Gourley GR. Neonatal cholestasis. *Semin Perinatol.* 2004;28:348–355.

58 Hyperbilirubinemia, Unconjugated

I. **Problem.** An infant's indirect (unconjugated) serum bilirubin level is 10 mg/dL. The exact definition of a physiologic range and management of indirect hyperbilirubinemia is complex and based on many factors, including gestational age (GA), postnatal age, birthweight, disease state, risk factors, degree of hydration, nutritional status, and ethnicity. **Total serum bilirubin (TSB)** is the sum of direct (conjugated) and indirect (unconjugated) and can be measured in the blood. The **indirect bilirubin** is calculated by subtracting the direct bilirubin from the total bilirubin. **Transcutaneous bilirubin (TcB)** is a measurement of total serum bilirubin from an instrument that uses reflectance measurements on the skin and correlates well with the laboratory TSB value.

II. **Immediate questions**

A. **How old is the infant? What is the gestational age? High indirect serum bilirubin levels during the first 24 hours of life are never physiologic.** Hemolytic disease (Rh isoimmunization or ABO incompatibility), congenital infection (eg, rubella, toxoplasmosis), sepsis, occult hemorrhage, and polycythemia are likely causes. The age and gestation of the infant help determine the bilirubin level at which phototherapy should be initiated. The risk of unconjugated hyperbilirubinemia is inversely proportional with GA. In premature infants, hyperbilirubinemia is usually more severe and lasts longer.

B. **Is the infant being breast-fed? Breast-feeding jaundice (early onset)** occurs within the first week of life and is probably associated with decreased production or decreased intake of breast milk resulting in caloric deprivation. **Breast milk jaundice (late onset)** usually occurs after the first week of life into the second to third week. It is secondary to the increased intestinal absorption of bilirubin by the enzyme B glucuronidase, and there may be a familial association. There is a correlation between bilirubin levels and epidermal growth factor concentrations in infants with breast milk jaundice. This may explain the reason for jaundice in these neonates.

C. **What is the family ethnicity?** The incidence of neonatal jaundice is increased in infants of Native American Indian, Inuit, Mediterranean (Greece, Turkey, Sardinia), Sephardic Jewish, Nigerian, and Eastern Asian descent. Native Greeks have a higher incidence than Greeks in the United States. The incidence is lower in African Americans. Glucose-6-phosphate dehydrogenase (G6PD) deficiency is more common in many of these groups and may be partially responsible. Immigration and intermarriage have increased the incidence of G6PD in the United States.

D. **Is the infant dehydrated?** With dehydration (or weight loss from birth >12%), fluid administration may lower the serum bilirubin level. Additional feedings should be given, if tolerated (milk-based formula is recommended in dehydrated breast-fed infants); otherwise, IV fluids should be given. It is recommended that mothers nurse their infants 8–12 times a day as a minimum for the first few days. For example, a 3-day-old infant is strictly breast-feeding, but his mother's milk has not yet "come in," so he has lost significant weight and becomes dehydrated. Adequate hydration is essential, but **excess hydration will not clear the bilirubin any more quickly, prevent hyperbilirubinemia, or decrease TSB.**

E. **Is the infant <35 weeks? If so, is the infant at greater risk for bilirubin toxicity?** Infants <35 weeks follow a different set of guidelines for phototherapy and exchange transfusion. Infants with a lower gestational age or a serum albumin <2.5 g/dL or a rapidly rising TSB (suggesting hemolytic disease) or those infants who are clinically unstable (blood pH <7.15, blood culture positive sepsis in the prior 24 hours, apnea and bradycardia requiring cardiorespiratory resuscitation [bagging and/or intubation] during the previous 24 hours, hypotension requiring pressor treatment during the previous 24 hours, or mechanical ventilation at the time of blood sampling) all need to have phototherapy or an exchange transfusion done at the lower level recommended.

III. **Differential diagnosis.** Indirect (unconjugated) bilirubin is derived mainly from hemoglobin metabolism and must be conjugated in the liver before it can be excreted in the bile, stool, or urine. It cannot be directly measured in the blood and is never present in urine. Jaundice in the newborn is caused by an increase in enterohepatic circulation, a decrease in the clearance of bilirubin, a decrease in conjugation and hepatic uptake, impaired bile flow, and an increase in production. (See also Chapter 100.)

A. **Common causes of indirect hyperbilirubinemia.** The majority of infants have hyperbilirubinemia in the first week of life. Differentiate physiologic from nonphysiologic hyperbilirubinemia. Timing onset and duration may aid in differentiating physiologic from nonphysiologic. The following are more likely associated with nonphysiologic indirect hyperbilirubinemia: onset <24 hours lasting >1–2 weeks, higher level requiring treatment, or if an infant is sick.

1. **Physiologic hyperbilirubinemia.** A normal response and can occur because of a shorter life span of red blood cells (RBCs) which causes an increase in bilirubin; a relative deficiency of uridine 5'-diphospho-glucuronosyltransferase (UGT), which causes a decrease in bilirubin clearance; decreased hepatic excretion; and an increase in enterohepatic circulation. It usually appears after the second day and peaks between the third and fifth days. The bilirubin level is usually <12 mg/dL but can rise up to 18 mg/dL and then decrease. It is not clinically significant and usually resolves within 1 week. **Exaggerated/severe physiologic jaundice** can occur where higher bilirubin levels occur and the hyperbilirubinemia lasts longer (ie, 2 weeks). Some factors associated with this include prematurity, severe weight loss, maternal diabetes, induction of labor with oxytocin, bruising of the infant, and breast-feeding. These infants may require treatment.

2. **Nonphysiologic hyperbilirubinemia**
   a. **Breast-feeding or breast milk jaundice.** Breast-feeding jaundice is due to dehydration from not taking in enough breast milk (13%). A substance in breast milk that blocks bilirubin elimination may also be present.
   b. **Infection (eg, congenital syphilis, viral, or protozoal infections).** Jaundice as the only sign of sepsis is rare. In one study of 171 newborns readmitted for a mean bilirubin of 18.8 mg/dL, no case of sepsis was identified.
   c. **Hemolysis related.** ABO incompatibility.
   d. **Increased bilirubin load from breakdown of RBCs.** Subdural hematoma, intraventricular hemorrhage in premature infants, cephalohematoma, excessive bruising, pulmonary hemorrhage, polycythemia, hyperviscosity.
   e. **Infant of a diabetic mother.**
   f. **Asphyxia/hypoxia.**
   g. **Respiratory distress syndrome.**
   h. **Hypoglycemia.**
B. **Less common causes of indirect hyperbilirubinemia**
   1. **Rh isoimmunization.** As a result of antenatal treatment of Rh-negative mothers with RhoGAM, this has become less frequent.
   2. **G6PD deficiency.** A late-rising bilirubin is seen. This is also more common in individuals of certain ethnic backgrounds (see Section I earlier).
   3. **Pyruvate kinase deficiency.**
   4. **Congenital spherocytosis, elliptocytosis, pyknocytosis.**
   5. **Syndromes.** Lucey-Driscoll (familial neonatal jaundice), Crigler-Najjar (type I and type II), and Gilbert syndrome.
   6. **Hypothyroidism/hypopituitarism.**
   7. **Hemoglobinopathy.** α- and γ-Thalassemia.
   8. **Early galactosemia or fructose intolerance.**
   9. **Medications.** Penicillin, oxytocin, sulfonamides, vitamin K, nitrofurantoin, novobiocin (not available in United States). Maternal use of naproxen, atazanavir, or methyldopa can cause a positive direct antiglobulin test and jaundice in the newborn. Maternal oxytocin and valium is a risk factor.
   10. **Disseminated intravascular coagulopathy.**
   11. **Intestinal (rare).** Obstruction, pyloric stenosis, ileus, or meconium plug.
IV. **Database**
   A. **History.** What is the infant's feeding regimen and frequency of voiding (hydration status)? Ask about jaundice in previous siblings and family ethnicity. Is there a familial history of significant hemolytic disease? Is there a history of light-colored stools or dark urine? Any maternal medication use?
   B. **Physical examination.** Attention to signs of bruising, cephalohematoma, or intracranial bleeding. Check for hepatosplenomegaly. The accumulation of bilirubin in body tissues produces jaundice (yellow skin) and scleral icterus. Jaundice is first seen in the face and progresses caudally to the trunk and extremities. Pressure on the skin often reveals jaundice. The **TSB can be estimated (not 100% reliable) by examining the skin of different areas of the body** for jaundice (face, ~5 mg/dL; upper chest, ~10 mg/dL; abdomen, ~12 mg/dL; palms and soles, usually >15 mg/dL). A complete neurologic examination should be performed, as bilirubin encephalopathy can occur. Look for signs such as poor feeding, lethargy, hypotonia, or seizures.
   C. **Laboratory studies.** Studies have questioned the need for extensive testing on any infant with possible hyperbilirubinemia. In normal and healthy term infants, few tests are necessary. It is useful to save cord blood for future testing if necessary.
      1. **Jaundiced infant of ≥35 weeks' gestational age.** These recommendations are based on the American Academy of Pediatrics (AAP) Subcommittee on Hyperbilirubinemia. All bilirubin levels should be interpreted based on infant's age in hours. See also the algorithm in Figure 58–1 for management of jaundice in the newborn nursery.

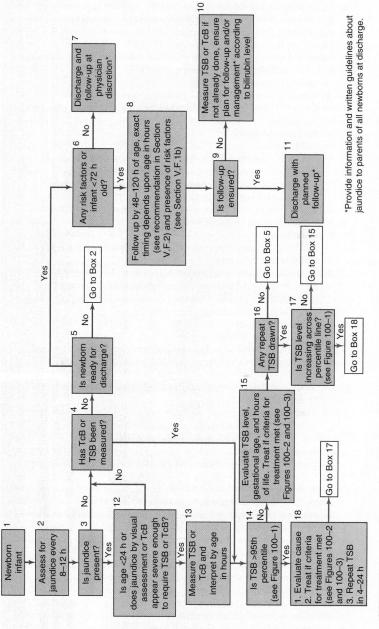

FIGURE 58-1. Algorithm for the management of jaundice in the newborn nursery. (*Reproduced with permission from Subcommittee on Hyperbilirubinemia. Management of hyperbilirubinemia in the newborn infant 35 or more weeks of gestation. Pediatrics. 2004;114:297–316.*)

a. **Infant jaundiced in the first 24 hours or the jaundice appears excessive for age: measure TSB and TcB.** TcB is determined by a portable transcutaneous instrument that measures the amount of yellow color in the skin, which correlates with the laboratory measurement of TSB.

b. **Infant is receiving phototherapy or TSB is rising rapidly and unexplained by history and physical examination.** Obtain:

  i. **Direct (conjugated) bilirubin.**

  ii. **Blood type and Coombs test.** If not obtained on the cord blood.

  iii. **Complete blood count (CBC) with differential and smear.** Observe RBC morphology.

  iv. **Reticulocyte count.**

  v. **G6PD level.**

  vi. **ETCOc if available.** ETCOc (end-tidal CO corrected for ambient CO) is a measurement of the rate of heme catabolism and rate of bilirubin production. It is used to confirm hemolysis and can help identify infants at risk for developing high bilirubin levels.

  vii. **Repeat TSB in 4–24 hours,** depending on infant's age and TSB level.

c. **TSB is approaching exchange levels (see Table 100–1) or is not responding to phototherapy:**

  i. **Reticulocyte count.** If anemia or hemolytic disease is suspected.

  ii. **G6PD level.**

  iii. **Albumin.** An albumin of <3.0 g/dL is a risk factor for lowering the threshold for phototherapy. Obtaining a serum albumin will allow you to calculate the bilirubin-to-albumin (B/A) ratio, which can help determine the need for exchange transfusion (see Figure 100–3).

  iv. **ETCOc.** See above.

d. **Direct bilirubin is elevated**

  i. **Evaluate for sepsis** including urinalysis and urine culture if indicated.

  ii. See Chapters 57 and 99 for more details on direct hyperbilirubinemia.

e. **Jaundice is present at 3 weeks or beyond, or if the infant is sick**

  i. **Total and direct bilirubin. If direct bilirubin is elevated,** evaluate for cholestasis.

  ii. **Thyroid screen (hypothyroidism) and galactosemia screen.** Does the infant have signs or symptoms of hypothyroidism?

2. **Jaundiced infant <35 weeks' gestation** (*controversial*). There are no formal guidelines for laboratory values for jaundiced infants <35 weeks. These are recommendations only. Follow institutional guidelines. (See also preceding tests for infant >35 weeks.)

a. **Total and direct serum bilirubin levels.** In preterm or ill infants, check levels every 12–24 hours depending on the rate of rise and until stable. In term infants, direct bilirubin is indicated only if jaundice is persistent or the infant is ill. In preterm infants, because of lack of data, there are no recommendations for an infant with an increase in direct bilirubin. Infants with a direct bilirubin >50% of the TSB require individual evaluation.

b. **CBC with differential.** If hemolytic disease, anemia, or infection is suspected.

c. **Mother's and infant's blood type with Rh determination.**

d. **Direct and indirect Coombs tests.** Used to detect in vivo or in vitro antibody-antigen reactions in hemolytic anemia.

e. **Reticulocyte count.** If the infant is anemic or hemolytic disease is suspected.

f. **Serum albumin.** If serum albumin is low, it is best to treat those infants at lower TSB levels.

g. **RBC smear.** Fragmented RBCs should be present in hemolysis.

h. **G6PD screen.** G6PD is more common in males and in infants of Mediterranean, African, Arabian, Asian, or Middle Eastern descent. The jaundice is late onset, and there is evidence of hemolysis (low hematocrit, high reticulocyte count, and a peripheral smear showing nucleated RBCs and other fragmented cells) or the response to phototherapy is poor.

   i. Hemoglobin electrophoresis. Used to rule out hemoglobinopathies (hemolytic anemia, thalassemia, sickle cell anemia, hemoglobin C disease).

D. **Imaging and other studies.** Usually unnecessary.

V. **Plan.** Based on gestational age, follow the guidelines for either >35 weeks versus <35 weeks. See also Chapter 100 for a detailed discussion.

A. **Phototherapy**

1. **Principles of phototherapy.** Bilirubin absorption of visible light in the blue region of the spectrum transforms unconjugated bilirubin (bound to albumin) into bilirubin "photoproducts," mostly isomers of bilirubin. The AAP Committee on Fetus and Newborn has recommended practice considerations for devices and the optimal administration of phototherapy in infants >35 weeks' gestation:

   a. Ensure that the phototherapy device fully illuminates the patient's body surface area. Maximum skin area should be exposed.

   b. Irradiance level of $\geq$30 $\mu W/cm^{-2}/nm^{-1}$ over waveband of 460–490 nm (blue-green region).

   c. Phototherapy should be implemented in a timely/urgent fashion.

   d. Briefly interrupt for feeding and other care.

   e. Measure bilirubin load reduction and discontinue when desired level reached. Beware of rebound increase in bilirubin.

2. **Phototherapy for the hospitalized infant of $\geq$35 weeks' gestation.** (See Figure 100–2.) Phototherapy is started when the TSB exceeds the line (or an option is to start 2–3 levels below the line) indicated for each category. The risk factors were selected because these conditions have a negative effect on the albumin binding of bilirubin, the blood–brain barrier, and the susceptibility of the brain cells to damage by bilirubin. When using this figure, follow these guidelines:

   a. **Use TSB.** Do not subtract direct bilirubin from the total.

   b. **Measure serum albumin.** If <3 g/dL, it is considered a risk factor. Lower the phototherapy threshold.

   c. **Other risk factors.** Isoimmune hemolytic disease, G6PD deficiency, asphyxia, significant lethargy, temperature instability, sepsis, acidosis, or albumin <3.0 g/dL.

   d. **Infants at low risk.** Infants who are $\geq$38 weeks and well.

   e. **Infants at medium risk.** Infants who are $\geq$38 weeks and have risk factors (see earlier). Other infants at medium risk involve those infants who are 35–37 6/7 weeks and well. It is optional to intervene at a lower TSB level for those infants who are closer than 35 weeks and at a higher level for those infants who are closer to 37 6/7 weeks.

   f. **Infants at high risk.** Infants who are 35–37 6/7 weeks with risk factors listed earlier.

3. **Phototherapy for the hospitalized infant < 35 weeks' gestation.** (See Table 100–1.) Due to the lack of evidence-based trials, the AAP has not published guidelines for infants <35 weeks. However a consensus-based recommendation has been published. Recently similar consensus guidelines have been published in other countries (Canada, Israel, Norway, South Africa, the Netherlands, the United Kingdom). When using this table, follow these guidelines:

   a. **Use the lower range number if the infant is at a greater risk for bilirubin toxicity. Risk includes** lower gestational age, serum albumin <2.5 g/dL, rapidly rising TSB (suggesting hemolytic disease), and those who are clinically unstable (see later).

   b. **When a decision is being made about the initiation of phototherapy or exchange transfusion, infants are considered to be clinically unstable if they have one or more of the following conditions:**

      i. Blood pH <7.15.

      ii. Blood culture positive sepsis in the prior 24 hours.

      iii. Apnea and bradycardia requiring cardiorespiratory resuscitation (bagging and/or intubation) during the previous 24 hours.

      iv. Hypotension requiring pressor treatment during the previous 24 hours.

      v. Mechanical ventilation at the time of blood sampling.

   c. **Increased mortality is observed in infants <1000 g treated by phototherapy.** Use less intensive levels of irradiance in these infants.

   d. **Infants <35 weeks. Special blue fluorescent lamps or light-emitting diode (LED) systems** that will deliver irradiance predominately in the 430–490-nm band are recommended. Fluorescent and LED light sources can be brought closer to the infant than halogen or tungsten lamps (burn risk).

   e. Discontinue phototherapy when TSB is 1–2 mg/dL below the initiation level for the infant's postmenstrual age.

  4. **If phototherapy is used, perform the following additional procedures:**

   a. Increase the maintenance infusion of IV fluids by 0.5 mL/kg/h if the infant weighs <1500 g and by 1 mL/kg/h if the infant weighs >1500 g (*controversial*). Excessive fluid administration will not decrease the bilirubin level, but some infants with high bilirubin levels are dehydrated and may need extra fluid. (*Note*: Water supplements to breast-fed infants do not reduce serum bilirubin. If supplementing breast-fed infants, use milk-based formula because it inhibits the enterohepatic circulation of bilirubin and helps decrease the level.) Maintaining adequate hydration and good urine output will help the efficacy of phototherapy because the by-products responsible for the decline in bilirubin are partially excreted in the urine.

   b. **Perform TSB testing every 6–12 hours.**

   c. **Attempt regular feedings if possible, and feed frequently.** Feeding inhibits the enterohepatic form of bilirubin and helps lower the serum bilirubin level. Studies indicate that increasing the frequency of breast-feeding will not have a significant effect on the serum bilirubin level in the first 3 days of life.

   d. **If the TSB rises.** Increase the irradiance or bring the infant closer to the phototherapy lamp or increase the body surface area of the infant exposed to phototherapy (above and below the infant, reflecting material around the incubator).

  5. **Phototherapy can be safely discontinued once serum bilirubin levels have fallen 1–2 mg/dL below the level at which phototherapy was initiated** (*controversial*). **There is no universal standard for discontinuing phototherapy.** Factors to consider when stopping phototherapy are the cause and the age at which it was initiated. A repeat TSB measurement is recommended on all infants within 24 hours of stopping phototherapy. Once phototherapy is stopped, the average bilirubin rebound in infants without hemolytic disease is <1 mg/dL.

  6. **If the TSB continues to rise or does not decrease on phototherapy.** Hemolysis may be present.

  7. **If the infant has an elevated direct bilirubin level and is receiving phototherapy.** Some of these infants may develop bronze baby syndrome. This is not a contraindication to phototherapy.

  8. **Congenital porphyria and use of medications that are photosensitizers.** Contraindications to phototherapy.

B. **Exchange transfusion.** (See Chapter 30.) Exchange transfusions should be performed only by trained personnel in a neonatal intensive care unit. There is considerable ***controversy*** concerning the exact level at which to initiate exchange transfusion.

  1. **Exchange transfusion for infants ≥35 weeks' gestation.** See Figure 100–3. This figure is based on guidelines from the AAP and displays the suggested levels for exchange transfusion (see lines) in jaundiced infants >35 weeks' GA despite phototherapy. When using this figure, follow these guidelines:

   a. Use TSB. Do not subtract direct bilirubin.

b. Risk factors. G6PD deficiency, asphyxia, sepsis, temperature instability, acidosis, isoimmune hemolytic disease, and lethargy that is significant.

c. The first 24 hours. (See dashed lines on Figure 100–3.) **Represent uncertainty** secondary to the wide range of clinical circumstances and a range of responses to phototherapy.

d. Immediate exchange transfusion. Indicated if the infant shows signs of bilirubin encephalopathy (hypertonia, arching, retrocollis, opisthotonos, fever, or high-pitched cry) even if the TSB is falling or if the TSB is 5 mg/dL above these lines in Figure 100–3.

e. Measure serum albumin and calculate bilirubin/albumin (B/A) ratio at which exchange transfusion should be considered. If an exchange transfusion is being considered, the serum albumin should be measured so the B/A ratio can be calculated and used with the TSB levels to help decide whether an exchange transfusion needs to be done. The ratio of B/A correlates with measured unbound bilirubin in newborns, which if elevated can be associated with kernicterus in sick preterm newborns and transient abnormalities in audiometric brainstem response in infants. See Figure 100–3.

2. **Exchange transfusion for infants <35 weeks.** See consensus guidelines in Table 100–1. Recommendations for exchange transfusion are only for those infants whose TSB levels are rising who are on intensive phototherapy to the maximal surface area. Exchange transfusion is recommended for any infant who shows signs of **acute bilirubin encephalopathy** (hypertonia, arching, retrocollis, opisthotonos, high-pitched cry), although these signs rarely occur in very low birthweight infants. Exchange transfusion is recommended at lower levels in those infants with hemolytic disease and at high risk as listed earlier.

C. Drug therapy

1. **Phenobarbital.** Effective in reducing the serum bilirubin level by increasing hepatic glucuronosyltransferase activity and conjugation of bilirubin. Often used to treat Crigler-Najjar type II and Gilbert syndrome. Studies indicate it is effective in reducing bilirubin levels during the first week of life. It is usually not helpful urgently because it takes a few days to become effective. Studies on the long-term effects of phenobarbital are needed. (For dosing, see Chapter 148.)

2. **Metal (tin [Sn] and zinc [Zn]) metalloporphyrins.** SnMP and ZnMP, respectively, decrease in the need for phototherapy in clinical trials. They work by decreasing the production of bilirubin by competitive inhibition of heme oxygenase. SnMP has been extensively studied and found to effectively reduce the need for phototherapy and exchange transfusion. These drugs are not approved by the US Food and Drug Administration, and their long-term safety needs further study.

3. **Albumin.** Given 1 g/kg IV over 2 hours can provide more binding sites for free bilirubin (*controversial*).

4. **IV immunoglobulin.** This has been effective in infants with Rh and ABO hemolytic disease and reduces the need for exchange transfusion in limited studies. Dose is 500 mg–1 g/kg over 2 hours, repeated in 12 hours if necessary. **AAP recommends this in isoimmune hemolytic disease if the TSB is rising despite phototherapy or the TSB is within 2–3 mg/dL of the exchange level.** AAP also suggests its use in other types of Rh hemolytic disease (anti-C and anti-E), even though data are limited. A recent study found that intravenous gamma globulin administration in infants with severe Rh hemolytic disease did not reduce the need for exchange transfusion. *Note:* An increased incidence of NEC has been found in term and late preterm infants with hemolytic disease who have been treated with intravenous immunoglobulin.

D. Breast-fed infants. The AAP does not recommend the interruption of breast-feeding in healthy term newborns with hyperbilirubinemia and encourages continued and frequent breast-feeding. Infants who require phototherapy should continue breast-feeding. They recommend mothers nurse their infants at least 8–12 times per day the first several days. They do not recommend routine supplementation of nondehydrated breast-fed infants with water or sugar water. **Supplementing with water or dextrose water does not lower the bilirubin level.** Different options are available, and the decision regarding which treatment option to use depends on the specific infant, whether phototherapy is indicated, the physician's judgment, and the family circumstances.

1. **If phototherapy is not recommended:**
    a. **Observation and follow serial TSB levels.**
    b. **Continue breast-feeding but supplement with formula,** while following serial TSB levels.
    c. **Interrupt breast-feeding and substitute formula,** while following serial TSB levels.

2. **If phototherapy is recommended:**
    a. **Continue breast-feeding, and administer phototherapy (AAP recommendation).** Supplementation with **expressed breast milk** is indicated if the infant's intake is inadequate, weight loss is excessive, or there is a question of dehydration. Although phototherapy does not reduce the serum bilirubin concentration in breast-fed infants as quickly as it does in formula-fed infants, it is still effective.
    b. **Continue breast-feeding, and administer phototherapy (AAP recommendation).** Supplementation with formula is indicated if the infant's intake is inadequate, weight loss is excessive, or there is a question of dehydration.
    c. **Interrupt breast-feeding temporarily and substitute formula and administer phototherapy (AAP optional recommendation).** This reduces bilirubin levels and improves the efficacy of phototherapy.

E. **Breast-fed infants with persistent jaundice after 2 weeks.** Approximately 30% of healthy term infants have persistent jaundice after 2 weeks of age. Treat as follows:
    1. **Observe.** If the physical examination is normal and pale stools or dark-yellow urine are not present.
    2. **Screen for congenital hypothyroidism.** A rare cause of direct hyperbilirubinemia.
    3. **If jaundice is still present after 3 weeks,** a urine bilirubin and total and direct serum bilirubin should be obtained. If elevated, it suggests direct hyperbilirubinemia (see Chapters 57 and 99).

F. **Follow-up should be provided for all neonates (especially those discharged <72 hours of age) to monitor for bilirubin-related problems.**
    1. **Perform a risk assessment of all infants before discharge.** The AAP recommends 2 clinical options used individually or in combination: the predischarge TSB or TcB and or a thorough evaluation of clinical risk factors. Recent studies state that combining these 2 offers the best estimate for predicting the risk of later hyperbilirubinemia.
        a. **Predischarge measurement of serum TSB or TcB level can then be plotted on the nomogram on Table 100–1.** This predicts subsequent significant hyperbilirubinemia. This table is for risk in well newborns at 36 weeks' GA with birthweight ≥2000 g or 35 weeks' GA with BW >2500 g.
            i. **TSB at discharge in the low-risk zone.** 0% risk of developing a TSB level >95th percentile.
            ii. **TSB at discharge in the low intermediate-risk zone.** 12 % risk of developing a TSB level >95th percentile.
            iii. **TSB at discharge in the high intermediate-risk zone.** 46% risk of developing a TSB level >95%.
            iv. **TSB at discharge in the high-risk zone.** 68% risk of developing a TSB level >95%.
        b. **Risk factors based on AAP recommendations in order of importance.** The greater the number of risk factors present, the greater the risk of significant hyperbilirubinemia. Certain risk factors before discharge were noted to be more

frequently associated with hyperbilirubinemia: breast-feeding, significant jaundice in a previous sibling, GA <38 weeks, and jaundice noted before discharge.

    i. **Decreased risk.** TSB or TcB in low-risk zone, gestational age ≥41 weeks, bottle feeding, black race, discharge after 72 hours.

    ii. **Minor risk factors.** Predischarge TSB or TcB in the high-intermediate risk zone, GA 37–38 weeks, jaundice before discharge, previous sibling with jaundice, macrosomic infant of a diabetic mother, maternal age ≥25 years, and male sex.

    iii. **Major risk factors.** Predischarge TSB or TcB in the high-risk zone, jaundice in the first 24 hours, blood group incompatibility with positive direct antiglobulin test (other known hemolytic disease, elevated ETCOc), GA 35–36 weeks, previous sibling who received phototherapy, cephalohematoma or significant bruising, exclusive breast-feeding (especially if nursing is not going well, with weight loss), east Asian race.

  c. **Key points**

    i. **Some newborns may require 2 follow-up visits, especially if the infant was discharged before 48 hours.** These can be between 24 and 72 hours and 72 and 120 hours.

    ii. **Infant with risk factors for hyperbilirubinemia.** Earlier and more frequent follow-ups are recommended.

    iii. **Infant with elevated risk and follow-up cannot be guaranteed.** May be necessary to delay discharge.

  2. **Follow-up schedules**

    a. **Infant discharged before age 24 hours.** Office follow-up by 72 hours.

    b. **Infant discharged between 24 and 47.9 hours.** Office follow-up by 96 hours.

    c. **Infant discharged between 48 and 72 hours.** Office follow-up by 120 hours.

  3. **Follow-up assessment.** Should include weight, intake, voiding and stooling pattern, and presence of jaundice. Use clinical judgment in deciding whether a TSB should be obtained.

Selected References

American Academy of Pediatrics. Subcommittee on hyperbilirubinemia. Clinical practice guideline: management of hyperbilirubinemia in the newborn infant 35 or more weeks of gestation. *Pediatrics.* 2004;114:297–316.

Bhutani VK; Committee on Fetus and Newborn; American Academy of Pediatrics. Phototherapy to prevent severe neonatal hyperbilirubinemia in a newborn infant 35 or more weeks of gestation. *Pediatrics.* 2011;128:e1046–e1052.

Maisels MJ, Watchko JF, Bhutani VK, Stevenson DK. An approach to the management of hyperbilirubinemia in the preterm infant less than 35 weeks of gestation. *J Perinatol.* 2012;32:660–664.

59 Hyperglycemia

I. **Problem.** The nurse reports an infant has a blood glucose level of 240 mg/dL. The incidence of hyperglycemia is higher in preterm than term infants (60–80% in extremely low birthweight [ELBW] infants). The definition and treatment of hyperglycemia is controversial. Following are some of the definitions used:

A. Whole blood glucose >120–125 mg/dL or a plasma glucose >145–150 mg/dL regardless of gestational or postnatal age or weight

B. Whole blood glucose >125 mg/dL in term and >150 mg/dL in preterm

C. Whole blood glucose >215 mg/dL (operational definition per Edmund Hey)

II. Immediate questions

A. **What is the serum glucose value on laboratory testing?** Bedside glucose testing using reagent strips is widely used for screening. It is best to confirm a serum glucose level from the laboratory before initiating treatment. Whole blood glucose measurements are 10–15% lower than plasma glucose.

B. **Is glucose being spilled in the urine (glucosuria/glycosuria)?** Glucosuria (glycosuria) is not reliable for hyperglycemia since it can occur at normal glucose blood levels. Mild hyperglycemia can also be associated with mild or no glucosuria. A trace amount of glucose in the urine is accepted as normal. If the **urinary glucose level is +1, +2, or greater, the renal threshold has been reached with an increased chance of osmotic diuresis.** Some institutions accept a urinary glucose level of +1 without treating the patient (*controversial*). Some authors suggest that the presence of >1+ glucosuria suggests osmolar changes and should be treated. *Note*: Each 18-mg/dL rise in blood glucose causes an increase in serum osmolarity of 1 mOsm/L.

C. **How much glucose is the patient receiving?** High glucose intake is a common cause of hyperglycemia in a preterm infant. Levels >10–12 mg/kg/min may result in hyperglycemia, and hyperglycemia may occur at lower levels if the infant is stressed. Normal initial maintenance glucose therapy in infants not being fed orally is 6–7 mg/kg/min on day 1 to 8–9 mg/kg/min on days 2 to 7. ELBW infants should be started at 4–6 mg/kg/min (see Chapter 12).

D. **Are there signs of stress?** Stressful situations like surgery may cause hyperglycemia by inducing a stress response (catecholamine mediated).

E. **Does the infant have necrotizing enterocolitis (NEC) or sepsis?** When an infant who has had normal glucose levels develops hyperglycemia and there is no change in IV fluids, or if an infant who is being fed only enterally suddenly develops hyperglycemia, suspect either sepsis or NEC. Hyperglycemia is seen more frequently **in fungal infections** than in bacterial infections. In Candida sepsis, infants may have a high blood sugar for 2–3 days before any other clinical signs appear.

F. **What is the birthweight of the infant?** Low birthweight is the most significant risk factor for hyperglycemia at any gestational age. The incidence is ~2% in infants >2000 g, 45% in infants <1000 g, and 80% in infants <750 g.

G. **Does the infant have any of the high-risk factors for hyperglycemia?** Risk factors include gestational age <37 weeks, postnatal age <72 hours, weight <2500 g (lower birthweight), hypoxia, infection, use of ionotrophs, lipid infusions, high glucose infusion rate, respiratory distress syndrome (RDS), and sepsis. These infants should have frequent monitoring of their blood sugars.

H. **What medications is the infant on?** Steroids (most common), vasoactive drugs, and methylxanthines can cause hyperglycemia.

III. **Differential diagnosis.** Hyperglycemia can cause hyperosmolarity, osmotic diuresis, and subsequent dehydration. Hyperglycemia is very common in ELBW and premature infants and is associated with an increase in mortality, white matter reduction on the magnetic resonance image (MRI) of the brain, intracranial hemorrhage, stage II/III NEC, risk of sepsis (if hyperglycemia occurs in the first few days after birth), retinopathy of prematurity (ROP) in ELBW infants, and developmental delay. Etiologies include excess administration or production, inadequate insulin secretion or insulin resistance, glucose intolerance, and defective glucoregulatory hormone control.

A. Factitious hyperglycemia

1. Blood drawn from an IV line containing glucose or a bolus was given when flushing a line.

2. False bedside hyperglycemia from a glucose meter. Some glucose meters will overestimate the serum glucose in an infant with galactosemia because of the

lack of specificity of the enzyme used by the assay. Always confirm with a serum sample if glucose meter is high.

B. **True hyperglycemia**

1. **Excess glucose administration** has a major role in hyperglycemia. Giving infants more glucose than what they can handle needs to be evaluated first. Incorrect calculation of glucose levels or errors in the formulation of IV fluids may cause hyperglycemia.

2. **Inability to metabolize glucose** may occur with prematurity or secondary to sepsis or stress. Most commonly, a tiny infant on total parenteral nutrition becomes hyperglycemic because of glucose intolerance.

3. **Impaired glucose homeostasis**

   a. **Extremely low birthweight infants (<1000 g).** These infants have greater fluid requirements because of their immature renal function and increased insensible water loss. This often leads to a high volume of fluid and administering too much glucose. They also may have insulin resistance, an immature insulin response, and are unable to stop gluconeogenesis when IV glucose is given.

   b. **Preterm infants/small for gestational age (SGA) infants.** Preterm infants receiving a glucose challenge show variable increases in insulin levels consistent with **insulin resistance**. This resistance may be related to immaturity or downregulation of peripheral receptors. Transient hyperglycemia can also be seen in **SGA infants** from impaired glucose homeostasis.

4. **Sepsis** can cause hyperglycemia. Suspect sepsis in a neonate who had normal glucose levels with no change in the rate or amount of IV glucose. The etiologies can include the stress response, a reduction in the peripheral utilization of glucose, or a decrease in release of insulin. Hyperglycemia is more frequent in fungal than bacterial sepsis in the neonate. Hyperglycemia may be the first sign in neonatal sepsis; in Candida sepsis it can appear 2 to 3 days before other signs.

5. **Hyperosmolar formula.** Ask how the formula was made. An inappropriate dilution can lead to a hyperosmolar formula, which in turn can cause transient neonatal glucose intolerance. Severe dehydration from gastroenteritis can lead to hypernatremia and hyperglycemia.

6. **Lipid infusion.** Infants who receive lipid infusion even with low rates of glucose administration may develop hyperglycemia. Lipids are emulsified in a Dextran solution. The lipid component may also cause a glycemic response and a decrease in peripheral glucose utilization, and may inhibit insulin's effect. One study found that giving lipid infusion increased plasma glucose concentrations by 24% over baseline values.

7. **Stress.** Pain, painful procedures (venipuncture, vascular cutdowns, and others), surgical procedures (during surgery and postoperative), NEC, acute intracerebral bleeding, hypoxia, catecholamine infusions, respiratory distress, and others can all cause hyperglycemia secondary to increased cortisol.

8. **Hypoxia** can cause increased glucose production.

9. **Medications** such as maternal use of diazoxide can cause hyperglycemia in the infant. Drugs used in infants that have been associated with hyperglycemia include caffeine, theophylline (slight increase), steroids (common), vasoactive drugs, and phenytoin. Prostaglandin E_1 has been associated with hyperglycemia in a case report.

10. **Neonatal diabetes mellitus.** It is a rare cause of diabetes and occurs when there is persistent hyperglycemia that lasts more than 2 weeks and requires insulin therapy. Neonatal diabetes occurs in infants <6 months old; it is not an autoimmune disease and is most commonly caused by genetic defects. Molecular analysis of chromosome 6 anomalies and the KCNJ11 and ABCC8 genes can provide a way of differentiating transient from permanent neonatal diabetes. **Infants with neonatal diabetes mellitus can have metabolic acidosis, ketosis, and glycosuria. There are 2 types:**

a. **Transient neonatal diabetes mellitus (TNDM)(50–60% of cases).** A developmental disorder of the production of insulin that resolves. It is primarily a genetic disorder (chromosome 6q24 anomalies and KATP channel defects). Most infants are SGA or have intrauterine growth restriction (IUGR); they present from 2 days to 6 weeks of age with hyperglycemia and require insulin therapy. It persists for more than 2 weeks and usually resolves by 3–4 months. Common findings are hyperglycemia, dehydration, glycosuria, polyuria, progressive wasting, hypoinsulinism, ketosis, metabolic acidosis and absent ketonuria, and normal or transiently low C-peptide levels in urine and serum. There is a positive family history in ~33% of cases. About half of these cases go on to develop insulin-dependent diabetes in adolescence or in adulthood.

b. **Permanent neonatal diabetes mellitus (PND or PNDM).** (Less common than TNDM.) It develops in the neonatal period and does not go into remission. Genetic mutations are common (KCNJ11, ABCC8, and INS genes). It is not associated with IUGR.

c. **Insulin-dependent (type 1) diabetes mellitus.** An autoimmune disease that occurs in children and adolescents.

11. **Idiopathic.** No identifiable cause is found; a diagnosis of exclusion.

IV. **Database**

A. **Physical examination and history.** Is the infant premature, SGA, or IUGR? Determine if there is a family history of diabetes and ask about maternal and infant medications. Infants with hyperglycemia usually have no obvious signs. Look for dehydration, weight loss, and fever. Evaluate for subtle signs of sepsis (eg, temperature instability, changes in peripheral perfusion) or changes in gastric aspirates if the infant is feeding. Look for signs of NEC.

B. **Laboratory studies**

1. **Initial studies**

a. **Serum glucose level.** Confirm any rapid bedside paper-strip test result with a serum glucose level. It is advisable to repeat serum blood glucose before treating.

b. **Urine dipstick testing for glucose.** High levels are a warning sign for osmotic diuresis.

c. **Complete blood count (CBC) with differential.** A screening test for sepsis.

d. **Blood, urine, and spinal cultures.** For sepsis workup if indicated.

e. **Serum electrolytes.** Hyperglycemia may cause osmotic diuresis, which may lead to electrolyte losses and dehydration. Monitor serum electrolyte levels in hyperglycemic patients.

f. **Arterial blood gas.** If concerned about hypoxia. Metabolic acidosis can be seen in sepsis and neonatal diabetes.

2. **Further studies**

a. **Serum ketones** can be positive in neonatal diabetes mellitus. **Ketonuria** can be absent or mild.

b. **Serum insulin level** is low to normal in transient neonatal diabetes mellitus and normal to high in sepsis.

c. **Serum or urine C-peptide levels** are low in transient neonatal diabetes.

d. **Molecular analysis of chromosome 6q24 anomalies and the KCNJ11 and ABCC8 genes** will help to differentiate transient from permanent neonatal diabetes mellitus.

e. **Genetic testing** can identify which types of permanent neonatal diabetes will respond to oral sulfonylurea therapy and which will require insulin.

C. **Imaging and other studies.** None are usually required; however, a **chest radiograph** may be useful in the evaluation of respiratory distress and sepsis and an **abdominal film** for NEC. **Head ultrasound** is recommended in premature infants to rule out a bleed.

V. **Plan.** The standard treatments of hyperglycemia are observation only or decrease the amount of glucose given or give insulin or a combination of glucose restriction and insulin. The most immediate risk is osmotic diuresis due to the glucose load. While treating hyperglycemia, maintain adequate nutrition for optimal postnatal growth because this relates to morbidity. **Cochrane review** states that large randomized trials are necessary to determine whether and how hyperglycemia should be treated. There was no evidence that treating hyperglycemia in very low birthweight (VLBW) infants would decrease mortality or morbidity rates. Recommended treatment is conservative since most cases are transient.

A. **Initial management.** Rule out factitious hyperglycemia. Make sure the infant is not receiving too much glucose. Try decreasing the amount of glucose. **Treat any underlying causes of hyperglycemia** (sepsis, hypoxia, pain, respiratory distress, stopping medications, checking formula dilution, and others).

B. **Excess glucose administration**

1. **Positive urinary glucose level.** The presence of ≥1+ glucosuria may increase the risk of osmolar changes. Decrease the concentration of dextrose in IV fluids or reduce the infusion rate gradually. The rate can be safely decreased by 1–2 mg/kg/min every 2–4 hours. Most infants who are not feeding initially require 5–7 mg/kg/min of glucose to maintain normal glucose levels. Monitor with bedside glucose testing every 4–6 hours, and check for glucose in the urine with each void.

2. **Negative urinary glucose level.** If glucose is being given to increase the caloric intake, it is acceptable to have a higher serum glucose level as long as glucose is not being spilled in the urine. Monitor with bedside glucose testing every 4–6 hours, and check for glucose in the urine with each void.

C. **Inability to metabolize glucose.** Sepsis should always be considered in an infant with hyperglycemia. If the CBC is suspicious or there are clinical signs of sepsis, it is acceptable to treat the infant for 3 days with antibiotics and stop if cultures are negative. Ampicillin and an aminoglycoside are usually given initially (for doses, see Chapter 148). **Treatment of infants unable to metabolize glucose for any reason is described next.**

1. **Decrease the concentration of glucose or the rate of infusion until a normal serum glucose level is present.** Do not use a solution that has a dextrose concentration of <4.7%. Such a solution is hypo-osmolar and could cause hemolysis, with resulting hyperkalemia.

2. **Feed as early if possible.** Either with hyperalimentation or enterally; both are associated with a decreased incidence of hyperglycemia. Even minimal enteral feeds induce insulin secretion. If the clinical situation is severe, feeding may not be possible.

3. **Insulin.** If hyperglycemia persists or if an osmotic diuresis occurs, insulin may be necessary. Levels vary widely on recommendations, but many will treat the infant with insulin if the blood glucose levels are at a level from 180 to 250 mg/dL (some recommend >300 mg/dL). Guidelines are institutional dependent and *controversial*. Insulin administration has been used in premature infants with success and has allowed more energy intake, promotes glucose tolerance, and promotes weight gain in these infants. Mortality (higher incidence of behavioral and neurologic problems at age 2) was higher in very preterm infants with hyperglycemia treated with insulin during the neonatal period. Early insulin therapy offers little clinical benefit in VLBW infants. **Cochrane review** does not support the routine use of insulin to prevent hyperglycemia in VLBW infants. Insulin therapy carries a risk of hypoglycemia. Several regimens are available for insulin dosing:

a. **Bolus infusion.** Insulin 0.05–0.1 U/kg/dose over 15–20 minutes every 4–6 hours PRN. Monitor glucose every 30 to 60 minutes. Consider infusion if bolus does not work after 2 to 3 doses.

b. **Continuous infusion (most common and preferred method).** Insulin loading dose of 0.05–0.1 U/kg/dose IV over 15–20 minutes, then maintenance

0.01–0.1 U/kg/h continuous IV infusion. Adding albumin to the bag to prevent insulin from adhering to the plastic tubing is now considered unnecessary. By flushing the tubing with an adequate amount (>25 mL) of the insulin-containing solution, all sites in the tubing will be saturated satisfactorily before beginning the infusion. Potassium should be added to the solution to limit hypokalemia. Bedside glucose testing must be performed every 30–60 minutes until the glucose is stable.

    c. **Insulin subcutaneously.** 0.1–0.2 U/kg/dose every 6–12 hours. Continuous IV insulin is preferred. Bedside glucose testing must be performed every 60 minutes until the glucose level is stable.

    d. **Early insulin therapy to prevent hyperglycemia.** Not recommended.

    e. **Amino acid and lipid administration.** Provides a substrate for gluconeogenesis and helps stimulate insulin release in infants receiving glucose.

    f. **Potassium and glucose levels need to be monitored when giving insulin therapy.** Insulin can cause hypokalemia and hypoglycemia.

D. **Transient or permanent neonatal diabetes mellitus**

  1. **Give IV or oral fluids** and monitor the urine output, blood pH, and serum electrolyte levels.

  2. **Give insulin** either by constant infusion or subcutaneously (see Section V.C.3). Monitor glucose levels with bedside testing every 4–6 hours. This disease usually resolves in days to months.

  3. **Continuous subcutaneous insulin infusion (CSII)** is used with an insulin pump and has been used in neonates with diabetes with less variability in glucose. Guidelines are lacking because of few cases where it has been used.

  4. **Oral sulfonylurea therapy** may be a useful treatment option for some patients where subcutaneous insulin might be difficult for some caregivers.

  5. **Repeat serum insulin values** to rule out permanent diabetes mellitus. Early genetic testing should be done.

  6. **KCNJ11- and ABCC8-related permanent neonatal diabetes** are responsive to oral sulfonylurea therapy. **GCK- and IPF1-related permanent neonatal diabetes** require insulin therapy.

  7. **Consult a pediatric endocrinologist.**

E. **Medications**

  1. **If the infant is receiving theophylline,** the serum theophylline level should be checked to detect possible toxicity, with resulting hyperglycemia. Other signs of theophylline toxicity include tachycardia, jitteriness, feeding intolerance, and seizures. If the level is high, the dosage must be altered or the drug discontinued.

  2. **With maternal use of diazoxide,** the infant may have tachycardia and hypotension as well as hyperglycemia. Toxicity in the infant is usually self-limited, and only observation is usually necessary.

  3. **Caffeine and phenytoin** should be adjusted or discontinued if possible.

  4. **Steroids.** Prolonged courses and pharmacologic dosing of corticosteroids are being used in some infants with chronic lung disease. When steroid use is deemed necessary, reducing the dose or frequency may limit the hyperglycemic effects.

F. **Hyperosmolarity.** Rehydration is necessary. If hyperglycemia is secondary to a hyperosmolar formula, stop the formula and give detailed instructions on how to make formula using powder or concentrated formula.

60 Hyperkalemia

I. **Problem.** The serum potassium level is 6.5 mEq/L in an extremely low birthweight infant. Normal potassium levels are generally between 3.5 and 5.5 mEq/L. Definitions can vary by weight, but most define hyperkalemia as >6 mEq/L in newborns. Hyperkalemia is common in extremely low birthweight infants. This is the most serious of electrolyte abnormalities because it can cause fatal arrhythmias. If electrocardiogram (ECG) changes relating to hyperkalemia are present, this is an emergency situation. (See Section V.B.)

II. **Immediate questions**

   A. **How was the specimen collected? What is the central serum potassium level? Is it a true level or factitious?** Blood obtained by heelstick or drawn through a tiny needle may yield falsely elevated potassium levels secondary to hemolysis. Clot formation can also cause falsely elevated potassium. The blood should not be obtained from a heparin-coated umbilical catheter (release of benzalkonium from a heparin-coated umbilical catheter can elevate the potassium reading). *Note:* Serum potassium level is 0.4 mEq/L higher than the plasma level.

   B. **Does the ECG show cardiac changes characteristic of hyperkalemia?** This may be the first indication of hyperkalemia. In neonates, serum potassium >6.7 mEq/L is associated with ECG changes. Early cardiac changes include tall, peaked, "tented" T waves, followed by loss or flattened P wave, widening QRS, ST-segment depression, bradycardia, sine wave QRS-T, first-degree atrioventricular block, ventricular tachyarrhythmias, and finally cardiac arrest if the potassium levels continue to increase.

      1. **Serum K 5.5–6.5 mEq/L.** Tall peaked T waves with a narrow base.
      2. **Serum K 6.5–8 mEq/L.** Tall peaked T waves, prolonged PR interval, loss or decreased P wave, amplified R wave, widening of QRS.
      3. **Serum K >8 mEq/L.** Absent P wave, wide bizarre diphasic QRS, progressive QRS widening merging with the T wave, bundle-branch blocks, ventricular fibrillation or asystole.

   C. **How much potassium is the infant receiving?** Normal amounts of potassium given for maintenance are 1–3 mEq/kg/d.

   D. **What are the blood urea nitrogen (BUN) and creatinine levels? What is the urine output and body weight?** Elevated BUN and creatinine suggest renal insufficiency. Another indication of renal failure is decreasing or inadequate urine output with weight gain.

   E. **Is there associated hyponatremia, hypoglycemia, and hypotension?** With low sodium and glucose, high potassium, and hypotension, consider adrenal insufficiency.

   F. **Does the infant have any of the common characteristics of premature newborns prone to hyperkalemia?** These include small for gestational age, female sex, severe respiratory distress syndrome, very low birthweight, requirement of exogenous surfactant, need for inotropic medications, and delayed feeding. Mildly elevated potassium (>5.6 mEq/L) and phosphate levels (>2 mEq/L) within 6 hours of birth may predict the development of hyperkalemia.

III. **Differential diagnosis.** True hyperkalemia can be caused by an increase in potassium intake (usually not a problem if kidneys able to excrete potassium), an increase in potassium release, a decrease or inability in potassium excretion by the kidneys, or by a shift of potassium into the extracellular space or an impaired aldosterone activity causing decreased renal excretion.

   A. **Pseudohyperkalemia is a falsely elevated potassium level (plasma potassium is normal).** It can be due to hemolysis (trauma causes destruction of red blood cells [RBCs] with leakage of potassium) during phlebotomy or heelstick or by drawing the sample proximal to an IV site infusing potassium. If an unspun sample is allowed to sit or if there is a delay in processing (after 2 hours), potassium release from the cells increase. Laboratory error (multiple processing variables) can also be a reason. **Thrombocytosis and leukocytosis** can lead to a false elevation of serum potassium levels because potassium leaks out of an increased number of white blood cells (WBCs) and platelets during clotting. The serum potassium increases by 0.15 mEq/L for every 100,000/mL elevation of the platelet count. Two rare genetic syndromes that can cause pseudohyperkalemia are **familial pseudohyperkalemia** and **hereditary spherocytosis**.

B. **True hyperkalemia**

1. **Common causes of hyperkalemia**

   a. **Increased potassium intake.** From excessive amount in IV fluids, excessive oral supplementation (as in excess KCL supplementation in a bronchopulmonary dysplasia/chronic lung disease infant), or medications containing potassium. Potassium supplements usually are not necessary on the first day of life and often are not necessary until day 3, with the typical requirement of 1–2 mEq/kg/d. This is rare cause because the kidneys usually excrete any excess potassium.

   b. **Pathologic hemolysis of RBCs.** May be secondary to intraventricular hemorrhage, use of a hypotonic glucose solution (<4.7% dextrose), sepsis (most commonly, *Pseudomonas*), intravascular hemolysis, cephalohematoma, bleeding, asphyxia, or Rh incompatibility.

   c. **Tissue necrosis and breakdown.** In certain disease states, such as necrotizing enterocolitis (NEC), tissue necrosis can occur and hyperkalemia may result. Trauma and severe hypothermia can cause rhabdomyolysis.

   d. **Renal failure/insufficiency.** Impaired kidney function can lead to hyperkalemia. Oliguria can cause decreased potassium clearance and hyperkalemia.

   e. **Immaturity-related nonoliguric hyperkalemia (NOHK).** Occurs in up to 50% of extremely low birthweight infants and is defined as a potassium level >6.5 mEq/L in the absence of acute renal failure/acute kidney injury or a serum potassium ≥7 mEq/L during the first 72 hours of life with urinary output ≥1 mL/kg/h. This occurs without potassium intake or oliguria. It can result from a shift of potassium from intracellular to extracellular space, immature renal tubular and glomerular functions, and a decreased response to aldosterone. Hyperkalemia is often associated with hyperglycemia as a result of insulin resistance and intracellular energy failure ("**hyperglycemia-hyperkalemia syndrome**").

   f. **Metabolic acidosis.** Causes potassium to move out of cells, resulting in hyperkalemia. For every 0.1-unit decrease in pH, the serum potassium increases ~0.3–1.3 mEq/L. Respiratory acidosis rarely causes significant hyperkalemia.

   g. **Dehydration.** Causes hyperkalemia. Volume depletion and congestive heart failure can cause renal hypoperfusion and therefore hyperkalemia.

   h. **Medications containing potassium.** May elevate the serum potassium level. Digoxin therapy can lead to hyperkalemia secondary to redistribution of potassium. K^+-sparing diuretics cause decreased potassium losses. Both propranolol and phenylephrine are associated with hyperkalemia. High glucose load can lead to hyperkalemia secondary to increases in plasma osmolality. Other medications, including tromethamine, indomethacin, angiotensin-converting enzyme inhibitors, β-blockers, heparin, trimethoprim, captopril, and nonsteroidal anti-inflammatory drugs are associated with hyperkalemia.

   i. **Adrenal insufficiency.** Seen **in congenital adrenal hyperplasia and bilateral adrenal hemorrhage.** In salt-losing congenital adrenal hyperplasia, infants have low serum sodium, chloride, and glucose; elevated levels of potassium; and hypotension. In bilateral adrenal hemorrhage, anemia, thrombocytopenia, and jaundice are seen, and bilateral adrenal masses are palpable.

Renal tubular hyperkalemia/hyperkalemic distal renal tubular acidosis type IV occurs secondary to hypoaldosteronism. Infants present with metabolic acidosis and hyperkalemia. It is seen in adrenal disorders (hypoaldosteronism, congenital adrenal hyperplasia) and obstructive uropathy, reduced renal mass, renal reflux, urinary tract infection, and pseudohypoaldosteronism.

j. **Decreased insulin levels.** Associated with hyperkalemia. Insulin drives potassium into cells; insulin deficiency can cause hyperkalemia.

k. **Transfusion-induced hyperkalemia.** Irradiation accelerates the leakage of potassium out of stored RBCs, which can induce the risk of transfusion-induced arrhythmias from hyperkalemia. Washing of irradiated RBCs reduces potassium and lactate loads. Exchange transfusion can also be a cause.

l. **Hyperosmolality.** Caused by inappropriately diluted formula/hyperosmolar amino acid solution/glucose infusions.

2. **Less common causes**

a. **Neonatal Bartter syndrome (a variant of this with *ROMK* mutation presents with early hyperkalemia).** It is a group of renal tubular disorders usually characterized by hypokalemic metabolic alkalosis.

b. **Hereditary hyperkalemic disorders.** Hereditary pseudohyperkalemia, hereditary hyperkalemic periodic paralysis, various types of hypoaldosteronism, hereditary tubular defects that cause hyperkalemia.

c. **Disorders that cause decreased renal excretion of potassium.** Addison disease, mineralocorticoid deficiency, primary hypoaldosteronism, aldosterone synthase deficiency, and pseudohypoaldosteronism.

IV. **Database**

A. **Physical examination.** The infant may exhibit no signs or can have bradycardia, ventricular fibrillation or other arrhythmias, or shock. Pay special attention to the abdomen for signs of NEC (ie, abdominal distention, decreased bowel sounds, and visible bowel loops). Evaluate for signs of underlying diseases. It is difficult to state an exact number when clinical signs will appear, but most agree when the serum potassium increases to >7 mEq/L. Signs can be polyuria, abdominal distention, lethargy. Muscle weakness occurs if >8 mEq/L but is hard to evaluate in a newborn. Tendon reflexes can be decreased.

B. **Laboratory studies**

1. **Immediate tests**

a. **Serum potassium level measured by a properly collected venous sample.** A repeat serum potassium level is usually recommended before treatment.

b. **Serum and urine electrolytes.**

c. **Complete blood count and differential.** To rule out sepsis and hemolysis.

d. **Serum ionized and total calcium levels.** Hypocalcemia may potentiate the effects of hyperkalemia. Maintain normal serum calcium concentrations.

e. **Serum pH and bicarbonate.** To rule out acidosis, which may potentiate hyperkalemia.

f. **BUN and serum creatinine levels.** May reveal renal insufficiency.

g. **Urine dipstick and specific gravity.** To assess renal status and blood and hemoglobin for tissue breakdown secondary to hemolysis. Examine for casts or sediment.

2. **Further testing**

a. **Serum cortisol, 17-OH progesterone 11B-hydroxylase, 21-hydroxylase levels** for congenital adrenal hyperplasia.

b. **Serum renin, angiotensin, and aldosterone** for hypoaldosteronism.

C. **Imaging and other studies**

1. **Abdominal radiograph** if NEC is suspected.

2. **ECG** may reveal the cardiac changes characteristic of hyperkalemia and provides a baseline study (see Section II.B).

V. Plan. First, confirm the potassium level through a repeat STAT serum sample. **Document any ECG changes, and if present, this is a medical emergency and needs to be treated immediately (see later).**

A. **Important considerations**

1. **Stop all potassium intake.** IV fluids, oral supplements, potassium-containing medications.

2. **Check the calculation of potassium in the IV fluids.** Verify that excess potassium was not given.

3. **Correct hypovolemia using isotonic saline.** To promote tubular secretion of potassium.

4. **Treat the specific cause. Renal failure** can be treated with fluid restriction. If **adrenal insufficiency** exists, replacement therapy is indicated.

5. **Monitor ECG changes during therapy.**

6. **Preterm infants.** The combination of insulin and glucose as a treatment has more immediate results and is preferred over the treatment with Kayexalate.

7. *Remember:* Calcium prevents cardiac arrhythmias by stabilizing the cell membrane of the myocardium; it does nothing to the serum potassium. **Insulin and glucose, albuterol, and sodium bicarbonate** decrease the serum potassium level by moving potassium into cells, which reduces the risk of immediate complications but does not remove potassium from the body. **Furosemide, sodium polystyrene (Kayexalate), and dialysis (exchange transfusion, peritoneal dialysis)** remove potassium from the body by renal excretion, gastrointestinal loss, or removal by dialysis.

B. **Hyperkalemia with ECG changes.** Arrhythmia from hyperkalemia is difficult to treat. The usual steps of defibrillation, epinephrine, or even antiarrhythmic drugs will not work without lowering the potassium level. *Note:* Calcium only protects the myocardium and does not decrease the serum potassium. First, give calcium to protect the heart, and then give medications to lower serum potassium levels but not total body stores, and then give medications to cause potassium excretion and lower total body stores.

1. **Stop administration of potassium in IV fluids.** Consider stopping any potassium-containing medications or medications known to induce hyperkalemia (see Section III.H).

2. **Protect the heart from the toxic effects of potassium with calcium (does not lower potassium).** It stabilizes the myocardium and lowers the threshold potential to protect against arrhythmias. Administer slow IV infusion over 10 minutes, optimally through a central line, not a scalp IV. Observe the ECG while infusing the medication. **Improvement in the ECG should occur within 1–5 minutes.** Once the arrhythmia or ECG changes disappear, the bolus can be stopped. This only decreases myocardial excitability. It is necessary to give a medication immediately that will begin to decrease potassium. If the infant is on digoxin therapy, remember that calcium therapy can worsen digoxin toxicity and a slower infusion may be necessary. **Calcium gluconate 10% (100–200 mg/kg/dose) IV diluted in appropriate fluid and given over 10–30 minutes can be used.**

3. **Start a medication to reduce serum potassium levels.** Sodium bicarbonate, glucose and insulin, and β-adrenergic agonists cause cellular intake of potassium. Sodium bicarbonate has an immediate onset; glucose, insulin, and albuterol take a minimum of 15 minutes to work. Deciding which one to use depends on your unit's preference. **For premature infants,** most agree that **insulin and glucose** is the first-line therapy. **One recommendation** is to give sodium bicarbonate or insulin and glucose or albuterol until the potassium is down, then give either Lasix or Kayexalate.

a. **Sodium bicarbonate can be used even when blood pH is normal** (*controversial*). Use debated and not recommended as monotherapy or with caution in premature infants. Cochrane review stated that results are equivocal (buffers acid by raising pH). Some suggest using only in life-threatening hyperkalemia or not at all. Correct the base deficit by using the following formula:

$$NaHCO_3 \text{ (mEq)} = 0.3 \times \text{weight (kg)} \times \text{base deficit (mEq/L)}$$

Or give 1–2 mEq/kg over 10–30 minutes intravenously (works in 5–10 minutes). Inducing alkalosis drives potassium ions into the cells. In very tiny infants, sodium bicarbonate may have associated risks. Avoid rapid infusion of sodium bicarbonate to decrease the risk of intraventricular hemorrhage. If the infant is intubated, hyperventilation can cause respiratory alkalosis (0.1-unit pH increase causes a 0.6-mEq/L decrease in serum K). This may decrease cerebral perfusion.

    b. Insulin and glucose. Insulin drives potassium into the cells. Insulin must be given with glucose to avoid hypoglycemia. The usual dose is 0.1–0.2 U/kg/h insulin in combination with a continuous infusion of 0.5 g/kg/h of dextrose. Adjust infusion rates based on serum glucose and potassium concentrations. Time to onset 15–30 minutes. Monitor the glucose levels.

    c. β-Adrenergic agonists (*controversial*). Drive potassium into the cell. They have a rapid onset of action. The most commonly used medication is albuterol nebulized 0.1–0.5 mg/kg/dose (minimum dose 2.5 mg) every 2–6 hours as needed. Nebulized albuterol is effective in premature neonates.

C. Hyperkalemia without ECG changes. Treatment is recommended when serum potassium is >6–6.5 mEq/L (*controversial*). Deciding which medication to use is dependent on your institution.

    1. Stop administration of potassium in IV fluids. Consider stopping any potassium-containing medications or medications known to induce hyperkalemia (see Section III.H).

    2. Cardiac monitoring with frequent ECGs.

    3. Check the serum potassium frequently (ie, every 1–2 hours) until stable.

    4. Furosemide (Lasix). Enhances potassium excretion in the urine and can be given if **renal function is adequate**; the usual dose is 1 mg/kg IV every 12 hours (*controversial*). It takes 5–10 minutes to work. Value is limited in renal failure, with higher doses required. Useful in hyperkalemia associated with congestive heart failure and hypoaldosteronism .

    5. Inhaled albuterol (*controversial*). See Section V.B.3c.

    6. Sodium polystyrene sulfonate (Kayexalate), a potassium-exchange resin, can be given. It removes potassium from the gut (1 g of resin removes ~1 mEq of potassium) in exchange for sodium. (Sorbitol free is recommended in neonates as sorbitol can cause bowel necrosis and sodium retention.) The usual dose is 1 g/kg/dose orally every 6 hours or rectally every 2–6 hours. Rectal route is preferred as it has faster onset of 1–2 hours (not effective by 4 hours in a Cochrane review). Administered orally, it lowers the potassium level slowly and therefore is of limited value acutely. **This therapy should not be used in extremely low birthweight infants because of risk of irritation, concretions, hemorrhagic colitis, gastrointestinal hemorrhage, colonic necrosis, sodium overload, and NEC.** This treatment can cause an increase in sodium and calcium. Repetitive rectal use can cause local bleeding. Do not use with obstructive bowel disease and infants with decreased gut motility (risk of intestinal necrosis).

D. Persistent hyperkalemia. Continuous infusion of insulin with glucose is recommended. Infants with chronic kidney disease may require low potassium diet, alkali treatment, exchange resins, and peritoneal dialysis.

E. Refractory hyperkalemia. If all of these measures fail to lower the potassium level, other measures, such as **exchange transfusion** with freshly washed packed RBCs reconstituted with plasma or **peritoneal dialysis,** must be considered. These methods work immediately and are very effective but are limited by the time and complexity involved. If hyperkalemia is secondary to cell breakdown, exchange transfusion is preferred.

F. Treatment and prevention of nonoliguric hyperkalemia of extremely low birthweight infants. Potassium should not be administered in the first days of life until good urinary output is established and serum potassium is normal and not rising.

Potassium levels should be monitored every 6 hours in the first few days of life. Early administration of amino acids (first day of life) may stimulate endogenous insulin secretions and prevent the need for insulin infusion. Continuous insulin IV infusion may be necessary. Cochrane review has no recommendations for treatment of hyperkalemia in nonoliguric hyperkalemia in preterm infant, except that **insulin and glucose is preferred over Kayexalate.**

Selected Reference

Vemgal P, Ohlsson A. Interventions for non-oliguric hyperkalaemia in preterm neonates. *Cochrane Database Syst Rev.* 2012;CD005257.

61 Hypertension

I. **Problem.** An infant has a systolic blood pressure (BP) of >95 mm Hg. Normal blood pressure values depend on the infant's gestational age, postnatal age, and birthweight. **Hypertension is commonly defined as a BP >2 standard deviations above normal** values for age and weight, but other definitions exist. The Task Force on Blood Pressure Control in Children defines hypertension as 95% percentile or above on 3 separate occasions. For a rapid reference of blood pressure ranges for premature and term infants see Table 65–1, page 446. For estimated BP levels at the 95th and 99th percentiles in infants after 2 weeks of age see Table 61–1. For other detailed BP values see Appendix C. Normal blood pressure increases with birthweight, gestational age, and postconceptional age.

II. **Immediate questions**

A. **How was the BP taken?** Verify that the BP reading is correct and the hypertension is real. As the first reading is usually the highest, it is best to take 2–3 confirmatory measurements. BP rises when the infant is feeding, sucking, or in an upright position. BP is lower in the prone versus supine position. Measure when the infant is calm. Most BP data is from measurements taken from the right arm.

   1. **Blood pressure cuff size** is important; it should encircle two-thirds of the length of the upper extremity. If the cuff is too narrow, the BP will be falsely elevated. **The American Academy of Pediatrics (AAP) recommendations for BP cuff bladder width are as follows:** newborn—4 cm; infant—6 cm. **For length:** newborn—8 cm; infant—12 cm. Maximum arm circumference: newborn—10 cm; infant—15 cm.

   2. **BP reading from an indwelling catheter** (radial or umbilical artery) is the most accurate (gold standard) of all methods. If measurements are taken by means of an umbilical artery catheter (UAC), be certain that the catheter is free of bubbles or clots and the transducer is calibrated; otherwise, erroneous results will occur.

   3. **Automated oscillometric devices** (electronic pressure sensor), common in the neonatal intensive care unit (NICU), can give lower pressures than intra-arterial catheters.

   4. **BP protocols** have been established to standardize blood pressure measurement in infants. One suggested by Nwankwo is to measure BP 1.5 hours after feeding or medical intervention, with the infant asleep or in a quiet state and lying prone or supine. Place an appropriate-sized cuff on the right upper arm, and let the infant rest undisturbed after cuff placement for 15 minutes. Measure by oscillometric device, and do 3 successive BP readings at 2-minute intervals.

Table 61–1. ESTIMATED BLOOD PRESSURE LEVELS AT THE 95TH AND 99TH PERCENTILES IN
INFANTS AFTER 2 WEEKS OF AGE

	Postconceptional Age in Weeks									
	26	28	30	32	34	36	38	40	42	44
95th percentile (systolic/ diastolic)	72/50	75/50	80/55	83/55	85/55	87/65	92/65	95/65	98/65	105/68
99th percentile (systolic/ diastolic)	77/56	80/54	85/60	88/60	90/60	92/70	97/70	100/70	102/70	110/73

Data from Dionne JM, Abitbol CL, Flynn JT. Hypertension in infancy: diagnosis, management and
outcome. *Pediatr Nephrol.* 2012;27(1):17–32. Epub 2011 Jan 22. Review. Erratum in: *Pediatr Nephrol.*
2012;27(1):159–160.

5. The AAP does not recommend universal screening but states it is important to screen blood pressure in those infants in whom coarctation of the aorta or renal disease is suspected.

B. **Is an umbilical artery catheter in place, or has one been in place in the past?** Incidence of hypertension is ~ 9% with a UAC. Umbilical artery catheters are associated with an increased incidence of renovascular hypertension. The hypertension is probably related to the thrombus formation at the time of line placement. The following conditions are risk factors for thrombus formation in the aorta: bronchopulmonary dysplasia/chronic lung disease (BPD/CLD), patent ductus arteriosus, hypervolemia, and certain central nervous system (CNS) disorders. Improved catheters and the use of heparin have helped decrease the incidence of thrombus formation. Hypertension appears with equal frequency in high versus low catheters.

C. **Are signs of hypertension present?** Infants with hypertension may be asymptomatic or manifest the following: irritability, tachypnea, cyanosis, seizures, lethargy, increased tone, apnea, abdominal distention, fever, and mottling. They may also have congestive heart failure (CHF), failure to thrive, GI problems, and respiratory distress.

D. **What is the BP in the extremities?** The BP in a healthy infant should be higher in the legs than in the arms. If the pressure is lower in the legs, **coarctation of the aorta** may be the cause of the hypertension. Coarctation of the aorta is the most common heart malformation that causes hypertension in a neonate.

E. **What is the birthweight, gestational age, and postnatal age of the infant?** Normal BP values increase with increasing birthweight, gestational age, and postconceptional age. Values rise ~1–2 mm Hg/d during the first week of life and then ~1–2 mm Hg/wk over the next 6 weeks.

F. **Is the infant in pain or agitated?** Pain from an invasive procedure, crying, agitation, or suctioning can cause a transient rise in BP. The systolic pressure can be 5 mm Hg lower in sleeping infants.

G. **Does the infant have BPD/CLD or an intraventricular hemorrhage?** Infants with BPD/CLD have a significant problem with hypertension (6% up to 40%). It often occurs after discharge from the nursery. Infants with an intraventricular hemorrhage (3% incidence) also have an increased risk of hypertension.

H. **Does the infant have any risk factors that would be associated with the development of hypertension?** Chronic lung disease, respiratory distress syndrome (RDS), prematurity, extremely low birthweight (ELBW), UAC placement, maternal hypertension, antenatal steroids, acute renal failure (acute kidney injury) in the postnatal period, and treatment with indomethacin are all associated with the development of hypertension in a neonate.

I. **Were recent boluses of fluids or blood products given?** Fluid overload is a common iatrogenic cause of hypertension, especially in infants with decreased urine output.

J. **Was there maternal drug use (cocaine or heroin)?** Maternal drug use of cocaine and heroin has been associated with hypertension in their newborn infants.

III. **Differential diagnosis.** Hypertension is rare in the healthy term newborn infant. The incidence is from 0.2–3% (healthy newborn) to 40% (in infants with chronic lung disease). **Hypertension in newborns is primarily of renal origin** (renovascular and renal parenchymal diseases). **BPD/CLD is the most common nonrenal cause.**

A. **Common causes of hypertension.** See Table 61–2 for comprehensive list.

1. **Renal causes/vascular causes**

a. **Renal artery stenosis.** The infant is hypertensive from birth. This accounts for 20% of the cases of hypertension in infants. It can be secondary to fibromuscular dysplasia. Congenital rubella infection can cause arterial calcification and renal artery stenosis.

b. **Renal artery thrombosis.** Most commonly related to **umbilical artery catheterization**, this is a relatively common cause of hypertension. The thrombi embolize to the kidneys causing infarction and increased release of renin.

c. **Renal vein thrombosis.** Seen in hypovolemic or asphyxiated infants, infants of diabetic mothers, and infants with coagulopathies. Signs are hypertension, gross hematuria, thrombocytopenia, and a flank mass.

d. **Renal failure.** Postnatal acute renal failure (acute kidney injury) is associated with hypertension. Acute tubular necrosis (ATN) secondary to perinatal asphyxia or sepsis is a common cause.

e. **Congenital renal disease.** Autosomal dominant or autosomal recessive polycystic kidney disease can present in the neonate with hypertension and enlarged kidneys. **Ureteropelvic junction obstruction** can activate the renin-angiotensin system and cause hypertension.

2. **Bronchopulmonary dysplasia/chronic lung disease (BPD/CLD) is the most common cause of nonrenal hypertension in the neonate.** Approximately 13–43% of patients with BPD/CLD have hypertension. The origin is unclear but is probably multifactorial (increased renin activity and catecholamine secretion and chronic hypoxemia may be associated with chronic lung disease). **The majority of these infants develop hypertension after being discharged from the hospital.**

3. **Coarctation of the aorta.** A common cause of hypertension in newborns. Occurs with an increased incidence in Turner syndrome.

4. **Neurologic.** Increased intracranial pressure and seizures can cause episodic hypertension. Intraventricular hemorrhage can cause increased intracranial pressure.

5. **Medications.** Such as corticosteroids (antenatal and postnatal), theophylline, caffeine, adrenergic agents, and ocular phenylephrine. Maternal use of cocaine can cause damage to the kidneys. **Drug withdrawal** from heroin can cause hypertension.

6. **Fluid/electrolyte overload.**

7. **Pain or agitation.** This usually causes episodic hypertension.

8. **Other.** Extracorporeal membrane oxygenation/extracorporeal life support (ECMO/ECLS) (up to 50% of infants), abdominal surgery (closure of an abdominal wall defect).

IV. **Database**

A. **History.** Evaluate maternal factors: Was cocaine or heroin used during pregnancy, or were antenatal steroids used? Does the infant have a predisposing illness that would account for the hypertension, eg, BPD/CLD, CNS disorder, PDA? Evaluate the current medication list, and determine if the infant has a UAC?

B. **Physical examination.** In most infants, hypertension is discovered on vital signs with no overt signs. **Life-threatening presentations** can include congestive heart

Table 61–2. **CAUSES OF HYPERTENSION IN NEWBORNS**

Cardiac	Coarctation of the aorta (thoracic), aortic arch interruption, hypoplastic aorta
Drugs: infant	Glucocorticoids (dexamethasone), theophylline, caffeine, vitamin D intoxication, indomethacin, pancuronium (prolonged use), high dose of adrenergic agents, phenylephrine eye drops, doxapram, opiate withdrawal
Drugs: maternal	Cocaine (may harm neonatal kidney and cause withdrawal) and heroin (causes withdrawal), antenatal steroid administration (***controversial***)
Endocrine	Adrenal hemorrhage/hematoma, adrenogenital syndrome, congenital adrenal hyperplasia, Cushing syndrome, primary hyperaldosteronism, hyperthyroidism/Graves disease, pseudohyperaldosteronism type II, familial hyperaldosteronism type II, Gordon syndrome
Metabolic	Hypercalcemia
Neurologic	Elevated intracranial pressure secondary to intracranial hemorrhage, hydrocephalus, meningitis or subdural hemorrhage/hematoma, seizures, subdural hematoma, familial dysautonomia, drug withdrawal (opiate), neural crest tumor, cerebral angioma
Pain/agitation	Usually causes episodic hypertension
Pulmonary	BPD/CLD, pneumothorax (rare)
Renal parenchymal diseases (acquired)	Acute tubular necrosis, cortical and medullary necrosis, interstitial nephritis, hemolytic uremic syndrome, nephrolithiasis/nephrocalcinosis, obstructive uropathy (eg, tumor or stones), pyelonephritis, glomerulonephritis, perirenal hematoma or urinoma, renal failure/renal insufficiency, renal infection
Renal parenchymal diseases (congenital)	Polycystic kidney disease (autosomal recessive or dominant), multicystic-dysplastic kidney disease, hypoplastic/dysplastic kidney, congenital nephrotic syndrome, unilateral renal hypoplasia, tuberous sclerosis, renal tubular dysgenesis, obstructive uropathy (posterior urethral valves, ureteropelvic junction obstruction), congenital mesoblastic nephroma
Renovascular/vascular	Renal artery thrombosis (UAC related), renal artery stenosis, renal vein thrombosis, mid aortic syndrome (abdominal coarctation), congenital rubella syndrome (causes arterial calcification), idiopathic arterial calcification, renal artery compression, hypoplastic aorta, abdominal aorta aneurysm, aortic thrombosis, thrombosis of the ductus arteriosus, intimal hyperplasia, mechanical compression of one or both arteries (abdominal mass or tumor)
Syndromes/malformation syndromes	Noonan, Williams, Turner, Liddle (glucocorticoid remediable aldosteronism), and Cockayne syndromes; neurofibromatosis; tuberous sclerosis complex
Tumors (compression of renal vessels or produce vasoactive substances)	Wilms tumor, mesoblastic nephroma, neuroblastoma, nephroblastoma, pheochromocytoma
Miscellaneous	Birth asphyxia, closure of abdominal wall defects (eg, omphalocele or gastroschisis), abdominal surgery, ECMO/ECLS, essential hypertension, iatrogenic (volume overload secondary to excess administration of sodium or IV fluids), idiopathic, total parenteral nutrition (TPN) related, infantile polyarteritis nodosa, maternal hypertension, environmental cold or noise stress

failure with cardiogenic shock or seizures or few or no signs. Some infants present with apnea, feeding difficulties, failure to thrive, irritability, lethargy, unexplained tachypnea, and mottling of the skin. Check for tachycardia and flushing for hyperthyroidism.

1. **Check the femoral pulse in both legs,** which are absent or decreased in coarctation of the aorta. Check blood pressure in all 4 extremities (blood pressure discrepancies between the upper and lower extremities, arterial hypertension in the upper extremities with normal to low blood pressure in the lower extremities).
2. **Are there any dysmorphic features** that would indicate a genetic syndrome that would explain the hypertension? Consider Turner, Noonan, Williams, or Liddle syndrome.
3. **Do a complete cardiac examination** to rule out congestive heart failure. Is there a heart murmur? Is there cyanosis? Is there tachycardia? Is there mottling and signs of vasomotor instability?
4. **Respiratory.** Is there tachypnea or cyanosis?
5. **Examine the abdomen** for masses and to determine the size of the kidneys. Is there abdominal distension? An enlarged kidney or flank mass may indicate tumor, polycystic kidneys, obstruction, or renal vein thrombosis. An epigastric bruit can indicate renal artery stenosis.
6. **Examine the genitalia** to rule out congenital adrenal hyperplasia.
7. **Neurologic signs** may include apnea, lethargy, tremors, seizures, asymmetric reflexes, or hypertonicity.

C. **Laboratory studies.** Few tests are usually needed and should be dictated by history and physical examination. **Basic tests should include CBC and platelet count, serum electrolytes, and serum calcium.** Abnormal sodium and potassium suggests endocrine causes. Elevated white blood cell count can be seen in pyelonephritis. High calcium validates hypercalcemia. Assessment of renal function is important and is as follows:

1. **Assessment of renal function** with the following:
   a. **Serum creatinine and BUN.** Elevation suggests renal insufficiency, which may be associated with hypertension.
   b. **Urinalysis.** Red blood cells in the urine suggests obstruction, infection, or renal vein thrombosis.
   c. **Urine culture.** To evaluate for urinary tract infection (UTI) including pyelonephritis.
   d. **Serum electrolytes and carbon dioxide.** A low serum potassium level and a high carbon dioxide level suggest primary hyperaldosteronism.
   e. **Urine protein/creatinine ratio, urine albumin/creatinine ratio.** To evaluate significant proteinuria and renal parenchymal disease.
2. **Other useful tests in selected infants**
   a. **Plasma renin levels (plasma renin activity [PRA])** may be elevated in patients with renovascular disease. Levels will be low in primary hyperaldosteronism. Rarely elevated in normal infants, PRA can be falsely elevated because of medications such as aminophylline. Direct renin assay has been used, but normal neonatal values are not readily available.
   b. **Thyroid studies (thyroid-stimulating hormone [TSH], free T_4)** to rule out hyperthyroidism.
   c. **Serum cortisol.**
   d. **Serum aldosterone.**
   e. **Urine vanillylmandelic acid (VMA)/homovanillic acid (HVA).** Twenty-four-hour urinary catecholamines to evaluate for pheochromocytoma or neuroblastoma.
   f. **Urinary 17-hydroxysteroid and 17-ketosteroid levels** to evaluate for Cushing syndrome and congenital adrenal hyperplasia.
   g. **Urine toxicology screen.**
   h. **Coagulation panel.**

D. Imaging and other studies
  1. **Chest radiograph.** May help in those infants with congestive heart failure and those with a murmur. Cardiomegaly can be seen.
  2. **Renal/abdominal ultrasonography. Preferred screening test in neonates** and should be done in all hypertensive infants to detect abdominal masses, assess adrenals, and check for renal vein thrombosis as well as kidney obstruction. **Color Doppler flow ultrasonography** can be used to screen for arterial or venous problems (thrombosis). Infants who had a UAC should have their aorta and renal arteries studied for thrombi.
  3. **Cranial ultrasonography.** To rule out intraventricular hemorrhage.
  4. **Echocardiography.** If a disease such as coarctation is suspected or to evaluate end-organ damage caused by hypertension (eg, left ventricular hypertrophy or decreased contractility).
  5. **Further studies.** The following procedures and studies are sometimes necessary to further evaluate the infant with hypertension:
      a. **Angiography** to evaluate renovascular disease, or **venacavography** to evaluate renal vein thrombosis. This is most commonly done through the umbilical artery catheter. **Renal angiography/scan** helps quantitate the function of each kidney. **Magnetic resonance angiography (MRA) is the gold standard for renal vascular hypertension** and is recommended in infants >3 kg.
      b. **Abdominal CT scan** if needed to obtain more specific anatomic information on an abdominal mass.
      c. **Voiding cystourethrography** if urinary tract pathology is possible.
      d. **Radionuclide imaging (nuclear scan)** can show renal perfusion abnormalities. It can also show decreased renal blood flow and increased isotope concentration in the abnormal kidney. A **dimercaptosuccinic acid (DMSA) renal scan** can rule out arterial infarctions.
      e. **Renal biopsy** to rule out any intrinsic renal disease.

V. Plan
  A. **General.** First treat any obvious or correctable underlying cause of hypertension. Stop medications or adjust inotropic infusions if they are causing hypertension. Correct fluid overload by decreasing fluids and administering diuretics. Always check volume status and restrict sodium and fluid intake. Administer pain medications if necessary. Remove UAC if possible. Treat hypercalcemia. Hormone replacement should be started in those infants with endocrine disorders. Consultation with a pediatric cardiologist is recommended.
  B. **Drug therapy.** (See Chapter 148.) To guide drug therapy, determine whether the hypertension is **mild, moderate, or life threatening. Note that treatment thresholds are unclear, and many of the recommendations are *controversial.*** More studies are necessary to establish guidelines in preterm infants. Many infants will require more than one medication. **Some experts believe that any asymptomatic infant with hypertension with no end-organ involvement should only be observed.**
  1. **Life-threatening hypertension.** See Table 61–1. If BP is extremely high (>99th percentile) this is considered a hypertensive crisis with or without signs (CHF, cardiogenic shock, seizures). Avoid too rapid of a decrease in the BP, as this may cause cerebral ischemia and hemorrhage. Monitor the BP every 10 minutes. The medications chosen depend on your institutional guidelines. **With life-threatening hypertension, continuous intravenous infusions are preferred, as these can be titrated, and the BP should begin to fall within 15 minutes to an hour.**
      a. **Nicardipine.** A calcium channel blocker, it is often considered a **drug of choice** because of its advantages and few side effects (reflex tachycardia). Initial dose is 0.5 mcg/kg/min constant IV infusion (see also Chapter 148).
      b. **Labetalol.** An α- and β-blocker. Relative contraindications are heart failure and BPD/CLD. Dose is 0.4–1 mg/kg/h IV infusion (3 mg/kg/h maximum).

    c. **Esmolol.** A short-acting β-blocker. Dose is 50 mcg/kg/min, increased by 25–50 mcg/kg/min every 5 minutes until target blood pressure reached (200 mcg/kg/min maximum).

    d. **Sodium nitroprusside.** A vasodilator. It is difficult to use but has a very short half-life, so its effect can be quickly reversed. Dose is 0.25–0.5 mcg/kg/min IV infusion. Titrate every 20 minutes to the desired response. Use for >72 hours or in infants with renal failure. It can cause thiocyanate toxicity. Usual dose is 3 mcg/kg/min; rarely >4 mcg/kg/min. Maximum is 8–10 mcg/kg/min.

    e. **Fenoldopam mesylate.** A new selective dopamine 1 receptor agonist. Widely studied in children over 5 kg and up to 12 years, it has been used for inadequate urine output after neonatal cardiopulmonary bypass.

2. **Moderate hypertension.** See dosing in Chapter 148.

    a. Begin diuretics first such as furosemide, hydrochlorothiazide, or chlorothiazide.

    b. Add a second-line drug (eg, hydralazine or propranolol) if necessary. Choice of drug depends on your institution; propranolol is the most extensively used β-blocker and has a low risk of side effects.

    c. If a third drug is needed with propranolol. Hydralazine can be added.

    d. Give captopril alone or with a diuretic. This drug is contraindicated in infants with bilateral renovascular disease. Angiotensin-converting enzyme (ACE) inhibitors also may result in hypotensive events at initiation of therapy and after long-term use. Oliguria and some neurologic complications have been reported after captopril use; therefore, use cautiously.

3. **Mild hypertension.** Usually managed by observation (recommended) or oral medications. **Simple observation** is best for asymptomatic patients with no readily identifiable cause and is supported in recent reviews. If needed, **diuretics** (such as chlorothiazide or hydrochlorothiazide) are preferred over furosemide because of fewer electrolyte disturbances. They work well in cases of volume overload but may cause hypotension when used with other agents. Spironolactone is a potassium-sparing diuretic that can also be considered.

4. **Patients with mild to moderate hypertension who cannot tolerate oral therapy because of gastrointestinal (GI) problems.** These are good candidates for **IV bolus** or intermittently administered IV agents:

    a. **Diuretics** such as IV furosemide. Monitor electrolytes.

    b. **Hydralazine** (vasodilator) dose is 0.1–0.5 mg/kg/dose IV bolus every 6–8 hours (2 mg/kg/dose maximum). Side effects include tachycardia.

    c. **Labetalol** dose is 0.2–0.5 mg/kg/dose over 2–3 minutes IV intermittent bolus. Range: 0.2–1.0 mg/kg/dose, maximum 20 mg/dose. Side effects include heart failure. Avoid in BPD/CLD patients.

5. **Long-term oral antihypertensive medications.** These are typically used in infants with moderate to severe hypertension who are ready to go on long-term oral therapy. Medication choice depends on your institution's preference. See Chapter 148 for more detailed information. The most common classes recommended are ACE inhibitors, α/β- and β-blockers, calcium channel blockers, vasodilators, and diuretics. Start all medications at the lowest dose.

    a. **ACE inhibitors.** Do not use if renal vascular disease is suspected.

        i. **Captopril.** A commonly used oral drug but because of the concern of renal development problems, especially in premature infants, it is preferred in infants at least 38 to 40 weeks (some state 44 weeks). Contraindicated in hyperkalemia, unilateral renal disease, and hyperkalemia.

        ii. **Enalapril.** Start with 0.04–0.1 mg/kg/d every 24 hours. Close monitoring is recommended.

        iii. **Lisinopril.** 0.07–0.6 mg/kg/d.

    b. **β-Blockers, α/β-blockers.** Do not use in infants with BPD/CLD.

        i. **Propranolol** (β-blocker). This is the most commonly used β-blocker and should not be used in infants with BPD/CLD.

    ii. **Labetalol** (α/β-blocker). Avoid in infants with BPD/CLD.

    iii. **Carvedilol** (α/β-blocker). May be good to use in heart failure. Start with 0.1 mg/kg/dose.

  c. **Vasodilators**

    i. **Hydralazine.** May cause increase in heart rate and flushing.

    ii. **Minoxidil.** Most useful for refractory hypertension. Dose: 0.2–5 mg/kg/d divided 3 times a day.

  d. **Calcium channel blockers**

    i. **Amlodipine.** Due to its slow onset, it is useful in chronic hypertension. Dose is 0.1–0.3 mg/kg/d divided twice a day.

    ii. **Isradipine.** Optimal dosing is difficult for smaller preemies due to the drug's ability to be made into a stable suspension. Dose is 0.05–0.15 mg/kg divided 4 times a day.

    iii. **Nifedipine.** May cause tachycardia and rapid temporary drops in blood pressure and is not used long term because of side effects. It is also difficult to administer in small doses (best to avoid). Dose is 0.2 mg/kg/dose.

  e. **Diuretics.** Diuretics are good for hypertension with BPD/CLD. Monitor electrolytes.

    i. **Hydrochlorothiazide.**

    ii. **Chlorothiazide.**

    iii. **Spironolactone** (aldosterone antagonist) can cause hyperkalemia.

  6. **Neonatal renovascular hypertension.** Enalaprilat (IV dicarboxylate containing ACE inhibitor) has been used with some success but has to be used with extreme caution. Side effects are oliguric acute renal failure (acute kidney injury) and prolonged hypotension, and use may be limited because of these side effects.

C. **Surgical intervention.** Used for urinary tract obstruction, certain tumors (Wilms and neuroblastoma), unilateral renal vein thrombosis, renal arterial stenosis, rare cases of polycystic kidney disease, and coarctation of the aorta.

Selected References

Dionne JM, Abitbol CL, Flynn JT. Hypertension in infancy: diagnosis, management and outcome. *Pediatr Nephrol.* 2012;27(1):17–32. Epub 2011 Jan 22. Review. Erratum in: *Pediatr Nephrol.* 2012;27(1):159–160.

Nwankwo MU, Lorenz JM, Gardiner JC. A standard protocol for blood pressure measurement in the newborn. *Pediatrics.* 1997;99(6):E10.

Pejovic B, Peco-Antic A, Marinkovic-Eric J. Blood pressure in non-critically ill preterm and full-term neonates. *Pediatr Nephrol.* 2007;22(2):249–257.

62 Hypoglycemia

I. **Problem.** An infant has a "low blood glucose level" on bedside glucose testing. The American Academy of Pediatrics (AAP) Committee on Fetus and Newborn states that the "**absolute definition of hypoglycemia as a specific value or range cannot be given, as no evidence-based studies can define what clinically relevant neonatal hypoglycemia is.**" Therefore, it is challenging to address treatment for hypoglycemia, as it is not possible to define a single blood glucose level that requires intervention in every newborn. Because blood glucose is lower in the first 12–24 hours after birth, some clinicians use a lower target number in the first 24 hours of life to define hypoglycemia.

Treatment decisions depend on the clinical situation and infant characteristics. *Note:* Aggressive screening and treatment is recommended because hypoglycemia is linked to poor neurodevelopmental outcome. Incidence varies depending on many factors, including gestational age and cause, but is ~15%.

    A. **At-risk late preterm (34–36 6/7 weeks) and term infants (small for gestational age [SGA], infants of diabetic mothers [IDMs], large for gestational age [LGA]).** AAP guidelines recommend treatment for low blood sugar in the following settings:

      1. Symptomatic infants at any age with a plasma glucose <40 mg/dL.

      2. Asymptomatic infants (**birth to 4 hours**) with a plasma glucose <40 mg/dL.

      3. Asymptomatic infants (4–24 hours) with a plasma glucose <45 mg/dL.

    B. AAP guidelines recommend a target plasma glucose of ≥45 mg/dL before routine feeding.

    C. **Preterm infants <34 weeks. Plasma glucose <45 mg/dL** (*controversial*; best to use your institutional guidelines). No guidelines have been established for premature infants with literature stating ranges **40–50 mg/dL.**

    D. Infants with documented hyperinsulinemic states. Value of <**60 mg/dL** is considered hypoglycemic (*controversial*).

  II. Immediate questions

    A. **Has the value been repeated, and has a serum blood glucose sample been sent to the laboratory?** Reagent strips can give incorrect values and be quite inaccurate in the low range (<40–50 mg/dL). Test strips can vary 10–20 mg/dL from the actual level of properly collected plasma glucose. **Never diagnose or treat hypoglycemia based on these screening reagent strips alone.** Always send a serum sample to the laboratory before starting treatment. **Bedside glucose meters (use only FDA cleared for testing in neonates) are sufficiently accurate and precise for in-hospital use** but only as screening devices. Remember, in infants with a high hematocrit a false low glucose may occur, and with galactosemia a false high glucose will occur. *Note:* Plasma glucose is 10–18% higher than serum glucose.

    B. **Does the mother have any risk factors that would increase her infant's risk of hypoglycemia, such as gestational or insulin-dependent diabetes?** Approximately 40% of IDMs have hypoglycemia. Throughout pregnancy, diabetic mothers can have episodes of hyperglycemia, resulting in fetal hyperglycemia. This fetal hyperglycemia induces pancreatic β cell hyperplasia, which in turn results in hyperinsulinism. After delivery, hyperinsulinism persists, and hypoglycemia results. An infant of an obese mother without glucose intolerance can also increase the risk in the infant. Infants born to mothers who had preeclampsia, or received glucose infusion during delivery, or were on oral terbutaline are also at increased risk.

    C. **Is the infant at risk for hypoglycemia?** Prematurity, intrauterine growth restriction (IUGR), LGA/SGA, IDMs, hypothermia, hypoxia/asphyxia, postexchange blood transfusion, illness (respiratory distress, sepsis), and polycythemia can increase the risk of hypoglycemia. If the mother received an intrapartum glucose infusion, was on β-blockers, or was on oral hypoglycemic agents, then the infant will also be at risk.

    D. **How much glucose is the infant receiving?** Glucose requirement depends on the gestational age, weight, and how many days old the infant is. The normal initial glucose requirement in term infants during the first 24 hours of life is 5–8 mg/kg/min. In extremely low birthweight infants, it is usually lower at 4–6 mg/kg/min. If the glucose order was not calculated on the basis of body weight, the infant may not be getting enough glucose. (For glucose calculations, see Chapter 9.)

    E. **Is the infant demonstrating signs of hypoglycemia?** Infants can have documented hypoglycemia and show no outward signs. There is no pathognomonic sign of hypoglycemia, and many of these signs can be seen in other disorders (sepsis, central nervous system disease, congenital heart disease, severe respiratory distress syndrome, renal and liver failure, adrenal insufficiency, metabolic disorders). These may include irritability, tremors, jitteriness, lethargy, floppiness, apnea, poor feeding, cyanosis, exaggerated Moro reflex, eye rolling, tachypnea, seizures, and weak or high-pitched cry. If these signs disappear with treatment and normalization of the glucose level, then they can most likely be attributed to hypoglycemia and not another disorder. Seizures and coma usually occur with severe, prolonged, and repetitive hypoglycemia.

III. **Differential diagnosis.** Hypoglycemia is often classified as **transient** (lasting a few days or longer up to a few weeks to months) or **persistent. Hypoglycemia can be caused** by hyperinsulinemia (transient or persistent), decreased production of glucose, decreased/depleted glycogen stores, or increased utilization of glucose.

   A. **Transient hypoglycemia.** The majority of hypoglycemia in the newborn period is transient and lasts only a few days. It is very common in infants whose feeding is delayed. Some cases of transient hypoglycemia may last longer than a few days (few weeks to months). These cases are caused by hyperinsulinemia and are acquired from perinatal stress and not genetic. The pathophysiology is unclear. These cases may include infants with birth asphyxia, maternal toxemia, prematurity, SGA, and neonates with fetal distress. **Common causes of transient hypoglycemia include the following:**

      1. **Intravenous (IV) issues.** Abrupt cessation of hypertonic glucose infusion in the neonate or infiltration of the IV is a common cause.
      2. **Insufficient caloric intake or delayed onset of feeding.**
      3. **Insulin dosing issues.**
      4. **Umbilical artery catheter near vessels supplying the pancreas (celiac and superior mesenteric arteries).** Stimulates insulin release.
      5. **Maternal intrapartum glucose administration.**
      6. **Maternal drug therapy.** Insulin, oral antidiabetic medications (sulfonylureas, glinides, gliptin), β-blockers (propranolol, labetalol), terbutaline, ritodrine, chlorothiazide, chlorpropamide.
      7. **LGA, SGA, IUGR infant.**
      8. **Infant of gestational or insulin-dependent (IDM) diabetic mother, infant of an obese mother without glucose intolerance.**
      9. **Postmature, premature infant.**
      10. **Infection, sepsis.**
      11. **Shock.**
      12. **Respiratory distress.**
      13. **Perinatal stress.**
      14. **Asphyxia or hypoxic-ischemic encephalopathy.**
      15. **Hypothermia/hyperthermia.**
      16. **Polycythemia/hyperviscosity.**
      17. **Erythroblastosis fetalis.**
      18. **Postresuscitation or exchange transfusion.**
      19. **Congenital heart disease.**
      20. **Indomethacin infusion.**
      21. **Idiopathic (no identified cause).**

   B. **Persistent hypoglycemia.** Usually defined as hypoglycemia lasting for more than 7 days or in infants who require higher amounts of glucose (>10–12 mg/kg/min) to maintain a normal glucose level for over a week. Some define hypoglycemia as persistent if it continues into infancy (>1 month). Because some types of transient hypoglycemia can persist past 1 month, persistent hypoglycemia is typically used to describe the more severe hypoglycemia that is caused by rarer causes such as congenital hyperinsulinemia, endocrine disorders, or inborn errors of metabolism.

      1. **Hyperinsulinism**
         a. **Congenital hyperinsulinism (HI).** (Older terminology includes nesidioblastosis, idiopathic hypoglycemia of infancy, persistent hyperinsulinemic hypoglycemia of infancy, and hyperinsulinemic hypoglycemia of infancy.) HI is an inappropriate or excessive amount of insulin secreted by the pancreatic islet β cells caused by a group of genetic disorders. It is the **most common cause of persistent hypoglycemia.** Mutations in the ABCC8 and KCNJ11 genes account

for 60–75% of the cases and are the most common cause. Incidence is from 1 per 2500 to 1 per 50,000.

   i. **Genetic causes.** Genetic abnormalities in several genes cause congenital forms of hyperinsulinism.

      (a) **Potassium–adenosine triphosphate (KATP) hyperinsulinemia.** Most common type of genetic hyperinsulinism with a diffuse and focal (more common) histological form. It is caused by mutations in the ABCC8 and KCNJ11 genes. Most of the mutations are recessive and cause severe hypoglycemia, unresponsive to medical treatment. The few dominant mutations cause milder hypoglycemia and respond to diazoxide.

      (b) **Glutamate dehydrogenase HI (GDH-HI) (hyperinsulinism-hyperammonemia syndrome).** Second most common type and is caused by a mutation in glutamate dehydrogenase 1 gene. It presents later (after 6 months) and is a milder form of hypoglycemia.

      (c) **Glucokinase (GCK) mutations.** These can cause hyperinsulinism from easy to very difficult to manage.

      (d) **SCHAD-HI.** Caused by short-chain 3-hydroxyacyl coenzyme A dehydrogenase (HADH) genetic defect. It causes mild to severe hypoglycemia.

      (e) **Others causes.** HNF4A, UCP2, and SLC16A1 genetic mutations.

   ii. **Focal lesions of insulin-producing tumors.** Include B-cell adenoma or islet adenomatosis. B-cell hyperplasia/dysplasias include adenoma spectrum, sulfonylurea receptor defect. Insulinoma is rare in children.

   iii. **Syndromes associated with hyperinsulinemia (syndromic hyperinsulinemia).** Most common is Beckwith-Wiedemann syndrome (hypoglycemia, macroglossia, visceromegaly, omphalocele, ear creases/pits, renal abnormalities, macrosomia). Others include hyperinsulinism/hyperammonemia syndrome, Perlman, Kabuki, Ondine, Costello, Usher type Ic, Simpson-Golabi-Behmel, and Sotos syndromes.

   iv. **Congenital defects of glycosylation.** Inherited defects of protein glycosylation. Two types (type Ia and Ib) with many subsets can cause hypoglycemia. CDG-Ia can present with heart defect/malformation, cerebellar atrophy/hypoplasia, and retinitis pigmentosa.

   v. **Insulin resistance syndromes.** These can cause hyperinsulinemic fasting hypoglycemia and can be genetic or autoimmune.

2. **Endocrine disorders.** Hormone deficiency disorders (rare) caused by deficiencies in cortisol, epinephrine, glucagon, and growth hormone (GH). Some of these disorders may have coexisting hyperinsulinemia.

  a. **Growth hormone deficiency (isolated).**

  b. **Adrenal insufficiency (cortisol deficiency).** Congenital adrenal hyperplasia, X-linked adrenal hypoplasia, adrenal hemorrhage, adrenogenital syndrome.

  c. **Congenital hypopituitarism.** Due to hypoplasia or aplasia of the anterior pituitary.

  d. **Congenital adrenocorticotropic hormone (ACTH) deficiency or familial glucocorticoid deficiency.**

  e. **Very rare.** Midline central nervous malformations such as congenital optic nerve hypoplasia, congenital hypothyroidism, glucagon deficiency, and epinephrine deficiency.

3. **Inborn errors of metabolism.** Hypoglycemia is more commonly seen in disorders of carbohydrate metabolism or fatty acid oxidation but may be seen in disorders of amino acid metabolism, organic acidurias, and respiratory chain defects.

  a. **Disorders of carbohydrate metabolism.** These include galactosemia, hereditary fructose intolerance, and glycogen storage diseases. Hypoglycemia may be the predominant finding in hepatic glycogen storage disorders (most common IEM associated with hypoglycemia). Hepatic glycogen storage disorders have hypoglycemia most commonly during fasting. Galactosemia and hereditary fructose intolerance (after sucrose in diet) both have hypoglycemia.

b. **Fatty acid oxidation defects.** Present with isolated nonketotic hypoglycemia or may also have hyperammonemia, metabolic acidosis, and elevated transaminases. The most common is medium-chain acyl-CoA dehydrogenase (MCAD) deficiency. Others include long-chain 3-OH acyl-CoA dehydrogenase (LCHAD) deficiency and carnitine deficiency disorders.

c. **Disorders of amino acid metabolism.** Hereditary tyrosinemia and maple syrup urine disease are disorders of amino acid metabolism that can present with hypoglycemia.

d. **Disorders of organic acidurias that may present with hypoglycemia.** Methylmalonic acidemia, propionic acidemia glutaric acidemia type II, 3-hydroxy-3-methylglutaric aciduria.

e. **Respiratory chain defects (oxidative phosphorylation deficiency).** May present only with hypoglycemia.

4. **Glucose transporter deficiency syndrome. Neurohypoglycemia** is a rare condition in which the infant lacks the transport protein (glucose transporter 1) that causes glucose to be transported across the brain.

IV. Database

A. **History and physical examination.** Evaluate the infant for signs of hypoglycemia (see Section II.E).

1. **Suggestive diagnostic findings.** Are there signs of sepsis or shock? Is there dysmorphism which may suggest a syndrome? Is the infant plethoric (polycythemia)? Does the infant have ambiguous genitalia (congenital adrenal hyperplasia)? Is there a midline defect and a micropenis (panhypopituitarism)? Are cataracts present (galactosemia and intrauterine infections)? Does the urine smell like maple syrup (inborn error of metabolism)? Is the growth abnormal (IUGR/SGA and LGA)? Is there a large liver (Beckwith-Wiedemann syndrome, galactosemia, fructosemia)? Is the infant macrosomic? Most infants will be macrosomic. Does the infant have hairy pinna (suggests IDM)? Infantile spasms (rare) can be seen in hyperinsulinemic hypoglycemia. Infants with congenital forms of hyperinsulinism may have facial dysmorphism (high forehead, small nasal tip and short columella, square face). Infants can also present with seizures.

2. **Specific findings for syndromic hyperinsulinemia. Beckwith-Wiedemann syndrome**: large for gestational age, large protruding tongue, large prominent eyes, creases in ear lobes, low set ears, abdominal wall defect, undescended testicles, diastasis recti; **Perlmann syndrome**: fetal gigantism, heart defect/malformation, risk of Wilms tumor, deep set eyes, depressed nasal bridge, agenesis of the corpus callosum; **Costello syndrome**: heart defect/malformation, cutis laxa (loose folds of skin), large mouth; **Usher syndrome type 1C**: intestinal malformation, deafness, retinitis pigmentosa; **Sotos syndrome**: LGA, skeletal malformation, heart defect/malformation; **Timothy syndrome**: syndactyly, heart defect/malformation, long QT syndrome; **Kabuki syndrome**: skeletal malformation, urinary tract anomalies, heart defect/malformation, intestinal malformation; **Simpson-Golabi-Behmel syndrome**: widely spaced eyes, macrostomia (large mouth), LGA, skeletal malformation, heart defect/malformation, intestinal malformation, tumor risk, corpus callosum agenesis, cerebellar atrophy/hypoplasia, deafness.

B. **Laboratory studies**

1. **AAP guidelines for hypoglycemia screening.** See Figure 62–1.

a. **Asymptomatic**

i. **Healthy term infants after normal pregnancy and delivery (no clinical symptoms and no risk).** No screening or monitoring necessary. Screen only term infants who have clinical signs or at risk.

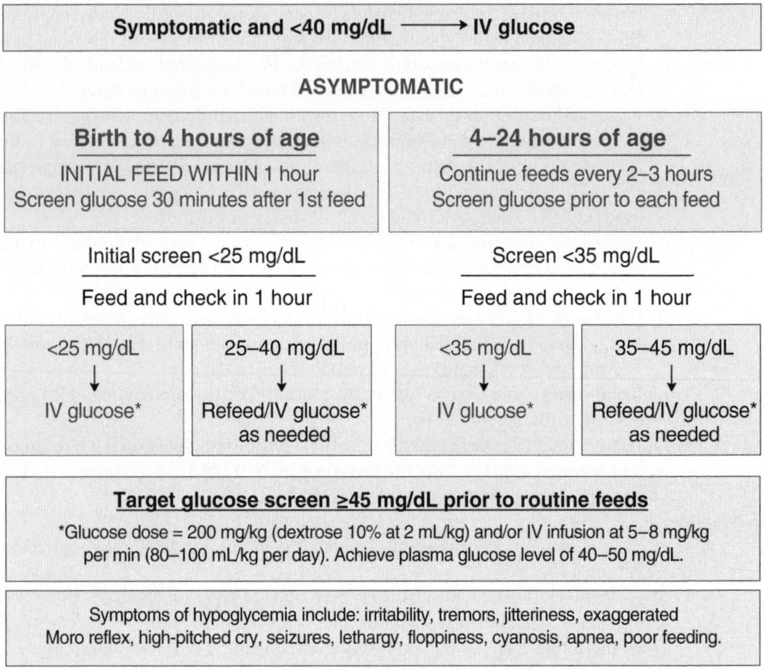

Symptomatic and <40 mg/dL ——→ IV glucose

ASYMPTOMATIC

Birth to 4 hours of age	**4–24 hours of age**
INITIAL FEED WITHIN 1 hour	Continue feeds every 2–3 hours
Screen glucose 30 minutes after 1st feed	Screen glucose prior to each feed

Initial screen <25 mg/dL	Screen <35 mg/dL
Feed and check in 1 hour	Feed and check in 1 hour

<25 mg/dL	25–40 mg/dL	<35 mg/dL	35–45 mg/dL
↓	↓	↓	↓
IV glucose*	Refeed/IV glucose* as needed	IV glucose*	Refeed/IV glucose* as needed

Target glucose screen ≥45 mg/dL prior to routine feeds
*Glucose dose = 200 mg/kg (dextrose 10% at 2 mL/kg) and/or IV infusion at 5–8 mg/kg per min (80–100 mL/kg per day). Achieve plasma glucose level of 40–50 mg/dL.

Symptoms of hypoglycemia include: irritability, tremors, jitteriness, exaggerated Moro reflex, high-pitched cry, seizures, lethargy, floppiness, cyanosis, apnea, poor feeding.

FIGURE 62–1. Screening for and management of postnatal glucose homeostasis in late-preterm (LPT 34–36 6/7 weeks), term small-for-gestational age (SGA) infants, and infants who were born to mothers with diabetes (IDM)/large-for-gestational age (LGA) infants. LPT and SGA (screen 0–24 hours), IDM and LGA ≥34 weeks (screen 0–12 hours). IV indicates intravenous. (*Reprinted with permission from Committee on Fetus and Newborn, Adamkin DH. Postnatal glucose homeostasis in late-preterm and term infants. Pediatrics. 2011;127:575–579.*)

ii. **At-risk late preterm or term infant.** Screen based on risk factors. IDM can be hypoglycemic as early as 1 hour after birth, SGA or LGA infants can be hypoglycemic by 3 hours of age, but can be hypoglycemic for 10 days after birth.

(a) **Screening the asymptomatic at-risk infant.** Should include **blood glucose** within the first few hours of birth and continued through multiple feeding cycles. They should be fed by 1 hour of age and screened 30 minutes after the feeding.

(b) **IDM and LGA infants ≥ 34 weeks.** Continue screening for IDM and LGA for 12 hours and maintain a plasma glucose >40 mg/dL.

(c) **Late preterm infants and term SGA.** Screen before each feeding for at least 24 hours. Feed every 2–3 hours. After 24 hours if glucose still <45 mg/dL, continue screening before each feeding.

b. **Symptomatic.** Any infant with clinical signs that suggest hypoglycemia needs a STAT blood glucose **immediately (within minutes).**

2. **Laboratory recommendations for infants <34 weeks.** There are no formal guidelines for these infants. Bedside glucose levels should be monitored frequently in these infants until a stable blood gas level is achieved. One recommendation is to screen on admission, then at 2, 4, 6, 12, 24, and 48 hours of age. Follow your institutional guidelines.

a. Initial studies for transient hypoglycemia
  i. Serum glucose level to confirm the bedside rapid determination.
  ii. CBC with differential to evaluate for sepsis and to rule out polycythemia.
3. Studies for persistent hypoglycemia for all infants. Draw any necessary labs at the time of hypoglycemia determination. There are multiple tests that can be performed, but the primary goal is to determine whether the infant has hyperinsulinemia.
  a. Initial studies
    i. Serum glucose and insulin (I/G level). Serum insulin will be high at the time of hypoglycemia with hyperinsulinemia, with some authors obtaining serum glucose and insulin to determine the ratio of insulin to glucose (I/G). A normal I/G is <0.30. A level >0.30 suggests a hyperinsulinemic cause of hypoglycemia.
    ii. Serum ketones. Low to absent in the presence of hyperinsulinemia and high in GH and cortisol deficiency.
    iii. β-Hydroxybutyrate and free fatty acids. Decreased levels can indicate excessive insulin.
    iv. Serum lactate. This can be elevated in metabolic defects.
    v. Serum ammonia. To rule out hyperinsulinism/hyperammonemia syndrome.
    vi. C peptide levels. Elevated in hyperinsulinemia and insulinoma.
    vii. Insulin-like growth factor binding protein (IGF-BP1). Decreased in hyperinsulinemia.
    viii. Increased serum insulin, C peptide, and proinsulin level and decreased glucose, free fatty acids, ketones, and IGF-BP1 can diagnose congenital hyperinsulinism.
  b. Critical labs to diagnose hyperinsulinism if associated with hypoglycemia
    i. Plasma insulin >2 μU/mL.
    ii. Plasma free fatty acids <1.5 mmol/L.
    iii. Plasma β-hydroxybutyrate <2 μmol/L.
    iv. Glucagon challenge 0.03 mg/kg IV >25–40 mg/dL rise in blood sugar.
  c. To differentiate a metabolic defect from hypopituitarism, and hyperinsulinism. Obtain data set of laboratory determinations before and 15 minutes after the parenteral administration of glucagon (0.3 mg/kg/dose). These include serum glucose, ketones, free fatty acids, lactate, alanine, uric acid, insulin, growth hormone, cortisol, glucagon, T_4, and thyroid-stimulating hormone (TSH). The results are interpreted as shown in Table 62–1.
  d. Other tests. Serum pH (metabolic disorders), cortisol and ACTH (adrenal insufficiency), growth hormone levels (growth hormone deficiency), blood ammonia (galactosemia, hyperinsulinism/hyperammonemia), T_4 and TSH (hypothyroidism), blood lactate levels (glycogen storage disorders), urine ketones and reducing substances or amino acids and organic acids (inborn error of metabolism), free fatty acid levels (fatty acid oxidation defect), plasma acylcarnitines (3-hydroxyacyl-CoA dehydrogenase [HADH] deficiency).
  e. Genetic testing. To diagnose any inherited syndromes.
C. Imaging and other studies
  1. Ultrasound/computed tomography (CT) of the pancreas to look for adenoma.
  2. Echocardiogram may show hypertrophic cardiomyopathy in infants with transient (IDM) hyperinsulinism.
  3. Electrospray ionization tandem mass spectrometry can identify inborn errors of metabolism more rapidly (see Chapter 101).
  4. Fluorine 18-L dihydroxyphenylalanine positron emission tomography ([18] F-DOPA PET/CT) allows preoperative localization of the focal lesion, allowing surgical resection.

Table 62–1. DIAGNOSIS OF PERSISTENT HYPOGLYCEMIA BEFORE AND AFTER PARENTERAL GLUCAGON ADMINISTRATION

Variable	Hyperinsulinism Before	Hyperinsulinism After	Hypopituitarism Before	Hypopituitarism After	Metabolic Defect Before	Metabolic Defect After
Glucose	↓	↑↑↑	↓	↑/N	↓	↓/N
Ketones	↓	↓	N/↓	N	↑	↑
Free fatty acids	↓	↑	N/↓	N	↑	↑
Lactate	N	N	N	N	↑	↑↑
Alanine	N	?	N	N	↑	↑↑
Uric acid	N	N	N	N	↑	↑↑
Insulin	↑↑	↑↑↑	N/↑	↑	N	↑
Growth hormone	↑	↓	↓	↓	↑	↑
Cortisol	↑	↓	↓ᵃ	↓ᵃ	↑	↑
TSH and T$_4$	N	N	↓ᵃ	↓ᵃ	N	N

N, normal or no change; ↑, elevated; ↓, lowered; ?, unknown; TSH, thyroid-stimulating hormone; T$_4$, thyroxine.
ᵃResponse may vary depending on the degree of hypopituitarism.

V. **Plan**

   A. **Overall plan.** There are many different recommendations on treatments. It is best to follow the guidelines of your institution. AAP recommendations for at-risk preterm and term infants and also suggested recommendations for preterm infants <34 weeks are noted here. The overall goal is to maintain normoglycemia. Infants at risk for hypoglycemia and those with established hypoglycemia should have glucose screening every 1–2 hours until glucose levels are stable and then every 4 hours. Once the glucose level is stable, the next step is to determine why the patient is hypoglycemic. Sometimes the cause is obvious, as in the case of an infant of a diabetic mother or one with IUGR. If the cause is not obvious, further workup is necessary.

      1. **AAP recommendations for at-risk late preterm and term infants (>34 weeks).** Signs of hypoglycemia include jitteriness, cyanosis, seizures, apneic episodes, tachypnea, weak or high-pitched cry, floppiness or lethargy, poor feeding, and eye rolling. (See Figure 62–1.)

         a. **Symptomatic infants.** If blood glucose <40 mg/dL, treat with IV glucose. Give 2 mL/kg of D10 at a rate of 1 mL/min. Then a continuous infusion of 5–8 mg/kg/min (80–100 mL/kg/d) to achieve a plasma glucose of 40–50 mg/dL.

         b. **Asymptomatic infants.** See Figure 62–1.

         c. **If glucose levels cannot be maintained at >45 mg/dL (on 5–8 mg/kg/min of D10W) after 24 hours.** Consider hyperinsulinemic hypoglycemia and send a serum insulin with plasma blood glucose when the bedside blood glucose is <40 mg/dL. Consultation with endocrinology should be obtained.

      2. **Recommendations for preterm infants <34 weeks** *(controversial)*

         a. **Asymptomatic hypoglycemia treatment is** *controversial.* One treatment approach is presented here. Some clinicians treat with early feeding based on glucose level, clinical status, and the gestational and postnatal age of the infant. Others rely on plasma blood level (usually <25 mg/dL) and treat all such infants with parenteral glucose. Follow your own institution's guidelines.

            i. **Draw a blood sample and send it to the laboratory for a STAT baseline plasma glucose level.**

            ii. **Infants with a plasma glucose <25 mg/dL. Insert an IV and start a glucose infusion of 5–8 mg/kg/min** (specific calculation in Chapter 9), even if the infant is not showing signs of hypoglycemia (***controversial***). Initially, glucose levels should be checked every 30 minutes until stable. The infusion should be increased until normoglycemia is achieved. A bolus of glucose in the asymptomatic infant is contraindicated because it is thought to result in rebound hypoglycemia (***controversial***).

    iii. **Infants with a plasma glucose 25–45 mg/dL.** If there are no risk factors for hypoglycemia and the infant is clinically stable, an early feeding (gavage if necessary) of 5% dextrose in water or formula can be given. The glucose levels are monitored every 30–60 minutes until stable and then every 4 hours. If the glucose remains low, an IV line should be started with a glucose infusion of 5–8 mg/kg/min.

  b. **Symptomatic hypoglycemia (transient).** See symptoms earlier. Treatment of symptomatic hypoglycemia with parenteral glucose is common although ***controversial***.

    i. **Draw a sample for a STAT baseline plasma glucose level.**

    ii. **Insert an IV and start a glucose infusion.** Infuse a mini-bolus (usually not associated with rebound hypoglycemia in this setting) of 2 mL/kg of a 10% glucose solution at a rate of 1.0 mL/min. Then start a continuous infusion of glucose (5–8 mg/kg/min or 80–100 mL/kg/d) and increase the rate as needed to maintain a normal blood glucose (>40–50 mg/dL). The level should be monitored every 30–60 minutes until stable. **The highest concentration of glucose that can be infused through a peripheral catheter is 12.5%.** One study found that 12.5% dextrose in water (DW) was preferred over 10% DW in sick preterm infants weighing 1500–2500 g. If a more concentrated solution is required, a central catheter is needed. Higher concentrations are hypertonic and may damage the veins. Also, if there is difficulty starting an IV catheter, an umbilical venous catheter can be placed emergently.

3. **If an IV is not available, glucagon** (see Chapter 148) **can be given to infants with adequate glycogen stores.** This may be particularly effective in IDMs and less effective in infants who have growth retardation or who are SGA because of poor muscle mass and glycogen stores. The dose is 0.02–0.30 mg/kg/dose, not to exceed 1.0 mg total dose. It may be given subcutaneously or intramuscularly while vascular access is being attempted.

4. **Transient hyperinsulinemia that lasts longer than a few days (up to 2–3 months).** These infants have a high glucose requirement (>20 mg/kg/min). They respond well to diazoxide therapy and usually require it transiently.

5. **Persistent hypoglycemia.** Defined as hypoglycemia persisting or recurring over >7 days. It also occurs when the infant requires >12 mg/kg/min to maintain a normal glucose. The management of these infants can be complicated, as they can have fluid overload and cardiac failure. Many require a central line to deliver high levels of glucose. Some will require a gastrostomy for frequent feedings. **Endocrinology and possible surgical consultation** should be obtained.

  a. Continue IV glucose and increase the rate of IV glucose to 16–20 mg/kg/min. Rates >20 mg/kg/min are usually not helpful. If it is evident at this point that the infant still has problems with hypoglycemia, medications to treat the hypoglycemia should be started.

    i. **Corticosteroids.** Formerly used in the treatment of persistent hypoglycemia. Some units are still using corticosteroids as first-line therapy. It is no longer recommended because of side effects and is now only used if there is evidence of adrenal insufficiency. (See dosage in Chapter 148).

    ii. **The following medications can be tried.** It is not necessary to stop the previous agent when trying a new medication. **Choice of treatment** can be variable and depends on the institution. **Knowledge of the genetic subtype can guide treatment.** Infants with GLUD1, HNF4A, HADH, GCK, and

UCP2 mutations respond better to diazoxide than those with ABCC8 and KCNJ11 mutations. The type caused by paternal ABCC8/KCNJ11 mutation is focal and may respond to surgery. **Infants with transient hyperinsulinemia from perinatal stress and syndromic hyperinsulinemia also respond to diazoxide.** See Chapter 148 for dosages.

(a) Diazoxide. **First treatment of choice.** Initial 10 mg/kg/d PO in divided doses every 8 hours. Range is 5–15 mg/kg/d divided every 8 hours. **Chlorothiazide** is often used with this for its synergistic effect and to decrease retention of fluid. Diazoxide is started for a trial of 5 days. Responsiveness is based on absence of hypoglycemia on normal feedings and during a 4-hour fast. If nonresponsive, octreotide is tried next.

(b) Octreotide. A long-acting analog of somatostatin; preferred over somatostatin because the latter has a very short half-life. It can be used if the infant is nonresponsive to diazoxide. The starting dose is 2–10 mcg/kg/d, subcutaneously divided every 6–12 hours, or by continuous IV infusion. Doses up to 40 mcg/kg/d divided every 6–8 hours can be used. It has been used long term in combination with feeding.

(c) Glucagon. Used if the infant has good glycogen stores. Usually only given in temporary situations (eg, waiting for IV/central line access, waiting for surgery, used with octreotide in short-term stabilization of infants with hyperinsulinemia.) Dose is 0.02–0.30 mg/kg/dose IV, intramuscularly, or subcutaneously. May repeat in 20 minutes (1 mg maximum dose).

(d) Nifedipine. It has been used in some infants, but because of severe hypotension and lack of long-term experience, it is not used often.

(e) Medications for endocrine deficiency disorders. **Growth hormone** should be used if there is a GH deficiency. **Epinephrine** can be used in epinephrine deficiency. **Zinc protamine glucagon** is indicated for infants with glucagon deficiency. **Glucose transporter deficiency syndrome** is treated with a ketogenic diet.

b. Pancreatic surgery. Considered if medical treatment does not work. It is also recommended for those infants with **focal lesions** (partial pancreatectomy) and some infants with diffuse lesions such as β-cell hyperplasia (subtotal pancreatectomy). A few infants may require a total pancreatectomy to control their hyperinsulinemia.

B. Specific treatment plans

1. Neonatal hyperinsulinism. Pancreatectomy (removes at least 95% of the organ) is usually necessary. Partial pancreatectomy can be done when hypersecretion is shown to be confined to a small area of the pancreas. Studies have shown that some cases of congenital hyperinsulinemia have been managed effectively with diazoxide and octreotide for decades.

2. Congenital hypopituitarism. Usually responds to administration of cortisone and IV glucose. Administration of human GH may be necessary. (For dosages, see Chapter 148.)

3. Metabolic defects

a. Type I glycogen storage disease. Frequent small feedings, avoiding fructose or galactose, may be beneficial.

b. Hereditary fructose intolerance. Begin a fructose-free diet.

c. Galactosemia. Begin a galactose-free diet immediately on suspicion of the diagnosis.

Selected Reference

Committee on Fetus and Newborn, Adamkin DH. Postnatal glucose homeostasis in late-preterm and term infants. *Pediatrics.* 2011;127:575–579.

63 Hypokalemia

I. **Problem.** The nurse reports a serum potassium of 2.8 mEq/L. Normal serum potassium values vary with technique used by the laboratory but are usually between **3.5 and 5 mEq/L.** Hypokalemia is defined as a serum potassium <3.5 mEq/L. Mild hypokalemia is 3.0–3.5 mEq/L. Moderate hypokalemia is 2.5–3.0 mEq/L; severe hypokalemia is <2.5 mEq/L. Severe hypokalemia can cause cardiac arrhythmias.

II. **Immediate questions**

A. **What is the central serum potassium?** If a low value is obtained by heelstick, central values should be obtained because they may actually be lower than values obtained by heelstick because of the hemolysis of red blood cells. **Was the sample sent immediately to the lab?** If a sample sat for hours in a warm area, pseudohypokalemia can occur.

B. **Is the infant on diuretics? Are potassium-wasting medications or digitalis being given?** Hypokalemia in a neonate usually occurs from chronic diuretic use. Hypokalemia may cause significant arrhythmias if digitalis is being administered.

C. **How much potassium is the infant receiving?** Normal maintenance doses are 1–2 mEq/kg/d.

D. **Are there any gastrointestinal (GI) losses from diarrhea, a naso-gastric/orogastric (NG/OG) tube, or ileostomy?** Loss of large amounts of GI fluids can cause hypokalemia. Severe vomiting can also cause hypokalemia such as in infantile hypertrophic pyloric stenosis.

E. **What is the infant's magnesium level? Hypomagnesemia** can cause hypokalemia. Consider this diagnosis if the hypokalemia does not correct despite potassium supplementation.

III. **Differential diagnosis.** Hypokalemia can be caused by a prolonged inadequate intake of potassium, gastrointestinal losses, renal losses, and transcellular shifts or redistrubution. GI and renal losses are more common. **Medications (diuretics) are the most common cause in the neonatal intensive care unit (NICU).**

A. **Pseudohypokalemia** can occur if the blood sample sits too long in a warm environment, with a very high white blood cell (WBC) count (uptake of potassium by abnormal WBC), or from a heelstick sample.

B. **True hypokalemia (total body deficit)**

1. **Inadequate intake (rare)** of either maintenance infusion or oral intake of potassium. For a further discussion, see Chapter 9.

2. **Gastrointestinal losses**

a. **Loss of fluid via nasogastric tube (common).** Unreplaced electrolyte loss from NG tube or excess drainage from ileostomy.

b. **Diarrhea.** Congenital chloride diarrhea, any gastrointestinal fistula, short bowel syndrome.

c. **Vomiting.** May cause hypokalemia such as infantile hypertrophic pyloric stenosis with vomiting.

d. **Medications.** Kayexalate causes fecal potassium loss.

3. **Renal losses**

a. **Medications**

i. **Diuretic use** especially long-term therapy with any thiazide or loop diuretic is the most common medication-related cause.

ii. **Steroids and steroid-like medications.**

iii. **Antibiotics.** High-dose penicillin, ampicillin, carbenicillin, vancomycin. Combined treatment of aminoglycosides and vancomycin can cause tubular disturbances in extremely low birthweight (ELBW) infants with renal tubular wasting of potassium.

      iv. Magnesium depletion medications such as amphotericin B and aminoglycosides. Amphotericin B can cause direct renal tubular damage with potassium loss.

    b. Any cause of polyuria

    c. Renal tubular losses

      i. Renal tubular acidosis (RTA). Type 1 and 2.

      ii. Hypomagnesemia. Exacerbates potassium loss by increasing distal potassium secretion.

      iii. Bartter syndrome (neonatal). A rare form of potassium wasting, secondary to chloride channel abnormality. **Pseudo-Bartter syndrome** presents with the same clinical and biological characteristics as Bartter syndrome but without the primary renal tubule abnormalities. **Congenital hypokalemia with hypercalciuria** resembles Bartter syndrome.

      iv. Other syndromes. Liddle, Gitelman, and Fanconi syndromes.

  4. Transcellular shifts of potassium from serum to cells

    a. Alkalosis (metabolic or respiratory) drives potassium into cells, causing hypokalemia. An increase in pH by 0.1 unit causes a decrease in the serum potassium by 0.6 mEq/L. The decrease is less in respiratory than in metabolic alkalosis.

    b. Insulin therapy causes intracellular uptake of potassium.

    c. Medications that cause an increase in intracellular uptake of potassium include β-adrenergic agonists (such as epinephrine, decongestants, bronchodilators, tocolytic drugs) and xanthine derivatives (theophylline, caffeine). Overdose related: insulin, verapamil.

    d. Hypothermia can drive potassium into cells and lower the plasma potassium concentration.

    e. Endocrinopathies causing potassium loss (less common)

      i. Congenital adrenal hyperplasia. 11B-hydroxylase deficiency accounts for ~5–10 % of cases and causes hypertension, hypokalemic alkalosis, and salt retention.

      ii. Primary hyperaldosteronism/Conn syndrome. Hypertension, hypokalemia, and suppressed renin activity are the 3 laboratory hallmarks of this disease. **Secondary hyperaldosteronism** can occur from renal artery stenosis, renin-secreting tumors, and coarctation of the aorta.

      iii. Cushing syndrome. Hyperfunction of the adrenal cortex in infants is usually caused by a functioning adrenocortical tumor.

      iv. Syndrome of apparent mineralocorticoid excess (AME). This can be congenital and causes hypokalemia.

      v. Hyperthyroidism.

IV. Database

  A. Physical examination. Mild hypokalemia may not cause any signs. Symptoms of low potassium can include musculoskeletal (weakness, decreased tendon reflexes, paresthesias, paralysis), GI (nausea, vomiting, diarrhea, ileus), and central nervous system (CNS) signs (lethargy). These are difficult to evaluate in an infant. In severe hypokalemia, the infant can have lethargy; an ileus (abdominal distension and hypoactive bowel sounds); cardiac arrhythmias (rare unless <2.5 mEq/L); flaccid or diaphragmatic paralysis; and bradycardia with cardiovascular collapse. In hypertrophic pyloric stenosis in infants, an enlarged pylorus, or **"pyloric olive"** may be felt 23% of the time (best felt during or at the end of a feeding).

  B. Laboratory studies

    1. Repeat the serum potassium level to confirm value.

    2. Spot-check urinary electrolytes. Perform periodic spot-checks of urinary potassium levels to determine whether urinary losses are high. Not accurate with recent diuretic use.

    3. Serum electrolytes and creatinine. To evaluate renal status and other electrolyte abnormalities.

4. **Blood gas levels.** An alkalosis may cause or aggravate hypokalemia (ie, as hydrogen ions leave the cells potassium ions enter the cells, causing decreased serum potassium levels). **Treatment of acidosis may worsen hypokalemia.**
5. **Serum magnesium.** To rule out hypomagnesemia.
6. **Drug screen.** If the infant is on any medication that can cause hypokalemia it is best to check the levels. Check digoxin level if the patient is on a digitalis preparation. Hypokalemia can potentiate digitalis-induced arrhythmias.
7. **Serum adrenocorticotropic hormone (ACTH), cortisol, renin activity, and aldosterone levels.** To evaluate for Cushing, adrenal hyperplasia, and Conn syndromes.
8. **Serum insulin and C-peptide tests.** To evaluate for hyperinsulinism.
C. **Imaging and other studies**
1. **Abdominal radiograph.** If ileus is suspected.
2. **Abdominal ultrasound.** In infants in whom pyloric stenosis is suspected, the diagnostic procedure of choice. Also check for adrenal tumor or hyperplasia.
3. **Electrocardiography (ECG).** The ECG may appear normal in hypokalemia or may show conduction defects. If hypokalemia is present and the infant is unstable, an ECG may show conduction defects such as prominent U wave with prolonged QT interval, flattening or biphasic of the T wave, and a depressed ST segment. Ventricular and atrial arrhythmias may also develop. The U-wave appearance may mimic atrial flutter. Note that these ECG findings are also seen in hypomagnesemia. Digitalis toxicity is increased with low potassium.
4. **Magnetic resonance image (MRI).** MRI of the head to rule out pituitary tumor if indicated.
V. **Plan**
A. **General measures.** Hypokalemia is increasing in neonatal intensive care units because of the widespread use of diuretics. The goal of treatment is to increase the potassium intake so that normal blood levels are maintained. Short-term intravenous (IV) potassium administration may cause damage to the veins and occasionally hyperkalemia, as potassium does not rapidly equilibrate. Rapid correction is not recommended because of hyperkalemia risk with potential cardiac complications. Corrections are given slowly, often over 24 hours. If too large a bolus is given, cardiac arrest may result. Serum potassium levels should be monitored every 4–6 hours until correction is achieved. Once levels reach high normal, decrease the amount of potassium given. The majority of cases can be corrected by increasing daily potassium intake by 1 or 2 mEq/kg/d.
1. **If alkalosis is present,** correct before potassium correction (see page 331).
2. **If the infant is acidotic,** potassium acetate or citrate salts can be given. Treatment of acidosis may worsen hypokalemia.
3. **Correct low magnesium,** see page 977.
B. **Emergency treatment of life-threatening cardiac arrhythmias or potassium <2.5 mEq/L.** IV potassium accompanied by ECG monitoring. Never give a bolus; only in extreme emergencies consider giving 0.5–1 mEq/kg/dose over 1 hour in a central line with continuous ECG monitoring (maximum dose rate: 1 mEq/kg/h).
C. **Symptomatic hypokalemia.** (Not life threatening.) Should be treated with IV potassium. This can be done by increasing the amount in the IV fluids (preferred) or a correction over 24 hours:

Potassium deficit (mEq/L) = (Normal potassium − Observed potassium) × Body weight in kg × 0.3

D. **Mild hypokalemia.** May resolve without treatment. If the infant is on oral feeds, oral supplementation with potassium chloride may be given, usually 2–3 mEq/kg/d in 3 to 4 divided doses (diluted with feedings), adjusted depending on serum potassium levels.
E. **Hypokalemia with hypovolemia.** IV fluid with potassium chloride (KCL) is indicated.
F. **Specific measures.** Any specific defects (ie, renal defects, adrenal disorders, and certain metabolic problems) require specific evaluation and therapy.

1. **Inadequate maintenance infusion of potassium.** Calculate the normal maintenance infusion of potassium that should be given and increase the amount accordingly (normal maintenance infusion is 1–2 mEq/kg/d, usually only necessary after the first day of life).
2. **Abnormal potassium losses**
   a. **Medications.** If the infant is receiving potassium-wasting medications, increase the maintenance dose of potassium (eg, patients with bronchopulmonary dysplasia on long-term furosemide therapy). Oral supplementation with potassium chloride may be given, 1–2 mEq/kg/d in 3 to 4 divided doses (with feedings), adjusted depending on serum potassium levels. It was once thought that a potassium-sparing diuretic decreased the amount of potassium supplementation; however, a randomized study showed that serum electrolytes sodium and potassium were not affected by the addition of spironolactone.
   b. **Gastrointestinal losses**
      i. **Severe diarrhea correction.** Withhold oral feedings to allow the gut to rest and give IV potassium (initial dose of KCl, 1–2 mEq/kg/d). Serum potassium levels are monitored, and the IV dose is adjusted.
      ii. **Nasogastric drainage/severe vomiting.** This amount should be measured each shift and replaced mL/mL with 1/2 normal saline with 10–20 mEq of KCl/L.
      iii. **Pyloric stenosis.** Correct dehydration if present and if surgery is indicated.
   G. **Renal loss of potassium.** Other than induced by medications.
      1. **Bartter syndrome.** Potassium supplementation is given orally with a starting dosage of 2–3 mEq/kg/d, which is increased as necessary to maintain a normal serum potassium level. Certain forms respond to indomethacin.
      2. **Hyperaldosteronism.** Surgery and dexamethasone therapy may be indicated.
      3. **Cushing syndrome.** Medication and possible surgery.
      4. **Renal tubular acidosis types 1 and 2.** Alkaline therapy and potassium supplementation if needed.
   H. **Redistribution of potassium**
      1. **Alkalosis.** Determine the cause of metabolic or respiratory alkalosis and treat the underlying disorder. Treat the alkalosis before increasing potassium intake.
      2. **Medications.** Should be discontinued if possible or alternatives used that do not affect potassium (see Section III.B.3a).

64 Hyponatremia

I. **Problem.** An infant has a serum sodium of 127 mEq/L, below the normal accepted value of 135 mEq/L. The incidence of hyponatremia is greater than hypernatremia in premature infants. Evidence now shows it is a serious condition in very preterm infants (<33 weeks' gestation), who have large variations of the serum sodium concentration, as they are at risk for poor neuromotor outcome at 2 years. Preterm infants with an increased risk of hyponatremia from sodium restriction show impaired growth and worse neurodevelopment at 10–13 years of age. Hyponatremia is also a risk factor for sensorineural hearing loss, intracranial hemorrhage, and cerebral palsy. Hyponatremia in infants who experienced perinatal birth asphyxia are at risk for an increased mortality.

II. **Immediate questions**
   A. **Is there any seizure activity?** Seizure activity can be seen in patients with extremely low serum sodium levels (usually <120 mEq/L). **This is a medical emergency, and urgent intravenous (IV) sodium correction is needed.**

B. **How much sodium and free water is the patient receiving? Is weight gain or loss occurring?** Be certain that an adequate amount of sodium is being given and that free water intake is not excessive. The normal amount of sodium intake is 2–4 mEq/kg/d. Weight gain with low serum sodium levels is most likely a result of volume overload, especially in the first day or two of life, when weight loss is expected.

C. **What is the urine output?** With syndrome of inappropriate secretion of antidiuretic hormone (SIADH), urine output is decreased. If the urine output is increased (>4 mL/kg/h), perform a spot check of urine sodium to determine whether urinary sodium losses are high.

D. **What medications is the infant receiving? Are renal salt-wasting medications being given?** Diuretics such as furosemide may cause hypovolemic hyponatremia. Other medications that cause hyponatremia include theophylline, carbamazepine, chlorpromazine, indapamide, amiodarone, and selective serotonin reuptake inhibitors. Most of these cause SIADH (euvolemic hyponatremia). Morphine and barbiturates can also cause hyponatremia.

E. **Did the mother receive hypotonic IV fluids or an excessive amount of oxytocin? Was the mother hyponatremic in the intrapartum period?** If so, the infant can have hyponatremia at birth. Infants of mothers with hyponatremia can have low levels of sodium after delivery.

F. **Is the infant <1 week old (early-onset hyponatremia) or is the infant in the third to fourth week of life (late-onset hyponatremia)? Early-onset hyponatremia** may be due to free water excess from either increased maternal free water in labor or perinatal nonosmotic release of vasopressin (occurs in perinatal asphyxia, respiratory distress syndrome, bilateral pneumothoraces, intraventricular hemorrhage [IVH], and with certain medications). It can also occur from too much free water given or not enough sodium intake in fluids. **Late-onset hyponatremia** is usually from inadequate sodium intake or excessive renal losses. Late onset can also be from excessive antidiuretic hormone (ADH) release, renal failure, or edema causing retention of free water, but it is less common. Preterm infants >28 weeks have a high fractional excretion of sodium.

III. **Differential diagnosis.** When considering the differential, determine whether the value is real. Certain conditions can cause pseudohyponatremia. Is the amount of sodium given adequate? Then you need to decide whether the hyponatremia is caused by deficit of total body sodium or an excess of free water. Is there an inability to excrete water? Is there an excessive sodium loss? Have medications caused the hyponatremia? The cause dictates the form of treatment. **The most frequent cause of hyponatremia in the neonate is hypotonic hyponatremia (dilutional) caused by excessive fluid administration or retention of free water.**

A. **Pseudohyponatremia.** This can be caused by hyperlipidemia, hyperproteinemia, or hyperglycemia. In hyperglycemia, for every 100 mg/dL the glucose is above 100, the sodium falls 1.6 mEq/L. A spurious result can also occur from a diluted sample drawn from an indwelling catheter with a low sodium fluid.

B. **Inadequate sodium intake.** Maintenance sodium is usually 2–4 mEq/kg/d.

C. **Hyponatremia with extracellular fluid (ECF) excess (hypervolemia).** This occurs with excess of ECF. There is a positive water balance. The total body sodium and total body water are increased. ECF is very increased, resulting in edema and weight gain. Causes include the following:

1. **Congestive heart failure**
2. **Sepsis with decreasing cardiac output**
3. **Neuromuscular paralysis with fluid retention (eg, pancuronium)**
4. **Renal failure**
5. **Liver failure (cirrhosis)**
6. **Nephrotic syndrome**
7. **Necrotizing enterocolitis (late)**
8. **Indomethacin therapy (can cause water retention)**

D. **Hyponatremia with hypovolemia (ECF deficit).** This occurs with a deficit of ECF and can be caused by either renal losses or extrarenal losses. The total body sodium and total body water and ECF are all decreased.
1. **Renal losses (spot urinary Na >20 mEq/L)**
   a. **Diuretics**
   b. **Renal disorders**
      i. **Renal immaturity.** Neonates can have immature kidneys. Preterm infants are prone to hyponatremia because of a lower glomerular filtration rate, lower proximal tubular reabsorption of sodium, and an increase arginine vasopressin level when sick. Often very low birthweight infants show increased renal tubular sodium and water loss causing hyponatremia.
      ii. **Salt-losing nephropathy.**
      iii. **Acute/chronic renal failure.**
      iv. **Renal tubular acidosis.**
      v. **Obstructive uropathy.** This can cause high urinary losses of sodium.
      vi. **Bartter and Fanconi syndromes.**
      vii. **Hypertension-hyponatremia syndrome in neonates caused by reno-vascular pathology.** Renal ischemia from renal microthrombi can be the cause. Suspect if umbilical artery catheter has been placed and unilateral renal arterial stenosis is present.
   c. **Mineralocorticoid deficiency (adrenal salt-wasting disorders)**
      i. **Addison disease**
      ii. **Hypoaldosteronism**
      iii. **Congenital adrenal hyperplasia**
      iv. **Pseudohypoaldosteronism**
      v. **Hypopituitarism**
   d. **Cerebral salt-wasting syndrome.** Occurs when there is loss of sodium in the urine and is secondary to acute or chronic damage to the central nervous system (hemorrhage, increased intracranial pressure). Extracellular volume is decreased and blood urea nitrogen, albumin, and hematocrit are increased.
   e. **Osmotic diuresis from hyperglycemia (rare in neonates), hyperosmolality.**
2. **Extrarenal losses (urinary Na <20 mEq/L)**
   a. **Gastrointestinal (GI) losses** such as vomiting, diarrhea, nasogastric tubes.
   b. **Third spacing of fluids.** Ascites, pleural effusion, ileus, necrotizing enterocolitis, sloughing of skin.
   c. **Radiant warmer skin loss.**
E. **Hyponatremia with normal ECF.** Total body water is increased, total sodium is normal or a slightly decreased, ECF is minimally increased but no edema.
1. **Excessive IV fluids, free water, or using diluted (hypotonic) formulas.** A common cause of the hyponatremia in a neonate. Maternal fluid overload (with glucose-only sodium-free solutions) or maternal water intoxication is also a cause of hyponatremia in a newborn. This is associated with a low urine-specific gravity and high urine output.
2. **SIADH.** Occurs more commonly in CNS disorders such as IVH, hydrocephalus, birth asphyxia, and meningitis, but may also be seen with lung disease (pneumothorax and positive pressure ventilation). SIADH is often seen in critically ill premature and term neonates. It can also be seen in association with pain and with medications such as opiates, carbamazepine, barbiturates, theophylline, and thiazides.
3. **Endocrine related.** Hypothyroidism or hypoadrenalism.
F. **Drug-induced hyponatremia.** Diuretics (used frequently with bronchopulmonary dysplasia/chronic lung disease [BPD/CLD]) can lead to sodium losses. Indomethacin causes water retention (dilutional hyponatremia). SIADH can be due to medications, as noted previously. Infusion of mannitol or hypertonic glucose can cause hyperosmolality with salt wasting. Maternal medication use (diuretics, infusion of oxytocin and glucose) can cause hyponatremia in the infant.

IV. Database
  A. Evaluate the bedside chart
      1. **Check for weight loss or gain.** Weight gain is more likely to be associated with dilutional hyponatremia. Weight loss is seen with hyponatremia with decreased ECF.
      2. **Check fluid intake and output over a 24-hour period.** Normally, infants retain two-thirds of the fluid administered, and the rest is lost in the urine or by insensible loss. If the input is much greater than the output, the patient may be retaining fluid, and dilutional hyponatremia should be considered.
      3. **Assess the urine output and specific gravity.** A low urine output with a high specific gravity is more commonly seen with SIADH. In excessive fluid, one sees a low urine-specific gravity and a high urine output.
  B. **History and physical examination.** Are there maternal factors present (hypotonic IV fluids or an excessive amount of oxytocin) or was there maternal hyponatremia in the intrapartum period? Note signs of seizure activity (abnormal eye movements, jerking of the extremities, and tongue thrusting). Is there a bulging fontanel, any lethargy? Check for edema, a sign of volume overload (renal failure, congestive heart failure). Decreased skin turgor and dry mucous membranes are seen in dehydration. Is the infant in shock? Does the infant have genital hyperpigmentation (congenital adrenal hyperplasia)? Is there virilization or ambiguous genitalia in a female infant or hypospadias in a male (3-β-hydroxysteroid dehydrogenase deficiency)?
  C. Laboratory studies
      1. Specific tests
          a. Serum sodium and osmolality
          b. Urine spot sodium, osmolality, and specific gravity
          c. Serum electrolytes, creatinine, and total protein to assess renal function
      2. See Table 64-1 for diagnosis specific laboratory results
          a. Volume overload (dilutional hyponatremia)
              i. **Excess IV fluids.** Increased urine output and decreased urine osmolality and (decreased) low specific gravity.
              ii. **Other** (congestive heart failure or paralysis with fluid retention). Decreased urine output and increased urine specific gravity.
          b. Increased sodium losses
              i. **Renal losses, with diuretics and adrenal insufficiency.** Increased urine output and urine Na$^+$ and decreased urine osmolality and specific gravity.
              ii. **Skin and GI losses and with third spacing.** Decreased urine output and sodium and increased urine osmolality and specific gravity.
          c. **SIADH.** The diagnosis is made by documenting the following on simultaneous laboratory studies: low urine output, urine osmolality greater than serum osmolality, low serum sodium level and low serum osmolality, and

Table 64-1. **HYPONATREMIA AND LABORATORY FINDINGS IN SPECIFIC DIAGNOSES**

	Urine Output	Urine Sodium	Urine Osmolality	Urine-Specific Gravity
Excess IV fluids	Increased		Decreased	Decreased
SIADH	Decreased	Increased	Increased	Increased
GI/skin/third spacing	Decreased	Decreased	Increased	Increased
Renal loss	Increased	Increased	Decreased	Decreased
Fluid retention	Decreased			Increased

IV, intravenous; SIADH, syndrome of inappropriate secretion of antidiuretic hormone; GI, gastrointestinal.

high urinary sodium level and high specific gravity. A plasma ADH concentration and a plasma concentration of atrial natriuretic peptide can be obtained. If they show a high ADH concentration in the presence of low serum osmolality and elevated urinary osmolality, the diagnosis is confirmed.

D. **Imaging and other studies.** None usually needed. Ultrasound of the head or brain magnetic resonance imaging (MRI) may reveal IVH as a cause of hyponatremia secondary to SIADH.

V. **Plan.** Treatment is essential, and effort should be made to keep sodium in the normal range especially in the preterm infant, as hyponatremia can cause future problems.

A. **Emergency measures. If the infant is having hyponatremia-induced seizures as a result of low sodium (usually <120 mEq/dL), hypertonic saline solution (3% sodium chloride) should be given.** Hyponatremic seizures usually stop with a correction of only 3–5 mEq/L. Rapid corrections (especially in chronic hyponatremia or a >8 mEq/L increase in serum sodium over 24 hours) can cause brain damage (**central pontine myelinolysis**). Suspect this in a neonate who, in the course of the correction, develops cranial nerve dysfunction and quadriparesis. MRI shows a round lesion in the central pontine area. **Once symptoms resolve** and the serum sodium is >120 mEq/dL, a slow correction can be given over 24 hours (not to exceed 8 mEq/L/d). There is ***controversy*** regarding the rate and how it should be given. Follow institutional guidelines.

1. **IV push over 15 minutes (1–3 mL/kg of 3% NaCl [513 mEq of sodium/L]).** This method should be reserved for those patients who have seizures, those with repeated apnea requiring intubation, or refractory status epilepticus from hyponatremia (***controversial***).

2. **Hourly correction.** 2 mL/kg/h of 3% NaCl can be given (should raise the sodium concentration by 2 mmol/L/h) until the sodium is >120 mmol/L.

3. **24-hour correction.** The total body deficit can be calculated (see below) and half of that is given over 12–24 hours.

4. **Anticonvulsant therapy.** Medication should be considered if seizures persist after 3% normal saline is given. ***Note:*** Use of anticonvulsants may not be effective and can be associated with apnea.

B. **General management.** Always treat the underlying disorder.

1. **Hyponatremia with hypervolemia.** Sodium and water restriction.

2. **Hyponatremia with hypovolemia.** Volume expansion with sodium and water to replace losses.

3. **Hyponatremia with normal ECF.** Water restriction.

C. **Specific management**

1. **Volume overload (dilutional hyponatremia).** Treated with fluid restriction. The total maintenance fluids can be decreased by 20 mL/kg/d, and serum sodium levels should be monitored every 6–8 hours. The underlying cause must be investigated and treated.

2. **Inadequate sodium intake**

a. **The maintenance sodium requirement for term infants is 2–4 mEq/kg/d and higher in premature infants.** Calculate the amount of sodium the patient is receiving, using the equations in Chapter 9. Readjust the IV sodium intake if it is the cause of hyponatremia.

b. **If the infant is receiving oral formula only, check the formula being used.** Low-sodium formulas such as Similac PM 60/40 or breast milk (which is low in sodium) may contribute to hyponatremia. Use of supplemental sodium chloride or a formula with higher sodium content may be necessary.

c. **Calculate the total sodium deficit using the following equation.** The result will be the amount of sodium needed to correct the hyponatremia. Usually, **only half of this amount** is given over 12–24 hours.

$$(\text{Desired sodium } [130\text{–}135 \text{ mEq/L}] - \text{Infant's sodium value}) \times$$
$$(\text{Weight } [kg] \times 0.6) = \text{Total sodium deficit}$$

3. **Increased sodium losses.** Treat the underlying cause and increase the sodium administered to replace the losses.

4. **Drug-induced hyponatremia.** If a renal salt-wasting medication such as furosemide is being given, serum sodium levels will be low even though an adequate amount of sodium is being given in the diet. An increase in sodium intake may be required, as is often the case in infants with BPD/CLD who are receiving diuretics. Most are also receiving oral feedings, so an oral sodium chloride supplement can be used. Start with 1 mEq 3 times per day with feedings and adjust as needed. Some infants may require 12–15 mEq/d. Sodium levels should be kept in the low 130s because higher levels may result in fluid retention when diuretics are used. Indomethacin-induced hyponatremia is treated with fluid restriction.

5. **SIADH. The cause of SIADH is usually obvious; if it is not, further investigation is needed** (eg, ultrasonography of the head or chest radiograph to rule out lung disease). During treatment, monitor the serum sodium, osmolality, and urine output to determine whether the patient is responding.
   a. **Seizures present or serum sodium is <120 mEq/L**
      i. **Hypertonic saline solution (3% sodium chloride).** See Section V.A.
      ii. **Lasix.** 1 mg/kg IV every 6 hours.
      iii. **Anticonvulsant therapy can be considered** (*controversial*). A case report successfully used phenytoin for a neonate with SIADH and refractory hyponatremic seizures.
      iv. **Fluid restriction.** Usually 40–60 mL/kg/d free water.
   b. **Serum sodium is >120 mEq/L without seizures:**
      i. **Fluid restriction.** Usually 40–60 mL/kg/d. This regimen does not allow for fluid loss that accompanies the use of a radiant warmer or phototherapy.
      ii. **Lasix** can also be used.

References

Baraton L, Ancel PY, Flamant C, Orsonneau JL, Darmaun D, Rozé JC. Impact of changes in serum sodium levels on 2-year neurologic outcomes for very preterm neonates. *Pediatrics.* 2009;124:e655–e661. DOI:10.1542/peds.2008-3415.

Moritz ML, Ayus JC. Hyponatremia in preterm neonates: not a benign condition. *Pediatrics.* 2009;124:e1014. DOI:10.1542/peds.2009-1869.

65 Hypotension and Shock

I. **Problem.** The nurse reports that an infant may be hypotensive and is showing signs of shock. Hypotension (diminished blood pressure [BP]) is distinct from shock, a clinical syndrome of inadequate tissue perfusion with the clinical signs noted in Section II.B. While hypotension frequently accompanies shock, there is no consensus on the exact definition of hypotension in the neonate. Normal BP values for extremely premature infants are also debated. Data are conflicting for the exact BP that requires treatment for every gestational, postnatal age, and infant weight. Some define hypotension as a BP >2 standard deviations below normal for age or below the fifth percentile. For a rapid reference for premature and term infants BP ranges, see Table 65–1 and for more detailed BP values, see Appendix C.

Table 65–1. RAPID REFERENCE BLOOD PRESSURE RANGES IN PREMATURE INFANTS ACCORDING TO BODY WEIGHT AND TERM INFANTS BASED ON BIRTH (DETAILED BLOOD PRESSURE VALUES ARE FOUND IN APPENDIX C)

Birthweight (g)	Mean (mm Hg)	Systolic (mm Hg)	Diastolic (mm Hg)
Premature infants			
501–750	38–49	50–62	26–36
751–1000	35.5–47.5	48–59	23–36
1001–1250	37.5–48	49–61	26–35
1251–1500	34.5–44.5	46–56	23–33
1501–1750	34.5–45.5	46–58	23–33
1751–2000	36–48	48–61	24–35
Term infants			
Day 1	31–63	46–94	42–57
Day 2	37–68	46–91	27–58
Day 3	36–70	51–93	26–61
Day 4	41–65	60–88	34–57

Based on data from Hegyi T, Carbone MT, Anwar M, et al. Blood pressure ranges in premature infants: I. The first hours of life. *J Pediatr.* 1994;124:627; and Kent A, Kecskes Z, Shadbolt B, Falk MC. Normative blood pressure data in the early neonatal period. *Pediatr Nephrol.* 2007;22:1335–1341.

II. **Immediate questions**

A. **What method of measurement was used?** If a BP cuff was used, be certain that it was the correct width (ie, covering two-thirds of the upper arm). A cuff that is too large gives falsely low readings. If measurements were obtained from an indwelling arterial catheter, a "dampened" waveform suggests air in the transducer or tubing or a clot in the system, and the readings are inaccurate (see also page 420).

B. **Are signs of shock present?** Signs of shock include tachycardia, poor/reduced perfusion, prolonged capillary refill time (>3–4 seconds), respiratory distress, poor tone, poor color, cold extremities (with a normal core temperature), lethargy, narrow pulse pressure, apnea and bradycardia, tachypnea, metabolic acidosis, and weak pulse.

C. **Is the urine output acceptable?** Normal urine output is ~1–2 mL/kg/h and is decreased in shock due to decreased renal perfusion. If the BP is low but the urine output is adequate, aggressive treatment may not be necessary as renal perfusion is adequate. (**Note:** An exception involves the infant with septic shock and hyperglycemia with osmotic diuresis.)

D. **Is there a history of birth asphyxia?** Birth asphyxia may be associated with myocardial dysfunction and cardiogenic shock.

E. **At the time of delivery, was there maternal bleeding** (eg, abruptio placentae or placenta previa) or was clamping of the cord delayed? These factors may be associated with loss of blood volume in the infant.

III. **Differential diagnosis. Types of shock are hypovolemic, cardiogenic, distributive** (septic, neurogenic, adrenal, anaphylactic), **obstructive,** and **dissociative.** Some of the causes are in more than one category. **Note:** Some inborn errors of metabolism resulting in hypoglycemia or hyperammonemia can mimic the presentation of shock in a newborn (eg, galactosemia, maple syrup urine disease, and others). (See Chapter 101.)

A. **Hypovolemic shock.** The **most common type of shock in a neonate** and results from an inadequate blood volume and can be secondary to hemorrhagic shock (antepartum or postpartum blood loss) or nonhemorrhagic shock (fluid and electrolyte losses). The **majority of very low birthweight (VLBW) infants** that are hypotensive are not hypovolemic.

1. Antepartum/intrapartum blood loss (often associated with asphyxia)
   a. Abruptio placentae.
   b. Placenta previa.
   c. Twin-twin transfusion.
   d. Fetomaternal hemorrhage.
   e. Others. Difficult delivery, umbilical cord tear, birth injuries (rupture of spleen and liver).
2. Postpartum blood loss
   a. Coagulation disorders (disseminated intravascular coagulation [DIC], coagulopathies).
   b. Vitamin K deficiency
   c. Iatrogenic causes (eg, loss of an arterial catheter).
   d. Birth trauma (eg, liver injury, adrenal hemorrhage, intraperitoneal hemorrhage).
   e. Pulmonary hemorrhage.
   f. Intracranial hemorrhage.
   g. Circumcision wound. Frenular artery bleed with death as the quantity of blood loss in diaper was concealed.
3. Fluid and electrolyte losses. Volume depletion is common in premature infants. Besides insensible water loss and diuretic use, sepsis, heat stress, vomiting, diarrhea, gastrointestinal (GI) abnormalities, and iatrogenic are other causes.

B. Cardiogenic shock. Inadequate tissue perfusion secondary to myocardial dysfunction. It implies primary failure of the heart as a pump and is relatively uncommon in the neonate.

1. Severe birth asphyxia can cause low cardiac output.
2. Metabolic problems (eg, severe hypoglycemia [infant of diabetic mother], hypocalcemia, acidemia) can cause decreased cardiac output with a decrease in BP. Adrenal insufficiency and inborn errors of metabolism can present with cardiac involvement including congestive heart failure, arrhythmias, cardiomyopathy, and conduction disturbances.
3. Congenital heart disease with left-sided obstructive lesions are the most common to present with shock after the patent ductus arteriosus (PDA) closes: hypoplastic left heart syndrome, congenital aortic stenosis, coarctation of the aorta, interruption of the aortic arch, and others with systemic outflow obstruction. Other congenital heart diseases can present with shock but are not as common.
4. Cardiomyopathies.
5. Persistent pulmonary hypertension.
6. PDA in a premature infant can cause cardiac failure and hypotension. Extremely low birthweight (ELBW) infants often present only with hypotension without a murmur.
7. Arrhythmias/dysrhythmias can cause a decrease in cardiac output. Examples include supraventricular tachycardia (SVT), ventricular tachycardia, ventricular fibrillation, complete atrioventricular (AV) block, atrial flutter, and others.
8. Infectious agents (bacterial, viral, or protozoan) can cause myocarditis and myocardial dysfunction in addition to septic shock.

C. Distributive shock includes septic, neurogenic, adrenal, anaphylactic, and others. There are abnormalities within the vascular beds that can cause blood volume to be distributed inadequately to organs and tissues. There is not a definite volume loss but inappropriate vasodilatation, dysfunction of the endothelium with a capillary leak, loss of vascular tone, or a combination of the above. Because the intravascular fluid volume is maldistributed, signs of shock appear. **The most common form of distributive shock in the neonate is sepsis.**

1. **Septic shock.** Endotoxemia occurs, with release of vasodilator substances and resulting hypotension. It usually involves gram-negative organisms such as *Escherichia coli, Klebsiella* spp., *Enterobacter, Pseudomonas,* and *Proteus* but can also occur with gram-positive organisms. Viruses such as herpes simplex and enteroviruses can also cause septic shock. Fungal infections such as Candida primarily occur in ELBW infants and can cause sepsis and shock. DIC can be a consequence of sepsis.

2. **Neurogenic shock.** Rare in neonates, this is secondary to decreased sympathetic activity and leads to a lack of vascular tone and vasodilation with decreased tissue perfusion. Birth asphyxia and intracranial hemorrhage can both cause hypotension.

3. **Anaphylactic shock.** Very rare in neonates, this is caused by a hypersensitivity response. There is vasodilation, increased capillary permeability, and fluid shifts with severe hypotension and circulatory collapse. Typical causes include food (through breast milk), cow's milk, formulas, medications (β-lactam antibiotics), penicillin (PCN), antipyretics (ibuprofen and neuromuscular blockers), intravenous immune globulin, hepatitis B immune globulin (HBIG; mom was a hepatitis B virus [HBV] carrier), parenteral nutrition, hepatitis B vaccine, cold exposure, latex, vaccinations, and idiopathic anaphylaxis, and all have been reported in infants.

4. **Adrenal shock.** Caused by endocrine disorders; complete 21-hydroxylase deficiency and adrenal hemorrhage are the most common. Suspect adrenogenital syndrome with low serum sodium, high serum potassium, and hypotension.

5. **Other causes of abnormal peripheral vasoregulation.** Necrotizing enterocolitis (NEC), extracorporeal membrane oxygenation/extracorporeal life support (ECMO/ECLS), respiratory distress syndrome (RDS), major surgery, asphyxia, and hydrops fetalis, and others.

D. **Obstructive shock.** Any obstruction of venous blood return (tension pneumothorax, pericardial tamponade, diaphragmatic hernia, severe pulmonary interstitial emphysema, air embolism, specific obstructive congenital heart disease [critical aortic stenosis, coarctation of the aorta, hypoplastic left heart syndrome, interrupted aortic arch, and others]).

E. **Dissociative shock.** Inadequate oxygen-releasing capacity such as in severe anemia or methemoglobinemia.

F. **Drug-induced hypotension.** Drugs such as tolazoline, tubocurarine, nitroprusside, sedatives, magnesium sulfate, digitalis, and barbiturates may cause vasodilation and a drop in BP. Transient hypotension has been seen after exogenous surfactant administration.

G. **Extreme prematurity and hypotension.** Hypotension is very common in ELBW infants (60–100% at 24–26 weeks) and VLBW infants (40% at 27–29 weeks). Hypotension in this group of infants is rarely secondary to hypovolemia and more likely due to adrenocortical insufficiency, poor vascular tone, immature catecholamine responses, and transient left ventricular dysfunction. Hypotension with evidence of end-organ dysfunction in ELBW infants is associated with intraventricular hemorrhage/periventricular leukomalacia (IVH/PVL). Blood pressure usually improves spontaneously during the first 24 hours in an ELBW infant. In VLBW infants in the first 3 days of life a mean arterial pressure <30 mm Hg or a mean arterial pressure with a number less than the gestational age in weeks of the infant is used to define hypotension (eg, mean BP <27 for a 27-week neonate). See Appendix Figure C–1 for mean blood pressure for infants <1000 g.

IV. **Database**

A. **Physical examination.** Particular attention is given to signs of blood loss (eg, intracranial or intra-abdominal bleeding), sepsis, or clinical signs of shock (cool extremities, mottling of the skin, tachycardia, decreased urine output). Anaphylaxis in an infant is hard to diagnose. Sudden onset of lethargy or hypotonia can be seen. Normal

Table 67–1. **TIME OF FIRST STOOL BASED ON A STUDY OF 500 TERM AND PRETERM INFANTS**

Hours	Preterm Infants (%) (majority >32 wk)[a]	Full-Term Infants (%)	Post-Term Infants (%)
Delivery room (0)	5.0	16.7	32
1–8	32.5	59.5	68
9–16	63.8	91.1	88
17–24	76.3	98.5	100
24–48	98.8	100.0	—
>48	100.0	—	—

Percentages are cumulative. Preterm: only 3 infants <32 weeks in the study.
Data from Clark DA. Times of first void and stool in 500 newborns. *Pediatrics.* 1977;60:457.

meconium can be passed and then a decrease or no stools occur. If a stool has never been passed, imperforate anus or some degree of lower intestinal obstruction may be present. Table 67–1 shows the time after birth at which the first stool is typically passed.

B. **What is the gestational age and birthweight of the infant?** An inverse relationship between gestational age, birthweight, and meconium passage exists. Premature and very low birthweight (VLBW) infants commonly have a delayed passage of stool because of immaturity of interstitial cells of the colon, increased viscosity of meconium (preemies have lack of water in stool), and lack of triggering effect of enteral feeds on gut hormones when the patient is maintained NPO. Studies show the older the gestational age, the shorter time to the first stool. Delayed meconium passage can be as high as 80% in VLBW infants. Remember that failure of a full-term or post-term infant to pass meconium within 24 hours may signify an intestinal obstruction. In preterm infants it may not.

C. **Were maternal drugs used that could cause a paralytic ileus with delayed passage of stool?** Magnesium sulfate, which is used to slow the premature onset of labor, may cause paralytic ileus. Narcotics for pain control or use of heroin by the mother may also cause delayed passage of stool in the neonate. Antenatal betamethasone exposure leads to earlier stool passage, and antenatal exposure to magnesium sulfate has conflicting results—some studies show it does not affect the timing of the first stool in premature infants and others state it was associated with delayed stool passage.

D. **Are there any other congenital abnormalities and associated syndromes?** Hirschsprung disease is associated with trisomy 21, neurofibromatosis, Waardenburg syndrome, multiple endocrine neoplasia (MEN) type 2, central hypoventilation syndrome, and cardiac septal defects.

III. **Differential diagnosis**

A. **Constipation.** This is just in infants who have already passed a stool and then fail to pass one. Infants have a mean of 4 stools per day during the first week of life; this gradually decreases to a mean average of 1.7 per day at age 2 years. Some breast-fed infants do not have stools for several days.

B. **Bowel obstruction.** Infants with distal small bowel (ileum) or colonic obstruction can present with abdominal distension and delayed passage of meconium. **Small bowel obstruction** usually presents with bilious vomiting with or without abdominal distension, and meconium can be passed, but it usually progresses to a decrease or no stools. **Large bowel obstruction** usually presents with **abdominal distension and no stools.**

1. **Large bowel obstruction**

a. **Meconium plug syndrome.** An obstruction in the lower colon and rectum caused by meconium. It is a transient form of distal colonic or rectal obstruction. Incidence is 1 in 500–1000 newborns. (***Note:*** A rectal biopsy should be considered in all these patients because they have an increased incidence [10–15%] of Hirschsprung disease.) Meconium plug syndrome is more common in infants of diabetic mothers (small left colon syndrome) and in premature infants (microcolon of prematurity).

   b. **Small left colon syndrome.** A functional distal bowel obstruction in which the plug extends to the splenic flexure, caused by transient dysmotility in the descending colon. Usually seen in term infants. Approximately 50% have a history of maternal diabetes, and most don't pass meconium in the first 24 hours of life. The others have sepsis, hypoglycemia, hypothyroidism, or increased magnesium. **Microcolon of prematurity** is the preterm equivalent of small left colon syndrome. Functional abnormality with failure of the small bowel contents to pass into the colon in utero. The majority of mothers had toxemia and magnesium sulfate.

   c. **Hirschsprung disease (congenital aganglionic megacolon).** Accounts for ~15% of infants who have delayed passage of stool. It occurs in 1 in 4000 live births. A functional obstruction is caused by aganglionosis of cells in Meissner and Auerbach plexus in the rectum and variable amounts of the distal colon. The affected segment of colon and rectum are aperistaltic. Typically the infant is full term and presents with delayed passage of meconium. Sixty to ninety percent of infants with Hirschsprung disease fail to pass meconium in the first 24–48 hours of life. It has a sex-dependent penetrance (4 males to 1 female) and 8% of patients have Down syndrome. It is more common in white males.

   d. **Anorectal malformations (1 in 4000–8000 infants)** such as imperforate anus (or anal atresia), which can be high or low type with a fistula or anal stenosis. An infant with an imperforate anus may pass meconium if a fistula exists. There are a high percentage of associated anomalies with anal atresia (70%). One example is the VATER/VACTERL (**v**ertebral defects, **a**nal atresia, **t**racheo**e**sophageal fistula, and **r**adial or **r**enal dysplasia/**v**ertebral defects, **a**nal atresia, **c**ardiac defects, **t**racheoesophageal fistula with **e**sophageal atresia, **r**enal defects and radial upper **l**imb hypoplasia) association. **Anal stenosis** can occur and may present with a small, tight anus, sometimes with a dot of meconium present.

2. **Small bowel obstruction**

   a. **Meconium ileus.** Occurs when meconium becomes obstructed in the terminal ileum. It can present with a failure to pass meconium. It occurs in 15% of newborns with cystic fibrosis (CF); 90% of patients with meconium ileum have CF and thus should be tested for it. It is the most common presentation of CF in the neonatal period.

   b. **Intestinal atresias.** Atresias most commonly occur in the ileum, followed by the duodenum, jejunum, and then colon. Bilious emesis, abdominal distension, and failure to pass meconium are seen; jaundice is possible.

   c. **Other small bowel obstructions.** (Duodenal atresia, malrotation and volvulus, and meconium peritonitis.) Usually meconium is passed and then they progress to a decrease or no stools.

3. **Adhesions.** Postoperatively, such as after surgery for necrotizing enterocolitis (NEC), there is a 30% chance of having adhesions.

4. **Rare causes. Colonic stenosis/atresia:** The colon is the least common site of stenosis and atresia. See dilated proximal intestine on radiograph. **Hypoganglionosis:** a reduced number of ganglion cells; presents with symptoms similar to Hirschsprung disease and can occur with Hirschsprung disease. **Neuronal intestinal dysplasia type A** is hypoplasia or aplasia of the sympathetic innervation of the myenteric plexus and mucosa, with inflammation of the mucosa; it presents with symptoms similar to Hirschsprung disease. **Megacystis-microcolon intestinal hypoperistalsis syndrome (Berdon syndrome)** has urinary retention, dilated small bowel, microcolon, megacystis (giant bladder), and hydronephrosis. Pathology reveals that ganglion cells are present.

C. **Other causes/associations**
1. **Prematurity/VLBW infants.** (See Section II.B.) Delayed passage of meconium is common. Immature colon and delayed first feeding with patent ductus arteriosus (PDA), respiratory distress syndrome (RDS), mechanical ventilation, and uteroplacental insufficiency is associated with delayed passage in VLBW infants. These infants usually do not have abdominal distension or bilious nasogastric aspirates.
2. **Infection. Sepsis is the most common infection causing delayed passage.** Other infections that can result in intestinal dysfunction include pneumonia/enterovirus infection/omphalitis/peritonitis.
3. **Respiratory distress syndrome.** Infants with RDS can have delayed gastric emptying which can cause dysmotility of the intestine.
4. **Electrolyte abnormalities.** Hypokalemia, hyponatremia, hypercalcemia, and hypermagnesemia. Fetal hypoglycemia can also impair neonatal intestinal motility.
5. **Maternal medications.** Magnesium sulfate, ganglionic blocking agents or illicit drugs (opiates, heroin), neuroleptics, antidepressants.
6. **Infant medications.** Theophylline, opiates, narcotic analgesic therapy.
7. **Hypothyroidism (most common).** Other endocrinopathies—adrenal insufficiency, hyperparathyroidism, adrenal bleeding.
8. **Ileus.** This can cause a delayed passage of stool.
9. **Idiopathic.**
10. **Other less common causes.** Congestive heart failure, hyperbilirubinemia, renal vein thrombosis, hypovolemia, PDA, embolism/thrombosis.

IV. **Database**
A. **Prenatal history may reveal abnormalities on the fetal ultrasound.** Polyhydramnios can be seen in jejuno-ileal atresia. Extraluminal meconium calcifications can be seen with meconium ileus. The classic double bubble of duodenal atresia can be seen on prenatal ultrasound.
B. **Physical examination.** Special attention to the abdomen is important. First, inspect the anus (eg, 5th digit probe, rectal thermometer, or soft feeding tube). If patency is in question, consult with surgery on the best way to further evaluate. Check for abdominal distention or rigidity, bowel sounds, and evidence of a mass. A rectal examination will also determine whether muscle tone is adequate, and it may reveal hardened stool in the rectum. Infants with Hirschsprung disease typically have a distended abdomen (63–91% of neonates) and bilious vomiting (19–37%).
C. **Laboratory findings**
1. **Complete blood count (CBC) with differential and blood culture** to rule out sepsis. A urine culture under sterile conditions should also be done.
2. **Urinary drug screening** on both mother and infant to detect maternal use of narcotics.
D. **Imaging and other studies**
1. **Plain film abdominal radiographs.** A flat plate and upright film of the abdomen should be obtained to look for ileus or bowel obstruction in any infant who has not passed a stool within 48 hours of birth. The radiograph does not tell if it is small or large bowel obstruction. Typically, dilated loops of bowel, air-fluid levels, and no air in the rectum will be seen. With Hirschsprung disease or meconium plug, distention of the colon with multiple air-fluid levels is seen.
   a. **Hirschsprung disease.** Gas and stool in the colon.
   b. **Meconium plug.** Distension of the small and large intestine, usually no air-fluid levels are seen. Distal obstruction with absence of air in the rectum can be seen.
   c. **Meconium ileus.** Distended bowel, some air-fluid levels. Right lower abdomen: meconium and air with ground glass appearance.
   d. **Small left colon syndrome.** Dilated intestinal loops and air-fluid levels.
2. **Contrast enema. Abdominal radiographs with contrast enema** should be obtained in all cases of delayed passage of stool if the patient is symptomatic.

These will help define the disease process and may be therapeutic. **Microcolon** is a radiologic finding of an abnormally small caliber of colon and usually means distal ileal obstruction: ileal atresia, colonic atresia, colon aganglionosis, volvulus, duplication.

    a. **Hirschsprung disease.** A transition zone is seen with marked dilatation, presence of barium after 24 hours.

    b. **Meconium plug syndrome.** The contrast enema is a diagnostic test for meconium plug syndrome because it shows the outline of meconium and meconium plugs.

    c. **Meconium ileus.** Microcolon is seen.

    d. **Meconium obstruction of prematurity.** Meconium plugs are seen in a small microcolon, with distal ileum obstruction. Can see distal ileum impacted with meconium.

    e. **Small left colon syndrome.** Short colon with lack of tortuosity. A transition zone can be seen.

3. **Anorectal manometry (ARM).** Using an anorectal micromanometric sleeve assembly, it records changes in anal pressure during and after rectal distension. If ganglion cells are present, a fall in anal pressure is seen. In Hirschsprung disease there is absent rectosphincteric reflex. Use of this test is difficult to perform and time-consuming, and requires patience in neonates. Serial manometry may prevent the need for rectal biopsy. Premature infants after 30 weeks' gestation have normal anorectal pressures and have a normal anorectal reflex.

4. **Full-thickness rectal biopsy/renal suction biopsy.** Either by suction anal biopsy or transanal wedge resection is the gold standard for diagnosis of Hirschsprung disease. Histology demonstrates the absence of ganglion cells and presence of acetyl cholinesterase–positive hypertrophic nerve fibers.

5. **Rectosigmoid index (RSI).** The diameter of the rectosigmoid colon and can be used to help diagnose Hirschsprung disease.

6. **Serum proteins.** Three specific protein markers have been identified for Hirschsprung disease, which will allow for early screening and diagnosis, but are not in use yet.

V. **Plan**

  A. **Rule out and treat any underlying etiologies** such as electrolyte abnormalities, infection, hypothyroidism, respiratory distress syndrome, medications in the mother or infant, and others.

  B. **Premature infants. Need to rule out pathologic cause versus normal delayed passage of stool.** As meconium passage can be delayed in infants who are premature and have a low birthweight, delayed passage of stool does not always predict gastrointestinal (GI) disease. It is best to only do a diagnostic workup for intestinal obstruction in those premature infants with other signs of GI disease (eg, progressive abdominal distension and vomiting).

  C. **Term infants** with delayed passage need to be evaluated earlier as failure to pass meconium in a term infant is highly suspicious for intestinal obstruction.

  D. **Specific treatment plans**

    1. **Constipation**

      a. **Digital rectal stimulation is the first step.**

      b. **Glycerin suppositories** can be used if digital rectal stimulation is unsuccessful. Enemas are not recommended. Mineral oil or stimulant laxatives are also not recommended. Saline irrigation is used in some NICUs.

    2. **Anorectal abnormality. Imperforate anus.**

      a. **Obtain immediate pediatric surgical consultation.**

      b. **Insert a double-lumen nasogastric (NG) tube for decompression.**

      c. **Look for other congenital anomalies.** Genitourinary tract abnormalities are frequently seen with imperforate anus.

3. Bowel obstruction
   a. Meconium plug
      i. Contrast enema. Performed using an agent such as Omnipaque 240 to verify meconium plug. In infants with this problem, the study usually reveals a normal-sized colon with filling defects.
      ii. If meconium plug is verified by contrast enema. Repeated water-soluble enemas are usually given every 4–6 hours.
      iii. Acetylcysteine (Mucomyst) enema. If water-soluble enemas are ineffective, a dilute 4% solution of acetylcysteine and water can be used as an enema to break down the meconium so the plug can be passed.
      iv. If normal stooling occurs. Monitor closely.
      v. If an abnormal pattern of stooling recurs. Further workup (eg, rectal biopsy) is necessary to rule out Hirschsprung disease, which ultimately will be diagnosed in half of these patients.
   b. Meconium ileus
      i. Contrast enema may reveal microcolon. Evidence of perforation, volvulus, or atresia may also be seen.
      ii. Obstruction can be treated with Mucomyst enemas (see Section V.D.3a.iii). Adequate fluid and electrolyte replacement must be given.
      iii. Antegrade agents in NG tube (N-acetylcysteine [NAC] or Gastrografin) have been entertained by some, but there is a potential for side effects and a lack of studies.
      iv. Operative management may be necessary in patients not relieved by enemas with passage of meconium within several hours.
   c. Hirschsprung disease
      i. Fluid resuscitation, rectal irrigation, and antibiotics are important to initially treat the enterocolitis and decrease the risk of mortality.
      ii. Initial radiograph shows marked gaseous distension of colon with undilated rectum.
      iii. Contrast enema usually shows a distal narrowed, aganglionic segment leading to a dilated proximal segment. A transition zone, irregular colonic contractions, irregular mucosa, and an abnormal rectosigmoid index (RSI) all suggest Hirschsprung disease.
      iv. Rectal biopsy, the definitive diagnosis, is performed to confirm aganglionosis.
      v. Surgical repair with a 2- or 3-stage procedure. Colostomy is usually indicated once the diagnosis is confirmed.
   d. Adhesions. Surgery is usually necessary to lyse the adhesions if a trial of nasogastric decompression fails.
   e. Incarcerated hernia. This is a surgical emergency.
   f. Malrotation
      i. Contrast enema reveals an abnormally placed cecum.
      ii. Surgical correction is necessary.
   g. Volvulus
      i. Contrast enema reveals obstruction at the midtransverse colon.
      ii. Surgery should be an immediate intervention.
   h. Intussusception. Hydrostatic reduction is attempted. If unsuccessful, surgery with operative reduction or resection is done.
   i. Duodenal atresia. Decompression with nasogastric suction and surgery.
   j. Small left colon syndrome. Contrast enema is done and is usually diagnostic and therapeutic. Surgery is indicated if the obstruction is recurrent or if there is a perforation.
   k. Microcolon of prematurity. Contrast enema examination, close observation of infants with possibility of surgical intervention if there are complications.

      l. **Meconium obstruction of prematurity.** Diluted contrast enema is the gold standard for diagnosis and treatment. Surgical management may be necessary if spontaneous intestinal perforation occurs or worsening of symptoms.

    m. **Ileus caused by sepsis**

        i. **Broad-spectrum antibiotics** are initiated after a sepsis workup is performed (see Chapter 130). Intravenous ampicillin and gentamicin are usually recommended. Vancomycin may be substituted for ampicillin if staphylococcal infection is suspected (for dosages, see Chapter 148).

       ii. **A nasogastric tube** should be placed to decompress the bowel. The infant should not be fed enterally.

    n. **Ileus caused by NEC.** See Chapter 113.

    o. **Ileus caused by hypokalemia**

        i. **Treat underlying metabolic abnormalities.** Correct potassium levels if low (see Chapter 63).

       ii. **Place a nasogastric tube to rest the bowel.**

  4. **Prematurity.** Conservative treatment is usually recommended in infants who are not vomiting but have progressive abdominal distention, even if microcolon is seen. Treatment consists of a low osmolality water-soluble contrast enema for passage of the stool. Consult a pediatric radiologist for appropriate contrast enema to be used.

  5. **Hypothyroidism.** If the serum T_4 and TSH levels confirm the presence of hypothyroidism, thyroid replacement therapy is indicated. Consult with an endocrinologist before starting therapy. See Chapter 140.

68 No Urine Output in 24 Hours

  I. **Problem.** Urine output has been scant or absent for 24 hours. One hundred percent of healthy premature, full-term, and post-term infants void by 24 hours of age. **Oliguria** is defined as urine output <1.0 mL/kg/h for 24 hours. **Anuria** is defined as absence of urine output usually by 48 hours of age. **Oliguria** is one of the **clinical hallmarks** of **renal failure.** Decreased urine output can be from mild dehydration or acute renal failure (ARF) or acute kidney injury (AKI). ARF/AKI is an acute renal dysfunction and occurs when there is a decrease in glomerular filtration rate, an increase in creatinine and nitrogenous waste products with the loss of ability to regulate fluid and electrolytes. Incidence of neonatal ARF/AKI is around 6–24%. There is a high percentage of ARF/AKI in very low birthweight infants, infants postcongenital heart surgery, infants on extracorporeal membrane oxygenation/extracorporeal life support (ECMO/ECLS) (especially with a congenital diaphragmatic hernia), and infants with perinatal depression.

  II. **Immediate questions**

    A. **Is the bladder palpable?** If a distended bladder is present, it is usually palpable. A palpable bladder suggests there is urine in the bladder. **Credé maneuver** (manual compression of the bladder) may initiate voiding, especially in infants receiving medications causing muscle paralysis.

    B. **Has bladder catheterization been performed?** Catheterization determines whether urine is present in the bladder. It is commonly done in more mature infants.

    C. **What is the blood pressure?** Hypotension can cause decreased renal perfusion and urine output. Hypertension may indicate renal/renovascular disease (if severe, suspect renal artery or venous thrombosis).

    D. **Has the infant ever voided? Did the infant void and was it not recorded on the bedside chart?** If the infant has never voided, consider bilateral renal agenesis,

Table 68–1. **TIME OF FIRST VOID BASED ON A STUDY OF 500 TERM AND PRETERM INFANTS**

Hours	Full-Term Infants (%)[a]	Preterm Infants (%)[a]
Delivery room (0)	12.9	21.2
1–8	51.1	83.7
9–16	91.1	98.7
17–24	100.0	100.0

[a]Percentages are cumulative.
Data from Clark DA. Times of first void and stool in 500 newborns. *Pediatrics.* 1977;60:457.

renovascular accident, or obstruction. Table 68–1 shows the time after birth at which the first voiding occurs. Remember: voiding can be missed (occurred in the delivery room or with the parents and was not recorded). Approximately 13–21% of infants void in the delivery room.

E. **Did the mother have oligohydramnios?** One of the etiologies of oligohydramnios (decrease in amniotic fluid) can be caused by a decrease in fetal urine production. This can be caused by renal problems such as decreased renal perfusion, obstructive uropathy, and congenital absence of renal tissue (renal agenesis, cystic dysplasia, and ureteral atresia).

F. **Is there gross hematuria?** Gross hematuria suggests intrinsic renal disease.

G. **What medications was the mother on during her pregnancy?** Certain medications (eg, angiotensin-converting enzyme [ACE] inhibitors, nonsteroidal anti-inflammatory drugs [NSAIDS]), if given to the mother during her pregnancy, may interfere with fetal nephrogenesis which can result in fetal renal injury and lead to acute kidney injury in the newborn. ACE inhibitors during pregnancy can cause renal tubular dysgenesis in the infant.

H. **Does the infant have a congenital renal disease? Did the prenatal ultrasound suggest kidney disease?** Acute renal failure in the newborn may have a prenatal onset. Renal agenesis, renal dysplasia, polycystic kidney disease, and congenital nephrotic syndrome, or any obstruction can all cause acute renal failure in the newborn.

I. **Did the mother have diabetes?** Infants of diabetic mothers have an increased risk of renal anomalies (renal agenesis, hydronephrosis, and ureteral duplication).

III. **Differential diagnosis.** A delay in urination can be from mild dehydration or ARF/AKI. For a complete discussion of ARF/AKI, see Chapter 123.

A. **Mild dehydration.** An infant may have decreased urination the first couple of days of life, especially if the infant is breast-feeding. Inadequate breast milk production can cause dehydration. Laboratory findings are usually normal or may show a minimal change.

B. **Acute renal failure/acute kidney injury.** Definitions vary and can be based on serum creatinine (see Section IV.C.1). ARF/AKI can be caused by prerenal, renal, and postrenal causes.

1. **Prerenal failure (most common type).** Normal kidneys with inadequate or decreased renal blood flow (perfusion). This leads to decreased renal function. **Renal hypoperfusion** can be caused by a **true volume depletion** (hemorrhage, dehydration, third space losses) or a **decreased effective blood volume** (a disease process that results in decreased perfusion to the kidney such as congestive heart failure or cardiac tamponade). Common causes in the neonatal intensive care unit (NICU) are

a. **Hemorrhage (perinatal or postnatal).**

b. **Dehydration.**

c. **Sepsis.** Renal failure occurs in 26% of neonates with septic shock.

d. **Necrotizing enterocolitis.**

e. **Respiratory distress syndrome.**

f. **Shock and hypotension.**

g. **Gastrointestinal losses.**

h. **Third space losses.**

i. **Cardiac.** Congestive heart failure, patent ductus arteriosus, congenital heart disease/cardiac surgery, pericarditis, cardiac tamponade.

j. **Polycythemia** can cause a decrease in GFR, oliguria, hematuria, and renal vein thrombosis.

k. **Infants requiring ECMO/ECLS** can experience fluid overload and decreased renal blood flow.

l. **Hypoalbuminemia.**

m. **Medications.** Any medications that can decrease renal blood flow can lead to prerenal disease. These include indomethacin, NSAIDS, aminoglycosides, amphotericin, adrenergic drugs (phenylephrine eye drops), and ACE inhibitors (captopril).

2. **Intrinsic renal disease (kidney injury).** This occurs due to structural renal damage to the tubules, glomeruli, or interstitium. Most often it is renal tubular dysfunction caused by an acute insult. Acute tubular necrosis (ischemic, drug, or toxin induced), glomerular lesions, and vascular lesions make up most of intrinsic renal failure.

a. **Acute tubular necrosis.** Most common cause of intrinsic renal disease and can be secondary to shock, dehydration, toxins, perinatal asphyxia, cardiac surgery, ischemic or hypoxic insults, drug induced or IV contrast media. Perinatal asphyxia is the most common cause of acute tubular necrosis. There is a large percentage of infants with severe perinatal asphyxia who have renal failure (25% of cases are oliguric and 15% are anuric). **Prolonged prerenal failure** that is not treated will progress to acute tubular necrosis.

b. **Interstitial nephritis.** Either drug induced or idiopathic.

c. **Congenital renal anomalies.** Renal tubular dysgenesis, renal agenesis (Potter syndrome), polycystic kidney disease, congenital nephrotic syndrome, hypoplastic or dysplastic kidneys.

d. **Infections.** Acute pyelonephritis, sepsis, gram-negative infections, candidiasis, and congenital infections (toxoplasmosis, cytomegalovirus, syphilis).

e. **Vascular lesions.** Bilateral renal artery thrombosis or bilateral renal vein thrombosis. Ischemic or hypoxic insults (twin-to-twin transfusion, abruptio placentae, or perinatal asphyxia) can cause renal cortical necrosis.

f. **Nephrotoxic medications.** Some **nephrotoxic medications** commonly used in the NICU include aminoglycosides, vancomycin, acyclovir, NSAIDS, IV contrast media, ACE inhibitors (eg, captopril, enalapril), and amphotericin B. Nephrotoxic ARF/AKI is usually associated with aminoglycoside antibiotics and NSAIDS that are used to close a patent ductus arteriosus. Diuretics may increase the nephrotoxicity of other medications (eg, NSAIDS).

g. **Endogenous toxins (rare).** Uric acid (uric acid nephropathy), myoglobin, free hemoglobin.

3. **Postrenal causes.** (Where urine is formed but not passed.) More common in newborn infants than older infants. Caused by a mechanical or functional obstruction to the flow of urine. The obstruction can be in the upper tract such as bilateral ureteropelvic junction obstruction or lower tract such as posterior urethral valves.

a. **Neurogenic bladder** from myelomeningocele or medications such as pancuronium or heavy sedation.

b. **Obstruction for any reason in a solitary kidney.**

c. **Meatal stenosis (usually males).**

d. **Bilateral ureteral obstruction** (bilateral ureteropelvic junction obstruction).

e. **Urethral stricture.**

f. **Posterior urethral valves (males only)** may also be complicated by bladder rupture.

g. **Extrinsic compression** (eg, sacrococcygeal teratoma).

h. **Drugs.** Certain medications (eg, acyclovir and sulfonamides) can precipitate within the tubules and cause obstruction.

i. **Systemic candidiasis with bilateral ureteropelvic fungal bezoar formation** (fungal balls causing obstruction).

j. **Spontaneous rupture of the bladder** with anuric renal insufficiency.

k. **Occult ureteropelvic junction obstruction** presenting as anuria.

l. **Imperforate hymen (female)** causing hydrometrocolpos, anuria, and bilateral hydronephrosis.

IV. **Database**

A. **Prenatal and maternal history.** Review for oligohydramnios, genetic renal disorders, list of maternal medications. Was there any risk of infection? Did bleeding occur during the delivery? Did perinatal asphyxia occur? Was there maternal hypovolemia?

B. **Physical examination.** First, determine the state of hydration. Is the infant dehydrated? Is there evidence of congestive heart failure? Is the infant edematous? Does the infant have hypertension/hypotension? Examination of the abdomen may reveal bladder distention (bladder outlet obstruction), abdominal masses, or ascites (ruptured obstructed urinary tract). Signs of renal disorders (eg, Potter facies [low-set ears, inner canthal crease]) should be noted. Dysmorphic features suggestive of renal disease include single umbilical artery, hypospadias, anorectal abnormalities, vertebral anomalies, abnormal ears, and esophageal atresia. Urinary ascites may be seen with posterior urethral valves. Oligohydramnios suggests possible renal problems.

1. **Prerenal.** Signs of volume depletion (tachycardia and hypotension).

2. **Intrinsic renal.** Edema, signs of congestive heart failure, hypertension. Palpable kidneys may mean polycystic kidney, hydronephrosis, or tumors.

3. **Postrenal.** Poor urinary stream, enlarged bladder, and dribbling of urine; urinary ascites with rupture.

C. **Laboratory studies.** The following laboratory tests can help establish the diagnosis in cases of low urine output. Interpret the results as outlined in Table 123–1. Remember blood urea nitrogen (BUN) and creatinine levels will reflect maternal function shortly after birth.

1. **Serum creatinine is used to define ARF/AKI and multiple definitions exist.**

a. **Persistent elevation of serum creatinine** or a serum creatinine ≥1.5 mg/dL is diagnostic of acute renal failure (if maternal renal function normal).

b. **Definition and staging for ARF/AKI based on serum creatinine proposed by Jetton and Askenazi:**

i. **No ARF/AKI.** No change in serum creatinine or an increase <0.3 mg/dL from a previous trough level.

ii. **Stage 1 ARF/AKI.** An increase in serum creatinine of 0.3 mg/dL or 1.5 to 2 times from the previous trough level.

iii. **Stage 2 ARF/AKI.** An increase in the serum creatinine by 2 to 3 times from the previous trough level.

iv. **Stage 3 AFR/AKI.** A serum creatinine ≥ 2.5 mg/dL, or a 3 times increase from the previous trough level, or the need for dialysis.

2. **Serum electrolytes and blood urea nitrogen also help to evaluate renal function.** An increased BUN and BUN/serum creatinine >20 are seen in prerenal oliguria. BUN/creatinine ratio of 10–15 can be seen in intrinsic renal damage. Electrolytes can be abnormal, especially potassium (hyperkalemia) with renal failure.

3. **Complete blood and platelet count.** An abnormal complete blood count can be seen in sepsis. Thrombocytopenia or polycythemia can be seen in bilateral renal vein thrombosis.

4. **Urinalysis.** Most likely normal in prerenal disease and urinary tract obstruction. May reveal white blood cells, suggesting a urinary tract infection. Red blood cells, tubular cells, and proteinuria suggest intrinsic renal disease.

Erythrocyte casts are seen in glomerulonephritis. Protein in the urine can indicate glomerular disease. Epithelial casts and brown granular casts can be seen in acute tubular necrosis.

5. **Arterial blood pH.** A metabolic acidosis can be seen in anything that causes hypovolemia, hypoperfusion, or hypotension, such as sepsis.

6. **Urinary indices.** See Table 123–1. Osmolality, urine sodium, urine-to-plasma creatinine ratio, fractional excretion of sodium, and renal failure index can help in the evaluation of deciding if the renal failure is prerenal or intrinsic.

7. **Urinary neutrophil gelatinase-associated lipocalin levels at birth.** May be able to predict renal function earlier than serum creatinine in very low birthweight infants.

D. **Imaging and other studies**

1. **Renal ultrasonography with Doppler flow studies of the abdomen and kidneys** will rule out urinary tract obstruction and help evaluate for other renal, congenital disorder, or vascular abnormalities. **Doppler examination** of renal blood flow can diagnose renal vascular thrombosis.

2. **Abdominal radiograph studies** may reveal ascites or masses. Spina bifida or an absent sacrum suggests neurogenic bladder.

3. **Voiding cystourethrography** can help diagnose lesions of the lower tract that cause obstruction if bladder outlet obstruction is suspected. It can also rule out vesicoureteral reflux.

4. **Radionuclide renal scanning** may be helpful in obstruction.

V. **Plan.** For management of renal failure, see Chapter 123.

A. **Decreased urine output, no evidence of renal failure based on laboratory findings or clinical examination.** For mild **dehydration** only an increase in fluids (IV) or feedings may be necessary. For an infant only on breast-feeding who is dehydrated, supplement breast-feeding with formula.

B. **Initial evaluation if renal failure suspected**

1. **Bladder catheterization.** This is done to see if urine is being made and to rule out lower urinary tract obstruction. It will not help in renal dysfunction or upper urinary tract obstruction. It may be helpful to keep an indwelling catheter in short term for strict intake and output (I&O).

2. **Evaluation of laboratory and ultrasound results.** Based on the laboratory results and ultrasound, one should be able to identify whether the infant has prerenal, renal, or postrenal failure.

3. **Fluid challenge for diagnosis and initial management.** A fluid challenge can be given in an infant without evidence of heart failure or volume overload (10–20 mL/kg of normal saline IV over 1–2 hours). If no response, this can be repeated once. An increase in urine output of ≥1 mL/kg/h indicates a **prerenal cause.** No response suggests **intrinsic renal disease.**

4. **Discontinue or restrict potassium from IV fluids.** Restrict intake of phosphates.

5. **Evaluate the infant's medications.** Adjust doses if necessary. Discontinue any nephrotoxic medications. **If nephrotoxic medications** cannot be discontinued, reduce the dose or use the minimal effective dose if possible.

6. **Strict I&O should be done.** Weight the infant every 12 hours.

7. **For hypotension.** Dopamine may increase renal perfusion.

C. **Prerenal failure.** The goal is to restore and maintain adequate renal perfusion. Because the kidneys are normal, prerenal failure is reversible once renal perfusion is restored.

1. **Treat the specific cause** (eg, sepsis, NEC, and others).

2. **Provide volume resuscitation to restore renal perfusion.** Depending how much fluid was given during the fluid challenge, another fluid challenge may be necessary to achieve euvolemia. Usual dose is 10–20 mL/kg over 1–2 hours of isotonic saline solution.

3. **Maintain adequate volume maintenance and replacement for any losses.**

4. **Dopamine.** Use of inotropic agents may be indicated in prerenal failure caused by hypoxia, acidosis, or indomethacin or in infants who develop hypotension. Renal dose of dopamine (1–3 mcg/kg/min) to improve renal perfusion is advocated by some, but no studies show that it improves survival. It increases urine output but does not prevent renal dysfunction or death. Cochrane review states that there is not enough evidence to give dopamine to prevent renal dysfunction specifically in indomethacin-treated preterm infants.

5. **Furosemide.** May be indicated if there is oliguria and volume overload. Diuretics can help in fluid management but do not change the course of ARF/AKI. Furosemide (1–2 mg/kg/dose) can increase urine flow but limit doses due to ototoxicity, especially if there is no response noted.

D. **Intrinsic renal disease.** Supportive measures and treatment of the specific cause. Recovery and prognosis depends on the etiology.

1. **Pediatric nephrology consultation.**

2. **Discontinue any nephrotoxic medications.**

3. **Restrict fluid intake, and only replace insensible losses plus urine output.** Consider potassium intake restriction.

4. **Follow serum sodium, potassium, calcium and phosphate, and acid-base balance.** Infants with ARF can have hyponatremia (usually dilutional), hyperkalemia, hypocalcemia, hyperphosphatemia, and metabolic acidosis.

5. **Consider low-dose dopamine to increase renal blood flow** (*controversial*). See Section V.C.4.

6. **Consider diuretics (furosemide, etc.) if fluid overload.** Limit doses due to ototoxicity. See Section V.C.5.

7. **Follow blood pressure.** Mild hypertension can occur.

E. **Postrenal**

1. **Urologic/pediatric surgical consultation.**

2. **If obstruction is distal to the bladder.** Perform initial bladder catheterization. Surgical vesicostomy may be indicated.

3. **If obstruction is proximal to the bladder.** Urologic surgical intervention should be considered (eg, nephrostomy tubes or cutaneous ureterostomy).

4. **Neurogenic bladder.** Initially managed with catheterization.

5. **Medications.** Medications that cause urinary retention should be discontinued.

6. **Consider urinary tract infection prophylaxis with antibiotics.**

F. **Renal replacement therapy (RRT).** Peritoneal dialysis (preferred method for neonates), hemodialysis, and hemofiltration with or without dialysis are considered only after medical management fails. RRT can be used in infants on ECMO with ARF/AKI and fluid overload. Indications include severe hyperkalemia, severe acidosis, severe hyponatremia, severe hypocalcemia, hyperphosphatemia, uremia, inadequate nutrition, and severe volume overload.

References

Andreoli SP. Acute kidney injury in children. *Pediatr Nephrol.* 2009;4(2):253–263.

Bridges BC, Selewski DT, Paden ML, et al. Acute kidney injury in neonates requiring ECMO. *NeoReviews.* 2012;13(7):e428.

Chan CMJ, Williams, DM, Roth KS. Kidney failure in infants and children. *Pediatr Rev.* 2002;23(2):47–60.

Chua AN, Sarwal MM. Acute renal failure management in the neonate. *NeoReviews.* 2005;6:e369–e376.

Jetton JG, Askenazi DJ. Update on acute kidney injury in the neonate. *Curr Opin Pediatr.* 2012;24(2):191–196.

Zappitelli M, Selewski DT, Askenazi, DJ. Nephrotoxic medication exposure and acute kidney injury in neonates. *NeoReviews.* 2012;13(7):e420.

69 Pneumoperitoneum

I. **Problem.** A pneumoperitoneum (an abnormal collection of free air in the peritoneal cavity) is seen on an abdominal radiograph. The air can be secondary to perforation of the gastrointestinal (GI) tract (most common), from the respiratory tract, or secondary to iatrogenic causes. Necrotizing enterocolitis (NEC) with perforation is the most common cause of a pneumoperitoneum in the neonate. **A neonate with a pneumoperitoneum requires immediate evaluation and treatment, as early recognition is important in successful management.**

II. **Immediate questions**

A. **Is a tension pneumoperitoneum present?** An emergency situation, this occurs when there is a large amount of air that impairs diaphragmatic excursion. A tension pneumoperitoneum can cause significant lung compression, severe respiratory distress, compression of the vena cava, and impaired venous return with cardiovascular compromise. If present, an emergency therapeutic paracentesis should be done (see Chapter 37).

B. **Are signs of pneumoperitoneum present?** These findings can include abdominal distention (most common sign), respiratory distress, deteriorating blood gas levels, and a decrease in blood pressure.

C. **Were signs of necrotizing enterocolitis (NEC) present before?** If so, the pneumoperitoneum is most likely to be associated with GI tract perforation. Bowel perforation typically occurs at a median interval of 1 day after clinical presentation of NEC.

D. **Are any signs of air leak present?** If a pneumomediastinum, pulmonary interstitial emphysema, or pneumothorax is present, the peritoneal air collection may be of respiratory tract origin.

E. **Is mechanical ventilation being used?** High peak inspiratory pressures (PIPs) greater than a mean of 34 cm H_2O can be associated with a pneumoperitoneum.

F. **Did the infant recently undergo abdominal surgery or an invasive procedure such as paracentesis?** Intra-abdominal air is normal in the immediate postoperative period and usually resolves without treatment. Paracentesis can perforate a hollow organ.

III. **Differential diagnosis.** A pneumoperitoneum most commonly develops **secondary to perforation of the GI tract** (spontaneous, secondary from underlying GI disease, or traumatic), **from the chest** (respiratory causes: air leak with or without mechanical ventilation), **or from no known cause** (no respiratory or GI cause found), or a **normal immediate postoperative finding.** In a neonate, unless the infant is on high ventilator settings and has an air leak **the cause is GI perforation until proven otherwise.** Some classify pneumoperitoneum into **medical (nonsurgical)** versus **surgical.**

A. **Pneumoperitoneum associated with GI perforation**

1. **Spontaneous perforation.** (No demonstrable cause: no obvious gastrointestinal disease, no evidence of trauma or obstruction.) This is the second most common cause of GI perforation in neonates (most common is due to NEC). **Proposed etiologies** include local ischemia in the perinatal period (from asphyxia or shock) or from noncommunication of right and left gastroepiploic arteries, trauma during pregnancy or delivery, sepsis, prematurity, excessive gastric acidity, lack of intestinal cajal cells (gastric perforation), maternal use of steroids or cocaine, or congenital defects in the muscular wall of the stomach. Spontaneous perforation occurs most commonly in the terminal ileum in premature infants (spontaneous intestinal perforation [SIP]) or in the stomach (preterm and term infants); rarely occurs elsewhere in the GI tract.

a. **Spontaneous gastric perforation.** Occurs most commonly between the 2nd and 7th days of life in both full-term and preterm infants. It is more common in males and African American babies. Infants present with sudden abdominal distension, respiratory distress, vomiting, lethargy, and a massive pneumoperitoneum. Perinatal stress, prematurity, and postnatal steroid use are risk factors. Many of these infants have sepsis.

b. **Spontaneous intestinal perforation (SIP).** Occurs primarily in the terminal ileum (rarely in the jejunum and colon) in infants under 28 weeks' gestational age (GA), with low birthweight <1500 g (2–3%) and <1000 g (5%). Median age of presentation is 7 days, and it is more common in males. Prematurity and early steroid therapies are risk factors. Early postnatal exposure of indomethacin combined with steroids increases the risk of SIP. SIP is frequently associated with systemic candidiasis or coagulase-negative *Staphylococcus*. It does not have the clinical signs that NEC has (see Chapter 131).

c. **Spontaneous colonic perforations.** These can occur but are very rare. They are more common in preterm infants and very difficult to diagnose. Signs include significant abdominal and scrotal distension, vomiting, cyanosis, respiratory distress, and tachypnea. Most infants have a massive pneumoperitoneum.

d. **Other perforations.** Isolated perforations can occur elsewhere in the intestine, including the appendix, cecum, and Meckel diverticulum.

e. **Medications associated with spontaneous perforation include indomethacin and steroids.** A meta-analysis of the effect of early treatment (<96 hours) with high doses of steroids for chronic lung disease showed an increased risk of spontaneous GI perforation. **Gastro-duodenal perforation** has been associated with steroid therapy. Combined therapy (early postnatal indomethacin and glucocorticoids) increases the risk of SIP.

f. **Other causes. Following exchange transfusion,** perforation of small and large intestine can occur. **Embolic phenomenon secondary to umbilical artery catheter** can also contribute to perforation.

2. **Secondary perforations.** These are caused by an underlying disease: obstruction in the gastrointestinal tract or secondary to a gastrointestinal disease process.

a. **NEC is the most common cause of secondary perforation.** Mortality is high (>60%). Conflicting data exist on whether indomethacin increases the risk of NEC with intestinal perforation. The most common affected areas are the terminal ileum and ascending colon, although any part of the GI tract may be involved. Perforation occurs most commonly in the terminal ileum (ileocecal) region.

b. **Gastrointestinal obstruction.** Causes increasing intraluminal pressure and the perforation occurs proximal to the obstruction. It can occur anywhere in the gastrointestinal tract. Causes include any gastrointestinal atresia (esophageal atresia with tracheoesophageal [TE] fistula, duodenal/pylorus atresia, small/large intestine or anal atresia, and others), meconium ileus/plug, duplication cyst, small left colon syndrome, obstructive bands, Hirschsprung disease, and anorectal malformations (imperforate anus, incarcerated hernia, and others). Bowel perforation occurs in ~3–4% of infants with Hirschsprung disease.

c. **Gastritis or peptic ulcer disease.** Perforation can be the initial presentation of ulcer disease. Perforations of the stomach (most common), duodenum, pylorus, or esophagus can occur.

d. **Other rare causes.** Malrotation with midgut volvulus, omphalocele, ruptured appendix, gastroschisis, mesenteric thrombosis, perforated Meckel diverticulum, idiopathic gastric necrosis, and pneumatosis cystoides intestinalis.

3. **Traumatic perforations.** An iatrogenic pneumoperitoneum caused by an intervention. Most gastric perforations are secondary to naso-/orogastric (NG/OG) placement or vigorous bag-and-mask/positive pressure ventilation.

a. **Normal transient finding** following laparotomy or laparoscopy.

b. **Nasogastric tube trauma.** Most gastric perforations are along the greater curvature due to trauma by vigorous NG/OG tube placement. Use of soft silastic feeding tubes may reduce this risk. An NG in an unusual position on x-ray (eg, right upper quadrant) indicates a possible perforation.

   c. **Intubation trauma.** During an intubation, the endotracheal tube (ETT) can be inadvertently placed in the esophagus and then through the posterior wall of the stomach. If the ETT on chest x-ray (CXR) is seen more distally than expected, consider intubation trauma.

   d. **Bag-and-mask/positive pressure ventilation.** Traumatic **gastric perforation** can occur from vigorous bag-and-mask ventilation or be due to positive pressure ventilation.

   e. **Neonatal rectal perforations of the sigmoid colon or rectum** can be caused by a rectal thermometer or rectal tubes. Because of the shape of the neonatal rectum, when a rectal thermometer is placed to a depth of 2 cm, it impinges on the anterior wall. Insert a rectal thermometer <2 cm. An attempt to push it any further may result in perforation. Enema-induced perforations occur in the anterior wall of the rectum or rectosigmoid.

   f. **Improperly performed suprapubic bladder aspiration or paracentesis** can perforate a hollow organ.

   g. **Umbilical vein catheterization** can cause perforation of Meckel diverticulum.

   h. **Aerophagia (swallowing air) secondary to prolonged crying** may cause gastric perforation. (There is a case report on an infant who had a circumcision with prolonged crying that may have caused a gastric rupture.)

B. **Pneumoperitoneum associated with a respiratory disorder (eg, pulmonary interstitial emphysema [PIE], pneumomediastinum, or pneumothorax).** A pulmonary air leak, with or without mechanical ventilation, can extend below the diaphragm resulting in a pneumoperitoneum. It can be secondary to barotrauma in ventilated neonates with severe respiratory disease. A thoracic leak can dissect transdiaphragmatically to the abdomen. **An infant can have a pneumoperitoneum from thoracic air dissection without a pneumothorax or pneumomediastinum.** Possibly an undetectable pulmonary rupture can occur with dissection into the peritoneal cavity. If there is a posterior pneumomediastinum, an air leak is probably the cause of the pneumoperitoneum.

C. **Benign neonatal pneumoperitoneum with no known cause.** There is no evidence of GI or respiratory pathology. Pulmonary rupture with a thoracic leak may not be apparent.

D. **Pseudopneumoperitoneum.** Occurs when there is a subphrenic lucency with no free intraperitoneal air. It can be from a subphrenic fat pad, linear atelectasis, abnormal subphrenic shape, subphrenic abscess, or **Chilaiditi syndrome** (interposition of a portion of the colon between the liver and diaphragm), which can present with respiratory distress. Gas can be seen between the liver and hemidiaphragm. This is gas-filled transverse colon. X-ray shadows can also cause a (false) radiographic pneumoperitoneum. A **mimicked pneumoperitoneum** includes a case report of transplacental passage of a nonionic contrast agent that resulted in opacification of the fetal bowel that mimicked a pneumoperitoneum.

IV. **Database**

A. **Physical examination.** Clinical evaluation may not help differentiate if the pneumoperitoneum is of respiratory or GI tract origin. The examination should focus on the pulmonary and abdominal aspects. **Abdominal distention (most common sign) and elevation of the diaphragm with increasing respiratory difficulty are hallmarks of pneumoperitoneum.** Other symptoms include bilious vomiting, tachypnea, rectal bleeding, and failure or delay to pass meconium. Is there respiratory compromise or unexplained tachypnea? Large amounts of air in the abdominal cavity can impair diaphragmatic excursion and lung compression. Cardiovascular compromise can occur secondary to compression of the vena cava and impaired venous return. Feeding intolerance and poor activity can also be present. Are there increased gastric residuals? Is there a bluish-black discoloration of the abdominal wall (with SIP but not NEC)? **Scrotal swelling** may indicate gastric perforation (pneumoscrotum). It can occur without significant abdominal distension. A pneumoscrotum can be secondary to a gastric perforation, perforation of Meckel diverticulum, perforation of ileum secondary to atresia, or after aggressive resuscitation or mechanical ventilation.

B. **Laboratory studies**

1. **Complete blood count (CBC) and serum electrolytes.** Elevation of the white blood cell count or a left shift may signify a GI tract perforation. Hyponatremia can be seen with NEC secondary to third spacing of fluid. Thrombocytopenia also can be seen.

2. **Arterial blood gas levels.** May reveal hypoxemia and increasing Pco_2 levels. Metabolic acidosis can be seen with peritonitis.

3. **Blood culture.** Should be obtained if bowel perforation or sepsis is suspected. Infants with bowel perforation can have a positive blood culture. In one study, 18 out of 30 infants had a positive blood culture (*Escherichia coli* was the most common organism).

4. **C-reactive protein.** Correlates with the inflammatory response and may be increased in NEC.

5. **Coagulation studies.**

C. **Imaging and other studies**

1. **Transillumination of the abdomen** with a cold fiber-optic light source, can be done and acts as a useful tool for diagnosis, especially if radiographs are not readily available.

2. **Radiographs.** Small amounts of air can be missed on a routine film; some infants have air but it cannot be seen on x-ray. Repeat radiographs frequently if air is suspected. Simple observation of free air is often sufficient, particularly if the air leak is large (see Figure 11–22). Supine films (some infants are too sick for an upright) are usually done. A massive pneumoperitoneum suggests gastric or colonic perforation.

   a. **Supine anterior-posterior radiograph of the chest and abdomen.** The chest may show signs of air leak syndrome (pneumomediastinum or pneumothorax) if it is suspected that the intraperitoneal air is from the respiratory tract. The abdomen may show signs of NEC (pneumatosis intestinalis or portal venous gas; see Figures 11–23 and 11–24) or ileus. Air-fluid levels in the peritoneal cavity usually indicate ileus. SIP will have a pneumoperitoneum without pneumatosis intestinalis or portal venous gas. **X-ray findings pathognomonic of a pneumoperitoneum:**

      i. **Right upper quadrant sign.** The most common finding is the presence of right upper quadrant subdiaphragmatic free air (collection of gas in the right upper quadrant adjacent to the liver, gas in the anterior subhepatic space).

      ii. **Doge's cap sign.** Air between the right kidney and liver. It is often the first sign and appears as an oval or triangular gas shadow.

      iii. **Cupola sign.** An inverted cup-shaped lucency (dome) of air accumulation that appears over the lower thoracic spine near the posterior part of the heart.

      iv. **Rigler sign (double wall sign).** Gas is seen on both sides of the bowel wall (the outer and inner walls of the bowel are seen). Normally only the inner wall of the bowel is seen. If the mean wall thickness of the bowel is >1 mm, it is a positive sign. If the thickness is ≤1 mm, it may be a false positive.

      v. **Falciform ligament sign.** Gas outlining the falciform ligament.

      vi. **Football sign.** A large oval radiolucency (gas outlining the peritoneal cavity) in the shape of an American football. It can also include when the falciform ligament is seen in the center as a vertical strip surrounded by gas (the radiographic appearance of pneumoperitoneum outlining the falciform ligament was renamed falciform ligament sign; see previous text). It appears as a white streak, which is surrounded by the oval lucency of a pneumoperitoneum. The football sign is most frequently seen in infants with spontaneous or iatrogenic gastric perforation.

vii. **Inverted V sign.** Gas outlines the medial umbilical folds (umbilical arteries) on the supine radiograph.

viii. **Saddle bag sign.** Spleen and liver are displaced downward toward the midline.

ix. **Arcade sign.** Air is seen between bowel loops and creates triangular-shaped areas of gas.

x. **A gasless abdomen.** May represent a perforation if there is no bowel gas to go into the peritoneal cavity (it is walled off).

b. **Left lateral decubitus radiographic study of the abdomen.** With the right side up, it is the best examination for the detection of free abdominal air; air (seen as a homogeneous lucency or streak-like lucencies) is seen over the liver if a perforation has occurred. This is also done to show smaller leaks not appreciated on the anteroposterior (AP) abdominal film. A lateral decubitus radiograph should be serially taken when NEC is suspected. Lateral decubitus studies have been shown to be more sensitive in detecting a pneumoperitoneum than upright view studies.

c. **Upright view of the chest abdomen.** **This will show air below the diaphragm** but is rarely done because of the difficulty in positioning a sick infant.

3. **Ultrasound or color Doppler ultrasonography of the abdomen** can be used to diagnose NEC by visualizing pneumatosis intestinalis and portal venous air, and can be obtained to assess ascites. The presence of particulate matter probably indicates perforation. Complex ascites (ascites with debris) verifies bowel perforation. Extraluminal calcifications usually indicate intrauterine intestinal perforation with intraperitoneal extravasation of meconium. It can also be used to diagnose NEC. (Central echogenic focus with hypoechoic rim can indicate necrotic bowel or presence of intermittent gas bubbles in the portal venous system and liver). **Color Doppler studies** can detect bowel necrosis.

4. **Paracentesis, diagnostic.** See Chapter 37.

a. **Air.** Air obtained by paracentesis may be tested for its oxygen level. If the baby is receiving oxygen supplementation and the oxygen level is high (greater than room air, 0.21 FIO_2), the air is probably from a respiratory tract leak. If the oxygen if similar to room air or lower, the air is probably from the GI tract.

b. **Fluid (peritoneal lavage).** Fluid may be obtained by paracentesis if the diagnosis is still undetermined. If green or brownish fluid is obtained, especially if bacteria are present on the Gram stain, the air is probably of GI tract origin. A microscopic smear of the fluid for white blood cells, if present, suggests peritonitis.

V. **Plan**

A. **Emergency measures.** For **tension pneumoperitoneum,** an emergency therapeutic paracentesis must be done to reduce the pressure and allow the diaphragm to mobilize (see Chapter 37).

B. **General measures.** Place a double-lumen tube (replogle) on low suction. This allows one lumen for drainage of fluid and the other as an air vent.

C. **Sepsis evaluation and antibiotics if indicated.**

D. **Differentiate surgical from nonsurgical pneumoperitoneum to guide treatment.** If the cause of the pneumoperitoneum is in doubt, attempts to distinguish pneumoperitoneum from GI perforation and that of pulmonary air leak can be done by the following:

1. **Contrast studies.** A low-osmolality, water-soluble contrast medium (eg, metrizamide) can be given through a nasogastric tube. If there is a pneumoperitoneum secondary to a GI perforation, contrast material will pass into the peritoneal cavity and confirm the diagnosis. **Barium should never be used because of the morbidity of barium peritonitis.**

2. Measurement of Po_2 in peritoneal air. See Section IV.C.4a.
3. Presence of air leak in the chest. Increases the chance it is from an air leak.

E. Specific measures

1. **Pneumoperitoneum of GI tract origin.** Stop all feedings, insert NG/OG tube to decompress the abdomen, provide supportive care (respiratory and circulatory support: correct hypoxia and acidosis, correct dehydration, correct any electrolyte disturbance), correct any coagulopathy, administer IV antibiotics, and call for an immediate surgical consult. **Optimal surgical management is controversial.** The debate is whether the infant needs to go to the operating room for a primary laparotomy or have primary peritoneal drainage. It is best to discuss options with the surgeon and make the decision based on each individual patient.

   a. **Surgical management with exploratory laparotomy has been the traditional therapy.** Unless the pneumoperitoneum is of a known iatrogenic origin (eg, postoperative), **immediate surgical evaluation** is often necessary. Exploratory laparotomy is often the treatment of choice. Preoperative management includes

      i. **Preoperative laboratory values** should be available.
      ii. **The infant should be stabilized** as much as possible before being taken to the operating room.
      iii. **IV antibiotics** should be started. Choice depends on the institution but should include broad spectrum antibiotics with anaerobic coverage.
      iv. **The surgical team may request a study with a water-soluble contrast medium given through the nasogastric tube** to try to localize the perforation.
      v. **Laparotomy** with primary repair or laparoscopy. "Mini laparotomy" is a newer bedside option.

   b. **Primary peritoneal drainage with conservative management is used selectively. Some suggest this for infants with the following:** perforation without peritonitis, a normal abdominal examination or mild abdominal distension, normal blood gases and platelets, minimal free air, and no air-fluid levels on x-ray. **Others suggest** this for isolated perforations or for infants who may be too sick for anesthesia and surgery. Recent studies have shown that primary peritoneal drainage was more effective than primary laparotomy in infants with NEC. Conservative management includes

      i. **NPO, fluids, and antibiotics.** Make infant NPO, start IV fluids, total parenteral nutrition (TPN), blood transfusion if indicated, and IV antibiotics.
      ii. **Primary peritoneal drainage (PPD) (closed abdominal drainage)** is done at the bedside; peritoneal drain is removed when the drainage resolves.
      iii. **Close observation** and frequent physical examinations, serial radiographs, and follow-up laboratory evaluations are required.
      iv. **Delayed laparotomy** may be required in many of these infants if they fail to improve clinically (increasing need for respiratory support, increasing inotrope requirement, increasing abdominal distension), or have persistent intestinal obstruction. Continued acidosis or free air that persists may also signify the need for laparotomy. Reviews have found that 38–74% infants required a delayed laparotomy.

2. **Pneumoperitoneum of respiratory tract origin.** The pulmonary air leak should be treated first if this is the cause of the pneumoperitoneum.

   a. **Asymptomatic patients.** Observation is often the treatment of choice, with follow-up radiographic studies usually performed every 8–12 hours but more frequently if the patient's clinical course changes.
   b. **Symptomatic patients.** Emergency paracentesis can be performed with treatment of coexisting pneumothorax if present. Review the ventilator settings to avoid high pressures that will contribute to the problems.

3. **Traumatic pneumoperitoneum**
   a. **Pneumoperitoneum.** A pneumoperitoneum caused by rectal thermometers, NG/OG placement, suprapubic bladder aspiration, umbilical venous lines, enemas, attempted intubation, or paracentesis may require surgical exploration.
   b. **Postlaparotomy or laparoscopy.** A pneumoperitoneum associated with an uncomplicated surgical procedure will resolve spontaneously over several days.
4. **Benign neonatal pneumoperitoneum with no known cause.** Depending on the infant and his or her clinical examination, observation with conservative management, primary peritoneal drainage, or surgical exploration may be indicated.

70 Pneumothorax

I. **Problem.** An infant may have a pneumothorax (an abnormal accumulation of air or gas in the pleural space, between the visceral and parietal pleura). It can develop spontaneous or be secondary to trauma. A pneumothorax occurs more often in the neonatal period than any other time in life.

A. **Spontaneous pneumothorax**
   1. **Primary spontaneous pneumothorax (PSP).** Occurs when there is no obvious precipitating factor, no clear cause, it is idiopathic, without lung disease. Familial spontaneous pneumothorax is a rare cause in neonates.
   2. **Secondary spontaneous pneumothorax (SSP).** Occurs from underlying lung disease (respiratory distress syndrome [RDS], meconium aspiration syndrome [MAS], and others).

B. **Traumatic pneumothorax**
   1. **Iatrogenic** occurs from an accidental insult during a procedure such as central line placement or thoracentesis.
   2. **Positive pressure ventilation (mechanical or noninvasive ventilation)** can cause barotrauma.
   3. **Chest trauma** can occur when blunt or penetrating trauma occurs to the chest (rare in neonate).

C. **Tension pneumothorax.** A life-threatening condition that occurs when air is trapped in the pleural cavity under positive pressure. Air goes into the pleural cavity during inspiration, but no air is allowed to escape during expiration. It acts as a 1-way valve. Because air is trapped, intrathoracic positive pressure rises, lung volume decreases, and pressure compresses the mediastinum and causes a shift, with increased pulmonary vascular resistance. This results in an increase in central venous pressure, decrease in venous return to the heart, and a decrease in cardiac output. This causes displacement of mediastinal structures and cardiopulmonary compromise.

D. **Persistent pneumothorax.** A pneumothorax that persists >7 days in the absence of mechanical problems.

II. **Immediate questions**
A. **Are symptoms of tension pneumothorax present?** A tension pneumothorax occurs when air is trapped in the pleural cavity under positive pressure. **A tension pneumothorax presents as a medical emergency, and the patient's status will deteriorate acutely.** The following signs may be seen with tension pneumothorax: cyanosis, hypoxia, tachypnea, a sudden decrease in heart rate with bradycardia, a sudden increase in systolic blood pressure followed by narrowing pulse pressure and hypotension, an asymmetric chest (bulging on the affected side), distention of the abdomen (secondary to downward displacement of the diaphragm), decreased breath sounds on the affected side, and shift of the cardiac apical impulse

(most consistent finding) away from the affected side. A cyanotic upper half of the body with a pale lower half can be seen.

B. **Is the patient asymptomatic?** An asymptomatic pneumothorax is present in 1–2% of neonates. It occurs more frequently in males and term and post-term infants. It is usually unilateral. Most of these cases are discovered on chest radiograph at admission. Up to 15% of these infants were meconium stained at birth.

C. **Is mechanical ventilation being used?** The incidence of pneumothorax in patients receiving positive-pressure ventilation is 15–30%. A life-threatening tension pneumothorax may result from mechanical ventilation.

D. **Are there risk factors for a pneumothorax?** Neonates delivered between 30 and 36 weeks, moderately preterm, or term by caesarean section have a higher incidence of pneumothorax. The following are associated with an increased risk: male infant, low birthweight, premature, meconium-stained amniotic fluid, vacuum extraction, a low 1-minute Apgar score, ventilator treatment, perinatal asphyxia, cardiopulmonary resuscitation, transient tachypnea, RDS, MAS, pneumonia, pulmonary hypoplasia, urinary tract anomalies, infants who were resuscitated at birth, continuous positive airway pressure, and positive pressure ventilation. α_1-Antitrypsin deficiency may play a role in some cases of spontaneous pneumothorax of the newborn.

III. **Differential diagnosis. Radiologically,** the differential diagnosis can include pneumomediastinum, congenital lobar emphysema, atelectasis with compensatory hyperinflation, congenital diaphragmatic hernia, congenital cystic adenomatoid malformation, and a large pulmonary cyst. **Clinically,** it can present as any process that causes respiratory distress, and it is important to exclude other causes of respiratory distress in a neonate: RDS, endotracheal tube obstruction/displacement, aspiration, congenital heart disease, asphyxia, congenital diaphragmatic hernia (CDH), congenital cystic adenomatoid malformation (CCAM), or pleural effusions. **Sudden rapid deterioration in a neonate** can be from a tension pneumothorax, pneumopericardium, or a massive pericardial effusion/cardiac tamponade (umbilical venous catheter).

A. **Pneumothorax**
1. **Symptomatic pneumothorax (includes tension vs nontension pneumothorax). Nontension symptoms:** irritability, grunting, pallor cyanosis, restlessness, apnea, mild tachypnea, respiratory distress. **Tension symptoms are noted in Section II.A previously.**
2. **Asymptomatic pneumothorax.**
3. **Persistent pneumothorax.**

B. **Pneumomediastinum.** Air in the mediastinal space that may be confused with a true pneumothorax. On the radiograph, mediastinal air can elevate the lobes of the thymus (called "angel wing" or "spinnaker sail" sign), and the air can also track within the extrapleural space and outline the inferior aspect of the heart ("continuous diaphragm sign"). See Figure 11–19.

C. **Congenital lobar emphysema.** A rare anomaly of lung development that presents with respiratory distress and pulmonary lobar hyperinflation. Overdistention of one lobe secondary to air trapping occurs most commonly (47–50%) in the left upper lobe. Other lobe involvement is right upper lobe (20%), right middle lobe (28%), and lower lobes (rare). The causes of congenital lobar emphysema are multifactorial.

D. **Atelectasis with compensatory hyperinflation.** Compensatory hyperinflation may appear as a pneumothorax on a chest radiograph.

E. **Pneumopericardium. In neonates, pneumopericardium and tension pneumothorax can both present as sudden and rapid clinical deterioration.** In pneumopericardium, the blood pressure drops, heart sounds are distant or absent, and pulses are muffled or absent. Massive abdominal distention can also be seen. In tension pneumothorax, the blood pressure may initially increase, but then hypotension follows. The chest radiograph easily differentiates the two. A pneumopericardium has a halo of air around the heart (see Figure 11–18). **The more common event is a tension pneumothorax.** If one is unsure and time does not permit radiographic verification, quick transillumination can be done. If not available or unsure of results, it is better to insert a needle in the chest on the suspected side. If no response, then a needle should be inserted on the other side. If there is still no response, then the diagnosis of pneumopericardium should be considered.

F. **Congenital diaphragmatic hernia (CDH).** A developmental defect in the diaphragm allows the abdominal viscera to protrude into the chest, which causes pulmonary hypoplasia and decreased pulmonary vasculature and dysfunction of the surfactant system. Ninety percent are on the left side. CDH is often mistaken as a left tension pneumothorax. Presents with respiratory distress, cyanosis, and circulatory insufficiency. It can be hard to differentiate a left-sided pneumothorax from a typically left-sided CDH. With CDH, the abdomen is scaphoid, and the spleen cannot be palpated. There can be a mediastinal shift on radiograph. If chest tubes are placed, there is a risk of perforating the herniated viscus.

G. **Congenital cystic adenomatoid malformation (CCAM).** This rare congenital abnormality of the lung results from abnormal embryogenesis and reduced alveolar growth. The infants present with respiratory distress. Tachypnea and cyanosis can be presenting signs that are similar to a pneumothorax. Many of these are detected on ultrasound prenatally. A chest radiograph usually identifies the mass containing air-filled cysts. (See Chapter 135.)

H. **Congenital pulmonary cysts.** These are space occupying, involve one or more lobes, have atelectasis of the adjacent lobe, and have symptoms similar to pneumothorax.

IV. **Clinical findings**

A. **Physical examination.** Specific findings are discussed in Section II.A. Transillumination is a useful rapid bedside technique in neonates (see Section IV.C and Chapter 40).

B. **Laboratory studies.** Blood gas levels may show decreased Pao_2 and increased Pco_2, with resultant respiratory acidosis.

C. **Imaging and other studies**

1. **Transillumination** of the chest is a rapid bedside method to identify a pneumothorax. **Always verify the diagnosis of pneumothorax by a chest radiograph if time permits.** The room lights are lowered, and a fiber optic transilluminator is placed along the posterior axillary line on the side on which pneumothorax is suspected. If a pneumothorax is present, the chest "lights up" on that side. The transilluminator may be moved up and down along the posterior axillary line and may also be placed above the nipple. Transilluminate both sides of the chest and then compare the results. If severe subcutaneous edema is present, transillumination may be falsely positive. Premature infants with pulmonary interstitial emphysema may also have a false-positive transillumination. Large infants with thick chest walls do not transilluminate well.

2. **Chest radiographs** are the method of choice for diagnosing pneumothorax. Early pneumothoraces are difficult to diagnose. Early on, there is separation of lung from the chest wall with no lung markings in that space. In infants there is a tendency of pleural air to cloak diaphragmatic and mediastinal surfaces. A pleural line is often not seen, but a well-defined costophrenic sulcus (deep sulcus sign) can be observed. The following films will aid the diagnosis:

a. **Anteroposterior (AP) view of the chest** (see Figure 11–20) will show the following:

   i. **A shift of the mediastinum** away from the side of pneumothorax (with tension pneumothorax).

   ii. **Depression of the diaphragm** on the side of the pneumothorax (with tension pneumothorax).

   iii. **Displacement of the lung** on the affected side away from the chest wall by a radiolucent band of air.

b. **Cross-table lateral view** will show a rim of air around the lung ("pancaking"). It will *not* help to identify the affected side. **You must have an AP film to identify the side of the pneumothorax.** This film must be considered together with the AP view to identify the involved side. Pleural air tends to collect anteriorly and may require the CT or lateral decubitus view.

    c. **Lateral decubitus view (shot through the AP position)** will detect even a **small pneumothorax** not seen on a routine chest radiograph. The infant should be positioned so the side of the suspected pneumothorax is up (eg, if pneumothorax is suspected on the left side, the film is taken with the left side up).

3. **Ultrasound examination of the lungs.** The absence of lung sliding (grainy appearance) and comet tails (normal pleura reflecting sound waves) confirms the **ultrasound diagnosis of a pneumothorax.** The sensitivity and specificity of ultrasound is 100% and 93% for a complete pneumothorax, and 79% and 100% for a radio-occult pneumothorax. As a bedside tool, this is useful to diagnose a pneumothorax.

4. **Transcutaneous carbon dioxide (tcpCO$_2$) reference percentiles with changes over time** can indicate a pneumothorax or a blocked or misplaced endotracheal tube.

5. **Echocardiography and renal ultrasound** may be indicated in spontaneous pneumothorax in term infants, as some of these infants can have renal and cardiac anomalies.

V. **Plan**

A. **Symptomatic pneumothorax**

1. **Tension pneumothorax. Symptomatic (tension) pneumothorax is an emergency!** A 1- to 2-minute delay could be fatal. If a tension pneumothorax is suspected, act immediately. It is better to treat in this setting, even if it turns out that there is no pneumothorax. There is no time for x-ray confirmation. If the patient's status is deteriorating rapidly, a needle or catheter over needle can be placed for aspiration, followed by formal chest tube placement. There is no specific sign that distinguishes a tension from a nontension pneumothorax. Signs of a tension pneumothorax from above can also occur in a nontension pneumothorax, except the signs and symptoms are more severe in a tension pneumothorax.

    a. **Needle aspiration (see Figure 70–1) can be done as an emergency.** Often times this is all that is necessary if the infant is not on a ventilator. If on a ventilator, a chest tube placement may need to be followed by needle aspiration.

        i. The site of puncture should be at the second intercostal space along the midclavicular line on the suspected side of pneumothorax. Cleanse this area with antibacterial solution. The **fourth intercostal space at the anterior axillary line** can also be used (needle would be inserted above the fifth rib).

        ii. Connect a 23- or 25-gauge butterfly needle or a 22- or 24-gauge catheter over needle (Angiocath) to a 10–20-mL syringe with a stopcock attached.

        iii. Palpate the third rib at the midclavicular line. Insert the needle (perpendicular to the chest surface) over the top of the third rib at the second intercostal space, and advance it until air is withdrawn from the syringe. Have an assistant hold the syringe to withdraw the air. The needle may be removed before the chest tube is placed if the infant is relatively stable, or it may be left in place for continuous aspiration while the chest tube is being placed. If an Angiocath is used, the needle can be removed and the catheter left in place.

    b. **Chest tube placement is discussed in Chapter 27.** This is necessary in most infants on mechanical ventilation with a tension pneumothorax.

    c. **If the infant does not improve with a chest tube.** Suspect extrapleural air leaks such as a pneumoretroperitoneum, which has been reported in infants with pneumothorax. **If air is still present on the radiograph, consider these causes:** obstruction of the tube with blood or pleural fluid, disconnected drainage tube, ineffective water seal, new air leak, or a lung perforation.

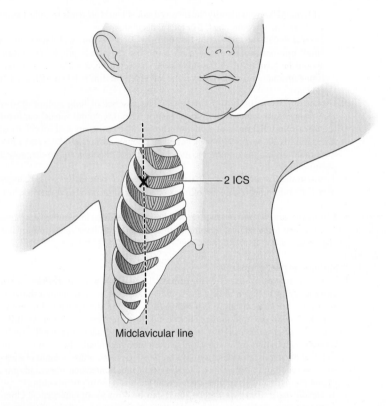

FIGURE 70–1. Site of emergency needle aspiration for tension pneumothorax is puncture at the second intercostal space (ICS) along the midclavicular line.

      2. Nontension pneumothorax. Depending on the infant, oxygen supplementation, needle aspiration, chest tube placement, or conservative management (oxygen, close observation) is done.

      a. Mild symptoms. Some require observation only.

      b. Symptomatic spontaneous pneumothorax (not on ventilator). Needle aspiration and possible chest tube placement. In one study the majority of infants did not require a needle aspiration or chest tube and could be managed with supplemental oxygen or close observation.

      c. Symptomatic spontaneous pneumothorax (on the ventilator). Needle aspiration and chest tube placement. Some infants on a ventilator who have a pneumothorax could be treated conservatively without a chest tube, but they usually are more mature, on lower ventilator settings, and had better gases at the time of the pneumothorax as compared with the infants who required a chest tube.

B. Asymptomatic pneumothorax

    1. If positive-pressure mechanical ventilation is being used:

      a. Needle aspiration/chest tube. A chest tube will probably need to be inserted because the ventilator pressure will prevent resolution of the pneumothorax, and tension pneumothorax may develop. Sometimes **needle aspiration is all**

that is needed. If a pneumothorax develops in a patient who is ready to be extubated, clinical judgment must be used in deciding whether a chest tube should be placed.

    b. **Expectant management.** Recent studies are showing that some select infants on a ventilator can be managed without a chest tube.

  2. **If positive-pressure mechanical ventilation is not being administered and there is no underlying lung pathology, these may be considered.**

    a. **Close observation with follow-up chest radiographs every 8–12 hours or sooner if the infant becomes symptomatic.** The pneumothorax will likely resolve within 24–48 hours.

    b. **Nitrogen washout therapy** (*controversial*). Allows a more rapid resolution of the asymptomatic pneumothorax but is infrequently used due to the toxicity of 100% oxygen. The infant receives 100% oxygen for 8–12 hours; less nitrogen is able to enter the lungs, and at the same time absorption of nitrogen from the extrapleural space is increased and then exhaled. The total gas tension is decreased, which also facilitates absorption of nitrogen by the blood. The method should be used only in full-term infants in whom retinopathy of prematurity will not be a problem. **Some NICUS give only enough oxygen to maintain a pulse oximetry reading >90% and have found resolution to be similar to the hyperoxic group.**

C. **Persistent pneumothorax.** Generally defined as a pneumothorax that persists >7 days in the absence of mechanical problems. Sometimes infants who have chest tubes still have air leaks that persist for more than a week. These infants have episodes of instability when air reaccumulates; some require a new or replacement chest tube and an increase in their ventilator settings. These are treated to decrease the complications associated with air leaks (air embolus, hypotension, intracranial hemorrhage). The following have been used:

  1. **High-frequency oscillatory ventilation (HFOV) or high-frequency jet ventilation (HFJV)** can be used due to lower mean airway pressures.

  2. **Unilateral lung intubation** has been reported as an efficient and relatively safe therapy for pneumothorax. Duration of therapy should be a minimum of 48 hours.

  3. **Fibrin glue,** such as CryoSeal C (ThermoGenesis Corp., Rancho Cordova, CA), has been injected in the chest tube with a marked reduction in the air leak. Risks include hypercalcemia, localized tissue necrosis, bradycardia, diaphragmatic paralysis, and pneumothorax on the contralateral side. More studies are needed before this treatment can be routinely recommended.

D. **Pneumomediastinum.** May progress to a pneumothorax or pneumopericardium. Close observation is required.

E. **Congenital lobar emphysema.** If asymptomatic, conservative management with observation. If symptomatic or respiratory failure is occurring, the treatment is usually surgical excision of the affected lobe.

F. **Atelectasis with compensatory hyperinflation**

  1. **Chest physiotherapy and postural drainage should be initiated.** Chest physiotherapy should be used with caution in premature infants. A study showed an association with intraventricular hemorrhage and porencephaly in extreme premature infants.

  2. **Treatment with bronchodilators is indicated.**

  3. **Positioning the infant with the affected (hyperinflated) side down may speed resolution.**

  4. **Bronchoscopy.** May be necessary with mucous plug.

G. **Pneumopericardium.** This should be treated emergently by pericardiocentesis (see Chapter 38).

H. **Cystic adenomatoid malformation or congenital cyst.** Surgery is the treatment of choice.

71 Polycythemia

I. **Problem.** The hematocrit (Hct) is 68% in a newborn. **Polycythemia** is defined as a venous hematocrit above 65% or a hemoglobin >22 g/dL. Polycythemia occurs in 2–4% of newborns and is rare in premature infants <34 weeks' gestation. The current definition and management of neonatal polycythemia is empirical and not evidence based. Polycythemia may result in an increase in blood viscosity, which causes a reduction in blood flow, acidosis, hypoglycemia, tissue hypoxia, and an increase in microthrombi formation. **Hyperviscosity** is defined as a viscosity value >14 centipoise (shear rate of 11.5 seconds) and is also defined as 2 standard deviations greater than the norm. **Polycythemia hyperviscosity syndrome (PHS)** is the symptom complex that involves polycythemia, hyperviscosity, and the symptoms that accompany it. Forty seven percent of polycythemic infants have hyperviscosity. Twenty-four percent of infants with hyperviscosity have polycythemia.

II. **Immediate questions**

A. **What is the central hematocrit (Hct)?** In blood obtained by heelstick, the Hct may be falsely elevated by up to 5–20%. Treatment should **never** be initiated based on heelstick Hct values alone; a central (peripheral venous phlebotomy) Hct is needed. If the sample is from the umbilical vein or radial artery, the upper limit of normal is 63%. The hematocrit in a newborn peaks at 2 hours of age and then decreases to a baseline by 24 hours of age. A micro-centrifuge hematocrit can be 2% higher than hematocrit by a hematology analyzer.

B. **Does the infant have symptoms of polycythemia?** Many infants with polycythemia are asymptomatic. Symptoms of hypoperfusion correlate more with viscosity than the hematocrit. One study found that **feeding problems and lethargy** were the most common symptoms. There are many signs of polycythemia, most of them nonspecific, which can include the following:

   1. **Central nervous system.** Lethargy, hypotonia, irritability, jitteriness, weak sucking reflex, vomiting, seizures, tremulousness, apnea, sleepiness, exaggerated startle, tremors, and cerebrovascular accidents.

   2. **Cardiovascular.** Heart murmurs, congestive heart failure, cyanosis, plethora, tachycardia, cardiomegaly, and prominent vascular markings on chest radiograph.

   3. **Respiratory.** Respiratory distress, tachypnea, and cyanosis.

   4. **Gastrointestinal.** Poor feeding, poor sucking, vomiting, and necrotizing enterocolitis (NEC).

   5. **Renal.** Proteinuria, oliguria, hematuria, renal vein thrombosis and decreased glomerular filtration rates, and transient hypertension.

   6. **Hematologic.** Thrombocytopenia, hepatosplenomegaly, thrombosis, disseminated intravascular coagulation (rare), and elevated reticulocyte count.

   7. **Metabolic.** Hypoglycemia (most common; 12–40%), hypocalcemia (1–11%), and increased jaundice (hyperbilirubinemia).

   8. **Skin.** Plethora or ruddiness.

   9. **Genitourinary (GU).** Testicular infarcts or priapism (majority are idiopathic).

C. **Is the mother diabetic?** Poor maternal control of diabetes during pregnancy leads to chronic fetal hypoxia, which may result in increased neonatal erythropoiesis. Infants of diabetic mothers have a 25 to >40% incidence of polycythemia. Infants of mothers with gestational diabetes also have an increased incidence (30%) of polycythemia.

D. **What is the infant's age?** The Hct normally rises after birth and reaches a peak at 2 hours of age, and then slowly decreases and stabilizes by 12 to 24 hours of age.

E. **Is the infant dehydrated?** Dehydration may cause hemoconcentration, resulting in a high Hct. It usually occurs in infants >48 hours old.

F. **Does the mother live at a high altitude?** Infants born to mothers at high altitudes have a higher incidence of polycythemia.

G. **Is the infant at high risk for polycythemia?** Infants that are small for gestational age, post-term infants, infants of diabetic mothers, infants with twin to twin transfusion, and infants with chromosomal abnormalities (Down syndrome, trisomy 13 and 18) have an increased risk for polycythemia.

III. **Differential diagnosis.** See also Chapter 122.

A. **Falsely elevated Hct.** Most often occurs when blood is obtained by heelstick.

B. **Dehydration.** Also called "relative polycythemia," it is associated with weight loss and decreased urine output (sensitive indicators of dehydration). Hemoconcentration secondary to dehydration is suspected if >8–10% of the birthweight has been lost. It usually occurs on the second or third day of life.

C. **Primary polycythemia (very rare in newborns).** Occurs when there is a problem with the production of red blood cells (excess production) in the bone marrow and occurs from inherited and acquired mutations. **Polycythemia vera, idiopathic erythrocytosis,** and **primary familial and congenital polycythemia** are examples.

D. **Secondary polycythemia.** Caused by an increase in the production of erythrocytes secondary to either fetal transfusions or placental insufficiency.

1. **Fetal transfusions.** Placental transfusion (hypertransfusion) occurs with delayed cord clamping (the most common cause in term infants). Clamping the cord >3 minutes after delivery can increase the blood volume by 30%, as can twin-twin transfusion, maternal–fetal blood transfusion, stripping the cord, and holding the infant with an intact cord 15–20 cm below the mother at delivery. Intrapartum asphyxia can cause blood volume to shift from the placenta to the fetus and cause polycythemia. Oxytocin administration can increase the volume of placental transfusion.

2. **Iatrogenic polycythemia.** Caused by overtransfusion of red cells.

3. **Intrauterine hypoxia.** Increased red blood cells (RBCs) are produced as a compensatory mechanism for intrauterine hypoxia. It may be caused by **placental insufficiency.**

    a. **Infant.** Intrauterine hypoxia may be seen in postmature, intrauterine growth restricted, or small for gestational age infants; preeclampsia/eclampsia; and infants with perinatal asphyxia.

    b. **Mother.** Maternal smoking, chronic or recurrent abruptio placentae, maternal hypertension, and severe maternal heart, pulmonary, or primary renovascular disease may also cause intrauterine hypoxia. Heavy maternal alcohol intake can be a cause. Severe maternal diabetes can cause reduced placental blood flow or pregnancy at high altitudes.

4. **Other causes/associations**

    a. **Infant of a diabetic mother** has a 22–29% incidence of polycythemia. This occurs with gestational and insulin-dependent diabetes and is due to increased erythropoiesis.

    b. **Chromosomal or congenital abnormalities.** Down syndrome (trisomy 21; 15–33%), trisomy 13 (8%), trisomy 18 (17%), fumarate hydratase deficiency, and Beckwith-Wiedemann syndrome.

    c. **Thyroid disorders.** Neonatal thyrotoxicosis and congenital hypothyroidism.

    d. **Congenital adrenal hyperplasia.**

    e. **Large for gestational age infants.**

    f. **Maternal use of propranolol.**

    g. **Sepsis.**

5. **Idiopathic.** No specific cause found.

IV. **Database**

A. **Physical examination.** Evaluate for possible dehydration. The mucous membranes will be dry. Increased skin turgor is usually not seen. True polycythemia is often, but not always, associated with visible skin changes. Ruddiness, plethora, or "pink-on-blue" or "blue-on-pink" coloration may be evident. In males, priapism may be seen secondary to sludging of red blood cells. Clinical signs are listed in Section II.B. Hypothermia is a sign of polycythemia.

B. **Laboratory studies.** The American Academy of Pediatrics (AAP) does not recommend universal screening for polycythemia, but it does recommend it for high-risk infants (infant of diabetic mother [IDM], infants with placental insufficiency).

 1. **Hct in cord blood >56% can predict polycythemia at 2 hours of age (*controversial*).**
 2. **Central Hct (venous or arterial) is essential.** Typically recommended at 2, 12, and 24 hours of age.
 3. **Serum glucose.** Hypoglycemia is commonly seen with polycythemia.
 4. **Complete blood count (CBC) with differential and platelets.** Thrombocytopenia can accompany polycythemia. Disseminated intravascular coagulation (DIC) is rare.
 5. **Serum bilirubin.** Infants with polycythemia can have problems with hyperbilirubinemia because of the increased turnover of red blood cells.
 6. **Sodium and blood urea nitrogen.** If dehydration is being considered. They are usually high, or higher than baseline values, with dehydration present.
 7. **Urine specific gravity >1.015 is usually seen with dehydration.**
 8. **Blood gas should be obtained to rule out inadequate oxygenation.**
 9. **Calcium.** Hypocalcemia can also be seen but is uncommon.

C. **Imaging and other studies.** These studies are usually not needed acutely.

 1. **Chest radiograph.** Cardiomegaly, increased pulmonary vascular markings, and pleural effusions may be seen on chest radiography.
 2. **Electrocardiogram (ECG) and electroencephalogram (EEG).** An abnormal ECG and EEG can be seen, but these tests are not routinely indicated. An ECG can show right ventricular hypertrophy and right and left atrial hypertrophy.
 3. **Echocardiogram.** Shows increased pulmonary resistance and decreased cardiac output.

V. **Plan.** (See also Chapter 122.) Treatment is *controversial*. Routine use of partial exchange transfusion (PET) is not recommended or supported. It is important to rule out other causes such as sepsis.

A. **Preventive measures.** Early cord clamping (clamping within 10 seconds vs clamping later) in high-risk infants caused fewer manifestations of polycythemia. This may be an effective way to prevent polycythemia in at-risk infants. Holding the infant at the level of the introitus at the time of delivery may also help minimize the maternal-to-fetal transfusion. Late cord clamping up to 2 minutes can be beneficial (improved Hct, improved iron levels and iron stores, and a decrease in anemia) in term infants, but there is a risk of polycythemia and jaundice, with a need for phototherapy. Cochrane review stated that delayed cord clamping (30–120 seconds) resulted in fewer transfusions and a decrease in intraventricular hemorrhage (IVH) in preterm infants.

B. **Falsely elevated Hct (>65%).** If the confirmatory central Hct is normal, no further evaluation is needed. If the central Hct is high, either dehydration or polycythemia is present.

C. **Hemoconcentration secondary to dehydration.** If the infant is dehydrated but does not have symptoms or signs of polycythemia, a trial of rehydration over 6–8 hours can be attempted. The type of fluid used depends on the infant's age and serum electrolyte status and is discussed in Chapter 9. Usually, 130–150 mL/kg/d is given. The Hct is checked every 6 hours and usually decreases with adequate rehydration.

D. **True polycythemia.** Treatment is usually based on whether or not the infant is symptomatic. The AAP states that there is no evidence that partial exchange transfusion affects the long-term outcome of the infant.

 1. **Asymptomatic infants**
  a. **Central Hct of 65–70%** and the infant is asymptomatic, only close observation and hydration (enteral or intravenous) may be needed. Many of these patients respond to increased fluid therapy; increased fluids of 20–40 mL/kg/d can be

attempted. The central Hct must be checked every 4–6 hours. About 25% of infants with an Hct of 60–64% have hyperviscosity.

b. **Central Hct >70%.** Treatment is *controversial*. Evaluate each case individually and follow your institutional guidelines. Some recommendations in the literature include

    i. **Central Hct of >70–75%** and the infant is asymptomatic, *controversy* exists as to whether a PET should be done. Hydration can be considered. Some advocate IV fluids be given and feedings withheld until Hct is <70%. Liberal IV fluid therapy can be associated with problems in preterm infants.

    ii. **Central Hct >75%.** Traditionally, neonatologists would do a partial exchange transfusion with the Hct >75%. PET should be considered if repeated Hct remains >75%.

2. **Symptomatic infants.** Some authorities recommend that any infant with polycythemia and symptoms should be treated. The goal of PET is to decrease blood viscosity and improve end-organ perfusion. *Controversy* exists but some recommendations are

a. **Central Hct >65%** in the **symptomatic** infant. Partial exchange transfusion should be performed (*controversial*). To calculate the volume that must be exchanged, use the following formula (blood volume = 80 mL/kg):

$$\text{Volume of exchange (mL)} = \frac{\text{Estimated blood volume (mL)} \times \text{Weight (kg)} \times (\text{Observed Hct} - \text{Desired Hct})}{\text{Observed Hct}}$$

Desired Hct is usually <60%, with a goal of decreasing it to 50–55%. PET may be administered via an umbilical venous catheter (UVC). **Care must be taken not to place the catheter in the liver** (see Chapter 44). A high umbilical artery catheter (UAC) or a peripheral intravenous catheter can also be used. **Normal saline is preferred in most institutions,** as crystalloids are as effective as colloids in PET. Crystalloids do not carry the risk of infection or anaphylaxis and are cheaper and more readily available. Plasmanate, 5% albumin, and fresh frozen plasma (FFP) can be used but are not recommended. Colloid products have also been associated with NEC. Serial Hct levels should be obtained after transfusion. The PET procedure is discussed in detail in Chapter 30. **Use these guidelines when performing PET:**

    i. Aliquots should not exceed 5 mL/kg and should be removed or delivered over 2–3 minutes.

    ii. Removal of blood can be from any arterial or venous line. Arterial lines are not recommended for infusion.

    iii. If there is both a UAC and a UVC, withdraw blood from the UAC while giving the replacement fluid through the UVC.

    iv. If only a UVC is in place, use the push-pull method: pull out the blood, and then push in the replacement fluid. **Never remove >5 mL/kg.** Isovolumetric method through 2 vessels is preferred.

    v. If you have a UVC, UAC, and peripheral venous catheter in, you can use either the UAC or UVC for blood withdrawal and then use the peripheral line for replacement fluid. Removal from the UVC and infusion in the peripheral venous catheter did not result in NEC in one study.

3. **Symptomatic infant with a central Hct of 60–65%.** If all other disease entities are ruled out, these infants may indeed be polycythemic and hyperviscous. Management is *controversial*. Use clinical judgment and institutional guidelines to decide whether or not these infants should have a partial exchange transfusion.

4. Restrictive management of neonatal polycythemia follows a more conservative approach. Hct of 65–69%: no treatment. Hct of 70–75%: IV fluids and no feedings until Hct is <70%. Hct ≥76% or in symptomatic neonates: use PET. A review demonstrated that the groups did not differ in morbidities or hospital stay, nor was there an increase in risk of short-term complications.

E. Observe for complications of polycythemia and disorders that are more common in polycythemic infants.

1. Apnea.
2. Hypocalcemia, hypoglycemia, electrolyte abnormalities.
3. Thrombocytopenia.
4. Hyperbilirubinemia.
5. Neurologic. Seizures, stroke, cerebral vein thrombosis.
6. Vascular. Vasospasms, peripheral gangrene.
7. Cardiac. Arrhythmia, congestive heart failure.
8. GI
   a. Necrotizing enterocolitis (NEC) risk is increased in neonates with hyperviscosity who received a partial exchange transfusion via a UVC with colloid (FFP, albumin, or Plasmanate). The development of NEC in these infants may be related to PET with colloid, not the polycythemia.
   b. Ileus, spontaneous intestinal perforations, intestinal atresia.
9. Genitourinary. Renal failure, renal vein thrombosis, testicular infarcts, priapism.
10. Air embolism.

F. Follow-up data. Polycythemia and hyperviscosity syndrome treated by PET can be associated with significant complications (increased risk of NEC) and may be associated with an earlier improvement in symptoms. Further research is needed to assess the impact on newborns, as there is conflicting (*controversial*) literature.

1. PET decreases viscosity and ameliorates most symptoms but does not significantly improve long-term neurologic outcomes. However, decreased IQ scores and lower achievement were reported in infants with hyperviscosity syndrome who were not treated with PET.
2. PET improves microcirculation in polycythemic neonates. Near infrared spectroscopy showed increased cerebral oxygenation and decreased fractional tissue oxygen extraction.
3. PET has been shown to improve cerebral blood flow velocity and decrease pulmonary vascular resistance, and may normalize cerebral hemodynamics.
4. There is no evidence of improvement in long-term neurologic outcome or early neurobehavioral assessment scores following PET in symptomatic or asymptomatic infants.
5. Polycythemic infants are at risk for speech abnormalities and for fine/gross motor delays.
6. Umbilical vein partial exchange transfusion with colloid increases the risk of NEC.
7. Intrauterine fetal hypoxia is related to polycythemia and the impaired long-term outcome.
8. Coexisting hypoglycemia may worsen the long-term outcome.
9. Cochrane review states no proven benefit to PET in infants with polycythemia who are well or who have minor symptoms. PET may increase the risk of NEC. It notes that the risk and benefits of PET are not clear at this time.

Selected References

Mimouni FB, Merlob P, Dollberg S, Mandel D. Neonatal polycythaemia: critical review and a consensus statement of the Israeli Neonatology Association. *Acta Paediatr.* 2011;100(10):1290–1296.

Morag I, Strauss T, Lubin D, Schushan-Eisen I, Kenet G, Kuint J. Restrictive management of neonatal polycythemia. *Am J Perinatol.* 2011;28(9):677–682.

Rabe H, Reynolds GJ, Diaz-Rosello JL. Early versus delayed umbilical cord clamping in preterm infants. *Cochrane Database Syst Rev.* 2004;(4). DOI:10.1002/14651858.CD003248.pub2.

72 Poor Perfusion

I. **Problem.** You receive a report that an infant "doesn't look good" or looks "mottled." Other descriptions may include a "washed-out appearance" or "poor perfusion."

II. **Immediate questions**

   A. **What is the age of the infant?** Hypoplastic left heart syndrome may cause poor perfusion and a mottled appearance. It may be seen at days 1–21 of life (more commonly at day 2 or 3). In an infant <3 days old, **sepsis** may be a cause. Associated risk factors for sepsis are premature rupture of membranes, maternal infection, and fever.

   B. **What are the vital signs?** If the temperature is lower than normal, cold stress or hypothermia associated with sepsis may be present. Hypotension may cause poor perfusion (see normal blood pressure values in Table 65–1 and Appendix C). Decreased urine output (<2 mL/kg/h) may indicate depleted intravascular volume or shock.

   C. **Is the liver enlarged? Are metabolic acidosis, poor peripheral pulse rate, and a gallop present?** These problems are signs of failure of the left side of the heart (eg, hypoplastic left heart syndrome). Poor perfusion occurs because of reduced blood flow to the skin.

   D. **If mechanical ventilation is being used, are chest movements adequate and are blood gas levels improving?** Inadequate ventilation can result in poor perfusion. Pneumothorax may also be a cause.

   E. **Are congenital anomalies present?** Persistent cutis marmorata (see Section III.A.12) may be seen in Cornelia de Lange syndrome and in trisomy 18 and 21. **Chromosome 22q11 deletion syndrome** can present with abnormal vascular tone with hypotension. **Cornelia de Lange syndrome** consists of multiple congenital anomalies: a distinctive facial appearance, pre- and postnatal growth deficiency, feeding problems, psychomotor delay, behavioral problems, and malformations that mainly involve the upper extremities.

III. **Differential diagnosis**

   A. **More common causes**

   1. **Sepsis.**
   2. **Cold stress/hypothermia.** In general, a skin temperature <36.5°C.
   3. **Hypotension** usually with shock.
   4. **Hypoventilation.**
   5. **Pneumothorax.**
   6. **Hypoglycemia** can mimic hypoxemia, and poor perfusion can be seen.
   7. **Polycythemia with hyperviscosity.** Infants have sluggish capillary refill and poor peripheral perfusion.
   8. **Acute hemorrhagic anemia** due to acute blood loss can present with symptoms of hypovolemia including poor perfusion, hypotension, tachycardia, and pallor. A decrease in peripheral perfusion occurs with a 10% loss of blood volume.
   9. **Necrotizing enterocolitis (NEC).**
   10. **Left-sided obstructive heart disease.** Newborns with critical left-sided obstructive lesions (ductal-dependent systemic circulation) generally appear normal at birth, and when the ductus arteriosus begins to close, they have cardiac failure

with systemic hypoperfusion (poor perfusion with cold, clammy, mottled skin), poor peripheral pulses, increasing metabolic acidosis, and shock. Cyanosis may not be seen until later. One study showed that the majority of infants presented with shock, approximately one-third presented with heart failure, and a small percentage presented with profound cyanosis. These diseases include hypoplastic left heart syndrome (HLHS), critical aortic stenosis (AS), coarctation of the aorta (COA) (with or without septal defect), and interrupted aortic arch (IAA). When the ductus closes, infants with COA and IAA have hypoperfusion of the lower half of the body, and infants with AS and HLHS have hypoperfusion of the entire systemic circulation.

11. **Infant of substance-abusing mother.** Mottling can be a sign of neonatal abstinence.

12. **Cutis marmorata.** A marbling, red/blue, lacy, reticulated mottling pattern on the skin. It may occur in healthy infants especially when exposed to cold stress (immature neurologic and vascular system). It may also indicate poor perfusion in septic infants. Persistent mottling (persistent cutis marmorata) can occur in hypothyroidism, central nervous system dysfunction, and some congenital syndromes (Cornelia de Lange, Edward [trisomy 18] and Down [trisomy 21]). **Cutis marmorata telangiectatica** congenita is a rare vascular malformation (see Chapter 6). See Plate 1.

B. **Less common causes**

1. **Enteroviral/viral or fungal infection.** Presents with poor perfusion and overwhelming sepsis.

2. **Periventricular hemorrhage/intraventricular hemorrhage (PVH/IVH).** Presentation varies but can present with extreme signs, including sudden onset of poor perfusion, pallor, and hypotonia.

3. **Subgaleal hemorrhage (rare).** Most commonly associated with a vacuum evacuation or forceps delivery. It progresses after birth and can have a massive amount of blood.

4. **Inborn errors of metabolism.** Present with a history of deterioration with poor perfusion. Organic acidemia, urea cycle defects, and certain disorders of amino acid metabolism can present with poor perfusion, lethargy, and other symptoms.

5. **Seizures.**

6. **Hematologic.** Bleeding disorders.

7. **Adrenal problems.** Congenital adrenal hyperplasia, Addison disease, adrenal hemorrhage.

8. **Renovascular hypertension.** Presents with apnea, irritability, and mottling of the skin.

9. **Gastrointestinal problems.** NEC, perforation, volvulus.

10. **Systemic air embolism.** Symptoms are sudden and include mottling of the skin with pallor.

11. **Chronic pain.** Infants experiencing chronic pain can exhibit decreased and poor perfusion with cool extremities.

IV. **Database**

A. **Physical examination.** Note the temperature and vital signs and look for signs of sepsis. The cardiovascular and pulmonary examinations are important because they may suggest cardiac problems or pneumothorax. Does the infant have an S3 gallop with or without a cardiac murmur (left-sided obstructive ductal-dependent heart lesion)? Signs of trisomy 18 include micrognathia and overlapping digits. Signs of trisomy 21 include a single palmar transverse crease and epicanthal folds. Look for scalp swelling to rule out subgaleal hemorrhage. Abdominal distension can be seen with gastrointestinal problems.

B. **Laboratory studies**

1. **Complete blood count (CBC) to evaluate for sepsis or decreased/increased hematocrit.** To evaluate for polycythemia or blood loss.

2. **Blood gas.** These studies reveal inadequate ventilation or the presence of acidosis, which may be seen in sepsis or NEC. Persistent metabolic acidosis can be seen in subgaleal hemorrhage.
3. **Blood glucose levels.** To rule out hypoglycemia.
4. **Cultures.** If sepsis is suspected, a complete workup should be considered, especially if antibiotics are to be started. This workup includes cultures of blood, urine, and spinal fluid (if indicated). If enteroviral infection is suspected, send for viral cultures.
5. **Polymerase chain reaction.** Studies of stool and cerebrospinal fluid and nasopharyngeal or throat swab for enterovirus and other viruses.
6. **Inborn errors of metabolism.** See Chapter 101 for appropriate tests.
C. **Imaging and other studies**
1. **Transillumination of the chest** (see Chapter 27, Section III.B and Chapter 40) can be performed quickly to help determine whether or not a pneumothorax is present.
2. **Chest radiograph** if pneumonia, pneumothorax, congenital heart lesion, or hypoventilation is suspected. In left-sided heart lesions, the radiograph shows cardiomegaly with pulmonary venous congestion (except in hypoplastic left heart syndrome, in which the size of the heart may be normal). If a view taken during lung expansion shows that the lungs are down only to the sixth rib or less, hypoventilation should be considered. With hyperventilation, lung expansion is down to the ninth or tenth rib. See Figure 11–15 for radiograph of pneumonia. See Figure 11–20 for radiograph showing a pneumothorax.
3. **Abdominal radiograph** if NEC is suspected. See Figure 11–23 for a radiograph showing pneumatosis intestinalis seen in NEC. Air can be seen with a perforation. Obstruction can be seen with malrotation with volvulus.
4. **Echocardiography** should be performed if a congenital heart lesion is suspected. In hypoplastic left heart syndrome, a large right ventricle and a small left ventricle are seen on the echocardiogram, and there is failure to visualize the mitral or aortic valve. In aortic stenosis, the echocardiogram reveals a deformed aortic valve. In coarctation of the aorta, it reveals decreased aortic diameter. In venous air embolism, one can see acute obstruction of the right ventricle outflow tract.
5. **Head ultrasound** to rule out intraventricular bleed. Optimal imaging for subgaleal hemorrhage is by computed tomography (CT) or magnetic resonance imaging.
6. **Karyotyping or molecular genetic testing** if trisomy 18 or 21 or a deletion is suspected. Cornelia de Lange syndrome has mutations in the NIPBL and SMC3 genes.
7. **CT of the head** to look for intracranial air bubbles if systemic air embolism suspected.
V. **Plan**
A. **Immediate plan.** An initial quick workup should be performed. While checking vital signs and quickly examining the patient, order a STAT blood gas and a chest radiograph. Initiate oxygen supplementation and transilluminate the chest if a pneumothorax is suspected. Send a STAT CBC and differential and blood culture.
B. **Specific plans**
1. **Sepsis.** Full cultures and empirical antibiotic therapy may be started at the discretion of the physician.
2. **Cold stress.** Gradual rewarming is necessary, usually at a rate of ≤1°C/h. It can be accomplished by means of a radiant warmer or incubator or a heating pad. (See Chapter 7.)
3. **Hypotension or shock.** If the blood pressure is low because of depleted intravascular volume, give crystalloid (normal saline), 10 mL/kg intravenously for 5–10 minutes. (See Chapter 65.)
4. **Hypoventilation.** If suspected, it may be necessary to increase the pressure being given by the ventilator. The amount of pressure must be decided on an

individual basis. One method is to increase the pressure by 2–4 cm H_2O and then obtain blood gas levels in 20 minutes. Another method is to use bag-and-mask ventilation, observing the manometer to determine the amount of pressure needed to move the chest. (See Chapter 46.)

5. **Pneumothorax.** See Chapter 70.
6. **Hypoglycemia.** See Chapter 62.
7. **Polycythemia.** See Chapters 71 and 122.
8. **Anemia secondary to acute blood loss.** See Chapter 82.
9. **NEC.** See Chapter 113.
10. **Left-sided obstructive heart lesions.** Initial stabilization with respiratory support (endotracheal intubation and mechanical ventilation if poor respiratory effort and hypoxemia), volume resuscitation, inotropic support with dopamine for low cardiac output, and correction of metabolic acidosis. Immediate cardiac consultation. PGE_1 is considered before diagnosis is confirmed if ductal-dependent systemic blood flow is suspected. The infant should be stabilized and transferred to a pediatric cardiac center. Surgery is usually indicated in all these patients. For a full discussion of cardiac abnormalities, see Chapter 89.
11. **Cutis marmorata.** If this condition is secondary to cold stress, treat the patient as described in Section V.B.2. If the condition persists, consider formal genetic testing for various syndromes noted. Thyroid studies will be necessary if hypothyroidism is suspected. If CNS dysfunction is suspected, this should be evaluated further.
12. **Periventricular hemorrhage/intraventricular hemorrhage (PVH/IVH).** Initial supportive care (maintain blood pressure, stabilize blood gases, transfuse if necessary, treat for seizures, etc.). After stabilization, close follow-up is required. Serial lumbar punctures may be necessary. (See also Chapter 104.)
13. **Subgaleal hemorrhage.** Early recognition, appropriate resuscitation, supportive care as in volume replacement, blood transfusion, and coagulation factors if necessary. Pressure wrapping of the head is *controversial*.
14. **Inborn errors of metabolism.** See Chapter 101.
15. **Seizures.** See Chapter 129.
16. **Hematologic problems.** Blood transfusions and diagnosing and treating the specific bleeding disorder are necessary.
17. **Adrenal insufficiency.** Blood volume replacement and steroid therapy are usually necessary.
18. **Renovascular hypertension.** Usually treated with aggressive medical management.
19. **Intestinal problems.** See Chapters 113 and 131.
20. **Enteroviral infections.** Supportive management. See Chapter 92.
21. **Systemic air embolism.** Supportive cardiac and respiratory care. One hundred percent oxygen therapy, hyperbaric oxygen.
22. **Chronic pain.** See Chapter 14.

73 Postdelivery Antibiotics

I. **Problem.** Two infants are born within the last hour. One infant's mother had premature rupture of membranes (PROM) but no antibiotics. The other infant's mother was pretreated with antibiotics for a positive group B *Streptococcus* (GBS) culture taken at 36 weeks. Should a sepsis workup be done, and should antibiotics be started in either of these newborns?

Early-onset sepsis (EOS) occurs within the first 3 days of life and is vertically transmitted (ascending organisms from the birth canal) and can occur from ruptured membranes, inhaling or swallowing infected amniotic fluid, or an amniotic fluid leak before or during labor. Sepsis in the first 3 days of life is a leading cause of morbidity and mortality among preterm infants. The incidence of sepsis is 1–10 in 1000 live births and 1 in 250 live premature births, with GBS being the most common pathogen followed by *Escherichia coli*. Black preterm infants have the highest incidence and case fatality. Since the institution of Centers for Disease Control and Prevention (CDC) guidelines, the incidence of early-onset GBS has decreased by 80%. Late-onset sepsis is discussed in Chapter 130, and infections of premature infants with prolonged hospital stays may require a different workup and antibiotic choice. **This on-call problem focuses on postdelivery antibiotics for early-onset or suspected sepsis.** The **American Academy of Pediatrics (AAP)** has a practical evidence-based approach to managing infants with suspected and culture-proven early-onset sepsis.

II. Immediate questions

A. **Are there any major risk factors for early-onset sepsis? Major risk factors** are preterm birth, low birthweight (risk factor most associated with early-onset sepsis), rupture of membranes (ROM) >18 hours, maternal colonization with GBS (if inadequate intrapartum therapy), or maternal chorioamnionitis (defined as maternal fever ≥38.0°C [≥100.4°F] and a minimum of 2 of the following: maternal white blood cell [WBC] count >15,000 mm^3, maternal tachycardia [>100 beats/min], fetal tachycardia [>160 beats/min], uterine tenderness, foul odor of the amniotic fluid).

B. **Are there any other maternal risk factors for sepsis in the infant?** Other risk factors include African race, maternal malnutrition, recently acquired sexually transmitted disease/sexually transmitted infection (STD/STI), maternal age <20 years, low socioeconomic status, and asymptomatic maternal bacteriuria. Maternal history of a previous infant with GBS infection also increases the risk of sepsis.

C. **Are there other intrapartum risk factors for sepsis in the infant?** These include maternal infection, any untreated or incompletely treated infection of the mother, and maternal fever without identifiable cause. The use of fetal scalp electrodes in the intrapartum period increases the risk of infection in the infant. Meconium-stained amniotic fluid and traumatic delivery are also risk factors.

D. **Are there any other neonatal risk factors involved?** Other risk factors include male sex, low Apgar scores, severe depression at birth with intubation and resuscitation, perinatal asphyxia, twin birth, and presence of the metabolic disorder galactosemia (increased risk of gram-negative sepsis).

E. **How long before delivery did the membranes rupture?** ROM that occurs >18 hours before birth is associated with an increased incidence of infection in the neonate.

F. **Was the infant monitored during labor?** Fetal tachycardia (>160 beats/min), especially sustained, and decelerations (usually late) can be associated with neonatal infection. Prolonged duration of intrauterine monitoring is a risk factor for early-onset group B streptococcal disease.

G. **Did the mother have a cerclage for cervical incompetence?** Cerclage increases the risk of infection in the infant. Preterm PROM occurs in 38% of women with cerclage in place. Retention of cerclage for more than 24 hours after PROM was found to prolong pregnancy for more than 48 hours, but also to increase maternal chorioamnionitis and neonatal mortality from sepsis.

H. **Are signs of sepsis present in the infant?** Signs of sepsis are nonspecific and can include apnea and bradycardia, temperature instability (hypothermia or hyperthermia), feeding intolerance, tachypnea, jaundice, cyanosis, poor peripheral perfusion, hypoglycemia, lethargy, poor sucking reflex, increased gastric aspirates, and irritability. Other signs include tachycardia, shock, vomiting, seizures, abnormal rash, abdominal distention, and hepatomegaly. Neonatal sepsis is associated with systolic and diastolic myocardial dysfunction. Bacteremia can also occur without clinical signs.

I. **Did the mother have epidural analgesia?** Studies have shown an increase in maternal intrapartum fever (15–20%) with the use of epidural analgesia. Because of this fever, an increase in sepsis evaluations and antibiotic treatment was found. However, the study did not find that epidurals caused infections or even increased the risk of infections.

J. **Was the mother tested for GBS, and did she receive antibiotics if she tested positive?** There are now specific guidelines to follow after delivery if the mother was treated for GBS.

K. **Did the mother have chorioamnionitis?** See definition above. Chorioamnionitis is a major risk factor for sepsis, and its incidence varies inversely with gestational age. Histological chorioamnionitis increases the chance of having markers of infection (increased C-reactive proteins and neutrophilia, bacterial colonization [by gastric lavage and ear swab] and congenital sepsis). Fourteen to twenty-eight percent of mothers who deliver preterm infants at 22 to 28 weeks have signs of chorioamnionitis. **Risk factors for chorioamnionitis** include spontaneous labor, low parity, multiple digital vaginal examinations, meconium-stained amniotic fluid, presence of genital tract microorganisms, long length of labor and membrane rupture, and internal fetal or uterine monitoring.

III. **Differential diagnosis**

A. **Culture-proven sepsis.** Cultures confirm sepsis diagnosis.

B. **Suspected sepsis.** An infant has nonspecific signs of sepsis or there is a high likelihood that the infant has sepsis based on clinical signs. Sepsis needs to be "ruled out" in the infant. From 18 to 33% of infants with negative blood cultures have sepsis confirmed at autopsy.

C. **Increased risk for sepsis.** The infant has risk factors (preterm birth, maternal colonization with GBS, rupture of membranes at >18 hours before birth, mother has signs of an intra-amniotic infection) that can increase the risk of early-onset sepsis.

D. **Infant at low risk for sepsis.** Newborns without the risk factors noted previously are at low risk of sepsis.

IV. **Database**

A. **Complete maternal, perinatal, and birth history.** This should be obtained and reviewed in an attempt to identify risk factors, as noted previously. Maternal history is just as important as the birth history. It is especially important to discuss the diagnosis of chorioamnionitis with the obstetrics (OB) department since it has major implications for the management of the newborn.

B. **Physical examination.** Observe for signs of sepsis (see above). Clinical observation is important. One study found that affect, peripheral perfusion, and respiratory status were key predictors in sepsis compared with feeding patterns, level of activity, and level of alertness. The maternal clinical examination should be reviewed with the obstetrics and gynecology (OB/GYN) service. **Early-onset sepsis can occur in infants who appear healthy at birth.**

C. **Laboratory studies**

1. **Complete blood count (CBC) with differential.** A single WBC count is not helpful when compared to serial tests. Timing of the CBC is important; an early CBC is not recommended. CBC at 4–6 to 12 hours is optimal, after the inflammatory response has occurred. The incidence of sepsis is increased only when the WBC count and absolute neutrophil count is low. Some recommend interval likelihood ratios to be used to interpret CBC instead of using normal ranges.

   a. **Normal total WBC.** The total leukocyte count is a very unreliable indicator of neonatal infection. Normal WBC counts may be seen in as many as 50% of culture-proven sepsis cases. A normal WBC count does not rule out sepsis, but a normal WBC is a better negative predictor of sepsis.

   b. **Abnormally low or high WBC count is worrisome.** Values <6000 cells/mm^3 or >30,000 cells/mm^3 in the first 24 hours of life are abnormal. A band neutrophil count >20% is abnormal. Only half of infants with WBC <5000 cells/mm^3 or WBC >20,000 cells/mm^3 have positive blood cultures (BCs). Septic infants

Table 73–1. NEONATAL NEUTROPHIL INDICES REFERENCE RANGES FOR LATE PRETERM AND TERM INFANTS (PER MM³) AT LOW ALTITUDE

Variable	Birth	12 Hours	24 Hours	48 Hours	72 Hours	>120 Hours
Absolute total neutrophil count[a]	1800–5400	7800–14,400	7200–12,600	4200–9000	1800–7000	1800–5400
Total immature neutrophil count[b]	≤1120	≤1440	≤1280	<800	<500	<500
I:T ratio[c]	<0.16	<0.16	<0.13	<0.13	<0.13	<0.12

[a]Total count includes mature and immature forms.
[b]Includes all neutrophils except segmented ones.
[c]Ratio of total immature neutrophil count divided by absolute total neutrophil count (I:T), ratio of immature to total neutrophils.
Based on data from Manroe BL, Weinberg AG, Rosenfeld CR, Browne R. The neonatal blood count in health and disease: I. Reference values for neutrophilic cells. *J Pediatr.* 1979;95:89.

with a WBC count <5000 cells/mm³ are more likely to have bacterial meningitis.

c. **Neutropenia can be a good marker for sepsis** because it occurs only in sepsis, asphyxia, inborn errors of metabolism (IEMs), hemolytic disease, and pregnancy-induced maternal hypertension. The neutropenia ranges depend on gestational age (WBC count increases with gestational age), type of delivery (vaginal births have higher WBC counts than cesarean section without labor), type of sample (arterial samples give lower WBC counts than venous samples), and altitude (WBC counts are higher at higher altitudes). Results from Manroe (Table 73–1) are for late preterm and term infants at low altitudes <500 ft. Results from Schmutz et al are for preterm to term infants at higher altitudes, ~4800 ft.

   i. **Total neutrophil count** is more sensitive than the total leukocyte count but too often is normal in cases of infection. It peaks in 12 hours, and it has a poor sensitivity and poor predictive accuracy for early-onset sepsis. See Tables 73–1 and 73–2 for Manroe data. For **high altitude (Schmutz data),** the lower and upper limits of normal for neutrophils at birth are

   (a) **<28 weeks' gestation.** 500–8000/mm³.
   (b) **28–36 weeks' gestation.** 1000–10,500/mm³.
   (c) **>36 weeks' gestation.** 3500–18,000/mm³.

Table 73–2. REFERENCE RANGES FOR NEUTROPHIL COUNTS IN VERY LOW BIRTHWEIGHT INFANTS (<1500 G)

Age	Absolute Total Neutrophil Count (mm³) (min to max)
Birth	500–6000
18 hours	2200–14,000
60 hours	1100–8800
120 hours	1100–5600

Based on data from Mouzinho A, Rosenfeld CR, Sánchez PJ, Risser R. Revised reference ranges for circulating neutrophils in very-low-birth-weight neonates. *Pediatrics.* 1994;94:76.

Peak values are seen 6–8 hours after birth. The lower and upper limits of normal at that time are
   (a) <28 weeks' gestation. 1500–41,000/mm³.
   (b) 28–36 weeks' gestation. 3500–25,000/mm³.
   (c) >36 weeks' gestation. 7500–28,500/mm³.

   ii. Total immature neutrophil count has poor sensitivity but better positive predictive value. See Table 73–1.
   iii. Ratio of immature to total neutrophils (I:T) has the highest sensitivity for early-onset neonatal sepsis. The greatest value relies in its negative predictive value; the likelihood of infection is minimal if the I:T ratio is normal. In the majority of healthy preterm infants at <32 weeks (96%), the I:T ratio is <0.22. The total neutrophil count can be calculated, and normal reference ranges can be found in Tables 73–1 and 73–2.

2. Peripheral blood cultures are the gold standard for diagnosis of sepsis. Small specimen volumes decrease the sensitivity (minimum of 1 mL per single bottle, aerobic culture only recommended). Antibiotic removal device bottles should be used if the mother has received any antibiotics. Acceptable ways to obtain blood culture in a neonate: peripheral vein, arterial puncture, newly placed intravenous catheter, umbilical artery catheter (UAC) immediately after placement. Umbilical venous catheter (UVC) at delivery is also acceptable if the cord is adequately prepared.

3. Urine culture is no longer recommended in infants <72 hours of age in an early-onset sepsis workup. More appropriately done for late-onset sepsis workup.

4. Gastric aspirates. Gram stain is of limited value and not recommended. WBCs in the gastric aspirate represent maternal response and do not correlate with sepsis in the neonate.

5. Body surface cultures (axilla, external ear canal, umbilical stump, groin) are not recommended.

6. Lumbar puncture (LP) for cerebrospinal fluid (CSF) examination is *controversial*. The AAP recommends that a LP be done with positive blood culture, if the infant deteriorates or does not respond on antibiotic therapy, and in infants whose lab data or clinical course suggests bacterial sepsis. Approximately 13% of infants with early-onset sepsis will also have meningitis. Infants with bacteremia have a risk of meningitis of 23%. Blood cultures can be negative in 38% of infants with meningitis. Infants with respiratory distress syndrome (RDS) and high-risk, healthy-appearing infants are at low risk of meningitis.

7. Tracheal aspirate. May be of benefit for Gram stain and culture if performed immediately after endotracheal tube placement. Some advocate this only if pneumonia is suspected or volume of secretions increases, or in overwhelming newborn EOS. Tracheal aspirates done after several days of intubation are of no value.

8. Baseline serum glucose.

9. Arterial blood gas. To rule out metabolic acidosis.

10. Platelet count and coagulation studies to rule out thrombocytopenia and disseminated intravascular coagulation (DIC). A decreased platelet count is usually a late sign of sepsis. A low platelet count is a nonspecific and insensitive test for sepsis.

11. Erythrocyte sedimentation rates (ESRs). Increased with infection but have a very limited value in diagnosing or monitoring infection. A low value does not exclude the diagnosis of sepsis.

12. Acute phase reactants (C-reactive protein [CRP] and procalcitonin [PCT]). Used to identify infants with sepsis. CRP is a quantitative test. An increasing CRP is worrisome and is elevated in 50–90% of infants with sepsis. CRP increases at 6–8 hours and peaks at 24 hours. If CRPs remain normal, sepsis is unlikely.

The main interest in CRP is its negative predictive value if repeated over 1–3 days. No recommendations exist on using an elevated CRP to help determine duration of antibiotic therapy. **Serum procalcitonin** levels are elevated in sepsis and may be helpful as a marker for sepsis. It can also be elevated in RDS, asphyxia, intracranial hemorrhage, pneumothorax, and resuscitation. It has better sensitivity but is less specific than CRP. Serial PCT levels may be helpful in deciding duration of antibiotic therapy. The following is a list of predicted CRP and PCT levels with lower and upper limits in parentheses in term and preterm infants.

   a. CRP (term) in mg/dL. Birth: 0.1 (0.01–0.65); 21 hours: 1.5 (0.2–10.0); 56–70 hours: 1.9 (0.3–13); 96 hours: 1.4 (0.2–9).
   b. CRP (preterm) in mg/dL. Birth: 0.1 (0.01–0.64); 27–36 hours: 1.7 (0.3–11); 90 hours: 0.7 (0.1–4.7).
   c. Procalcitonin (term) in mcg/L. Birth: 0.08 (0.01–0.55); 24 hours: 2.9 (0.4–18.7); 80 hours: 0.3 (0.04–1.8).
   d. Procalcitonin (preterm) in mcg/L. Birth: 0.07 (0.01–0.56); 21–22 hours: 6.5 (0.9–48.4); 5 days: 0.10 (0.01–0.8).

13. Laboratory tests that could be helpful in screening for sepsis but are not routinely used. Lack of availability, lack of confirmatory studies, and wide variations in results.
   a. Cytokines. Interleukins (IL-1, IL-6, IL-8), soluble IL-2 receptor, and soluble tumor necrosis factor alpha (TNF-α) receptor have been identified; IL-6 has been studied the most. **Interleukins 6 and 8 are early sensitive markers of infection.** IL-6 is higher in infants with polycythemia.
   b. Neutrophil surface antigens. CD11b is a marker for early-onset sepsis.
   c. Urinary neutrophil gelatinase–associated lipocalin (NGAL). A promising biomarker for sepsis in neonates, it is elevated in sepsis, ischemia, hypoxia, and drug toxicity.
   d. Multiple markers. Using serial and multiple investigational markers showed the best reliability for predicting sepsis.
   e. Septic scoring systems. Usually include a battery of multiple laboratory tests (and sometimes clinical indicators of sepsis) where each test is given a number based on the result and the total score assesses the risk of sepsis. Institutions have devised their own septic scoring systems. Studies of scoring systems (using a combination of the laboratory tests mentioned previously) have shown that they all have limited value in screening for sepsis unless the score is high, with a negative panel being a better predictor than a positive panel. They may be helpful in deciding which healthy high-risk infants do not need antibiotics or whether antibiotics can be stopped.

D. Imaging and other studies
   1. Chest x-ray. With signs of respiratory infection, obtain a chest radiograph to rule out pneumonia.
   2. Echocardiography and Doppler imaging. To assess myocardial function. Infants with sepsis have systolic and diastolic myocardial dysfunction.
   3. Head ultrasound or magnetic resonance imaging (MRI). May be helpful in meningitis.

V. Plan
   A. General measures. For the majority of cases, a decision about whether an infant requires a sepsis workup and antibiotics is usually straightforward. These infants either are clinically sick or have a positive history of an increased risk for sepsis with clinical signs, thereby making the antibiotic decision easy. However, if an infant does not have a clear-cut history and clinical presentation, the decision is more difficult. One single test is often not helpful and it is necessary to "repeat, repeat, and repeat" the test. Once the decision is made to treat the infant, treatment usually involves at least 36–48 hours of antibiotics after obtaining cultures. The following guidelines can be used to help make the decision to treat:

1. **CDC recommendations should be followed if possible.** The CDC now recommends universal prenatal screening for vaginal and rectal GBS of all pregnant women at 35–37 weeks' gestation. The following are CDC recommendations for the management of **all newborns**. If antibiotics are given, use broad spectrum for the most common causes of sepsis (IV ampicillin for GBS and coverage for other organisms [*E. coli* and other gram-negative organisms]). When deciding antibiotics, check local antibiotic resistance patterns. If there are any signs of sepsis during the observation period, the infant should receive a full diagnostic evaluation. GBS prophylaxis is indicated if there are one or more of the following:

   a. Positive GBS vaginal rectal screening in late gestation (optimal at 35–37 weeks' gestation).

   b. **GBS status unknown at onset of labor** (culture not done, culture incomplete, or unknown results) with one or more intrapartum risk factors, including delivery <37 weeks' gestation, ROM ≥18 hours or intrapartum T ≥100.4°F (38.0°C), intrapartum nucleic acid amplification test (NAAT) positive for GBS.

   c. **GBS bacteriuria** during any trimester during the current pregnancy (intrapartum antibiotic prophylaxis [IAP] not indicated if culture and sensitivity [C/S] done before onset of labor with intact membranes).

   d. **History of a previous infant** with invasive GBS disease.

2. **CDC treatment plan for secondary prevention of early-onset GBS among all newborns (term and preterm).** See also Figure 130–1.

   a. **Any signs of sepsis.** Full diagnostic workup (CBC with differential and platelets, blood culture, chest x-ray [CXR] with abnormal respiratory signs, LP if stable enough to tolerate, and sepsis is strongly suspected). Give empiric antibiotics.

   b. **Well infant, mother with suspected chorioamnionitis.** Consultation with OB department is important to discuss level of clinical assessment of chorioamnionitis. Perform a limited evaluation: Do a blood culture at birth, CBC with differential, platelet count at birth and/or at 6–12 hours of life. Start empiric antibiotics.

   c. **Well infant, mother without chorioamnionitis, and GBS prophylaxis not indicated for the mother.** Routine clinical care. If signs of sepsis develop, do a full diagnostic evaluation and initiate antibiotics.

   d. **Well infant, GBS prophylaxis indicated for mother and she received adequate intrapartum GBS prophylaxis** (≥4 hours of IV penicillin, ampicillin, or cefazolin before delivery). Observe for 48 hours or more; no testing necessary. If signs of sepsis develop, do a full diagnostic evaluation and start antibiotics. Infant may go home after 24 hours if ≥37 weeks' gestation and discharge criteria have been met. **Well-appearing infants at gestational age (GA) of 35–36 weeks** do not routinely require diagnostic evaluations.

   e. **Well infant, mother had indication for GBS prophylaxis but did not receive adequate prophylaxis.**

      i. **Infant ≥37 weeks and ROM <18 hours.** Observe infant for 48 hours or more; no testing. Some recommend CBC and differential at 6–12 hours. If signs of sepsis develop, do a full diagnostic evaluation and start antibiotics.

      ii. **Infant <37 weeks or ROM ≥18 hours.** Limited evaluation (blood culture at birth, CBC with differential at birth and/or at 6–12 hours of life) with observation for 48 hours or more. Some experts recommend a CBC and differential at 6–12 hours. If signs of sepsis develop, do a full diagnostic evaluation and start antibiotics.

3. **The AAP guidelines** recognize the clinical challenges in this area. The concern of overtreatment is validated by recent data showing that prolonged antibiotic treatment >5 days in preterm infants had a higher incidence of NEC, late-onset sepsis, and mortality. **They have come up with management plans for neonates with suspected or proven early-onset bacterial sepsis.** When reviewing these specific guidelines, remember these key points. If the **mother was diagnosed**

with chorioamnionitis, it is important to talk to the obstetricians and confirm the diagnosis since it has major treatment implications for the infant. **Inadequate IAP** means the mother received another antibiotic (not penicillin, ampicillin, or cefazolin) or received the correct antibiotic but the duration was <4 hours.

a. **Any critically ill infant.** Requires a complete sepsis evaluation and antibiotics (even if there are no risk factors).

b. **Any mature infant without risk factors for infection with mild findings** (tachypnea with or without O_2 requirement). Observe for ~6 hours after birth. With improvement (tachypnea is resolving, O_2 requirement is decreasing), antibiotics are probably not indicated but continued observation is. With worsening clinical state, obtain cultures and start antibiotics empirically.

c. **Healthy-appearing, asymptomatic infant <37 weeks with one risk factor for sepsis.** For example, intrapartum antimicrobial prophylaxis indicated but inadequate or PROM ≥18 hours or chorioamnionitis.

   i. **Do blood culture at birth,** WBC and differential and optional CRP at age 6–12 hours.

   ii. **Start broad-spectrum antibiotics.** Now what?

     (a) **Blood culture positive.** Continue antibiotics. Lumbar puncture is indicated in any infant with a positive blood culture or if sepsis is highly suspected (based on clinical signs, response to treatment, or lab results).

     (b) **Blood culture negative, infant well, lab values abnormal.** Continue antibiotics in the infant for a total of 72 hours if mother received antibiotics during labor and delivery. If at 72 hours the physical examination is normal, the antibiotics can be discontinued.

     (c) **Blood cultures negative, infant well, lab values normal.** Discontinue antibiotics after 48 hours.

d. **Healthy-appearing, asymptomatic infant ≥37 weeks with risk factor of chorioamnionitis.**

   i. **Blood culture at birth,** WBC and differential and optional CRP at age 6–12 hours.

   ii. **Start broad-spectrum antibiotics.** Now what?

     (a) **Blood culture positive.** Continue antibiotics. Lumbar puncture is indicated in any infant with a positive blood culture or if sepsis is highly suspected (based on clinical signs, response to treatment, or lab results).

     (b) **Blood culture negative, infant well, lab values abnormal.** Continue antibiotics for a total of 48–72 hours in the infant if mother received antibiotics during labor and delivery. Discontinue antibiotics at 48–72 hours if the physical examination remains normal.

     (c) **Blood culture negative, infant well, lab values normal.** Discontinue antibiotics and discharge by 48 hours.

e. **Healthy-appearing, asymptomatic infant ≥37 weeks with risk factors for sepsis but not chorioamnionitis.** PROM ≥18 hours or intrapartum antimicrobial prophylaxis indicated but inadequate.

   i. **Observation without doing any lab tests.** Acceptable if observation is every 2–4 hours for a minimum of 24 hours.

   ii. **Or do lab tests.** Do WBC and differential and optional CRP at age 6–12 hours.

   iii. **No antibiotics necessary, observation.** Now what?

     (a) **Lab values abnormal.** Do blood culture. If the blood culture is negative and the infant is well then discharge by 48 hours.

     (a) **Lab values normal.** Infant well, discharge by 48 hours. Discharge at 24 hours is acceptable only if other discharge criteria are met, access to medical care is readily available, and there is an able person who can fully comply with instructions for home observation.

B. Antibiotic therapy

1. If the decision is to treat:

   a. Obtain cultures of the blood and spinal fluid if indicated. Lumbar puncture is indicated if there is a positive blood culture or sepsis is highly suspected based on clinical signs or lab values, or if infants do not respond to treatment. Any other cultures that seem appropriate should be sent to the laboratory (eg, if there is eye discharge, send a Gram stain and culture). Tracheal aspirate Gram stain and culture if pneumonia is suspected and there is an increase in tracheal secretions. (*Note:* Tracheal aspirates need to be obtained right after endotracheal tube placement to be of value in early-onset sepsis.)

   b. Ampicillin and gentamicin are the antibiotics most commonly used for empirical initial therapy in a newborn with sepsis. Once a pathogen is identified, use narrow therapy if possible unless synergism is necessary. If GBS is documented, penicillin G or ampicillin is given, but an aminoglycoside is often added for synergism. Recent reviews have documented that in infants (≥32 weeks' gestation), once-a-day gentamicin is superior to multiple doses a day because it achieves higher peak levels and avoids toxic trough levels. Third-generation cephalosporins are an alternative to gentamicin, but recent studies have shown resistance and increased candidiasis with use. Cefotaxime should only be used in infants with gram-negative meningitis. Cefotaxime and an aminoglycoside should be used in infants with gram-negative meningitis until susceptibility testing is back.

   c. If the cultures are positive, treat accordingly. Bacteremia without source: treat for 10 days. Uncomplicated GBS meningitis: treat for 14 days. Gram-negative meningitis: treat for 21 days or 14 days after obtaining a negative culture.

2. Discontinuing antibiotics is another *controversial* topic.

   a. See AAP management guidelines above for neonates with suspected or proven early-onset bacterial sepsis.

   b. Other recommendations

      i. If the cultures are negative, the patient is doing well, and the risk of sepsis low. Antibiotics may be stopped after 48 hours (for asymptomatic term infants, negative cultures after 36 hours may be sufficient). A normal I:T ratio and serial negative CRP might help determine whether antibiotics can be stopped because of their high negative predictive value. Use of procalcitonin concentrations may also be helpful in deciding when to stop antibiotics.

      ii. If the cultures are negative but the infant had signs of sepsis (clinical sepsis). Some clinicians treat the infant for 7–10 days.

C. Beyond antibiotic therapy

1. Immunoglobulin (Ig) therapy (*controversial*). Endogenous immunoglobulin synthesis begins at 24 weeks of life. Placental transfer of immunoglobulins does not occur until later and postnatal IgG levels decrease after birth. Studies show a reduction in mortality in proven infection but less reduction in suspected infection. In a recent review, intravenous immune globulin administration resulted in a 3% reduction in sepsis but was not found to not have any significant effect on mortality. The data do not support the routine use in sepsis. Some institutions give a single dose in infants with overwhelming sepsis.

2. Fresh frozen plasma. Its use is only indicated in disseminated intravascular coagulation, and no benefit has been shown in septic infants.

3. Granulocyte or neutrophil transfusions. Although benefits of granulocyte transfusions have been documented, there are potential serious side effects. Cochrane review states that there is not enough evidence to either support or refute the use in sepsis.

4. Cytokines. Granulocyte macrophage colony-stimulating factor (GM-CSF) and granulocyte colony-stimulating factor (G-CSF) stimulate bone marrow

neutrophils. Cochrane review states that there is not enough evidence to support the use of GM-CSF or G-CSF as treatment to reduce mortality or as prophylaxis.

5. **Double volume exchange transfusion.** Exchange transfusion with fresh whole blood is beneficial in severe or gram-negative neonatal sepsis, and it may be used as a last resort. Because of significant risks and that evidence from few prospective studies is not strong on the subject, many institutions have not advocated its use.

6. **Pentoxifylline.** Current evidence shows that pentoxifylline as an adjunct to antibiotics reduces mortality in neonatal sepsis and duration of hospitalization. The studies have been small, and the results need to be interpreted with caution. More research is needed.

7. **Selenium/melatonin supplementation.** More studies are needed before recommendations can be made.

8. **Lactoferrin.** Cochrane review states that there is no recommendation to use or refute the use in treatment of neonatal sepsis.

Selected References

Polin RA; Committee on Fetus and Newborn. Management of neonates with suspected or proven early-onset bacterial sepsis. *Pediatrics* 2012;129(5):1006–1015. Erratum to Pediatrics.

Prevention of Perinatal Group B Streptococcal Disease. *MMWR*. Revised guidelines from CDC, 2010. November 19, 2010/59(RR10);1–32. http://www.cdc.gov/mmwr/preview/mmwrhtml/rr5910a1.htm. Accessed September, 2012.

Sise ME, Parravicini E, Barasch J. Urinary neutrophil gelatinase–associated lipocalin (NGAL) identifies neonates with high probability of sepsis. *Pediatrics* 2012; 130(4):1053–1054.

74 Pulmonary Hemorrhage

I. **Problem.** Grossly bloody secretions are seen in the endotracheal tube (ETT). The incidence of pulmonary hemorrhage varies from 0.8 to 12 per 1000 live births. It can be as high as 50 per 1000 live births if high risk. The mortality rate can be as high as 50%. Survivors of pulmonary hemorrhage require longer ventilator support, and many will develop bronchopulmonary dysplasia/chronic lung disease. Others survivors may have an increase in cerebral palsy, cognitive delay, seizures, and periventricular leukomalacia. **Most cases of pulmonary hemorrhage are secondary to hemorrhagic pulmonary edema and not a true bleed.**

II. **Immediate questions**

A. **Are any other signs abnormal?** Typically, an infant with pulmonary hemorrhage is a ventilated low birthweight infant, often from a multiple birth, and 2–4 days old (usually in the first week of life). Late gestation infants with pulmonary hemorrhage usually have low 1- and 5-minute Apgar scores. The infant has a sudden deterioration: hypoxic, severe retractions, and may experience associated pallor, shock, apnea, bradycardia, and cyanosis.

B. **Is the infant hypoxic? Has a blood transfusion recently been given?** Hypoxia or hypervolemia (usually caused by over transfusion) may cause an acute rise in the pulmonary capillary pressure and lead to pulmonary hemorrhage.

C. **Is there bleeding from other sites?** If so, coagulopathy may be present, and coagulation studies should be obtained. Volume replacement with colloid or blood products may be needed.

D. **What is the hematocrit (Hct) of the endotracheal blood?** If the Hct is close to the venous Hct, it represents a true hemorrhage, and the blood is usually from trauma, aspiration of maternal blood, or bleeding diathesis. If the Hct is 15–20 percentage points lower than the venous Hct, the bleeding is likely hemorrhagic edema fluid. This is seen with the majority of cases of pulmonary hemorrhage (such as those secondary to patent ductus arteriosus [PDA], surfactant therapy, and left-sided heart failure; others discussed later).

E. **Has there been a recent procedure or has suctioning just taken place? Was surfactant recently given?** Vigorous suctioning, traumatic intubation, or chest tube insertion may be a cause. Surfactant can also be associated.

F. **Did the mother or infant have any risk factors for pulmonary hemorrhage?**
   1. **Maternal risk factors.** Breech delivery, maternal cocaine use, maternal hypertension during pregnancy, abruptio placentae, maternal antibiotic therapy, preeclampsia, possible previous pregnancy losses. (Antenatal steroids may be protective.)
   2. **Infant. Prematurity** is the most common factor. **Others include** respiratory problems (hypoxia, asphyxia, respiratory distress syndrome [RDS], meconium aspiration, pneumothorax, surfactant treatment, or any need for ventilator support), mechanical ventilation, PDA with left to right shunting, disseminated intravascular coagulation (DIC), cold injury, oxygen toxicity, urea cycle defects, multiple births, male sex, infections/sepsis, coagulopathy, hypothermia, polycythemia, intrauterine growth restriction, erythroblastosis fetalis, extracorporeal membrane oxygenation/extracorporeal life support, toxemia of pregnancy, surfactant therapy.
   3. **Infant near term or term.** Hypotension, requirement of positive pressure ventilation in the delivery room, meconium aspiration.

G. **Did the infant receive indomethacin?** Prophylactic indomethacin reduces the rate of early serious pulmonary hemorrhage; it reduced the rate of serious pulmonary hemorrhage by 35% but only in the first week. It is less effective after the first week of life in preventing serious pulmonary hemorrhage.

III. **Differential diagnosis**
   A. **Hemorrhagic pulmonary edema.** Fluid from the lungs is a mixture of plasma and blood with a low hematocrit. Its cause is not known and may be multifactorial. Causes may include stress and injury on pulmonary capillaries, fragile pulmonary capillaries, inadequate surface tension, acute left ventricular failure caused by asphyxia, and severe acidosis or other conditions that lead to capillary endothelium injury. A decrease in pulmonary vascular resistance can increase the left to right shunt through the PDA with increase in pulmonary blood flow. Surfactant decreases the pulmonary vascular resistance, increasing the left to right shunting across the PDA, with an increase in pulmonary blood flow with pulmonary edema and rupture of pulmonary capillaries. Other theories include surfactant dysfunction or intrauterine neutrophil activation in premature infants with RDS causing pulmonary hemorrhage.
   B. **Direct trauma to the airway.** Occurs due to nasotracheal or endotracheal intubation, vigorous suctioning, mechanical ventilation, or lung trauma during chest tube insertion.
   C. **Aspiration of gastric or maternal blood.** Often seen after cesarean or vaginal delivery. The majority of blood is usually obtained from the nasogastric tube, but blood may be seen in the ETT.
   D. **Coagulopathy.** May be due to sepsis, DIC, or congenital factors. The role of coagulation abnormalities is not the cause of pulmonary hemorrhage (as believed earlier) but found to exacerbate the degree of hemorrhage.
   E. **Other disorders associated with pulmonary hemorrhage**
       1. **Hypoxia/asphyxia.** Acute left ventricular failure due to asphyxia is a factor in pulmonary hemorrhage. Intrauterine and intrapartum asphyxia can be related to pulmonary hemorrhage. Resuscitation may exacerbate pulmonary hemorrhage.
       2. **Hypervolemia.** Over transfusion or fluid overload.

3. **Congenital heart disease or congestive heart failure** (especially in pulmonary edema caused by PDA). A PDA can cause a rapid increase in pulmonary blood flow. In one series, 60% of infants with pulmonary hemorrhage had a clinical PDA, with more than 90% of those with a pulmonary hemorrhage having a PDA of >1.6 mm in size.

4. **Pulmonary related.** RDS, pulmonary interstitial emphysema, pneumothorax, meconium aspiration, aspiration, and pneumonia (usually caused by gram-negative organisms). Pulmonary congestion (severely reduced left ventricular function in an asphyxiated or septic infant) can also be a factor. Diffuse pulmonary emboli can be a predisposing factor.

5. **Surfactant administration.** Pulmonary hemorrhage within hours of surfactant therapy and may be related to a rapid increase in pulmonary blood flow due to improved lung function. There is a significant relationship between pulmonary hemorrhage and a clinical PDA in surfactant-treated infants. Rescue surfactant therapy did not increase the risk of pulmonary hemorrhage, but prophylactic surfactant did.

6. **Hematologic disorders.** Severe Rh incompatibility, thrombocytopenia, hemorrhagic disease of the newborn (from failure to administer vitamin K).

7. **Prematurity, intrauterine growth restriction,** and/or multiple births.

8. **Severe hypothermia.**

9. **Infection/sepsis.** Overwhelming sepsis is seen in many cases of pulmonary hemorrhage and may be associated with the DIC that accompanies sepsis and the increased microvascular permeability seen. Pulmonary hemorrhage can occur from group B coxsackievirus and multiple infections with septicemia (congenital cytomegalovirus, *Haemophilus influenzae, Escherichia coli, Candida, Staphylococcus epidermis,* etc.).

10. **Urea cycle defects with hyperammonemia.** These infants typically have hepatomegaly, coagulopathy, and usually normal liver function tests except for hyperammonemia. Pulmonary bleeding is usually a terminal event in these infants.

11. **High concentrations of oxygen or oxygen toxicity.** Histologic evidence of oxygen toxicity has been associated with massive pulmonary hemorrhage.

12. **Airway hemangioma (rare).**

IV. **Database**

A. **Physical examination.** Typically, the infant is premature and has a sudden deterioration and bloody secretions from the airway. Clinical signs may vary from the infant being pale, limp, and unresponsive, to fighting the ventilator, to looking well. The infant can be cyanotic, bradycardia, apneic, gasping, hypotensive, agitated, hypoxic, or hypercapnic or have an increased work of breathing and require more ventilatory support. Note the presence of other bleeding sites, signs of pneumonia, infection, or congestive heart failure. Look for peripheral edema, hepatosplenomegaly, and murmur. Listen to the chest for decreased breath sounds. There can be a **prodrome of frothy reddish blood-tinged tracheal secretions** before pulmonary hemorrhage.

B. **Laboratory studies**

1. **Complete blood count with differential and platelet count.** With pneumonia, sepsis, or other infection, results of these studies may be abnormal. Thrombocytopenia may be seen. The Hct should be checked to determine whether excessive blood loss has occurred.

2. **Coagulation profile (prothrombin time [PT], activated partial thromboplastin time [PTT], thrombin time, D-dimers, fibrinogen level)** may reveal coagulation disorders or DIC.

3. **Arterial blood gas levels** detect hypoxia and increase in Pco_2, a decrease in oxygen, and metabolic acidosis. The oxygenation index can increase significantly after the hemorrhage.

4. **Apt test** if aspiration of maternal blood is suspected. (See Chapter 55.)

5. **Hct of the aspirate** may differentiate between hemorrhagic pulmonary edema and a true bleed (see earlier).

6. **Ammonia level** to evaluate for urea cycle defects.

C. Imaging and other studies
  1. Chest radiograph can be variable and nonspecific. It may indicate pneumonia, RDS, or congestive heart failure. With pulmonary hemorrhage, radiographic findings depend on whether the hemorrhage is focal (patchy, linear, nodular densities, or fluffy opacities) or massive (the film shows diffuse ground-glass opacities or a complete whiteout). The chest radiograph can also be clear.
  2. Lung ultrasonography can detect pulmonary complications of RDS by showing consolidations, but cannot differentiate between pneumonia, hemorrhage, or atelectasis.
  3. Echocardiogram to rule out left to right shunting through a PDA and ventricular function.

V. Plan
  A. Emergency measures. These methods are acceptable modes of treatment.
    1. Suction the airway initially (sometimes as often as every 15 minutes) until bleeding subsides. This is critical to reduce the risk of secretions blocking the airway. Use a 6.5F suction catheter for a 2.5-mm ETT and an 8.0F suction catheter for a 3.0- or 3.5-mm ETT. **Percussion should be used with caution and has no primary role in pulmonary hemorrhage.**
    2. Oxygen therapy should be given. If already given, increase the inspired oxygen concentration.
    3. If mechanical ventilation is not being used. Consider initiating its use.
    4. If already on a ventilator, increase the positive end-expiratory pressure to 6–8 cm H_2O (or higher if needed). This may cause tamponade of the capillaries, force edema back into the pulmonary vascular bed, and improve ventilation and oxygenation. Risks of positive end-expiratory pressure include hypercapnia and hyperventilation.
    5. Consider increasing the peak inspiratory pressure. Consider if bleeding does not subside to improve ventilation and raise the mean airway pressure.
  B. General measures
    1. Support and correct the blood pressure with volume expansion and colloids. (See Chapter 65.) Vasoactive medications may be necessary.
    2. Blood volume and Hct should be restored with packed red blood cell transfusions. The majority of these infants are not volume depleted and thus administering excessive fluid volume may only worsen the situation (increasing the left arterial pressure may increase the pulmonary edema). **Correct any underlying disorders of coagulation if present.**
    3. Correct acidosis by correcting hypovolemia, hypoxia, and low cardiac output. Bicarbonate infusion in certain select cases may be considered **if metabolic acidosis persists after** ventilation is adequate and volume restored, but is not routinely recommended (*controversial*).
    4. Treat any underlying disorder. Early recognition and treatment of PDA is essential, especially in extremely premature infants. Surgical treatment of the PDA should be considered. Treat sepsis/infection with antibiotics if indicated. Treat any asphyxia or coagulopathy.
  C. Other measures to consider if the preceding methods are not effective (*controversial*)
    1. ETT administration of epinephrine (0.1 mL/kg of 1:10,000) (*controversial*). This may cause constriction of the pulmonary capillaries. Epinephrine and/or 4% cocaine (4 mg/kg) may be a useful adjunct to increasing the mean airway pressure in the management of pulmonary hemorrhage. Epinephrine is often used clinically, even though the efficacy has not been proven in clinical trials.
    2. Consider high-frequency ventilation. It is not known if it has any benefits over conventional ventilation, but some studies suggest that high-frequency ventilation may improve survival. One review showed a 71% survival with the use of high-frequency ventilation (high-frequency jet ventilation, **high-frequency**

oscillatory ventilation [HFOV], and high-frequency flow interrupter were used in the review) after conventional ventilation failed. HFOV has been used as rescue therapy in some infants with massive pulmonary hemorrhage and showed dramatic improvements.

3. **Consider using a single dose of surfactant.** This has been reported to improve respiratory status based on the oxygenation index. Pulmonary hemorrhage can deactivate surfactant. Reviews note promising results, but a lack of randomized trials prevents this from being universally recommended. Cochrane review gives no recommendation based on randomized controlled studies.

4. **Steroids.** Because chronic inflammation was found on lung biopsies of infants with pulmonary hemorrhage, and more infants survived with pulmonary hemorrhage who had been on steroids, steroid use can be considered. Methylprednisolone 1 mg/kg every 6 hours during hospital stay and 1 mg/kg daily thereafter and discontinued after a 4-week period has been reported to be beneficial.

5. **Activated recombinant factor VII (rFVIIa).** Low-volume alternative to blood products and is effective as a pan-hemostatic agent. If platelets are given at the same time, the effect is enhanced. It has been used in very low birthweight infants when conventional ventilator management failed. There are a few positive studies, but the optimal dose has not been established. One dose of 50 mcg/kg twice per day 3 hours apart for 2–3 days was used successfully.

6. **Hemocoagulase.** Preterm infants treated with hemocoagulase (0.5 KU [Klobusitzky unit] through the ETT every 4–6 hours) until the hemorrhage stopped plus mechanical ventilation for pulmonary hemorrhage showed promising results; the duration of ventilation, pulmonary hemorrhage, and mortality were all decreased compared with controls. Due to potential risks of use and lack of quality studies, routine use is not recommended yet. Use as a last resort.

7. **Diuretics.** Some advocate diuretic therapy (furosemide 1 mg/kg) to treat fluid overload. Cochrane review states that it is not beneficial.

8. **Antibiotics.** May be necessary until infection ruled out.

D. **Specific targeted therapy**
   1. **Direct nasotracheal or endotracheal trauma.** If there is significant bleeding immediately after an endotracheal or nasotracheal intubation, trauma is the most likely cause; surgical consultation is indicated.
   2. **Aspiration of maternal blood.** If the infant is stable, no treatment is needed because the condition is typically self-limited.
   3. **Coagulopathy.** See Chapter 87.
      a. **Hemorrhagic disease of the newborn.** Vitamin K, 1 mg, administered intravenously with fresh-frozen plasma with active bleeding.
      b. **Other coagulopathies.** Transfusion of blood products and correction of coagulopathies is necessary. Fresh-frozen plasma, 10 mL/kg every 12–24 hours, may be given. If the platelet count is low, transfuse 1 unit and monitor closely. Monitor PT/PTT, platelet count, and fibrinogen level. DIC is managed as noted in Chapter 87.
   4. **PDA.** If the patient is hemodynamically significant, treat medically or surgically (see Chapter 118). Surgical treatment should be considered because indomethacin causes bleeding.
   5. **Sepsis.** Appropriate antibiotics should be started immediately.

Selected References

Cetin H, Yalaz M, Akisu M, Karapinar DY, Kavakli K, Kultursay N. The use of recombinant activated factor VII in the treatment of massive pulmonary hemorrhage in a preterm infant. *Blood Coagul Fibrinolysis.* 2006;17:213–216.

Olomu N, Kulkarni R, Manco-Johnson M. Treatment of severe pulmonary hemorrhage with activated recombinant factor VII (rFVIIa) in very low birth weight infants. *J Perinatol.* 2002;22:672–674.

Zahr RA, Ashfaq A, Marron-Corwin M. Neonatal pulmonary hemorrhage. *NeoReviews.* 2012;13:e302–e306.

75 Rash and Dermatologic Problems

I. **Problem.** A nurse calls you to tell you that an infant has a rash. A rash is any change of skin that affects its color, appearance, or texture. **Although the majority of rashes in newborns are benign and require no treatment, certain rashes require a workup and intervention.**

II. **Immediate questions**

A. **What are the characteristics of the rash?** Morphology of the lesion aids differential diagnosis. **Is it macular** (flat lesion <1 cm), **papular** (raised up to 1 cm), **nodular** (raised up to 2 cm), **vesicular** (raised, <1 cm, filled with clear fluid), **bullous** (raised, >1 cm, with clear fluid), or **pustular** (raised with purulent fluid)?

B. **Are there petechiae (tiny pinpoint red dots from broken blood vessels), purpura (large, flat area of blood under tissue), or ecchymosis (very large bruised area)?** All can result from intradermal bleeding and need to be differentiated from **erythema** (redness of the skin). With erythema, the redness is cleared when pressed and returns when you release. With pressure, petechiae, purpura, and ecchymosis do not blanch. Petechiae on the lower body after a breech delivery or upper body with a vertex presentation can be normal. If widespread, petechiae are considered abnormal. **Petechiae and purpura can signify thrombocytopenia and require a workup.**

C. **Is there a history of a congenital infection?** Obtain a thorough maternal history. TORCH (*t*oxoplasmosis, *o*ther, *r*ubella, *c*ytomegalovirus, *h*erpes simplex virus) infections are known to cause rashes. The **"blueberry muffin baby"** has widespread purpura and papules and can be seen in rubella (the term was first used to describe infants infected with rubella in the epidemic of 1960), cytomegalovirus (CMV; most common viral infection), and syphilis. Cutaneous extramedullary hematopoiesis causes the blueberry muffin rash. The blueberry muffin rash has historically been associated with congenital viral infections but can also be seen in blood disorders (hemolytic disease of the newborn, twin-to-twin transfusion, hereditary spherocytosis), vascular disorders (multiple hemangiomas, blue rubber bleb nevus, multiple glomangiomas, multifocal lymphangioendotheliomatosis), and malignancies (neuroblastoma, congenital leukemia cutis, Langerhans cell histiocytosis, and congenital rhabdomyosarcoma). See Chapter 141 and disease-specific chapters.

D. **Is the infant ill appearing?** A well infant with a rash suggests a benign rash. A febrile or ill-appearing infant with a rash requires a thorough workup to search specifically for an infectious cause.

E. **What medications did the mother receive during pregnancy and delivery? Is the mother breast-feeding and taking any medications?** Medications are a rare cause of rash in infants. Methimazole, an antithyroid medication, has been associated with aplasia cutis, a localized absence of skin on the scalp.

F. **Does the skin lesion make you think of a genetic disorder?** Skin lesions can be associated with genetic syndromes. **Blisters:** epidermolysis bullosa. **Brown, flat patches:** Neurofibromatosis. **Cutis marmorata:** Cornelia de Lange syndrome and in trisomies 18 (Edward syndrome) and 21 (Down syndrome). **Deficient hair and nails:** ectodermal dysplasias. **Scaly, thick skin:** ichthyoses. **Thin, fragile skin:** collagen disorders and hypoplasia of the dermis. **Unformed skin:** aplasia cutis congenita, Adams-Oliver and epidermolysis bullosa. **White skin and hair: piebaldism, tuberous sclerosis.**

III. **Differential diagnosis**

A. **Absence of part of the skin. Aplasia cutis congenita** consists of 9 groups of disorders based on the location and presence of other malformations that involve absence of part of the skin. It can be localized (most commonly on the scalp) or involve a large portion of the body (Plate 3).

B. **Skin and soft tissue infections in the neonatal intensive care unit (NICU).** These are common because preterm infants have fragile skin. Types of infections seen are **cellulitis, abrasions, and abscesses.** These usually occur where the skin has been traumatized (diaper areas, surgical incision sites, fetal scalp electrodes, venipuncture sites, heelstick sites, and others). The most common organism is *Staphylococcus aureus.* Methicillin-resistant strains are becoming more frequent. Skin and soft tissue infections involving surgical procedures (gastrointestinal [GI] tract) are caused more commonly by gram-negative rods and yeasts. **Omphalitis,** an infection of the umbilical stump and the area around it, can also occur and is usually caused by bacteria (gram negative or gram positive).

C. **Benign skin disorders/rashes that usually require no workup or intervention.** These rashes are very common.

1. **Erythema toxicum.** The most common newborn rash, it consists of erythematous macules with a central papule or pustule. It can be present at birth, typically appears within the first 48 hours, and may appear at up to 2 weeks of age. It is more common in full-term infants and more common on the trunk, extremities, and perineum. New lesions can appear after the initial onset and usually disappear after a week (Plate 4).

2. **Transient neonatal pustular melanosis.** These 2- to 5-mm pustules are usually present at birth on various sites, typically the face and sacrum of full-term infants. Pustules evolve and disappear within 48 hours, but can leave hyperpigmented macules that eventually resolve but may persist for months (Plate 5).

3. **Sebaceous gland hyperplasia.** Tiny yellow papules usually occurring on the cheeks and nose. Smaller and more yellow than milia.

4. **Milia.** Tiny (1-mm) white-yellow papules frequently present on the face, chin, and forehead and scalp. Caused by sebaceous retention cysts (Plate 6).

5. **Miliaria crystallina.** Obstruction of eccrine/sweat ducts. May appear on the scalp or face as vesicular or papular lesions with or without erythema. Exacerbated by heat and humidity, they resolve quickly when the infant is cooled.

6. **Miliaria rubra ("prickly heat").** One- to two-millimeter papules or papulopustules surrounded by small red areas. Miliaria pustulosis is a variant with more pustules and less erythema.

7. **Miliaria profunda.** Deep obstruction of the sweat ducts. White papules and edema that can prevent sweating, leading to hyperthermia.

8. **Acropustulosis of infancy.** Recurrent areas of pruritic vesicopustules develop on the palmar surface of the hand and plantar surface of the feet. Usually last 7–14 days (Plate 7).

9. **Seborrheic dermatitis.** Patchy redness and scales on the scalp (**"cradle cap"**), face, skin folds, and behind the ears.

10. **Neonatal acne.** Erythematous comedones, papules, and pustules. May be present at birth or develop during early infancy; may take several weeks/months for complete resolution (Plate 8).

11. **Sucking blister.** Vesicular or bullous lesions present at birth on fingers, lips, or hands; no associated erythema (distinguishes these from herpetic lesions).

12. **Subcutaneous fat necrosis.** Erythematous nodules and plaques occurring during the first few weeks of life and resolving by 2 months of age. Usually on areas of trauma (face, back, arms, legs, and buttocks). Hypercalcemia can occur if these lesions calcify (Plate 9).

13. **Nevus simplex ("stork bite," "salmon patch," "angel's kiss").** Pink macules that are dilated superficial capillaries, seen commonly at the nape of the neck, midforehead, and upper eyelids, but also on nose and upper lip, that usually fade within a year. The most common vascular malformation.

14. **Mongolian spot (dermal melanocytosis).** A blue-black macular discoloration at the base of the spine and on the buttocks but can occur elsewhere. More common in blacks (>90%) and Asians (81%); usually fades over several years. Extensive spots have been described in infants with GM1 gangliosidosis (Plate 10).

15. **Harlequin sign (color change, not Harlequin fetus).** Secondary to vasomotor instability, there is a sharp demarcation of blanching (one side of the body is red and the other is pale) that usually only lasts a few minutes.

16. **Infantile hemangioma.** A common vascular tumor (3–5% of all infants). More common in girls and preterm infants.

17. **Benign petechiae.** Nonblanching erythematous macules present on the lower body after a breech delivery or upper body with a vertex presentation.

D. **Rashes caused by infections.** These typically require intervention. The most common pathogens are *S. aureus*, *Streptococcus* spp., *Candida albicans*, and herpes simplex.

1. **Bacterial infections causing rashes**

   a. *Staphylococcus aureus*

      i. **Impetigo (nonbullous and bullous).** Usually present with intact vesicles then intact pustules rupture, erode, and dry out to form crusts often secondary to an infected umbilical wound.

      ii. **Staphylococcal scalded skin syndrome (SSSS).** Usually presents during the first week of life; starts with marked erythema of the face then spreads caudally and tends to be most severe in flexural areas. Lesions progress to bullae that are easily denuded (Plate 11).

   b. **Cutaneous streptococcal infections.** Uncommon, group A streptococcal infections can have an erysipelas-like eruption. Skin infections caused by group B are very rare. Vesiculopustular lesions, abscesses, and cellulitis (most common) have been reported.

   c. **Syphilis.** Usually macular or maculopapular eruptions (in congenital syphilis, infants present with vesicles, bullae, and erosions). Hemorrhagic bullae on the palms and soles are characteristic of syphilis.

   d. *Listeria monocytogenes.* Small (2- to 3-mm) cutaneous pinkish-gray granulomas are characteristic.

2. **Viral infections causing rashes**

   a. **Herpes simplex virus (HSV).** (Plate 12) See also Chapter 96.

      i. **Neonatal HSV.** Transmitted perinatally and occurs in 3 forms. Erythematous papules or vesicles progress into pustular clusters with intense erythema.

      ii. **Congenital HSV.** Acquired in utero and presents with vesicles that are apparent the first day of life. Typically associated with low birthweight, chorioretinitis, and microcephaly.

   b. **Varicella-zoster.** See also Chapter 147.

      i. **Congenital/fetal varicella syndrome.** Acquired in utero in the first/ second trimester. Infant is born with cicatricial scars.

      ii. **Congenital/perinatal/early neonatal varicella.** Acquired in utero late in third trimester or in the first few days postpartum. Infant presents with centripetal rash similar to postnatal rash in the first 10-12 days of life.

      iii. **Postnatally acquired chickenpox.** No transplacental infection. Infant presents with symptoms on days 12–28 of life. Typical chicken pox rash with centripetal spreading first on trunk, then face and scalp. All stages appear (red macules, clear vesicles, crusting). (Image 13)

   c. **CMV.** Most common congenital infection. The majority of cases are asymptomatic. If symptomatic, they can have multi-organ disease with petechiae and purpura and jaundice.

    d. Rubella. Can have petechiae, but if severe, may have bluish red papules ("blueberry muffin") that appear on the head and trunk and extremities.
  3. Fungal infections causing rashes
    a. *Candida albicans.* The most common fungal infection that causes problems in neonates is discussed here. Other species (*Candida parapsilosis, Candida lusitaniae, Candida glabrata,* etc.) are less common.
      i. Candida diaper dermatitis/oral candidiasis (thrush). Most common presentation of Candida infections in a normal infant. The diaper rash is usually erythematous with satellite pustules. Oral candidiasis can present with fussiness and refusal to take oral feedings, and is characterized by white patches in the oral cavity.
      ii. Congenital candidiasis. Acquired in utero, infants can either have cutaneous or systemic disease. **Congenital cutaneous candidiasis** presents with an extensive rash within 12 hours of birth. The rash consists of erythematous macules, diffuse papules and pustules. Unlike erythema toxicum, this rash frequently involves the palms and soles. In term infants there is desquamation of these lesions, which may mimic SSSS. Premature infants may present with a rash with variable presentation (pustules, vesicles, or a burn-like dermatitis with peeling) (Plate 14). In **congenital systemic candidiasis,** majority of infants do not have a rash but can present with pneumonia, meningitis, or other presentations. This is a very invasive infection with a high mortality rate, especially in very low birthweight infants.
    b. Aspergillus. This has been reported to cause cutaneous fungal infections but is rare.
      i. Primary cutaneous aspergillosis (PCA). Characterized by lack of involvement of organs except the skin at the time of diagnosis. Preterm infants are at risk for PCA because of vulnerability of their skin and immature host defenses. Risk factors include prematurity, neutropenia, prior use of antibiotics, and glucocorticoid administration. A plaque with an eschar is characteristic of PCA. Disruption of the skin occurs due to contaminated hand splints, skin maceration caused by oximeter sensor, or adhesive tape.
      ii. Secondary aspergillosis. Characterized by involvement of organs and a maculopapular eruption caused by thrombosis of small vessels.
  4. Parasitic infections that can cause a rash
    a. Scabies. An infestation with the mite *Sarcoptes scabiei* that has been reported in infants as young as 2 weeks. Infants tend to have widespread lesions often on the face and scalp (usually not seen in older patients who present with intertriginous locations). They can have papules, nodules, vesicles, and pustules.
    b. *Toxoplasma gondii* **infections.** Present with a generalized maculopapular rash.
E. Rashes that cause scaling. Usually benign and self-limited. Infectious and dietary etiologies need to be ruled out because they need immediate treatment. Genetic and immune etiologies can be considered later in the differential.
  1. Postmaturity. The majority of term and postmature infants normally shed their skin. The skin appears similar to parchment paper and peels off. This is a normal physiologic finding that requires no medical treatment.
  2. Seborrheic dermatitis. Usually seen on the scalp and flexure areas. It is a red erythematous rash with yellow scaling. Can be seen in the diaper area and is self-limiting.
  3. Fatty acid deficiency. Superficial scaling and desquamation can occur. Can be seen in fatty acid deficiency syndrome (where infants have decreased fat stores) or in fat malabsorption. Fatty acid replacement is necessary.
  4. Ichthyoses. May present as "harlequin fetus" or "collodion baby." Many types of ichthyoses are present. These are genetic disorders that cause severe thick, scaly skin sometimes with restricted movement. The infant can have a shiny, tight membrane covering at birth that can peel off. The skin is prone to cracking and secondary infection. Some of the ichthyoses are associated with sensorineural hearing defects; others are associated with neurological problems including seizures (Plate 15).

5. **Infantile eczema.** Scaling is present. Eczema is rarely seen in the newborn but is often seen in infants.
6. **Atopic dermatitis.** Red scaly and itchy rash; rarely seen in the newborn.
7. **Staphylococcal scalded skin syndrome.** See page 508.
8. **Psoriasis.** Seen as a diaper rash with dissemination (scaly patches beyond the diaper rash) or can present as erythroderma progressing to pustular psoriasis.
9. **Candida infections.** These can also cause redness and scaling (see earlier).
10. **Syphilis infections.** See page 508.
11. **Ectodermal dysplasias.** There are over 150 subtypes but the most common form is X-linked recessive hypohidrotic ectodermal dysplasia.
12. **Immunodeficiencies.** Infants with immunodeficiencies (acquired immune deficiency syndrome [AIDS], severe combined immunodeficiency, diffuse cutaneous mastocytosis, Wiskott- Aldrich syndrome, Langerhans cell histiocytosis) can have a red scaly rash.
13. **Neonatal lupus.** An immune-mediated disorder that is caused by maternally transferred autoantibodies (SSA/Ro, SSB/La, and/or U1RNP). Major manifestations are skin and cardiac (primary cause of congenital heart block). Skin findings are transient and usually start at a few weeks of age but can be present at birth. Two variants are papulosquamous and annular. Fifteen to twenty-five percent of cases have cutaneous manifestations. Typical rash is 0.5- to 3-cm annular erythematous papules with a central scale. Liver and hematologic involvement occurs in about 10% of cases (Plate 16).

F. **Rashes that cause blisters and bullae.** Infectious and dietary causes need to be ruled out because they require immediate treatment. Then less common causes can be evaluated.
1. **Epidermolysis bullosa.** A group of inherited diseases that cause blistering. Trauma induces the blisters. Congenital localized absence of skin is often noted at birth (Plate 17).
2. **Zinc deficiency dermatosis.** Presents as a blistering rash or more commonly an eczematous rash on the angle of the mouth, chin, or cheeks in a U-shaped distribution, and on the diaper area. It can be red and scaly, and can have a dark color at the periphery.
3. **Congenital herpes infection.** See above.
4. **Staphylococcal scalded skin syndrome (SSSS).** See above.
5. **Incontinentia pigmenti.** A rare X-linked dominant genetic disorder that is more common in females. It has 4 stages: stage 1 occurs at birth to 2 weeks—vesiculobullous (erythematous vesicles/bullae that occur linearly on the trunk, extremities, and scalp); stage 2 occurs 2–3 weeks after birth—verrucous; stages 3 and 4 occur later. Infants can also have neurologic, dental, and ophthalmologic abnormalities. *Note:* Stage 1 lesions can be confused with herpes simplex infection (Plate 18).
6. **Less common causes.** Genetic disorders, epidermolytic hyperkeratosis, toxic epidermal necrolysis, and bullous mastocytosis.

G. **Birthmarks.** The majority of birthmarks are benign and require no treatment. However, if there are many lesions present, this may signify an associated syndrome, or if very large they can be at risk for melanoma and have to be closely followed. Vascular lesions need to be evaluated as they may interfere with vital organs.
1. **Pigmented lesions**
   a. **Café-au-lait spots (macule).** Benign lesions that are oval or irregular with a light brown color. If they are >5 mm in diameter and there are more than 6, suspect an associated syndrome (think neurofibromatosis, Albright syndrome, Turner and Noonan syndrome, tuberous sclerosis, ataxia-telangiectasia).
   b. **Mongolian blue spot.** See page 508.
   c. **Congenital melanocytic nevus.** Small (<1.5 cm) and intermediate (<20 cm) in size are common with a small risk of malignant melanoma. Large congenital nevi (>20 cm) and giant congenital nevi (>40 cm) have a higher risk of

malignant transformation (5–15% risk). Giant congenital nevi also have a risk of neurocutaneous melanosis (Plate 19).

  d. **Nevus of Ota/Ito.** A blue or grayish area involving the orbital and zygomatic area common in Asians, and carries the risk of glaucoma. Unlike Mongolian spots, these do not fade.

 2. **Diffuse hyperpigmentation.** Not normal and can be secondary to Addison disease, biliary atresia, hepatic atresia, sprue, melanism, lentiginosis, porphyria, Hartnup disease, or idiopathic.

 3. **Hypopigmentation/hypopigmented lesions**
  a. **Diffuse or localized loss of pigment.** This can be secondary to phenylketonuria, Addison disease, trauma, postinflammation, or genetic.
  b. **Ash-leaf macules.** Small area of hypopigmentation, oval shaped and similar to the leaf of an ash tree; a marker for tuberous sclerosis.
  c. **Hypomelanosis of Ito.** Syndrome (primarily neurologic) with hypopigmented macule or linear/whorled pattern of hypopigmentation.
  d. **Partial albinism (piebaldism).** An autosomal dominant disorder of off-white macules on forehead, scalp, trunk, and extremities. This type of depigmentation can also be seen secondary to Addison disease, tuberous sclerosis, vitiligo, and Klein-Waardenburg syndrome.
  e. **Albinism.** Genetic disorders that cause abnormal melanin synthesis.

 4. **Vascular lesions**
  a. **Port wine stain (nevus flammeus).** This usually presents at birth on the face or extremities. It is a permanent capillary angioma. Rarely it is associated with Sturge-Weber syndrome, Klippel-Trenaunay syndrome, Parkes-Weber syndrome, or RASA-1 mutations (Plate 20).
  b. **Nevus simplex/salmon patch.** See page 508.
  c. **Hemangiomas.** Most common benign tumors of vascular endothelium of infancy and are more frequent in premature infants. Females are more likely to be affected, and they occur most commonly on the head and neck, followed by the trunk and limb.
   i. **Superficial ("strawberry") hemangioma.** A bright red tumor (of dilated mass of capillaries) that protrudes above the skin and can appear anywhere on the body. Usually does not require treatment unless it interferes with vital functions.
   ii. **Deep (cavernous) hemangioma.** More deep into the skin and bluish red; usually benign unless it interferes with vital organs.
   iii. **Mixed hemangioma.** This has both deep and superficial components.
   iv. **Benign neonatal hemangiomatosis.** Multiple congenital cutaneous hemangiomas that appear at birth or shortly after with spontaneous regression of lesions within the first 2 years of life.
   v. **Diffuse neonatal hemangiomatosis.** Multiple cutaneous hemangiomas plus hemangiomas of at least 3 separate organ systems. This disorder has a grave prognosis if not recognized and treated.

H. **Rashes that cause petechiae/purpura.** These may relate to birth trauma (considered "normal") or if generalized and recurring can signify a serious infection or hematologic etiology that needs immediate evaluation and treatment.

 1. **Birth trauma.** Petechiae on the lower body after a breech delivery or on the upper body with a vertex presentation can be normal. They do not recur.

 2. **Autoimmune disorders.** Neonatal lupus with maternal transmission of autoantibodies.

 3. **Thrombocytopenia.** Usually generalized scattered petechiae, particularly in response to minor trauma.

 4. **Neonatal alloimmune thrombocytopenia (NAIT).** An isoimmune reaction that can cause thrombocytopenia and severe bleeding, including intracranial bleeding.

5. **Maternal idiopathic thrombocytopenic purpura.** Approximately 80% of cases of thrombocytopenia are caused by autoimmune form.
6. **Coagulation factor deficiencies.** Petechiae and purpura are more common in thrombocytopenia, with large ecchymoses, muscle hemorrhages, and bleeding from heelsticks, venipuncture, and other sites more common with coagulation defects.
7. **Sepsis/infection related.** Usually caused by gram-negative bacterial sepsis (*Escherichia coli, Pseudomonas*). Listeriosis and aspergillosis also involved. Coxsackievirus can cause "blueberry muffin" lesions.
8. **Disseminated intravascular coagulation.** Main causes are sepsis, birth asphyxia, necrotizing enterocolitis (NEC), and respiratory distress syndrome (RDS). One can see petechiae on the skin and bleeding can occur from venipuncture sites and the GI tract.
9. **Purpura fulminans.** Symmetrical and well-defined lakes of confluent ecchymosis without petechiae, with sudden onset and development of hemorrhagic bullae and sudden death. Characteristic of meningococcal sepsis or other life-threatening infection.
10. **TORCH infections.** Toxoplasmosis, other infections (syphilis), rubella, cytomegalovirus, and herpes can all cause "blueberry muffin" lesions (widespread papules and purpura) (Plate 21).
11. **Maternal drugs.** Salicylates, steroids.
12. **Congenital leukemia cutis.** A rare disorder. Cutaneous leukemic infiltrates occur in 25–30% of infants with congenital leukemia. Infants can present with petechiae, purpura, firm blue violaceous lesions, purple nodules, hepatosplenomegaly, lethargy, pallor, and fever. Chloromas (nodular infiltrations of the skin that are solid collections of myeloblasts) look like red-purple papules and nodules (**blueberry muffin rash**) (Plate 21). Congenital leukemia can be associated with Down, Edward, and Patau syndromes. Can be confused with benign hemangiomatosis.

IV. Database
  A. **History.** Obtain thorough history from the mother and family, and a detailed history from the obstetric department. Is there a family history of skin disorders? Many skin disorders are genetic (ichthyoses, immunodeficiency, albinism). Asking about recent infections (varicella), early infections during the pregnancy (congenital infections), sexual history (syphilis), unusual travel destinations, and pet history (*T. gondii*) may provide some clues to the diagnosis. Does the mother have herpes? Did she have any unusual food products or undercooked food (*Listeria*)? What medications did the mother take?
  B. **Physical examination.** Check vital signs. Is the infant febrile or does the infant appear sick, suggesting an infection? Do not just examine the presenting rash, but check the entire body to see if there are signs of the rash anywhere else. The distribution of the rash may be characteristic. Frequent follow-up examinations may document any progression or resolution of the lesions. Examine the eye to check for chorioretinitis (TORCH infections). Hepatosplenomegaly may be seen in congenital TORCH infections.
  C. **Laboratory studies**
    1. **Sepsis evaluation** of labs if systemic infection suspected. **Aspirate appropriate** lesion fluid for bacterial culture, viral culture and polymerase chain reaction (PCR), and fungal cultures.
    2. **If active bleeding suspected,** send complete blood count with differential, platelet and reticulocyte count, TORCH titers, and sepsis workup.
    3. **Potassium hydroxide prep** if Candida/fungal infection suspected (reveals pseudohyphae).
    4. **Wright stain** of lesion fluid can show polymorphonuclear neutrophils with bullous impetigo and transient neonatal pustulosis and eosinophils with erythema toxicum. Wright stain of milia shows keratinocytes.

5. Mineral oil prep can show mites and ova with scabies.
6. PCR or direct fluorescent antibody (DFA) of cutaneous lesion if herpes suspected.
7. Skin biopsy is sometimes indicated, especially if the lesion is atypical.
8. Gram stain, culture of the purulent material of cellulitis/abscess. Gram stain of staph pustulosis will show gram-positive cocci and neutrophils.
9. Maternal and neonatal autoantibodies for lupus.
10. Coagulation studies. Platelet count, fibrinogen, prothrombin time (PT), and partial thromboplastin time (PTT).
11. Molecular cytogenetic analysis of DNA of skin biopsy if congenital leukemia suspected.

D. Imaging and other studies (rarely needed)
1. Computed tomography (CT) scan or contrast-enhanced magnetic resonance image (MRI) of the head to rule out calcifications if Sturge-Weber syndrome is suspected.
2. Ultrasound, echocardiography, and/or CT scans may be needed to manage hemangiomas.
3. Imaging studies may be necessary for larger defects of aplasia cutis congenita to rule out underlying bone or soft tissue defects.

V. Plan. As noted previously, the majority of rashes that occur in the neonate do not require treatment. **Pediatric dermatology consultation** is recommended for any unusual lesions. It is important to note that acyclovir is recommended early in cases of infants with a vesicular skin rash, even if the diagnosis of herpes is not confirmed.

A. Aplasia cutis congenita. Depending on the size and involvement, treatment includes medical (local includes cleaning, ointment, possible antibiotics), surgical (none if small; larger may require excision with closure, skin grafting, and other treatment), or both.

B. Skin and soft tissue infections (abscesses and/or cellulitis, omphalitis). Incision and drainage of **abscess** (if indicated) with local wound care. Send fluid for culture and sensitivity. An incision and drainage of the abscess may be adequate if the infant is not clinically ill. If the infant is clinically ill, a complete blood count (CBC) with differential and blood culture is usually done. Antibiotics (usually nafcillin) are started to cover for skin flora, unless methicillin-resistant *S. aureus* (MRSA) is suspected (use vancomycin). Lumbar puncture is done if the infant has any signs suspicious for meningitis. Infants with **cellulitis**, especially at IV sites, are usually treated with antibiotics based on culture or empirically with oxacillin or nafcillin and gentamicin. **Omphalitis** is treated with a full sepsis workup (including a lumbar puncture [LP]), and antibiotics (ampicillin and gentamicin) are started to cover both gram-positive and -negative organisms until culture and sensitivities come back.

C. Benign skin disorders. No treatment is necessary.

D. Rashes that are caused by infections. See specific infectious disease chapters for more details where appropriate.
1. *Staphylococcus aureus.* Systemic antibiotics.
2. *Streptococcus.* Cutaneous infection is usually group A, treated by penicillin.
3. Syphilis. See Chapter 138.
4. *Listeria monocytogenes.* Ampicillin and an aminoglycoside such as gentamicin (cephalosporins are not active).
5. Herpes simplex. Acyclovir 60 mg/kg/d IV divided twice daily for 14 days for SEM (skin, eyes, and/or mouth) disease only if there is no central nervous system (CNS) or disseminated disease.
6. Varicella. Acyclovir and VariZIG (see doses in Chapter 148) may decrease the severity of the course and improve outcome. Treatment must begin early in the course of the illness.
7. Cytomegalovirus (CMV). Ganciclovir (Cytovene) in adults; limited data in pediatrics. Parenteral ganciclovir and oral valganciclovir are being used but are

limited to use in those with symptomatic congenital CMV disease with CNS disease. See Chapter 90.

8. **Rubella.** Supportive management. See Chapter 128.

9. *Candida albicans.* Systemic antifungal medications such as amphotericin B to treat disseminated infection. Topical antifungals are used to treat isolated skin lesions. Thrush is treated by oral nystatin, 0.5 mL inside each cheek twice daily, for 10 days.

10. **Aspergillus.** Amphotericin B deoxycholate in high doses.

11. **Scabies.** Apply 5% permethrin cream topically. (*Note:* Permethrin is off label in neonates and may not be safe in very low birthweight infants.)

12. **Toxoplasmosis.** See Chapter 142.

E. **Rashes that cause scaling**

1. **Postmaturity.** No treatment is necessary.

2. **Seborrheic dermatitis.** Usually resolves by 1 year; supportive care.

3. **Fatty acid deficiency.** Replacement of fatty acids through IV lipid solutions or diet is necessary.

4. **Ichthyoses.** Aggressive supportive care, close monitoring of fluid and electrolytes, and meticulous skin care with the goal of preventing infections. Collodion babies frequently have temperature instability and excessive fluid loss.

5. **Infantile eczema.** Avoid any irritants; use protective creams such as zinc oxide in the diaper area. Short-term topical steroids may be needed.

6. **Atopic dermatitis.** Emollients and mild topical steroids are used.

7. **Staphylococcal scalded skin syndrome.** Antibiotics (IV penicillinase resistant, antistaphylococcal [eg, Cloxacillin]), supportive care, and attention to fluid and electrolyte management.

8. **Psoriasis.** Topical steroids and sometimes wet dressings are used.

9. **Candida.** See above.

10. **Syphilis.** See Chapter 138.

11. **Ectodermal dysplasias.** Supportive care with artificial tears.

12. **Immunodeficiencies.** See specific entity.

13. **Neonatal lupus erythematosus.** Thorough cardiac examination, liver function tests, and CBC. Apply protective sunscreen and avoid direct sunlight for 4 to 6 months. Topical steroids may be necessary.

F. **Rashes that cause blisters and bullae**

1. **Epidermolysis bullosa.** Meticulous skin care, infection prevention, and special attention to nutrition and feedings because of the problems with dysphagia from scarring.

2. **Zinc deficiency dermatosis.** Zinc supplementation.

3. **Congenital herpes.** See Chapter 96.

4. **Staphylococcal scalded skin syndrome.** See Section V.D.1.

5. **Incontinentia pigmenti.** No specific treatment for the cutaneous lesions.

G. **Birthmarks**

1. **Hyperpigmented lesions.** Most of these lesions require no treatment. If the lesions are large (>3 cm), removal is recommended. Giant hairy nevi are removed to prevent cancer development.

2. **Hypopigmented lesions.** Piebaldism is treated with cosmetic camouflage. Those with albinism should follow sun restriction guidelines and sunblock.

3. **Vascular lesions.** Many hemangiomas can be closely watched and left to regress. If treatment is necessary, steroid therapy, embolization, excision, occlusion, laser therapy, α-interferon, and radiotherapy are options. Port wine stains can be treated with laser therapy. Need to differentiate benign neonatal hemangiomatosis from diffuse neonatal hemangiomatosis as treatment is different.

H. **Rashes that cause petechiae and purpura.** These rashes usually require a thorough workup and treatment if there is a bleeding disorder. Infections are treated with antibiotics or antiviral agents. Platelet transfusion and replacement of coagulation factors may be necessary.

1. **Birth trauma.** No treatment is necessary.
2. **Autoimmune disorders such as maternal or neonatal lupus.** Cardiology examination to look for heart block is indicated.
3. **Thrombocytopenia, neonatal isoimmune thrombocytopenia (NAIT)/maternal idiopathic thrombocytopenic purpura (ITTP).** See Chapter 139.
4. **Coagulation factor deficiencies.** See Chapter 87.
5. **Sepsis/TORCH infections.** See Chapters 130 and 141.
6. **Disseminated intravascular coagulation (DIC).** See Chapter 87.
7. **Purpura fulminans.** Treat the underlying infection.
8. **Congenital leukemia.** The optimum treatment plan is unclear. Treatment consists of intensive combination therapy plus supportive care.

76 Sedation and Analgesia

I. **Problem.** An infant with pulmonary hypertension with extreme lability needs sedation. Should the infant be sedated, and which agent is available to use? An infant is having a bedside procedure. Should I use a local anesthetic?

II. **Immediate questions**

   A. **What is the indication for the sedation?** Agitation and movement by the infant during procedures such as extracorporeal membrane oxygenation/extracorporeal life support (ECMO/ECLS) can risk injury. Certain procedures (eg, magnetic resonance imaging [MRI]) mandate that the infant be immobilized, so sedation may be required. Infants with extreme lability on mechanical ventilation may benefit from sedation.

   B. **Why does the infant need analgesia?** If the newborn is to undergo minor procedures such as elective circumcision, local anesthesia is usually administered. For emergency procedures such as chest tube placement, the need for analgesia must be weighed against the delay of administering the analgesic agent.

   C. **If treating for agitation while an infant is on mechanical ventilation, is the infant adequately ventilated?** Hypoxia and inadequate ventilation can result in agitation, and sedation is dangerous in these situations.

   D. **Is sedation needed for a short period (ie, for a diagnostic procedure) or long term?** Certain medications are indicated for short-term sedation (ie, chloral hydrate) and should not be used long term.

III. **Differential diagnosis and indications**

   A. **Indications for analgesia.** Whether a newborn can experience pain remains in the philosophical realm, but they undeniably react to painful stimuli (nociception). Such stimuli elicit both clinical symptoms (eg, tachycardia, hypertension, and decreased oxygenation) and complex behavioral responses in term and preterm infants. By 23 weeks' gestation, the nervous system has developed sufficiently to enable the conduction of nociceptive stimuli from peripheral skin receptors to the brain. The development of the descending inhibiting pathways occurs at a later stage; therefore, the more immature infant may have an even lower threshold for noxious stimulus than at a later age. Neonates possibly have an increased sensitivity to pain compared with older age groups. During surgical interventions, the neonate, like the adult, mounts a hormonal response that consists of the release of catecholamines, β-endorphins, corticotropin, growth hormone, and glucagon as well as the suppression of insulin secretion. This response is reduced by prior administration of analgesia or anesthesia.

Although we do not know whether or not the neonate experiences psychological distress and lasting psychological sequelae, there are enough reasons to attempt to control exposure to pain as well as other unpleasant experiences.

1. Major surgical procedures such as ligation of the ductus arteriosus or laparotomy require major anesthesia. General anesthesia should be provided by inhalation of anesthetic gases or intravenous (IV) administration of narcotic agents. In all these conditions, **the use of paralytic agents without analgesia is absolutely contraindicated.**

2. Postoperative management
   a. Narcotic agents should always be included in the immediate postoperative period. Supplementary sedation is often provided by benzodiazepines or chloral hydrate, which are useful to combat agitation and potentiate the effect of opiates. It is important to remember that these sedative agents do not have any analgesic effect and, therefore, cannot be given alone to relieve pain.
   b. Other pain-relieving agents. IV paracetamol (acetaminophen) has been used in Europe for neonatal analgesia and is now available in the United States (Ofirmev). Its use may be helpful to reduce the dosage and frequency of opiate administration.

3. Minor surgical procedures. Analgesia for so-called "minor procedures" is mostly provided by local anesthesia, at times supplemented by small doses of opiates or sedative agents.
   a. Unless the infant's condition requires extreme urgent action, provide analgesia for procedures such as chest tube insertion and vascular cutdown.
   b. The need for analgesia for circumcision is becoming less controversial and is now widely accepted.
   c. The effectiveness and need for analgesia for more minor procedures such as lumbar puncture have not been demonstrated.

4. "Stressful" conditions. There is wide controversy with regard to providing analgesia or sedation in "stressful" conditions, akin to "anxiolysis" in the adult and pediatric population. The period during which mechanical ventilation and its related routine procedures are provided has been identified as the most frequent time when infants are being "stressed."

5. "Painful" conditions. Pain scores/scale have been proposed to provide a rational approach for assessing the need for and to monitor efficacy of pain management. Those scores are usually composites of measured behavioral, physiologic, and stress response. Seven pain scoring tools have found widespread use: the **Neonatal Infant Pain Scale (NIPS),** the **Children's Revised Impact of Event Scale (CRIES),** the **Premature Infant Pain Profile (PIPP),** the **Liverpool Infant Distress Scale (LIDS),** the **Distress Scale for Ventilated Newborn Infants (DVSNI),** the **Pain Assessment Tool (PAT),** and the **COMFORT scale.** The wide variety of these scores exemplify the lack of a gold standard.
   a. The arguments to favor analgesia or sedation for these situations are as follows:
      i. It reduces the level of various biochemical markers of stress such as blood levels of catecholamines, cortisol, and β-endorphin.
      ii. It lessens the duration of hypoxemia associated with endotracheal intubation and/or suctioning.
      iii. Additional argument for its use involves the difficulty in diagnosing discomfort and pain when the infant is under muscle paralysis.
   b. The arguments against such routine use of analgesia or sedation are as follows:
      i. The pharmacokinetic characteristics of narcotic agents in the preterm infant are variable and not always predictable.
      ii. The same assumed "safe" dose for some infants can, for others, result in severe toxicity (eg, hemodynamic and respiratory depression, toxic accumulation, leading to a transient comatose state).

      iii. The prolonged use (sometimes as little as 4 days) of narcotic and sedative agents is associated with the rapid development of tolerance, withdrawal, and encephalopathy and the requirement for higher ventilatory support in the early phase of respiratory distress syndrome. Furthermore, it often delays weaning from mechanical ventilation.

      iv. Treating for "agitation" by sedation can be dangerous when the former is the result of inadequate ventilation or hypoxemia. Therefore, before treating agitation, one must always ensure, by careful examination, that the endotracheal tube is not obstructed or misplaced and that adequate ventilating pressures are being used.

B. Indications for sedation

  1. **Extreme respiratory lability.** Infants who have demonstrated extreme respiratory lability develop hypoxemia rapidly with minimal handling. Infants with severe pulmonary hypertension and pulmonary vascular hyperreactivity are often candidates for sedation.

  2. **Therapeutic procedures.** When it is necessary to prevent the child from moving vigorously (eg, during ECMO/ECLS), sedation may be needed to prevent accidental dislodgment of the vascular cannulas.

  3. **Diagnostic procedures.** Procedures that require the child to be immobilized include imaging procedures such as MRI, cardiac catheterization, and occasionally computed tomography (CT).

  4. **Elective endotracheal intubation and rapid sequence intubation (RSI).** The question of premedicating neonates before nonemergent intubation has been debated in the past, and its use is on the rise. Various combinations of drugs have been proposed, including anticholinergic agents (to prevent reflex bradycardia), short-acting analgesics and/or hypnotic/sedative (to prevent pain and hypertension), and muscle relaxants (to decrease the time and number of attempt for successful intubation). See Table 29–2.

IV. Database

A. **Physical examination.** Before instituting any type of sedation or analgesia, there must be a clear diagnosis. The physical examination is directed at the underlying condition.

B. **Laboratory studies.** These are usually not needed, except in the context of the underlying disease.

C. **Imaging and other studies.** Such studies are usually not needed, except in the context of the underlying disease.

V. Plan

A. **General management.** Prevention of distress and pain should be a priority in the neonatal unit and in newborn nurseries. Measures to prevent or minimize stress in the neonate should include the following:

  1. Reduce noise (eg, close the incubator door gently).

  2. Protect the infant from intense light.

  3. Cluster blood drawings as much as possible.

  4. Use spring-loaded lancets for heelsticks.

  5. Replace tape with a self-adhesive bandage.

  6. Perform intratracheal suctioning only if indicated.

  7. Use adequate medication before invasive procedures.

B. **Specific agents**

  1. **Pharmacologic management provided by systemic analgesia**

    a. **Opiates.** All opiates may lead to respiratory depression and hypotension. Muscular rigidity is seen mostly with the synthetic opiates with rapid IV administration, such as fentanyl (>2 mcg/kg), sufentanil, and especially alfentanil. The risk of chest wall rigidity can be attenuated by slow administration (preferably over 3–5 minutes or at least 1–2 minutes). It can be treated with a muscle-relaxing agent (eg, pancuronium) and acutely reversed by naloxone (0.1 mg/kg).

      i. **Morphine sulfate.** The most commonly used opioid for sedation during mechanical ventilation. A loading IV dose of 50–200 mcg/kg is followed by IV infusion of 10–40 mcg/kg/h. The peak action occurs in 20 minutes and lasts for 2–4 hours in full-term infants and 6–8 hours in preterm infants. The use of morphine infusions reduces pain and stress in mechanically ventilated preterm infants at the expense of increasing the duration of mechanical ventilation. For shorter duration of sedation, only 50–100 mcg/kg (0.05–0.1 mg/kg) can be administered IV or intramuscularly (IM). The onset of action will occur only 5–10 minutes after IV administration of the drug and 10–30 minutes when given IM.

      ii. **Fentanyl (Sublimaze).** Frequently used in neonates for its ability to provide rapid analgesia. It has a faster onset (3–4 minutes) and shorter duration (30 minutes) of action and is 13–20 times more potent than morphine. Fentanyl blocks endocrine stress responses and prevents pain-induced increases in pulmonary vascular resistance, while hemodynamic stability is better preserved than with morphine because it causes less histamine release. For anesthesia, use IV bolus 10–50 mcg/kg, and for analgesia use 1–4 mcg/kg. In case of no IV access, it can be given IM, resulting in a slower onset of action (7–15 minutes). A continuous IV infusion of 1–3 mcg/kg/h may be used for ongoing sedation. Tolerance to opioid-induced analgesia and sedation occurs more rapidly than with morphine. A cumulative fentanyl dose of >2.5 mg/kg or a duration of infusion >9 days is predictive of opioid withdrawal syndrome.

      iii. **Remifentanil.** Give 1–3 mcg/kg IV. Its onset of action is almost immediate and last only 3–10 minutes.

      iv. **Sufentanil.** Give 0.2 mcg/kg over 20 minutes, then continuous IV, 0.05 mcg/kg/h.

   b. **Ketamine.** Ketamine is unique; it produces sedation, analgesia, and amnesia. It has a mild effect on the respiratory drive, increases blood pressure, produces bronchodilation, and can be used IV, IM, or enterally. It can provide anesthesia for a short duration at 0.5–2 mcg/kg per dose (IV). Use in the neonatal intensive care unit has been limited. It may be of value, possibly in combination with atropine sulfate, for sedation before endotracheal intubation. Infants with severe bronchopulmonary dysplasia and refractory bronchospasm may also benefit from the use of ketamine for its additional bronchodilatory effect.

   c. **Acetaminophen.** A loading dose of 20 mg/kg is recommended for initial IV or PO analgesia. Maintenance dose of 10 mg/kg is to be given every 12, 8, and 6 hours for postconceptional age <28, 28–36, and >36 weeks, respectively. Bioavailability is lower by the rectal route, requiring administration at a higher dose (30–45 mg/kg/d). The administration of the repeated dose should not exceed 48–96 hours. The new IV formulation (Ofirmev) requires extreme caution, as a 10-fold dosing error is facilitated by the preparation's concentration being formatted for adult use.

2. **Pharmacologic management provided by sedative-hypnotics**

   a. **Benzodiazepines.** Activate γ-aminobutyric acid receptors and produce sedation, anxiolysis, muscle relaxation, amnesia, and anticonvulsant effects. They may improve synchrony with assisted ventilation but offer little pain relief. Side effects include respiratory depression, hypotension, dependence, and occasional neuroexcitability, or clonic activity resembling seizures.

      i. **Midazolam (Versed)** has a rapid onset of action (1–2 minutes) and can produce apnea if given too rapidly. Its very short half-life (30–60 minutes) makes it a good choice for brief rapid sedation. Midazolam is given as a single dose, 50–100 mcg/kg, or by continuous infusion at a rate of 0.4–0.6 mcg/kg/min. Withdrawal may occur when given continuously for

>48 hours. Combining midazolam with opioids increases the incidence of adverse effects of both agents.

    ii. **Lorazepam (Ativan)** has a longer duration of action (8–12 hours) and may require less frequent dosing (50–100 mcg/kg every 8 hours).

  b. Thiopental. A short-acting oxybarbiturate, thiopental is used at a dose of 3–4 mg/kg for anesthetic induction in neonates. Its onset of action occurs within 30–60 seconds and lasts 5–30 minutes. Hypotension is more likely to occur when used in combination with fentanyl and/or midazolam. May be unavailable in some countries due to suspended manufacturing.

  c. Propofol. A nonbarbiturate anesthetic used for induction of anesthesia. It is lipophilic and rapidly equilibrates between plasma and brain with quick loss of consciousness (within 30 seconds) and short duration of action after a single bolus dose (3–10 minutes). Possible adverse effects are histamine release, apnea, hypotension, bradycardia, and bronchospasm. It often causes pain at injection site. Neonatal dosing has not yet been well established.

  d. Chloral hydrate. A sedative-hypnotic used primarily for short-term sedation. It is especially useful during diagnostic procedures such as CT and MRI. The onset of action is usually within 10–15 minutes. Administer 20–50 mg/kg every 6–8 hours rectally or orally for sedation. It should not be used long term.

  e. Oral pentobarbital (Nembutal). May produce fewer adverse effects than chloral hydrate when used for sedation for MRI or CT. The initial dose is 4 mg, which may be supplemented at aliquots of 2 mg/kg every 30 minutes to a maximum of 8 mg/kg.

3. Additional medications for premedication for nonemergency intubation (RSI)

  a. Muscle relaxants. Given to facilitate intubation and minimize the increase in intracranial pressure that occurs during awake intubation. Their adverse effects may include histamine release, tachycardia, hypertension/hypotension, and bronchospasm. Their effect scan be reversed by atropine and neostigmine. **The use of muscle relaxant for intubation should never be attempted without the presence of individuals well experienced with bag and mask ventilation technique.** As an alternative to bag and mask ventilation, appropriate size laryngeal mask airway has been used successfully in late preterm and term newborns.

    i. **Pancuronium.** Pancuronium 0.1 mg/kg IV has been has been widely used as a muscle relaxant in neonates. Although its onset of action is fast (1–3 minutes), its duration of action (40–60 minutes) makes it less desirable for RSI than the following.

    ii. **Vecuronium.** Vecuronium 0.1 mg/kg IV has a duration of action of 30–40 minutes.

    iii. **Rocuronium.** Rocuronium 0.6–1.2 mg/kg IV, a metabolite derivative of vecuronium, has a quicker onset to paralysis (1–2 minutes) and shorter duration (20–30 minutes).

    iv. **Succinylcholine.** Succinylcholine (1–2 mg/kg IV) is a neuromuscular depolarizing agent with the most rapid onset of action (20–30 seconds) and the shortest duration (4–6 minutes) of all muscle relaxants. If no IV access is available, it can be administered IM (2/mg/kg); this results in a longer onset of action (2–3 minutes) and duration (10–30 minutes) than when administered IV. **Succinylcholine is contraindicated in the presence of hyperkalemia or a family history of malignant hyperthermia.**

  b. Vagolytic agents. Prevent bradycardia during intubation and decrease bronchial and salivary secretions.

    i. **Atropine** 0.02 mg/kg IV or IM. Its onset of action is 1–2 minutes and the duration of action lasts 0.5–2 hours. Tachycardia occurs frequently.

    ii. **Glycopyrrolate** 4–10 mcg/kg IV. Tachycardia occurs less frequently than with atropine.

4. **Pharmacologic management provided by local analgesia**
   a. **Subcutaneous (SC) infiltration with lidocaine, 0.5–1% concentration.** Always use solution without epinephrine. Maximum dose (SC infiltration): 5 mg/kg or 1 mL/kg of 0.5% or 0.5 mL/kg of 1%.
   b. **Buffered lidocaine.** One part sodium bicarbonate with 10 parts 1% lidocaine; typically prepared in the hospital pharmacy. The pain associated with anesthetic infiltration is reduced by buffering the pH from 7.0 to 7.4.
   c. **Topical local anesthetics**
      i. **Lidocaine 2.5% and prilocaine 2.5% (EMLA cream).** This is a eutectic anesthetic mixture (ie, liquid at room temperature). A single dose of 0.5–1.25 g of EMLA cream applied under an occlusive dressing provides adequate local anesthesia 60–80 minutes later. In the term infant, it is an alternative to penile dorsal block for anesthesia during circumcision. The risk of methemoglobinemia (from prilocaine) may restrict its use to the full-term infant, and repeated doses should be avoided.
      ii. **Tetracaine 4% gel (Ametop).** Apply 1.5 g 30–60 minutes before the procedure. It has no risk of methemoglobinemia, but its repeated use may lead to contact dermatitis.
      iii. **4% Liposomal lidocaine cream (L.M.X.4 or Ela-Max).** Increasingly used in pediatrics for its rapid onset of action (20–30 minutes) and can be applied with (preferred) or without an occlusive dressing.
5. **Oral sucrose.** A disaccharide composed of fructose and glucose shown to promote calming behaviors and reduce distress associated with acute painful events. Gustatory inputs from the taste buds lead to cholecystokinin release in the brainstem, which activates descending inhibitory opioid. It is effective for the management of procedural pain in the neonate. Analgesic effects are present with doses as low as 0.1 mL of 24% sucrose. The usual dose is 0.5–1.5 mL of a 24% sucrose solution given by syringe or pacifier 2 minutes before procedures such as heelstick or venipuncture. The potential risk for fluid overload, hyperglycemia, and necrotizing enterocolitis should limit this method to infants >34 weeks' gestation. Other sweet-tasting liquids such as glucose, mother's milk, and saccharin are reported to be equally effective.
6. **Nonpharmacologic management.** Physical measures such as the use of swaddling, containment, or facilitated tucking as well as skin-to-skin contact with the mother ("kangaroo care") are likely to be efficacious in decreasing the noxious effect of the routine procedures (eg, heelstick) needed for the management of the sick infant. Nonnutritive sucking may be helpful. (See also Chapter 14.)

Selected References

De Lima J, Karmo KB. Practical pain management in the neonate. *Best Pract Res Clin Anaesthesiol.* 2010;24:291–307.

Kumar P, Denson SE, Mancuso TJ; Committee on Fetus and Newborn, Section on Anesthesiology and Pain Medicine. Premedication for nonemergency endotracheal intubation in the neonate. *Pediatrics.* 2010;125:608–615.

Lago P, Garetti E, Merazzi D, et al. Guidelines for procedural pain in the newborn. *Acta Paediatrica.* 2009;98:932–939.

Raeside L. Physiological measures of assessing infant pain: a literature review. *Br J Nurs.* 2011;20:1370–1376.

Stevens B, Johnston C, Taddio A, Gibbins S, Yamada J. The premature infant pain profile: evaluation 13 years after development. *Clin J Pain.* 2010;26:813–830.

van den Anker J, Tibboel D. Pain relief in neonates: when to use intravenous paracetamol. *Arch Dis Child.* 2011;96:573–574.

77 Seizure Activity

I. **Problem.** The nurse reports that an infant is having abnormal movements of the extremities consistent with seizure activity. Seizures in the neonate are common and are more prevalent during the neonatal period than any other time. Neonatal seizures may be harmful to the immature brain and may have adverse long-term neurodevelopmental outcomes. Incidence is 2.5–3.5 per 1000 in full term, and up to 22% in preterm. **Neonatal seizures are rarely idiopathic and are a common manifestation of a serious central nervous system disorder:** hypoxic ischemic encephalopathy (~30–50%; most common), intracranial hemorrhage (10–17%), metabolic abnormalities (hypocalcemia [6–15%]; hypoglycemia [6–10%]), central nervous system (CNS) infections (5–14%), infarction (7%), inborn errors of metabolism (3%), CNS malformations (5%), and unknown (10%).

II. **Immediate questions**

A. **Is the infant really seizing?** This question is very important and is often initially difficult to answer. Infants can have many unusual movements that may look like seizures but are not. It is sometimes difficult to distinguish these and an electroencephalogram (EEG) is often necessary. The following are common episodic movements that are not seizures.

1. **Jitteriness.** "Jitteriness" is sometimes confused with seizures. In a jittery infant, eye movements are normal (no ocular deviation), hands stop moving if they are grasped, and movements are of a fine nature (tremor-like, not clonic-like as in seizures). In an infant who is seizing, eye movements can be abnormal (eg, staring, blinking, nystagmoid jerks, or tonic horizontal eye deviation). The hands continue to move if grasped, and movements are of a coarser nature. The EEG is normal with jitteriness and abnormal with seizure activity.

2. **Benign neonatal sleep myoclonus.** Another benign condition that mimics seizures. This presents with rhythmic movements only during sleep. EEG shows no seizures.

3. **Benign myoclonus of early infancy (rare).** This involves muscle spasms of the head, neck, and extremities and eye blinking that resembles seizures.

4. **Benign shuddering attacks.** These events involve shuddering movements that consist of tremors and stiffening of the upper extremities.

5. **Neonatal dystonia/dyskinesia.** These abnormal movements can be associated with asphyxia, metabolic diseases, or maternal drug toxicity.

6. **Rapid eye movement (REM)-associated movements.** Infants can have rapid vertical and horizontal eye movements combined with twitches of the limbs to movements of the entire body.

7. **Sandifer syndrome.** Infants with gastroesophageal (GE) reflux can have spells of opisthotonic posturing and stiffening with staring and jerking of extremities. This can be secondary to pain from acidic material refluxing into the esophagus. They typically occur 30 minutes after eating.

8. **Benign paroxysmal torticollis.** Episodic head tilting to one side can occur with irritability and pallor.

9. **Dystonic drug reaction.** This can occur with an acute drug reaction. Metoclopramide can cause this.

10. **Opisthotonos can be seen.** There is prolonged arching of the back and normal eye movements. This can be secondary to meningeal irritation (Gaucher disease, kernicterus, aminoacidurias).

11. **Neonatal opsoclonus.** This is characterized by rapid oscillations of the eyes. It can be normal or seen in herpes simplex encephalitis or hypoxic ischemic encephalopathy (HIE).

12. **Other movements (motor automatisms).** Certain movements (stretching, sucking, pedalling, swimming, bicycling, intermittent oral buccal lingual movements, and tongue fasciculations) can be normal or represent a subtle seizure or represent brainstem release phenomena since they do not correlate with EEG seizure activity.

B. **Is there a history of birth asphyxia or risk factors for sepsis?** Asphyxia and sepsis with meningitis may cause neonatal seizures.

C. **Is the infant full term or preterm?** Term infants are more likely to have subtle seizures and seizures from asphyxia, and to develop seizures earlier. Preterm infants are more likely to have clonic seizures and seizures from peri-intraventricular hemorrhage, and to develop seizures later.

D. **Does the infant have any risk factors?** Low birthweight or small for gestational age.

E. **What is the blood glucose level?** Hypoglycemia is an easily treatable cause of seizures in the neonatal period.

F. **How old is the infant?** The age of the infant is often the best clue to the cause of the seizures. Common causes of seizures for specific ages are as follows:

1. **At birth.** Maternal anesthetic agents can cause severe tonic seizures typically in the first few hours of life, and they can occur at up to 6–8 hours of life. The anesthetic can be injected into the neonate accidently during delivery. Neonate presents with apnea, flaccidity, asphyxia, and seizures.

2. **Within 30 minutes to 3 days after birth.** Pyridoxine deficiency (B_6-dependent seizures). These infants can also have seizures in utero.

3. **Day 1 (first 24 hours).** Metabolic abnormalities such as hypoglycemia, hypocalcemia, HIE (presenting at 6–18 hours after birth and becoming more severe in the next 24–48 hours). Birth trauma (presents at 12 hours or more: primary subarachnoid hemorrhage, cerebral venous thrombosis, laceration of falx or tentorium with subdural hematoma), CNS intrauterine infections and sepsis, drug withdrawal, inadvertent local anesthetic toxicity, and pyridoxine dependency.

4. **24–72 hours.** Cerebral dysgenesis, vascular (cerebral infarct, intracerebral hemorrhage, cortical vein/sinus thrombosis), intraventricular hemorrhage (IVH), subarachnoid hemorrhage with cerebral contusion from birth trauma. Metabolic (hypocalcemia, hypoglycemia, hyponatremia, hypernatremia), glycine encephalopathy, urea cycle disorders, and aminoacidurias and organic aciduria. Drug withdrawal, pyridoxine dependency, incontinentia pigmenti, tuberous sclerosis meningitis, and therapeutic hypothermia.

5. **72 hours to 1 week.** Familial neonatal seizures, cerebral malformations, cerebral infarction, hypoparathyroidism, vascular events (venous thrombosis hemorrhage), kernicterus, glycine encephalopathy, urea cycle disorders, aminoacidurias and organic aciduria, tuberous sclerosis hypocalcemia, and TORCH infections.

6. **1–4 weeks (>1 week).** Late-onset hypocalcemia, peroxisomal disorders, cerebral dysgenesis, fructose dysmetabolism, Gaucher disease type 2, GM1 gangliosidosis type 1, herpes simplex virus (HSV) 2 encephalitis, ketotic hyperglycinemia, maple syrup urine disease (MSUD), tuberous sclerosis, urea cycle disorders, methadone withdrawal, and De Vivo syndrome (earliest seizures at 2 weeks of age, but typically in this range).

7. **Variable onset.** Stroke, sinus thrombosis, other developmental defects.

G. **Is there a family history of seizures?** If so, a genetic/inherited syndrome may be present and may suggest a good prognosis (benign familial infantile seizures).

H. **Are there any clues in the pregnancy, delivery, or postnatal history that would point to seizures?** Nulliparity, preeclampsia, gestational diabetes, obesity, smoking, and asthma increase the risk. Advanced maternal age and infants of African American mothers have a higher risk; infants of Asian and white Hispanic mothers have a lower risk than Caucasian mothers. Intrapartum risk factors are prolonged second stage of labor, fetal distress, catastrophic delivery, cesarean or operative vaginal delivery, maternal fever, TORCH infections, or history of rubella.

I. **Is the infant on therapeutic hypothermia protocol?** Seizures are common during the therapeutic hypothermia protocol. (See Chapter 39.)

III. **Differential diagnosis.** (See also Chapter 129 and Table 129-1.) The majority of newborns (75–90%) with seizures have an underlying etiology. **Seizure activity** may be secondary to:

A. **CNS abnormalities**

1. **Hypoxic-ischemic cerebral injury. This is the most common cause of neonatal seizures.** It can be secondary to prenatal (abruption placentae, fetal distress, cord compression), perinatal (fetal distress, maternal hemorrhage), and postnatal causes (persistent pulmonary hypertension [PPH], congenital heart disease, respiratory disease). Can be generalized, clonic, or more subtle. **Infants receiving therapeutic hypothermia have a high incidence of seizures.**

2. **CNS bleeds. Intracranial hemorrhage,** including subarachnoid (more common in term infants), germinal matrix, periventricular-intraventricular (mainly preterm), parenchymal (more common in premature infants), or subdural (more common in term infants). Infants born by vaginal delivery are more likely to have an intracranial hemorrhage. CNS trauma from a difficult delivery can contribute.

3. **Neonatal cerebral infarction (perinatal stroke).** A common cause of seizures in full-term infants (1 in 2300 to 1 in 5000). Its origin remains unclear (either thrombotic or embolic causes). Usually presents with focal seizures with cerebral artery or vein infarction. Focal cerebral ischemic lesions are rare in the term infant and present as focal seizures.

4. **Perinatal venous sinus thrombosis.** Presents with seizures, apnea, and irritability.

5. **Hydrocephalus.** Twenty percent of infants with periventricular or intraventricular hemorrhage develop posthemorrhagic hydrocephalus.

6. **Congenital/developmental abnormalities of the brain.** These can cause seizures. Often the infant has obvious anomalies of the face or head if developmental abnormalities are present. Most common are lissencephaly and holoprosencephaly.

7. **Hypertensive encephalopathy.**

8. **CNS trauma.** Usually there is a history of a difficult delivery.

9. **Neurocutaneous syndromes** such as tuberous sclerosis and incontinentia pigmenti.

B. **Electrolyte abnormalities**

1. **Hypoglycemia.** Infant of diabetic mother (IDM), pancreatic disease, glycogen storage disease.

2. **Hypocalcemia.** Neonates exposed to topiramate in utero or with chromosome 22q11 deletion can have hypocalcemic seizures. **Early hypocalcemia** (2–3 days) can occur in preterm infants with prenatal or perinatal insults. **Late hypocalcemia** (5–14 days) can occur from nutritional causes, maternal and neonatal hyperparathyroidism, or Di George syndrome.

3. **Hypomagnesemia, hyponatremia, or hypernatremia.**

C. **Infection**

1. **Meningitis, encephalitis, or abscess.** Bacterial meningitis (especially due to *Escherichia coli* and group B *Streptococcus*) is a common cause. Herpes simplex is the most common cause of nonbacterial encephalitis. Human parechoviruses can cause encephalitis and seizures.

2. **Sepsis.** Often due to *E. coli* and group B *Streptococcus*. Septicemia without meningitis can present with seizures.

3. **Congenital infections.** Toxoplasmosis, cytomegalovirus, herpes simplex, rubella, syphilis, coxsackievirus, acquired immune deficiency syndrome (AIDS).

D. **Neonatal drug withdrawal.** (See Chapter 103.) Seizures are an uncommon manifestation of withdrawal whose mechanism is unclear. Seizures occur in 2–11% of infants withdrawing from opiates. Infants can also have an abnormal EEG without seizures (30% in opiate withdrawal). Seizures can also occur in nonnarcotic withdrawal (alcohol, antidepressants, selective serotonin reuptake inhibitors [SSRIs], barbiturates, sedative hypnotics, cocaine).

E. **Inborn errors of metabolism.** (See Chapter 101.) Seizures are a common symptom in metabolic disorders. Seizure type or EEG findings are rarely specific for a particular metabolic disorder. Usually seen in infants after feeding and who are >72 hours of age. These include glycogen storage disease, galactosemia, organic acidemias, hereditary fructose intolerance, maple syrup urine disease, urea cycle disorders, nonketotic hyperglycinemia, disorders of amino acid metabolism, pyridoxine dependency, peroxisomal disorders, congenital disorders of glycosylation, fatty acid oxidation disorders, and respiratory chain defects.

1. **Pyridoxine-dependent seizures or pyridoxine-dependent epilepsy (PDE).** The majority are caused by a rare genetic mutation.

2. **Folinic acid responsive seizures.** Occur when there is an abnormality in the cerebrospinal fluid (CSF) neurotransmitter studies. Very rare disorder; <10 cases have been reported.

3. **De Vivo syndrome (GLUT-1 deficiency syndrome).** This is a rare condition that is caused by inadequate transport of glucose across the blood-brain barrier.

F. **Maternal anesthetic agents (rare cause).** If a local anesthetic (eg, mepivacaine) is accidentally injected into the infant's scalp during a pudendal, paracervical, or epidural block, seizures can occur at birth. Can verify by sending blood level of suspected agent.

G. **Drug toxicity.** Occurs from agents such as theophylline or caffeine.

H. **Polycythemia with hyperviscosity.**

I. **Genetic syndromes.** Those that can present with seizures include Zellweger syndrome, Smith-Lemli-Opitz syndrome, and others.

J. **Five early epileptic syndromes that can present in the newborn period (rare cause of neonatal seizures).** These infants can have a normal examination and appear well with recurrent seizures.

1. **Benign familial neonatal convulsions.** Usually present on the second or third day of life and are usually autosomal dominant or from a spontaneous mutation. Infants can have 10–20 seizures a day but usually "outgrow" them after 1–6 months with no long-term or recurring problems.

2. **Benign nonfamilial (idiopathic) neonatal seizures, otherwise known as "fifth day fits."** Usually start on days 4–6 and tend to be over in 24 hours. They are multifocal with no family history. The chance of having seizures later on is the same as in the general population.

3. **Early myoclonic epilepsy is a rare epileptic encephalopathy.** It presents within hours of birth with myoclonus and partial seizures. Infants usually die within the first 2 years of life and may have an underlying metabolic defect.

4. **Early infantile epileptic encephalopathy (Ohtahara syndrome).** A severe epileptic syndrome with an associated brain malformation.

5. **Malignant migrating partial seizures in infancy.** Occurs in 3 phases: first is sporadic focal seizures presenting from first day of birth; in the second phase, seizures become more frequent; and the third phase is seizure-free.

IV. Database

A. **History.** A detailed history may help diagnose seizure activity. Does the mother have gestational diabetes, have any sexually transmitted diseases/sexually transmitted infections (STDs/STIs), use any medications or drugs, or have a bleeding disorder, or have any history of epilepsy in the family? Is there a history of consanguinity (think inborn error of metabolism). The provider observing the activity should record a complete description of the event on the chart. Did the mother note hiccups in utero (nonketotic hyperglycemia)? Infants born by vaginal delivery are more likely to have intracranial hemorrhage than infants born by cesarean section.

B. **Physical examination.** Pay close attention to the neurologic status. Look at the scalp for evidence of injection during delivery. Is there macro/microcephaly? Recurrent apnea can be a manifestation of a seizure. Does the cutaneous examination reveal a vesicular rash (herpes, incontinentia pigmenti)? Look for dysmorphic features seen in Zellweger syndrome or Smith-Lemli-Opitz syndrome. Most seizures in the neonate are focal. Try to assess the type of seizures using the classification of Volpe:

1. **Clonic.** Primarily term infants with slow rhythmic movement. Focal or multifocal. Typically see one extremity (focal; best prognosis) or only one side of body.
2. **Tonic.** Usually generalized. Primarily preterm infants with sustained extension or flexion posturing. Typically involves one extremity or whole body with extension of arms and legs or stiffening of body. Eyes deviate upward and apnea is seen. Focal (less common) and generalized (more common).
3. **Myoclonic (rare).** Rapid flexion twitching or jerking movements. Typically one extremity or in several body parts. Can be focal, multifocal, or generalized. Rapid flexion or extension movements of extremities and carries a poor prognosis.
4. **Subtle seizures/autonomic seizures (motor automatisms).** Any alterations in neonatal behavior, motor functions, and autonomic function that are usually difficult to recognize and are overlooked. Examples include ocular movements, chewing, pedaling, or apnea. Some of these alterations may not represent seizure activity but brainstem release (automatic reflex behaviors released when the cerebral cortex is not functioning normally). If found in preterm infants it is more common and more likely to be seizure activity than if found in term infants. Recurrent apnea may rarely be a seizure manifestation (suspect this if no change in heart rate [no bradycardia] and there is tonic-clonic posturing).

C. **Laboratory studies.** Immediate laboratory tests should include a minimum of arterial blood gas, serum electrolytes, and complete blood count (CBC) with differential.

1. **Metabolic workup**
   a. **Serum glucose.** If bedside paper-strip testing is <40 mg/dL, obtain a central value.
   b. **Serum sodium.** To evaluate for hyponatremia or hypernatremia.
   c. **Serum ionized and total calcium levels.** Only an ionized calcium level is usually necessary, but if this cannot be done STAT, a total calcium should be ordered. Ionized calcium is the most accurate measurement of calcium.
   d. **Serum magnesium.**
2. **Infection workup**
   a. **CBC with differential.** A hematocrit also rules out polycythemia.
   b. **Blood, urine, and CSF cultures (for bacteria and viruses).** CSF polymerase chain reaction (PCR) for herpes simplex virus if suspected.
   c. **Serum immunoglobulin M (IgM) and IgM-specific TORCH titers.** The serum IgM titer may be elevated in TORCH infections.
3. **Urine drug screening.** If drug withdrawal is suspected.
4. **Theophylline or caffeine level.** If the infant is on this medication and toxicity is suspected.
5. **Blood gas levels.** To rule out hypoxia or acidosis.
6. **Coagulation studies.** If there is evidence of hemorrhage.
7. **Studies for inborn errors of metabolism.** Include serum ammonia (increased in urea cycle and organic acid metabolism defects), lactic acid (elevated in organic acid metabolism), CSF lactate, urine organic acids/serum amino acid assays. Urine for amino acids and 2,4-dinitrophenylhydrazine (DNPH) screening test (MSUD). Test serum and CSF for glycine (nonketotic hyperglycinemia.)
8. **Lumbar puncture.** If blood is in the CSF it may suggest an intraventricular hemorrhage (IVH). Cultures and rapid testing of the fluid should be done to diagnose infection (see Chapters 35 and 109). Check glucose for De Vivo syndrome and CSF neurotransmitters for folinic acid responsive seizures. Spinal fluid for glycine for nonketotic hyperglycemia, lactic acid for mitochondrial disorders, and neurotransmitters for hydroxyindoleacetic acid (HIAA) and homovanillic acid (HVA). Elevated ammonia level may indicate a urea cycle or organic acid metabolism defect.

D. **Imaging and other studies.** Immediate radiologic studies should include an ultrasound of the head and EEG.

1. **Ultrasound examination of the head.** This confirms periventricular-intraventricular hemorrhage (PV-IVH). *Note:* The coexistence of IVH and seizures does not necessarily mean the two are related.

2. **CT scan of the head.** To diagnose subarachnoid or subdural hemorrhage. It may also reveal a congenital malformation or cerebral infarction if suspected. Radiation exposure is a concern.

3. **Cranial magnetic resonance image (MRI).** A very sensitive test used to help determine the etiology of the seizures. It actually has greater sensitivity in identifying ischemic damage, intracranial hemorrhages, and brain malformations than computed tomography (CT) or ultrasound. Its disadvantage is that it is difficult to obtain in an unstable infant. **Magnetic resonance angiography and venography** is helpful in making the diagnosis of cerebral infarction. **Diffusion weighted imaging (DWI)** is helpful in early hypoxic injury.

4. **Electroencephalography (EEG).** It is usually not possible to perform an EEG during the episode of seizure activity. The EEG is rarely helpful in making a specific diagnosis. This study should be done at some time after seizure activity has been documented; it may confirm seizure activity, and it may also be used as a baseline study and may show changes consistent with the localization of the lesion in cerebral infarction. The interictal pattern is also helpful in predicting future seizure activity. Focal clonic seizures have a consistent EEG correlation; subtle seizures do not. **Polygraphic video EEG monitoring** can be done if infrequent neonatal seizures continue.

5. **Amplitude-integrated electroencephalography (aEEG).** Smaller portable units with only 2–4 scalp electrodes, instead of the usual 12–16. They also provide shorter, simpler readouts than the conventional EEG. These units detected most seizures in at-risk infants. aEEG has a high sensitivity and specificity by experienced users.

V. **Plan**

A. **General measures.** Once it is determined that the infant is having seizures, **immediate evaluation and possible treatment is necessary. Cochrane review** states that there is little evidence to support the use of any anticonvulsants currently used in neonates. Most evidence supports that recurrent seizures should be treated. Neurology consultation should be obtained. The following immediate measures should be taken:

1. **Rule out hypoxia by measurement of blood gases, and start oxygen therapy.** Assess the infant's airway and breathing. Intubation and mechanical ventilation may be necessary to maintain oxygenation and ventilation. Correct any metabolic acidosis.

2. **Check the glucose level.** A Dextrostix or Chemstrip-bG paper-strip test should be immediately done to rule out hypoglycemia while a STAT sample is sent to the laboratory for confirmation. If the paper-strip test shows low blood glucose, it is acceptable to give 10% glucose, 2–4 mL/kg IV push, before obtaining results from the laboratory.

3. **Obtain STAT serum calcium, sodium, and magnesium levels.** If these levels were low on earlier values and a metabolic disorder is strongly suspected as the cause of the seizures, it is acceptable to treat the infant before new laboratory values are available.

4. **Anticonvulsant therapy.** If hypoxia and all metabolic abnormalities have been treated, or if blood gas and metabolic workup values are normal, start anticonvulsant therapy. For detailed pharmacologic information, see Chapter 148.

   a. **Phenobarbital is the first-line drug.** Initially, 20 mg/kg is given as the loading dose, but additional doses of 5 mg/kg up to 40 mg/kg can be given if the seizures continue. Successful in <50% of patients.

   b. **If seizures persist.** Give **phenytoin (Dilantin)**, 20 mg/kg/dose, at a rate of 1 mg/kg/min or less. **Fosphenytoin may be preferred** at some centers (see dosage in Chapter 148) because it has been associated with fewer side effects than phenytoin (less hypotension, fewer cardiac abnormalities, and less soft tissue injury).
   c. **If seizures still persist.** The **third medication** used is a **benzodiazepine.** Respiratory depression can occur with these medications, but is usually not a problem because most infants are already on mechanical ventilation. Most institutions use **lorazepam.**
      i. **Lorazepam.** Given IV, can be repeated 4–6 times in a 24-hour period. It is advantageous to use over diazepam because it causes less sedation and respiratory depression. Dose is 0.05–0.1 mg/kg every 8–12 hours.
      ii. **Midazolam.** A short-acting benzodiazepine that can be given by a continuous infusion. See dose in Chapter 148.
      iii. **Diazepam.** Effective if given by a continuous infusion of 0.3 mg/kg/h. Another dose listed was 0.25 mg/kg every 6–8 hours.
      iv. **Some institutions** are using levetiracetam (Keppra) as the third choice, especially after pediatric neurology consultation.
   d. **If seizures persist and other causes have been ruled out.** Three disorders need to be considered because they are treatable:
      i. **Pyridoxine (B_6)-dependent seizures.** A trial of pyridoxine (vitamin B_6), 50–100 mg given IV with EEG monitoring, is now recommended. With pyridoxine dependency, the seizures stop quickly after the medication is given. Some institutions wait to give this after 3 medications have been given and failed; some try this after 2 medications have been given.
      ii. **Folinic acid responsive seizures (rare).** Obtain CSF neurotransmitter studies. Then folinic acid is given at 2.5 mg twice daily (up to 4 mg/kg/d initially) in 2 doses. After 24 hours of treatment, seizures may stop. Folinic acid can be given for 48 hours as a trial.
      iii. **De Vivo syndrome (glucose transporter deficiency).** Treatment is a ketogenic diet.
   e. **If seizures still persist.** The following salvage drugs may be used depending on institutional preference:
      i. **High-dose phenobarbital.** >30 mg/kg to achieve serum level >60 mcg/mL.
      ii. **Midazolam.** IV and has been given intranasally. IV dose is 0.2 mg/kg, then 0.1–0.4 mg/kg/h.
      iii. **Pentobarbital.** 10 mg/kg IV, then 1 mg/kg/h.
      iv. **Thiopental.** 10 mg/kg IV, then 2–4 mg/kg/h.
      v. **Clonazepam.** 0.1 mg/kg orally.
      vi. **Valproic acid.** 10–25 mg/kg, then 20 mg/kg/d in 3 doses.
      vii. **Levetiracetam (Keppra).** See dose in Chapter 148.
      viii. **Lignocaine.** 2 mg/kg IV with maintenance of 1–6 mg/kg/h.
      ix. **Paraldehyde.** Given rectally (IV preparation no longer available in the United States); used as a last effort.
      x. **Lidocaine.** 2 mg/kg IV, then 6 mg/kg/h with cardiac monitoring. New infusion doses have been used to decrease cardiac arrhythmias. Not recommended in infants who have been treated with phenytoin or who have congenital heart disease.
B. **Specific measures**
   1. **Hypoxic-ischemic injury.** Seizures secondary to birth asphyxia usually present at anywhere from 6–18 hours of age. Many infants will receive therapeutic hypothermia, in which the incidence of seizures is high.
      a. **Careful observation.** Required by the physician and nursing staff to detect seizure activity.

    b. Prophylactic phenobarbital. Used at some institutions (*controversial*). One study stated that the use of phenobarbital within 6 hours of birth in infants with hypoxic ischemic encephalopathy decreased the incidence of neonatal seizures. However, anticonvulsant therapy soon after birth to birth-asphyxiated infants cannot be recommended unless larger and more studies are done.

    c. Restrict fluids to ~60 mL/kg/d. Monitor serum electrolytes and urine output.

    d. If seizures begin. Follow the guidelines given in Section V.A.4. Optimal seizure treatment is *controversial* and many of the medications have limited efficacy.

2. **Hypoglycemia.** Treat and determine the cause, as outlined in Chapter 62.

3. **Hypocalcemia.** Give 100–200 mg/kg calcium gluconate slowly IV. Make certain that the infant is receiving maintenance calcium therapy (usually 50 mg/kg every 6 hours). Monitor the heart rate continuously, and confirm correct IV position. (See also Chapter 85.)

4. **Hypomagnesemia.** Give 0.2 mEq/kg magnesium sulfate IV every 6 hours until magnesium levels are normal or symptoms resolve. (See Chapter 107.)

5. **Hyponatremia.** See Chapter 64.

6. **Hypernatremia.** Treat the seizure activity as described in Section V.A.4. If hypernatremia is secondary to decreased fluid intake, increase the rate of free water. The amount of sodium needs to be decreased; it should be reduced over 48 hours to decrease the possibility of cerebral edema.

7. **Hypercalcemia.** Usual treatment plans include the following:

    a. Increase IV fluids by 20 mL/kg/d.

    b. Administer a diuretic (eg, furosemide [Lasix], 1–2 mg/kg/dose every 12 hours).

    c. Administer phosphate 30–40 mg/kg/d orally or IV.

    d. Glucocorticoids may be effective short term.

    e. Calcitonin but limited newborn experience.

8. **Infection.** If sepsis is suspected, a complete workup should be performed and empirical broad-spectrum antibiotic therapy initiated. Remember aminoglycosides have poor CSF penetration. Antiviral therapy (acyclovir) should be considered in infants >1 week of age or sooner if premature rupture of membranes for treatment of herpes simplex virus. Some institutions treat all infants with seizures empirically with acyclovir when there is a high index of suspicion of herpes infection. A complete septic workup includes white blood cell count with differential, blood culture, urine and serum antigen test, lumbar puncture, culture for bacteria and viruses (if indicated), and urinalysis and urine culture (if indicated). CSF polymerase chain reaction and surface cultures should be done if herpes is suspected.

9. **Drug withdrawal syndrome.** Supportive therapy and anticonvulsants are used. (See Chapter 103.)

10. **Subarachnoid hemorrhage.** Only supportive therapy is necessary. (See Chapter 104.)

11. **Subdural hemorrhage.** Only supportive therapy is necessary, unless the infant has lacerations of the falx and tentorium, for which rapid surgical correction is necessary. Hemorrhage over cerebral convexities is treated by subdural taps. (See Chapter 104.)

12. **CNS trauma.** In cases of depressed skull fracture, elevation of the bone may be necessary.

13. **Hydrocephalus.** Repeated lumbar taps may be necessary, or a shunt may be placed. (See Chapter 98.)

14. **Polycythemia.** Partial plasma exchange is often used. (See Chapters 71 and 122.)

15. **Cerebral infarction.** Supportive therapy and seizure therapy as noted above. Close follow-up is necessary because of possible neurologic sequelae (eg, hemiplegia, cognitive difficulties, delays in language acquisition, and developmental delay). Most cases have a normal outcome.

16. **Accidental anesthetic injection.** Vigorous ventilatory support and removal of the drug by diuresis or exchange transfusion is recommended. Seizure medications are usually not needed.

78 Traumatic Delivery

I. **Problem.** An infant is noted to have severe bruises after birth, and a nurse observes that the infant is not using his right arm. The birth was noted to be traumatic, and the nurse calls you to evaluate the infant. **Birth injuries** are injuries that occur during the birth process. The incidence is ~6–8 per 1000 live births (higher rates for infants >4500 g). Birth injuries occur from both vaginal and cesarean deliveries. Infants delivered by cesarean section are at risk for different types of birth trauma than infants delivered vaginally. Infants delivered by cesarean have a decreased risk of all birth trauma due to the decreased risk of clavicle fractures, brachial plexus, and scalp injuries.

II. **Immediate questions**
   A. **Are there any risk factors for a birth injury?** Certain factors predispose the infant to birth injuries. These include fetal macrosomia, prima gravida, small maternal stature, prolonged or very rapid labor, precipitous delivery, difficult fetal extraction, abnormal presentation (especially breech), vaginal breech delivery, cephalopelvic disproportion, maternal pelvic abnormalities, oligohydramnios, nuchal cord, very low birthweight infant, very large fetal size, fetal anomalies (osteogenesis imperfecta), use of forceps or vacuum extraction, and prematurity.
   B. **Is the injury so serious that it requires immediate attention?** The majority of birth injuries are not serious and do not require urgent treatment. Significant injuries requiring immediate intervention, such as abdominal organ injuries that present as shock and require surgery, need to be identified early.
   C. **Was forceps or vacuum extraction used during the delivery?** Studies suggest that the use of mid-forceps and vacuum extraction may increase the infant's risk of fractures and paralysis.

III. **Differential diagnosis (based on site of injury)**
   A. **Skin**
      1. **Petechiae.** Small (<3 mm) bruises that do not blanch on pressure. In birth trauma, petechiae are usually localized (eg, on the head, neck, upper chest area, and lower back). There is no associated bleeding, and no new lesions appear. If petechiae are diffuse, suspect thrombocytopenia or other systemic disease. If there is bleeding from venipuncture sites, suspect coagulation disorders or other diseases.
      2. **Ecchymosis.** A >1 cm bruise beneath the skin. Bruising can occur after a traumatic delivery, especially when labor is rapid or the infant is premature.
      3. **Abrasions or lacerations.** These can occur secondary to the use of a scalpel during a cesarean delivery. They usually occur on the buttocks, scalp, or thigh. Sometimes suturing is necessary.
      4. **Forceps injury.** Frequently, reddish linear marks are seen across both sides of the face.
      5. **Scalp electrode injury.** The site of insertion of the scalp electrode can sometimes become infected (1% of cases) and in premature infants can rarely cause severe bleeding.
      6. **Subcutaneous fat necrosis.** Typically involves the shoulders and the buttocks with a well-circumscribed lesion of the skin and underlying tissue. It usually appears between 6 and 10 days of age. Lesion size is 1–10 cm, it can be irregular and hard, and the overlying skin can be purple or colorless. (See Chapter 75 and Plate 9.)
   B. **Head**
      1. **Soft tissue injury.** Bruising and petechiae of the soft tissue can occur.
      2. **Extracranial injury.** See Chapter 6, Figure 6–1.
         a. **Caput succedaneum.** This is an area of generalized edema over the presenting part of the scalp during a vertex delivery and is associated with bruising and petechiae. **It crosses the midline of the skull** and suture lines. The bleeding

is external to the periosteum. Hyperbilirubinemia rarely develops. A **vacuum-induced caput occurs** during a delivery using a vacuum device.

b. **Cephalhematoma.** Incidence is 1.5–2.5% of all deliveries. This is caused by bleeding that occurs below the periosteum overlying one cranial bone (usually the parietal bone). **There is no crossing of the suture lines.** The overlying scalp is not discolored, and the swelling sometimes takes days to become apparent. The incidence of an associated skull fracture is 5% in unilateral lesions and 18% in bilateral lesions and is most often a linear fracture. Hyperbilirubinemia (sometimes significant if the lesion is extensive) may develop. Other complications such as meningitis and osteomyelitis can occur.

c. **Subgaleal hemorrhage (also called subaponeurotic hemorrhage).** A collection of blood in the soft tissue space under the aponeurosis but above the periosteum of the skull. Usually caused by forceps or vacuum with traction on the emissary veins. Diffuse swelling of the soft tissue, often spreading toward the neck and behind the ears, can be seen. Periorbital swelling is also evident. Associated signs include severe blood loss (potential to hold more than half the total blood volume), shock, anemia, hypotonia, seizures, and pallor. Rarely, a fatal complication of a traumatic birth.

3. **Intracranial injury.** Most common subdural hemorrhage (73%), then subarachnoid (20%), intracerebral (20%), intraventricular, then epidural hemorrhage. (See also Chapter 104.)

a. **Subdural hemorrhage.** Blood between the arachnoid membrane and dura. Infants present shortly after birth with stupor, seizures, a full fontanelle, unresponsive pupils, and coma.

b. **Subarachnoid hemorrhage.** Blood between the arachnoid membrane and pia mater. Usually asymptomatic, but seizures and other complications such as high bilirubin can be seen.

c. **Intraparenchymal hemorrhage**
   i. **Intracerebellar hematoma/cerebellar hemorrhage.** Associated with traumatic delivery and can present with apnea, unexplained motor agitation in preterm infants, bulging fontanel, and decreased hematocrit.
   ii. **Intracerebral hemorrhage.** This can occur from cranial birth trauma but is more commonly associated with other causes.

d. **Intraventricular hemorrhage.** Bleeding into the ventricular system; occurs secondary to prematurity. In the **term infant** it occurs secondary to birth trauma or asphyxia. Presents with apnea, lethargy, cyanosis, seizures, weak suck, and high-pitched cry.

e. **Epidural hemorrhage.** Blood between the skull and outside of the dura; very rare and one cause is the infant being dropped during delivery. Symptoms are similar to those of subdural hemorrhage; diagnosed by computed tomography (CT) or magnetic resonance imaging (MRI). Clinical manifestations are usually delayed, and it is often associated with skull fracture and cephalhematoma.

f. **Contusion bruise (cerebral and cerebellum) of the brain.** Presents with nonspecific neurologic dysfunction. CT shows punctate hemorrhages.

4. **Skull fracture.** These bone injuries are uncommon in neonates; most are linear and are associated with a cephalhematoma. Fractures at the base of the skull may result in shock. Occipital fractures can be associated with breech deliveries.

a. **Linear fracture.** A break that transverses the full thickness of the skull, is straight, and has no displacement. Usually no therapy is required.

b. **Depressed fracture.** A depressed fracture (ping-pong fracture) of the skull is caused by the bone (most commonly the parietal) being displaced inward. Depressed fractures are often visible and can result in seizures. It occurs from birth trauma but a congenital depressed fracture of the skull can also occur prenatally or in the absence of trauma.

      c. **Occipital osteodiastasis. Rare because of improved obstetric techniques.** Traumatic separation of the cartilaginous joint between the squamous and lateral portion of the occipital bone that results in a posterior fossa subdural hemorrhage associated with laceration of the cerebellum. There are 3 types: classic, fatal form, and less severe variant compatible with survival.

C. Facial

   1. **Fractures of the nose, mandible, maxilla, lacrimal bones, and septal cartilage.** These can often present as respiratory distress or feeding problems and require treatment. Urgent plastic surgery consultation is recommended.

   2. **Dislocations of the facial bones.** Nasal septal dislocation (the most common facial injury) can occur and presents as stridor and cyanosis. Facial bone and mandibular fractures can occur.

   3. **Facial nerve palsy.** This is the most common cranial nerve (cranial nerve VII) injury secondary to birth trauma. It is not increased in deliveries involving forceps, as previously believed. The nerve is injured at the point where it emerges from the stylomastoid foramen.

     a. **Central paralysis.** Involves the lower half or two-thirds of the contralateral side of the face. On the paralyzed side, the nasolabial fold is obliterated, the corner of the mouth droops, and the skin is smooth and full. When the infant cries, the wrinkles are deeper on the normal side, and the mouth is drawn to the normal side.

     b. **Peripheral paralysis.** Involves the entire side of the face. At rest, the infant has an open eye on the affected side. When the infant cries, the findings are similar to those with central paralysis.

D. Eye

   1. **Eyelids.** Edema and bruising can occur. Swollen eyelids should be forced open to examine the eyeball. Laceration of the eyelid can also occur.

   2. **Orbit fracture.** Rarely occurs. Immediate ophthalmologic evaluation is necessary if disturbances of the extraocular muscle movements and exophthalmos are evident. Severe injuries may result in death.

   3. **Horner syndrome.** Due to impaired sympathetic outflow with signs such as miosis, partial ptosis, enophthalmos, and anhidrosis of the ipsilateral side of the face. Delayed pigmentation of the ipsilateral iris can be seen as the child grows.

   4. **Subconjunctival hemorrhage.** A common finding that resolves without treatment.

   5. **Cornea.** Haziness can be secondary to edema or use of eye prophylaxis. With persistent haziness, suspect rupture of Descemet membrane.

   6. **External ocular muscle injuries** involving the third, fourth, and sixth cranial nerves.

   7. **Optic nerve injury.** Vision may be affected.

   8. **Intraocular hemorrhage**

     a. **Retinal hemorrhage.** Most commonly a flame-shaped or streak hemorrhage found near the optic disk. A subdural hemorrhage can cause preretinal and intraretinal hemorrhages.

     b. **Hyphemas.** Gross blood is seen in the anterior chamber.

     c. **Vitreous hemorrhage.** Indicated by floaters, absent red reflex, and blood pigment seen on slit-lamp examination by the ophthalmologist.

E. Ear. Ear injuries (abrasions, bruising, hematomas, avulsion, or laceration of the auricle) can occur, often due to forceps placed near the ears.

F. Nose. Nasal deformity (deformity of the nasal pyramid, soft tissue, and septum) can occur. It is increased in prolonged delivery, increased head circumference, and vaginal delivery. Fracture and dislocation can occur, and infants may have respiratory distress.

G. Vocal cord injuries. Although rare, they can occur as a result of excessive traction on the head during delivery and are caused by an injury to the recurrent laryngeal branch of the vagus nerve. Often associated with forceps in a difficult delivery, they can result in bilateral or unilateral vocal cord paralysis and may cause acute respiratory compromise.

1. **Unilateral paralysis.** Involves the recurrent laryngeal branch of one of the vagus nerves in the neck. Clinically, hoarseness (weak cry, abnormal voice) and mild to moderate stridor with inspiration are seen. Unilateral vocal cord paralysis is usually left sided because of the nerves' longer course and position for injury.

2. **Bilateral paralysis.** Caused by trauma to both recurrent laryngeal nerves. Symptoms at birth include respiratory distress, stridor, and cyanosis.

H. **Neck shoulder and chest injuries**

1. **Shoulder dystocia.** Occurs when the head is delivered and the shoulder gets stuck during delivery. Trauma to the neck can occur when the baby is delivered. The most common injury is brachial plexus injury, but the clavicle can be broken, or cord compression can occur.

2. **Clavicular fracture. The most common bone fracture during delivery.** If the fracture is complete, symptoms involve decreased or absent movement of the arm, gross deformity of the clavicle, pain response on palpation, localized crepitus, and an absent or asymmetric Moro reflex. Green-stick fracture usually presents with no symptoms, and the diagnosis is made because of callus formation at 7–10 days.

3. **Rib fractures.** Very rare.

4. **Brachial palsy.** Usually secondary to prolonged delivery of a macrosomic infant. The spinal roots of the fifth cervical through the first thoracic spinal nerves (brachial plexus) are injured during birth. This is usually unilateral and occurs twice as often on the right as the left. Obstetrical shoulder dystocia training was associated with a lower incidence of brachial plexus injury. (See Chapter 6.) There are 3 different presentations.

    a. **Duchenne-Erb palsy.** This involves the upper arm and is the most common type (~90% of cases). The fifth and sixth cervical roots are affected, and the arm is adducted and internally rotated. Moro reflex is absent (sometimes it can be asymmetric or weakened), but the grasp reflex is intact.

    b. **Klumpke palsy.** This involves the lower arm because the seventh and eighth cervical and first thoracic roots are injured; it is rare (2.5% of cases). The hand is paralyzed, the wrist does not move, and the grasp reflex is absent (ie, dropped hand). Cyanosis and edema of the hand can also occur. An ipsilateral Horner syndrome (ptosis, miosis, and enophthalmos) can be seen because of injury involving the cervical sympathetic fibers of the first thoracic root. Phrenic nerve paralysis with Klumpke palsy is evident.

    c. **Entire arm (global or total brachial plexus) paralysis.** The entire brachial plexus is damaged. The patient has a flaccid arm, hanging limply with no reflexes.

5. **Phrenic nerve paralysis.** Difficult breech delivery can rarely cause **diaphragmatic paralysis** and usually occurs along with upper brachial nerve palsy (75% of cases). It is associated with cyanosis, tachypnea, irregular respirations, and thoracic breathing with no bulging of the abdomen.

6. **Sternocleidomastoid muscle (SCM) injury (muscular or congenital torticollis).** A well-circumscribed, immobile mass in the mid-portion of the SCM that enlarges, regresses, and disappears. This results in a transient torticollis after birth. The head tilts toward the involved side, the chin is elevated and rotated, and the patient cannot move the head into normal position.

I. **Spinal cord injuries.** Rare and are caused by lateral or longitudinal stretching force of the neck or hyperextension or torsion of the fetal neck. Symptoms vary, depending on the location of the injury. Such injuries usually occur with breech deliveries or use of forceps. They can involve meningeal damage with epidural hemorrhage, spinal artery occlusion, vertebral artery injuries and occlusion, laceration of the spinal nerve roots and bruising, and laceration or complete transection of the cord. The higher the injury, the greater is the risk of respiratory problems.

1. **Infants with a high cervical lesion.** Usually have severe respiratory depression with paralysis at birth. Mortality is high.
2. **Upper or mid cervical lesions.** Usually present without symptoms but can have hypotonia. Mortality is high.
3. **Lesions in the seventh cervical to first thoracic roots.** Present with paraplegia and urinary and respiratory problems.
4. **Partial spinal cord injuries.** On neurologic examination, these infants have signs of spasticity.

J. **Abdominal organ injuries (uncommon).** These injuries should be suspected with shock, increasing abdominal circumference, anemia, and irritability. These infants can be asymptomatic for hours and then deteriorate acutely. Risk factors for these include macrosomia and breech presentation. **Intraperitoneal bleed needs to be ruled out in every infant** who presents with shock and abdominal distension. Paracentesis is essential.

1. **Liver hematoma/rupture.** The liver is the most common organ affected. Subcapsular hematomas are the most common lesion and are usually not easily diagnosed (subtle signs of blood loss include onset of jaundice, tachypnea, and poor feeding). Rupture of the hematoma presents with sudden circulatory collapse (a hematoma ruptures through the capsule).
2. **Splenic hematoma/rupture.** Signs are similar to rupture of the liver; blood loss and hemoperitoneum may be seen. Less frequent than hepatic injury.
3. **Adrenal hemorrhage.** Usually right sided and unilateral. Symptoms include fever, tachypnea, flank mass, pallor, cyanosis, poor feeding, shock, vomiting, and diarrhea.
4. **Renal/kidney trauma.** Similar to the other organ injuries with ascites, flank mass, and gross hematuria.

K. **Extremity injuries.** See also Chapter 115.

1. **Fractured humerus.** The second most common fracture during birth trauma. The arm is immobile, with tenderness and crepitation on palpation. Moro reflex is absent on the affected side.
2. **Fractured femur.** May occur secondary to breech delivery. Infants with congenital hypotonia are at risk. Deformity is usually obvious; the affected leg does not move, and there is pain with assisted movement.
3. **Fractured radius.** Rare.
4. **Epiphyseal displacement/dislocation.** Rarely seen, this usually involves the radial head but can also involve the humeral or femoral epiphysis. Examination reveals adduction, internal rotation of the affected arm, and poor Moro reflex. Palpate lateral and posterior displacement of the radial head.
5. **Sciatic nerve palsy.** Rare and can occur in breech deliveries. Prolonged labor and a forceful extraction of the leg is usually obtained from the history. Complete or partial paralysis can occur.
6. **Radial nerve palsy (rare).** Infants present with absent wrist and digital extension, but good shoulder and elbow function. Ecchymosis and fat necrosis may support a compression injury during labor.

L. **Genital injuries**

1. **Edema, bruising, and hematoma of the scrotum and penis.** Occur especially in large infants and with breech deliveries. Injury usually does not affect micturition.
2. **Testicular and epididymal injury.** Findings are scrotal swelling, with the infant experiencing vomiting and irritability. A **hematocele** can form if the tunica vaginalis testis is injured; the scrotum will not transilluminate. **Scrotal rupture** is only in case reports.

M. **Umbilical cord rupture.** This can occur from trauma from an operative vaginal delivery (forceps or vacuum device used). Hemorrhage with bradycardia and respiratory distress can occur.

IV. **Database**
  A. **Physical examination.** Details on the physical examination of the newborn are found in Chapter 6.
   1. **Skin.** Look for petechiae, bruising, and any lacerations. Check the side of the face for forceps marks. Look for and palpate any area that looks like fat necrosis.
   2. **Head.** Carefully examine the head for any evidence of a caput succedaneum, cephalhematoma, subgaleal hemorrhage, or fracture. Check to see whether the suture lines are crossed (differentiates between the caput succedaneum and cephalhematoma). Depressed skull fractures are obvious; others may require radiologic studies.
   3. **Face.** Examine the face at rest and during crying to look for any facial asymmetry (nerve palsy). Check for any signs of respiratory distress (stridor or cyanosis).
   4. **Eyes.** Examine the eyeball and the eyelid. Make sure that extraocular muscle movements are normal. Check for the red reflex.
   5. **Ears.** Examine the front and back of the ear, looking for lacerations, swelling, and hematomas.
   6. **Vocal cords.** Signs may include high-pitched cry or stridor. If injury is suspected, examine the vocal cords by direct laryngoscopy or use a flexible fiber optic laryngoscope.
   7. **Neck and shoulder injuries.** Carefully examine the neck and the shoulder. Check Moro and grasp reflexes. Examine the arm to see whether movement is normal. Check respirations, and note any thoracic breathing. Make sure the head rests in a normal position and is not tilted.
   8. **Spinal cord.** A careful and thorough neurologic examination should be done.
   9. **Abdomen.** Examine the abdomen, and check for ascites, masses, and increase in size.
   10. **Extremities.** Observe for movement and deformity.
   11. **Genitalia.** Examine the testes and the penis in males; transilluminate the scrotum.
  B. **Laboratory studies based on site of trauma**
   1. **Skin**
      a. **Platelet count.** A normal platelet count excludes neonatal thrombocytopenia.
      b. **Serum bilirubin test.** Hyperbilirubinemia may result from reabsorption of blood from extensive ecchymoses.
      c. **Serum hematocrit.** Anemia may result from severe ecchymoses.
   2. **Head**
      a. **Hematocrit.** Blood loss can occur, sometimes requiring transfusions, especially in subgaleal hemorrhage.
      b. **Serum bilirubin.** Significant hyperbilirubinemia may result from cephalohematoma.
   3. **Face.** Arterial blood gas may be indicated in those infants with respiratory distress. Nerve excitability or conduction tests are recommended if there is no improvement in the facial nerve palsy after 3–4 days.
   4. **Eyes, ears, or vocal cords.** No laboratory tests are usually required.
   5. **Neck and shoulder.** Arterial blood gas helps diagnose hypoxia associated with phrenic nerve paralysis.
   6. **Spinal cord.** The usual laboratory tests required for respiratory depression and shock, if indicated.
   7. **Abdomen.** Obtain hematocrit to rule out anemia and blood loss and urine dipstick to check for hematuria. Consider abdominal paracentesis with fluid sent to the laboratory for cell count with differential.
   8. **Extremities and genitalia.** No laboratory tests are usually needed.
  C. **Imaging and other studies**
   1. **Head.** Skull radiographs should be obtained to rule out the possibility of skull fractures. A CT scan can also be obtained and can be useful in the diagnosis of an intracranial hemorrhage.

2. **Face.** Radiographs and a cranial CT scan to help diagnose facial fractures.
3. **Eyes.** Radiographs, to rule out orbit fracture, may be indicated.
4. **Neck and shoulder**
   a. **Radiograph of the clavicle.** Necessary for confirmation of the diagnosis of fracture.
   b. **Radiograph of the chest for phrenic nerve paralysis.** Shows an elevated diaphragm.
   c. **Fluoroscopy.** Reveals elevation of the affected side and descent of the normal side on inspiration with phrenic nerve impairment. Opposite movements occur with expiration.
   d. **Ultrasound of the diaphragm.** Shows abnormal motion on the affected side.
   e. **MRI of the neck and spine.** Shows nerve root avulsion.
   f. **Electroencephalogram.** Reveals the extent of the denervation weeks after the injury.
5. **Spinal cord**
   a. **Cervical and thoracic spine radiographs.** These should be obtained.
   b. **MRI.** Most reliable method for diagnosing spinal cord injuries.
6. **Abdomen.** Abdominal ultrasound usually diagnoses liver and splenic rupture, adrenal hemorrhage, and kidney damage. An abdominal radiograph may reveal a stomach bubble displaced medially in splenic rupture.
7. **Extremities.** A radiograph of the extremities confirms the diagnosis.
8. **Genitalia.** Ultrasonography is diagnostic.

V. **Plan**

A. **Skin**

1. **Petechiae.** No specific treatment is necessary, as traumatic petechiae usually fade in 2–3 days.
2. **Subcutaneous fat necrosis.** The lesions require minimal pressure at the affected site and observation only. They disappear within a couple of months but may calcify. Closely monitor the first 6 weeks for symptomatic hypercalcemia (vomiting, fever, and weight loss with high serum calcium), which can occur. This can usually be treated with intravenous hydration, furosemide, and hydrocortisone therapy.
3. **Ecchymoses.** No specific treatment is necessary because they usually resolve within 1 week. Monitor for hyperbilirubinemia (reabsorption of blood from a bruised area), anemia (blood loss from bruising), and hyperkalemia.
4. **Lacerations and abrasions.** If superficial, the edges may be held together with butterfly adhesive strips. If deeper, they should be sutured with 7–0 nylon. Healing is usually rapid. Observe for infections, especially a scalp lesion and caput succedaneum.

B. **Head**

1. **Caput succedaneum.** No specific treatment is necessary, as it resolves within several days.
2. **Cephalhematoma.** Usually no treatment is necessary, and it resolves anywhere between 2 weeks and 3 months. CT or skull radiography may be necessary if neurologic symptoms or depressed skull fracture are present. In some cases, blood loss and hyperbilirubinemia can occur.
3. **Subgaleal hemorrhage.** If hypovolemic shock develops, it requires immediate treatment. Surgery is done if the bleeding does not subside. Death may occur. Look for coagulopathies and treat as needed.
4. **Intracranial hemorrhage.** Circulatory and ventilatory support are indicated in deteriorating conditions. (See also Chapter 104.)
   a. **Subarachnoid.** Resolution usually occurs without treatment.
   b. **Epidural.** Prompt surgical evacuation for large bleeds. Prognosis is good with early treatment.
   c. **Subdural.** Subdural taps are indicated to drain a large hematoma.

5. **Skull fracture.** Linear fractures do not require treatment. Depressed skull fractures can be treated conservatively or surgically. For a simple depressed skull fracture nonsurgical management is recommended. For larger and deeper depressions, vacuum extraction or surgery is required.

C. **Face**

1. **Facial nerve injury.** No specific therapy is necessary. Full resolution usually occurs within a few months. Neurology consult should be obtained if no improvement in 2–3 weeks.

   a. **Complete peripheral paralysis.** Cover the exposed eye with an eye patch and instill synthetic tears (1% methylcellulose drops) every 4 hours. This will prevent irritation from the dryness.

   b. **Electrodiagnostic testing.** May be beneficial in predicting recovery.

   c. **Surgery.** May be necessary in severe cases.

2. **Fractures. Maxilla, lacrimal, mandible, and nose fractures** require immediate evaluation. An oral airway is required, and surgical consultation is needed. The fractures must be reduced and fixated. Plastic surgery consultation recommended.

D. **Eyes**

1. **Eyelids.** Edema and bruising usually resolve within 1 week. Laceration of the eyelid may require microsurgery.

2. **Orbit fracture.** Immediate ophthalmologic consultation is required.

3. **Horner syndrome.** No treatment is necessary, and resolution usually occurs.

4. **Subconjunctival hemorrhage.** No treatment is necessary because the blood is usually absorbed within 1–2 weeks.

5. **Cornea.** Haziness disappears usually within 2 weeks. If persistent and if rupture of Descemet membrane has occurred, then a white opacity of the cornea will occur. This is usually permanent, and ophthalmologic input is essential.

6. **Intraocular hemorrhage**

   a. **Retinal hemorrhage.** Usually disappears within 1 week. No treatment is necessary.

   b. **Hyphema.** Usually resolves without treatment within 1 week.

   c. **Vitreous hemorrhage.** If resolution does not occur within 1 year, surgery must be considered.

E. **Ears**

1. **Abrasions and ecchymoses.** These injuries are usually mild and require no treatment, except for keeping the area clean. They resolve spontaneously.

2. **Hematomas.** Incision and evacuation may be indicated.

3. **Avulsion of the auricle.** Surgical consultation is required if cartilage is involved.

4. **Laceration of the ear.** Most of these can be sutured with 7–0 nylon sutures.

F. **Vocal cords**

1. **Unilateral paralysis.** Observe these infants closely. Keeping them quiet and giving small, frequent feedings decreases the risk of aspiration. This condition usually resolves within 4–6 weeks.

2. **Bilateral paralysis.** Intubation is required if there is airway obstruction. Ear, nose, and throat consultation and tracheostomy are usually required. The prognosis is variable.

G. **Neck and shoulder**

1. **Clavicular fracture.** Immobilization (pinning the infants sleeve to the shirt) helps to decrease pain, and the prognosis is excellent. Pain medication can be given.

2. **Brachial palsy.** Immobilization and physical therapy to prevent contractures until recovery of the brachial plexus. Recovery depends on the extent of the lesions and is usually good but may take many months. In Erb-Duchenne paralysis, one can see improvement in 2 weeks, and recovery is usually complete by 18 months. In Klumpke paralysis, prognosis is poorer and sometimes never complete. Muscle atrophy and contractures can occur. Orthopedic consultation is recommended early on.

3. **Phrenic nerve paralysis.** Treatment is usually supportive and nonspecific, and the prognosis is usually good. Some infants may require continuous positive airway pressure or mechanical ventilation. Most infants recover in 1–3 months.

4. **Sternocleidomastoid muscle injury.** Most recover spontaneously. Passive exercise may be indicated, and appropriate positioning of the infant is recommended. If it is not resolved within 1 year, surgery should be considered.

H. **Spinal cord.** Prognosis depends on the level and severity of the injury. Most infants with a severe spinal cord injury do not survive. Treatment is supportive, and some require intubation for respiratory problems. Specific therapy needs to be directed at the bladder, bowel, and skin because these present as ongoing problems.

I. **Abdomen.** Surgical consultation is needed, and the prognosis for all of these depend on early recognition and treatment. Early management strategies that increase survival include volume replacement and identifying and correcting coagulation disorders.

1. **Liver rupture.** Transfusion, laparotomy with evacuation of hematomas, and repair of any laceration.

2. **Splenic rupture.** Volume replacement with transfusion of whole blood and correction of coagulation disorders. Exploratory laparotomy, with preservation of the spleen if possible.

3. **Adrenal hemorrhage.** Management is supportive, with blood transfusion and intravenous steroids usually the only treatment.

4. **Kidney damage.** Use supportive measures. Surgery may be necessary if severe.

J. **Extremities**

1. **Fractured humerus.** Obtain an orthopedic consultation. Immobilize the arm for usually 2 weeks. Displaced fractures may require closed reduction and casting. The prognosis is excellent.

2. **Fractured femur.** Obtain an orthopedic consultation. Splinting is necessary. Displaced fractures may require closed reduction and casting. The prognosis is excellent.

3. **Epiphyseal displacement/dislocation.** Treatment is immediate reduction with immobilization of the arm for 8–10 days.

K. **Genitalia**

1. **Edema and bruising.** These usually resolve within 4–5 days, and no treatment is necessary.

2. **Testicular injury.** Urgent urologic or pediatric surgical consultation is necessary, as rupture may require surgical repair.

3. **Hematocele.** Elevate the scrotum with cold packs. Resolution occurs without other treatment, unless there is a severe underlying testicular injury.

79 Vasospasms and Thromboembolism

I. **Problem.** An infant with an indwelling umbilical artery catheter develops a vasospasm in one leg. The nurse notifies you that another infant with an indwelling umbilical line has no pulses in the lower legs with severely decreased perfusion. Infants are at a high risk for thromboembolism because of their immature hemostatic system and smaller vessel size, and the fact that they require frequent catheter use. The majority of neonatal thromboembolisms are iatrogenic from umbilical artery or venous catheters, indwelling central catheters, and peripheral arterial lines.

II. **Immediate questions**

A. **Can the catheter be removed?** Evaluate the need for the catheter. If the catheter can be removed, this is the treatment of choice. Vasospasm is most commonly related to the use of umbilical artery catheters (UACs), but it can also occur in other catheters such as radial artery catheters. Over 80% of venous thromboembolisms in newborns are secondary to central venous lines. Arterial thrombosis is less common than venous thrombosis. The incidence of UAC-related thrombosis is 14–35% by ultrasound, and up to 64% by angiography. In some cases of thrombosis, the catheter should not be removed so thrombolytic medication can be given through it.

   B. **Was a medication given recently through the catheter?** Most medications, if given too rapidly, can cause vasospasm.

   C. **How severe is the vasospasm?** Deciding on the severity of the vasospasm may dictate treatment choices (see Section IV.B.1 and 2).

   D. **Is there a pulse in the affected extremity?** A loss of pulse with a thrombus is a medical emergency.

   E. **Does the infant have any risk factors for thromboembolism?**

      1. **Maternal.** Autoimmune disorders, premature rupture of membranes (PROM), diabetes, preeclampsia, infertility, oligohydramnios, prothrombotic disorder, intrauterine growth restriction (IUGR), chorioamnionitis, family history of thrombosis, antiphospholipid or anticardiolipin antibodies.

      2. **Delivery.** Instrumentation, fetal heart rate (FHR) abnormalities, emergency cesarean section, traumatic delivery.

      3. **Neonate.** Central arterial catheters (most common risk factor for arterial thromboembolism), central venous catheters (one of the most common risk factors for venous thromboembolism), some congenital heart diseases, birth asphyxia, sepsis, small for gestational age (SGA), respiratory distress syndrome (RDS), polycythemia, necrotizing enterocolitis (NEC), pulmonary hypertension, dehydration, surgery, extracorporeal membrane oxygenation/extracorporeal life support (ECMO/ECLS), congenital renal vein defects, congenital nephrotic or nephritic syndrome, prematurity, hypotension, disseminated intravascular coagulation (DIC), impaired liver function, fluctuations in cardiac output, low cardiac output, prothrombotic disorders.

      4. **Inherited factors.** Protein C, protein S deficiency; factor V Leiden mutation; antithrombin deficiency; prothrombin gene G20210A mutation; elevated lipoprotein a levels; and others.

III. **Differential diagnosis**

   A. **Vasospasm.** A **muscular contraction (spasm)** of an **arterial** vessel, manifested by acute color change (white or blue) in the perfused extremity (upper or lower extremity, sometimes only on the toes or fingers). Occasionally, the color change extends to the buttocks and the abdomen. The change in color may be transient or persistent. It may be caused by prior injection of medication or a manifestation of thromboembolism/thromboembolic phenomenon. Arterial blood sampling can also be a predisposing factor.

   B. **Thromboembolism.** A **thrombus** is a blood clot formation in an artery or vein and can cause partial or complete obstruction. An **embolus** is a clot that is mobile and lodges in a blood vessel and may cause obstruction or vasospasm. Neonates are the most commonly affected age group with an incidence of ~41 cases in 100,000 per year. The initial sign is usually that the catheter does not work. One cannot infuse fluid or withdraw from the line. **Thrombosis can be iatrogenic (catheter related) or spontaneous (non–catheter related).**

   C. **Inherited thrombophilias.** Less commonly, thromboembolic phenomena are due to inherited or acquired thrombophilias. Positive family history, early onset of disease, and more than one thromboembolism are clues to an inherited thrombophilia. **Prothrombotic genetic mutations** do not appear to increase the risk of umbilical catheter–associated thrombosis.

      1. **Inherited.** Deficiencies of protein C, protein S, antithrombin III, factor V Leiden (heterozygous or homozygous). Also, prothrombin mutation G20210A, elevated

factor VIII, homocystinemia, elevated lipoprotein, fibrinogen abnormalities (dysfibrinogenemia and plasminogen abnormalities), dysplasminogenemia, and hypoplasminogenemia.

2. **Acquired.** Deficiencies of protein C, protein S, or antithrombin III; elevated factor VIII activity; antiphospholipid antibodies; lupus anticoagulant and anticardiolipin antibody. Placental transfer of antibodies can cause an acquired thrombophilia in the newborn. Newborns with sepsis have an increased and ongoing consumption of coagulation factors and platelets, with reduced levels of protein C.

3. **Neonatal purpura fulminans is rare and may be inherited or acquired.** If inherited, it is caused by a deficiency in protein C or S or antithrombin III and presents after birth with ecchymosis, venous and arterial thromboses, and DIC. The acquired form is usually in older infants but has been described in neonates. It is idiopathic or can occur secondary to a bacterial or viral infection that can result in a decrease in levels of protein C.

IV. **Database**

A. **History.** Obtain a detailed family history of any inherited clotting or other hematologic disorder. Did anyone in the family have any clotting disorders?

B. **Physical examination.** The severity of the vasospasm and thrombosis must be assessed because it dictates treatment. The areas of involvement, appearance of the skin over the involved areas, and pulses of the affected extremity are measures of severity. Compare the affected extremity with the other extremity. A handheld Doppler is useful to assess peripheral arterial flow. An acute scrotum (discoloration and pain upon palpation) can be caused by renal vein thrombosis.

1. **Severe vasospasm.** Involves a large area of one or both legs, the abdomen, or the buttocks. In the upper extremity, a severe vasospasm includes most of the arm and all of the fingers. The skin may be completely white. Decreased perfusion is present, and pulses of the affected extremity are weak but detectable.

2. **Less severe vasospasm.** Involves a small area of one or both legs (usually some of the toes and part of the foot). In the arm, it can involve part of the extremity and some fingers. The skin has a mottled appearance and pulses are present but can be diminished.

3. **Thrombosis.** If pulses are completely absent, an **arterial thrombosis**, which is a **medical emergency**, is likely. Persistent bacteremia and thrombocytopenia may be associated with thrombosis. **Venous thrombosis** is more common.

   a. **Venous thrombosis.** Iatrogenic venous thrombosis in the newborn occurs most commonly from an indwelling venous catheter (90% central venous pressure [CVP] or umbilical venous catheter [UVC]) or from a non–catheter related reason (most commonly renal vein thrombosis). **If from a catheter**, presentation includes difficulty infusing and withdrawing from the line. Other symptoms are persistent thrombocytopenia and persistent infection. **Sites in which a venous thrombosis can occur** are mesenteric, adrenal veins, hepatic veins, portal vein, femoral vein, inferior and superior vena cava, and cerebral sinuses.

      i. **Extremities (peripheral thrombosis).** Extremities are swollen, cyanotic, hyperemic, and discolored with distended superficial veins.

      ii. **Kidney. Renal vein thrombosis is the most common type of spontaneous venous thrombosis. Triad** of macroscopic hematuria, thrombocytopenia, and a palpable abdominal mass can be seen. Risk factors are perinatal asphyxia, dehydration, and maternal diabetes mellitus. Acute hypertension, proteinuria, and renal dysfunction can also occur. There is a higher male prevalence, usually unilateral (70%) or left kidney (64%), increased in premature infants, with a high level of thrombophilia.

      iii. **Inferior vena cava thrombosis.** Presents with palpable kidneys and hematuria. Edematous lower limbs, respiratory distress, and hypertension can also be seen.

  iv. **Superior vena cava thrombosis.** Common after repair of complex congenital heart disease.

  v. **Intracardiac thrombosis.** In infants with complex congenital heart disease from right atrial catheter placement. Right atrial thrombi can be life threatening and disseminate into lungs or obstruct the right pulmonary artery. Pericardial tamponade and symptoms of right heart failure are consequences.

  vi. **Central nervous system (CNS). Neonatal cerebral sinovenous thrombosis (CSVT)** is a rare multifactorial disease. It is most commonly caused by coagulopathy. Early signs within 48 hours of birth (respiratory distress, poor tone, asphyxia, fetal distress) or later signs (seizures, lethargy, fever, poor feeding, apnea) are typical. Most common sites are superior sagittal sinus, transverse lateral sinuses of the superficial venous system, and the straight sinus of the deep venous system. **Thalamic hemorrhage** suggests cerebral sinovenous thrombosis.

  vii. **Intestine. Neonatal portal vein thrombosis** is uncommon but is increasing. Risk is higher in neonates than in children. Clinical presentation is nonspecific or asymptomatic in 90%. Impaired liver function, portal hypertension, hepatomegaly, and splenomegaly can be seen. Umbilical catheterization, exchange transfusion, and sepsis and thrombophilia are all risk factors. **Mesenteric venous thrombosis** presents with gradual onset of abdominal pain with later signs once necrosis develops. Heme-positive stool is seen.

  viii. **Umbilical vein thrombosis.** Rare, and if it occurs, portal vein thrombosis should be ruled out.

 b. **Arterial thrombosis.** Less common than venous thrombosis. **Iatrogenic catheter-related** arterial thrombosis is usually from UAC, peripheral arterial line (PAL), and femoral artery catheters. It usually presents with line dysfunction, blanching or cyanosis of the extremity, sepsis, and persistent thrombocytopenia. **Spontaneous (not catheter-related)** arterial thromboses are rare but usually involve the iliac artery, left pulmonary artery, aortic arch, and descending aorta, and symptoms depend on the location. Neonatal arterial thrombosis can occur in the aorta and present as cyanotic heart disease such as coarctation of the aorta.

  i. **Aortic thrombosis.** Rare in newborns. UAC will stop working and blood pressure will be higher in the arms than in the legs. Decreased or no pulses in the lower extremities with color change and a decrease in perfusion, hematuria, hypertension, oliguria, and NEC can all be seen. Cytomegalovirus (CMV) infection can cause aortic arch thrombosis.

  ii. **Extremities (peripheral arterial thrombosis).** Radial, posterior tibial, and dorsalis pedis arterial lines are rarely associated with thrombosis. Weak or absent peripheral pulse, pallor of the extremities, coldness, and decreased perfusion of the extremity can be seen. Acute arterial occlusion in a limb in a newborn is rare. **Neonatal arterial thrombosis** at birth is very rare and has been reported in the left subclavian, axillary, and brachial arteries.

  iii. **Intestine (mesenteric thrombosis).** Bloody stools, bilious aspirates, abdominal pain, feeding intolerance, pneumatosis.

  iv. **Kidney (renal artery thrombosis).** Causes elevated blood pressure.

  v. **Lung (pulmonary embolism).** Very rare in neonates. It can be seen in infants with congenital heart disease with right heart failure, poor oxygenation, and ventilation/perfusion mismatch.

  vi. **CNS. Ischemic perinatal stroke (cerebral artery thrombosis)** most commonly occurs in the left hemisphere within the middle cerebral artery often secondary to indwelling intravascular catheters but can also be secondary to lupus anticoagulant. Placenta pathology may play a role in the etiology. Signs include seizures, lethargy, apnea, poor feeding, and hypotonia.

c. **Systemic air embolism (SAE).** In neonates, it is devastating and usually fatal. Most iatrogenic air emboli are venous and occur from central venous catheters (UVC, peripherally inserted central catheter [PICC]), but rarely can also occur from peripheral venous or arterial lines. A disconnected line is a common cause. Air embolism secondary to mechanical ventilation (barotrauma leads to systemic gas embolism) is rare but can occur in premature infants. Suspect embolism if air bubbles are in the infusion line. **Clinical symptoms** of systemic air embolism (SAE) are usually sudden and dramatic and can include pallor, cyanosis, hypoxemia, seizures, shock, bradycardia, respiratory distress, mottling of the skin, or neurologic deficits (if CNS emboli) such as paraplegia. Infants with cyanotic congenital heart disease are at a risk for **cerebral arterial gas embolism (CAGE)** from infusion lines.

4. **Inherited thrombophilias.** See Chapter 87.

C. **Laboratory studies.** Not usually needed for vasospasm. However, the following laboratory tests should be obtained if a thrombosis is suspected and clot-dissolving medication is to be used.

1. **Coagulation profile.** Prothrombin time (PT), activated partial thromboplastin time (aPTT), thrombin time, plasma fibrinogen concentration.
2. **Hematocrit.**
3. **Platelet count.** The thrombus itself and the use of heparin can cause thrombocytopenia.
4. **Genetic tests.** May be done at some point to evaluate congenital thrombophilia.
5. **CMV workup.** See Chapter 90.
6. **Workup for suspected prothrombotic disorder.** See Chapter 87.

D. **Imaging and other studies**

1. **A plain radiograph of the abdomen.** For catheter placement.
2. **Ultrasound or computed tomography (CT) of the head.** To evaluate for cerebrosinovenous thrombosis. Also to evaluate for intraventricular hemorrhage (IVH) before initiating thrombolytic therapy.
3. **Real-time ultrasonography with color Doppler flow imaging.** This can be used to diagnose thrombosis. It is the most common study used but can be unreliable. It can also be used to monitor the progress over time. Renal vein thrombosis shows enlarged echogenic kidneys and absence of flow in the main or arcuate renal veins.
4. **Contrast angiography (the gold standard).** Performed through the umbilical artery catheter and can be used to diagnose aortoiliac thrombosis. In several studies, this procedure was found to be the most effective diagnostic technique. A contrast study should be considered before administrating a fibrinolytic agent. Remember this test is difficult to perform in sick neonates.
5. **"Linograms."** Injecting radio-opaque dye directly into the line is sometimes done, but this method may also miss thrombosis.
6. **Contrast venography is considered the gold standard for diagnosing venous thrombosis.** Done by injection of contrast through peripheral vessels.
7. **Magnetic resonance (MR) angiography.** Recommended in ischemic neonatal stroke.
8. **MR venography.** Also done at some centers.
9. **Imaging for air embolism.** CT scan of the head for intracranial air bubbles. Echocardiogram of venous air embolism: acute obstruction of the right ventricular (RV) outflow tract secondary to air embolism (known as an "air lock").

V. **Plan.** Management of vasospasms is *controversial*. Management of thrombosis is largely based on treatment plans for older children and adults. Lack of organized studies in neonates adds to the problem. Current management protocols for thrombophilia can be obtained from the International Children's Thrombophilia Network (phone: 1-800-NO-CLOTS). The network was established as a free consultative service and to develop collaborative research studies.

A. **Key points**
  1. **Monitor for potential signs of vasospasm** or **thromboembolic complications** in all infants with any intravascular catheter.
  2. **Thromboembolism can occur in newborns** and produce little or no clinical symptoms.
  3. **Heparin is often added to neonatal infusions** as it prolongs patency, extends catheter life (UACs, UVCs, PICCs, peripheral arterial catheters), and may also decrease the incidence of thromboembolic occlusions. For extremely low birthweight infants, use the lowest dose. There are no randomized trials of heparin use in PICCs, but its use is common in neonatal intensive care units (NICUs). Heparin use in UVCs is *controversial* but the majority of NICUs use heparin in UVCs. Heparin is not used in peripheral intravenous lines. **Common recommendations:**
     a. **Central venous lines (UVC and PICC).** The American College of Chest Physicians Evidence-Based Clinical Practice Guidelines study recommends heparin in central venous access devices. They recommend UFH continuous infusion at 0.5 U/kg/h to maintain CVAD patency.
     b. **Peripheral arterial catheters.** The American College of Chest Physicians Evidence-Based Clinical Practice Guidelines study recommends UFH continuous infusion at 0.5 U/mL at 1 mL/h.
     c. **UACs.** Heparin (0.25–1 U/mL) for a total heparin dose of 25–200 U/kg/d to maintain patency. **Cochrane Review** notes the use of heparin (as low as 0.25 U/mL) is recommended to prolong the life of the catheter by decreasing the incidence of catheter occlusion. It does not decrease the incidence of aortic thrombosis. Heparinization of intermittent flushes alone is ineffective in preventing catheter occlusion. The **American Academy of Pediatrics** (AAP) recommends low doses of heparin (0.25–1.0 U/L) through the umbilical arterial catheter. The **American College of Chest Physicians Evidence-Based Clinical Practice Guidelines** (2012) recommends prophylaxis with a low-dose UFH infusion via the UAC (heparin concentration of 0.25–1 U/mL, total heparin dose of 25–200 U/kg/d to maintain patency.
  4. **Umbilical lines should be removed as soon as possible** as duration of both UACs and UVCs is a significant risk factor for thrombosis. The Centers for Disease Control and Prevention (CDC) recommend that UACs should not be left in place >5 days and umbilical venous catheters should be removed as soon as possible, but can be used up to 14 days.
  5. **High umbilical arterial catheters** have a lower incidence of thrombotic complications and a longer catheter life. Low umbilical arterial catheters are associated with an increased incidence of vasospasms and cyanosis. Cochrane Review and the American College of Chest Physicians Evidence-Based Clinical Practice Guidelines recommend high position for UACs.
  6. **Use a peripheral arterial line** over an umbilical artery catheter.
  7. **If there is difficulty infusing into the line,** consider a thrombotic event.
  8. **Heparinization of flush solution** without heparinization of the infusate is inadequate. Use of intermittent heparin flushes has no benefit over normal saline (NS) flushes.
  9. **Always use umbilical artery catheters** with a hole at the end and not the side, as the side hole may increase aortic thrombosis risk. Single-lumen construction is associated with a decrease in thrombosis.
  10. **The use of multiple lumen umbilical venous catheters** is associated with a decrease in the need for peripheral intravenous lines in the first week of life but with an increase in catheter malfunctions.
  11. **Heparin-bonded catheters versus polyvinyl chloride catheters** showed no difference in the incidence of aortic thrombosis or duration of patency.
  12. **A PICC line** has a lower incidence of thrombosis when compared to a central line. The highest incidence is in femoral lines.
  13. **Papaverine** was found to prolong the patency of peripheral arterial catheters in a study of neonates, with no difference in the incidence of IVH (*controversial*).

B. **Vasospasm.** Treatment is ***controversial***, and guidelines vary extensively. Check your institution's guidelines before initiating treatment. Use of heparin and thrombolytics is not uniformly recommended. If the vasospasm does not resolve with treatment and the tissue ischemia persists, rule out a vascular thrombosis. This can be secondary to a peripheral arterial line or umbilical artery catheter.

1. **Severe vasospasm of the leg/arm**
    a. **If possible, remove the catheter.** Spontaneous resolution is likely.
    b. **Warming the contralateral leg/arm.** Wrap the entire ***unaffected*** leg in a warm (not hot) washcloth. This measure should cause reflex vasodilatation of the vessels in the affected leg, and the vasospasm may resolve. Treatment should continue for 15–30 minutes before a beneficial effect is seen.
    c. **Gentle massage at the site of occlusion** can be attempted.
    d. **Topical nitroglycerin therapy** (*controversial*). (2% ointment, 4 mm/kg, applied as a thin film over the area.) Nitroglycerin has a direct vasodilating effect on vascular smooth muscle and improves circulation. Reports note one application but some repeat it every 8 hours for 2–27 days. Improvement was usually seen within 15–45 minutes. Observe for hypotension.
    e. **If it is not possible to remove the catheter (as in a tiny infant) and this is the only catheter.** Consider a **papaverine-containing solution** (60 mg/500 mL in 1/2 NS with 1.0 U/mL heparin) through the catheter as a continuous infusion for 24–48 hours (***controversial***). If the vasospasm resolves, the infusion may be stopped. If the vasospasm does not resolve, remove the catheter. **Exercise caution using this technique** in premature infants in the first few days of life where the incidence of developing an intracranial hemorrhage is high.
    f. **Lidocaine** has been used intra-arterially for vasospasm. Results are questionable, from dose-dependent issues to ***controversial*** antispasmolytic effect.
    g. **Intra-arterial lidocaine and papaverine** have been used successfully to treat a catheter-induced vasospasm during arterial catheterization (***controversial***, case reports only).

2. **Less severe vasospasm of the leg/arm**
    a. **If possible, remove the catheter.**
    b. **Warming the contralateral leg/arm.** Wrap the entire **unaffected** leg in a warm (not hot) washcloth. This measure should cause reflex vasodilatation of the vessels in the affected leg, and the vasospasm may resolve. Treatment should continue for 15–30 minutes before a beneficial effect is seen.
    c. **Gentle massage at the site of the occlusion** can be tried.
    d. **Papaverine** (*controversial*). A spasmolytic is an opium alkaloid that has a direct action on vascular smooth muscle. Dosing is 1 mg intramuscularly, in the unaffected leg. Papaverine is a mild vasodilator; the effect is apparent within 30 minutes.
    e. **Topical nitroglycerine** (*controversial*). Two percent ointment, 4 mm/kg, applied as a thin film over the area.
    f. **If it is not possible to remove the catheter (as in a tiny infant) and this is the only catheter.** Consider a papaverine-containing solution (60 mg/500 mL in 1/2 NS with 1.0 U/mL heparin) as above (***controversial***; see above).
    g. **Lidocaine/intra-arterial lidocaine and papaverine.** As above.

C. **Problems after vasospasm with peripheral tissue ischemia.** Ischemia can sometimes occur after a vasospasm. Even after a catheter has been removed, a persistent vasospasm or small emboli in distal end arteries can cause poor perfusion of an extremity. **Topical 2% nitroglycerin ointment** (4 mm/kg of body weight) can be applied to the ischemic area with resolution, with no adverse effects except mild episodes of decreased blood pressure (***controversial***).

D. **Thromboembolism.** If suspected and there is loss of pulses in the affected extremity, it is a **medical emergency.** Symptomatic thrombosis can lead to irreversible organ damage or loss of limbs or digits. The **most common treatments** are observation with supportive care, anticoagulation therapy with heparin or low molecular weight heparin, thrombolytic agents (clot-dissolving drugs, streptokinase, and tissue plasminogen activator), or surgery. Clot-dissolving drugs can cause severe bleeding and there are no current randomized trials comparing these treatments. Management is *controversial*. Treatment depends on the extent and severity of the thrombus. Management is identical for peripheral arterial thrombosis, venous thrombosis, and aortic thrombosis.

1. **Mild or minor thrombosis.** This can present with decreased limb perfusion, hypertension, and hematuria and can usually be treated with removal of the catheter, supportive care, and close ultrasonographic follow-up. Many of these resolve spontaneously.
2. **Moderate thrombosis.** This has all the findings of mild/minor thrombosis plus oliguria and congestive heart failure. Can be treated with systemic heparin therapy and with management of systemic hypertension.
3. **Major thrombosis.** Presents with all of the above plus major multi-organ failure. Should be treated aggressively with systemic heparin therapy, antithrombolytic agents, and supportive care. May require further evaluation for underlying hypercoagulative disorder.

E. **General guidelines for thrombosis treatment.** Treatment involves supportive care, observation only, thrombolytic and/or anticoagulant therapy, and surgery. (See also Chapter 87.)

1. **Supportive care**
   a. **Prompt removal of the catheter is indicated** unless it is needed to facilitate arteriography or thrombolytic drug infusion.
   b. **Treatment of volume depletion, electrolyte abnormalities, sepsis, thrombocytopenia, and anemia is essential.** Control hypertension and any coagulation deficiency or hypofibrinogenemia before initiation of treatment.
   c. **Emergency consultation with vascular surgery and pediatric hematology is recommended.**
   d. **Evaluate patients for intraventricular hemorrhage (IVH)** before initiating thrombolytic therapy. During treatment, ultrasounds of the head should be obtained at regular intervals.
   e. **Absolute contraindications for anticoagulant and thrombolytic therapy. If the infant has had CNS surgery or ischemia or birth asphyxia in the last 10 days,** or evidence of major active bleeding (gastrointestinal, pulmonary, or intracranial), invasive procedures within 3 days, or seizures within 48 hours, anticoagulant and thrombolytic therapy is contraindicated.
   f. **Relative contraindications for anticoagulant and thrombolytic therapy.** Hypertension, severe coagulation deficiency, platelet count <50 × 10⁴/μL (<100 × 10⁴/μL for ill neonates), fibrinogen concentration <100 mg/dL, international normalized ratio (INR) >2.

2. **Heparin therapy is recommended for clinically significant thrombosis with the purpose of preventing embolism or expansion of the clot. Low molecular weight heparins** are best because of the following advantages: reduced need for laboratory monitoring, subcutaneous dosing, longer half-life, decreased risk of osteopenia and heparin-induced thrombocytopenia, and decreased risk of hemorrhage. Monitor platelet counts if heparin is used. Obtain daily complete blood count (CBC) and aPTT. General recommendations are:
   a. **Low molecular weight heparin (LMWH) therapy using enoxaparin (Lovenox).** The treatment of choice in preterm neonates and most widely used in neonates. Other LMWH preparations include dalteparin and reviparin. For therapeutic treatment, <2 months of age, use enoxaparin 1.5 mg/kg/dose every 12 hours subcutaneously; if >2 months, 1.0 mg/kg/dose subcutaneously. Follow antifactor Xa levels 4–6 hours after dose (0.5–1 U/mL and adjust accordingly, or 0.5–0.8 U/mL in a sample taken 2–6 hours after subcutaneous injection). Adjust

as needed. Some studies suggest that preterm neonates require higher mean maintenance doses to achieve target levels (2.0 mg/kg every12 hours if preterm).

b. **Unfractionated (standard) heparin.** Load 75 U/kg IV over 10 minutes, then 28 U/kg/h maintenance through a dedicated IV line. (Premature infants: 25–50 U/kg/h over 10 minutes, then 15–20 U/kg/h). **Adjust based on aPTT 4 hours after initiation of after each dosing change** (target aPTT 60–85 seconds). Duration of therapy is generally 5–14 days. Always increase or decrease the infusion amount by 10%, depending on the aPTT. If the aPTT is >96 seconds, hold the heparin for 30–60 minutes and start at a lower infusion rate.

c. **If urgent reversal of unfractionated heparin effect is needed.** IV protamine can be given based on the total amount of heparin administered in the previous 2 hours. Stopping the infusion is usually sufficient for LMWH, and protamine is only partially effective.

3. **Warfarin therapy.** (Oral anticoagulant.) Not recommended in neonates (bleeding risk, difficulty in maintaining therapeutic doses, drug interactions including vitamin K content of the diet, tablet formulation).

4. **Thrombolytic drugs.** Do not use in milder cases, and few studies have been done in very preterm infants. With extensive thrombosis, life-threatening thrombosis, right atrial thrombosis, and the possibility of limb loss or organ damage, one of these drugs may be used. Treatment is ***controversial***, and it is best to follow institutional guidelines. When using thrombolytic therapy, maintain a platelet count >50–100 × 10^4 μL and fibrinogen >100 mg/dL using platelet transfusion and cryoprecipitate. Monitor PT/INR, partial thromboplastin time (PTT), and fibrinogen every 4 hours. If the catheter is still patent, the medications can be given through it. If the catheter is obstructed and needs to be removed, systemic therapy is used.

a. **Recombinant tissue plasminogen activator (tPA) (Alteplase)** has become the drug of choice (lowest risk of allergies, the shortest half-life, less manufacturing concerns). See Chapter 148 for dosage.

b. **Infusion of intra-arterial streptokinase** has been successful in some infants. Dose: 2000 U/kg IV over 30–60 minutes, 1000–2000 U/kg/h as continuous infusion for 6–12 hours. Lower doses (500 U/kg/h) have been effective. In one study of aortoiliac thrombosis, a dose of 50 U/kg/h given directly into the clot was effective. Because of systemic side effects (allergic and toxic reactions and bleeding), its use has declined.

c. **Urokinase** is no longer available in the United States but may be used in other countries. Dose: 4400 U/kg initial bolus dose IV over 10 minutes, then 4400 U/kg/h for 6–12 hours.

d. **Newer agents.** Both bivalirudin and argatroban (direct thrombin inhibitors) have been approved in adults and use in infants is evolving.

5. **Catheter-directed thrombolysis (CDT).** A sophisticated method in which the agent is injected into the thrombosis. In some reports it is superior to systemic thrombolytic therapy with fewer side effects. It is also used if neonates fail to respond to unfractionated heparin (UFH) therapy. **For a blocked central venous access device**, local thrombolysis is recommended after clinical assessment. **For neonates with limb-threatening or organ-threatening femoral artery thrombosis** who fail initial UFH therapy, thrombolysis is recommended. Drug of choice is tPA with a dose of 0.01–0.05 mg/kg/h.

6. **Surgery.** Immediate surgery has been successfully performed in neonates and may be indicated in the presence of an occluding embolism if thrombolysis is contraindicated for peripheral arterial occlusion. Guidelines are not well established. Surgical options include thrombectomy, microvascular reconstruction, vascular decompression through the use of a fasciotomy, mechanical disruption of the thrombus (medical thrombectomy), and amputation. If antithrombotic therapy is contraindicated, arteriotomy, embolectomy, and microvascular reconstruction is an option.

7. Specific treatment
   a. **Peripheral arterial catheter–related thromboembolism. Remove the catheter immediately. Symptomatic peripheral arterial catheter–related thromboembolism:** UFH anticoagulation with or without thrombolysis or surgical thrombectomy with microvascular repair with heparin therapy.
   b. **Central venous lines thrombosis.** Clinical assessment and local thrombolysis.
   c. **Acute femoral thrombosis.** Therapeutic doses of IV UFH as initial therapy or LMWH for a total of 5–7 days of anticoagulation. **For infants with limb-threatening or organ-threatening femoral artery thrombosis who fail to respond to UFH therapy and there are no contraindications**: thrombolysis. **With contraindications**: surgical intervention.
   d. **Renal vein thrombosis**
      i. **Unilateral (no renal impairment, no IVC extension).** Supportive care with close follow-up by radiology or anticoagulation in therapeutic doses for 6 weeks to 3 months. **Unilateral (with extension into inferior vena cava [IVC])**: anticoagulation for 6 weeks to 3 months.
      ii. **Bilateral (with renal impairment).** Anticoagulation or initial thrombolytic therapy with tPA, then long-term anticoagulation.
   e. **Cerebral sinovenous thrombosis (without significant intracranial hemorrhage).** Anticoagulation for 6 weeks to 3 months. **With significant intracranial hemorrhage**: anticoagulation or supportive care with radiologic monitoring, and anticoagulation if extension of the thrombus occurs.
   f. **First arterial ischemic stroke with no ongoing source of the cardioembolic source.** Supportive care. **With documented cardioembolic source**: anticoagulation recommended. **Recurrent arterial ischemic stroke**: anticoagulant or aspirin therapy.
   g. **Systemic air embolism.** Use caution in setting up infusion lines with complex parts; use of IV fluid filters may decrease air embolism. Treatment is supportive cardiac care and supportive respiratory care, with 100% oxygen therapy. Hyperbaric oxygen has been used in some cases.
   h. **Neonatal purpura fulminans/thrombophilias.** See Chapter 87.

Selected Reference

Monagle P, Chan AK, Goldenberg NA, et al. Antithrombotic therapy in neonates and children: Antithrombotic Therapy and Prevention of Thrombosis, 9th ed: American College of Chest Physicians Evidence-Based Clinical Guidelines. *Chest.* 2012;141(suppl 2): e737S–e801S.

80 ABO Incompatibility

I. **Definition.** Isoimmune hemolytic anemia may result when ABO incompatibility occurs between the mother and the newborn infant. This disorder is **most common with blood type A or B infants born to type O mothers.** The hemolytic process begins in utero and is the result of active placental transport of maternal isoantibody. In type O mothers, isoantibody is predominantly 7S-IgG (immunoglobulin G) and is capable of crossing the placental membranes. Because of its larger size, the mostly 19S-IgM (immunoglobulin M) isoantibody found in type A or type B mothers cannot cross. Symptomatic clinical disease, which usually does not present until after birth, is a compensated mild hemolytic anemia with reticulocytosis, microspherocytosis, and early-onset unconjugated hyperbilirubinemia.

II. **Incidence.** Risk factors for ABO incompatibility are present in 12–15% of pregnancies, but evidence of fetal sensitization (positive direct Coombs test) occurs in only 3–4%. Symptomatic ABO hemolytic disease occurs in <1% of all newborn infants but accounts for approximately two-thirds of observed cases of hemolytic disease in the newborn.

III. **Pathophysiology.** Transplacental transport of maternal isoantibody results in an immune reaction with the A or B antigen on fetal erythrocytes, which produces characteristic **microspherocytes.** This process eventually results in complete extravascular hemolysis of the end-stage spherocyte. The ongoing hemolysis is balanced by compensatory reticulocytosis and shortening of the cell cycle time, so that there is overall maintenance of the erythrocyte indices within physiologic limits. A paucity of A or B antigenic sites on the fetal (in contrast to the adult) erythrocytes and competitive binding of isoantibody to myriad other antigenic sites in other tissues may explain the often mild hemolytic process that occurs and the usual absence of progressive disease with subsequent pregnancies.

IV. **Risk factors**

   A. **A_1 antigen in the infant.** Of the major blood group antigens, the A_1 antigen has the greatest antigenicity and is associated with a greater risk of symptomatic disease. However, the hemolytic activity of anti-B antibodies is higher than those of anti-A and may produce a more severe disease in particular among infants of African American descent.

   B. **Elevated isohemagglutinins.** Antepartum intestinal parasitism or third-trimester immunization with tetanus toxoid or pneumococcal vaccine may stimulate isoantibody titer to A or B antigens.

   C. **Birth order.** Birth order is not considered a risk factor. Maternal isoantibody exists naturally and is independent of prior exposure to incompatible fetal blood group antigens. First-born infants have a 40–50% risk for symptomatic disease. Progressive severity of the hemolytic process in succeeding pregnancies is a rare phenomenon.

V. **Clinical presentation**

   A. **Jaundice.** Icterus is often the sole physical manifestation of ABO incompatibility with a clinically significant level of hemolysis. The onset is usually within the first 24 hours of life. The jaundice evolves at a faster rate over the early neonatal period than nonhemolytic physiologic pattern jaundice.

   B. **Anemia.** Because of the effectiveness of compensation by reticulocytosis in response to the ongoing mild hemolytic process, erythrocyte indices are maintained within a physiologic range that is normal for asymptomatic infants of the same gestational age. Additional signs of clinical disease (eg, hepatosplenomegaly

547

or hydrops fetalis) are extremely unusual but may be seen with a more progressive hemolytic process (see Chapter 127). Exaggerated physiologic anemia may occur at 8–12 weeks of age, particularly when treatment during the neonatal period required phototherapy or exchange transfusion.

VI. **Diagnosis.** Obligatory screening for infants with unconjugated hyperbilirubinemia includes the following studies:

   A. **Blood type and Rh factor in the mother and the infant.** These studies establish risk factors for ABO incompatibility.

   B. **Reticulocyte count.** Elevated values after adjustment for gestational age and degree of anemia, if any, support the diagnosis of hemolytic anemia. For term infants, normal values are 4–5%; for preterm infants of 30–36 weeks' gestational age, 6–10%. In ABO hemolytic disease of the newborn, values range from 10 to 30%.

   C. **Direct Coombs test (direct antiglobulin test).** Because there is very little antibody on the red blood cell (RBC), the direct Coombs test is often only weakly positive at birth and may become negative by 2–3 days of age. A strongly positive test is distinctly unusual and would direct attention to other isoimmune or autoimmune hemolytic processes.

   D. **Blood smear.** The blood smear typically demonstrates **microspherocytes, polychromasia** proportionate to the reticulocyte response, and **normoblastosis** above the normal values for gestational age. An increased number of nucleated RBCs in the cord blood could be a sign of ABO incompatibility.

   E. **Bilirubin levels (fractionated or total and direct).** Indirect hyperbilirubinemia is mainly present and provides an index of the severity of disease. The rate at which unconjugated bilirubin levels are increasing suggests the required frequency of testing, usually every 4–8 hours until values plateau.

   F. **Additional laboratory studies.** Supportive diagnostic studies may be indicated on an individual basis if the nature of the hemolytic process remains unclear.

      1. **Antibody identification (indirect Coombs test).** The indirect Coombs test is more sensitive than the direct Coombs test in detecting the presence of maternal isoantibody and identifies antibody specificity. The test is performed on an eluate of neonatal erythrocytes, which is then tested against a panel of type-specific adult cells.

      2. **Maternal IgG titer.** The absence in the mother of elevated IgG titers against the infant's blood group tends to exclude a diagnosis of ABO incompatibility.

VII. **Management**

   A. **Antepartum treatment.** Because of the low incidence of moderate to severe ABO hemolytic disease, invasive maneuvers before term is reached (eg, amniocentesis or early delivery) are usually not indicated.

   B. **Postpartum treatment**

      1. **General measures.** The maintenance of adequate hydration (see Chapter 9) and evaluation for potentially aggravating factors (eg, sepsis, drug exposure, or metabolic disturbance) should be considered.

      2. **Phototherapy.** Once a diagnosis of ABO incompatibility is established, phototherapy may be initiated before exchange transfusion is given. Because of the usual mild to moderate hemolysis, phototherapy may entirely obviate the need for exchange transfusion or may reduce the number of transfusions required. For guidelines on phototherapy, see Table 100–1 and Figure 100–2.

      3. **Exchange transfusion.** See Table 100–1 and Figure 100–3 for guidelines on exchange transfusion and Chapter 30 for exchange transfusion procedure.

      4. **Tin (Sn) porphyrin.** This can decrease the production of bilirubin and reduce the need for exchange transfusion and duration of phototherapy. It is an inhibitor of heme oxygenase, which is the enzyme that allows the production of bilirubin from heme. The dose of Stannsoporfin is 6 μmol/kg intramuscularly as a single dose given within 24 hours of birth with severe hemolytic disease, and it is available via compassionate use protocol.

5. **Intravenous immunoglobulin (IVIG).** By blocking neonatal reticuloendothelial Fc receptors and thus decreasing hemolysis of the antibody-coated RBCs, high-dose IVIG (1 g/kg over 4 hours) reduces serum bilirubin levels and the need for blood exchange transfusion with ABO or Rh hemolytic diseases. Caution should be used when considering treatment with IVIG as there are emerging reports of increased incidence of necrotizing enterocolitis in term and late-preterm infants with hemolytic disease of the newborn and isoimmune neonatal thrombocytopenia who were treated with IVIG.

6. **Synthetic blood group trisaccharides.** Their use is investigational; studies have shown a decrease in exchange transfusion rates in severe ABO hemolytic disease when A or B trisaccharides were administered.

VIII. **Prognosis.** For infants with ABO incompatibility, the overall prognosis is excellent. Timely recognition and appropriate management of the rare infant with aggressive ABO hemolytic disease may avoid any potential morbidity or severe hemolytic anemia and secondary hyperbilirubinemia and the inherent risks associated with exchange transfusion with the use of blood products.

Selected References

Figueras-Aloy J, Rodríguez-Miguélez JM, Iriondo-Sanz M, Salvia-Roiges MD, Botet-Mussons F, Carbonell-Estrany X. Intravenous immunoglobulin and necrotizing enterocolitis in newborns with hemolytic disease. *Pediatrics.* 2010;125:139–144.

Miqdad AM, Abdelbasit OB, Shaheed MM, Seidahmed MZ, Abomelha AM, Arcala OP. Intravenous immunoglobulin G (IVIG) therapy for significant hyper-bilirubinemia in ABO hemolytic disease of the newborn. *J Matern Fetal Neonat Med.* 2004;16:163–166.

Murray NA, Roberts IA. Haemolytic disease of the newborn. *Arch Dis Child.* 2007;92:83–88.

Poole J, Daniels J. Blood group antibodies and their significance in transfusion medicine. *Transfus Med Rev.* 2007;21:58–71.

Wagle S. Hemolytic disease of the newborn. http://emedicine.medscape.com/article/974349-overview. Accessed September 21, 2011.

81 Air Leak Syndromes

I. **Definition.** The **pulmonary air leak syndromes** (pneumomediastinum, pneumothorax, pulmonary interstitial emphysema [PIE], pneumatocele, pneumopericardium, pneumoperitoneum, and pneumoretroperitoneum) comprise a spectrum of diseases with the same underlying pathophysiology. Overdistention of alveolar sacs or terminal airways leads to disruption of airway integrity, resulting in dissection of air into extraalveolar spaces. Very rarely air can enter pulmonary vasculature (pulmonary veins) and cause **air embolus.** Air can also leak into the subcutaneous layers of the skin, especially skin of the chest, neck, and face, causing **subcutaneous emphysema.**

II. **Incidence.** The exact incidence of the air leak syndromes is difficult to determine. **Pneumothorax is the most common of the air leak syndromes,** reported to occur spontaneously in 1–2% of all neonates. The incidence increases in preterm infants to about 6%. The incidence also increases to 9–10% in infants with underlying lung disease (such as respiratory distress syndrome [RDS], meconium aspiration, pneumonia, and pulmonary hypoplasia) who are on ventilatory support, and in infants who had vigorous resuscitation at birth.

III. **Pathophysiology.** Overdistention of terminal air spaces or airways can result from uneven alveolar ventilation, air trapping, or injudicious use of alveolar-distending pressure in infants on ventilatory support. As lung volume exceeds physiologic limits, mechanical stresses occur in all planes of the alveolar or respiratory bronchial wall, with eventual tissue rupture. Air can track through the perivascular adventitia, causing PIE, or dissect along vascular sheaths toward the hilum, causing a pneumomediastinum. Rupture of the mediastinal pleura and into the thoracic cavity results in a pneumothorax. Pneumoretroperitoneum and pneumoperitoneum may occur when mediastinal air tracks downward to the extraperitoneal fascial planes of the abdominal wall, mesentery, and retroperitoneum and eventually ruptures into the peritoneal cavity.

A. Barotrauma. **The common denominator of the air leak syndromes is barotrauma.** Barotrauma results whenever positive pressure is applied to the lung. It cannot be avoided in the ill newborn infant needing ventilatory support, but its effects should be minimized. Peak inspiratory pressure (PIP), positive end-expiratory pressure (PEEP), inspiratory time (IT), respiratory rate, and the inspiratory waveform play important roles in the development of barotrauma. Contributing factors include high PIP, large tidal volume, and long IT. It is difficult to determine which of these parameters is the most damaging and which plays the largest role in the development of the air leaks.

B. **Other causes of lung overdistention.** Barotrauma is not the only cause of lung overdistention. **Atelectatic alveoli in RDS** may cause uneven ventilation and subject the more distensible areas of the lung to receive high pressures, placing them at risk for rupture. Small mucous plugs in the airway in meconium aspiration may cause gas trapping secondary to a ball-valve effect. Other events, such as inappropriate intubation of the right main stem bronchus, failure to wean after surfactant replacement therapy, and vigorous resuscitation or the development of high opening pressures with the onset of air breathing, can also lead to overdistention, with rupture of airway integrity at birth.

C. **Lung injury**
1. **Large tidal volume.** It has long been considered that lung injury is primarily a result of high-pressure ventilation (barotrauma). Although reports show variable relationships between airway pressures and lung injury, more recent studies support the concept that lung overdistention resulting from high maximal lung volume ("volutrauma") and transalveolar pressure, rather than high airway pressure, is the harmful factor.
2. **Atelectasis.** The alveolar units in patients with RDS are subjected to a cycle of recruitment and derecruitment. Strategies to decrease this mechanism of atelectatic trauma, optimizing lung recruitment and decreasing lung injury and severity of lung disease, lessen the risk for pulmonary air leak.

IV. **Risk factors**
A. **Ventilatory support.** The infants on ventilatory support, such as preterm infants and infants with underlying pulmonary disease, have an increased risk of developing one of the air leak syndromes. Various reports have indicated an incidence as high as 41%, and as low as 9% for infants receiving some form of mechanical ventilatory assistance. Factors that contribute to the development of air leak include high inspiratory pressure, large tidal volume, long inspiratory time, and excessive positive end-expiratory pressure.
B. **Meconium staining.** Other infants at risk include those who are meconium stained at birth. In these infants, meconium may be plugged in the airways, with resultant air trapping. During inspiration, the airway expands, allowing air to enter; however, during exhalation, there is airway collapse with resultant trapping of air behind the meconium plugs.
C. **Failure to wean after surfactant therapy.** Studies have shown that prophylactic use of surfactant therapy in infants at risk for RDS is associated with a decrease in

from displaced diaphragm. When compression of major veins and decreased cardiac output occur because of downward displacement of the diaphragm, signs of shock may be evident.

6. **Diagnosis.** A high index of suspicion is necessary for the diagnosis of pneumothorax.

  a. **Transillumination of the chest.** (See Chapters 40 and 70.) With the aid of transillumination, the diagnosis of pneumothorax may be made without a chest radiograph. A fiber-optic light probe placed on the infant's chest wall will illuminate the involved hemithorax. Although this technique is beneficial in an emergency, it should not replace a chest radiograph as the means of diagnosis.

  b. **Chest radiograph.** (See Figure 11–20.) Radiographically, a pneumothorax is diagnosed on the basis of the following characteristics:

    i. **Presence of air in the pleural cavity** separating the parietal and visceral pleura. The area appears hyperlucent with absence of pulmonary markings.

    ii. **Collapse** of the ipsilateral lobes.

    iii. **Displacement of the mediastinum** toward the contralateral side.

    iv. **Downward displacement of the diaphragm.** In infants with RDS, the compliance may be so poor that the lung may not collapse, with only minimal shift of the mediastinal structures. The AP radiograph may not demonstrate the classic radiographic appearance if a large amount of the intrapleural air is situated just anterior to the sternum. In these situations, the cross-table lateral radiograph will show a large lucent area immediately below the sternum, or the lateral decubitus radiograph (with the suspected side up) will show free air.

  c. **Transcutaneous carbon dioxide ($tcPco_2$).** Reference percentiles for $tcPco_2$ level and slope of the trended $tcPco_2$ over various time intervals have been used to detect the occurrence of pneumothorax preclinically. The area under the curve for 5 consecutive minutes with a 5-minute $tcPco_2$ slope >90th percentile shows good discrimination for a pneumothorax. False-positive results such as presence of a blocked or misplaced endotracheal tube may be encountered. If the problem with $tcPco_2$ persists after appropriately suctioning the endotracheal tube, a confirmatory radiograph should be ordered.

7. **Management.** Treatment of a pneumothorax depends on the clinical status of the infant. In infants without respiratory distress, continuous air leak, or need for assisted ventilation, close monitoring and observation may be all that is needed. The pneumothorax typically resolves in 1–2 days. If the pneumothorax affects <15% of a patient's hemithorax, the pneumothorax most likely will resolve spontaneously; otherwise, the air must be removed.

  a. **Oxygen supplementation.** In the term infant who is mildly symptomatic, an oxygen-rich environment is often all that is necessary. The inspired oxygen facilitates nitrogen washout of the blood and tissues and thus establishes a difference in the gas tensions between the loculated gases in the chest and those in the blood. A diffusion gradient results for resorption of the loculated gas and resolution of the pneumothorax. The pneumothorax usually resolves within 1–2 hours. This mode of therapy is not appropriate in the preterm infant because of the high oxygen levels needed for washout and resulting increase in oxygen saturation, making it unsuitable for premature infants with a high risk for retinopathy of prematurity.

  b. **Decompression.** In the symptomatic neonate or the neonate on mechanical ventilatory support, immediate evacuation of air is necessary. The technique is described in Chapter 70. Placement of a chest tube of appropriate size will eventually be necessary (see Chapter 27).

8. **Prognosis.** See Section VIII.

C. **Pulmonary interstitial emphysema**
  1. **Definition.** PIE is dissection of air into the perivascular tissues of the lung from alveolar overdistention or overdistention of the smaller airways.
  2. **Incidence.** This disorder arises almost exclusively in the very low birthweight infant on ventilatory support. It may also emerge in the extremely low birthweight infant without mechanical ventilation but receiving ventilatory support by CPAP. Although localized persistent PIE is rarely reported in infants not receiving ventilatory support, it must be considered in any infant with cystic lung lesions. PIE has been reported to occur in at least a third of infants <1000 g who have RDS on the first day of life and are receiving mechanical ventilator support. PIE frequently develops in the first 48–72 hours of life.
  3. **Pathophysiology.** PIE may be the precursor of all other types of pulmonary air leaks. With overdistention of the alveoli or conducting airways, or both, rupture may occur, and there may be dissection of the air into the perivascular tissue of the lung. The interstitial air moves in the connective tissue planes and around the vascular axis, particularly the venous ones. Once in the interstitial space, the air moves along bronchioles, lymphatics, and vascular sheaths or directly through the lung interstitium to the pleural surface. The extrapulmonary air is trapped in the interstitium (PIE), or it may extend and cause pneumomediastinum, pneumopericardium, or pneumothorax. PIE may exist in 2 forms, either localized (which involves 1 or more lobes) or diffuse (bilateral).
  4. **Risk factors.** See Section IV.
  5. **Clinical presentation.** The patient in whom PIE develops may have sudden deterioration accompanied by bradycardia and hypotension. More commonly, however, the onset of PIE is heralded by slow, progressive deterioration of arterial blood gas levels (hypoxemia, hypercarbia, acidosis) and the apparent need for increasing ventilatory support. Invariably, a diffusion block develops in these patients, with the alveolar membrane becoming separated from the capillary bed by the interstitial air. The response to increase ventilatory support in the face of poor arterial blood gas levels may lead to worsening of PIE and further clinical deterioration.
  6. **Diagnosis.** In infants with PIE, the chest radiograph generally reveals radiolucencies that are either linear or cyst-like. The linear radiolucencies vary in length and do not branch. They are seen in the periphery of the lung as well as medially and may be mistaken for air bronchograms. The cyst-like lucencies vary from 1.0 to 4.0 mm in diameter and can be lobulated. (See Figure 11–21.)
  7. **Management**
    a. **Lessening lung injury.** In general, once PIE is diagnosed, an attempt should be made to decrease ventilatory support and lessen lung trauma. Decreasing the PIP, decreasing the PEEP, or shortening the IT may be required. When decreasing these settings, some degree of hypercarbia and hypoxia may have to be accepted.
    b. **Positioning of the infant with the involved side down.** This has also proved beneficial in some cases of unilateral PIE.
    c. **Other treatments.** Suctioning of the endotracheal tube and manual positive pressure ventilation should be minimized. More invasive measures include selective collapse of the involved lung on the side with the worse involvement, with selective intubation or even the insertion of chest tubes before the development of pneumothorax. In cases of severe PIE, surgical resection of the affected lobe may be considered.
    d. **High-frequency ventilation (HFV).** Both high-frequency oscillatory ventilation (HFOV) and HFJV are used effectively in the treatment of PIE and other types of air-leak syndromes. Although these treatment modalities may improve survival of the infant with PIE, the long-term outcome remains uncertain.

COLOR INSERT

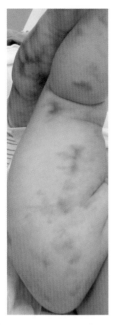

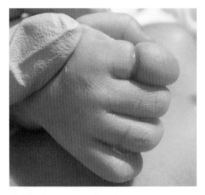

PLATE 1. Cutis marmorata telangiectatica congenita (CMTC). (*Reproduced with permission of Leslie Castelo-Soccio, MD, PhD, Children's Hospital of Philadelphia Division of Dermatology.*)

PLATE 2. Amniotic band syndrome. (*Reproduced with permission of Leslie Castelo-Soccio, MD, PhD, Children's Hospital of Philadelphia Division of Dermatology.*)

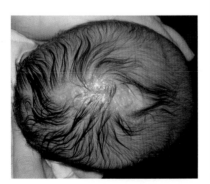

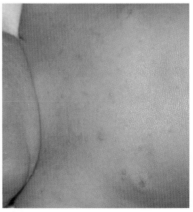

PLATE 3. Aplasia cutis congenita on scalp. (*Reproduced with permission of Leslie Castelo-Soccio, MD, PhD, Children's Hospital of Philadelphia Division of Dermatology.*)

PLATE 4. Erythema toxicum. (*Reproduced with permission of Leslie Castelo-Soccio, MD, PhD, Children's Hospital of Philadelphia Division of Dermatology.*)

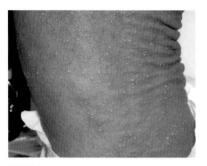

PLATE 5. Transient neonatal pustular melanosis. (*Reproduced with permission of Leslie Castelo-Soccio, MD, PhD, Children's Hospital of Philadelphia Division of Dermatology.*)

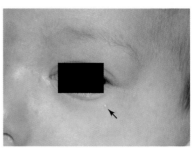

PLATE 6. Milia. (*Reproduced with permission of Leslie Castelo-Soccio, MD, PhD, Children's Hospital of Philadelphia Division of Dermatology.*)

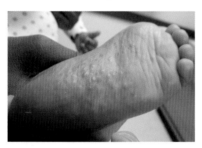

PLATE 7. Acropustulosis of infancy. (*Reproduced with permission of Leslie Castelo-Soccio, MD, PhD, Children's Hospital of Philadelphia Division of Dermatology.*)

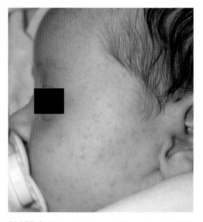

PLATE 8. Neonatal acne. (*Reproduced with permission of Leslie Castelo-Soccio, MD, PhD, Children's Hospital of Philadelphia Division of Dermatology.*)

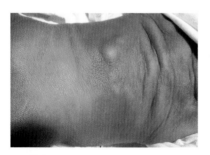

PLATE 9. Subcutaneous fat necrosis. (*Reproduced with permission of Leslie Castelo-Soccio, MD, PhD, Children's Hospital of Philadelphia Division of Dermatology.*)

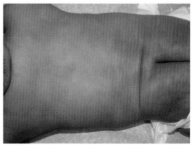

PLATE 10. Mongolian spots. (*Reproduced with permission of Leslie Castelo-Soccio, MD, PhD, Children's Hospital of Philadelphia Division of Dermatology.*)

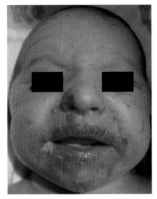

PLATE 11. Staphylococcal scalded skin syndrome (SSSS). (*Reproduced with permission of Leslie Castelo-Soccio, MD, PhD, Children's Hospital of Philadelphia Division of Dermatology.*)

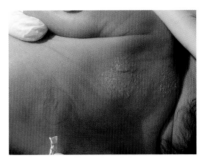

PLATE 12. Herpes simplex virus. (*Reproduced with permission of Leslie Castelo-Soccio, MD, PhD, Children's Hospital of Philadelphia Division of Dermatology.*)

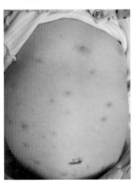

PLATE 13. Varicella zoster on the abdomen. (*Reproduced with permission of Leslie Castelo-Soccio, MD, PhD, Children's Hospital of Philadelphia Division of Dermatology.*)

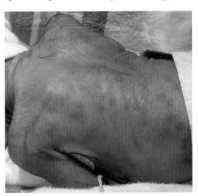

PLATE 14. Congenital cutaneous candidiasis. (*Reproduced with permission of Leslie Castelo-Soccio, MD, PhD, Children's Hospital of Philadelphia Division of Dermatology.*)

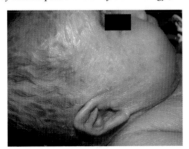

PLATE 15. Lamellar ichthyosis. (*Reproduced with permission of Leslie Castelo-Soccio, MD, PhD, Children's Hospital of Philadelphia Division of Dermatology.*)

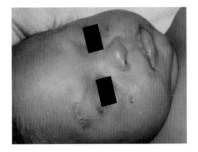

PLATE 16. Neonatal lupus. (*Reproduced with permission of Leslie Castelo-Soccio, MD, PhD, Children's Hospital of Philadelphia Division of Dermatology.*)

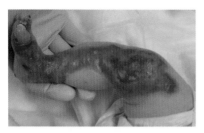

PLATE 17. Congenital absence of skin in epidermolysis bullosa, dominant dystrophic. (*Reproduced with permission of Leslie Castelo-Soccio, MD, PhD, Children's Hospital of Philadelphia Division of Dermatology.*)

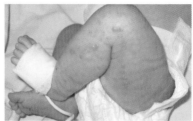

PLATE 18. Incontinentia pigmenti. (*Reproduced with permission of Jacek J. Pietrzyk, MD, PhD, Department of Pediatrics, Jagiellonian University Medical College, Krakow, Poland.*)

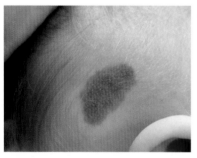

PLATE 19. Congenital melanocytic nevus of the scalp. (*Reproduced with permission of Leslie Castelo-Soccio, MD, PhD, Children's Hospital of Philadelphia Division of Dermatology.*)

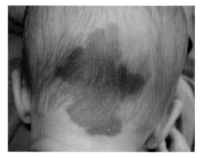

PLATE 20. Port wine stain. (*Reproduced with permission of Leslie Castelo-Soccio, MD, PhD, Children's Hospital of Philadelphia Division of Dermatology.*)

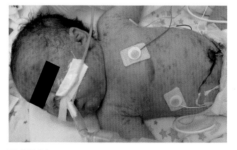

PLATE 21. "Blueberry muffin lesion" of congenital leukemia. Can also be seen in congenital viral infections (TORCH), blood and vascular disorders, and other malignancies. (*Reproduced with permission of Leslie Castelo-Soccio, MD, PhD, Children's Hospital of Philadelphia Division of Dermatology.*)

    8. Prognosis. See Section VIII.
  D. Pneumopericardium
    1. Definition. A pneumopericardium is air in the pericardial sac, which is usu-
    ally secondary to passage of air along pulmonary vascular sheaths. It is most
    often a complication of mechanical ventilation and can result in fatal cardiac
    tamponade.
    2. Incidence. A pneumopericardium is a rare occurrence and the least common
    form of pulmonary air leak in the neonatal period. The incidence in a study
    involving very low birthweight neonates was reported at 2%.
    3. Pathophysiology. **A pneumopericardium is usually preceded by pneumome-
    diastinum or other air leaks such as PIE or pneumothorax.** The mechanism
    by which pneumopericardium develops is probably due to passage of air along
    vascular sheaths. From the mediastinum, air can travel along the fascial planes
    in the subcutaneous tissues of the neck, chest wall, and anterior abdominal wall
    and into the pericardial space, causing pneumopericardium.
    4. Risk factors. See Section IV.
    5. Clinical presentation. The clinical signs of pneumopericardium range from
    asymptomatic to the full picture of cardiac tamponade. The first sign of
    pneumopericardium may be a decrease in blood pressure or a decrease in
    pulse pressure. There may also be an increase in heart rate with distant heart
    sounds.
    6. Diagnosis. A pneumopericardium has the most classic radiographic appearance
    of all the air leaks (see Figure 11–18). **A broad radiolucent halo completely
    surrounds the heart, including the diaphragmatic surface.** This picture is eas-
    ily distinguished from all the other air leaks by its extension completely around
    the heart in all projections.
    7. Management. Treatment of pneumopericardium is essential and requires the
    placement of a pericardial drain or repeated pericardial taps. Tube drainage
    is recommended for all neonates because of a high rate of reaccumulation (as
    much as 50% of the time). The procedure is described in Chapter 38. Successful
    pericardiocentesis in most instances should result in 75–80% survival.
    8. Prognosis. See Section VIII.
  E. Pneumoperitoneum. See also Chapter 69.
    1. Definition. A pneumoperitoneum is air in the peritoneal cavity that is usually
    caused by gastrointestinal perforation, but it can also be caused by air that has
    ruptured from the mediastinum into the peritoneum.
    2. Incidence. A pneumoperitoneum from passage of air into the chest is rare.
    It has been reported to occur in ~1% of mechanically ventilated children in
    intensive care units.
    3. Pathophysiology. A pneumoperitoneum in the newborn most commonly
    arises from a perforated hollow viscus or a preceding abdominal operation. It
    can also be secondary to ventilator-assisted pulmonary air leakage. Air from
    ruptured alveoli can flow trans-diaphragmatically along the great vessels and
    esophagus into the retroperitoneum. When air accumulates in the retroperito-
    neum, rupture into the peritoneal cavity can occur.
    4. Risk factors. See Section IV.
    5. Clinical presentation. Depending on the cause and severity, a pneumoperitoneum
    can present with or without associated abdominal findings. Because pneumoperi-
    toneum can occur as a result of pneumothorax, pneumomediastinum, and PIE,
    infants generally present with increasing signs of respiratory distress.
    6. Diagnosis. A pneumoperitoneum can be detected in radiographic films as free
    air under the diaphragm. (See Figure 11–22.)
    7. Management. Conservative management may be strongly considered if evi-
    dence of pulmonary air leak precedes or simultaneously appears with pneu-
    moperitoneum. See Chapter 37 for air removal technique.

8. **Prognosis.** See Section VIII.
F. **Pneumoretroperitoneum.** A pneumoretroperitoneum is the presence of air in the retroperitoneal space. **An isolated pneumoretroperitoneum is rare in neonates.** It can occur when massive intrathoracic pressure from a pneumothorax or pneumomediastinum causes free air to dissect into the retroperitoneal space from the chest. On radiograph, one sees air around the kidneys and in the perinephric space.
G. **Pneumatocele.** A pneumatocele represents subpleural or intraparenchymal cystic lesions in the lungs. They are thin-walled, air-filled cysts and mainly result from ventilator-induced lung injury in preterm infants. Pneumatoceles also can occur as a sequela of acute pneumonia. Causative agents include *Staphylococcus aureus*, *Streptococcus pneumoniae*, *Haemophilus influenzae*, and *Escherichia coli*. Most pneumatoceles are asymptomatic. They rarely require any surgical intervention. Traumatic pneumatoceles caused by positive pressure ventilation commonly resolve spontaneously; however, it is important to follow them closely, because high pressures during mechanical ventilation can cause a sudden increase in their size and result in a pneumothorax.
H. **Subcutaneous emphysema.** Subcutaneous emphysema occurs when an air leak dissects into tissues beneath the skin (tissue planes of the face, neck, and upper chest). It can be seen as a smooth bulging of the skin and detected by palpation of crepitus in the involved area. Usually it doesn't cause any clinical deterioration, but in extremely low birthweight infants, subcutaneous emphysema can result in compression of the airway. Subcutaneous emphysema is of clinical importance as it may signify a more serious underlying air leak.

Selected References

Agrons GA, Courtney SE, Stocker JT, Markowitz RI. Lung disease in premature neonates: radiopathologic correlation. *Radiographics.* 2005;25:1047–1073.

Berk DR, Varch LJ. Localized persistent pulmonary interstitial emphysema in a preterm infant in the absence of mechanical ventilation. *Pediatr Radiol.* 2005;35:1243–1245.

Corriea-Pinto J, Henriques-Coelho T. Neonatal pneumomediastinum and the spinnaker-sail sign. *N Engl J Med.* 2010;363:2145.

Davis C, Stevens G. Value of routine radiographic examination of the newborn, based on study of 702 consecutive babies. *Am J Obstet Gynecol.* 1930;20:73.

De Bie H, van Toledo-Eppinga L, Verbeke JI, van Elburg RM. Neonatal pneumatocele as a complication of nasal continuous positive airway pressure. *Arch Dis Child Fetal Neonatal Ed.* 2002;86:F202–F203.

Greenough A. Air leaks. In: Greenough A, Milner AD, eds. *Neonatal Respiratory Disorders.* London, UK: Oxford University Press; 2003:311–319.

Ibrahim H, Ganesam K, Mann G, Shaw NJ. Cause and management of pulmonary air leak in newborns. *Pediatr Child Health.* 2009;19:165–70.

Joseph L, Bromiker R, Toker O, Schimmel MS, Goldberg S, Picard E. Unilateral lung intubation for pulmonary air leak syndrome in neonates: a case series and a review of the literature. *Am J Perinatol.* 2011;28:151–156.

Joshi VH, Bhuta A. Rescue high-frequency jet ventilation versus conventional ventilation for severe pulmonary dysfunction in preterm infants. *Cochrane Database Syst Rev.* 2006;1:CD000437.

Korones S. Complications. In: Goldsmith J, Karotkin E, eds. *Assisted Ventilation of the Neonate.* 5th ed. Philadelphia, PA: Saunders Elsevier; 2011:407–414.

Lee C. Radiologic signs of pneumoperitoneum. *N Engl J Med.* 2010;362:2410.

Rojas MA, Lozano JM, Rojas MX, et al. Very early surfactant without mandatory ventilation in premature infants treated with early continuous positive airway pressure: a randomized controlled trial. *Pediatrics.* 2009;123:137–142.

Shaweesh J. Respiratory disorders in preterm and term infants. In: Martin RJ, Fanaroff AA, Walsh MC, eds. *Fanaroff & Martin's Neonatal-Perinatal Medicine Diseases of the Fetus and Infant.* 9th ed. Philadelphia, PA: Mosby Elsevier; 2011:1164–1166.

Stevens TP, Harrington EW, Blennow M, Soll RF. Early surfactant administration with brief ventilation vs. selective surfactant and continued mechanical ventilation for preterm infants with or at risk for respiratory distress syndrome. *Cochrane Database Syst Rev.* 2007;4:CD003063.

Yizhen JY, Arulkumaran S. Meconium aspiration syndrome. *Obstet Gynaecol Reproductive Med.* 2008;18:106–109.

82 Anemia

I. **Definition.** Anemia developing during the neonatal period (0–28 days of life) in infants of >34 weeks' gestational age is indicated by a central venous hemoglobin <13 g/dL or a capillary hemoglobin <14.5 g/dL.

II. **Incidence.** Anemia is the most common hematologic abnormality in the newborn. Specific incidence depends on the cause of the anemia.

III. **Pathophysiology**

   A. **Normal physiology. At birth, normal values for the central venous hemoglobin in infants of >34 weeks' gestational age are 14–20 g/dL,** with an average value of 17 g/dL. Reticulocyte count in the cord blood of infants ranges from 3–7%. The average mean corpuscular volume of red blood cells (RBCs) is 107 fL. Premature infants have slightly lower hemoglobin and higher mean corpuscular volume and reticulocyte counts. In healthy term infants, **hemoglobin values remain unchanged until the third week of life and then decline, reaching a nadir of 11 g/dL at 8–12 weeks.** This is known as the "physiologic anemia of infancy." In preterm infants, this decline is more profound, reaching a nadir of 7–9 g/dL at 4–8 weeks. This exaggerated physiologic anemia of prematurity is related to a combination of decreased RBC mass at birth, increased iatrogenic losses from laboratory blood sampling, shorter RBC life span, inadequate erythropoietin production, and rapid body growth. In the absence of clinical complications associated with prematurity, infants remain asymptomatic during this process.

   B. **Etiologies of anemia.** Anemia in the newborn infant results from 1 of 3 processes: **loss of RBCs, or hemorrhagic anemia,** the most common cause; **increased destruction of RBCs, or hemolytic anemia;** or **underproduction of RBCs, or hypoplastic anemia.**

      1. **Hemorrhagic anemia**

         a. **Antepartum period** (1 in 1000 live births)

            i. **Loss of placental integrity.** Abruptio placentae, placenta previa, or traumatic amniocentesis (acute or chronic) may result in loss of placental integrity.

            ii. **Anomalies of the umbilical cord or placental vessels.** Velamentous insertion of the umbilical cord occurs in 10% of twin gestations and almost all gestations with >3 fetuses. Communicating vessels (vasa praevia), umbilical cord hematoma (1 in 5500 deliveries), or entanglement of the cord by the fetus may also cause hemorrhagic anemia.

            iii. **Twin-twin transfusion.** Observed only in monozygotic multiple births. Monozygotic (MZ) twin pregnancies account for ~30% of spontaneously conceived twins. The occurrence of MZ twins is 0.4–0.45% of nonstimulated in vivo conceptions. The incidence of monochorionic twins is rising, owing to the increase in the use of assisted reproductive technology (ART). The use of ART has been associated with a 2- to 12-fold increase in the conception of MZ twins. In the presence of a monochorionic placenta, 13–33% of twin pregnancies are associated with twin-twin transfusion. The difference in hemoglobin concentration between twins is >5 g/dL. The anemic donor twin may develop congestive heart disease, whereas the recipient plethoric twin may manifest signs of the hyperviscosity syndrome. In utero laser photocoagulation, which interrupts the vascular connections on the chorionic plate, has improved the low survival rate for twin-twin transfusion diagnosed before 26 weeks' gestation.

b. **Intrapartum period**

   i. **Fetomaternal hemorrhage.** Fetomaternal hemorrhage is a common event during pregnancy, demonstrable in ~75% of gestations. The risk is increased with preeclampsia, with the need for instrumentation, and with cesarean delivery. In ~8% of pregnancies, the volume of the hemorrhage is >10 mL. Clinically significant fetomaternal hemorrhage has traditionally been set at a cutoff of 30 mL. At this cutoff, the incidence of fetomaternal hemorrhage has been estimated to be 3 per 1000 births. With bleeds >80 mL/kg, two-thirds of the fetuses may die before delivery. The severity of the fetomaternal hemorrhage is related to the size of the bleed in relation to the overall fetal blood volume, as well as the rate at which this blood is lost, and whether the event is acute or chronic.

   ii. **Cesarean delivery.** In elective cesarean deliveries, there is a 3% incidence of anemia. The incidence is increased in emergency cesarean deliveries.

   iii. **Traumatic rupture of the umbilical cord.** Rupture may occur if delivery is uncontrolled or unattended.

   iv. **Failure of placental transfusion.** Failure is usually caused by umbilical cord occlusion (eg, a nuchal cord or an entangled or prolapsed cord) during vaginal delivery. Blood loss may be 25–30 mL in the newborn.

   v. **Obstetric trauma.** During a difficult vaginal delivery, occult visceral or intracranial hemorrhage may occur. It may not be apparent at birth. Difficult deliveries are more common with large for gestational age infants, breech presentation, or difficult extraction.

c. **Neonatal period**

   i. **Enclosed hemorrhage.** Hemorrhage severe enough to cause neonatal anemia suggests obstetric trauma, severe perinatal distress, or a defect in hemostasis. See Figure 6–1.

      (a) **Caput succedaneum** is relatively common and may result in benign hemorrhage.

      (b) **Cephalhematoma** is found in up to 2.5% of births. It is associated with vacuum extraction and primiparity (5% risk of associated linear nondepressed skull fracture).

      (c) **Subgaleal (subaponeurotic) hemorrhage** is a rare but potentially lethal medical emergency caused by rupture of the emissary veins, which are connections between the dural sinuses and the scalp veins. Blood accumulates between the epicranial aponeurosis of the scalp and the periosteum. This potential space extends forward to the orbital margins, backward to the nuchal ridge, and laterally to the temporal fascia. In term infants, this subaponeurotic space may hold as much as 260 mL of blood. Subgaleal hemorrhage is most often associated with vacuum extraction and forceps delivery, but it may also occur spontaneously from an associated coagulopathy.

(d) Intracranial hemorrhage may occur in the subdural, subarachnoid, or subependymal space.

(e) Visceral parenchymal hemorrhage is uncommon. It is usually the result of obstetric trauma (eg, difficult breech extraction) to an internal organ, most commonly the liver but also the spleen, kidneys, or adrenal glands.

ii. Defects in hemostasis. Defects in hemostasis may be congenital, but more commonly hemorrhage occurs secondary to consumption coagulopathy, which may be caused by the following:

   (a) Congenital coagulation factor deficiency

   (b) Consumption coagulopathy

      (i) Disseminated congenital or viral infection

      (ii) Bacterial sepsis

      (iii) Intravascular embolism of thromboplastin (as a result of a dead twin, maternal toxemia, necrotizing enterocolitis, or others)

   (c) Deficiency of vitamin K–dependent coagulation factors (factors II, VII, IX, and X)

      (i) Failure to administer vitamin K at birth usually results in a bleeding diathesis at 3–4 days of age.

      (ii) Use of antibiotics may interfere with the production of vitamin K by normal gastrointestinal flora.

      (iii) Maternal ingestion of anticonvulsant (carbamazepine, phenytoin, and barbiturates but not valproic acid), antituberculosis agent (isoniazid, rifampicin), and vitamin K antagonists.

   (d) Thrombocytopenia. See Chapter 139.

      (i) Immune thrombocytopenia may be isoimmune or autoimmune.

      (ii) Congenital thrombocytopenia with absent radii is a syndrome frequently associated with hemorrhagic anemia in the newborn.

      (iii) Iatrogenic blood loss. Anemia may occur if blood loss resulting from repeated venipuncture is not replaced routinely. Symptoms may develop if a loss of >20% occurs within a 48-hour period.

2. Hemolytic anemia

  a. Immune hemolysis

    i. Isoimmune hemolytic anemia. Caused mostly by Rh incompatibility.

    ii. Autoimmune hemolytic anemia.

  b. Nonimmune hemolysis

    i. Bacterial sepsis may cause primary microangiopathic hemolysis.

    ii. Congenital TORCH (*t*oxoplasmosis, *o*ther, *r*ubella, *c*ytomegalovirus, and *h*erpes simplex virus) infections (see Chapter 141).

  c. Congenital erythrocyte defect

    i. Metabolic enzyme deficiency

      (a) Glucose-6-phosphate dehydrogenase (G6PD) deficiency

      (b) Pyruvate kinase deficiency

    ii. Thalassemia. Hemolytic anemia secondary to thalassemia is invariably associated with homozygous α-thalassemia and presents at birth. The disorders in β-thalassemia become apparent only after 2–3 months of age.

    iii. Hemoglobinopathy. May be characterized as unstable hemoglobins or congenital Heinz body anemia.

    iv. Membrane defects. Usually autosomal dominant.

      (a) Hereditary spherocytosis (1 in 5000 neonates) commonly presents with jaundice and less often with anemia.

        (b) **Hereditary elliptocytosis** (1 in 2500 neonates) rarely presents in the newborn infant.

    d. **Systemic diseases**

      i. Galactosemia

      ii. Osteopetrosis

    e. **Nutritional deficiency.** Vitamin E deficiency occurs with chronic malabsorption but usually does not present until after the neonatal period.

  3. **Hypoplastic anemia**

    a. **Congenital disease**

      i. Diamond-Blackfan syndrome (congenital hypoplastic anemia)

      ii. Atransferrinemia

      iii. Congenital leukemia

      iv. Sideroblastic anemia

    b. **Acquired disease**

      i. Infection. Rubella and syphilis are the most common causes.

      ii. Aplastic crisis.

      iii. Aplastic anemia.

IV. Risk factors. Prematurity, certain race and ethnic groups, and hereditary blood disorders (see Section III).

V. Clinical presentation

  A. **Symptoms and signs.** The 4 major forms of neonatal anemia may be demonstrated by determination of the following factors: age at presentation of anemia, associated clinical features at presentation, hemodynamic status of the infant, and presence or absence of compensatory reticulocytosis.

    1. **Hemorrhagic anemia.** Often dramatic in clinical presentation when acute but may be more subtle when chronic. Both forms have significant rates of perinatal morbidity and mortality if they remain unrecognized. Neither form has significant elevation of bilirubin levels or hepatosplenomegaly.

      a. **Acute hemorrhagic anemia.** Presents at birth or with internal hemorrhage after 24 hours. There is pallor not associated with jaundice and often without cyanosis (<5 g of deoxyhemoglobin) and unrelieved by supplemental oxygen. Tachypnea or gasping respirations are present. Vascular instability ranges from decreased peripheral perfusion (a 10% loss of blood volume) to hypovolemic shock (20–25% loss of blood volume). There is also decreased central venous pressure and poor capillary refill. Normocytic or normochromic RBC indices are present, with reticulocytosis developing within 2–3 days of the hemorrhagic event.

      b. **Chronic hemorrhagic anemia.** Presents at birth with unexplained pallor, often without cyanosis (<5 g of deoxyhemoglobin), and unrelieved by supplemental oxygen. Minimal signs of respiratory distress are present. The central venous pressure is normal or increased. Microcytic or hypochromic RBC indices are present, with compensatory reticulocytosis. The liver is often enlarged because of compensatory extramedullary erythropoiesis. Hydrops fetalis or stillbirth may occur with failure of compensatory reticulocytosis or intravascular volume maintenance.

      c. **Asphyxia pallida (severe neonatal asphyxia).** Not associated with hemorrhagic anemia at presentation. This disorder must be distinguished clinically from acute hemorrhage because specific immediate therapy is needed for each disorder. Asphyxia pallida presents at birth with pallor and cyanosis, which improves with supplemental oxygen delivery, respiratory failure, bradycardia, and normal central venous pressure.

    2. **Hemolytic anemia.** Jaundice is often seen before diagnostic levels of hemoglobin are obtained, in part because of the compensatory reticulocytosis that is invariably present. The infant usually presents with pallor after 48 hours of age. However, severe Rh isoimmune disease or homozygous α-thalassemia presents

at birth with severe anemia and, in many cases, hydrops fetalis. Unconjugated hyperbilirubinemia of >10–12 mg/dL, tachypnea, and hepatosplenomegaly may be seen with hemolytic anemia.

3. **Hypoplastic anemia.** Uncommon. It is characterized by presentation after 48 hours of age, absence of jaundice, and reticulocytopenia.

4. **Other forms of anemia**

a. **Anemia associated with twin-twin transfusion.** If chronic hemorrhage is occurring, there is often a >20% difference in the birthweights of the 2 infants, with the donor being the smaller twin.

b. **Occult (internal) hemorrhage**

i. **Intracranial hemorrhage.** Signs include a bulging anterior fontanel and neurologic signs (eg, a change in consciousness, apnea, or seizures).

ii. **Visceral hemorrhage.** Most commonly, the liver has been injured. An abdominal mass or distention is seen.

iii. **Pulmonary hemorrhage.** Partial or total radiographic opacification of a hemithorax and bloody tracheal secretions are seen. (See Chapter 74.)

B. **History**

1. **Anemia at birth**

a. **Hemorrhagic anemia.** There may be a history of third-trimester vaginal bleeding or amniocentesis. Hemorrhagic anemia may be associated with multiple gestation, maternal chills or fever postpartum, and nonelective cesarean delivery.

b. **Hemolytic anemia.** May be associated with intrauterine growth restriction (IUGR) and Rh-negative mothers.

2. **Anemia presenting after 24 hours of age** is often associated with obstetric trauma, unattended delivery, precipitous delivery, perinatal fetal distress, or a low Apgar score.

3. **Anemia presenting with jaundice** suggests hemolytic anemia. There may be evidence of drug ingestion late in the third trimester; IUGR; a family member with splenectomy, anemia, jaundice, or cholelithiasis; maternal autoimmune disease; or Mediterranean or Asian ethnic background.

VI. **Diagnosis**

A. **Obligatory initial studies**

1. **Hemoglobin**

2. **RBC indices**

a. **Microcytic or hypochromic RBC indices** suggest fetomaternal or twin-twin hemorrhage or α-thalassemia (mean corpuscular volume <90 fL).

b. **Normocytic or normochromic RBC indices** are suggestive of acute hemorrhage, systemic disease, intrinsic RBC defect, or hypoplastic anemia.

3. **Reticulocyte count (corrected).** An elevated reticulocyte count is associated with antecedent hemorrhage or hemolytic anemia. A low count is seen with hypoplastic anemia. The following formula is used:

Corrected reticulocyte count =

$$\frac{\text{Observed reticulocyte count} \times \text{Observed hematocrit}}{\text{Normal hematocrit for age}}$$

4. **Blood smear**

a. **Spherocytes** are associated with ABO isoimmune hemolysis or hereditary spherocytosis.

b. **Elliptocytes** are seen in hereditary elliptocytosis.

c. **Pyknocytes** may be seen in G6PD deficiency.

d. **Schistocytes or helmet cells** are most often seen with consumption coagulopathy.

      5. **Direct antiglobulin test (direct Coombs test).** This test is positive in isoimmune or autoimmune hemolysis.

  B. **Other selected laboratory studies**

      1. **Isoimmune hemolysis.** The blood type and Rh type should be determined and an eluate of neonatal cells prepared.

      2. **Fetomaternal hemorrhage.** The **Kleihauer-Betke test** should be performed. Using an acid elution technique, a maternal blood smear is stained with eosin. Fetal RBCs containing hemoglobin F resistant to acid elution stain darkly. Adult RBCs voided of their acid-sensitive hemoglobin A do not stain and appear as "ghost cells." A 50-mL loss of fetal blood into the maternal circulation shows up as 1% fetal cells in the maternal circulation. **ABO incompatibility between mother and infant results in an increased clearance rate of fetal cells from the maternal circulation, giving a falsely low result.** Conversely, the Kleihauer-Betke test may overestimate the extent of the hemorrhage, with maternal conditions leading to the overproduction of maternal hemoglobin F such as hereditary sickle-cell anemia, and β-thalassemia trait. Immunofluorescence flow cytometry is an alternative diagnostic test that circumvents some of the problems associated with the Kleihauer-Betke screen. This technology quantifies the number of fetal cells present by measuring the fluorescence intensity of monoclonal antibodies binding to hemoglobin F or to other surface antigens (eg, carbonic anhydrase) differentially expressed in fetal compared with adult erythrocytes. The College of American Pathologists has published a tool, accessible online at www.cap.org, which allows users to plug in the percentage of fetal cells observed by Kleihauer-Betke test or flow cytometry and the maternal height and weight to calculate the fetomaternal hemorrhage volume.

      3. **Congenital hypoplastic or aplastic anemia.** Bone marrow aspiration is usually indicated.

      4. **TORCH infection**

        a. Skull and long-bone films

        b. IgM levels

        c. Acute or convalescent serology

        d. Urine culture for cytomegalovirus

      5. **Consumption coagulopathy**

        a. Prothrombin time (PT) and partial thromboplastin time (PTT)

        b. Platelet count

        c. Thrombin time or fibrinogen assay

        d. Factor V and factor VIII levels

        e. Fibrin split products (D-dimers)

      6. **Occult hemorrhage**

        a. Pathologic examination of the placenta

        b. Cranial or abdominal ultrasonography will help identify the site of bleeding

      7. **Intrinsic RBC defect**

        a. RBC enzyme studies

        b. Analysis of the globin chain ratio

        c. Studies of RBC membrane

VII. **Management.** Treatment of neonatal anemia may involve, individually or in combination, simple replacement transfusion, exchange transfusion, nutritional supplementation, or treatment of the underlying primary disorder.

  A. **Simple replacement transfusion**

      1. **Indications**

        a. **Acute hemorrhagic anemia.**

        b. **Ongoing deficit replacement.**

        c. **Maintenance of effective oxygen-carrying capacity.** There are no universally accepted guidelines; however, those presented next are fairly representative of most common practice.

    i. Hematocrit <35% with severe cardiopulmonary disease (eg, intermittent positive-pressure ventilation with mean airway pressure >6 cm H_2O).

    ii. Hematocrit <30%

        (a) With mild to moderate cardiopulmonary disease (FIO_2 >35%, continuous positive airway pressure).

        (b) Significant apnea (>9–12 hours, or requiring bag-and-mask ventilation).

        (c) "Symptomatic anemia" weight gain <10 g/kg/d at full caloric intake and heart rate >180 beats/min persisting for 24 hours.

        (d) If undergoing major surgery.

    iii. Hematocrit <21%. Asymptomatic but with low reticulocyte count (<2%).

  2. **Emergency transfusion at birth only. Use type O, Rh-negative packed RBCs.**

    a. **Adjust the hematocrit to 50%.**

    b. **If a medical emergency exists,** blood that has not been cross-matched may be given; if time permits, blood may be cross-matched to the mother's blood.

    c. **Alternative replacement fluids** include normal saline, fresh-frozen plasma, and 5% albumin in saline. Timely infusion of packed RBCs or partial exchange transfusion should follow.

    d. **Perform umbilical vein catheterization** to a depth of 4–5 cm or until free blood flow is established (see Chapter 44).

    e. **Draw initial blood samples for diagnostic studies.** Obtain a complete blood count and differential, blood type and Rh type, direct Coombs test, and, if indicated, total bilirubin levels. In a medical emergency, transfusion may be started before the results of laboratory testing are known.

    f. **Infuse 10–15 mL/kg of replacement fluid over 10–15 minutes if emergency measures are needed.** Once the infant's status is stable, reassess the diagnostic studies, physical examination, and obstetric history.

    g. **Calculate the RBC volume.** Under controlled circumstances or if simple transfusion is indicated, calculate the volume of packed RBCs needed to achieve the desired increase in RBC mass (see page 452). **The volume of a single transfusion should not exceed 10–20 mL/kg.**

B. **Exchange transfusion**

  1. Indications

    a. Chronic hemolytic anemia or hemorrhagic anemia with evidence of tissue hypoxia (poor perfusion, metabolic acidosis, oliguria)

    b. Severe isoimmune hemolytic anemia with circulating sensitized RBCs and isoantibody

    c. Consumption coagulopathy

  2. **Technique.** See Chapter 30 for the technique of exchange transfusion in neonates.

C. **Nutritional replacement**

  1. **Iron.** Iron replacement is useful in the following situations:

    a. **Fetomaternal hemorrhage** of significant volume.

    b. **Chronic twin-twin transfusion** (in the donor twin).

    c. **Incremental external blood loss** (if unreplaced).

    d. **Preterm infant** (<36 weeks' gestational age).

  2. **Folate.** Especially with serum levels <0.5 ng/mL.

    a. **Premature infants** weighing <1500 g or <34 weeks' gestational age.

    b. **Chronic hemolytic anemias** or conditions involving "stress erythropoiesis."

    c. **Infants receiving phenytoin (Dilantin).**

  3. **Vitamin E.** Preterm infants of <34 weeks' gestational age, unless they are being breast-fed.

D. Prophylactic
   1. Recombinant human erythropoietin (r-HuEPO) (*controversial*). High doses of erythropoietin are capable of increasing neonatal erythropoiesis and have very little adverse side effect. It decreases the requirement for "late" transfusions (those required past the age of 2–3 weeks); it will not compensate for the anemia secondary to phlebotomy losses. Its use in the very low birthweight infant continues to be *controversial* because the severity of anemia in this group can be more effectively minimized by a restrictive policy for blood sampling and the use of micromethods in the laboratory. The need for transfusions is also reduced when a consistent "protocolized" approach for transfusions is available in the neonatal intensive care unit. It has been also argued that what needs to be avoided, more than the transfusion itself, is the exposure to multiple donors. The allocation of a single donor for each high-risk infant, for a 42-day period, is the most effective way to reach that former goal. Early and late strategies have been used for erythropoietin treatment. (See doses in Chapter 148.)
      a. Early. Starting on day 1 or 2, 1200–1400 U/kg/wk. r-HuEPO is added to the total parenteral nutrition solution, and 1 mg/kg/d of iron is added.
      b. Late. 500–700 U/kg/wk given 3–5 times per week subcutaneously. Supplemental oral iron needs to be provided at 3 mg/kg/d in 3 divided doses. The iron dose is increased to 6 mg/kg/d as soon as the infant is tolerating full enteral feeds.
   2. Nutritional supplementation
      a. Elemental iron. 1–2 mg/kg/d, beginning at 2 months of age and continuing through 1 year of age.
      b. Folic acid. 1–2 mg/wk for preterm infants; 50 mcg/d for term infants.
      c. Vitamin E. 25 IU/d until a corrected age of 4 months is reached.
E. Treatment of selected disorders
   1. Consumption coagulopathy
      a. Treat the underlying cause (eg, sepsis).
      b. Give blood replacement therapy. Perform exchange transfusion or give fresh-frozen plasma, 10 mL/kg every 12–14 hours. Platelet concentrate, 1 U, may be used as a substitute for plasma transfusion.
      c. Perform coagulation studies. Monitor the PTT, PT, and fibrinogen and D-dimers levels and the platelet count.
   2. Immune thrombocytopenia
      a. Isoimmune thrombocytopenia
         i. Consider performing cesarean delivery if the diagnosis has been confirmed and there is an older sibling with immune thrombocytopenia (75% risk of recurrence).
         ii. Give maternal washed platelets when indicated for bleeding diathesis in an infant with a platelet count <20,000–30,000 µL. Exchange transfusion may be used as an alternative.
         iii. Corticosteroid therapy and intravenous immune globulin are *controversial*.
      b. Autoimmune thrombocytopenia
         i. Cesarean delivery. Consider if the maternal platelet count is <100,000 µL or the fetal platelet count is <50,000 µL.
         ii. Use of corticosteroids is *controversial*. Under the conditions just mentioned, consider giving corticosteroids to the mother several weeks before delivery. Transfusion of random donor platelets may be given when indicated.
VIII. Prognosis. Depends on the underlying cause, its severity, and how acutely the anemia develops.

Selected References

Alpay F, Sarici SU, Okutan V, Erdem G, Ozcan O, Gökçay E. High-dose intravenous immuno-globulin therapy in neonatal immune haemolytic jaundice. *Acta Paediatr.* 1999;88:216–219.

American Academy of Pediatrics. Commentary: neonatal jaundice and kernicterus. *Pediatrics.* 2001;108:763.

Bell E, Strauss RG, Widness JA, et al. Randomized trial of liberal versus restrictive guidelines for red blood cell transfusion in preterm infants. *Pediatrics.* 2005;115:1685–1691.

Bifano EM, Curran TR. Minimizing donor blood exposure in the neonatal intensive care unit: current trends and future prospects. *Clin Perinatol.* 1995;22:657.

Bishara N, Ohls RK. Current controversies in the management of the anemia of prematurity. *Semin Perinatol.* 2008;33:29–34.

Blanchette VS, Rand ML. Platelet disorders in newborn infants: diagnosis and management. *Semin Perinatol.* 1997;21:53.

Blau J, Calo JM, Dozor D, Sutton M, Alpan G, La Gamma EF. Transfusion-related acute gut injury: necrotizing enterocolitis in very low birth weight neonates after packed red blood cell transfusion. *J Pediatr.* 2011;158:403–409.

Brugnara C. The neonatal erythrocyte and its disorder. In: Nathan DG, Orkin S, eds. *Hematology of Infancy and Childhood.* 7th ed. Philadelphia, PA: Saunders; 2008.

Christensen RD. Association between red blood cell transfusions and necrotizing enterocolitis. *J Pediatr.* 2011;158:349–350.

Crowley M, Kirpalani H. A rational approach to red blood cell transfusion in the neonatal ICU. *Curr Opin Pediatr.* 2010;22:151–157.

Kirpalani H, Whyte RK, Andersen C, et al. The Premature Infants in Need of Transfusions (PINT) study: a randomized, controlled trial of a restrictive (low) versus liberal (high) transfusion threshold for extremely low birth weight infants. *J Pediatr.* 2006;149:301–307.

Liley HG. Immune hemolytic disease of the newborn. In: Nathan DG, Orkin S, eds. *Hematology of Infancy and Childhood.* 7th ed. Philadelphia, PA: Saunders; 2008.

Nopoulos PC, Conrad AL, Bell EF, et al. Long-term outcome of brain structure in premature infants: effects of liberal vs restricted red blood cell transfusions. *Arch Pediatr Adolesc Med.* 2011;165:443–450.

Valieva OA, Strandjord TP, Mayock DE, Juul SE. Effects of transfusions in extremely low birth weight infants: a retrospective study. *J Pediatr.* 2009;155:331–337.

Wylie BJ, D'Alton ME. Fetomaternal hemorrhage. *Obstet Gynecol.* 2010;115:1039–1051.

83 Apnea

I. **Definition.** Apnea is common in preterm neonates and is a significant clinical problem. It is manifested by an unstable respiratory rhythm, reflecting the immaturity of the respiratory control system. Apnea can also be secondary to other pathological conditions, which need to be excluded before the diagnosis of apnea of prematurity is assumed. In contrast, periodic breathing is a benign condition and does not merit any treatment. Apnea is defined as cessation of breathing that lasts for at least 20 seconds and is accompanied by bradycardia, oxygen desaturation, or cyanosis.

A. **Central apnea.** Characterized by total cessation of inspiratory effort with no evidence of obstruction.

B. **Obstructive apnea.** Infant tries to breathe against an obstructed airway resulting in chest wall motion without air flow throughout the entire apneic episode.

C. **Mixed apnea.** Consists of obstructed respiratory efforts usually followed by central apnea. Purely obstructive apnea in the absence of a positional problem is probably uncommon.

D. **Periodic breathing.** Periodic breathing is a normal breathing pattern followed by apnea for 5 to 10 seconds without change in heart rate or skin color. Periodic breathing consists of breathing for 10 to 15 seconds followed by apnea for 5 or 10 seconds, without change in heart rate or skin color, and the net effect may be hypoventilation. It is due to an imbalance between the effect of peripheral and central chemoreceptors on ventilatory drive. Periodic breathing in premature infants is often due to excessive stimulation by the chemoreceptors, thus promoting an imbalance. Prevalence of periodic breathing approaches 100% in preterm infants <1000 g. It is more frequent during active sleep. The prognosis is good, and it is **controversial** whether periodic breathing is associated with an increased risk for apnea of prematurity.

II. **Incidence.** The incidence of apnea and periodic breathing in the term infant has not been adequately determined. More than 50% of infants weighing <1500 g and 90% of infants weighing <1000 g have apnea. Mixed apnea is the most common type (50%), followed by central (40%), and then obstructive (10%).

III. **Pathophysiology.** Apnea of prematurity is a developmental disorder and reflects a "physiological" rather than "pathological" immature state of respiratory control.

A. **Fetal to neonatal transition.** The postnatal rise in Pao_2 somewhat diminishes the response of peripheral chemoreceptors, resulting in a brief delay in the onset of spontaneous breathing. This effect is increased when neonates are exposed to 100% oxygen during resuscitation. The immature respiratory pattern and chemoreceptor function in premature infants may delay this postnatal adjustment, given fewer synaptic connections and less myelination of the immature brainstem.

B. **Ventilatory response to hypoxia.** A transient increase in respiratory rate and tidal volume that lasts for 1–2 minutes followed by a late sustained decrease in spontaneous breathing. This unique response to hypoxia may last for several weeks in response to hypoxic episodes after birth. This late hypoventilatory depression associated with delayed postnatal respiratory adjustment occurs in premature infants. Peripheral chemoreceptor stimulation secondary to hypocapnia after hyperventilation may also contribute to apnea.

C. **Ventilatory response to laryngeal chemoreflex.** The laryngeal chemoreflex is mediated through the superior laryngeal nerve afferents and is assumed to be a protective reflex. An exaggerated response brought about during feedings may also contribute to apneic episodes.

D. **Neurotransmitters and apnea.** Increased sensitivity to inhibitory neurotransmitters such as GABA (γ-aminobutyric acid), adenosine, serotonin, and prostaglandins may be related to apnea.

E. **Genetic variability and apnea.** Genetic and environmental factors may lead to apnea. Heritability of apnea of prematurity was 87% among same-gender twins. The congenital hypoventilation syndrome, defined by a lack of CO_2 responsiveness during sleep, is thought to occur due to the mutation of developmental transcription factor Phox2b. Severe depletion of neurons of the respiratory group of muscles was observed in experimentation animals due to the above mutation.

F. **Sleep-related apnea.** Most apnea occurs during active sleep. Preterm infants are asleep 80% of time, and 50% of sleep is active. This relationship lasts until 6 months of age. During active sleep there is a low-voltage electrocortical state, decreased arousal from sleep, decreased muscular tone, absence of upper airway adductor activity, and decreased respiratory drive. Irregular breathing and inspiratory chest wall distortion associated with decreased ventilatory drive causes slight elevation in arterial Pco_2. The ventilatory response to hypoxia and ventilatory sensitivity to CO_2 is more depressed during active sleep. Activation of serotonin-containing neurons that are part of the arousal system of the brainstem decreases by nearly half during slow-wave sleep and become nearly silent during rapid eye movement (REM) sleep via activation of GABAergic inputs.

G. **Siblings with sudden infant death syndrome (SIDS).** The collaborative home monitoring evaluation (CHIME) study showed that the incidence of apnea was the same in siblings of SIDS and normal term infants.

H. **Gastroesophageal reflux (GER) and apnea.** Studies have shown no temporal relation between GER and apnea. A decreased lower esophageal sphincter tone and increased GER following apnea have been documented, but apnea also occurs before reflux events. Apnea with desaturation events can lead to relaxation of the gastroesophageal junction and may explain the presence of formula often found in the pharynx of infants suctioned during an apneic event. Studies have shown that anti-reflux medications do not reduce apnea and bradycardia.

IV. **Risk factors**
   A. **Physiologic immaturity of the respiratory center.** This condition is usually present after 1–2 days of life, and is often referred to as **apnea of prematurity (AOP).**
   B. **Secondary causes**
      1. **Neurologic.** Birth trauma, meningitis, intracranial hemorrhage, seizures, perinatal asphyxia, congenital myopathies or neuropathies, placental transfer of narcotics, magnesium sulfate ($MgSO_4$), or general anesthetics.
      2. **Pulmonary.** Surfactant deficiency, pneumonia, pulmonary hemorrhage, obstructive airway lesions, pneumothorax, hypoxemia, and hypercarbia.
      3. **Cardiac.** Cyanotic congenital heart disease, hyper- or hypotension, congestive heart failure, patent ductus arteriosis, increased vagal tone, and prostaglandin therapy.
      4. **Gastrointestinal.** GER and necrotizing enterocolitis (NEC).
      5. **Hematologic.** Anemia.
      6. **Hypothermia or hyperthermia.**
      7. **Metabolic.** Acidosis, hypoglycemia, hypocalcemia, and hypo- or hypernatremia.
      8. **Inborn errors of metabolism.**
      9. **Sepsis.**

V. **Clinical manifestations.** It is difficult to separate clinical manifestations of apnea from consequences of apnea. Symptoms and signs depend on the duration and frequency of apnea and most are related to hypoxia. Other clinical manifestations depend on the etiology of apnea such as feeding intolerance, lethargy, temperature instability, jitteriness, poor feeding, central nervous system (CNS) depression, irritability, desaturation, tachypnea, tachycardia, bradycardia, hypotonia, and seizures.

VI. **Diagnosis**
   A. **History and physical examination** must include a review of maternal risk factors, medications, birth history, and feeding intolerance. Physical examination should include a search for abnormal neurological signs and signs of sepsis.
   B. **Laboratory studies**
      1. Complete septic workup (eg, complete blood count [CBC], appropriate cultures)
      2. Screening for metabolic disorders
   C. **Imaging and other studies**
      1. **Imaging** to evaluate for atelectasis, pneumonia, air leak, and NEC, and cranial ultrasound to detect intracranial hemorrhage or congenital abnormalities.
      2. **Electroencephalogram (EEG)** to rule out seizures, as apnea may be the sole presentation of seizures.
      3. **Polysomnography** determines the type of apnea in relation to sleep cycles of the infant.

VII. **Management.** Treatment strategies of apnea of prematurity should be based on modulating an unstable respiratory rhythm into a more stable one. (See Chapter 47.)

A. **Pharmacologic management**
   1. **Methylxanthine therapy.** Caffeine, theophylline, and aminophylline have been used as respiratory stimulants to decrease apnea of prematurity. Both caffeine and theophylline are an effective treatment for AOP. Initially, theophylline was the standard of treatment and required close monitoring of serum levels. Since the U.S. Food and Drug Administration (FDA) approval of caffeine for infant use, it has largely replaced theophylline as the first drug for AOP management. Methylxanthines increase minute ventilation, improve CO_2 sensitivity, decrease hypoxic depression, enhance diaphragmatic activity, and decrease periodic breathing. Enhancing the CO_2 sensitivity may be an important component of its effectiveness. Common side effects include tachycardia, feeding intolerance, emesis, jitteriness, restlessness, and irritability. Toxic effects may produce arrhythmias and seizures. Methylxanthines increase metabolic rate and oxygen consumption and have a mild diuretic effect. Caffeine has substantially fewer side effects, is better tolerated, and has a high therapeutic index when compared to theophylline. Caffeine has a long half-life, which makes for a convenient once-a-day dosing regimen, and monitoring of caffeine levels at the recommended dosing is seldom necessary. See Chapter 148 for dosage regimens.
   2. **Doxapram.** Doxapram is a potent nonspecific respiratory stimulant. It stimulates peripheral chemoreceptors at low dose and central chemoreceptors at high dose. Small doses are used for the treatment of AOP. Doxapram increases tidal volume and minute ventilation. Studies have shown the effectiveness of doxapram in reducing apnea when refractory to methylxanthines. As a result of poor absorption, it is used as a continuous intravenous infusion. Side effects include an increase in blood pressure, abdominal distension, irritability, jitteriness, increased gastric residuals, and emesis. See Chapter 148 for dosage regimens.

B. **Nonpharmacologic management**
   1. **Evidence based**
     a. **Prone, head elevated positioning.** The chest wall is stabilized and thoracoabdominal asynchrony is reduced in prone position. Prone position along with head elevated tilt position showed reduction in apnea and bradycardia. The effect of head position on bradycardia and intermittent hypoxia is less pronounced in infants already receiving other treatment for apnea of prematurity.
     b. **Continuous positive airway pressure (CPAP).** CPAP at 4–6 cm H_2O has proven to be a safe and effective therapy of apnea of prematurity. It is effective in obstructive apnea rather than central apnea. Effectiveness of CPAP is related to maintaining airway patency and its splinting effects. CPAP delivers a continuous distending pressure via the infant's pharynx to the airway to prevent both pharyngeal collapse and alveolar atelectasis, thereby enhancing functional residual capacity, reducing work of breathing, improving oxygenation, and decreasing bradycardia. CPAP decreases periodic breathing and apnea.
     c. **Flow through nasal cannula.** Both high and low flow through nasal cannula can be a useful adjunct therapy in some infants with apnea who are already receiving methylxanthines. High flow produces a distending pressure, especially in very low birthweight infants. It is a variable form of treatment and depends on factors such as flow rate, nasal leak, and mouth closure. Airway pressure cannot be readily monitored while on nasal cannula.
     d. **Synchronized nasal ventilation.** An extension of CPAP is administration of nasal intermittent positive pressure ventilation (N-IPPV). It has been suggested to be more effective over CPAP in preventing extubation failure.

2. Other interventions with unclear efficacy
   a. **Orogastric versus nasogastric feeding tube placement.** A nasogastric tube increases nasal resistance by 50%; therefore, orogastric feeding tubes are sometimes preferred in preterm infants with apnea.
   b. **Kangaroo mother care (KMC).** Studies have shown that infants receiving KMC had decreased episodes of apnea and bradycardia. The effect of KMC in improvement of apnea and bradycardia is the same as that seen with prone positioning.
   c. **Keeping environmental temperature at the lower end of the thermoneutral range.** Increase in body temperature in infants enhances the instability of the breathing pattern. Overheating should be avoided, but there is no significant data to recommend a specific environmental temperature that may be used to reduce the incidence of AOP.
   d. **Oscillating waterbed and tactile stimulation.** Synchronization of respiration may be achieved between the infant's own breathing rhythm and an external rhythm generator (eg, an inflatable mattress connected to a respirator). This synchronization is better beyond 35 weeks gestational age (GA) when AOP is no longer a major issue, so this intervention was largely abandoned. Recently stochastic mechanosensory stimulation using actuators embedded in a specially designed mattress for subcutaneous stimulation have been shown to decrease in the duration of oxygen desaturation.
   e. **Olfactory stimulation.** Olfactory stimulation modulates the infant's respiratory pattern, particularly during active sleep when apnea is more common. Introduction of a pleasant odor into the incubator reduces the incidence of apnea and bradycardia. A study was done in smaller group for a period of 24 hours.
   f. **Red blood cell transfusion.** An increase in respiratory drive resulting from increased tissue oxygenation is one of the proposed mechanisms for red cell transfusion to ameliorate AOP. There is insignificant evidence to recommend transfusion to treat AOP in anemic infants. Data on the effect of blood transfusion in treating AOP is conflicting, though it was not associated with apnea frequency, but it was associated with increased risk of bronchopulmonary dysplasia/chronic lung disease (BPD/CLD) and NEC.
   g. **Oxygen administration.** Application of low flow oxygen results in reduced rate of intermittent hypoxia and apnea. Oxygen toxicity should be considered while using this modality of treatment.
VIII. **Discharge planning and follow-up**
   A. **Consider stopping caffeine at 34 weeks postmenstrual age.**
   B. **More aggressive approach** is to stop when infant is apnea-free for a period of 7 days irrespective of age.
   C. **If asymptomatic for 5 days after stopping methylxanthines,** the child may be discharged without further therapy.
   D. **Considerations for home apnea monitoring**
      1. Persistent, symptomatic apnea at >36 weeks postmenstrual age
      2. History of a severe, apparently life-threatening event and abnormal polysomnography
      3. Technology-dependent infant (eg, home mechanical ventilation)
      4. Home oxygen administration
      5. Central hypoventilation syndromes
IX. **Prognosis.** Apnea of prematurity resolves with maturation. The physiological basis for resolution of apnea is believed to be myelination of the brainstem. Poor neurodevelopmental outcome is associated with a delay in myelination in infants with apnea of prematurity. Otherwise, in most infants apnea resolves without the occurrence of long-term deficiencies.

Selected References

Carroll JL, Agarwal A. Development of ventilatory control in infants. *Paediatr Resp Rev.* 2010;11:199–207.

Jalal M, Martin RJ. Neonatal apnea: what's new? *Pediatr Pulmonol.* 2008;43:937–944.

Lorch SA, Srinivasan L, Escobar GJ. Epidemiology of apnea and bradycardia resolution in premature infants. *Pediatrics.* 2011;128:e366–e373.

Mathew OP. Apnea of prematurity: pathogenesis and management strategies *J Perinatal.* 2011;31:302–310.

Schmidt B, Roberts RS, Davis P, et al. Long-term effects of caffeine therapy for apnea of prematurity. *N Engl J Med.* 2007;357(19):1893–1902.

Slocum C, Arko M, Di Fiore J, Martin RJ, Hibbs AM. Apnea, bradycardia and desaturation in preterm infants before and after feeding. *J Perinatol.* 2009;29(3):209–212.

84 Bronchopulmonary Dysplasia/Chronic Lung Disease

I. **Definition.** Classic bronchopulmonary dysplasia (BPD) is a neonatal form of chronic pulmonary disorder that follows a primary course of respiratory failure (eg, respiratory distress syndrome [RDS], meconium aspiration syndrome) in the first days of life. It is sometimes referred to as **chronic lung disease** (CLD) of prematurity. A **"new" form of BPD** has been described in extremely low birthweight infants. This occurs in infants who initially had none or modest initial ventilatory and oxygen needs. **BPD is defined as persistent oxygen dependency up to 28 days of life.** The severity of BPD-related pulmonary dysfunction in early childhood is more accurately predicted by an oxygen dependence at 36 weeks' postmenstrual age (PMA) in infants <32 weeks' gestational age (GA) and at 56 days of age in infants with older GA. BPD is thus classified at this later postnatal age according to the type of respiratory support required to maintain a normal arterial oxygen saturation (89%).

   A. **Mild BPD.** Infants who have been weaned from any supplemental oxygen.

   B. **Moderate BPD.** Infants who continue to need up to 30% oxygen.

   C. **Severe BPD.** Infants whose requirements exceed 30% and/or include continuous positive airway pressure or mechanical ventilation.

II. **Incidence.** The incidence of BPD is influenced by many risk factors, the most important of which is lung maturity. The incidence of BPD increases with decreasing birthweight and affects ~30% of infants with birthweights <1000 g. The large variability in rates among centers is partly related to differences in clinical practices, such as criteria used for the management of mechanical ventilation.

III. **Pathophysiology.** A primary lung injury is not always evident at birth. The secondary development of a persistent lung injury is associated with an abnormal repair process and leads to structural changes such as arrested alveolarization and pulmonary vascular dysgenesis.

   A. **The major factors contributing to BPD are as follows:**

      1. **Inflammation.** Central to the development of BPD. An exaggerated inflammatory response (alveolar influx of numerous proinflammatory cytokines as well as macrophages and leukocytes) occurs in the first few days of life in infants in whom BPD subsequently develops.

      2. **Mechanical ventilation.** Volutrauma/barotrauma is one of the key risk factors for the development of BPD. Minimizing the use of mechanical ventilation by

the use of early nasal continuous positive airway pressure, noninvasive ventilatory support (nasal intermittent positive pressure ventilation), and early use of methylxanthines (caffeine) has led to fewer days of mechanical ventilation and to lesser use of postnatal steroids.

3. Oxygen exposure. **Classic BPD** observed before the availability of exogenous surfactant treatment was always associated with prolonged exposure (>150 hours) to an F_{IO_2} >60%. Hyperoxia can have major effects on lung tissue, such as proliferation of alveolar type II cells and fibroblast, alterations in the surfactant system, increases in inflammatory cells and cytokines, increased collagen deposition, and decreased alveolarization and microvascular density. Today, in the postsurfactant era, exposure to prolonged high oxygen is limited, and a new form of BPD is being observed. For this **"new" BPD**, the association between persistent need for mechanical ventilation and supplemental oxygen in the first 2 weeks of life is not as dominant as in the past. For instance, a third of the preterm infants receiving either supplemental oxygen or intermittent positive pressure ventilation at 14 days did not develop BPD, whereas 17% of the infants in room air at 14 days of age did. Nevertheless, aiming for Spo_2 in the range of 85–93% rather than >92% has led to a decrease in the need for supplemental oxygen at 36 weeks' PMA in this postsurfactant era. The advantages off keeping Spo_2 at the lower range, for BPD (and retinopathy of prematurity) prevention, needs to be carefully weighed against the possibility that keeping Spo_2 in the range of 85–89% may be associated with higher mortality.

B. Pathologic changes. Compared with the presurfactant era, lungs of infants currently dying from BPD have normal-appearing airways, less fibrosis, and more uniform inflation. However, these lungs have deficient septation, leading to fewer and larger alveoli with possible reduced pulmonary capillarization that may lead to pulmonary hypertension.

IV. Risk factors. Major risk factors are prematurity, white race, male sex, chorioamnionitis, tracheal colonization with *Ureaplasma*, and the increased survival of the extremely low birthweight infant. Other risk factors are RDS, excessive early intravenous fluid administration, symptomatic patent ductus arteriosus (PDA), sepsis, oxygen therapy, vitamin A deficiency, and a family history of atopic disease.

V. Clinical presentation. BPD is usually suspected in infants with progressive and idiopathic deterioration of pulmonary function. Infants in whom BPD develops often require oxygen therapy or mechanical ventilation beyond the first week of life. Severe cases of BPD are usually associated with poor growth, pulmonary edema, and a hyperreactive airway.

VI. Diagnosis
A. Physical examination
1. General signs. Worsening respiratory status is manifested by an increase in the work of breathing, in oxygen requirement, or in apnea-bradycardia, or in a combination of these signs.
2. Pulmonary examination. Retractions and diffuse fine rales are common. Wheezing or prolongation of expiration may also be noted.
3. Cardiovascular examination. A right ventricular heave, single S_2, or prominent P_2 may accompany cor pulmonale.
4. Abdominal examination. The liver may be enlarged secondary to right-sided heart failure or may be displaced downward into the abdomen secondary to lung hyperinflation.
B. Laboratory studies. These studies are intended to rule out differential diagnosis such as sepsis or PDA during the acute nature of the disease and to detect problems related to BPD or its therapy.
1. Arterial blood gas levels. Frequently reveal carbon dioxide retention. However, if the respiratory difficulties are chronic and stable, the pH is usually subnormal (pH ≥7.25).

2. **Electrolytes.** Abnormalities of electrolytes may result from chronic carbon dioxide retention (elevated serum bicarbonate), diuretic therapy (hyponatremia, hypokalemia, or hypochloremia), or fluid restriction (elevated urea nitrogen and creatinine), or all 3.

3. **Complete blood count and differential.** To diagnose neutropenia or an elevated white blood count in sepsis.

4. **Urinalysis.** Microscopic examination may reveal the presence of red blood cells, indicating a possible nephrocalcinosis as a result of prolonged diuretic treatment.

C. **Imaging and other studies.** To detect problems related to BPD or its therapy.

1. **Chest radiograph.** Radiographic findings may be quite variable. Most frequently, BPD appears as **diffuse haziness and lung hypoinflation** in infants who were very immature at birth and have persistent oxygen requirements. In other infants, a different picture is seen, reminiscent of that originally described by Northway: **streaky interstitial markings, patchy atelectasis intermingled with cystic area, and severe overall lung hyperinflation.** Because those findings persist for a prolonged period, new changes (eg, a secondary infection) are difficult to detect without the benefit of comparison to previous radiographs. (See Figure 11–17 for an example of BPD.)

2. **Renal ultrasonography.** Radiologic studies of the abdomen should be considered during diuretic therapy to detect the presence of nephrocalcinosis. It should be performed when red blood cells are present in the urine.

3. **Electrocardiography and echocardiography.** Indicated in nonimproving or worsening BPD. Electrocardiograms and echocardiograms could detect cor pulmonale and/or pulmonary hypertension, manifested by right ventricular hypertrophy and elevation of pulmonary artery pressure with right axis deviation, increased right systolic time intervals, thickening of the right ventricular wall, and abnormal right ventricular geometry.

VII. **Management**

A. **Prevention of BPD**

1. **Prevention of prematurity and RDS.** Therapies directed toward decreasing the risk of prematurity and lowering the incidence of RDS include improving prenatal care and antenatal corticosteroids.

2. **Reducing exposure to risk factors.** Successful measures should include minimizing exposure to oxygen by limiting $SpaO_2$ to 90–95%, ventilation strategies that minimize the use of excessive tidal volume (above 4–6 mL/kg), prudent administration of fluids, aggressive closure of PDA (*controversial*), and adequate nutrition. **Early surfactant replacement therapy may be beneficial, but the avoidance of intubation and mechanical ventilation with the initiation of continuous positive airway pressure (CPAP) shortly after birth may prove to be an effective preventive strategy.**

3. **Vitamin A.** Low blood levels of vitamin A seen in extremely low birthweight infants have been associated with increased risk of BPD. Vitamin A supplementation, 5000 IU administered intramuscularly 3 times per week for 4 weeks, significantly reduced the rate of BPD. Its effects were modest. One additional infant survived without BPD for every 15 extremely low birthweight infants treated; however, no long-term beneficial respiratory or neurodevelopmental outcomes have been found.

4. **Caffeine.** Methylxanthines decrease the frequency of apnea and allow for shorter duration of mechanical ventilation, leading to a reduced rate of BPD.

5. **Inhaled nitric oxide (iNO).** Its use to prevent BPD remains *controversial*. Although inhaled nitric oxide has been shown in animal models to reduce pulmonary vascular tone and prevent lung inflammation, its clinical benefits remain equivocal and do not justify the cost. At present, routine use of iNO for preterm infants at risk for BPD is not recommended.

B. **Treatment of BPD.** Once BPD is present, the goal of management is to prevent further injury by minimizing respiratory support, improving pulmonary function, preventing cor pulmonale, and emphasizing growth and nutrition.

1. **Respiratory support**
   a. **Supplemental oxygen.** Maintaining adequate oxygenation is important in the infant with BPD to prevent hypoxia-induced pulmonary hypertension, bronchospasm, cor pulmonale, and growth failure. However, the least-required oxygen should be delivered to minimize oxygen toxicity. Spo_2 should be monitored during the infant's various activities, including rest, sleep, and feeding, and should be maintained in the range of 90–95%. Infrequent blood gas measurements are important for the assessment of trends in pH, $Paco_2$, and serum bicarbonate, but they are of limited use in monitoring oxygenation because they provide information about only one point in time.
   b. **Positive-pressure ventilation.** Mechanical ventilation should be used only when clearly indicated. Similarly, inspiratory pressure needs to be limited at the expense of tolerating $Paco_2$ of 50–60 mm Hg (*controversial*). Nasal CPAP can be useful as an adjunctive therapy after extubation.

2. **Improving lung function**
   a. **Fluid restriction.** Restricting fluid to 120 mL/kg/d is often required. It can be accomplished by concentrating proprietary formulas to 24 cal/oz. Increasing the caloric density further to 27–30 cal/oz may require the addition of fat (eg, medium-chain triglyceride oil or corn oil) and carbohydrate (eg, Polycose) to avoid excessive protein intake.
   b. **Diuretic therapy.** See Chapter 148 for dosing.
      i. **Furosemide.** Furosemide (1–2 mg/kg every 12 hours, orally or intravenously) is a potent diuretic that is particularly useful for rapid diuresis. It is associated with side effects such as electrolyte abnormalities, interference with bilirubin-albumin binding capacity, calciuria with bone demineralization and renal stone formation, and ototoxicity. When used as a chronic medication, Na^+ and K^+ supplementation are often required.
      ii. **Bumetanide.** Bumetanide 0.015–0.1 mg/kg daily or every other day, orally or intravenously. When administered orally, 1 mg of bumetanide (Bumex) has a diuretic effect similar to that of 40 mg of furosemide. Whereas furosemide's bioavailability is 30–70%, bumetanide's bioavailability is >90%. Bumetanide produces side effects similar to those of furosemide, except that it may produce less ototoxicity and less interference with bilirubin-albumin binding.
      iii. **Chlorothiazide and spironolactone.** When used in doses of 20 mg/kg/d (chlorothiazide) and 2 mg/kg/d (spironolactone), a good diuretic response can often be achieved. Although less potent than furosemide, this combination is often better suited for chronic management because it has relatively fewer side effects. It may be the diuretic combination of choice when the calciuric effect of furosemide has led to the development of nephrocalcinosis.
   c. **Bronchodilators.** See doses in Table 8–3.
      i. **β_2-Agonists.** Inhaled β_2-agonists (eg, albuterol) produce measurable acute improvements in lung mechanics and gas exchange in infants with BPD exhibiting symptoms of increased airway tone. Their effect is usually time limited. Because of their side effects (eg, tachycardia, hypertension, hyperglycemia, and possible arrhythmia), their use should be limited to the management of acute exacerbations of BPD. **Xopenex** (levalbuterol) is a nonracemic form of albuterol recently introduced in pediatric and adult populations. Its experience in newborns is limited. Its potential

advantages are better and it has longer efficacy; hence lower doses have a therapeutic effect, enabling a significant reduction in the adverse effects associated with racemic albuterol. If bronchodilators are being used long term, a frequent reevaluation of their benefit is essential.

ii. **Anticholinergic agents.** The best studied and most available inhaled quaternary anticholinergic is **ipratropium bromide** (nebulized Atrovent). Its bronchodilatory effect is more potent than that of atropine and similar to that of albuterol. Combined albuterol and ipratropium therapy has a larger effect than either agent alone. Unlike atropine, systemic effects do not occur because of its poor systemic absorption.

iii. **Methylxanthine.** The beneficial actions of theophylline include smooth airway muscle dilation, improved diaphragmatic contractility, central respiratory stimulation, and mild diuretic effects. It appears to improve lung function in BPD when levels are maintained at >10 mcg/mL. Side effects are fairly common and may include central nervous system (CNS) irritability, gastroesophageal reflux, and gastrointestinal irritation. Prevention of apnea rather than bronchodilation is the major reason for infants with BPD to receive a methylxanthine treatment (mostly caffeine).

d. **Corticosteroids.** Although very efficient, the use of postnatal steroids should be limited to infants who are at high risk for mortality secondary to severe lung disease and who cannot be weaned from mechanical ventilation after 7 days of age. Parents should be informed that the use of postnatal steroids could be associated with impaired brain and somatic growth and increased incidence of cerebral palsy. Although dexamethasone has been the most studied postnatal steroids to treat BPD, various therapy regimens using milder types of steroids have been proposed, hoping to decrease the observed adverse effects. However, the beneficial effects of these mild steroids on extubation, duration of mechanical ventilation, BPD, and death have not been prospectively studied.

i. **Dexamethasone.** Initiate at >7 days of age at 0.25 mg/kg twice daily for 3 days and then gradually taper by 10% every 3 days for a total course of 42 days. It is one of the original regimens that have proven efficacious in the treatment of BPD. Decrease brain growth and increased incidence of cerebral palsy has been associated with dexamethasone treatment. Its early use (<7 days) increases the risk of spontaneous gastrointestinal perforation, in particular when used in conjunction with prostaglandins inhibitor such as indomethacin. Other side effects include infection, hypertension, gastric ulcer, hyperglycemia, adrenocortical suppression, lung growth suppression, and hypertrophic cardiomyopathy. Lower doses and shorter duration of dexamethasone have been attempted to decrease its undesirable effects.

ii. **Methylprednisolone (Solu-Medrol).** A corticosteroid with much weaker genomic activity than dexamethasone, methylprednisolone has almost similar nongenomic activity and thus possibly fewer CNS and somatic side effects. In a pilot study, methylprednisolone, 0.6, 0.4, 0.2 mg/kg/dose every 6 hours, respectively, for 3 consecutive days, followed by betamethasone, 0.1 mg/kg orally every other day for a total of 21 days, was found to have similar beneficial effects and fewer side effects (eg, periventricular leukomalacia, hyperglycemia) than dexamethasone. These findings still need to be confirmed by large randomized controlled trials.

iii. **Hydrocortisone.** Hydrocortisone 5 mg/kg/d divided every 6 hours for 1 week, and then gradually tapered for the following 2–5 weeks. In contrast to infants treated with dexamethasone, when compared with controls, hydrocortisone therapy has not been associated with adverse neurodevelopmental outcome or with brain abnormalities on magnetic resonance imaging in long-term follow-up studies up to 5–8 years of age.

     iv. **Prednisolone.** Prednisolone 2 mg/kg/d orally divided twice per day for 5 days, then 1 mg/kg/dose orally daily for 3 days, and then 1 mg/kg/dose every other day for 3 doses has been used to wean from oxygen therapy before discharge home.

     v. **Nebulized corticosteroids.** Nebulized corticosteroids (eg, beclomethasone, 100–200 mcg 4 times/day) produced fewer side effects than oral or parenteral forms but are much less efficacious in the treatment of BPD.

   3. **Growth and nutrition.** Because growth is essential for recovery from BPD, adequate nutritional intake is crucial. Infants with BPD frequently have high caloric needs (120–150 kcal/kg/d or more) because of increased metabolic expenditures. Concentrated formula is often necessary to provide sufficient calories and prevent pulmonary edema. In addition, specific micronutrient supplementation, such as antioxidant therapy, may also enhance pulmonary and nutritional status.

 C. **Discharge planning.** Oxygen can often be discontinued before discharge from the neonatal intensive care unit. However, home oxygen therapy can be a safe alternative to long-term hospitalization. The need for home respiratory, heart rate, and oxygen monitoring must be decided on an individual basis but is generally recommended for infants discharged home on oxygen. Synagis (palivizumab, humanized monoclonal antibodies against respiratory syncytial virus [RSV]) should be given monthly (15 mg/kg administered intramuscularly) throughout the RSV season. All parents should be instructed in cardiopulmonary resuscitation.

 D. **General care.** Care plans for older infants with BPD should include adapting their routine for home life and involving the parents in their care. Immunizations should be given at the appropriate chronologic age. Periodic screening for chemical evidence of rickets and echocardiographic evidence of pulmonary hypertension is recommended. Assessment by a developmental specialist and occupational or physical therapist, or both, can be useful for prognostic and therapeutic purposes.

VIII. **Prognosis.** The prognosis for infants with BPD depends on the degree of pulmonary dysfunction and the presence of other medical conditions. Most deaths occur in the first year of life as a result of cardiorespiratory failure, sepsis, or respiratory infection or as a sudden, unexplained death.

 A. **Pulmonary outcome.** The short-term outcome of infants with BPD, including those requiring oxygen at home, is surprisingly good. Weaning from oxygen is usually possible before their first birthday, and they demonstrate catch-up growth as their pulmonary status improves. However, in the first year of life, rehospitalization is necessary for ~30% of patients for treatment of wheezing, respiratory infections, or both. Although upper respiratory tract infections are probably no more common in infants with BPD than in normal infants, they are more likely to be associated with significant respiratory symptoms. Most adolescents and young adults who had moderate to severe BPD in infancy have some degree of pulmonary dysfunction, consisting of airway obstruction, reactive airway disease, and hyperinflation.

 B. **Neurodevelopmental outcome.** Children with moderate to severe BPD appear to be at an increased risk for adverse neurodevelopmental outcome compared with comparable infants without BPD. Neuromotor and cognitive dysfunction appears to be more common. In addition, children with BPD may be at higher risk for significant hearing impairment and retinopathy of prematurity. They are also at risk for later problems, including learning disabilities, attention deficits, and behavior problems.

Selected References

Cerny L, Torday JS, Rehan VK. Prevention and treatment of bronchopulmonary dysplasia: contemporary status and future outlook. *Lung.* 2008;186:75–89.

Ehrenkranz RA, Walsh MC, Vohr BR, et al. Validation of the National Institute of Health consensus definition of bronchopulmonary dysplasia. *Pediatrics.* 2005;116:1353–1360.

Jobe A, Bancalari E. Bronchopulmonary dysplasia. *Am J Respir Crit Care Med.* 2001;163:1723–1729.

Jobe AH. The new bronchopulmonary dysplasia. *Curr Opin Pediatr.* 2011;23:167–172.

Kinsella JP, Greenough A, Abman SH. Bronchopulmonary dysplasia. *Lancet.* 2006;367: 1421–1431.

Kugelman A, Durand M. A comprehensive approach to the prevention of bronchopulmonary dysplasia. *Pediatr Pulmonol.* 2011;46:1153–1165.

Rademaker KJ, de Vries LS, Uiterwaal CS, Groenendaal F, Grobbee DE, van Bel F. Postnatal hydrocortisone treatment for chronic lung disease in the preterm newborn and long-term neurodevelopmental follow-up. *Arch Dis Child Fetal Neonatal Ed.* 2008;93:F58–F63.

85 Calcium Disorders (Hypocalcemia, Hypercalcemia)

Abnormalities of calcium (Ca^{+2}) and magnesium (Mg^{+2}) metabolism are not infrequent occurrences among infants admitted for neonatal intensive care. Moreover, the disturbances of Ca^{+2} may be mirrored by Mg^{+2}, or conversely, as in hypocalcemia and hypomagnesemia. Infants of diabetic mothers (IDMs) and infants with intrauterine growth restriction (IUGR) may present with low serum levels of either Ca^{+2} or Mg^{+2}, or both. Serum values for Ca^{+2} and Mg^{+2} above or below accepted normal values are of concern in any infant and warrant further clinical studies. (See also Chapter 107.)

I. **Hypocalcemia**

   A. **Definition.** Hypocalcemia is likely the most common disorder of either Ca^{+2} or Mg^{+2} in newborn infants and affects both preterm and term infants. Hypocalcemia is determined as either **total serum calcium (tCa) or ionized calcium (iCa).** Clinical chemistry values for serum levels vary by units (ie, mEq/L, mmol/L, or mg/dL), by gestational age, and by day of age following the immediate newborn period. Reference textbooks reflect considerable variance of serum values for Ca^{+2} and Mg^{+2}. Interpretation of serum values for any given patient is dependent on recognition of one's institution laboratory values and range of acceptable values.

   A **generally accepted value for hypocalcemia** is <2.0 mmol/L (<8.0 mg/dL) for a term infant or <1.75 mmol/L (<7.0 mg/dL) for a preterm infant. A typical range of normal values for a term newborn can be 2.25–2.65 mmol/L (9.0–10.6 mg/dL) throughout the first week of life. Preterm infant tCa levels closely parallel those for term infants. Of greater significance is the ionized fraction of Ca^{+2}. It is the active physiological component and is dependent on the interaction of tCa^{+2}, normal acid-base status, and normal serum albumin. Typical iCa^{+2} values for term infants over the first 72 hours of life are 1.24 (1.13–1.35) mmol/L to 1.22 (1.08–1.36) mmol/L (4.88–4.96 mg/dL). Preterm infant mean values are similar for 24 and 72 hours: 1.21–1.28 mmol/L (4.84–5.12 mg/ dL). Interestingly, preterm infants slightly increase their iCa^{+2} levels, whereas term infants experience a slight decline. **Ionized calcium levels of <4 mg/dL are considered hypocalcemic.**

   B. **Incidence.** Hypocalcemia is likely the most common disorder of either Ca^{+2} or Mg^{+2} in newborn infants, and it affects both preterm and term infants. It occurs in up to 30% of infants with birthweight <1500 g. Late-onset hypocalcemia is more common in developing countries where cow's milk or formulas with phosphate concentrations are used.

   C. **Pathophysiology.** Ionized Ca^{+2} is the biologically important form of calcium. The tCa^{+2} levels have been repeatedly shown to not be predictive of iCa^{+2} levels.

Therefore, tCa^{+2} levels are unreliable as criteria for true hypocalcemia. In premature infants, it has been shown that tCa^{+2} levels as low as ≤ 6 mg/dL correspond to iCa^{+2} levels >3 mg/dL.

D. **Risk factors**

1. **Early-onset neonatal hypocalcemia.** During the third trimester of pregnancy, the human fetus receives at least 120–150 mg/kg/d of elemental Ca^{+2} via the umbilical cord. Most of this Ca^{+2} is readily incorporated into the newly forming bones. After delivery, this massive supply of Ca^{+2} is suddenly stopped, and Ca^{+2} must be given enterally.

   a. A full-term infant receiving 100–120 mL of normal formula would be receiving 50–60 mg/kg/d of Ca^{+2} orally. Despite this drop in supply, full-term infants tolerate the change well and do not become hypocalcemic.

   b. Premature (especially <28 weeks) or sick infants often become hypocalcemic during the first 3 days of life. Total serum Ca^{+2} levels can drop to <7 mg/dL and occasionally fall below 6 mg/dL.

   c. Calcium levels (both iCa^{+2} and tCa^{+2}) usually return to normal within 48–72 hours regardless of whether supplemental Ca^{+2} is given. Immunoreactive parathyroid hormone (iPTH) is often low at birth but rises to higher levels within 24–72 hours after delivery. Intravenous Ca^{+2} supplementation suppresses this increase in iPTH, thus some centers for neonatal care do not use IV calcium supplementation.

2. **Perinatal stress.** Term or preterm infants who have asphyxia and acidosis present with hypocalcemia. Resuscitation and the use of alkali to correct acidosis (bicarbonate therapy) may have multiple effects resulting in hypocalcemia (eg, lower iCa^{+2} levels, decreased Ca^{+2} flux from bones, relative hyperphosphatemia secondary to increased circulating endogenous phosphorous following postasphyxial renal impairment). Additional factors include meconium aspiration syndrome, compromised placental blood flow, sepsis, and shock. Of special note is alkalosis secondary to hyperventilation and hypocarbia postresuscitation. The combination of bicarbonate infusions and hypocarbia can induce an alkalosis with profound hypocalcemia.

3. **Infant of diabetic mother (IDM).** Onset of hypocalcemia is usually early (1–3 days) and may recur throughout the first week. The mechanism for IDM hypocalcemia is unknown. Related factors that have been identified are increased calcitonin levels, decreased bone Ca^{+2} flux, hypomagnesemia, hypoparathyroidism, and hyperphosphatemia. The occurrence and severity of IDM hypocalcemia follows the severity of maternal diabetes and the prenatal management for euglycemic control.

4. **Intrauterine growth restriction (IUGR).** Sporadic hypocalcemia occurs and may be associated with one or more of the known complications of IUGR (eg, hypoglycemia, asphyxia, meconium aspiration, hypothermia, polycythemia, and placental insufficiency).

5. **Nutritional deprivation.** Infants unable to take enteral feeds by 3 days of age will need calcium supplementation. Breast milk or calcium-enriched formulas provide adequate Ca^{+2} intake. Because hypocalcemia is related to hypomagnesemia, both elements require supplementation to prevent secondary suppression of parathormone recurrence of hypocalcemia.

6. **Hypomagnesemia.** May be secondary to maternal gestational magnesium losses or to impaired intestinal uptake. Hypomagnesemia frequently occurs with hypocalcemia and must be looked for in any at-risk infant.

7. **Congenital abnormalities.** The DiGeorge sequence with absence of parathyroid glands and related craniofacial and cardiac anomalies often presents with hypocalcemia.

8. **Maternal hyperparathyroidism.** This causes transient hypoparathyroidism in the infant due to fetal parathyroid suppression.

9. **Other therapeutic modalities.** Include furosemide-induced hypercalciuria; citrated blood transfusions, which reduce iCa^{+2} due to a citrate-calcium complex and an alkalosis following metabolism of citrate; and inadequate prenatal vitamin D supplementation of the mother or the infant during the first 6 months of life. Maternal use of anticonvulsants like phenobarbital can cause increased hepatic catabolism of vitamin D, resulting in maternal vitamin D deficiency and subsequent neonatal hypocalcemia.

E. **Clinical presentation**

  1. **Early-onset hypocalcemia (first week of life)**
     a. Apnea
     b. Stridor
     c. Irritability, jitteriness, tremors, or hyperreflexia
     d. Clonus, tetany, or seizures
     e. Arrhythmia secondary to prolonged QT interval

  2. **Late-onset hypocalcemia (anytime after first week)**
     a. Lethargy, apnea
     b. Feeding intolerance
     c. Abdominal distention
     d. Bone demineralization, increased alkaline phosphatase
     e. Skeletal fractures

  3. **Paradoxically, neonatal hypocalcemia may be asymptomatic.** Only an index of suspicion on the basis of risk factors will lead to a correct diagnosis.

F. **Diagnosis**

  1. **Laboratory studies**
     a. **Total and ionized Ca^{+2} levels** should be available for the neonatal intensive care unit (NICU) patient. Serum tCa of <1.75 mmol/L (7.0 mg/dL) is usually diagnostic of hypocalcemia. Confirmation is afforded by iCa levels of <1.10 mmol/L (4.4 mg/dL). See previous definition for range of normal values for both tCa and iCa.
     b. **Serum magnesium levels** of <1.5 mg/dL are indicative of hypocalcemia as they often follow one another.
     c. **Elevated alkaline phosphatase levels.**
     d. **Urinary calcium losses** of >4 mg/kg/24 h are indicative of hypercalciuria.
     e. **Testing for vitamin D metabolites, parathyroid hormone (PTH) level, calcitonin, and genetic screening** (eg, Microarray for 22q deletion) should also be considered to find the etiology of hypocalcemia.

  2. **Imaging studies for bone demineralization, metaphyseal lucencies, and rib and long bone fractures** may be helpful for late hypocalcemia. More acutely, the absence of a thymic shadow on chest radiograph will suggest the DiGeorge sequence. For late-onset hypocalcemia and rickets, DEXA scan and quantitative ultrasonography using broadband ultrasonographic measurement, speed of sound (SOS), or bone transmission time have been employed to assess bone density.

  3. **Electrocardiographic studies** will identify arrhythmias due to QT interval changes.

G. **Management**

  1. **Acute treatment.** Reserved for symptomatic hypocalcemic infants with apneic spells, seizures, or cardiac failure with arrhythmia. Dosage is 100–200 mg/kg of 10% calcium gluconate *slowly* by peripheral IV over 15–20 minutes with constant cardiac monitoring (see Chapter 148 for dosing information).

  2. **Maintenance treatment.** For infants with limited enteral intake or who are dependent on parenteral calcium intake, an intravenous dosage of 45 mg/kg/d of elemental calcium with a calcium-phosphate ratio ranging from 1.3:1.0 to 2:1 is adequate for promoting both calcium and phosphate retention. Parenteral nutrition is usually started by day 2 or 3 of life. Intrauterine calcium source is

~140 mg/kg/d of elemental calcium. Parenteral fluids cannot approximate the intrauterine level of Ca^{+2} intake without some precipitation in solution. Therefore, early and continuous maintenance treatment is essential until milk or formula feeds can be successfully initiated.

3. **Vitamin D supplementation.** Should be started along with parenteral nutrition at 400 IU/d.

4. **Intravenous calcium administration.** This is not without some risk for complications. The potential problems include extravasation of calcium solution and resulting subcutaneous calcium deposition with limited joint movement, sloughing of skin, nephrocalcinosis, cardiac arrhythmias with prolonged QT intervals, or bradycardia if Ca^{+2} gluconate is given too quickly. Use of umbilical artery or vein is *not* recommended for administration of calcium solutions.

5. **Hypocalcemia secondary to blood/exchange transfusions.** This may require supplementation with Ca^{+2} gluconate. See Chapter 148 for dosing information and Chapter 30 for recommendations and dosage guidelines.

6. **Hypocalcemia secondary to diuretic therapy.** Infants receiving loop diuretics have an increased urinary loss of calcium. This loss can be demonstrated by urine calcium-creatinine ratio (>0.21–0.25). If hypercalciuria exists, an attempt should be made to substitute furosemide or bumetanide with chlorothiazide, or use in combination. Thiazide diuretics cause calcium retention and tend to offset the calciuric effect of loop diuretics. Caution is needed to guard against excessive potassium losses while compensating for diuretic effects on calcium.

H. **Prognosis.** No long-term effects of hypocalcemia treated in the neonatal period are seen as attributable to known adverse neurobehavioral or neurological outcomes of preterm or sick term infants. Decreased bone mineralization and the development of nephrocalcinosis are seen as long-term complications of calcium disorders. See Chapter 116 for more information on long-term hypocalcemia outcomes. Both hypocalcemia and hypomagnesemia have a generally good outcome if diagnosed promptly and treated adequately. The exception is a clinical presentation that includes seizures for either hypocalcemia or hypomagnesemia. Follow-up studies have suggested a 20% or greater incidence of neurological abnormalities.

II. **Hypercalcemia**

A. **Definition.** Hypercalcemia is defined as an **iCa^{+2} serum level >1.35 mmol/L (5.4 mg/dL)** for any infant, irrespective of a tCa serum level of more or less than 2.75 mmol/L (11.0 mg/dL). The iCa^{+2} level is the physiologically active component of serum Ca^{+2} and thus the most important determination. Although tCa^{+2} is indicative of hypercalcemia at levels >2.75 mmol/L, it is not a reliable measure.

B. **Incidence.** Uncommon and a specific occurrence rate is unknown. It occurs much less often in infants than adults.

C. **Pathophysiology.** Hypercalcemia may be due to parathyroid-related causes or to mechanisms unrelated to the parathyroid. A number of cases of hypercalcemia have recently been reported in neonatal units due to subcutaneous fat necrosis following therapeutic hypothermia as treatment for hypoxic ischemia encephalopathy. A number of cases of hypercalcemia are related to clinical management by way of excessive supplementation of vitamins A or D, calcium salts, or thiazide diuretics. A rare condition due to polymorphisms of calcium-sensing receptors can also result in hypercalcemia. Two forms involving calcium receptors are familial hypocalciuric hypercalcemia and neonatal hyperparathyroidism.

D. **Risk factors**

1. **Congenital hyperparathyroidism**

   a. **Primary.** Due to genetic defects as either familial hypocalciuria, hypercalcemia, or severe neonatal hyperparathyroidism.

   b. **Secondary.** Due to maternal hypoparathyroidism.

2. **Maternal hypocalcemia**

3. **Subcutaneous fat necrosis**

4. Therapeutic hypothermia
5. Idiopathic infantile hypercalcemia
6. William syndrome
7. Hypophosphatasia
8. Subcutaneous fat necrosis
9. Hyper- or hypothyroidism
10. Malignancy (very rare in the newborn)
11. Distal renal tubular acidosis, Jansen metaphyseal chondrodysplasia
12. Iatrogenic
   a. Hypophosphatemia due to inadequate dietary intake of phosphorus, especially in preterm infants
   b. Excessive vitamin D intake
   c. Excessive calcium intake
   d. Thiazide diuretics
   e. Extracorporeal life support
E. **Clinical presentation.** Mostly hypercalcemia is asymptomatic unless severe hypercalcemic levels have been reached and signs as described below appear.
   1. Feeding intolerance, constipation, failure to thrive
   2. Polyuria, dehydration
   3. Hematuria, nephrocalcinosis, nephrolithiasis
   4. Lethargy, hypotonia, seizures (rare, only in the most severe hypercalcemia)
   5. Bradycardia, short QT interval, hypertension
F. **Diagnosis**
   1. Laboratory studies
      a. Serum calcium for levels as given previously
      b. Serum total protein and albumin-globulin ratio for hypoproteinemia
      c. Blood gases for acid-base status
      d. Serum phosphorus for hypophosphatemia
      e. Urine calcium and phosphorus
      f. Parathyroid hormone, 25-hydroxy (OH) vitamin D, 1,25-OH vitamin D
      g. Thyroid studies
      h. Alkaline phosphatase for hypophosphatasia
      i. Serum creatinine
   2. Imaging studies
      a. Renal ultrasound for calcifications
      b. Long bone x-rays for demineralization secondary to hyperparathyroidism, or osteosclerotic lesions secondary to hypervitaminosis
G. **Management.** Treatment depends on the cause and severity of hypercalcemia. Hypercalcemia is usually mild, and a conservative approach is prudent. Immediate steps are to calculate calcium and vitamin D intake, and correct excess doses or discontinue. After hypercalcemia has been resolved, dietary calcium, phosphorus, and vitamin D intakes can be recalculated and administered according to basic daily requirements. An endocrine consult is recommended.
   1. Acute symptomatic hypercalcemia
      a. Discontinue any parenteral intake of calcium.
      b. Increase fluid intake as IV normal saline.
      c. Augment calcium loss (calciuria) using furosemide with intravenous saline intake; exercise caution to monitor urine output and serum electrolytes.
   2. Less acute but severe hypercalcemia. Consider:
      a. Calcitonin (limited newborn/neonatal experience).
      b. Glucocorticoids are effective on a short-term basis, but are not recommended.
      c. Intravenous bisphosphonates are promising (limited newborn/neonatal experience). Recently there have been some case reports of successful use of bisphosphonates in neonates for therapy of hypercalcemia occurring in infants receiving therapeutic hypothermia due to hypoxic ischemic encephalopathy (HIE).

3. **Refractory hypercalcemia.** In extreme situations, parathyroidectomy has been the last resort.

H. **Prognosis.** Hypocalcemia generally has good outcome if diagnosed promptly and treated adequately. The exception is a clinical presentation that includes seizures. Follow-up studies have suggested 20% or greater incidence of neurological abnormalities. If unrecognized and not treated, it may result in renal and central nervous system damage.

Selected References

Barrett H, McElduff A. Vitamin D and pregnancy: an old problem revisited. *Best Pract Res Clin Endocrinol Metab.* 2010;24(4):527–539.

Christensen SE, Nissen PH, Vestergaard P, Mosekilde L. Familial hypocalciuric hypercalcaemia: a review. *Curr Opin Endocrinol Diabetes Obes.* 2011;18(6):359–370.

Dupuy O, Aubert P, Dumuis ML, Bordier L, Mayaudon H, Bauduceau B. Hyperparathyroidism during pregnancy: dangerous association for the mother and her infant. *Rev Med Interne.* 2010;31(11):e9-e10.

Forsythe RM, Wessel CB, Billiar TR, Angus DC, Rosengart MR. Parenteral calcium for intensive care unit patients. *Cochrane Database Syst Rev.* 2008;(4):CD006163.

Hakan N, Aydin M, Zenciroglu A, et al. Alendronate for the treatment of hypercalcaemia due to neonatal subcutaneous fat necrosis. *Eur J Pediatr.* 2011;170(8):1085–1086; author reply, 1087 (Epub April 13, 2011).

Jacques R, Mohamed M, Mario D. Disorders of calcium, phosphorus and magnesium metabolism. In: Martin RJ, Fanaroff AA, Walsh MC, eds. *Fanaroff & Martin's Neonatal-Perinatal Medicine: Diseases of the Fetus and Infant.* 9th ed. Philadelphia, PA: Elsevier Mosby; 2011: 1523–1555.

Jatana V, Gillis J, Webster BH, Adès LC. Deletion 22q11.2 syndrome—implications for the intensive care physician. *Pediatr Crit Care Med.* 2007;8:459–463.

Patra S, Singh V, Pemde HK, Chandra J. Case series of neonatal hypocalcemia due to pseudo-hypoparathyroidism. *J Pediatr Endocrinol Metab.* 2010;23(10):1073–1075.

Strohm B, Hobson A, Brocklehurst P, Edwards AD, Azzopardi D; UK TOBY Cooling Register. Subcutaneous fat necrosis after moderate therapeutic hypothermia in neonates. *Pediatrics* 2011;128(2):e450–e452.

86 Chlamydial Infection

I. **Definition.** *Chlamydia trachomatis* is an obligate intracellular small Gram-negative bacterium that possesses a cell wall, contains DNA and RNA, and can be inactivated by several antimicrobial agents. It is the most common cause of sexually transmitted genital infections. It may cause urethritis, cervicitis, and salpingitis in the mother. In the infant, it can cause conjunctivitis and pneumonia.

II. **Incidence.** The prevalence of *C. trachomatis* in pregnant women varies from 2–15%. The risk of infection to infants born to infected mothers is high; conjunctivitis occurs in 25–50% and pneumonia in 5–20%. In the Netherlands, where prenatal screening is not routine, one study showed *C. trachomatis* to be responsible for 64% of all cases of neonatal conjunctivitis.

III. **Pathophysiology.** *Chlamydia trachomatis* subtypes B and D through K cause the sexually transmitted form of the disease and the associated neonatal infection. They frequently cause a benign subclinical infection. The infant acquires infection during vaginal delivery through an infected cervix. Infection after cesarean delivery is rare and usually occurs with early rupture of amniotic membranes; however, infection associated with intact membranes has been reported. Population-based studies suggest that maternal *C. trachomatis* infection is associated with an increased risk of preterm delivery and premature rupture of membranes.

IV. **Risk factors.** Risk is inversely proportional to gestational age. Risk factors include vaginal delivery of an infant with an infected mother and cesarean delivery with early rupture of the amniotic membranes of an infected mother.

V. **Clinical presentation**

   A. **Conjunctivitis.** See Chapter 53.

   B. **Pneumonia.** This is one of the most common forms of pneumonia in the first 3 months of life. The respiratory tract may be directly infected during delivery. Approximately half of infants presenting with pneumonia have concurrent or previous conjunctivitis. Pneumonia usually presents at 3–11 weeks of life. The infants experience a gradual increase in symptoms over several weeks. Initially, there is often 1–2 weeks of mucoid rhinorrhea followed by cough and increasing respiratory rate. More than 95% of cases are afebrile. The cough is characteristic, paroxysmal, and staccato, and it interferes with sleeping and eating. Approximately a third of infants have otitis media. Preterm infants may present with apneic spells. *Chlamydia trachomatis* has been isolated from tracheal secretions of preterm infants with pneumonia in the first week after birth.

VI. **Diagnosis**

   A. **Laboratory studies**

      1. **Tissue culture.** Because chlamydiae are obligate intracellular organisms, culture specimens must contain epithelial cells. **Culture of the organism** is the **gold standard** for diagnosing neonatal conjunctivitis and pneumonia. The specificity and sensitivity of culture is nearly 100% with adequate sampling and transport. Material should be obtained from the tarsal conjunctiva (for conjunctivitis) or from nasopharyngeal aspiration or deep suctioning of the trachea (for suspected pneumonia).

      2. **Nucleic acid amplification tests (NAAT).** These use methods to amplify *C. trachomatis* DNA or RNA sequences. Currently available tests are polymerase chain reaction (Amplicor), transcription-mediated amplification (Aptima Combo 2), and strand displacement amplification (ProbeTec). These tests are approved by the U.S. Food and Drug Administration (FDA) to be used in adults (largely replaced tissue culture as the diagnostic method of choice), but no sufficient data are available in infants.

      3. **Antigen detection tests.** Include **direct fluorescent antibody** and **enzyme immunoassay** tests. These tests appear to be sensitive and specific when used with conjunctival specimens, but the sensitivity with nasopharyngeal samples is poor. These tests are used infrequently and have largely been replaced by **NAAT**.

      4. **Serum anti-chlamydial antibody (IgM) concentration.** Difficult to determine and not widely available. In children with pneumonia, a titer >1:32 is diagnostic of infection.

      5. **Other tests.** In cases of pneumonia, the white blood cell count is normal, but there is **eosinophilia** in 70% of cases. Blood gas measurements show mild to moderate hypoxemia.

   B. **Imaging and other studies.** In cases of pneumonia, the chest radiograph may reveal hyperexpansion of the lungs, with bilateral diffuse interstitial or alveolar infiltrates.

VII. **Management.** Isolation precautions for all infectious diseases, including maternal and neonatal precautions, breast-feeding, and visiting issues, can be found in Appendix F.

A. **Prevention.** In high-risk populations, identification and treatment of infected mothers can prevent disease in the infant. The U.S. Centers for Disease Control and Prevention (CDC) recommends that all pregnant women be screened for chlamydia at the first prenatal visit. Women under age 25 and those at increased risk for chlamydial infection should have repeat testing in the third trimester. Infants born to mothers known to have untreated chlamydial infection should be monitored clinically. Prophylactic antimicrobial treatment is no longer recommended because the efficacy of such therapy is unknown. Additionally, oral erythromycin, the agent most commonly used, is associated with significant risk for **infantile hypertrophic pyloric stenosis (IHPS)**.

B. **Conjunctivitis.** Treated with oral erythromycin base or ethylsuccinate (50 mg/kg/d in 4 divided doses) for 14 days. Topical therapy is ineffective and unnecessary.

C. **Pneumonia.** Also treated with erythromycin, 50 mg/kg/d in 4 divided doses for 14 days. This not only shortens the clinical course but decreases the duration of nasopharyngeal shedding. Because the efficacy of erythromycin therapy is ~80%, a second course may be required, and follow-up of infants is recommended. Limited data on **azithromycin** therapy for treatment of *C. trachomatis* infections in infants suggest that dosing of 20 mg/kg as a single daily dose for 3 days may be effective. The mother and her sexual partner(s) should be evaluated and treated. **IHPS** may occur when infants are treated with erythromycin in the first 2 weeks of life. Because alternative therapies for *C. trachomatis* in the newborn are not well studied, the American Academy of Pediatrics and CDC continue to recommend erythromycin to treat neonatal chlamydia infection. Parents should be informed about the signs and potential risks of developing IHPS. Cases of IHPS after the use of oral erythromycin should be reported to MedWatch, the FDA Safety Information and Adverse Event Reporting Program. No isolation measures are necessary.

VIII. **Prognosis.** Infants who are diagnosed and treated early generally recover. Experimental studies suggest that neonatal chlamydial pneumonia, especially in preterm neonates, may cause airway hyperreactivity and respiratory dysfunction that continues into adulthood.

Selected References

American Academy of Pediatrics. Chlamydial trachomatis. In: Pickering LK, Baker CJ, Kimberlin DW, Long SS, eds. *Red Book: 2012 Report of the Committee on Infectious Diseases.* 29th ed. Elk Grove Village, IL: American Academy of Pediatrics; 2012:253–259.

Darville T. Chlamydial infections. In: Remington JS, Klein JO, Wilson CB, Nizet V, Maldonado Y, eds. *Infectious Diseases of the Fetus and Newborn Infant.* Philadelphia, PA: Elsevier Saunders; 2011:600–606.

Jupelli M, Murthy AK, Chaganty BK, et al. Neonatal chlamydial pneumonia induces altered respiratory structure and function lasting into adult life. *Lab Invest.* 2011;91:1530–1539.

Maheshwai N. Are young infants treated with erythromycin at risk for developing hypertrophic pyloric stenosis? *Arch Dis Child.* 2007;92:271–273.

Rours IG, Hammerschlag MR, Ott A, et al. Chlamydia trachomatis as a cause of neonatal conjunctivitis in Dutch infants. *Pediatrics.* 2008;121:e321–326.

Workowski KA, Berman S; Centers for Disease Control and Prevention (CDC). Sexually transmitted diseases treatment guidelines, 2010. *MMWR Recomm Rep.* 2010; 59:1–110.

87 Coagulation Disorders

Bleeding and thrombosis are the 2 extremes of the physiological process of coagulation disorders. Despite major differences in the levels of individual components of the hemostatic system, neonatal coagulation is equal to or somewhat more rapid than that observed in adults. This suggests the existence of a delicately balanced hemostatic system in neonates, with uncommon bleeding or thrombosis in healthy term infants. However, a number of perinatal or neonatal conditions can disrupt this balance and increase the risk for either hemorrhage or thrombus formation. The presence of bleeding in a healthy term or late preterm infant, especially in an infant with a normal platelet count, is strongly suggestive of a congenital bleeding disorder. **Hemophilia A and B and von Willebrand disease** account for 95–98% of congenital bleeding disorders.

Principles of Hemostasis

I. **Normal physiology of hemostasis**

   A. **The primary phase.** The production of the platelet plug. This involves platelet adhesion (to the injured vessel's subendothelium) and their activation mediated by platelet surface glycoprotein (Ib, IIb/IIa) and von Willebrand factor (vWF).

   B. **The secondary phase.** Results in the formation of a cross-linked fibrin clot. Coagulation proteins (factor XII to V) circulating as inactive precursor forms (zymogens) are converted to active forms through limited proteolysis. These activated proteins then further activate other zymogen factors in a chain reaction. Ultimately, the activation of factors V and X leads to cleavage of prothrombin (factor II) to thrombin (factor IIa). Cleavage of fibrinogen (factor I) to fibrin (factor Ia) by thrombin results in the formation of the blood clot.

   C. **The third phase.** Modulates and limits the interactions of activated platelets and the clotting cascade (and Ca^{+2}) that give rise to a clot. This includes the removal of activated factors (through the reticuloendothelial system) and the control of activated procoagulants by natural antithrombotic pathways (antithrombin III, protein C, protein S). Furthermore, restoration of vessel patency is triggered by the fibrinolytic pathway that generates plasmin from plasminogen. This is stimulated by tissue plasminogen activator and limited by α_2-antiplasmin and plasminogen activator inhibitor (PAI). Plasmin is a proteolytic enzyme that degrades fibrin into fibrin split products such as D-dimers. Defects in fibrinolytic factors that result in excessive plasmin generation can lead to bleeding.

II. **Newborn hemostasis**

   A. **Neonatal platelets** are reported to be hypo-reactive; however, this deficiency is balanced by increased vWF activity, resulting in overall normal platelet function.

   B. **Factor VIII, factor V, fibrinogen, and factor XIII levels are normal at birth.**

   C. **Vitamin K–dependent (factors II, VII, IX, and X) and contact factors (XI and XII) are reduced to about 50% of normal adult values** and are further reduced in preterm infants. Similarly, concentrations of the naturally occurring anticoagulants antithrombin, protein C, and protein S are low at birth. As a consequence, both thrombin generation and thrombin inhibition are reduced in the newborn period.

   D. **Neonatal fibrinolytic activity is intact,** despite the decreased concentrations and functional activity of plasminogen. Very low levels of histidine-rich glycoprotein (a physiologic inhibitor of plasminogen binding) and delayed inactivation of neonatal plasmin partially compensate for the reduced plasmin capacity. On the other hand, the increased plasma levels of PAI may explain the high rate of thromboembolic phenomena associated with intravascular devices in newborns. Most coagulation factors reached adult levels by 6 months of life with the exception of protein C levels, which remain low until later in childhood.

III. **Hemostatic testing in neonates.** Correct interpretation of coagulation tests in the newborn is fraught with difficulties. The following precautions are needed for the appropriate interpretation of neonatal coagulation testing.

   A. **Gestational and postnatal age reference ranges.** Vital to adequately interpret coagulation results in preterm and term neonates (Table 87–1).

   B. **A free-flowing blood specimen.** Needs to be obtained from an atraumatic venipuncture. Samples obtained through intravascular catheters may be contaminated with heparin as it adheres tightly to the walls of the tubing. This sample contamination with trace amounts of heparin will result in a prolonged activated partial thromboplastin time (aPTT) and sometimes prothrombin time (PT), unless heparin is degraded in the specimen. Additionally, small clots can form within the catheter or at the tip, resulting in consumption of clotting factors and alteration of coagulation testing. Difficult venipuncture can hamper sample integrity and lead to platelet clumping that produces a falsely low platelet count.

   C. **Special sample tubes should be prepared for coagulation testing in infants with a hematocrit >55% or <25%.** This allows for a correct amount of anticoagulant to be added to the blood sample (citrate-to-blood ratio of 1:9). Similarly, an insufficient filling of adequately citrated tube (<80%) can produce falsely prolonged coagulation time.

   D. **A stepwise approach to the neonate with suspected coagulation disorders is key to a correct diagnosis.**

      1. **Initial screening.** Consists of a complete blood count (CBC) with platelets, PT/international normalized ratio (INR), aPTT, and fibrinogen level.

      2. **Prolonged PT.** Reflects decreased plasma concentrations of vitamin K–dependent factors.

      3. **Prolonged aPTT.** Results from decreased plasma levels of contact factors (V and VIII to XI) as well.

      4. **Bleeding neonate who has no laboratory abnormality.** Factor XIII and α_2-antiplasmin activity should be assessed.

      5. **D-dimers.** Elevated as an acute phase reaction in all patients with infection or systemic inflammatory response syndrome (SIRS). A negative D-dimer assay is relatively accurate in ruling out thrombosis.

IV. **Bleeding disorders in neonates**

   A. **Clinical presentation.** Persistent oozing from the umbilical stump, excessive bleeding from peripheral venipuncture/heelstick sites, large caput succedaneum and cephalhematoma or subgaleal hemorrhage occurring without significant birth trauma history, and prolonged bleeding following circumcision are common presentations of neonatal bleeding disorders. The presence of an intracranial hemorrhage in a term or late preterm infant without history of birth trauma should be investigated for possible coagulation defect. Gastrointestinal bleeding must be distinguished from swallowed maternal blood (see page 387). Pulmonary hemorrhages are most frequently hemorrhagic pulmonary edema not associated with specific coagulation anomaly. Similarly, major abdominal organ bleeding such as liver or spleen are more often related to traumatic injury or local lesion (such as teratoma) than any coagulopathy.

   B. **Maternal, family, and neonatal history.** A history of any prior pregnancies and their outcomes can be a clue for disorders such as neonatal alloimmune thrombocytopenia. Maternal medication use can also lead to immune-mediated thrombocytopenia. Parental ethnic background and whether there is consanguinity are significant. However, absence of family history for a bleeding disorder cannot exclude occurrence of severe bleeding disorders. Perinatal complications can result in coagulation activation and disseminated intravascular coagulation (DIC). Although giving vitamin K to neonates is almost a universal routine, it is still important to ascertain that the vitamin K was indeed administered.

   C. **Physical examination.** An otherwise normal neonate with thrombocytopenia is suggestive of alloimmune thrombocytopenia. Skeletal abnormalities such as absence of

Table 87–1. REFERENCE VALUES FOR COAGULATION STUDIES IN HEALTHY FULL-TERM AND PRETERM INFANTS DURING THE FIRST 30 DAYS OF LIFE

Tests	Healthy Full Term (Mean ± SD)			Healthy Preterm (30–36 wk) Infant: Mean (range)		
	Day 1	Day 5	Day 30	Day 1	Day 5	Day 30
PT (seconds)	13.0 ± 1.43	12.4 ± 1.46	11.8 ± 1.25	13 (10.6–16.2)	12.5 (10.0–15.3)	11.8 (10.0–13.6)
aPTT (seconds)	42.9 ± 5.80	42.6 ± 8.62	40.4 ± 7.42	53.6 (27.5–79.4)	50.5 (26.9–74.1)	44.7 (26.9–62.5)
TCT (seconds)	23.5 ± 2.38	23.1 ± 3.07	24.3 ± 2.44	24.8 (19.2–30.4)	24.1 (18.8–24.4)	24.4 (18.8–29.9)
Fibrinogen (g/mL)	2.83 ± 0.58	3.12 ± 0.75	2.70 ± 0.54	2.43 (1.50–3.73)	2.8 (1.60–4.18)	2.54 (1.50–4.14)
Factor II (U/mL)	0.48 ± 0.11	0.63 ± 0.15	0.68 ± 0.17	0.45 (0.20–0.77)	0.57 (0.29–0.85)	0.57 (0.36–0.95)
Factor V (U/mL)	0.72 ± 0.18	0.95 ± 0.25	0.98 ± 0.18	0.88 (0.41–1.44)	1 (0.46–1.54)	1.02 (0.48–1.56)
Factor VII (U/mL)	0.66 ± 0.19	0.89 ± 0.27	0.90 ± 0.24	0.67 (0.21–1.13)	0.84 (0.30–1.38)	0.83 (0.21–1.45)
Factor VIII (U/mL)	1.00 ± 0.39	0.88 ± 0.33	0.91 ± 0.33	1.11 (0.50–2.13)	1.15 (0.53–2.05)	1.11 (0.50–1.99)
vWF (U/mL)	1.53 ± 0.67	1.40 ± 0.57	1.28 ± 0.69	1.36 (0.78–2.10)	1.33 (0.72–2.19)	1.36 (0.66–2.16)
Factor IX (U/mL)	0.53 ± 0.19	0.53 ± 0.19	0.51 ± 0.15	0.35 (0.19–0.65)	0.42 (0.14–0.74)	0.44 (0.13–0.80)
Factor X (U/mL)	0.40 ± 0.14	0.49 ± 0.15	0.59 ± 0.14	0.41 (0.11–0.71)	0.51 (0.19–0.83)	0.56 (0.20–0.92)
Factor XI (U/mL)	0.38 ± 0.14	0.55 ± 0.16	0.63 ± 0.13	0.3 (0.08–0.52)	0.41 (0.13–0.69)	0.43 (0.15–0.71)
Factor XII (U/mL)	0.53 ± 0.29	0.47 ± 0.18	0.49 ± 0.16	0.38 (0.10–0.66)	0.39 (0.09–0.69)	0.43 (0.11–0.75)
Prekallikrein (U/mL)	0.37 ± 0.16	0.48 ± 0.14	0.57 ± 0.17	0.33 (0.09–0.57)	0.45 (0.26–0.75)	0.59 (0.31–0.87)
HMW-K (U/mL)	0.54 ± 0.24	0.74 ± 0.28	0.77 ± 0.22	0.49 (0.09–0.89)	0.62 (0.24–1.00)	0.64 (0.16–1.12)
Factor XIIIa (U/mL)	0.79 ± 0.26	0.94 ± 0.25	0.93 ± 0.27	0.7 (0.32–1.08)	1.01 (0.57–1.45)	0.99 (0.51–1.47)
Factor XIIIb (U/mL)	0.76 ± 0.23	1.06 ± 0.37	1.11 ± 0.36	0.81 (0.35–1.27)	1.1 (0.68–1.58)	1.07 (0.57–1.57)
Plasminogen (U/mL)	1.95 ± 0.35	2.17 ± 0.38	1.98 ± 0.36	1.7 (1.12–2.48)	1.91 (1.21–2.61)	1.81 (1.09–2.53)

SD, standard deviation.
Adapted and reproduced, with permission, from Andrew M, Monagle PT, Brooker L. *Thromboembolic Complications During Infancy and Childhood*. Hamilton, Ontario: BC Decker; 2000.

thumb or radii are important clues for conditions such as thrombocytopenia with absent radii or Fanconi anemia. Cardiac defects may be associated with factor V deficiency. Delayed cord separation and persistent oozing from the umbilical stump is typical for infants with defective fibrinogen production or function and factor XIII deficiency. Acquired consumptive coagulopathy is generally a secondary event in a "sick" acting infant. Bacterial or viral infection and metabolic disorders (such as tyrosinemia) are a few of the conditions that need to be then considered.

Inherited Bleeding Disorders: Hemophilia A and B

I. **Definition.** Hemophilia A and B are inherited as sex-linked (X chromosome) recessive traits and are characterized by deficiencies of factor VIII or IX. However, one-third of cases will occur in the absence of a positive family history. Factor VIII deficiency is 5 times as common as factor IX deficiency.

II. **Incidence.** Hemophilia A occurs in 1 per 5000 males, and hemophilia B occurs in 1 per 25,000 males; very rare in females.

III. **Pathophysiology.** Deficiency of factor VIII or IX interferes with coagulation cascade.

IV. **Risk factors.** Male sex, family history of hemophilia or bleeding disorders.

V. **Clinical presentation.** The pattern of hemophilia-associated bleeding differs from that seen in older children. Hemarthroses are rare and many bleeds are iatrogenic in origin (eg, oozing or hematoma following venipuncture or vitamin K IM administration, prolonged bleeding following circumcision). Major bleeding, both intracranial (mostly subdural) and extracranial, is also occasionally seen. **Severe factor VIII deficiency (factor VIII activity <1%)** is the most common congenital coagulation disorder to present in the neonatal period. A third of cases will present with bleeding manifestations during the first month of life.

VI. **Diagnosis.** Screening coagulation test shows a prolonged aPTT while PT and platelets counts are within normal range. Factor VIII normally approaches adult level at birth, thus a low level reliably diagnoses hemophilia A. On the other hand, the diagnosis of moderate hemophilia B requires testing beyond the neonatal age as factor IX levels are low at birth (≈15%), reaching adult values at 2–6 months.

VII. **Management**

A. **The treatment for hemophilia A or B is recombinant factor VIII or factor IX concentrate, respectively.** Fresh frozen plasma should be used only in the instance of acute hemorrhage when confirmatory testing is not yet available.

B. **Desmopressin (DDAVP) has been used for mild hemophilia A and for von Willebrand disease type 1 or 2 to increase release of factor VIII and vWF from endothelial stores.** The antifibrinolytic agents ε-aminocaproic acid (Amicar) and tranexamic acid can be used in mucocutaneous bleeding to stabilize the fibrin clot and retard fibrinolysis. These agents are contraindicated in hematuria because of concerns about obstruction of urine flow by thrombi.

VIII. **Prognosis.** In most Western countries, people with hemophilia have a life expectancy not different from that of the male population without hemophilia. The optimal schedule for lifelong prophylaxis treatment continues to be *controversial* and onerous, and the development of inhibitors to factor VIII is still a major unresolved problem.

Inherited Bleeding Disorders: von Willebrand Disease

von Willebrand Disease (vWD) rarely presents during the neonatal period, because healthy neonates have higher plasma concentrations of von Willebrand factor (vWF) activity and an increased proportion of high-molecular-weight vWF multimers compared with adults. The condition is divided into 3 types. Type 3, an autosomal recessive disorder where vWF concentrations are almost absent, is the only type presenting with severe neonatal bleeding.

Inherited Bleeding Disorders: Isolated Factor II, VII, X, VIII, or XIII Deficiencies

Isolated factor II, VII, X, VIII, or XIII deficiencies can present in the neonatal period. These rare coagulation deficiencies have an autosomal recessive inheritance (except factor XIII) and present with abnormal coagulation screening tests.

Acquired Bleeding Disorders: Hemorrhagic Disease of the Newborn

 I. **Definition.** Vitamin K deficiency bleeding in the newborn.
 II. **Incidence.** Rare in the United States with routine administration of vitamin K.
 III. **Pathophysiology.** Vitamin K, a fat-soluble vitamin, is required for γ-carboxylation of glutamic acid residues on precursors of vitamin K–dependent coagulation proteins (factors II, VII, IX, X, C, and S). Vitamin K exists in 2 forms: vitamin K_1 or phylloquinone (the plant form of the vitamin) and vitamin K_2, a series of compounds synthesized by bacteria and referred to as menaquinones. In contrast to human milk, infant formula contains large amounts of vitamin K (10 vs 65–100 mcg/L). Newborn infants are at risk for vitamin K deficiency because of vitamin K's poor placental transfer, insufficient endogenous production from the intestinal bacterial flora prior to complete colonization of the neonatal colon, and inadequate dietary intake among solely breast-fed infants.
 IV. **Risk factors.** Additional risk factors are liver disease, cholestasis, and maternal short-gut syndrome.
 V. **Clinical presentation**
   A. **Mild vitamin K deficiency.** Manifests as an isolated prolongation of PT, with more severe deficiency characterized by prolongation of aPTT. The diagnosis can be confirmed by high serum level of abnormal form of prothrombin (PIVKA-II).
   B. **Early vitamin K deficiency bleeding (VKDB).** Occurs in the first 24 hours among infants born to mothers on oral anticoagulants, anticonvulsants, or anti-tuberculosis therapy and presents generally as serious bleeding such as intracranial hemorrhage (ICH).
   C. **Classic disease.** Presents between days 1 and 7 with gastrointestinal bleeding, ICH, skin bruising, and bleeding following circumcision and tends to occur in infants who did not receive vitamin K at birth and are breast-fed or receiving inadequate overall milk intake. In the absence of vitamin K prophylaxis, the incidence of classic VKDB is 0.25–1.7%.
   D. **Late VKDB.** Presents between 2 and 12 weeks of life. These infants are exclusively breast-fed infants who received none or only one oral dose of vitamin K, or have an associated disease process that interferes with the absorption or supply of vitamin K (intestinal malabsorption defects, cholestatic jaundice, cystic fibrosis, biliary atresia, α_1-antitrypsin deficiency). The majority of cases of late VKDB, whose incidence is 4–7 per 100,000 births, present with ICH.
 VI. **Diagnosis.** No routine test is diagnostic. Increased PT with normal platelets and fibrinogen levels are typical.
 VII. **Management**
   A. **Infants who present with a non–life-threatening bleed only need to be treated with vitamin K_1** given slowly by IV/SQ (no intramuscular [IM] injection) at a dose of 250–300 mcg/kg to restore PT to 30–50% of its normal value within an hour.
   B. **Treatment of serious bleeding** includes fresh frozen plasma (FFP) (20 mL/kg), a prothrombin complex concentrate (50 U/kg), or recombinant factor VIIa (100 mcg/kg).

C. **The American Academy of Pediatrics recommends** that all infants receive 1 mg of IM vitamin K on the first day of life (0.3 mg for infants <1000 g and 0.5 mg for infants >1000 g but <32 weeks). This single parenteral dose prevents both classic and late VKDB.

D. **The safety of IM vitamin K was questioned** because of its reported possible association with increased incidence of childhood cancer. Subsequent studies have disproved this risk. Nevertheless, an alternative oral regimen of 2 mg dose at birth followed by a 1 mg dose given weekly for 3 months has been suggested. Its efficacy has not been well established.

VIII. **Prognosis.** Depends on the severity and location of the bleeding.

Acquired Bleeding Disorders: Disseminated Intravascular Coagulation

I. **Definition.** Disseminated intravascular coagulation (DIC) is the result of excessive and inappropriate activation of the hemostatic system related to exposure of blood to a source of tissue factor. It is a secondary manifestation of an underlying problem such as bacterial or viral infection, asphyxia, or necrosis.

II. **Incidence.** The most common causes of DIC in the newborn are sepsis, severe respiratory distress syndrome, asphyxia, and necrotizing enterocolitis.

III. **Pathophysiology.** Massive thrombin generation with widespread fibrin deposition and consumption of coagulation proteins and platelets leads to multiple organ dysfunction.

IV. **Risk factors.** Concurrent bacterial or viral infection, asphyxia, or necrosis.

V. **Clinical presentation.** The presence of DIC in a neonate without any evidence of sepsis or history of asphyxia should warrant the evaluation for a capillary hemangioma.

VI. **Diagnosis.** The diagnosis of DIC is made in an ill neonate with thrombocytopenia, prolonged PT and aPTT, reduced fibrinogen, and increased D-dimers.

VII. **Management**

A. **The most important therapeutic intervention is to treat the underlying cause of the DIC.**

B. **Focus on the acute hematologic management is to support adequate hemostasis to limit hemorrhage.** This is usually achieved with platelet transfusions, FFP, or cryoprecipitate, with a goal of maintaining platelets >50,000–100,000/μL, PT <3 seconds above the upper limit of normal, and fibrinogen >100 mg/dL.

C. **Anticoagulant therapy is not generally used.** The benefit has not proved to outweigh the added risk for hemorrhage.

D. **The use of activated protein C is** *controversial* **(increased risk of ICH).**

E. **Recombinant factor VIIa (rFVIIa; 40–300 mcg/kg).** This has been used successfully to treat severe bleeding in infants with DIC. In the presence of endothelial damage, rFVIIa binds to exposed tissue factor to activate factor X and thus generate thrombin. The potential for thrombotic complications makes its use limited to life-threatening hemorrhagic situations.

VIII. **Prognosis.** Related to the underlying cause of the DIC.

Acquired Bleeding Disorders: Liver Disease

Vitamin K–dependent factors (II, VII, IX, and X) as well as factor V are synthesized by the liver, and hepatic damage can result in their lower levels. The diagnosis of acute liver disease should include elevated liver enzymes, direct hyperbilirubinemia, and elevated ammonia concentration. A low factor VII associated with low factor V will distinguish between vitamin K deficiency and hepatic dysfunction. A normal factor VIII may differentiate between liver disease and DIC where all clotting factors are depleted. On the other hand, liver disease may trigger DIC and ascites may lead to a loss of all clotting factors.

Acquired Bleeding Disorders: Extracorporeal Membrane Oxygenation/ Extracorporeal Life Support Related

Systemic anticoagulation with heparin is performed during the duration of extracorporeal membrane oxygenation/extracorporeal life support (ECMO/ECLS) to minimize the potential for clotting within the circuit. Monitoring to prevent bleeding complications is essential. This is done by the activated coagulation time (ACT), a rapid, whole blood point-of-care test. Patients are usually maintained close to a target time of 200 seconds.

Thromboembolic Disease in Neonates

Thrombotic complications are more frequent in neonates than in any other pediatric age group. Depending on the type of thrombosis and screening methods used, incidence of 0.5 events per 10,000 live births or 2.4 clinically apparent events (excluding stroke) per 1000 neonatal intensive care unit (NICU) admissions have been reported.

Arterial Thrombosis: Perinatal and Prenatal Arterial Ischemic Stroke

   I. Definition. An arterial ischemic stroke (AIS) is a cerebrovascular event occurring between 28 weeks of gestation and 28 days of birth with radiological or pathological evidence of focal arterial infarction of the brain.
  II. Incidence. The incidence of cerebral arterial occlusion may range from 0.5–1 per 1000 live births. Most occur within the middle cerebral artery of the left hemisphere.
 III. Pathophysiology. Paradoxical embolism (through the foramen ovale) from the fetal placental circulation is believed to be the most common etiology. Clotting activation originating from the placenta could release thrombin or small fibrin clots into the fetal circulation.
  IV. Risk factors. Twin-to-twin transfusion syndrome, fetal heart rate abnormality, and hypoglycemia are independent risk factors.
   V. Clinical presentation. Approximately 60% of the cases are perinatal AIS and present with symptoms in the first few days of life, chiefly seizures and apnea. **AIS is the second most common underlying etiology of neonatal seizures in the full-term newborn.** Presumed prenatal stroke, asymptomatic at birth, presents with asymmetrical motor development, hemiplegia, or seizures several months postnatally.
  VI. Diagnosis. Magnetic resonance imaging (MRI) with diffusion weighted imaging is the most sensitive technique for the early detection of acute cerebral infarction. Magnetic resonance angiography allows for the detection of thrombosed cerebral vessels. Cranial ultrasound has a poor sensitivity for the detection of AIS.
 VII. Management. In adults with AIS, recombinant tissue plasminogen activator (rTPA) has shown efficacy in restoring cerebral blood flow when delivered within 3 hours of its onset. In the neonate with AIS, the determination of time of onset is challenging, and there is currently no evidence for the efficacy of any form of anticoagulation treatment.
VIII. Prognosis. Many newborns with symptomatic AIS appear clinically normal after recovery from the acute event. On follow-up, one-third will exhibit hemiparesis and another third cognitive abnormalities affecting speech and language.

Arterial Thrombosis: Iatrogenic/Spontaneous Arterial Thrombosis

   I. Definition. Arterial thrombosis is classified as catheter related or non-catheter related.
  II. Incidence. Spontaneous arterial thrombosis is extremely rare. The incidence of catheter (mostly umbilical arterial catheter [UAC])–related thrombosis has been reported as being as high as 30% depending on the method used for diagnosis (such as ultrasound,

angiography). The incidence of major clinical symptoms attributable to UAC thrombus is ~1–5% of catheterized infants.

III. **Pathophysiology.** Arterial thrombosis usually involves the aorta and tends to mimic congenital heart disease (such as coarctation). Iatrogenic arterial thrombosis is mainly related to complications from indwelling catheters.

IV. **Risk factors.** Presence of UACs and peripheral arterial catheters.

V. **Clinical presentation.** Findings suggestive of an acute thrombosis include line dysfunction, extremity blanching and/or cyanosis, decreased pulse, and persistent thrombocytopenia.

VI. **Diagnosis.** Ultrasound Doppler is the method more frequently used in sick preterm infants, although contrast angiography may be more accurate when feasible.

VII. **Management**

A. **Suspicion or confirmation of an arterial thrombosis.** Warrants prompt removal of the catheter unless local instillation of TPA into the thrombus is contemplated.

B. **Recommendations for UAC-related thrombosis.** Treat with heparin. rTPA thrombolysis may be attempted for life-, limb-, or organ-threatening conditions (see page 595).

VIII. **Prognosis.** Most symptomatology attributed to thrombus formation will resolve with prompt removal of the catheter.

Arterial Thrombosis: Purpura Fulminans

I. **Definition.** Purpura fulminans (PF) is a rare syndrome of diffuse intravascular thrombosis and hemorrhagic infarction of the skin that is rapidly progressive and often fatal.

II. **Incidence.** The incidence of severe protein C deficiency is 1 per 1,000,000 live births.

III. **Pathophysiology.** Based on severe genetic (or acquired) protein C and/or protein S deficiency. Acquired PF may result from conditions triggering acute reduction of protein C activity such as bacterial infection.

IV. **Risk factors.** Protein C deficiency.

V. **Clinical presentation.** Extensive venous and arterial thrombosis with ecchymosis is present soon after delivery and can result in skin necrosis.

VI. **Diagnosis.** Laboratory tests yield results consistent with DIC (thrombocytopenia, hypofibrinogenemia, and increased PT and aPTT) and show no measurable protein C or S.

VII. **Management.** Early treatment is paramount for successful outcome and consists of FFP, protein C concentrate, or activated protein C and lifelong anticoagulation.

VIII. **Prognosis.** Purpura fulminans is associated with a high mortality rate.

Venous Thrombosis: Cerebral Sinovenous Thrombosis

I. **Definition.** Cerebral sinovenous thrombosis (CSVT) typically involves the thrombosis of cerebral veins or the dural sinus with cerebral parenchymal lesions or central nervous system (CNS) dysfunction.

II. **Incidence.** The incidence of CSVT has been reported as 0.4 per thousand live births.

III. **Pathophysiology.** Thrombophilic factors (Table 87–2) may play a role in perinatal stroke. The superior and lateral sinuses are the most frequently involved vessels, and up to 30% of cases have venous infarction with subsequent hemorrhage.

IV. **Risk factors.** Often associated with perinatal asphyxia, coagulopathy, maternal diabetes, and infection.

V. **Clinical presentation.** The symptoms of cerebral sinovenous thrombosis are those of a perinatal stroke and include seizures, apnea, and lethargy.

VI. **Diagnosis.** Diagnosis of CSVT is best made through diffusion MRI and MR venography.

Table 87–2. THROMBOPHILIC CONDITION MARKERS FOR THROMBOPHILIA AND PREVALENCE IN HEALTHY POPULATION

Condition/Marker	Testing Methods	Prevalence (%)
Genetic		
Factor V Leiden mutation	PCR	4–6
Prothrombin G20210A mutation	PCR	1–2
Elevated plasma lipoprotein (a)	ELISA	
Acquired or genetic		
Antithrombin deficiency	Chromogenic (functional) assay	0.019
Protein C deficiency	Chromogenic (functional) assay	0.023
Protein S deficiency	ELISA for free protein S antigen	0.037
Elevated factor VIII	One-stage clotting assay (aPTT based)	
MTHR enzyme gene mutation	Hyperhomocysteinemia	9
Maternal lupus	ELISA for antiphospholipid antibodies	
Activate protein resistance	Clotting assay (aPPT based)	

aPTT, activated partial thromboplastin time; ELISA, enzyme-linked immunosorbent assay; PCR, polymerase chain reaction.
Adapted and reproduced, with permission, from Goldenberg NA, Bernard TJ. Venous thromboembolism in children. *Hematol Oncol Clin North Am.* 2010;24:151–166.

VII. **Management.** Heparin anticoagulation is indicated only when there is evidence of thrombus propagation, multiple emboli, or a severe prothrombotic state, but is contraindicated in the presence of intracerebral hemorrhage.

VIII. **Prognosis.** Based on extent of cerebral defect.

Venous Thrombosis: Upper and Lower Venous System Deep Vein Thrombosis

I. **Definition.** Thrombus in a major vein in the upper or lower extremity with or without central extension.

II. **Incidence.** The true incidence of neonatal deep vein thrombosis (DVT) is difficult to determine and many central venous lines (CVLs) related to venous thrombosis are clinically "silent." Thrombosis and infection have been reported to occur in 2–22% of neonates with indwelling CVLs with a higher incidence reported in studies applying regular ultrasound screening.

III. **Pathophysiology.** Infants are at increased risk of thrombosis, with indwelling catheters further increasing the risk of venous thrombosis.

IV. **Risk factors.** Nearly one-third of cases are associated with systemic infection, while prematurity is also correlated with higher prevalence of DVT. Other risk factors may include polycythemia, dehydration, repair of congenital heart disease, and hypoxia and parenteral nutrition.

V. **Clinical presentation.** Upper or lower venous DVT in neonates may present as swelling and discoloration of the associated limb, swelling of the face and head, chylothorax, and superior vena cava syndrome. Thrombocytopenia may be present.

VI. **Diagnosis.** Doppler ultrasound is the technique most frequently used for confirmation of neonatal DVT, although a venogram might be a more sensitive diagnostic method.

VII. **Management**
   A. **Suspicion or confirmation of a venous thrombus.** This warrants prompt catheter removal. However, due to the risk for emboli, delaying CVL removal until 3 to 5 days after the start of anticoagulant therapy may be considered (*controversial*).

B. Anticoagulation and thrombolytic treatment is equally *controversial*. The decision needs to take into account the degree of threat to limbs or vital organs.
C. Role of thrombophilia screening in neonatal DVT. In light of its poor yield and the low risk and predictability of DVT recurrences, this remains ***controversial*** as well.
VIII. **Prognosis.** Short-term morbidities include pulmonary embolism and neonatal stroke from emboli or brain hemorrhagic infarction.

Venous Thrombosis: Right Atrial Thrombosis

I. **Definition.** Thrombosis of the superior vena cava (SVC) with extension into the right atrium.
II. **Incidence.** Right atrial thrombosis (RAT) accounts for 6% of all neonatal thromboses.
III. **Pathophysiology.** Despite early administration of aspirin, this has become a common complication in infants undergoing repair of complex congenital heart disease. There is a strong association of the location of the catheter tip in the right atrium and the development of RAT.
IV. **Risk factors.** The most important is an indwelling CVL. Other associated risk factors include prematurity, administration of parenteral nutrition (PN), sepsis, and congenital heart disease.
V. **Clinical presentation.** More than half of the cases are asymptomatic and are detected incidentally during echocardiography performed for other reasons such as investigation for a persistent infection focus. The remaining cases may present with respiratory distress, new heart murmur, heart failure symptoms, or tachyarrhythmia.
VI. **Diagnosis.** The diagnostic method of choice for RAT is echocardiography. Documentation of the size, mobility, and shape of the thrombus, as well as the concomitant cardiac function are essential in helping to decide on treatment and predict outcome.
VII. **Management**
A. **Asymptomatic and hemodynamically stable infants** with small, immobile RATs may need no treatment except close echocardiography follow-up.
B. **For symptomatic patient** or RATs that are large, mobile, pedunculated, or snake shaped, treatment should include systemic anticoagulation therapy.
C. **Thrombolytic therapy or surgical embolectomy** may be indicated in life-threatening conditions.
VIII. **Prognosis.** Thrombolytic therapy in preterm infant with infective endocarditis carries a high risk for intracranial hemorrhage.

Venous Thrombosis: Renal Vein Thrombosis

I. **Definition.** It is most common cause of non–catheter-associated thrombosis and usually presents in the first week of life.
II. **Incidence.** Renal vein thrombosis (RVT) accounts for up to 10% of venous thromboses in newborns.
III. **Pathophysiology.** Unilateral left-sided RVTs are the most common.
IV. **Risk factors.** Risk factors for the development of RVT include perinatal asphyxia, dehydration, maternal diabetes, and male sex.
V. **Clinical presentation.** The classic clinical triad of RVT includes hematuria, palpable abdominal mass, and thrombocytopenia. Other features include hypertension, proteinuria, and renal impairment. Patients with thrombus extension and caval occlusion may also develop bilateral lower limb edema.
VI. **Diagnosis.** The diagnosis of RVT is usually made via ultrasound (US) with Doppler. Ultrasonographic features of RVT include enlarged, echogenic kidneys with attenuation or loss of corticomedullary differentiation. Color flow Doppler shows absence of flow in the main or arcuate renal veins.
VII. **Management.** The treatment for RVT is ***controversial***. Renal outcomes appear to be similar between supportive treatment and anticoagulation therapy. Similar proportions

of affected kidneys that received supportive care or received anticoagulation became atrophic on follow-up. Possible exceptions to exclusive supportive treatment may include the following:

A. **Low molecular weight heparin (LMWH) therapy** for unilateral renal vein thrombosis with inferior vena cava extension for 6 weeks to 3 months. (See page 596.)

B. **Bilateral RVT with caval extension** may warrant thrombolytic therapy. (See page 597.)

VIII. **Prognosis.** Acute complications of RVT include adrenal hemorrhage, extension of the clot into the inferior vena cava (IVC), renal failure, hypertension, and death. Chronically, cortical or segmental infarction of the affected kidney and/or hypertension is common.

Venous Thrombosis: Portal Vein Thrombosis

I. **Definition.** Thrombus in the portal vein usually associated with umbilical vein catheterization.

II. **Incidence.** The incidence of portal vein thrombosis (PVT) has been reported as 3.6 per 1000 NICU admissions. The incidence of PVT in neonates associated with the insertion of umbilical venous catheters (UVCs) varies between 1 and 43% depending on imaging protocols.

III. **Pathophysiology.** Hypercoagulability of the newborn coupled with UVC entering the liver in an area of relatively low flow.

IV. **Risk factors.** Risk factors include umbilical infection as well as position of the tip of UVC. The UVC tip should be kept outside the low flow portal venous system and placed at the level of inferior vena cava/right atrium, or below the level of the umbilical-portal confluence. Its position needs to be ascertained by imaging.

V. **Clinical presentation.** Most thromboses in the portal venous system are clinically silent and spontaneously resolved within a short period of time after catheter removal.

VI. **Diagnosis.** Large studies have shown that PVT can usually be detected by ultrasound within the first week of a UVC insertion.

VII. **Management.** Use of anticoagulation is *controversial* (see Prognosis). For dosing see page 595.

VIII. **Prognosis.** Long-term outcome of neonatal PVT and whether anticoagulation has any benefit in the outcome is unknown. Left lobe atrophy and portal hypertension are the most important sequelae. PVT is the major cause of extrahepatic portal hypertension in children, and a history of neonatal umbilical venous catheterization is frequently found among those children.

Venous Thrombosis: Thrombophilia

I. **Definition.** Thrombophilia is a term used to describe known inherited or congenital blood coagulation disorders that may predispose to thrombosis.

II. **Incidence.** Rare.

III. **Pathophysiology.** Conditions that predispose to thrombophilia are noted in Table 87-2. Despite a high prevalence of multiple thrombophilic gene mutations, the majority of neonates with these traits do not develop thrombosis.

IV. **Risk factors.** Central venous and arterial catheters constitute the greatest acquired risk for the development of thromboembolic events (TEs) in neonates in addition to those noted in Table 87-2.

V. **Clinical presentation.** Thrombophilia should be considered in any neonate who presents with thrombotic events or extensive thrombosis in the absence of identifiable environmental risk factors (intravascular catheter, neonatal sepsis, or shock).

VI. **Diagnosis.** The evaluation of a neonate with a significant TE for a prothrombotic disorder is *controversial*.

VII. **Management.** See below.
VIII. **Prognosis.** Neonates with multiple traits of thrombophilia and symptomatic thrombosis are at an increased risk for thrombus recurrence, although those usually occur in the setting of other comorbidities, such as infection, surgery, or trauma.

Management of Thrombosis: General Guidelines

The optimal treatment modality for neonates with thrombosis is *controversial*. Information on treatment of neonatal thrombosis is limited to case reports and small case series. Dosing information is often extrapolated from children or adult data. Available options include observation, anticoagulation, thrombolytic therapy, and surgical thrombectomy. Treatment should be limited to clinically significant thrombosis with the goal of preventing clot expansion or embolism.

I. Unfractionated heparin (UFH)
   A. Pharmacology
      1. UFH is a heterogeneous mixture of negatively charged glycosaminoglycans with a molecular weight ranging from 5000 to 30,000 kDa. The anticoagulant properties are via conformational change in antithrombin (AT), converting it to a more efficient (1000-fold) inhibitor of factors IIa, IXa, Xa, XIa, and XIIa.
      2. The anticoagulant activity of heparin is variable because of the differential clearance of the various sizes of heparin moieties, as well as its propensity to bind to other positively charged noncoagulation proteins, as well as to platelets and endothelial surfaces.
      3. The most important anticoagulant actions of heparin are the potentiation of AT inhibition of thrombin (IIa) and factor Xa.
   B. Dosage. See Table 87–3.
      1. The half-life of UFH, secondary to increased clearance, is short in neonates. Infants with the most significant thromboses demonstrate the highest clearance.
      2. The efficacy of UFH might be decreased in neonates because of the physiologically low antithrombin plasma concentration. Antithrombin supplementation with FFP is sometimes suggested.
      3. Neonates require continuous intravenous therapy. Higher doses than those used in older patients are required to achieve therapeutic adult aPTT levels. Anticoagulation is recommended for 10–14 days.
   C. Monitoring
      1. The goal for anticoagulation is to maintain aPTT at 1.5–2 times the upper limit of age values. When feasible, anti–factor Xa level monitoring is preferable with its level kept at 0.3–0.7 U/mL.
      2. Following the initial dose, anti–factor Xa or aPTT level are assessed 4 or 6 hours later, respectively, and once daily thereafter. If the level of anticoagulation is below or above target values, the test is repeated 4–6 hours after appropriate dose adjustment. In general, a 10% rate adjustment is made when levels are inappropriate. An additional 50 U/kg may be given if aPTT is <50 seconds.

Table 87–3. **DOSAGE OF UNFRACTIONATED HEPARIN IS MODULATED ACCORDING TO POSTCONCEPTIONAL AGE**

Postconceptional Age	<28 Weeks	28–37 Weeks	>37 Weeks
Loading dose IV over 10 minutes	25 U/kg	50 U/kg	10 U/kg
Maintenance dose IV	15 U/kg/h	15 U/kg/h	28 U/kg/h

3. A CBC, platelet count, and coagulation screening (including aPTT, PT, and fibrinogen) should be performed before starting UFH therapy. Platelet count and fibrinogen levels should be repeated daily for 2–3 days once therapeutic levels are achieved and twice weekly thereafter.

D. Complications
   1. The most important adverse effect from heparin therapy is bleeding. A 2% risk has been reported in term infants, and the risk is higher among preterm infants.
   2. Accidental overdose of UFH is a major safety issue. This occurs when an inappropriately diluted, supposedly low-dose UFH is used to flush a vascular access device.
   3. Heparin-induced thrombocytopenia (HIT) rarely occurs in neonates.
   4. Treatment of hemorrhage
      a. Usually, due to the UFH's short half-life, it only requires cessation of the infusion.
      b. If bleeding continues following cessation of the infusion. A full coagulation assessment should be performed and hemostatic deficiencies replaced as indicated.
      c. Protamine. One milligram of protamine will neutralize 100 U of UFH. The amount to be administered is according to the time elapsed since the last heparin injection. A full neutralizing amount is to be given if that time was <30 minutes. This dose is reduced by 50% for every hour past the last time heparin had been given. A repeat aPTT is required 15 minutes later.

E. Advantages over LMWH
   1. Because of its short half-life, it can be used as the first-line agent in patients whose anticoagulation may need to be stopped rapidly.
   2. Antidote (protamine sulfate) is available.
   3. At doses below 100 U/kg, its elimination is unaffected by renal dysfunction.

II. Low molecular weight heparin
A. Pharmacology
   1. LMWH is a glycosaminoglycan of smaller molecular weight (2000–8000 kDa) than UFH. As such it lacks a binding site for thrombin.
   2. Primary action of LMWH. To potentiate the antithrombin inhibition of factor Xa with little effect on the antithrombin inhibition of thrombin. Consequently, aPTT is unaffected at therapeutic LMWH doses.

B. Dosage of LMWH (enoxaparin)
   1. Dosing recommendations for enoxaparin. 1.7 mg/kg every 12 hours in term neonates and 2.0 mg/kg every 12 hours in preterm neonates.
   2. LMWH can be administered by subcutaneous injection. Frequent needle pricks can be minimized with the use of an extremely low dead space subcutaneous catheter (Insuflon TM). Local bruising, induration, and leakage occur in 10% of neonates.

C. Monitoring. See Table 87–4.
   1. LMWH works largely by inhibiting factor Xa, thus dosing must be titrated to anti–factor Xa activity and not to the aPTT.
   2. The goal of treatment is to maintain an anti–factor Xa level of 0.5–1.0 U/mL.
   3. Levels should be obtained 4 hours after the second dose and then weekly.

D. Advantage over UFH. Low molecular weight heparin (specifically, enoxaparin) has become an increasingly popular alternative to UFH following studies in adults that demonstrated at least comparable efficacy and safety.
   1. Pharmacokinetics of LMWH are more predictable, making the need for monitoring less frequent.
   2. Lesser risk of bleeding complications.
   3. LMWH is given subcutaneously, which eliminates the requirement for intravenous access.

Table 87–4. **LMWH (ENOXAPARIN) ADJUSTMENT** [a]

Anti–Factor Xa Level (U/mL)	Hold Next Dose	Dose Change
>0.35	No	Increase by 25%
0.35–0.49	No	Increase by 10%
0.5–1.0	No	No change
1.1–1.5	No	Decrease by 20%
1.6–2.0	3 hours	Decrease by 30%
>2.0	Until anti–factor Xa 0.5/mL	Decrease by 40%

[a]A repeat anti–factor Xa needs to be measured after every individual adjustment.
Modified and reproduced, with permission, from Andrew M, de Veber G. *Pediatric Thromboembolism and Stroke Protocols*. Hamilton, Ontario: BC Decker; 1997.

    4. **LMWH has a lesser risk of heparin-induced thrombocytopenia** as well a reduced risk of osteoporosis that is associated with long-term use of UFH.

III. **Thrombolytic therapy.** The goal of thrombolytic therapy is to degrade fibrin and dissolve the fibrin clot. Systemic thrombolytic therapy should be strongly considered for clots that have a high risk of morbidity and mortality. The rate of vascular patency following anticoagulant therapy in older children has been reported at 50%; following thrombolysis, it is >90%.

  A. **Pharmacology**

    1. **Recombinant tPA,** which facilitates conversion of plasminogen to plasmin to enhance degradation of fibrin, fibrinogen, and factors V and VII; it is the most commonly used agent.

    2. **Systemic tPA is effective** when administered within 2 weeks of symptomatic clot onset and is only partially effective beyond 2 weeks.

    3. **Direct instillation of potent thrombolytic agents into clots via an infusion catheter** has been shown to result in significant increases in vessel patency rates in adults. It also carries the potential advantage of less exposure to the bleeding risks of systemic thrombolysis.

  B. **Dosage.** Based on a limited number of studies, the following protocol is proposed:

    1. **Systemic low doses.** Starting dose of 0.06 mg/kg/h with possible escalation up to 0.24 mg/kg/h over the next 48–96 hours.

    2. **Alternatively use one of the following local treatments:**

      a. **Bolus.** Initial dose of 0.5 mg/kg for 15 minutes to be followed by 0.1–0.4 mg/kg/h for a maximal period of 72 hours

      b. **Single dose.** 0.7 mg/kg over 30–60 minutes

    3. **Repeat echocardiogram/Doppler** every 6–8 hours to assess the presence of the clot to guide the escalation of thrombolytic treatment or its cessation.

    4. **Heparin.** Because thrombolysis does not inhibit clot propagation or directly affect hypercoagulability, simultaneous treatment with low-dose UFH (5–10 U/kg/h) or LMWH (0.5 mg/kg bid) is recommended.

    5. **Plasminogen supplementation.** Prolonged thrombolytic therapy is likely to exhaust the low plasminogen neonatal supplies more readily than in adults. With thrombolytic therapy lasting over 24 hours, consideration should be given to either monitoring plasminogen concentrations or empiric infusion of FFP (10–20 mL/kg) to optimize thrombolysis.

    6. **Fibrinogen.** Fibrinogen concentration decreases by 25–50% in response to systemic thrombolytic therapy. If fibrinogen concentrations are <100 mg/mL, dose reductions of the thrombolytic agent and infusion of replacement therapy in the form of cryoprecipitate or fresh frozen plasma should be considered.

    7. **Platelet counts.** Need to be maintained over 50,000.

8. D-dimer and fibrinogen degradation product (FDP) plasma concentrations are expected to increase as a response to effective thrombolytic action.
9. Daily head sonograms.
10. Avoid IM injections and urinary catheterizations.
C. Exclusion criteria for tissue plasminogen activator (TPA) thrombolysis
1. Major surgery or CNS bleeding within 10 days
2. Major asphyxial event within 7 days (usually birth asphyxia)
3. An invasive procedure within 72 hours
4. Seizures within 48 hours
D. Adverse effects
1. Bleeding complications have been reported in nearly two-thirds of pediatric patients; half of those patients required replacement blood transfusions.
2. Most frequently, bleeding is at sites of invasive procedures. Gastrointestinal, pulmonary, and intraventricular hemorrhages are reported in about 1% of term infants and 14% of preterm infants.
3. The frequency and severity of bleeding may be dose and duration (<6 hours) dependent.
4. Concurrent low-dose heparin treatment and FFP (10 mL/kg) given a half hour before each TPA infusion may lessen those bleeding risks.
IV. Surgical thrombectomy. The small size of neonatal blood vessels, the rarity of thrombosis in neonates, and the severity of illness in neonates with thrombosis preclude the use of surgical thrombectomy in the majority of neonates. However, with the use of microsurgical techniques combined with thrombolytic regimens, thrombectomy has been successfully used in neonates in isolated cases.

Selected References

Andrew M. The relevance of developmental hemostasis to hemorrhagic disorders of newborns. *Semin Perinatol.* 1997;21:7.

Bernard T, Goldenberg NA. Pediatric arterial ischemic stroke. *Hematol Oncol Clin North Am.* 2010;24:167.

Goldenberg NA, Manco-Johnson MJ. Pediatric hemostasis and use of plasma components. *Clin Haematol.* 2006;19:143.

Hartmann J, Hussein A, Trowitzsch E, Becker J, Hennecke KH. Treatment of neonatal thrombus formation with recombinant tissue plasminogen activator. *Arch Dis Child Fetal Neonatal Ed.* 2001;85:F18.

Jordan LC, Rafay MF, Smith SE, et al. Antithrombotic treatment in neonatal cerebral sinovenous thrombosis. *J Pediatrics.* 2010;156:704.

Lau K, Stoffman JM, Williams S, et al. Neonatal renal vein thrombosis: review of the English-language literature between 1992 and 2006. *Pediatrics.* 2007;120:e278.

Malowany J, Knoppert DC, Chan AK, Pepelassis D, Lee DS. Enoxaparin use in the neonatal intensive care unit: experience over 8 years. *Pharmacotherapy.* 2007;27:1263.

Monagle P, Chan A, Chalmers E, Michelson AD. Antithrombotic therapy in children. *Chest.* 2004;126;645S.

Raffini L. Thrombolysis for intravascular thrombosis in neonates and children. *Curr Opin Pediatr.* 2009;21:14.

Ramenghi L, Govaert P, Fumagalli M, Bassi L, Mosca F. Neonatal cerebral sinovenous thrombosis. *Semin Fetal Neonatal Med.* 2009;14:278.

Torres-Valdivieso MJ, Cobas J, Barrio C, et al. Successful use of tissue plasminogen activator in catheter-related intracardiac thrombus of a premature infant. *Am J Perinatology.* 2003;20:91.

Wang M, Hays T, Balasa V, et al. Low-dose tissue plasminogen activator thrombolysis in children. *J Pediatr Hematol Oncol.* 2003;25:379.

88 Common Multiple Congenital Anomaly Syndromes

I. **Definition. A congenital anomaly** is defined as a structural defect, present at birth and different from the norm. These anomalies can be further divided into **major anomalies** that require medical and surgical care (eg, congenital heart defect, cleft palate, meningomyelocele) and **minor anomalies** that do not have medical significance (eg, single palmar crease, epicanthal folds, fifth digit clinodactyly). Anomalies themselves can be classified based on the developmental process involved in their formation. Well-defined types of anomalies include malformations, deformations, disruptions, dysplasias, syndromes, associations, and sequences (Table 89–1). It is also important to understand that these may not be entirely mutually exclusive. Table 89–1 provides an overview of congenital anomalies that are associated with congenital heart disease, and Table 89–2 reviews the teratogens associated with some of these lesions.

II. **Incidence.** Among newborns, ~1–3% have more than one major congenital anomaly recognized at birth. These infants often have longer hospital stays and have increased mortality rates. Malformations can cause >20% of neonatal deaths.

III. **General approach to diagnosis.** In the management of multiple congenital anomaly (MCA) syndromes, the neonatologist must deal with complex clinical issues calling for a wide range of diagnostic skills. Without a correct diagnosis of MCA syndrome, many available forms of therapy go underused and others may be tried, although they will be relatively ineffective. Furthermore, unrealistic counseling may be given about prognosis and recurrence risk. Only a few common MCA syndromes are life-threatening in the neonatal period. It is important to note, however, that **malformations are the most common cause of death at this critical point** in the life span. Table 88–2 lists symptoms and signs that should alert the clinician to the possibility of cryptogenic malformations or disorders. Obviously, if overt malformations are present, an MCA syndrome will be immediately recognized and diagnostic efforts will shortly follow. However, if external features of the disorder are subtle or nonspecific and the usual procedures associated with intensive newborn support have been started, findings may go unrecognized early. Each manifestation listed in Table 88–2 is more common in infants with MCA syndromes. Underlying etiologies for MCA syndromes include chromosomal abnormalities, monogenic disorders, multifactorial disorders, and unknown. The diagnostic approach to MCA syndromes in neonates is no different from that in older children. Because so many of these children are intubated with multiple lines and tubes, detailed assessment of physical characteristics can be challenging. Clinical photographs are essential, especially when a clinical geneticist is not available locally. If specialists in these fields are not available, a telephone call to a university medical center for expert advice is often useful. If the infant is critically ill and suspicion for a MCA syndrome is present, looking for other major malformations is important (eg, echocardiogram, renal/abdominal ultrasound, brain imaging). **The basis for diagnosis of an MCA syndrome in a neonate involves a combination of defining the physical manifestations and diagnostic genetic testing.** Diagnostic problems can also occur because immediate efforts tend to emphasize therapy. Nevertheless, diagnosis will often facilitate or guide therapy more efficiently.

IV. **Genetic testing**

A. **Comparative genomic hybridization (CGH) or chromosomal microarray analysis (CMA).** A new but now well-established cytogenetic technique that can be used to detect chromosomal deletions or duplications. CGH/CMA is a fluorescent

Table 88–1. TYPES OF CONGENITAL ANOMALIES

Malformation: The morphologic defect of an organ or larger region of the body resulting from an intrinsically abnormal developmental process. A primary defect.

Deformation: An alteration in shape and or structure, caused by biomechanical forces that distort otherwise normally developing structure. A secondary defect.

Disruption: A structural defect resulting from an extrinsic insult to an originally normal developmental process.

Dysplasia: An abnormality in the organization or differentiation of cells within a specific tissue type that results in clinically apparent structural changes.

Syndrome: A recognizable pattern of anomalies considered to have a specific cause.

Association: A nonrandom, statistically significant association of multiple anomalies for which no specific etiology has been described.

Sequence: A pattern of multiple anomalies derived from a single abnormality followed by a cascade of secondary effects.

technique that compares a reference standard DNA to the patient's DNA. Depending on the laboratory and specific platform used, comparisons are made at hundreds to thousands of regions across the entire genome to assess for copy number differences between the 2 samples. CGH/CMA assesses for common microdeletion and microduplication regions, subtelomeric regions, and pericentromeric regions. This test is not only capable of diagnosing described chromosomal abnormalities, but it can also detect novel changes. Recently CGH/CMA testing has replaced high-resolution karyotyping as first-tier testing for infants with MCA.

B. **High-resolution karyotype.** This test typically involves the analysis of chromosomes obtained from white blood cells present in a peripheral blood sample and is unaffected by a red blood cell transfusion. This process can take up to 2 weeks for completion. Differences in chromosomal number, large chromosomal deletions or duplications, and translocations can be detected with this test. This test remains the standard for confirming a well-recognized clinical phenotype (eg, Down syndrome), but has been replaced by CGH/CMA as the first-line test for infants with MCA.

Table 88–2. SYMPTOMS AND SIGNS IN NEONATES THAT MIGHT INDICATE A MULTIPLE CONGENITAL ANOMALY SYNDROME

Prenatal
Oligohydramnios
Polyhydramnios
Decreased or unusual fetal activity
Abnormal fetal problem/position

Postnatal
Abnormalities of size: small for gestational age or large for gestational age, microcephaly or macrocephaly, large or irregular abdomen, small chest, limb-trunk disproportion, asymmetry
Abnormalities of tone: hypotonia, hypertonia
Abnormalities of position: joint contractures, fixation of joints in extension, hyperextension of joints
Midline aberrations: hemangiomas, hair tufts, dimples or pits
Problems of secretion, excretion, or edema: no urination, no passage of meconium, chronic nasal or oral secretions, edema (nuchal, pedal, generalized, ascites)
Symptoms: unexplained seizures, resistant or unexplained respiratory distress
Metabolic disorders: resistant hypoglycemia, unexplained hypo- or hypercalcemia, polycythemia, hyponatremia, thrombocytopenia

        4. Associated anomalies. Include renal anomalies and an increased risk of mortality associated with Wilms tumor and hepatoblastoma. The estimated risk for tumor development in children with BWS is 7.5%. This increased risk for neoplasia seems to be concentrated in the first 8 years of life. Tumor development is uncommon in affected individuals >8 years of age.

IX. Teratogenic malformation syndromes

    A. Fetal alcohol syndrome (FAS). The incidence is estimated to be 1–2 per 1000 live births. Features include prenatal and postnatal growth deficiency, irritability in infancy, microcephaly, short palpebral fissures, smooth philtrum with thin and smooth upper lip, joint anomalies, and congenital cardiac defects. Brain development and function are the most serious consequences of prenatal alcohol exposure.

    B. Fetal hydantoin (Dilantin) syndrome. When taken during pregnancy, it results in a 2- to 3-fold increased risk for congenital malformations. Approximately 5–10% of exposed fetuses manifest the embryopathy. Features include mild to moderate prenatal growth deficiency, microcephaly, wide anterior fontanelle, low-set hairline, hirsutism, hypertelorism, strabismus, broad, depressed nasal bridge, cleft lip and palate, digit and nail hypoplasia, and umbilical and inguinal hernias. Similar craniofacial features are also associated with prenatal exposure to carbamazepine, Mysoline, and phenobarbital.

    C. Fetal valproate syndrome was described when an association was made between maternal ingestion of valproic acid and neural tube defects. Additional anomalies of fetal valproate syndrome include narrow bifrontal diameter, epicanthal folds; telecanthus; midface hypoplasia; broad, low nasal bridge with a short nose; long philtrum; micrognathia; long, thin fingers; congenital heart defects; genitourinary anomalies; and clubfeet.

    D. Fetal Accutane (isotretinoin) syndrome. Caused by the maternal use of isotretinoin, an active metabolite of vitamin A, for severe cystic acne. An estimated 25% of fetuses exposed to isotretinoin have a major malformation. Fetal anomalies include congenital heart defects, hydrocephalus, microcephaly, cranial nerve deficits, microtia, and a cleft palate. Pregnancy should wait until 2 years posttreatment with isotretinoin. Ingestion of large amounts of vitamin A may result in the same adverse effects to the fetus.

    E. Diabetic embryopathy. Children born to insulin-dependent diabetic mothers have a 2- to 3-fold risk for congenital malformations. The cardiovascular, genitourinary, and central nervous systems are the most frequently affected systems. Cardiovascular anomalies include ventricular septal defect, transposition of great arteries, single umbilical artery, and situs inversus. Anomalies of the genitourinary system consist of renal agenesis and hypospadias, and anomalies of the central nervous system include spina bifida and anencephaly.

    F. Infants of mothers with myotonic dystrophy vary in their clinical presentation from mild hypotonia and feeding problems to severe respiratory insufficiency causing death. Other abnormalities include a history of polyhydramnios and decreased fetal movement, multiple joint contractures, clubfeet, and facial weakness. The mutation identified to be the cause of myotonic dystrophy is a trinucleotide-containing cytosine-thymidine-guanosine that undergoes expansion in females with each transmission from an affected mother to a child. The severity of symptoms and onset of disease increases with transmission of this disorder to family members in subsequent generations.

    G. Infectious (prenatal) diseases. Infectious diseases such as toxoplasmosis, rubella, and, cytomegalovirus can result in anomalies including microcephaly, macrocephaly, hydrocephalus, and congenital heart defects. **Toxoplasmosis** is the most common cause of congenital infections, with an occurrence rate of 0.5–2.5% of all live births. (See Chapter 142.)

Selected References

Aase JM. *Diagnostic Dysmorphology*. New York, NY: Plenum; 1990.

Bishara N, Clericuzio C. Common dysmorphic syndromes in the NICU. *NeoReviews.* 2008;9:e29–e38.

Gorlin RJ, Cohen MM Jr, Henneken RCM, eds. *Syndromes of the Head and Neck.* 4th ed. New York, NY: Oxford University Press; 2001.

Jones KL. *Smith's Recognizable Patterns of Human Malformation.* Philadelphia, PA: Elsevier Saunders; 2006.

Lalani SR, Hefner MA, Belmont JW, Davenport LHS. CHARGE syndrome. *GeneReviews.* 2009. www.genetests.org. Accessed September, 2011.

McDonald-McGinn DM, Emanuel BS, Zacka EH. 22q11.2 deletion syndrome. *GeneReviews.* 2005. www.genetests.org. Accessed September, 2011.

Morris CA. Williams syndrome. *GeneReviews.* 2006. www.genetests.org. Accessed September, 2011.

Schinezel A. *Catalogue of Unbalanced Chromosome Aberrations in Man.* 2nd ed. New York, NY: Walter de Gruyter; 2001.

Shuman C, Beckwith JC, Smith AC, Weksberg R. Beckwith-Wiedemann syndrome. *GeneReviews* 2010. www. genetests.org. Accessed September, 2011.

Weijerman ME, de Winter JP. Clinical practice. The care of children with Down syndrome. *Eur J Pediatr.* 2010;169:1445–1452.

Weiner J, Sharma J, Lantos J, Kilbride H. How infants die in the neonatal intensive care unit: trends from 1999 through 2008. *Arch Pediatr Adolesc Med.* 2011;165:630–634.

89 Congenital Heart Disease

The diagnostic dilemma of the newborn with congenital heart disease must be resolved quickly because therapy may prove lifesaving for some of these infants. Congenital heart disease occurs in ~1% of live-born infants. Nearly half of all cases of congenital heart disease are diagnosed during the first week of life. In patients with complex congenital heart disease, neonatal hospital mortality can be as high as 7%. These patients have a high frequency of multiple congenital anomalies, syndromes, low birthweight, and prolonged length of stay. The most frequently occurring anomalies seen during this first week are patent ductus arteriosus (PDA), D-transposition of the great arteries, hypoplastic left heart syndrome (HLHS), tetralogy of Fallot (TOF), and pulmonary atresia.

   I. Classification. Symptoms and signs in newborns with heart disease permit grouping according to levels of arterial oxygen saturation based on the 100% oxygen test (see the following). Further classification (based on other physical findings, laboratory testing) facilitates delineation of the exact cardiac lesion present.

   A. Cyanotic heart disease. Infants with cyanotic heart disease are usually unable to achieve a Pao_2 of >100 mm Hg after breathing 100% inspired oxygen for 10–20 minutes (hyperoxia test).

   B. Acyanotic heart disease. Infants with acyanotic heart disease achieve Pao_2 levels of >100 mm Hg under the same conditions as noted in Section I.A.

   II. Cyanotic heart disease. See Figure 89–1. (See Chapter 51.)

   A. Hyperoxia test. Because of intracardiac right-to-left shunting, the newborn with cyanotic congenital heart disease (in contrast to the infant with pulmonary

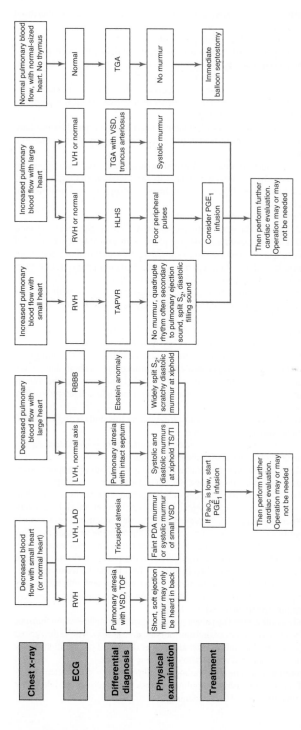

FIGURE 89–1. Cyanotic congenital heart disease (Pao$_2$ <100 mm Hg in 100% Fio$_2$). ECG, electrocardiography; HLHS, hypoplastic left heart syndrome; LAD, left axis deviation; LVH, left ventricular hypertrophy; PDA, patent ductus arteriosus; PGE$_1$, prostaglandin E$_1$; RBBB, right bundle branch block; RVH, right ventricular hypertrophy; TAPVR, total anomalous pulmonary venous return; TGA, transposition of the great arteries; TI, tricuspid incompetence; TOF, tetralogy of Fallot; TS, tricuspid stenosis; VSD, ventricular septal defect.

disease) is unable to raise the arterial saturation, even in the presence of increased ambient oxygen.

1. **Determine Pao$_2$** while the infant is on room air.
2. **Give 100% oxygen for 10–20 minutes** by mask, hood, or endotracheal tube.
3. **Obtain an arterial blood gas level** while the infant is breathing 100% oxygen.
4. **Interpret results** based on Section I.

B. **Cyanosis.** Care must be taken in evaluating cyanosis by skin color because polycythemia, jaundice, racial pigmentation, or anemia may make clinical recognition of cyanosis difficult. See pages 364–365.

C. **Murmur.** The infant with cyanotic congenital heart disease often does not have a distinctive murmur. The most serious of these anomalies may not be associated with a murmur at all.

D. **Other studies.** Cyanotic infants may be further classified on the basis of pulmonary circulation on chest radiograph and electrocardiographic findings.

E. **Diagnosis and treatment.** Figure 89–1 outlines the diagnosis and treatment of cyanotic heart disease.

F. **Specific cyanotic heart disease abnormalities**

1. **D-transposition of the great arteries (D-TGA).** This is the most common cardiac cause of cyanosis in the first year of life, with a male-to-female ratio of 2:1. The aorta comes from the right ventricle and the pulmonary artery from the left ventricle, with resultant separate systemic and pulmonary circuits. With modern newborn care, the 1-year survival rate is ~90%.

   a. **Physical examination.** Typical infant is large and vigorous, with cyanosis but little or no respiratory distress. There may be no murmur or a soft, systolic ejection murmur.

   b. **Chest radiograph.** This study may be normal, but typically it reveals a very narrow upper mediastinal shadow ("egg on a stick" appearance).

   c. **Electrocardiography (ECG).** There are no characteristic ECG findings.

   d. **Echocardiography is diagnostic.** Typical findings include branching of the anterior great vessel into the innominate, subclavian, and carotid vessels and branching of the posterior great vessel into the right and left pulmonary arteries.

   e. **Cardiac catheterization.** Like echocardiography, this study is diagnostic and often therapeutic, as outlined next.

   f. **Treatment.** If severe hypoxia or acidosis occurs, urgent balloon atrial septostomy can be done under echocardiogram guidance in the nursery. Cardiac catheterization with balloon septostomy and subsequent arterial switch operation are methods of treatment. Prostaglandin E$_1$ (PGE$_1$) may increase shunting.

2. **Tetralogy of Fallot (TOF).** Tetralogy of Fallot is characterized by 4 anomalies: pulmonary stenosis, ventricular septal defect, overriding aorta, and right ventricular hypertrophy (RVH). There is a slight male predominance. Cyanosis usually signifies complete or partial atresia of the right ventricular overflow tract or extremely severe pulmonary stenosis with hypoplastic pulmonary arteries. The degree of right ventricular outflow obstruction is inversely proportional to pulmonary blood flow and directly proportional to the degree of cyanosis. Tetralogy of Fallot with absent pulmonary valve may present with respiratory distress or poor feeding (because of compression of the esophagus or bronchi by the large pulmonary arteries).

   a. **Physical examination.** The patient is cyanotic with a systolic ejection murmur along the left sternal border. Loud murmurs are associated with more flow across the right ventricular outflow tract and milder degrees of desaturation. Softer murmurs are associated with less flow and more hypoxia.

   b. **Chest radiograph.** The chest radiograph film reveals a small, often "boot-shaped" heart, with decreased pulmonary vascular markings. A right aortic arch is seen in ~20% of these infants.

      c. **ECG.** The ECG may be normal or may demonstrate RVH. The only sign of RVH may be an upright T wave in V_4R or V_1 after 72 hours of age.

      d. **Echocardiography.** Usually diagnostic, with an overriding aorta, ventricular septal defect (VSD), and small right ventricular outflow tract.

      e. **Treatment.** Pulmonary blood flow may be ductal dependent with severe cyanosis and may respond to ductal dilation using PGE_1 (see Chapter 148). This measure allows more flexibility for planning cardiac catheterization and surgical correction. Surgery (shunting or total correction) may be considered.

III. **Acyanotic heart disease (Figure 89-2)**

  A. **Hyperoxia test.** See Section II.A.

  B. **Murmur.** The infant who is not cyanotic will have either a heart murmur or symptoms of congestive heart failure.

  C. **Diagnosis and treatment.** See Figure 89-2.

  D. **Specific acyanotic heart disease abnormalities**

    1. **Ventricular septal defect (VSD).** The most common congenital heart abnormality with equal sex distribution. Murmurs can be heard at birth but typically appear between 3 days and 3 weeks of age. Congestive heart failure is unusual before 4 weeks of age but may develop earlier in premature infants. Symptoms and physical findings vary with patient age and defect size. Spontaneous closure occurs in half of the patients. Surgical correction is reserved for large, symptomatic VSDs only.

    2. **Atrial septal defect (ASD).** Not an important cause of morbidity or mortality in infancy. Occasionally, congestive heart failure can occur in infancy but not usually in the neonatal period.

    3. **Endocardial cushion defects.** Include ostium primum–type ASD with or without a cleft mitral valve and an atrioventricular (AV) canal. These defects are commonly associated with multiple congenital anomalies, especially Down syndrome. If marked AV valve insufficiency is present, the patient may have congestive heart failure at birth or in the neonatal period.

      a. **Physical examination.** On physical examination, a systolic murmur resulting from AV valve insufficiency may be heard. Cyanosis may be present but is often not severe. Infants with severe pulmonary artery hypertension may have little or no murmur.

      b. **Chest radiograph.** Variable findings may include a dilated pulmonary artery or a large heart secondary to atrial dilatation.

      c. **ECG.** Left axis deviation (left superior vector) is *always* found; the PR interval may be long, or there may be an RSR' pattern in V_4R and V_1.

      d. **Echocardiography.** Usually diagnostic; the echocardiogram usually demonstrates a common AV valve with inlet VSD or a defect in the septum primum with an abnormal mitral valve.

      e. **Treatment.** Congestive heart failure is treated with diuretics and digoxin (for dosages, see Chapter 148); early cardiac catheterization with corrective surgery may be needed to prevent pulmonary vascular obstructive disease.

IV. **Hypoplastic left heart syndrome (HLHS).** Occurs in both cyanotic and acyanotic forms. In 15% of cases, the foramen ovale is intact and thus prevents mixing at the atrial level, causing cyanosis. Infants with mixing at the atria are acyanotic. HLHS accounts for 25% of all cardiac deaths during the first week of life.

  A. **Physical examination.** The infant is typically pale and tachypneic, with poor perfusion and poor to absent peripheral pulses. A loud single S_2 is present, usually with a gallop and no murmur. There is hepatomegaly, and metabolic acidosis is usually present by 48 hours of age.

  B. **Electrocardiogram.** Demonstrates small or absent left ventricular forces.

  C. **Chest radiograph.** Moderate cardiomegaly is present, often with a large main pulmonary artery shadow.

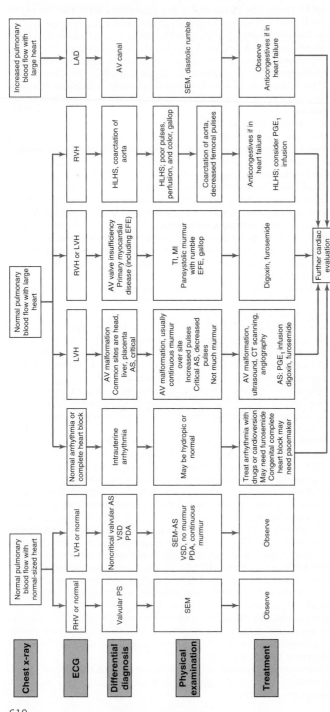

FIGURE 89-2. Acyanotic congenital heart disease (Pao$_2$ >100 mm Hg in 100% Fio$_2$). AS, aortic stenosis; AV canal, atrioventricular canal; AV malformation, arteriovenous malformation; AV valve, atrioventricular valve; CT, computed tomography; ECG, electrocardiogram; EFE, endocardial fibroelastosis; HLHS, hypoplastic left heart syndrome; LAD, left axis deviation; LVH, left ventricular hypertrophy; MI, myocardial infarction; PDA, patent ductus arteriosus; PGE$_1$, prostaglandin E$_1$; PS, pulmonary stenosis; RVH, right ventricular hypertrophy; SEM, systolic ejection murmur; TI, tricuspid incompetence; VSD, ventricular septal defect.

D. **Echocardiography.** A diagnostic study demonstrates a small or slit-like left ventricle with a hypoplastic ascending aorta.

E. **Treatment.** Systemic blood flow is ductal dependent; therefore, PGE_1 is of value. Oxygen should not be given, as the resultant dilatation of the pulmonary vessels increases pulmonary blood flow. Respiratory compromise and subsequent dilatation and reduced right ventricular (RV) function are undesired effects of oxygen administration. In fact, infants with HLHS and pulmonary overcirculation may require oxygen concentrations <21%. Frequent monitoring of blood gases and lactate is required preoperatively. Surgical correction is done in 3 stages. The first is palliation (the Norwood procedure), redirecting the blood flow so that the right ventricle serves as the "systemic ventricle" and a surgically constructed "shunt" provides pulmonary blood flow. Some surgeons prefer to do a Sano modification of the Norwood, which involves placing a Gore-tex tube from the RV to the main pulmonary artery (MPA). Successful outcome is influenced by gestational age (term infants do much better than preterm infants) and the presence of other major anomalies. The second stage usually consists of a hemi-Fontan or bidirectional Glenn operation, routing superior vena cava blood to the lungs and closing the systemic-to-pulmonary artery shunt. The third stage (the Fontan procedure) directs remaining systemic venous return directly to the pulmonary circulation. Neonatal cardiac transplantation is a second option, but shortage of organs is a significant deterrent. Compassionate care (keeping the infant comfortable until death) may be appropriate in some instances.

V. **Associated anomalies and syndromes.** (Table 89–1) A discussion of heart disease in neonates would not be complete without the inclusion of common multiple congenital

Table 89–1. **CONGENITAL ANOMALIES ASSOCIATED WITH HEART DEFECTS**

Congenital Anomaly	Heart Defect
Chromosomal anomaly	
Trisomy 21 (Down syndrome)	Atrioventricular canal, ventricular septal defect
Trisomies 13, 15, and 18	Ventricular septal defect, patent ductus arteriosus
Syndrome associated with 4p–	Atrial septal defect, ventricular septal defect
Syndrome associated with 5p– (Cri du Chat syndrome)	Variable
XO (Turner syndrome)	Coarctation of aorta, aortic stenosis
Syndromes with predominantly skeletal defects[a]	
Ellis-van Creveld syndrome	Atrial septal defect, single atrium
Laurence-Moon-Biedl syndrome	Tetralogy of Fallot, ventricular septal defect
Carpenter syndrome	Patent ductus arteriosus, ventricular septal defect
Holt-Oram syndrome	Atrial septal defect, ventricular septal defect
Fanconi syndrome	Patent ductus arteriosus, ventricular septal defect
Thrombocytopenia–absent radius syndrome	Atrial septal defect, tetralogy of Fallot
Syndromes with characteristic facies[a]	
Noonan syndrome (long arm of chromosome 12)	Pulmonary stenosis
DiGeorge syndrome (chromosome 22 deletion)	Tetralogy of Fallot, aortic arch anomalies
Smith-Lemli-Opitz syndrome	Ventricular septal defect, patent ductus arteriosus
de Lange syndrome	Tetralogy of Fallot, ventricular septal defect
Goldenhar syndrome	Tetralogy of Fallot, variable
Williams syndrome	Supravalvular aortic stenosis, peripheral pulmonary artery stenosis
Asymmetric crying facies	Variable

[a]Not all infants with these syndromes have heart defects.

anomaly (MCA) syndromes associated with heart defects. Many times, recognition of MCA syndromes facilitates identification of the heart defect. Syndromes that tend to present after the newborn period have not been included. See Chapter 88 for a complete discussion of anomalies and syndromes.

VI. **Teratogens and heart disease.** Several teratogens associated with congenital heart disease have been identified (Table 89–2), although there is not a 100% relationship between exposure and heart defects. A history of teratogen exposure may help in the diagnosis.

VII. **Abnormal situs syndromes.** Syndromes of abnormal situs are associated with congenital heart disease. For example, an infant with situs inversus totalis and dextrocardia has the same incidence of congenital heart disease as the general population. If, however, there is disparity between thoracic and abdominal situs, the incidence of congenital heart disease is >90%. (Check the chest radiograph to see that the cardiac apex and the stomach bubble are on the same side. Both should be on the left.) Some of these syndromes involve bilateral left-sidedness (two bilobed lungs or multiple spleens) and complex cyanotic congenital heart disease, whereas others have bilateral right-sidedness (two trilobed lungs or an absent spleen) and complex cyanotic congenital heart disease.

VIII. **General principles of management**
   A. **Fetal echocardiography**
      1. **General considerations.** Fetal echocardiography is now possible in many centers. The optimal gestational age to perform echocardiography is between 18 and 24 weeks when structural abnormalities and arrhythmias can be detected. With early detection of cardiac abnormalities, arrangements can be made for delivery at a center with pediatric cardiac and surgical facilities. If the anomaly is not consistent with life, some families may elect termination of pregnancy.
      2. **Indications.** See Table 89–3.
         a. **Maternal factors.** Oligohydramnios or polyhydramnios, diabetes, collagen vascular disease, teratogen exposure, or a previous child with congenital heart disease.

Table 89–2. TERATOGENS ASSOCIATED WITH HEART DEFECTS

Teratogen	Heart Defect
Drugs	
Alcohol	Ventricular septal defect, tetralogy of Fallot, atrial septal defect
Anticonvulsants	Variable, ventricular septal defect, tetralogy of Fallot
Retinoic acid	Aortic arch anomalies
Lithium	Ebstein anomaly of the tricuspid valve
SSRIs	Slightly increased risk septal defects
Environmental agents	
Irradiation	Variable
High altitude	PDA; others variable
Maternal factors	
Diabetes	Variable
Maternal lupus	Complete (3rd degree) AV block
Maternal PKU	Ventricular septal defect, coarctation
Infections	
Rubella syndrome	PDA, peripheral pulmonary stenosis
Parvovirus, coxsackie	Cardiomyopathy
Other viruses	Variable

AV, atrioventricular; PDA, patent ductus arteriosus; PKU, phenylketonuria.

Table 89–3. **INDICATIONS FOR FETAL ECHOCARDIOGRAM**

Maternal conditions
Diabetes
Collagen vascular disease
Maternal drug/teratogen exposure

Family conditions
History of congenital heart disease
History of chromosomal or genetic abnormalities

Fetal conditions
Abnormal fetal heart rate
Suspected cardiac malformation on screening ultrasonogram
Presence of other malformations on ultrasonogram
Oligo- or polyhydramnios
Evidence of hydrops fetalis
Intrauterine growth restriction

b. **Fetal factors.** Suspected cardiac abnormality on obstetric ultrasound examination, pleural fluid, pericardial fluid, heart rate abnormalities, intrauterine growth retardation, or other abnormality on obstetric ultrasound examination.

c. **Genetic factors.** Familial history of chromosomal disorders or congenital heart disease.

B. **Emergency therapy.** Once the specific lesion has been identified as emergent, a decision about therapy must be made. As an example, if confronted with a very cyanotic infant with no murmur, a normal chest radiograph, and a normal ECG, and it is believed that the diagnosis of D-transposition of the great arteries is likely, it is necessary to prepare for a **balloon septostomy**.

C. **Prostaglandins.** As a general principle, if an infant is cyanotic and has decreased pulmonary blood flow, the Pao$_2$ will be improved by promoting flow through the ductus arteriosus via a drip of **prostaglandin E$_1$** (alprostadil or Prostin VR Pediatric). Maintaining patency of the ductus will enable stabilization of the infant and subsequent catheterization or surgery to be planned on an urgent rather than emergent basis. Similarly, if poor peripheral pulses and acidosis from poor perfusion are present, infusion of prostaglandin, using the same dose, will open the ductus arteriosus and allow right ventricular blood flow to augment the systemic circulation. This measure is beneficial in critical aortic stenosis, coarctation of the aorta, and HLHS. (For dosage and other pharmacologic information, see Chapter 148.)

D. **Antiarrhythmic drugs.** Rapid arrhythmias may occur during intrauterine life or after delivery. Arrhythmias are a cause of fetal hydrops and intrauterine death; most often, the rhythm disturbance is a rapid supraventricular tachycardia with a 1:1 ventricular response. Occasionally, atrial flutter with 2:1 block presents before or just after birth. Some anti-arrhythmia medications given to mothers can cross the placenta, enabling fetal treatment. **Digitalis** and **propranolol** have been successful antiarrhythmic agents in newborns, but treatment with adenosine or electrical cardioversion (see Chapter 28) is also sometimes necessary. Digitalis is contraindicated in Wolff-Parkinson-White syndrome.

E. **Pacemaker.** Fetal hydrops can result from congenital complete heart block. If cardiovascular demise is imminent, delivery and **temporary transvenous ventricular pacing may be lifesaving**. It should be followed by urgent surgical placement of a permanent pacemaker. Mothers may have anti-Rho or anti-LA antibodies.

F. **Other imaging techniques.** While magnetic resonance imaging (MRI) is enjoying increasing utility in the identification of congenital heart disease in children, MRI of the neonatal heart is of limited utility. The rapid heart rate of neonates makes gaiting for image acquisition very difficult. Computed tomography (CT) and CT angiography (CTA) may help identify anomalies of pulmonary venous return. CTA has become the gold standard of evaluation of vascular rings, but these do not usually present in the immediate neonatal period.

G. **Other considerations.** Optimal care of the infant prior to and immediately after heart surgery determines overall outcome. A perfectly executed corrective procedure cannot succeed without support of the infant postoperatively. Drugs that manipulate pulmonary vascular resistance (nitric oxide [NO], sildenafil, oxygen) and have a favorable influence on cardiac output and its distribution are required more often than not. Milrinone as an afterload reducer is often used and can be transitioned to the oral enalapril. Nesiritide (Natrecor), a recombinant form of human B-type natriuretic peptide, has both vasodilation and diuretic properties and can be safely used for shorter periods of time than milrinone. Levosimendan, a calcium-sensitizing agent, has inotropic and vasodilator effects. Studies with small numbers of infants/neonates have, to date, shown no advantage of levosimendan over milrinone in low cardiac output states following open-heart surgery. Milrinone use after surgical ductal ligation treats hemodynamic instability, facilitating central nervous system and gut perfusion.

Selected References

Allan LD, Sharland GK, Milburn A, et al. Prospective diagnosis of 1,006 consecutive cases of congenital heart disease in the fetus. *J Am Coll Cardiol.* 1994;23:1452.

Alwan S, Reefhuis J, Rasmussen S, et al. Use of selective serotonin-reuptake inhibitors in pregnancy and the risk of birth defects. *N Engl J Med.* 2007;356;2584–2692.

Ballard RA, Wernosky G. Cardiovascular system. In: Taeusch HW, ed. *Avery's Diseases of the Newborn.* Philadelphia, PA: Elsevier Saunders; 2005:779–901.

Brooks PA, Penny DJ. Management of the sick neonate with suspected heart disease. *Early Hum Dev.* 2008;84(3):155–159.

Dallopiccola B, Marino B, Digilio MC, Mingarelli R, Novelli G, Giannotti A. A Mendelian basis of congenital heart defects. *Cardiol Young.* 1996;6:264–271.

Dorfman AT, Marino BS, Wernovsky G, et al. Critical heart disease in the neonate: presentation and outcome at a tertiary care center. *Pediatr Crit Care Med.* 2008;9(2):193–202.

Hofer LE, Freynschlag R, Leitner-Penedr G, et al. *Levosimendan versus Milrinone after Corrective Open-Heart Surgery in Infants.* Clinical trial NCT00549107. Leitz, Germany.

Jenkins PC, Flanagan MF, Sargent JD, et al. A comparison of treatment strategies for hypoplastic left heart syndrome using decision analysis. *J Am Coll Cardiol.* 2001;38:1181.

Paradisi M, Jiang X, McLachlan J, et al. Population pharmacokinetics and dosing regimen design of milrinone in preterm infants. *Arch Dis Child Fetal Neonatal ED.* 2007;92: F204–F209.

Pendersen LH, Henriksen TB, Vestergaard M, et al. Selective serotonin reuptake inhibitors in pregnancy and congenital malformations: population based cohort study. *BMJ* 2009;339:b3569.

Perry LW, Neill CA, Ferencz C, Rubin JD, Loffredo CA. Infants with congenital heart disease: the cases. In: Ferencz C, Loffredo CA, Rubin JD, Magee CA, eds. *Epidemiology of Congenital Heart Disease: The Baltimore-Washington Infant Heart Study 1981–1989.* Mt. Kisco, NY: Futura; 1993:63–62

Rosenthal A. Hypoplastic left heart syndrome. In: Moller JH, Hoffman JIE, eds. *Pediatric Cardiovascular Medicine.* New York, NY: Churchill Livingston; 2000.

Simsic JM, Reddy VS, Kanter KR, et al. Use of nesiritide (human B-type natriuretic peptide) in infants following cardiac surgery. *Pediatr Cardiol.* 2004;25:668–670.

Soufia M, Aoun J, Gorsane M, et al. SSRIs and pregnancy: a review of the literature. *Encephale* 2010;36(6):513–516.

Tobias JD. B-type natriuretic peptide: diagnostic and therapeutic applications in infants and children. *J Intensive Care Med.* 2011;26:183–195.

90 Cytomegalovirus

I. **Definition.** Cytomegalovirus (CMV) is a DNA virus and a member of the herpesvirus group (human herpesvirus 5).

II. **Incidence.** CMV is the **most common cause of congenital infection** in the United States and occurs in ~0.2–2.2% of all live births. This results in ~40,000 new cases in the United States per year.

III. **Pathophysiology.** CMV is a ubiquitous virus that may be transmitted in secretions, including saliva, tears, semen, urine, cervical secretions, blood (white blood cells), and breast milk. The seroprevalence increases with age and is influenced by many factors, such as hygienic circumstances, socioeconomic factors, breast-feeding, and sexual contacts. In addition to **transplacental infection**, CMV may also be transmitted to the infant **intrapartum** (through exposure to CMV in cervical secretions), via **breast milk,** and via **blood transfusion** of seropositive blood to an infant whose mother is seronegative. CMV infection acquired during delivery or via breast milk has no effect on future neurodevelopmental outcome in full-term infants. There is no definite evidence of CMV transmission among hospital personnel.

In developed countries, CMV seroprevalence varies inversely with socioeconomic status, with 40–80% of women of childbearing age in the United States having serologic evidence of past CMV infection. Seroconversion and initial infection can occur around the time of puberty, and shedding of the virus may continue for a long time. CMV can also become latent in white blood cells and reactivate periodically. In addition, a seropositive individual can be infected by a different strain of CMV.

Maternal reinfection by new strains of CMV has been recognized recently as a major source of congenital infection in a highly CMV-immune maternal population like that of Brazil. Reactivation and reinfection are grouped as a "nonprimary" infection. CMV is capable of penetrating the placental barrier as well as the blood–brain barrier. During early pregnancy, CMV has a **teratogenic potential** in the fetus. CMV infections may result in neuronal migration disturbances in the brain. Both **primary** and **nonprimary** maternal CMV infection can lead to transmission of the virus to the fetus. When primary maternal infection occurs during pregnancy, the virus is transmitted to the fetus in ~35% of cases. Infection in early pregnancy causes more severe fetal infection with significant CNS sequelae. During nonprimary infection, transmission rate is only 0.2–1.8%. Even though the risk for congenital infection is high after primary maternal infection, nonprimary infection is responsible for 75% of the overall burden of congenital CMV infection.

More than 85% of infants born with CMV have a subclinical infection. Symptomatic infants are usually born to women with a primary infection. **Symptomatic infants have a mortality rate of 20–30%.** When the placenta becomes infected with CMV after a primary maternal infection, its ability to provide oxygen and nutrients to the developing fetus becomes impaired. This leads to placental enlargement due to viral **placentitis and revascularization**. Although not completely elucidated, placental tissue damage occurs due to direct tissue injury by persistent CMV replication, ischemic tissue damage due to vasculitis with viral infection of endothelial cells, and tissue damage by immune complex deposition. Eventual fetal viremia leads to fetal multiorgan involvement. The primary target organs are the CNS, eyes, liver, lungs, and kidneys.

Characteristic histopathologic features of CMV include focal necrosis, inflammatory response, formation of enlarged cells with intranuclear inclusions (cytomegalic cells), and the production of multinucleated giant cells. A sepsis-like illness has been described in premature infants.

IV. **Risk factors.** CMV infection in neonates is associated with nonwhite race, lower socioeconomic status, drug abuse, and neonatal intensive care unit admittance. Premature infants are more often affected than full-term infants. Transfusion with unscreened blood is an additional risk factor for neonatal disease. Risk factors for primary CMV infection during pregnancy include prolonged exposure to young children (daycare workers, multiparous women) and sexual contact (young maternal age, greater numbers of sexual partners, abnormal cervical cytology, and having a sexually transmitted infection during pregnancy).

V. **Clinical presentation**

A. **Prenatal presentation.** Pregnant women who acquire primary CMV may develop a mononucleosis-like illnesses (<25% of the time). Maternal screening is currently not recommended routinely. Fetal anomalies consistent with congenital CMV infection that can be detected on prenatal ultrasound examination include fetal growth restriction, cerebral periventricular echogenicity or calcifications, cerebral ventriculomegaly, microcephaly, polymicrogyria, cerebellar hypoplasia, hyperechogenic fetal bowel, hepatosplenomegaly, amniotic fluid abnormalities, ascites and/or pleural effusion, and placental enlargement. Prenatal magnetic resonance imaging (MRI), especially to evaluate brain anomalies, is being used increasingly. Amniocentesis to perform polymerase chain reaction (PCR) for CMV DNA in amniotic fluid is the preferred diagnostic approach for identifying an infected fetus. Amniocentesis is most sensitive when done after 21 weeks of gestation and after 6 weeks from maternal infection/exposure.

B. **Postnatal presentation**

1. **Subclinical infection.** Occurs in 85–90% of cases. Despite being asymptomatic at birth, these infants are at risk for sensorineural hearing loss (SNHL) during the first 6 years of life.

2. **Low birthweight.** Maternal CMV infection is associated with low birthweight and small for gestational age infants, even when the infant is not infected.

3. **Classic CMV inclusion disease.** Occurs in 10–15% of the cases and consists of intrauterine growth restriction, hepatosplenomegaly with jaundice, abnormal liver function tests (LFTs), thrombocytopenia with or without purpura, and severe central nervous system (CNS) involvement (CNS and sensory impairments are seen in 50–90% of symptomatic newborns). Neurologic complications include microcephaly, intracerebral calcifications (most characteristically in the subependymal periventricular area), chorioretinitis, and progressive SNHL (10–20% of cases). Other symptoms include hemolytic anemia and pneumonitis. The most severely affected infants have a mortality rate of ~30%. Deaths are usually due to hepatic dysfunction, bleeding, disseminated intravascular coagulation, or secondary bacterial infection. Factors associated with poor outcome in symptomatic infants include microcephaly, abnormal findings on head computed tomography (CT), and increased viral load.

4. **Late sequelae.** Approximately 10–20% of children with congenital CMV infections, regardless of symptoms, exhibit neurologic damage at follow-up. SNHL occurs in 22–65% of symptomatic and 6–23% of asymptomatic infants. CMV-related SNHL may be present at birth or occur later in childhood. Repeated auditory evaluation during the first 5 years of life is strongly recommended. Visual impairment and strabismus are common in children with clinically

symptomatic CMV infection. Visual complications may occur, usually secondary to chorioretinitis, pigmentary retinitis, macular scarring, optic atrophy, and central cortical defects.

VI. **Diagnosis**
   A. **Laboratory studies**
      1. **Culture for demonstration of the virus.** The **gold standard** for the diagnosis of congenital CMV is urine or saliva culture obtained before 3 weeks of age. Most urine specimens from infants with congenital CMV are positive within 48–72 hours, especially if shell vial tissue culture techniques are used. Shell vial assay detects CMV-induced antigens by monoclonal antibodies, allowing for identification of the virus within 48 hours compared with the standard tissue culture, which takes 2–4 weeks. Studies evaluating a rapid assay for detection of CMV in saliva as a screening method for congenital infection have shown it to be at least as sensitive a method for detecting congenital infection as for detection of viruria (viruses in the urine). Given that saliva can be collected with less difficulty and expense, it may eventually replace the current use of urine screening.
      2. **Polymerase chain reaction (PCR).** PCR for CMV DNA is as sensitive as a urine culture for the detection of CMV infection. PCR has been used successfully in retrospective diagnosis of congenital CMV beyond 3 weeks of age through CMV DNA analysis of dried blood spots (Guthrie cards). The sensitivity of CMV DNA detection by PCR assay of dried blood spots is low, limiting use of this type of specimen for widespread screening for congenital CMV. A positive PCR assay result from a neonatal dried blood spot confirms congenital infection, but a negative result does not rule it out it.
      3. **Serologic tests.** Serologic tests based on the detection of immunoglobulin M (IgM) should not be used to diagnose congenital CMV because they are less sensitive and more subject to false-positive results than culture or PCR. Only 70% of neonates infected with congenital CMV have IgM antibodies at birth.
      4. **Other laboratory tests.** Other lab tests that are indicated in the workup include complete blood count, LFTs, disseminated intravascular coagulation panel and cerebrospinal fluid analysis, culture, and PCR.
   B. **Imaging and other studies.** Ultrasound or CT scans of the head may demonstrate characteristic periventricular calcifications in addition to other abnormalities (see prenatal presentation earlier). Brain MRI is preferred over other modalities because it is likely to identify most of the brain anomalies associated with congenital CMV.

VII. **Management**
   A. **Prevention and treatment of maternal infection during pregnancy.** Possible approaches to preventing and treating congenital CMV infections during pregnancy include changes in hygienic behavior for seronegative pregnant women, administration of CMV hyperimmune globulin (HIG) to pregnant women with a primary infection, administering antiviral therapy to women with primary infection, and vaccines administered to girls or women well before pregnancy or during pregnancy. With regard to **hygienic** measures, epidemiologic studies have shown that instructing mothers who are pregnant on frequent hand washing; wearing gloves for specific child-care tasks; avoiding kissing children under age 6 on the mouth or cheek; not sharing food, drinks, or oral utensils (eg, fork, spoon, toothbrush, pacifier) with young children; and cleaning toys, countertops, and other surfaces that come into contact with children's urine or saliva reduces their chances of acquiring congenital CMV infection. To test the efficacy of **HIG,** a multicenter nonrandomized study in Italy enrolled pregnant women with primary congenital CMV infection diagnosed before 21 weeks' gestation. The study demonstrated that HIG (100 U/kg) given monthly until delivery reduces congenital infection in the newborn infants (16% vs 40%) compared with mothers who refused therapy. HIG

was safe, and therefore this therapy should be considered for mothers diagnosed with primary CMV during the first half of gestation. Use of antiviral therapy for the infected pregnant woman has not been studied in controlled trials. The most effective preventive strategy is developing a **vaccine** against CMV. Recently, a vaccine targeted toward CMV envelope glycoprotein B, an antigen that typically induces a serum antibody response, was tested in a phase 2 clinical trial. This vaccine has been shown to be immunogenic with an acceptable risk profile. Other trials are underway.

B. **Antiviral agents.** No antiviral agent is yet approved for treatment of congenital CMV infection. **Ganciclovir** has been used to treat infants who have symptomatic disease. In a randomized, placebo-controlled, phase III clinical trial in infants with congenital CMV and CNS involvement, treatment with intravenous ganciclovir (6 mg/kg/dose, administered every 12 hours) for 6 weeks at a dose of 6 mg/kg/d resulted in improved hearing compared with controls after 6 months of follow-up. In addition, 68% of controls had deterioration of hearing at 1-year follow-up compared with 21% of treated children. During therapy, the viral excretion in urine decreases but returns to near pretreatment levels after cessation of therapy. The antiviral therapy may suppress virus replication temporarily but may not prevent long-term sequelae. No effect on long-term neurodevelopmental outcome (>2 years) has been reported yet. Ganciclovir was associated with significant side effects, especially neutropenia, which occurred in 60% of the recipients. Based on the results of this study, some experts suggest that ganciclovir therapy may be offered to CMV-infected neonates who manifest CNS disease for prevention of hearing impairment. Another possible indication is chorioretinitis, which involves the macula and may result in blindness. A third possible indication is the critically ill preterm infant who acquires the infection natally (intrapartum) or postnatally. Such infants have life-threatening CMV infection manifested by pneumonitis, hepatitis, or encephalitis, and ganciclovir may modify the course of the disease. **Valganciclovir** is a prodrug of ganciclovir that is suitable for oral administration. Valganciclovir administered orally to young infants at 16 mg/kg/dose, twice daily, provides the same systemic ganciclovir exposure as does intravenous ganciclovir at 6 mg/kg/dose. Small observational studies from Europe on using valganciclovir to treat congenital CMV are encouraging. In the United States, oral valganciclovir is being evaluated in clinical trials conducted by the National Institute of Allergy and Infectious Diseases Collaborative Antiviral Study Group.

VIII. **Prognosis.** Congenital CMV is the leading cause of SNHL regardless of the seroprevalence in the population. For symptomatic infants at birth, mortality is up to 30%, and up to 90% will have late complications (intellectual or developmental impairment, hearing loss, spasticity). Factors associated with poor developmental outcome include intrauterine growth restriction, microcephaly, urine and cerebrospinal fluid viral load, and presence of CNS abnormalities on brain imaging studies (CT or MRI). Visual impairment develops in 10–20% of symptomatic newborns. With asymptomatic, congenitally infected infants, the prognosis is uncertain, but they are at a risk for SNHL (up to 20% by 6 years of age).

Selected References

American Academy of Pediatrics. Cytomegalovirus infection. In: Pickering LK, Baker CJ, Kimberlin DW, Long SS, eds. *Red Book: 2012 Report of the Committee on Infectious Diseases.* 29th ed. Elk Grove Village, IL: American Academy of Pediatrics; 2012:275–280.

Boppana SB, Ross SA, Shimamura M, et al. Saliva polymerase-chain-reaction assay for cytomegalovirus screening in newborns. *N Engl J Med.* 2011;364:2111–2118.

Doneda C, Parazzini C, Righini A, et al. Early cerebral lesions in cytomegalovirus infection: prenatal MR imaging. *Radiology.* 2010;255:613–621.

Enders G, Daiminger A, Bäder U, Exler S, Enders M. Intrauterine transmission and clinical outcome of 248 pregnancies with primary cytomegalovirus infection in relation to gestational age. *J Clin Virol.* 2011;52:244–246.

Lazzarotto T, Guerra B, Gabrielli L, Lanari M, Landini MP. Update on the prevention, diagnosis, and management of cytomegalovirus infection during pregnancy. *Clin Microbiol Infect.* 2011;17:1285–1293.

Leruez-Ville M, Vauloup-Fellous C, Couderc S, et al. Prospective identification of congenital cytomegalovirus infection in newborns using real-time polymerase chain reaction assays in dried blood spots. *Clin Infect Dis.* 2011;52:575–581.

Lombardi G, Garofoli F, Stronati M. Congenital cytomegalovirus infection: treatment, sequelae and follow-up. *J Matern Fetal Neonatal Med.* 2010;23(suppl 3):45–48.

Lombardi G, Garofoli F, Villani P, et al. Oral valganciclovir treatment in newborns with symptomatic congenital cytomegalovirus infection. *Eur J Clin Microbiol Infect Dis.* 2009;28:1465–1470.

Pass RF, Zhang C, Evans A, et al. Vaccine prevention of maternal cytomegalovirus infection. *N Engl J Med.* 2009;360:1191–1199.

Ross SA, Arora N, Novak Z, Fowler KB, Britt WJ, Boppana SB. Cytomegalovirus reinfections in healthy seroimmune women. *J Infect Dis.* 2010;201:386–389.

Sabbaj S, Pass RF, Goepfert PA, Pichon S. Glycoprotein B vaccine is capable of boosting both antibody and CD4 T-cell responses to cytomegalovirus in chronically infected women. *J Infect Dis.* 2011;203:1534–1541.

Wang C, Zhang X, Bialek S, Cannon MJ. Attribution of congenital cytomegalovirus infection to primary versus non-primary maternal infection. *Clin Infect Dis.* 2011;52:e11–e13.

Yamamoto AY, Mussi-Pinhata MM, Boppana SB, et al. Human cytomegalovirus reinfection is associated with intrauterine transmission in a highly cytomegalovirus immune maternal population. *Am J Obstet Gynecol.* 2010;202:297.e1–e8.

91 Disorders of Sex Development

I. **Definition.** Ambiguous genitalia are present when the sex of an infant is not readily apparent after examination of the external genitalia. If the appearance resembles neither a male with a normal phallus and palpable testes nor a female with an unfused vaginal orifice and absence of an enlarged phallic structure, the genitalia are ambiguous, and investigation before gender assignment is indicated. The recent trend has been to refer to these disorders as **disorders of sex development** (DSDs) because many of the other terms used are considered pejorative by some patients and professionals. Also, the term **"atypical genitalia"** instead of "ambiguous genitalia" has been suggested. New definitions and classifications are also being proposed in this already very complex area. For the purpose of this on-call manual, the embryology and pathophysiology are reviewed as relevant to the initial evaluation and treatment of patients in the neonatal period.

II. **Incidence.** The quoted incidence of ambiguous genitalia varies according to the source and is likely somewhat variable for different ethnic groups; it appears to be ~1 in 5000. Congenital adrenal hyperplasia is often considered the most common cause with an incidence quoted from 1 in 14,000 to 1 in 28,000, followed by androgen insensitivity and mixed gonadal dysgenesis. Hypospadias has a frequency of about 1 in 300 births, but only a minority of these patients has a disorder of sex development (usually presenting with hypospadias in combination with cryptorchidism).

III. **Embryology.** The early fetus, regardless of the genetic sex (XX or XY), is bipotential and can undergo either male or female differentiation. The innate tendency of the embryo is to differentiate along female lines.

   A. **Development of the gonads.** Gonadal development occurs during the embryonic period (the third through the seventh to eighth weeks of gestation).

   1. **Testicular differentiation.** Gonadal differentiation is determined by the absence or presence of the Y chromosome. If the **Y chromosome** (more specifically, the sex-determining region of the Y or *SRY* gene) is present, the gonads differentiate as testes. The testes then produce and release testosterone, which is converted to dihydrotestosterone (DHT) in the target organ cells by 5α-reductase. DHT induces male differentiation of the external genitalia (see Section III.B.1). The testes descend behind the peritoneum and normally reach the scrotum by the eighth or ninth month.

   2. **Ovarian differentiation.** In the female fetus, where the Y chromosome/*SRY* gene is absent, the gonads form ovaries (even in 45,X Turner syndrome, histologically normal ovaries are present at birth). As ovaries do not produce testosterone, female differentiation proceeds. Two X chromosomes are needed for differentiation of the primordial follicle. If part or all of the second X chromosome is missing, ovarian development fails, resulting in atrophic, whitish, streaky gonads by 1–2 years of age.

   B. **Development of external genitalia.** This part of sexual differentiation occurs in the fetal period, beginning in the seventh week of gestation, and proceeds up to the 14th week (about 16 weeks after the last menstrual period).

   1. **Normal male.** At ~9 weeks postconceptional age, in the presence of systemic androgens (especially DHT), masculinization begins with lengthening of the anogenital distance. The urogenital and labioscrotal folds fuse in the midline (beginning caudally and progressing anteriorly), leading to the formation of the scrotum and the penis.

   2. **Normal female.** In the female fetus, the anogenital distance does not increase. The urogenital and labioscrotal folds do not fuse and instead differentiate into the labia majora and minora. The urogenital sinus divides into the urethra and the vagina.

IV. **Pathophysiology**

   A. **Virilization of female infants (female pseudohermaphroditism).** Many neonates with disorders of sex development belong to this group. They have a 46,XX karyotype, are *SRY* negative, and have exclusively ovarian tissue. The degree of masculinization of the female newborn depends on the potency of the androgenic stimulation to which she is exposed, the stage of development at the time of initial exposure, and the duration of exposure.

   1. **The most common cause** of excess fetal androgens is an autosomal recessively inherited **enzymatic deficiency in the cortisol pathway,** leading to excessive corticotropin (adrenocorticotropic hormone [ACTH]) stimulation with **congenital adrenal hyperplasia (CAH)** and excessive production of adrenal androgens (dehydroepiandrosterone and androstenedione) and testosterone (Figure 91–1). Most common is **21-hydroxylase deficiency,** which causes inadequate cortisol levels, leading to excessive ACTH stimulation (through feedback to the hypothalamus and pituitary), adrenal hyperplasia, and excessive production of adrenal androgens (dehydroepiandrosterone and androstenedione) and testosterone, producing virilization. **Two forms of CAH are seen in neonates, depending on the associated relative or absolute aldosterone deficiency: a simple virilizing form and a salt-losing form.** In the first form, the salt loss is mild and adrenal insufficiency tends not to occur, except in stressful circumstances. In the second, adrenal insufficiency occurs under basal conditions and tends to manifest in the neonatal period or soon thereafter as an adrenal crisis. The electrolyte status of all infants

with 21-hydroxylase deficiency should be monitored because the extent of virilization is not a reliable indicator of the degree of adrenal insufficiency. **11-Hydroxylase enzyme deficiency** is less common and associated with salt retention, volume expansion, and hypertension.

2. **Other, less common causes.** Virilizing maternal or fetal tumors or maternal androgen ingestion or topical use.

B. **Inadequate virilization of male infants (male pseudohermaphroditism).** This condition is caused by inadequate androgen production or incomplete end-organ response to androgen. These patients have a 46,XY karyotype and exclusively testicular tissue. These abnormalities are rare, and most require extensive laboratory investigation before a final diagnosis can be confirmed.

1. **Decreased androgen production.** This can be caused by one of several rare enzyme defects, which are inherited in an autosomal recessive manner. Some of these defects also cause cortisol deficiency and **nonvirilizing adrenal hyperplasia**, and others are specific to the testosterone pathway. Other causes of decreased androgen production include **deficiency of Müllerian-inhibiting substance** (the most common presentation is a male infant with inguinal hernias that contain a uterus or fallopian tubes); **testicular unresponsiveness to human chorionic gonadotropin (hCG) and luteinizing hormone (LH)**; and **anorchia** (absent testes caused by loss of vascular supply to the testis during fetal life). The association of **microphallus/micropenis** and **hypoglycemia** suggests a **pituitary deficiency** with absence of gonadotropins, ACTH, or growth hormone.

2. **Decreased end-organ response to androgen.** Also referred to as **testicular feminization**, can be caused by a defect in the androgen receptor or an unknown defect with normal receptors. It can be total (labial testes with otherwise normal-appearing female genitalia) or, more commonly, partial (incomplete virilization of a male).

3. **5α-Reductase deficiency.** Results in failure of the external genitalia to undergo male differentiation because of the lack of DHT (see Figure 91–1). The outcome

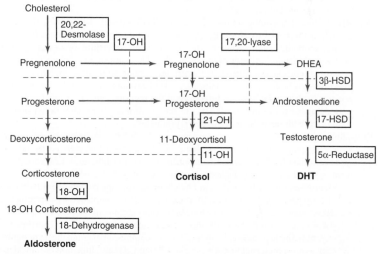

FIGURE 91–1. Adrenal metabolic pathways relevant to normal sex development. 11-OH, 11-hydroxylase; 17-OH, 17-hydroxylase; 18-OH, 18-hydroxylase; 21-OH, 21-hydroxylase; 3β-HSD, 3β-hydroxysteroid dehydrogenase; 17-HSD, 17-hydroxysteroid dehydrogenase (17-ketosteroid reductase); DHEA, dehydroepiandrosterone; DHT, dihydrotestosterone.

is a neonate with female or atypical genitalia but with a 46,XY karyotype, normally developed testes, and male internal ducts.

C. **Disorders of gonadal differentiation**
   1. **True hermaphroditism.** The presence of both a testis and an ovary (or ovotestes) in the same individual is a rare cause of ambiguous genitalia. Most individuals with true hermaphroditism have a 46,XX karyotype, but mosaics of 46,XX/45,X/46,XY/multiple X/multiple Y have all been reported. The appearance of the genitalia is variable; fertility is poor.
   2. **Gonadal dysgenesis**
      a. **Pure gonadal dysgenesis.** Characterized by the presence of a streak gonad bilaterally (complete gonadal dysgenesis) or unilaterally (partial gonadal dysgenesis). It is important to distinguish the X-chromosomal from the Y-chromosomal form because the streak gonads in the Y-positive patients carry a significant **risk for tumor development**.
      b. **Mixed gonadal dysgenesis.** Characterized by the presence of a unilateral functioning testis and a contralateral streak gonad. All patients have a Y chromosome and some degree of virilization of the external genitalia. Mixed gonadal dysgenesis is associated with a high incidence of **gonadal malignancy** in mid to late childhood.

D. **Chromosome abnormalities, syndromes, and associations.** In general, chromosomal abnormalities do not usually lead to genital abnormalities. However, disruption of normal sex development has been reported occasionally in **trisomies 13 and 18, triploidy, and a number of other chromosomal anomalies**. Single-gene disorders and syndromes such as **Smith-Lemli-Opitz syndrome, Rieger syndrome, CHARGE syndrome** (*c*oloboma, *h*eart defects, choanal *a*tresia, *r*etarded growth and development, *g*enital abnormalities, and *e*ar anomalies), **camptomelic dysplasia**, and others can also be associated with external sexual ambiguity (>90 syndromes with "ambiguous genitalia" were found in a search of a syndrome database). **VATER/VACTERL** (*v*ertebral, *a*nal, *t*racheal, *e*sophageal, *r*enal dysplasia/*v*ertebral defects, *a*nal atresia, *c*ardiac malformations, *t*racheoesophageal fistula, *r*enal dysplasia, and *l*imb abnormalities) association can include abnormally developed genitalia.

V. **Risk factors.** The etiology of disorders of sex development is developmental/genetic. Therefore, there are no definite behavioral risk factors, but a history of relatives with genital anomalies, abnormal pubertal development, infertility, or neonatal/infant deaths could be an indicator of increased risk. The question of whether techniques of assisted reproduction, especially in vitro fertilization with intracytoplasmic sperm injection, may be associated with disorders of sex development and other birth defects remains *controversial* because the abnormalities reported could also be related to the underlying cause of infertility leading to the use of these techniques rather than an association with the process of assisted reproduction.

VI. **Clinical presentation.** Note that the American Academy of Pediatrics issued a policy statement on the evaluation of the newborn with developmental anomalies of the external genitalia in 2000. In 2006, after an International Conference on Intersex, a "Consensus Statement on the Management of Intersex Disorders" was published (see Selected References).

A. **History.** A careful history should be obtained from the parents. **Family history** of early neonatal deaths (a death in early infancy accompanied by vomiting and dehydration may be secondary to CAH), consanguinity of the parents (increased risk for autosomal recessive disorders), and female relatives with amenorrhea and infertility (male pseudohermaphroditism or chromosomal anomalies) are significant, as are **maternal history** of virilization or CAH and ingestion or topical use of drugs during pregnancy (particularly androgens or progestational agents).

B. **Physical examination**
   1. **General examination.** A general examination should address the presence of any of the following: dysmorphic features (syndromes and chromosomal

abnormalities), hypertension or hypotension, areolar hyperpigmentation, and signs of dehydration (as signs of CAH).

2. **Genitalia. Gonads**: The number, size, and symmetry of gonads should be evaluated. Palpable gonads below the inguinal canal are usually testes. Ovaries are not found in scrotal folds or in the inguinal region. However, the testes may be intra-abdominal. **Phallus length**: Measured from the pubic ramus to the tip of the glands, a stretched penile length in a full-term infant should be ≥2.0 cm. Reference values for premature infants have been established; ethnic background may influence penile length. **Urethral meatus**: Look for hypospadias (usually accompanied by chordee). **Labioscrotal folds**: Findings can range from unfused labia majora, variable degrees of posterior fusion, and bifid scrotum to fully fused, normal-appearing scrotum. The presence of a vaginal opening or urogenital sinus should be determined. A rectal examination, to determine presence of a uterus, may be considered.

VII. **Diagnosis**
   A. **Laboratory studies**
      1. **Initial evaluation.** An important test in the initial evaluation is the **chromosome analysis**. Most cytogenetic laboratories can now provide preliminary results of a karyotype in a few days. **Fluorescent in situ hybridization techniques (FISH)** allow even faster determination of the sex chromosome status; X- and Y-specific probes are available. Buccal smears are unreliable and therefore obsolete. The remainder of the diagnostic evaluation depends on the sex chromosome status. Blood for **basic biochemical studies** can be obtained at the same time as the karyotype, including 17-hydroxyprogesterone (17-OHP), testosterone, dihydrotestosterone, sodium, and potassium levels. Other tests may be necessary, depending on the results of the karyotype. Biochemical tests are therefore discussed in the context of the different chromosomal constellations.

      2. **Normal 46, XX karyotype.** This finding implies virilization of a genetic female and is caused by excessive maternal or fetal androgen. If the mother is not virilized, the infant almost always has **virilizing adrenal hyperplasia**. To confirm the diagnosis, measure the following:
         a. **17-hydroxyprogesterone (17-OHP).** This is the immediate precursor to the enzyme defect in 21-hydroxylase enzyme deficiency and a precursor one step further removed in 11-hydroxylase enzyme deficiency. In infants with either defect, the serum or plasma level of 17-OHP will be 100–1000 times the normal infant level. Note that the 17-OHP level may be somewhat elevated in normal infants within the first 24 hours of life; a repeat level several days later may be indicated while fluid and electrolyte balance is monitored. 17-OHP is now measured by many newborn screening programs in the United States and other countries as a screening for CAH.
         b. **Daily serum measurements of sodium and potassium.** Infants with 21-hydroxylase enzyme deficiency usually have relative or absolute aldosterone deficiency and begin to demonstrate hyperkalemia at days 3–5 and hyponatremia 1–2 days later. If hyperkalemia becomes clinically significant before the 17-OHP result is available, empirical treatment with intravenous saline, cortisol, and fludrocortisone may be needed (for dosages, see Section VIII.B.1a and b).
         c. **Serum testosterone.** About 3% of infants with ambiguous genitalia are true hermaphrodites, and most have a 46,XX karyotype. If the 17-OHP is not elevated and there is no maternal virilization, a high testosterone level suggests hermaphroditism or fetal testosterone-producing tumor.

      3. **Normal 46,XY karyotype.** The differential diagnosis of an **incompletely virilized genetic male** is extremely complex and includes in utero testicular damage, defects of testosterone synthesis, end-organ resistance, and an enzymatic

defect in the conversion of testosterone to dihydrotestosterone. The laboratory evaluation is correspondingly complex and usually proceeds through a number of steps.

    a. Testosterone (T) and dihydrotestosterone (DHT). These hormone levels should be measurable and are higher in newborns than later in childhood. In the male pseudohermaphrodite, testosterone is low in any defect in testosterone production. The T-to-DHT ratio should be between 5:1 and 20:1 when expressed in similar units. A high T-to-DHT ratio suggests 5α-reductase deficiency (see also Section VII.A.3c). **Androstenedione** levels are measured to diagnose **17-ketosteroid reductase deficiency.**

    b. LH and follicle-stimulating hormone (FSH). These hormones are also higher in infancy than they are in childhood. A diagnosis of gonadotropin deficiency is suspected if these values are low in a reliable assay but can be confirmed in infancy only if there are **other pituitary hormone deficits** (see Section VII.A.3d). Note that growth hormone and ACTH deficiency are manifested in the newborn period as **hypoglycemia.** In primary gonadal defects and some androgen-resistant states, LH and FSH are elevated.

    c. hCG stimulation test. hCG is administered to stimulate gonadal steroid production when testosterone values are low (as in gonadotropin deficiency or a defect in testosterone synthesis). Recommendations vary, and the test should be performed under the guidance of a specialist. In general, a dose of 500–1000 U every day or every other day for 3 doses may be given. Then testosterone and DHT are measured again to evaluate the gonadal response. A rise in the testosterone level confirms the presence of Leydig cells and, by implication, testicular tissue. In patients with 5α-reductase deficiency, the basal T-to-DHT ratio may be normal but elevated after hCG stimulation. It is wise to obtain enough blood after hCG injection to measure other steroid intermediates if the testosterone is low. Considering the complexity of male pseudohermaphroditism, the restrictions in drawing blood from newborns, and the fact that many specific tests can be performed only in special laboratories, involvement of a pediatric endocrinologist in the planning and interpretation of these tests is crucial. In any case, it is always advisable to ask the initial processing laboratory to freeze any remaining serum or plasma.

    d. Assessment of pituitary function. If gonadotropin deficiency due to impairment of pituitary function is suspected (eg, microphallus/micropenis combined with hypoglycemia), thyroid function tests, growth hormone levels, ACTH stimulation test, and imaging studies of the pituitary gland may be indicated.

  4. Abnormal karyotype. Mixed gonadal dysgenesis with a dysplastic gonad may be present in infants with abnormal karyotype and abnormal genitalia. Hormone studies are unlikely to be revealing in this scenario. Note that a normal karyotype from peripheral white blood cells does not exclude mosaic chromosomal abnormalities, and there is a limit in the resolution of conventional karyotypes. **Special genetic testing (FISH analysis, genome microarray analysis, or specific DNA analysis)** may be needed. These techniques may allow detection of *SRY* gene material in 46,XX phenotypic males and be useful in determining whether Y material is present in a 45,X individual, placing the patient at risk for gonadoblastoma.

B. Radiographic studies

  1. Ultrasonography to evaluate adrenal and pelvic structures. Although a uterus is sometimes palpable on rectal examination shortly after birth (because of enlargement in response to maternal estrogen), ultrasonography seems less invasive. The presence and localization of gonads may also be clarified by ultrasonography. Adrenal ultrasonography is sufficiently sensitive to determine adrenal abnormalities in the majority of patients with untreated adrenal hyperplasia.

2. Contrast studies to outline the internal anatomy (sinography, urethrography, vesicocystoureterography, and intravenous urography) may be indicated in complex cases and before reconstructive surgery.

3. Magnetic resonance imaging (MRI) has been used to evaluate patients with disorders of sex development but, at least in the neonatal period, sensitivity may only be marginally improved over ultrasound.

VIII. Management

A. General considerations. The presence of any disorders of sex differentiation is likely to cause significant emotional and social stresses and anxieties for the family. It is very important to protect the privacy of child and parents while diagnostic studies are in progress. A multidisciplinary team should assist the patient and family throughout the diagnostic process and beyond. Once a diagnosis has been established, gender should be assigned (see Section IX) and a team of specialists should supervise medical treatment (steroid replacement, gonadal removal, reconstructive surgery, etc.) and treatment of psychosocial aspects. **Circumcision should be delayed in any infant with a DSD until completion of multidisciplinary evaluation and gender assignment.**

1. Early interactions with the parents and general care. As soon as the abnormality is noted, a physician responsible for the infant should be identified and the parents should be informed. During the initial counseling of the family, gender neutral terms such as "your infant" should be used; gender-specific pronouns should be avoided. A phrase often recommended in this situation is to refer to the genitalia as "incompletely developed." Parents should be informed that it is not possible without further tests to identify the sex of their child. Meet with the parents as soon as possible to discuss the situation in more detail (the delivery room is usually not appropriate for an in-depth discussion). The feelings, impressions, and biases perceived at the time parents first learn about the diagnosis of a sex differentiation disorder often persist. Examining the infant with the parents may be beneficial, but any attempts to identify the sex of the child on the basis of appearance should be resisted, although there is likely to be great pressure to do so from parents, relatives, and hospital personnel. It is important not to complete the birth certificate or make any reference to gender in any of the permanent medical records of the mother or the child. It may be advisable to isolate the child and parents from the inquiries of certain nonessential hospital personnel and the community, but any actions implying that the condition is shameful or should be "hidden" must be avoided. Parents may want to delay sending out birth announcements and telling anyone outside the immediate family that the infant has been born until a gender assignment has been made. Be aware that many children live the majority of their lives in the community of their birth, and confusion about gender assignment because of premature release of information may have long-term consequences. Parents should be reassured that in most cases the gender will be determined as soon as test results are available, and some specialists discourage the use of unisex/epicene names in the early neonatal period.

2. Early referral. It is advisable to seek consultation from a specialist in the evaluation of children with disorders of sex differentiation (the first specialist involved is often a pediatric endocrinologist) as soon as feasible. It is usually not appropriate to discharge a child from the nursery before a detailed evaluation is done. In most cases, a complete diagnosis, assignment of the sex of rearing, and a plan for future treatment can be accomplished before discharge.

B. **Medical management in the neonatal period and early infancy**
   1. **Congenital adrenal hyperplasia.** The most immediate concern in a neonate with abnormal genitalia is whether CAH is present. The onset of adrenal insufficiency occurs between days 3 and 14 in 50% of affected patients. All forms of adrenal hyperplasia have absolute or relative cortisol deficiency and require early diagnosis and replacement therapy to prevent potential life-threatening complications such as vascular collapse.
      a. **Glucocorticoid therapy.** Should be initiated as soon as possible. Maintenance cortisol replacement therapy is often given orally. **Hydrocortisone** is the oral preparation of choice. (See Chapter 148.) Initial doses usually range from 10 to 20 mg/m^2/d given as 3 divided doses and often require adjustments for growth and during periods of stress. Alternatively, intramuscular **cortisone acetate** is sometimes used in children <6 months of age out of concern that oral hydrocortisone may be absorbed erratically in these infants. Supervision of replacement therapy and long-term follow-up with a pediatric endocrinologist is advised; institutional practices may vary.
      b. **Mineralocorticoid therapy.** Fludrocortisone acetate at a dose of 0.05–0.1 mg daily (given orally) is often used. Unlike hydrocortisone, the dose of fludrocortisone does not change with increase of body size or during stress. Some endocrinologists also recommend sodium supplementation (1–5 mEq/kg/d).
   2. **Incompletely virilized genetic male.** Treatment with **depo-testosterone** might be considered by the team of specialists depending on the results of the diagnostic evaluation.
IX. **Prognosis, gender assignment, long-term care.** Discussion surrounding issues of gender assignment are beyond the scope of this book. In general, the sex of rearing should be determined only after diagnostic evaluation by a specialist team. In the past, gender assignment had been approached as though individuals are psychosexually neutral at birth and as though healthy psychosexual development is related to the appearance of the external genitals. However, these beliefs have been challenged. It is now believed that prenatal and early exposure of the brain to androgens, if present, influences gender-specific behavioral patterns and sexual identity in addition to the external appearance of the genitalia or their future function. Considering the significance of the decision for the affected patient's emotional, physical, and reproductive health, a highly specialized multidisciplinary team of pediatricians, urologists, endocrinologists, geneticists, psychiatrists, and others is needed, and each case must be approached individually. Specialized treatment centers should provide long-term care to optimize prognosis. The Consortium on Disorders of Sex Development maintains a website with clinical guidelines and information for families (www.dsdguidelines.org), as do many other support groups such as the Intersex Society of North America (www.isna.org), the Congenital Adrenal Hyperplasia Support and Education (CARES) Foundation (www.caresfoundation.org), and others.

Selected References

Achermann JC, Hughes IA. Disorders of sexual differentiation. In: Melmed S, Polonsky KS, Larsen PR, Kronenberg HM, eds. *Williams' Textbook of Endocrinology.* 12th ed. Philadelphia, PA: Saunders; 2011.

Ahmed SF, Rodie M. Investigation and initial management of ambiguous genitalia. *Best Pract Res Clin Endocrinol Metab.* 2010;24:197.

American Academy of Pediatrics Committee on Genetics. Evaluation of the newborn with developmental anomalies of the external genitalia. *Pediatrics.* 2000;106(1):138–141.

Antal Z, Zhou P. Congenital adrenal hyperplasia: diagnosis, evaluation and management. *Pediatr Rev.* 2009;30:e49.

Barbaro M, Wedell A, Nordenström A. Disorders of sex development. *Semin Fetal Neonatal Med.* 2011;16:119.

Chavhan GB, Parra DA, Oudjhane K, Miller SF, Babyn PS, Pippi Salle FL. Imaging ambiguous genitalia: classification and diagnostic approach. *RadioGraphics.* 2008;28:1891.

Chi C, Chong LH, Kirk, NE. Ambiguous genitalia in the newborn. *NeoReviews* 2008;9:e78.

Diamond DA, Yu RN. Sexual differentiation: normal and abnormal. In: McDougall WS, Wein AJ, Kavoussi LR, et al., eds. *Campbell-Walsh Urology.* 10th ed. Philadelphia, PA: Saunders; 2011.

Hewitt JK, Warne GL. Management of disorders of sex development. *Pediatric Health.* 2009;3:51.

Houk CP, Hughes IA, Ahmed SF, Lee PA; Writing Committee for the International Intersex Consensus Conference Participants. Summary of consensus statement on intersex disorders and their management. International Intersex Consensus Conference. *Pediatrics.* 2006;118(2):753–757.

Hughes IA. Congenital adrenal hyperplasia: 21-hydroxylase deficiency in the newborn and during infancy. *Semin Reprod Med.* 2002;20(3):229–242.

Hughes IA. Disorders of sex development: a new definition and classification. *Best Pract Res Clin Endocrinol Metab.* 2008;22(1):119–134.

Hyun G, Kolon TF. A practical approach to intersex in the newborn period. *Urol Clin North Am.* 2004;31(3):435–443.

Lee PA, Houk CP, Ahmed SF, Hughes IA; International Consensus Conference on Intersex organized by the Lawson Wilkins Pediatric Endocrine Society and the European Society for Paediatric Endocrinology. Consensus statement on management of intersex disorders. *Pediatrics.* 2006;118(2):e488–e500.

Vidal I, Gorduza DB, Haraux E, et al. Surgical options in disorders of sex development (DSD) with ambiguous genitalia. *Best Pract Res Clin Endocrinol Metab.* 2010;24:311.

Warne GL. Long-term outcome of disorders of sex development. *Sex Dev.* 2008;2:268.

92 Enteroviruses and Parechoviruses

I. **Definition.** Enteroviruses and parechoviruses are a large group of viral pathogens represented by 2 different genera of the family *Picornaviridae*. They are all of a single strand of RNA in a capsid of individually distinct polypeptides. The capsid proteins impart antigenicity and facilitate transfer of RNA into the cells of newly infected hosts.

   A. **Enteroviruses.** The genus of **enteroviruses** traditionally consisted of 5 groups, each with well-known human infant pathogenicity: coxsackie A viruses, coxsackie B virus, echoviruses, numbered enteroviruses, and polio virus. The new classification (based on viral genomic structure) of the enterovirus genus has 4 species: human enteroviruses (HEV) A, B, C, and D. Although they were reclassified, virus serotypes continue to use their original name.

   B. **Parechoviruses.** The genus of **human parechoviruses (HPeVs)** is made up of 16 described types but 8 sequenced human parechovirus types. Types 1 and 2 were formerly thought to be human enteroviruses 22 and 23, but after the discovery of capsid proteins distinctly different from those of the genus enterovirus, they have been relegated to a single genus. To date, only types 1–3 have been identified in neonatal sepsis-like viral syndromes. HPeV4–6 are associated with gastrointestinal and respiratory symptoms in young infants. Genotypes are continuing to be characterized and identified.

II. **Incidence**

A. **Enteroviruses.** Enteroviruses are of worldwide distribution and produce human illness of varying severity, from mild coryza to life-threatening multisystem disease. The diseases have some seasonal variation such as summer-fall in temperate zones but of little variation in the more tropical regions of the world.

Of special interest to neonatologists is the now well-established enteroviral transplacental passage, enteroviruses detected in breast milk, and vertical passage of enteroviruses within first-degree family members without clinical signs of illness. Enteroviral illnesses are transmitted by the fecal–oral route and, to a lesser extent, respiratory droplets. Incubation periods are typically 3–6 days. All subgroups of enteroviruses are linked to nursery and neonatal intensive care unit (NICU) outbreaks of enteroviral diseases.

Numerous outbreaks of nonpolio neonatal enterovirus have been reported for newborn nurseries, NICUs, and maternity units over the past 3 decades. Overall incidence for newborn and neonatal infants is variable. The Centers for Disease Control and Prevention (CDC) have reported from the National Enterovirus Surveillance System, 2006–2008, that coxsackie B1 virus (CVB1) accounted for 17% of all reported enterovirus isolates. In contrast, from 1970–2005, they had only accounted for 2.3% of cases. During this time there was also an increase in reports of neonatal morbidity and 5 cases of neonatal death in the United States.

B. **Parechoviruses.** During 2006–2008 surveillance, HPeV type 1 was the most common isolate of that genus, but only accounted for <2% of identified enteroviral suspect specimens. More recently, a report from Edinburgh, Scotland, for enterovirus surveillance from 2006–2010 revealed an incidence of 2.8% for HPeV, but for infants <3 months of age, HPeV type 3 was the predominant isolate (22–25%).

III. **Pathophysiology**

A. **Enteroviruses.** Human enteroviruses manifest disease in nearly all body systems. Paradoxically, signs of disease can be mild to nearly nonexistent or life-threatening within the same serotype. Host susceptibility seems to be the distinguishing factor. For the great majority of children and adults, enteroviral illnesses are mild, but for the neonate, a more susceptible host, enteroviruses can cause serious multiorgan dysfunction and death. Some human enteroviruses are more pathogenic than others. Examples of the more serious infections by nonpolio enterovirus serotypes are echo 11, coxsackie B3, coxsackie A9, coxsackie B1, and enterovirus 71.

1. **Echo virus 11.** This has been particularly associated with neonatal fatalities. Most pathologic findings have been extensive hepatic necrosis with adrenal hemorrhage and acute tubular necrosis as less frequent additional findings.

2. **Coxsackievirus B3 (CVB3).** Neonatal infections have been marked by hepatitis, disseminated intravascular infection, fever, thrombocytopenia, and intracranial hemorrhage. CVB3 has also been closely associated with antenatal maternal infection and positive virus cultures from placenta, cord, and infant tissues at death. All circumstances suggested transplacental viral passage.

3. **Coxsackievirus A9 (CVA9).** Although much less common than CVB3, it has a more protean spectrum of neonatal morbidity. It may present as aseptic meningitis, a nonspecific sepsis-like illness, myocarditis, pneumonia, or disseminated intravascular coagulation.

4. **Coxsackievirus B1 (CVB1).** Until recently, this has been a fairly uncommon strain. In 2006, for the first time, CVB1 became the most commonly reported enterovirus and remained so through 2008. In 2007 there was a significant increase in neonatal disease, including febrile illness, hepatitis, coagulopathy, meningitis, respiratory distress, and myocarditis. In 2007, in 4 of 5 cases of neonatal death, mothers had chorioamnionitis or febrile illness near the time of delivery.

5. **Enterovirus 71.** This has been less frequently reported but has been identified with aseptic meningitis, encephalitis, acute flaccid paralysis, and secondary

pulmonary hemorrhage and cardiopulmonary collapse. Community-wide outbreaks in 2003 and 2005 in Denver, Colorado, revealed involvement of infants ≥4 weeks of age with most having central nervous system (CNS) disease.

B. **Parechovirus.** Parechovirus infections are now recognized as an agent for nursery outbreaks of diarrhea coupled with respiratory illnesses. Several cases of more severe illness have been reported, including meningoencephalitis, neonatal sepsis-like disease, hepatitis, and coagulopathy. Other conditions have included myocarditis and conjunctivitis. Parechoviruses occur in association with other conditions (hemorrhage hepatitis syndrome, necrotizing enterocolitis, myocarditis, herpangina, and febrile illness), but further studies are needed to link them.

1. **HPeV1 (previously echovirus 21).** Most common HPeV identified. Usually asymptomatic or mild gastrointestinal (GI) or respiratory symptoms. Very rarely it can cause myocarditis, paralysis, and CNS involvement (encephalitis and paralysis).
2. **HPeV2 (previously echovirus 22).** Rare GI symptoms but can have respiratory tract and GI infections with otitis media.
3. **HPeV3.** Aseptic meningitis, sepsis-like disease with more severe disease (neonatal sepsis, meningitis, encephalitis with white matter injury, and hepatitis). Also associated with gastroenteritis, respiratory illness, and transient paralysis. Fatal cases have been reported.
4. **HPeV4, 5, and 6.** HPeV4 was first isolated from an infant with a fever and feeding problems. These are associated with GI and respiratory symptoms in younger infants. HPeV6 has been associated with flaccid paralysis.

IV. **Risk factors**

A. **Infants born to mothers** who have symptoms of enterovirus/parechovirus around the time of the delivery have a higher chance of being infected. In 2010, a study of 242 pregnant Taiwanese women affected by herpangina during their pregnancy had a significantly higher risk for infants being low birthweight, small for gestational age, or preterm.

B. **Risk of severe infection** is higher if the infant is infected during the first 2 weeks of life.

V. **Clinical presentations.** HPeV infections may mimic HEV infections. When evaluating an infant and looking at clinical signs, it is not possible to distinguish neonatal parechovirus from an enterovirus infection.

A. **Enteroviruses.** The clinical presentations of nonpolio enterovirus diseases are varied and overlap with the many subspecies and serotypes. In neonates, the signs that suggest an enteroviral outbreak in a nursery might include a cluster of infants with similar findings of coryza, morbilliform rash, low-grade fever, or cough. The latter is a most unusual occurrence in neonates, prompting close observation and investigation. A sepsis-like illness is frequently ascribed to enteroviral illnesses. Sepsis evaluation is often negative, but findings of lethargy, poor feeding, and fever are hallmarks suggesting sepsis. It can also cause hepatitis, coagulopathy, pneumonia, meningoencephalitis, and myocarditis. Hemophagocytic lymphohistiocytosis and severe enteroviral infection can be difficult to distinguish based on clinical presentation and cerebrospinal fluid findings.

B. **Parechoviruses.** May mimic the presentation of enteroviruses. The majority of infants with HPeV1 and 2 have mild GI and respiratory syndromes. HPeV serotype 3 has been associated with severe neonatal infection, including CNS infection. The most common clinical presentation of HPeV3 is a sepsis-like syndrome. In one study, parechovirus CNS infection was found to be more common in male infants during the late summer or autumn season. Symptoms included irritability, fever, and a nonspecific rash. Infants with parechoviruses may present with an acute distended abdomen accompanied by an erythematous rash, low C-reactive protein, and low lymphocyte count and have been associated with small clusters of patients with necrotizing enterocolitis.

VI. **Diagnosis**
   A. **Enteroviruses.** Polymerase chain reaction (PCR) is readily available in commercial laboratories but lacks specificity for serotyping. Advanced PCR techniques are required to further identify most enterovirus subspecies. PCR is both more rapid and more sensitive than cell culture. Some serotypes are difficult to isolate from cerebrospinal fluid, but can be readily isolated from either throat or rectal swab. Cell culture had been the standard method for isolation and diagnosis, but specific serotype identification requires expensive neutralization assays or genomic sequencing. Several serotypes cannot be grown effectively in culture. Specimens for cell culture or PCR assays should include cerebrospinal fluid, blood, urine, nasal swabs, throat swabs, and stool specimens. Real-time PCR assay for enterovirus RNA allows shorter turnover time for the detection.
   B. **Parechoviruses.** Current enterovirus specific testing does not detect parechovirus infection because of the genetic differences between the two. The best diagnostic tests are PCR primers that have been developed by the CDC that detect all known parechoviruses. White matter injury has been visualized with a cranial ultrasound and magnetic resonance imaging with diffusion weighted imaging in infants with HPeV3 with encephalitis. Many of the parechoviruses do not grow well in cell culture. A direct PCR of stool samples can be obtained.

VII. **Management.** No specific therapy for human enteroviruses or parechoviruses exists. Overall care involves supportive measures, close observation for organ-specific disease (eg, meningitis, myocarditis), and diagnostic testing to confirm infection. In cases of severe neonatal disease, high-dose human immune globulin has been suggested, but depending on antibody per lot of immune globulin, efficacy varies. Prophylactic immune globulin has been reported to be helpful in controlling hospital nursery outbreaks of enterovirus disease. Observation for bacterial colonization and secondary infection is appropriate, especially for staphylococcal disease. If fulminate hepatic disease is present, oral neomycin therapy to minimize gut flora may be beneficial. Currently the safety and efficacy of the antiviral drug pleconaril is being studied in neonatal viremia.

VIII. **Prognosis.** The illness is usually mild and recoverable. Mortality is increased with the more severe forms of the infection.

Selected References

American Academy of Pediatrics. Enterovirus (nonpoliovirus) and parechovirus infections. In: Pickering LK, Baker CJ, Kimberlin DW, Long SS, eds. *Red Book: 2012 Report of the Committee on Infectious Diseases.* 28th ed. Elk Grove Village, IL: American Academy of Pediatrics; 2012:315–318.

Bangalore H, Ahmed J, Bible J, Menson EN, Durward A, Tong CY. Abdominal distention: an important feature in human parechovirus infection. *Pediatr Infect Dis J.* 2011;30:260–262.

Centers for Disease Control and Prevention. Increased detections and severe neonatal disease associated with coxsackie virus B1 infection–United States, 2007. *MMWR Morb Mortal Wkly Rep.* 2010;59:1577–1580.

Chen Y-H, Lin HC, Lin HC. Increased risk of adverse pregnancy outcomes among women affected by herpangina. *Am J Obstet Gynecol.* 2010;203:49.e1–e7.

Cherry JD. Enteroviruses and parechoviruses. In: Remington JS, Klein JO, Wilson CB, Nizet V, Maldonado Y, eds. *Infectious Diseases of the Fetus and Newborn Infant.* 6th ed. Philadelphia, PA: Elsevier Saunders; 2006:783–822.

Harvala H, McLeish N, Kondracka J, et al. Comparison of human parechovirus and enterovirus detection frequencies in cerebrospinal fluid samples collected over a 5-year period in Edinburgh: HPev type 3 identified as the most common picornavirus type. *J Med Virol.* 2011;83:889–896.

Levorson R. Human parechovirus-3 infection, emerging pathogen in neonatal sepsis. *Pediatr Infect Dis J.* 2009;2:545–547.

Sedmak G, Nix WA, Jentzen J, et al. Infant deaths associated with human parechovirus infection in Wisconsin. *Clin Infect Dis.* 2010;50:357–361.

Selvarangan R, Nzabi M, Selvaraju SB, Ketter P, Carpenter C, Harrison CJ. Human parechovirus 3 causing sepsislike illness in children from Midwestern United States. *Pediatr Infect Dis J.* 2011;30:238–242.

Verboon-Maciolek MA, Krediet TG, Gerards LJ, de Vries LS, Groenendaal F, van Loon AM. Severe neonatal parechovirus infection and similarity with enterovirus infection. *Pediatr Infect Dis J.* 2008;27:241–245.

93 Eye Disorders of the Newborn

I. **Eye examination.** The infant's first eye examination is performed sometime after birth and prior to discharge home. The extent of the examination should be appropriate to the infant's condition. This initial selective screening examination assesses structural development of the eyes and the relationship of the eyes to the overall facies. In addition, reactivity of the pupils and the red reflex are assessed. The eye examination also provides a good opportunity to observe an infant's resting state and his or her ability to transition from one state to another. Observations that give information about the infant's general well-being and maturity include apparent awareness and visual interest in the surroundings as opposed to abnormal staring or absent visual fixation. In otherwise healthy infants, assessment of visual acuity is delayed until early childhood when cooperation with the eye examination can be expected. Normal findings that resolve include edema, eversion, bruising, hemorrhage, and nevus simplex. (See also Chapter 6.)

The **American Academy of Pediatrics (AAP) recommends an age-appropriate assessment in the newborn period:** ocular history, vision assessment (ability to fix and follow objects after 3 months of age), external inspection of the eyes and lids (conjunctiva, sclera, cornea, iris, and lids), ocular motility assessment, pupil examination (equal, round, and reactive to light), red reflex examination (should be bright reddish-yellow, or light gray in brown-eyed infants, and identical in both eyes). Newborns should be evaluated for cataracts, ptosis, and corneal opacities. Any abnormalities on examination should be referred to a pediatric ophthalmologist. **Infants at high risk of eye problems** (premature, significant neurological or developmental difficulties, metabolic or genetic diseases, positive family history of congenital cataracts, retinoblastoma, any systemic diseases associated with eye abnormalities) should be referred for a specialized eye examination by a pediatric ophthalmologist.

II. **Basic eye information.** Structure and function of the eye are dynamic processes that begin early in pregnancy and continue throughout childhood. In term infants, the eye and visual pathway system are immature with most neonates being far-sighted. During early school age, they become more nearsighted. Binocularity is established by 3–4 months of age. By 4–5 months, infants can fixate on an image with both eyes simultaneously with a steady gaze; the ability to distinguish color begins at ~5 months. Visual acuity in infants ranges from 20/400 to 20/50. The optic nerve is completely myelinated by 2 years of age and visual acuity reaches 20/40 by that time.

The pupils are small with undeveloped reflexes until about 5 months of age. Transient nystagmus is common in infants <6 months. Extraocular muscle function is poorly coordinated for the first 6 months of life, resulting in intermittent convergent strabismus. Accommodation and convergence should be established by 24 months. There is little pigment in the iris at birth; pigmentation of the eye is complete by 6–12 months of age. The lacrimal apparatus is not fully developed at birth. Neonates don't produce tears until ~4–6 weeks of age. Both corneal and blink reflexes are present at birth. The eye size reaches adult proportion by about 8 years of age.

III. **Amblyopia**
   A. **Definition.** Amblyopia is a reduction in corrected visual acuity in the absence of organic eye disease. It results from unequal visual stimulation during the sensitive period of visual development and is the most common cause of monocular vision loss in children.
   B. **Incidence.** Estimated prevalence is 2–5% in the United States. This condition affects 2–3 out of every 100 children.
   C. **Pathophysiology.** Amblyopia may be caused by any condition that affects normal visual development or use of the eyes. There are 3 major etiologies for amblyopia in the neonate.
      1. **Strabismus.** This is the preference of one eye when the visual axes are misaligned and is the most common contributing factor. It develops whether it is from esotropia, exotropia, or hypertropia.
      2. **Refractive errors.** Amblyopia resulting from refractive errors can be divided into 2 types: anisometropic and isometropic. Anisometropic amblyopia results from significant inequality of the refractive errors in each eye, blunting the development of the visual pathway in the affected eye. Isometropic amblyopia occurs when the refractive errors in the 2 eyes are equal.
      3. **Deprivation.** The least common condition, congenital or early-acquired opacity, causes deprivation amblyopia. This can be the most severe and damaging type. Cataracts, corneal lesions, or ptosis blocks or distorts the retinal image formation. This can affect one or both eyes and may develop as early as 2–4 months.
   D. **Risk factors.** Low birthweight, prematurity, familial factors, and certain congenital anterior lens opacities with significant anisometropia.
   E. **Clinical presentation.** Strabismus is recognized as a consistently deviating eye in the first few months after the newborn period. Diagnosis is made during the newborn or early infant eye examination or when there is evidence of reduced visual acuity that cannot be explained by physical abnormalities.
   F. **Management.** Treatment is individualized depending on the cause. The treatment for strabismus is patching of the preferred eye or surgical correction. Refractive amblyopia is treated with patching or glasses. Surgical interventions are needed for deprivation amblyopia.
   G. **Prognosis.** It is critical that these be diagnosed and treated as early as possible. Most vision loss is preventable or reversible with the right intervention for the individual etiology. The recovery depends on the maturity of the visual connections, the length of deprivation, and the age at which therapy is begun.

IV. **Anophthalmos/microphthalmos**
   A. **Definition.** Anophthalmos is absence of ocular tissue in the orbit. Microphthalmos describes an eye that measures <15 mm in diameter after birth.
   B. **Incidence.** The prevalence of anophthalmos and microphthalmos are generally estimated to be 3 and 14 per 100,000 births, respectively. The combined prevalence may be up to 30 per 100,000 births.
   C. **Pathophysiology.** Anophthalmos is caused by failure of development of either optic vesicle or regression after initiation of vesicle development. May occur in isolation or as part of a syndrome.

    D. **Risk factors.** Advanced maternal age, multiple births, prematurity, and low birthweight.

    E. **Clinical presentation.** Either the presence of no eye tissue or a small orbit. Diagnosis is made by inspection, palpation, and imaging. Ultrasound is commonly used to determine length of the globe in microphthalmia. Computed tomography (CT) and magnetic resonance imaging (MRI) can facilitate diagnosis of anophthalmia. Detectable function may be present in microphthalmic cases.

    F. **Management.** Conservative approaches include refracting the eyes and treating any underlying amblyopia. In unilateral cases, the "good" eye must be protected and any visual deficit managed appropriately. Reconstructive surgical interventions allow for growth of the orbit and prevention of soft tissues and orbit hypoplasia.

    G. **Prognosis.** Visual development depends on the degree of retinal development and other ocular characteristics in microphthalmic patients. Therapy is aimed at maximizing existing vision and enhancing cosmetic appearance rather than improving sight.

V. **Coloboma**

    A. **Definition.** Colobomas are cleft-shaped fissures in the eyelid, iris, ciliary body, retina, choroid, or optic nerve. They are usually restricted to the iris.

    B. **Incidence.** Ocular colobomas occur in 1 per 2077 live births.

    C. **Pathophysiology.** Incomplete embryologic closure of fetal fissures that may be associated with persistence of hyaloid vessels and papillary membrane.

    D. **Risk factors.** The majority are sporadic, but there is an increased incidence in infants with trisomy 13 and infants with CHARGE syndrome (*c*oloboma, *h*eart defects, choanal *a*tresia, *r*etarded growth and development, *g*enital abnormalities, and *e*ar anomalies), or as a result of maternal ingestion of LSD or thalidomide. Familial colobomas are autosomal dominant.

    E. **Clinical presentation.** A keyhole-shaped defect that may be seen in a variety of optic structures.

    F. **Management.** Indicated in a severe defect or when an eyelid coloboma prevents adequate lid closure.

    G. **Prognosis.** Dependent on the location of the coloboma. A coloboma in the iris would not affect vision. A coloboma that includes the optic nerve, the macula, and other parts of the retina can cause legal blindness.

VI. **Congenital cataracts**

    A. **Definition.** A nonspecific reaction to a change in the lens metabolism leading to lens opacification.

    B. **Incidence.** Estimates are 1.2–6.0 cases per 10,000 in the United States.

    C. **Pathophysiology.** Any process that alters the glycolytic pathway or epithelial cell mitosis of the avascular lens causes cataracts.

    D. **Risk factors.** About 25% of the cases are hereditary; the most frequent mode of transmission is autosomal dominant; about one-third of cases occur sporadically.

        1. **Metabolic causes.** Hypoglycemia, hypoparathyroidism, mannosidosis, maternal diabetes, galactosemia, hypocalcemia, and vitamin A or D deficiency.

        2. **Congenital infections.** Infants with rubella, herpes simplex, and varicella can have congenital cataracts.

        3. **Other causes.** In utero radiation exposure and associations with specific genetic syndromes (trisomy 21, Stickler, Smith-Lemli-Opitz).

    E. **Clinical presentation.** The newborn presents with a white papillary reflex or leukocoria. Cataracts in infants may be transient and disappear spontaneously within a few weeks. Lens opacities may be isolated or associated with other eye anomalies or systemic conditions. Cataracts seen with congenital rubella are characteristically total or near-total opacities in a smaller than normal lens. Abnormalities of the retinal pigment, "salt and pepper" changes, are typically seen.

    F. **Management.** The initial workup includes the many causes and associations. Maternal and infant history direct laboratory evaluation. An ophthalmologic slit lamp confirms the presence of a cataract. If the cataract directly threatens vision, then prompt surgical removal is indicated to avoid legal blindness from deprivation amblyopia. Infants will require significant visual rehabilitation.

1. **Optical devices are used to provide focus** after the lost lens. Contact lenses are used early.

2. **Occlusion therapy of the better eye** to reverse amblyopia may be necessary. Length of treatment ranges from 1 to 8 weeks in infants <1 year of age.

G. **Prognosis.** Cataracts lead to varying degrees of visual impairment from blurred vision to blindness, depending on the extent and location of the opacity.

VII. **Congenital glaucoma**

A. **Definition.** Increased ocular pressure in the aqueous humor that eventually causes damage to the optic nerve.

B. **Incidence.** It is estimated to affect <1% of all children.

C. **Pathophysiology.** Primary congenital glaucoma is caused by structural abnormalities of the eye drainage channels. Secondary causes include retinopathy of prematurity, persistent fetal vasculature, congenital rubella, and homocystinuria.

D. **Risk factors.** Males are found to have a higher incidence of the disease, comprising ~65% of cases. The disease is typically autosomal recessive. Infants with galactosemia, lysosomal storage disorders, and peroxisomal disorders can all present with glaucoma.

E. **Clinical presentation.** Corneal cloudiness, photophobia, lacrimation, buphthalmos, and eye rubbing.

F. **Management.** Diagnosis is made by measuring ocular pressure. Periodic monitoring of ocular pressure and vision is necessary. Infants usually require surgery to increase drainage.

G. **Prognosis.** Early intervention is preferred as there is increased risk for blindness if left untreated.

VIII. **Conjunctivitis.** See Chapter 53.

IX. **Nasolacrimal duct obstruction.** See also Chapter 53.

A. **Definition.** Congenital obstruction of the nasolacrimal duct.

B. **Incidence.** This common abnormality is found in 2–6% of all newborns.

C. **Pathophysiology.** The obstruction is caused by an imperforate membrane at the end of the nasolacrimal duct.

D. **Risk factors.** Children with Down syndrome, craniosynostosis, Goldenhar sequence, clefting syndromes, hemifacial microsomia, or any midline facial anomaly are at an increased risk for congenital nasolacrimal duct obstruction.

E. **Clinical presentation.** The signs of obstruction are an increase of mucus or mucopurulent discharge and epiphora. The periocular skin is sometimes chapped. The globe is usually white. Pressure over the lacrimal sac produces a reflux of mucoid or mucopurulent material from the punctum.

F. **Management.** Treatment consists of initial observation for resolution followed by probing of children with persistent duct obstruction. Medical management includes observation, lacrimal massage, and treatment with topical antibiotics.

G. **Prognosis** for resolution is good.

X. **Congenital ptosis**

A. **Definition.** A unilateral or bilateral decrease in the vertical distance between the upper and lower eyelids.

B. **Incidence.** The frequency of congenital ptosis in the United States has not been reported. However, in 70% of known cases, only one eye is affected.

C. **Pathophysiology.** Due to dysfunction of the levator palpebrae muscle.

D. **Risk factors.** It may be transmitted as an autosomal dominant condition or caused by third-nerve palsy.

E. **Clinical presentation.** Ptosis can affect one or both eyes. With partial dysfunction the eyelid droops; with complete dysfunction of the muscle, there is no elevation of the eyelid during an upward gaze. Infants with mild unilateral ptosis should be evaluated for Horner syndrome.

   F. **Management.** Infants should be monitored every 3–12 months for signs of amblyopia. Surgical correction of congenital ptosis can be undertaken at any age depending on the severity of the disease. Earlier intervention may be required if significant amblyopia or ocular torticollis are present.

   G. **Prognosis.** Repair of congenital ptosis can produce excellent functional and cosmetic results. Of patients who require surgical intervention, 50% or more may require repeat surgery in 8–10 years following the initial surgery. With careful observation and treatment, amblyopia can be treated successfully.

XI. **Chalazion**

   A. **Definition.** Chronic granulomatous inflammation of the meibomian glands developing away from the lid margins.

   B. **Incidence.** Unknown.

   C. **Pathophysiology.** This is caused by a blockage in one of the ducts that drains the glands.

   D. **Risk factors.** Males and females are equally affected.

   E. **Clinical presentation.** A nontender, firm nodule is seen deep within the eyelid; usually centered on an eyelash; usually not seen in neonates.

   F. **Management.** Small, asymptomatic chalazia can be ignored. Treatment includes massage, moist heat, and topical mild steroid drops. Management of infected chalazia includes antibiotics, heat, and possible incision and drainage.

   G. **Prognosis for resolution is good.**

XII. **Retinoblastoma**

   A. **Definition.** A cancerous tumor of the retina.

   B. **Incidence.** Retinoblastoma affects 1 in every 15,000–30,000 live babies that are born in the United States. It is the most frequent tumor of the eye.

   C. **Pathophysiology.** In all cases, it is caused by an abnormality in chromosome 13, which is responsible for controlling retinal cell division.

   D. **Risk factors.** The majority of families have no family history, though there is an increased risk of transmission once in the family. It affects children of all races and both boys and girls.

   E. **Clinical presentation.** The majority of infants present with a white papillary reflex (leukocoria). Other signs are strabismus, poor vision, enlarged pupils, or inflammation of tissue around the eye. Most cases (75%) involve only one eye.

   F. **Management.** Diagnosis is made during an ophthalmologic examination under general anesthesia. Treatment is customized for each patient. Enucleation of the affected eye has been standard treatment of this tumor, though intraoptical chemotherapy is currently being used in some institutions. Radiation, laser therapy, cryotherapy, laser reduction, and chemoreduction are also used.

   G. **Prognosis.** Long-term prognosis is good. Most children with retinoblastoma survive. In the United States, nearly 98% of children survive, but not so in less advanced countries where about 50% of children die from tumor spread. Long-term ocular and pediatric examinations are advised for the child.

Selected References

American Academy of Ophthalmology. Amblyopia summary benchmarks for preferred practice pattern guidelines. http://one.aao.org/CE/PracticeGuidelines/PPP_Content.aspx?cid=930d01f2-740b-433e-a973-cf68565bd27b. Accessed November 2, 2011.

Committee on Practice and Ambulatory Medicine, Section on Ophthalmology. American Association of Certified Orthoptists; American Association for Pediatric Ophthalmology and Strabismus; American Academy of Ophthalmology. Eye examination in infants, children, and young adults by pediatricians. *Pediatrics.* 2003;111(4):902–907.

Donahue R. Pediatric strabismus. *N Engl J Med.* 2007;356:1040.

Haddad MA. Causes of visual impairment in children: a study of 3,210 cases. *J Pediatr Ophthalmol Strabismus.* 2007;44:232.

Nakamura KM, Diehl NN, Mohney BG. Incidence, ocular findings, and systemic associations of ocular coloboma: a population-based study. *Arch Ophthalmol.* 2011;129:67.

Pai A, Mitchell P. Prevalence of amblyopia and strabismus. *Ophthalmology.* 2010;117:2042.

Verma AS, Fitzpatrick DR. Anophthalmia and microphthalmia. *Orphanet J Rare Dis.* 2007;2:47.

94 Gonorrhea

I. **Definition.** Infection with *Neisseria gonorrhoeae* (**a Gram-negative oxidase-positive diplococcus**) is a reproductive tract infection that is an important infection in pregnancy because of transmission to the fetus or neonate.

II. **Incidence.** In 2010, the reported rate of gonorrhea in the United States was ~ 1 per 1000. The incidence is highest in females 15 through 24 years of age. If routine ophthalmic prophylaxis was not used, it is estimated that a third of newborn infants born to infected mothers would become infected.

III. **Pathophysiology.** *Neisseria gonorrhoeae* primarily affects the endocervical canal of the mother. The infant may become infected during passage through an infected cervical canal or by contact with contaminated amniotic fluid if rupture of membranes has occurred. Coinfection with *Chlamydia trachomatis* is frequent, and human immunodeficiency virus (HIV) transmission is enhanced in the presence of gonorrhea.

IV. **Clinical presentations**

A. **Ophthalmia neonatorum (neonatal conjunctivitis).** The most common clinical manifestation is gonococcal ophthalmia neonatorum. This occurs in 1–2% of cases of positive maternal gonococcal infection despite appropriate eye prophylaxis. For a description of this disease, see Chapter 53.

B. **Gonococcal arthritis.** The onset of gonococcal arthritis can occur at any time from 1–4 weeks after delivery. It is secondary to gonococcemia. The source of bacteremia has been attributed to infection of the mouth, nares, and umbilicus. The most common sites are the knees and ankles, but any joint may be affected. The infant may present with mild or moderate symptoms. Drainage of affected joint and antibiotics are mandatory.

C. **Amniotic infection syndrome.** Occurs when there is premature rupture of membranes, with inflammation of the placenta and umbilical cord. The infant may have clinical evidence of sepsis. This infection is associated with a high mortality rate.

D. **Sepsis and meningitis.** See Chapters 130 and 109, respectively.

E. **Scalp abscess.** Usually secondary to intrauterine fetal monitoring.

F. **Other localized infections.** Other infections involving mucus membranes like the pharynx, vagina, urethra, and anus has been described.

V. **Diagnosis**

A. **Mother.** Endocervical scrapings should be obtained for culture.

B. **Infant**

1. **Gram stain.** Gram stain of any exudate should be performed.

2. **Culture.** Material may be obtained by swabbing the eye or nasopharynx or the orogastric or anorectal areas. Blood should be obtained for culture. Cultures for concomitant infection with *Chlamydia trachomatis* should also be done. Gonococcal cultures from nonsterile sites (eg, the pharynx, rectum, and vagina) should be done using selective media.

3. **Lumbar puncture with spinal fluid studies.** Cell count, protein, culture, Gram stain, and others should be ordered.

VI. **Management.** Isolation precautions for all infectious diseases, including maternal and neonatal precautions, breast-feeding, and visiting issues, can be found in Appendix F.

   A. **Hospitalization.** Infants with clinical evidence of ophthalmia neonatorum, scalp abscess, or disseminated infection should be hospitalized. Complete sepsis evaluation including lumbar puncture should be performed. Tests for concomitant *C. trachomatis,* congenital syphilis, and HIV infection should be done. Results of the maternal tests for hepatitis B surface antigen should be confirmed.

   B. **Antibiotic therapy.** For dosages, see Chapter 148.

      1. **Maternal infection.** Most infants born to mothers with gonococcal infection do not experience infection; however, because there have been some reported cases, it is recommended that newborns receive a single injection of ceftriaxone. Although treatment failure after cephalosporin therapy is rare in the United States, minimum inhibitory concentrations to cephalosporins are increasing. Treatment failures have been reported more frequently from Asian countries. The mother and her sexual partner(s) should be evaluated (and treated) for other sexually transmitted infections, including HIV infection.

      2. **Nondisseminated infection.** Includes ophthalmia neonatorum; treatment is ceftriaxone given once. Alternative treatment for ophthalmia is cefotaxime as a single dose. Infants with ophthalmia should have their eyes irrigated with saline immediately and at frequent intervals until the discharge is eliminated. Topical antibiotics are inadequate and unnecessary with systemic therapy. Infants with conjunctivitis should be hospitalized and evaluated for disseminated infections (sepsis, arthritis, meningitis).

      3. **Disseminated infection. For arthritis and septicemia:** Ceftriaxone or cefotaxime for 7 days. **For meningitis:** Ceftriaxone or cefotaxime for 10–14 days. Use Cefotaxime if the infant has hyperbilirubinemia.

   C. **Isolation.** All infants with gonococcal infection should be placed in contact isolation until effective parenteral antimicrobial therapy has been given for 24 hours. See Appendix F.

VII. **Prognosis.** Excellent if treatment is started early.

Selected References

American Academy of Pediatrics. Gonococcal infections. In: Pickering LK, Baker CJ, Kimberlin DW, Long SS, eds. *Red Book: 2012 Report of the Committee on Infectious Diseases.* 29th ed. Elk Grove Village, IL: American Academy of Pediatrics; 2012:336–344.

Babl FE, Ram S, Barnett ED, Rhein L, Carr E, Cooper ER. Neonatal gonococcal arthritis after negative prenatal screening and despite conjunctival prophylaxis. *Pediatr Infect Dis J.* 2000;19:346–349.

Embree JE. Gonococcal infections. In: Remington JS, Klein JO, Wilson CB, Nizet V, Maldonado Y, eds. *Infectious Diseases of the Fetus and Newborn Infant.* 7th ed. Philadelphia, PA: Elsevier Saunders; 2011:516–523.

95 Hepatitis

Hepatitis may be produced by many infectious and noninfectious agents. Typically, viral hepatitis refers to several clinically similar diseases that differ in cause and epidemiology. These include hepatitis A, B, C, D (delta), E, and G. Chronic lifelong infection has only been documented with hepatitis B (HBV) and hepatitis C (HCV) virus.

Table 95–1. **HEPATITIS TESTING**

Specific Test	Description
HAV	Etiologic agent of "infectious" hepatitis
Anti-HAV	Detectable at onset of symptoms; lifetime persistence
Anti-HAV-IgM	Indicates recent infection with HAV; positive up to 4–6 months postinfection
Anti-HAV-IgG	Signifies previous HAV infection; confers immunity
HBV	Etiologic agent of "serum" hepatitis
HBsAg	Detectable in serum; earliest indicator of acute infection or indicative of chronic infection if present >6 months
Anti-HBs	Indicates past infection with and immunity to HBV, passive antibody from HBIG, or immune response from HBV vaccine
HBeAg	Correlates with HBV replication; high-titer HBV in serum signifies high infectivity; persistence for 6–8 weeks suggests a chronic carrier state
Anti-HBe	Presence in carrier of HBsAg suggests a lower titer of HBV and lower risk of transmitting HBV
HBcAg	No commercial test available; found only in liver tissue
Anti-HBc	Identify people with acute, resolved, or chronic HBV infection (not present after immunization); high titer indicates active HBV infection; low titer presents in chronic infection
Anti-HBc-IgM	Recent infection with HBV positive for 4–6 months after infection; detectable in "window" period after surface antigen disappears
Anti-HBc-IgG	Appears later and may persist for years if viral replication continues
HCV	Etiologic agent of hepatitis C
Anti-HCV	Serologic determinant of hepatitis C infection

anti-HAV, antibody to HAV (IgG and IgG subclasses); anti-HAV-IgG, IgG class antibody to HAV; anti-HAV-IgM, IgM class antibody to HAV; anti-HBc, antibody to HBcAg; anti-HBc-IgG, IgG class antibody to HBcAg; anti-HBc-IgM, IGM class antibody to HBcAg; anti-HBe, antibody to HBeAg; anti-HBs, antibody to HBsAg; anti-HCV, antibody to hepatitis C; HBeAg, hepatitis B e antigen; HBcAg, hepatitis B core antigen; HBsAg, hepatitis B surface antigen; HBV, hepatitis B virus; HCV, hepatitis C virus; IgM and IgG, immunoglobulins M and G.

The differential diagnosis of newborn liver disease includes idiopathic neonatal hepatitis (giant cell), biliary atresia, metabolic disorders, antitrypsin deficiency, cystic fibrosis, iron storage disease, and other infectious agents that cause hepatocellular injury (eg, cytomegalovirus [CMV], herpes simplex, rubella, varicella, toxoplasmosis, *Listeria monocytogenes*, syphilis, and tuberculosis, as well as bacterial sepsis, which can cause nonspecific hepatic dysfunction). Table 95–1 outlines various hepatitis panel tests useful in the management of this disease. Isolation precautions for all infectious diseases, including maternal and neonatal precautions, breast-feeding, and visiting issues, can be found in Appendix F.

Hepatitis A

I. **Definition.** Hepatitis A (**infectious hepatitis**) is caused by a nonenveloped 27-nM RNA virus that is a member of the Picornaviridae family (HAV). It is transmitted by the fecal-oral route. A high concentration of virus is found in stools of infected persons, especially during the late incubation and early symptomatic phases. Children, especially neonates, may excrete HAV for a more prolonged period than has been noted in adults. HAV RNA was detected in neonatal stool samples for 4–5 months in 23% of infants diagnosed with HAV infection. Incubation period is 15–50 days. There is no chronic carrier state.

II. **Incidence.** The true incidence of HAV infection in neonates is unknown. The overall incidence of HAV infection in the U.S. population decreased significantly after the introduction of HAV vaccine (26,150 cases/year from 1980–1999 to 5683 cases/year in 2004).

III. **Pathophysiology.** In addition to fecal-oral transmission, parenteral transmission is possible via blood transfusion. Maternal-infant transmission appears to be very rare; however, both intrauterine and perinatal transmissions have been documented in case reports. The risk of transmission is limited because the period of viremia is short, and fecal contamination does not occur at the time of delivery. Occasional outbreaks of HAV infection in neonatal intensive care units have been reported, presumably from neonates infected through transfused blood who subsequently transmitted HAV to other neonates and staff. Severe disease in otherwise healthy infants is rare.

IV. **Risk factors.** The newborn infant born to an infected mother whose symptoms began between 2 weeks before and 1 week after delivery is at risk. Risk factors for postnatal acquisition of HAV include poor hygiene, poor sanitation, contact with an infected individual (which can be nosocomial), and recent travel to a developing country where the disease is endemic.

V. **Clinical presentation.** Most infants (>80%) are asymptomatic, with mild abnormalities of liver function.

VI. **Diagnosis**

   A. **Immunoglobulin M antibody to hepatitis A virus (anti-HAV-IgM).** Present during the acute or early convalescent phase of disease. In most cases it becomes detectable 5–10 days after exposure and can persist for up to 6 months after infection. **Anti-HAV-IgG** appears in the convalescent phase, remains detectable, and confers immunity. Research laboratories also can detect virus in blood or stool by means of reverse transcriptase polymerase chain reaction (RT-PCR).

   B. **Liver function tests (LFTs).** Characteristically, the transaminases (alanine transaminase [ALT] and aspartate transaminase [AST]) and serum bilirubin levels (total and direct) are elevated, whereas the alkaline phosphatase level is normal.

VII. **Management**

   A. **Immune serum globulin (ISG).** 0.02 mL/kg IM should be given to the newborn whose mother's symptoms began between 2 weeks before and 1 week after delivery. If an outbreak of hepatitis A is documented in the nursery, postexposure prophylaxis with ISG should be given to susceptible health care workers as well as exposed neonates who may have close contact with infectious secretions. ISG offers >85% protection against symptomatic infection.

   B. **HAV vaccine.** Two inactivated hepatitis A vaccines, Havrix and Vaqta, are available in the United States. They are recommended for all children (1–18 years old). If given within 2 weeks of exposure, HAV vaccine has similar efficacy to ISG in preventing symptomatic infection in adults and children over 2 years of age.

   C. **Isolation.** The infant should be isolated with enteric precautions.

   D. **Breast-feeding.** Not contraindicated.

VIII. **Prognosis** for HAV-infected infants is favorable. Less than 20% are clinically symptomatic after infection. Chronic carrier state does not exist.

Hepatitis B

I. **Definition.** Hepatitis B (**serum hepatitis**) is caused by a DNA-containing, 42-nM-diameter hepadnavirus. It has a long incubation period (45–160 days) after exposure.

II. **Incidence.** Each year in the United States, ~20,000 infants are born to HBV-infected pregnant women, and without immunoprophylaxis ~5500 would become chronically infected. As a result of universal immunization against HBV, the incidence of acute HBV infection among U.S. children decreased by 98% between 1990 and 2010.

III. **Pathophysiology.** In the fetus and neonate, transmission has been suggested by the following mechanisms:

    A. Transplacental transmission. Either during pregnancy or at the time of delivery secondary to placental leaks. This is rare and accounts for <25% of neonatal infection.

    B. Natal transmission. By exposure to HBV in amniotic fluid, vaginal secretions, or maternal blood; accounts for 90% of neonatal infections. The role of the mode of delivery in the transmission of HBV from mother to infant has not been fully determined.

    C. Postnatal transmission. By fecal-oral spread, blood transfusion, or other mechanisms.

IV. **Risk factors**

    A. Factors associated with higher rates of HBV transmission to neonates include the following:

        1. The presence of HBeAg and absence of anti-HBe in maternal serum: attack rates of 70–90%, with up to 90% of these infants becoming chronic carriers. In HBeAg-negative and HBsAg-positive mothers, the transmission rate is 5–20%; however, those infants are at risk for acute hepatitis and acute fulminant hepatitis.

        2. Asian racial origin, particularly Chinese, with attack rates of 40–70%.

        3. Maternal acute hepatitis in the third trimester or immediately postpartum (70% attack rate).

        4. Higher-titer HBsAg in maternal serum (attack rates parallel the titer).

        5. Antigenemia present in older siblings.

    B. Factors not related to transmission include the following:

        1. The particular HBV subtype in the mother.

        2. The presence or absence of HBsAg in amniotic fluid.

        3. The presence or titer of anti-HBc in cord blood.

V. **Clinical presentation.** Maternal hepatitis B infection has not been associated with abortion, stillbirth, or congenital malformations. Prematurity has occurred, especially with acute hepatitis during pregnancy. Fetuses or newborns exposed to HBV present a wide spectrum of disease. Because of the long incubation period, the infants do not present in the neonatal period. Even after the neonatal period, they are rarely ill; jaundice appears <3% of the time. Various clinical presentations include the following:

    A. Mild transient acute infection

    B. Chronic active hepatitis with or without cirrhosis

    C. Chronic persistent hepatitis

    D. Chronic asymptomatic HBsAg carriage

    E. Fulminant fatal hepatitis B (rare)

    F. Hepatocellular carcinoma in older children and young adults

VI. **Diagnosis**

    A. Differential diagnosis. Major diseases to consider include biliary atresia and acute hepatitis secondary to other viruses (eg, hepatitis A, CMV, rubella, and herpes simplex virus).

    B. Liver function tests (LFTs). ALT and AST levels may be markedly increased before the rise in bilirubin levels.

    C. Hepatitis panel testing. See Table 95–1.

        1. **Mother.** Test for HBsAg, HBeAg, anti-HBe, and anti-HBc.

        2. **Infant.** Test for HBsAg and anti-HBc-IgM. Anti-HBc-IgM is highly specific for establishing the diagnosis of acute infection and is the only marker of acute infection during the "window" period. Most infants demonstrate antigenemia by 6 months of age, with peak acquisition at 3–4 months. Nucleic acid amplification testing (NAAT), gene-amplification techniques (eg, polymerase chain reaction assay, branched DNA methods), and hybridization assays are available to detect and quantify HBV DNA. Cord blood is not a reliable indicator of neonatal infection because contamination could have occurred with

antigen-positive maternal blood or vaginal secretions and possible noninfectious antigenemia from the mother.

VII. **Management**

A. **HBsAg-positive mother.** If the mother is HBsAg positive, regardless of the status of her HBe antigen or antibody, the infant should be given hepatitis B immune globulin (HBIG), 0.5 mL IM, within 12 hours after delivery. Additionally, hepatitis (HB) vaccine is given at birth, at 1 month, and at 6 months of age. If the first dose is given simultaneously with HBIG, it should be administered at a separate site, preferably in the opposite leg. For preterm infants weighing <2 kg, this initial dose of vaccine should not be counted in the required 3-dose schedule, and the subsequent 3 doses should be initiated when the infant is 30 days old. HBIG and HB vaccinations do not interfere with routine childhood immunizations. No specific antiviral therapy exists for acute HBV, or for infants <1 year of age; however, U.S. Food and Drug Administration (FDA) licensure of interferon for pediatric patients 1 year of age or older does exist for chronic HBV. Consultation with an infectious disease specialist is recommended for clinical monitoring and treatment of HBV-positive infants.

B. **Infant born to mother whose HBsAg status is unknown.** Test the mother as soon as possible. While awaiting the results, give the infant HB vaccine within 12 hours of birth. If the mother is found to be HBsAg positive, the infant should receive HBIG (0.5 mL) within 7 days of birth. If the infant is preterm and the maternal HBsAg status cannot be determined within the initial 12 hours after birth, HBIG should be given as well as HB vaccine.

C. **Isolation.** Precautions are needed in handling blood and secretions.

D. **Breast-feeding.** HBsAg has been detected in breast milk of HBsAg-positive mothers but only with special concentrating techniques. Studies have shown that, with appropriate immunoprophylaxis (HBIG and HB vaccine), breast-feeding of infants of chronic HBV carrier mothers pose no additional risk for the transmission of the hepatitis B virus. Therefore, breast-feeding should be encouraged.

E. **Vaccine efficacy.** The overall protective efficiency rate in neonates given HB vaccine and HBIG is ~90%. The World Health Organization recommends that all countries add HB vaccine to their routine childhood immunization programs. Such programs (in Taiwan) have been shown to lower the incidence of chronic HBsAg carrier state, fulminant hepatic failure, and hepatocellular carcinoma. Infants born to HBsAg-positive women should be tested for anti-HBs and HBsAg after completion of the immunization series at 9–18 months of age. Infants with anti-HBs concentrations <10 mIU/mL and who are HBsAg negative should receive 3 additional doses of HB vaccine.

F. **Prevention of HB vaccine failure.** Failure of combined immunoprophylaxis (HBIG and HB vaccine) occurs in ~5% infants born to HBsAg-positive mothers. Often these infants are HBsAg positive at birth, suggesting the infection is already established in utero. Their mothers may have acquired the infection in the third trimester and/or have a high viral load at time of delivery. For this select group of patients, maternal treatment with lamivudine or HBIG in the third trimester may further reduce the transmission rate to 1–2%.

VIII. **Prognosis.** The majority of perinatally infected infants remain clinically healthy. Approximately 30–50% develop persistently elevated values on liver function tests. About 5% have moderately severe histopathologic changes on liver biopsy. Late complications including cirrhosis and hepatocellular carcinoma are rare.

Hepatitis C

I. **Definition.** Hepatitis C virus (HCV) is a small, single-stranded, enveloped RNA virus that is a member of the Flaviviridae family. It is responsible for 20% of all cases of acute hepatitis.

II. **Incidence.** Estimates of HCV seroprevalence in children have ranged from 0.2 to 0.4%. The true incidence of neonatal HCV is unknown.

III. **Pathophysiology.** Hepatitis C is transmitted primarily by parenteral means. Historically, exposure to blood and blood products was the most common source of infection; however, because of screening tests to exclude infectious donors, the risk of HCV is <0.01% per unit transfused. Seroprevalance among pregnant women has been estimated to be 1–2%. Vertical perinatal transmission of HCV is ~5%. Intrauterine infection accounts for 30–50% of the cases; the rest is presumably acquired intrapartum. Serum antibody to HCV (anti-HCV) and HCV RNA have been detected in colostrum, but the risk of HCV transmission is similar in breast-fed and bottle-fed infants.

IV. **Risk factors**
A. **Maternal human immunodeficiency virus (HIV)-HCV coinfection.** Associated with a 2- to 3-fold increase in risk of transmission.
B. **Maternal HCV viremia.** Correlates with transmission. However, viremia levels fluctuate considerably over time and no "safe level" can be defined below which transmission never occurs.
C. **Gender.** Girls are twice as likely to be infected as boys.
D. **Prolonged rupture of membrane and delivery complications.** Rupture of membranes more than 6 hours before delivery is associated with an increased risk of perinatal transmission of HCV. However, **mode of delivery** (ie, cesarean delivery) does not seem to offer any protection except if the mother is coinfected with HIV.
E. **Maternal intravenous drug use.** Several studies have shown that the maternal history of intravenous drug use increase the risk for perinatal transmission of HCV.

V. **Clinical presentation.** The average incubation period is about 6–7 weeks, with a range of 2–26 weeks. Infants with acute hepatitis C typically are asymptomatic or have a mild clinical illness. Approximately 65–70% of patients experience chronic hepatitis (carriers), 20% cirrhosis, and 1–5% hepatocellular carcinoma.

VI. **Diagnosis** of HCV infection in infants can be made by detecting **anti-HCV IgG** in serum after 12–18 months of age. Testing for anti-HCV IgG earlier may detect maternal transplacentally acquired antibodies. For earlier diagnosis, NAAT to detect **HCV RNA** can be performed as early as 2 months of age. NAATs carry a low sensitivity if used at birth. All children born to HCV-infected women need to be tested with NAAT at 2–3 months of age and again at 6 months of age. Two positive tests are highly suggestive of infection. Regardless of NAAT testing, anti-HCV IgG needs to be done at 12–18 months. LFTs may be elevated and fluctuate widely over time. The interval between exposure to HCV or onset of illness and detection of anti-HCV IgG may be 5–6 weeks. Infants born to anti-HCV mothers may test positive for passively acquired antibody for up to 18 months. Assays for anti-HCV IgM are not available.

VII. **Management**
A. **If the mother was infected during the last trimester.** The risk of transmission to the infant is highest. Immune globulin prophylaxis is not recommended. Despite intensive research in the field, it does not appear that a vaccine against hepatitis C will be available in the foreseeable future.
B. **Breast-feeding.** Advise mothers that transmission of HCV by breast-feeding has not been documented. According to guidelines of the Centers for Disease Control and Prevention and the American Academy of Pediatrics, maternal HCV infection is not a contraindication to breast-feeding. Mothers who are HCV positive and choose to breast-feed should consider abstaining if their nipples are cracked or bleeding.
C. **Treatment.** The FDA has approved the use of both pegylated and nonpegylated interferon alfa 2b in combination with ribavirin for the treatment of HCV in children 3–17 years of age. No specific therapy is currently recommended for HCV-positive infants; consultation with a pediatric infectious disease specialist should be sought for clinical monitoring and evaluation for possible antiviral therapy.

Children with HCV seem to have a higher sustained virologic response compared with adults, with fewer adverse events. All infants with chronic HCV infection should be immunized against hepatitis A and hepatitis B because of the very high rate of severe hepatitis if coinfection with hepatitis A or B virus develops.

VIII. **Prognosis.** A study from Italy looking at 10-year follow-up after putative exposure (56.2% perinatal) to HCV in untreated patients showed undetectable viremia in 7.5%, persistent viremia in 92%, and decompensated cirrhosis in 1.8%. The few children with chronic HCV infection who cleared viremia spontaneously were more likely to have genotype 3. Of infants treated, 27.9% achieved a sustained virologic response. Risk factors for end-stage liver disease included perinatal exposure, maternal drug use, and infection with HCV genotype 1a. Children with such features should be considered for early treatment.

Hepatitis D

Hepatitis D virus (HDV), also known as *delta hepatitis*, is a defective RNA virus that cannot survive independently and requires the helper function of DNA virus hepatitis B. Therefore, it occurs either as coinfection with hepatitis B or as superinfection of a hepatitis B carrier. Transmission from mother to newborn infant is uncommon. Prevention of hepatitis B infection prevents hepatitis D. There are, however, no available treatments to prevent HDV in HBsAg carriers before or after exposure. Management should be similar to that for hepatitis B infection (see prior discussion). Diagnosis of HDV is based on the detection of antibody to HDV (anti-HDV) by radioimmunoassay or enzyme immunoassay. HDV testing should be assessed in known carriers of hepatitis B because coinfection may lead to acute or fulminant hepatitis or a more rapid progression of chronic hepatitis.

Hepatitis E

Hepatitis E virus (HEV) is a nonenveloped, positive sense, single-stranded RNA virus. Transmission is by fecal-oral route. HEV is not transmitted readily from person to person so, unlike HAV, familial clusters of disease are unusual. Unlike other viral hepatitis, HEV is found in wild and domestic animals, especially in swine. HEV infection is particularly common in the Indian subcontinent, where some studies have shown HEV to be the most common etiology for acute viral hepatitis. In the United States, HEV infection is uncommon and generally occurs in travelers returning from endemic areas or swine workers. However, seroprevalence is higher than expected based on clinical disease, possibly because of exposure to infected animals. HEV commonly causes an acute illness with jaundice, malaise, fever, and arthralgia. Hepatitis E is clinically indistinguishable from hepatitis A. It is rarely symptomatic in children <15 years old. There is a very high maternal mortality when HEV is acquired during pregnancy, especially during the third trimester. Mother-to-infant transmission is high (50–100%). Fetal loss or early neonatal mortality is also significant. Commercial kits are now available to detect anti-HEV IgG and IgM. Definitive diagnosis may be made by demonstrating viral RNA in serum or stool by RT-PCR. The only treatment is supportive. A recombinant HEV phase III clinical trial in adults was recently completed and demonstrated the vaccine to be safe and highly effective; however, the vaccine is not available outside the research setting.

Hepatitis G

Hepatitis G virus (HGV), or GBV-C, is a positive, single-stranded RNA virus that has been classified in the family Flaviviridae. Despite extensive study, HGV has not been identified as a causative agent of any type of liver disease or any other known clinical condition. The virus is transmitted by parenteral exposure to blood and blood products from HGV-infected persons. The prevalence of HGV RNA in blood donors ranges from 1–4%. Coinfection with HCV and HIV is common, and HGV may be protective against HIV progression in adults.

Vertical transmission has been documented, with transmission rates of ≥60%. No biochemical or clinical signs of hepatitis are observed in HGV-infected infants.

Selected References

American Academy of Pediatrics. Hepatitis A-E. In: Pickering LK, Baker CJ, Kimberlin DW, Long SS, eds. *Red Book: 2012 Report of the Committee on Infectious Diseases.* 29th ed. Elk Grove Village, IL: American Academy of Pediatrics; 2012:361–398.

Bortolotti F, Verucchi G, Cammà C, et al. Long-term course of chronic hepatitis C in children: from viral clearance to end-stage liver disease. *Gastroenterology.* 2008;134:1900–1907.

Chang MH. Hepatitis B virus infection. *Semin Fetal Neonatal Med.* 2007;12:160–167.

Davison SM, Mieli-Vergani G, Sira J, Kelly DA. Perinatal hepatitis C virus infection: diagnosis and management. *Arch Dis Child.* 2006;91:781–785.

Emerson SU, Purcell RH. Hepatitis E. *Pediatr Infect Dis J.* 2007;26:1147–1148.

Fischler B. Hepatitis C virus infection. *Semin Fetal Neonatal Med.* 2007;12:168–173.

Hill JB, Sheffield JS, Kim MJ, Alexander JM, Sercely B, Wendel GD. Risk of hepatitis B transmission in breast-fed infants of chronic hepatitis B carriers. *Obstet Gynecol.* 2002;99:1049–1052.

Indolfi G, Resti M. Perinatal transmission of hepatitis C virus infection. *J Med Virol.* 2009;81:836–843.

Karnsakul W, Schwarz KB. Hepatitis. In: Remington JS, Klein JO, Wilson CB, Nizet V, Maldonado Y, eds. *Infectious Diseases of the Fetus and Newborn Infant.* Philadelphia, PA: Elsevier Saunders; 2011:800–811.

Patra S, Kumar A, Trivedi SS, Puri M, Sarin SK. Maternal and fetal outcomes in pregnant women with acute hepatitis E virus infection. *Ann Intern Med.* 2007;147:28–33.

Resti M, Jara P, Hierro L, et al. Clinical features and progression of perinatally acquired hepatitis C virus infection. *J Med Virol.* 2003;70(3):373–377.

Rosenblum LS, Villarino ME, Nainan OV, et al. Hepatitis A outbreak in a neonatal intensive care unit: risk factors for transmission and evidence of prolonged viral excretion among preterm infants. *J Infect Dis.* 1991;164:476–482.

Shi Z, Yang Y, Ma L, Li X, Schreiber A. Lamivudine in late pregnancy to interrupt in utero transmission of hepatitis B virus: a systematic review and meta-analysis. *Obstet Gynecol.* 2010;116:147–159.

Shrestha MP, Scott RM, Joshi DM, et al. Safety and efficacy of a recombinant hepatitis E vaccine. *N Engl J Med.* 2007;356:895–903.

Stapleton JT. GB virus type C/hepatitis G virus. *Semin Liver Dis.* 2003;23:137–148.

Towers CV, Asrat T, Rumney P. The presence of hepatitis B surface antigen and deoxyribonucleic acid in amniotic fluid and cord blood. *Am J Obstet Gynecol.* 2001;184:1514–1518.

Wirth S, Pieper-Boustani H, Lang T, et al. Peginterferon alfa-2b plus ribavirin treatment in children and adolescents with chronic hepatitis C. *Hepatology.* 2005;41:1013–1018.

Withers MR, Correa MT, Morrow M, et al. Antibody levels to hepatitis E virus in North Carolina swine workers, nonswine workers, swine, and murids. *Am J Trop Med Hyg.* 2002;66:384–388.

Zanetti AR, Tanzi E, Romanó L, et al. Multicenter trial on mother-to-infant transmission of GBV-C virus. The Lombardy Study Group on Vertical/Perinatal Hepatitis Viruses Transmission. *J Med Virol.* 1998;54:107–112.

96 Herpes Simplex Viruses

I. **Definition.** Herpes simplex viruses (HSV-1 and HSV-2) are enveloped, double-stranded DNA viruses. They are part of the herpes group, which also includes cytomegalovirus, Epstein-Barr virus, varicella zoster virus, and human herpes virus (HHV-6 and HHV-7). HSV infection is among the most prevalent of all viral infections encountered by humans.

II. **Incidence.** A study from the United States found an overall incidence of 9.6 per 100,000 births in 2006. Separately, a range of 1 per 3000 to 1 per 20,000 is given for an overall incidence in newborn infants for 2012. Seroprevalence of HSV-1 and HSV-2 in pregnant women in the United States is ~63% and 22%, respectively.

III. **Pathophysiology.** Two serologic subtypes can be distinguished by antigenic and serologic tests: HSV-1 (usually affects face and skin above the waist) and HSV-2 (genitalia and skin below the waist). Three quarters of neonatal herpes infections are secondary to HSV-2. HSV-1, however, can be the cause of maternal genital herpes infections in 9% of the cases, and its rate appears to be increasing. HSV infection of the neonate can be acquired at 1 of 3 times: intrauterine, intrapartum, or postnatal. Most infections (85%) are acquired in the intrapartum period as ascending infections with ruptured membranes (4–6 hours is considered a critical period for this to occur) or by delivery through an infected cervix or vagina. An additional 10% of infected neonates acquire the virus postnatally (eg, from someone shedding HSV from the mouth who then kisses the infant). The final 5% of neonatal HSV infections occur in utero. The usual portals of entry for the virus are the skin, eyes, mouth, and respiratory tract. Once colonization occurs, the virus may spread by contiguity or via a hematogenous route. The incubation period is from 2–20 days. Three general patterns of neonatal HSV infection are recognized: **disease localized to the skin, eyes, and mouth (SEM)**; **central nervous system (CNS) disease** (with or without SEM involvement); and **disseminated disease** (which also may include signs of the first 2 groups). Maternal infection can be classified as either *first-episode* or *recurrent* infections. First-episode infections are further classified as either *primary* or *first-episode nonprimary* based on type-specific serologic testing. *Primary infections* are those in which the mother is experiencing a new infection with either HSV-1 or HSV-2 and has not already been infected with the other virus type. *First-episode nonprimary* infections are those in which the mother has a new infection with one virus type, usually HSV-2, but has antibodies to the other virus type, usually HSV-1. Infants born vaginally to mothers with a true primary infection are at highest risk, with a transmission rate of 50%. Those born to a mother with a first-episode nonprimary infection are at a somewhat lower risk of 30%. The lowest risk (<2%) infants are those who are born to a mother with recurrent infections. Maternal antibody is not always protective in the fetus.

IV. **Risk factors.** The risk of genital herpes infection may vary with maternal age, socioeconomic status, and number of sexual partners. Only ~12% of pregnant women who test seropositive for HSV-2 give a clinical history suggestive of the disease. The first-episode infection may stay "active" with asymptomatic cervical shedding for as long as 2 months. Besides a first-episode infection (primary or nonprimary), additional risk factors for neonatal HSV infection include the use of a fetal-scalp electrode and maternal age <21 years.

V. **Clinical presentation.** Congenital in utero HSV infection is rare and is associated with high rate of fetal demise; it shares clinical features such as microcephaly, hydrocephalus, and chorioretinitis with other congenital infections. In addition, skin ulcerations or scarring and eye damage are commonly noted. The neonatal disease is commonly acquired intrapartum. It may be localized or disseminated. Humoral and cellular immune mechanisms appear important in preventing initial HSV infections or limiting their spread. Infants with disseminated and SEM disease generally present at 10–12 days of life, whereas patients with CNS disease usually present at 16–19 days of life. More than 20% of infants with disseminated disease and 30–40% of infants with encephalitis never have skin vesicles (Plate 12).

A. **SEM disease.** In the era of acyclovir therapy, HSV disease localized to the skin, eyes, or oral cavity accounts for ~45% of the cases. **Skin lesions** vary from discrete vesicles to large bullous lesions and denuded skin. It typically involves the presenting part (eg, vertex) and sites of skin trauma (eg, scalp electrodes). There is skin involvement in 80–85% of SEM cases. **Ulcerative mouth lesions** (~10% of SEM cases) with or without cutaneous involvement can be seen. **Ocular findings** include keratoconjunctivitis and chorioretinitis (see Chapter 53). Without treatment, there is a high risk of progression to encephalitis or disseminated disease.

B. **Disseminated disease** carries the worst prognosis with respect to mortality and long-term sequelae. Patients commonly present with fever, lethargy, apnea, and a septic shock–like picture, including respiratory collapse, liver failure, neutropenia, thrombocytopenia, and disseminated intravascular coagulation (DIC). Approximately half of these cases also have localized disease as described previously, and 60–75% have CNS involvement. More than 20% of infants with disseminated disease will not develop any cutaneous vesicles during the course of their illness. Recognition of the disseminated HSV disease is often delayed. It should be suspected in any infant presenting with a sepsis-like picture associated with thrombocytopenia, elevated hepatic enzymes, and cerebrospinal fluid (CSF) pleocytosis. Infants with disseminated HSV infection account for 25% of all cases of neonatal herpes infection.

C. **CNS disease** accounts for ~30% of neonatal HSV infection. CNS involvement can present with or without SEM lesions. Clinical manifestations include seizures (focal and generalized), lethargy, irritability, tremors, poor feeding, temperature instability, and a bulging fontanelle. These infants usually present at 16–19 days of age, and 30–40% have no herpetic skin lesions. CSF findings are variable and typically show a mild pleocytosis, increased protein, and a slightly low glucose.

VI. **Diagnosis.** Diagnosis of neonatal HSV infection can be challenging, and the diagnosis is often delayed. Early manifestations are subtle and nonspecific (especially for the disseminated form). The maternal history is often not helpful.

A. **Laboratory studies**

1. **Viral cultures.** Isolation of HSV by culture remains the definitive diagnostic method of documenting HSV infection. Skin or mucous membrane lesions or surfaces (mouth, nasopharynx, conjunctivae, and anus) are scraped and transferred in appropriate viral transport media on ice. Swab specimens from mouth, nasopharynx, conjunctivae, and anus can be obtained with a single swab ending with the anus and placed in one viral transport media tube. With the exception of CNS involvement, the important information gathered from such cultures is the presence or absence of the replicating virus, rather than its precise location. Preliminary results may become available in 24–72 hours. Positive cultures obtained from any of these sites more than 12–24 hours after birth indicate viral replication and, therefore, are suggestive of infant infection rather than merely contamination after intrapartum exposure.

2. **Polymerase chain reaction (PCR).** PCR is an important tool in the diagnosis of HSV infection. PCR has been used to detect HSV DNA in **CSF** and **blood** specimens. PCR is especially useful for the diagnosis of HSV encephalitis. Overall sensitivities of CSF PCR in neonatal HSV disease have ranged from 75 to 100% with overall specificities ranging from 71 to 100%. Negative CSF PCR does not exclude the diagnosis of HSV CNS disease; it may be negative early in the course

of the disease or if the test is done after antiviral therapy has been given for a few days. PCR is especially important in monitoring therapy of CNS disease, with discontinuation of therapy only when PCR is negative.

3. **Immunologic assays.** Immunologic assays to detect HSV antigen in lesion scrapings, usually using monoclonal anti-HSV antibodies in either an enzyme-linked immunosorbent assay or fluorescent microscopy assay, are very specific and 80–90% sensitive.

4. **Liver function tests (LFTs).** Whole-blood sample for measuring LFTs, especially alanine aminotransferase, is recommended. HSV characteristically invade the liver and cause hepatocellular damage.

5. **Serologic tests.** These are not helpful in the diagnosis of neonatal infection but are helpful in diagnosing and classifying maternal disease (primary versus secondary).

6. **Lumbar puncture.** Should be performed in all suspected cases. CSF may be normal early in the course of the disease but typically will show a mononuclear cell pleocytosis, normal or moderately low glucose, and mildly elevated protein. Red blood cells are not notably increased in HSV CNS disease. PCR should always be performed on CSF.

B. **Imaging and other studies**

1. **Brain imaging with computed tomography (CT) or preferably magnetic resonance imaging (MRI).** Recommended in all infants with HSV CNS disease. Findings include parenchymal brain edema or attenuation, hemorrhage, and destructive lesions, especially in the temporal lobe.

2. **Electroencephalogram (EEG).** Should be performed in all neonates suspected to have CNS involvement (seizures, abnormal CSF, abnormal neurologic examination). EEG is often abnormal very early in the course of the CNS disease; it may show focal or multifocal epileptiform discharges before abnormal changes are detected by CT or MRI.

VII. **Management**

A. **Antepartum.** The history of genital herpes in a pregnant woman or in her partner(s) should be solicited and recorded in the prenatal record. If a positive history is obtained, the following steps may be taken:

1. **Antiviral therapy. Acyclovir** or **valacyclovir** may be given to pregnant women who have a primary episode of genital HSV as well as to women with an active infection (primary or secondary) near or at the time of delivery. Multiple trials showed that prophylactic acyclovir beginning at 36 weeks' gestation reduces the risk of clinical HSV recurrence at delivery, cesarean delivery, and HSV viral shedding at delivery. Valacyclovir in randomized studies also demonstrated similar results. These studies did not identify any neonatal side effects from maternal suppressive therapy. These infants will need to be monitored closely because the risk of neonatal HSV infection is not totally eliminated. See dosing in Chapter 148.

2. **If there are no visible lesions** at the onset of labor or prodromal symptoms, vaginal delivery is acceptable.

3. **Delivery by cesarean is recommended** in women who have clinically apparent HSV infection. Debate exists if membranes have already been ruptured for >4 hours. Most experts still recommend cesarean delivery. All neonates delivered by cesarean should be monitored closely because neonatal HSV infections have occasionally occurred despite delivery before the membranes rupture.

4. **The ultimate preventive strategy** might be the development of a vaccine to prevent HSV infection in the pregnant woman and her newborn infant. An inactivated glycoprotein-D-adjuvant vaccine has been evaluated and shown to be 70% effective in seronegative women (for both HSV-1 and HSV-2), but it is not effective in men or seropositive women.

B. **Neonatal treatment**
   1. **Infants born to mothers with a genital lesion.** If it is a known recurrent lesion and the infant is asymptomatic, the infection rate is 1–3%. Educate the parents regarding the signs and symptoms of early herpes infection. Consider surface (screening) cultures of the infant at 12–24 hours of age. Treat if symptoms develop or if the culture is positive. If the maternal infection is primary, or the first episode nonprimary, the risk to the infant is high (57% for primary and 25% for the first-episode nonprimary), and most clinicians recommend empirical acyclovir therapy after cultures have been obtained. Serologic testing of the mother will help classify the mother's infection (recurrent, primary, or first episode nonprimary).
   2. **Pharmacologic therapy.** Neonates with HSV disease should be treated with **intravenous acyclovir at 60 mg/kg/d**, divided, every 8 hours (20 mg/kg/dose). The dosing interval of intravenous acyclovir may need to be increased in premature infants, based on their creatinine clearance. Duration of therapy is 21 days for patients with disseminated or CNS disease and 14 days for those with SEM disease. All patients with CNS involvement should have a repeat lumbar puncture at the end of intravenous acyclovir therapy to determine whether CSF is PCR negative. Those infants who remain PCR positive should receive intravenous acyclovir therapy until PCR negativity is achieved. Absolute neutrophil counts should be followed twice weekly during the course of therapy. Lower dose acyclovir is associated with a higher morbidity and mortality and should be avoided. Trifluridine is the treatment of choice for ocular HSV infection in the neonate.

      Oral acyclovir suppressive therapy is recommended for 6 months after treatment of acute neonatal HSV disease. In particular, improved neurodevelopmental outcome has been observed with suppressive therapy after HSV CNS disease. Moreover, suppressive therapy has been associated with reduced recurrences of skin lesions after other forms of HSV. The oral acyclovir dose is 300 mg/m^2/dose 3 times per day for 6 months.
C. **Breast-feeding.** The infant may breast-feed as long as no breast lesions are present on the mother, and the mother should be instructed in good hand washing technique.
D. **Parents with orolabial herpes.** Parents should wear a mask when handling the newborn and should not kiss or nuzzle the infant.
VIII. **Prognosis.** Antiviral therapy, especially high-dose acyclovir (60 mg/kg/d) has greatly reduced **mortality** for neonatal HSV infection. In the preantiviral era, 85% of patients with disseminated neonatal HSV disease died by 1 year of age, as did 50% of patients with CNS disease. With current antiviral therapy, 12-month mortality has been reduced to 29% for disseminated disease and 4% for CNS disease. Predictors of mortality include disease severity (pneumonia, DIC, seizures, and hepatitis), virus type (HSV-1 in systemic disease, HSV-2 in CNS disease), and prematurity. Systemic infection in premature infants is associated with near 100% mortality. Improvements in **morbidity** rates have not been as dramatic as with mortality. The proportion of survivors of disseminated neonatal HSV disease who have normal neurologic development has increased from 50% in the preantiviral era to 83% today. In the case of CNS disease, morbidity in survivors has not changed, with only ~30% developing normally by 12 months of age. Persistently positive CSF PCR after 4 weeks of acyclovir therapy is associated with poor neurodevelopmental outcome. In contrast to the disseminated or CNS disease, morbidity after SEM disease has dramatically improved during the antiviral era, with <2% of acyclovir recipients having developmental delays. Survivors of neonatal HSV infections should undergo **developmental assessments** regularly. Cutaneous recurrences are relatively common (~50%), especially for SEM disease. Suppressive oral acyclovir therapy may have a role in decreasing cutaneous recurrences and improves neurodevelopmental outcome.

Selected References

ACOG Committee on Practice Bulletins. ACOG Practice Bulletin. Clinical management guidelines for obstetrician-gynecologists. No. 82 June 2007. Management of herpes in pregnancy. *Obstet Gynecol.* 2007;109:1489–1498.

American Academy of Pediatrics. Herpes simplex. In: Pickering LK, Baker CJ, Kimberlin DW, Long SS, eds. *Red Book: 2012 Report of the Committee on Infectious Diseases.* 29th ed. Elk Grove Village, IL: American Academy of Pediatrics; 2012:363–373.

Caviness AC, Demmler GJ, Selwyn BJ. Clinical and laboratory features of neonatal herpes simplex virus infection: a case-control study. *Pediatr Infect Dis J.* 2008;27:425–430.

Centers for Disease Control and Prevention. Seroprevalence of herpes simplex virus type 2 among persons aged 14-49 years: United States, 2005-2008. *MMWR Morb Mortal Wkly Rep.* 2010;59:456–459.

Corey L, Wald A. Maternal and neonatal herpes simplex virus infections. *N Engl J Med.* 2009;361:1376–1385.

Flagg EW, Weinstock H. Incidence of neonatal herpes simplex virus infections in the United States, 2006. *Pediatrics.* 2011;127:e1–e8.

Malm G. Neonatal herpes simplex virus infection. *Semin Fetal Neonatal Med.* 2009;14:204–208.

Roberts S. Herpes simplex virus: incidence of neonatal herpes simplex virus, maternal screening, management during pregnancy, and HIV. *Curr Opin Obstet Gynecol.* 2009;21:124–130.

Thompson C, Whitley R. Neonatal herpes simplex virus infections: where are we now? *Adv Exp Med Bio.* 2011;697:221–230.

97 Human Immunodeficiency Virus

I. **Definition.** Two types of HIV cause disease in humans: HIV-1 and HIV-2. These are enveloped RNA cytopathic lentiviruses belonging to the family Retroviridae. Infection is most commonly secondary to HIV-1. HIV-2 is rare in the United States but more common in West Africa. HIV results in a broad spectrum of disease, with **AIDS** representing the most severe end of the clinical spectrum.

II. **Incidence.** The Joint United Nations Program on HIV/AIDS estimated that 33.3 million people worldwide were infected with HIV-1 at the end of 2009. More than 95% of the total cases reside in developing countries. In the same year, an estimated 370,000 children contracted HIV during the perinatal and breast-feeding period, down from 500,000 in 2001 (down 24%). This drop reflects the fact that access to services for preventing the mother-to-child transmission (MTCT) of HIV has increased. On the other hand, the estimated number of children living with HIV increased to 2.5 million worldwide in 2009, mainly due to a decrease in AIDS-related mortality as antiretroviral drugs (ARDs) becomes more available. Currently, the Centers for Disease Control and Prevention (CDC) estimates that each year, 215–370 infants with HIV infection are born in the United States; this is a significant drop from 1650 in 1991.

III. **Pathophysiology.** HIV-1 is particularly tropic for CD4$^+$ T cells and cells of monocyte or macrophage lineage. After infection of the cell, viral RNA is uncoated and a double-stranded DNA transcript is made. This DNA is transported to the nucleus and integrated into the host genome DNA. There is eventual destruction of both the cellular and humoral arms of the immune system. As well, HIV-1 gene products or cytokines elaborated by infected cells may affect macrophage, B-lymphocyte, and T-lymphocyte function.

Hypergammaglobulinemia caused by HIV-induced polyclonal B-cell activation is often detected in early infancy. Disruption of B-cell function results in poor secondary antibody synthesis and response to vaccination. A small proportion (<10%) of patients will develop panhypogammaglobulinemia. Additionally, profound defects in cell-mediated immunity occur, allowing a predisposition to opportunistic infections such as fungus, *Pneumocystis jiroveci* pneumonia (PCP), and chronic diarrhea. The virus can also invade the central nervous system and produce psychosis and brain atrophy.

IV. Risk factors

A. **High-risk mother.** Any infant born to a high-risk mother is at risk. High-risk mothers include intravenous (IV) drug users, hemophiliacs, spouses of hemophiliacs, spouses of bisexual males, those with a history of exchanging sex for money or drugs, sex partners of HIV-infected persons, and those who were diagnosed with sexually transmitted disease/sexually transmitted infection (STD/STI) during pregnancy. Several mechanisms/predisposing factors for viral transmission exist, including maternal disease state, fetal exposure to infected maternal body fluids, depressed maternal immune response, and breast-feeding. **Maternal plasma HIV RNA level is the best single predictor of MTCT risk.** Other risk factors include mode of delivery, duration of rupture of membranes (the risk increases with each hour increase in the duration), prematurity and low birthweight, cervical-vaginal viral load, low $CD4^+$ cell count, maternal symptomatic HIV disease/AIDS, viral subtype, and host genetic factors. Most MTCT occurs intrapartum, with smaller proportions of transmission occurring in utero and postnatally through breast-feeding. MTCT may occur in utero, intrapartum, or postpartum through breast-feeding. Transplacental infection has been proven by evidence of infection in aborted first-trimester fetal tissues as well as isolation of HIV-1 in blood samples obtained within 48 hours of birth. Potential routes of infection include mixture of maternal and fetal blood and infection across the placenta when its integrity is compromised (eg, placentitis [syphilitic] and chorioamnionitis).

B. **Blood transfusion.** Screening of blood donors has reduced but has not totally eliminated the risk because some newly infected persons are viremic but seronegative for 2–4 months, and because some infected persons (5–15%) are seronegative. The current risk of transmission of HIV per unit transfused is 1 in 2 million. (See also Chapter 17.)

C. **Breast milk.** Breast-feeding is the predominant means of postnatal HIV transmission to infants and accounts for an estimated one-third to one-half of all MTCT events in breast-feeding populations. According to a 2007 report from the World Health Organization (WHO), ~200,000 infants worldwide become infected annually with HIV through breast-feeding. HIV-1 RNA and proviral DNA have been detected in both the cell-free and cellular portions of breast milk. Colostrum viral load appears to be particularly high. Risk from breast milk is highest when maternal primary infection occurs within the first few months after delivery. In areas where infant formula is accessible, affordable, safe, and sustainable, avoidance of breast-feeding has represented one of the main components of prevention efforts of MTCT of HIV-1 for many years. Complete avoidance of breast-feeding by HIV-1–infected women has been recommended by the American Academy of Pediatrics (AAP) and CDC and remains the only means by which prevention of breast-feeding transmission of HIV-1 can be absolutely ensured. In resource-limited countries where local sanitary conditions are poor and access to infant formulas is limited, the 2010 WHO guidelines recommend **exclusive** breast-feeding in combination with **maternal** or **infant** antiretroviral prophylaxis to minimize HIV transmission from the mother and to optimize the benefits of breast-feeding for the infant. Exclusive breast-feeding is associated with a lower risk of postnatal transmission compared to mixed breast-feeding and formula feeding. In areas where ARDs are available, infants should receive daily nevirapine prophylaxis until 1 week after human milk consumption stops.

D. **Premastication.** Possible transmission of HIV-1 by caregivers who premasticate food for infants has been described in 3 cases in the United States. HIV-1–infected caregivers should be asked and counseled not to premasticate food for infants.

V. **Clinical presentation.** Disease progression after vertical HIV-1 infection is highly variable.

  A. **Incubation period.** The onset of symptoms is ~12–18 months of age for untreated, perinatally infected infants in the United States; however, some may become ill in the first few months of life (15–20%).

  B. **Signs and symptoms.** The newborn is usually asymptomatic or may have low birthweight, weight loss, or failure to thrive (if infected in utero). The frequency of different opportunistic pathogens among HIV-infected children decreased significantly with the application and widespread use of **highly active antiretroviral therapy (HAART).** In the pre-HAART era, serious bacterial infection, herpes zoster, disseminated *Mycobacterium avium* complex (MAC), PCP, and candidiasis were common. History of a previous AIDS-defining opportunistic infection was a predictor of developing a new infection. In the HAART era, descriptions of opportunistic infections among HIV-infected children have been limited because of the substantial decreases in morbidity and mortality among children receiving HAART. Nonspecific features of HIV infection include hepatosplenomegaly, lymphadenopathy, and fever. Neurologic disease may be either static (delayed attainment of milestones) or progressive, with impaired brain growth, failure to reach milestones, and progressive motor deficits. Common computed tomography (CT) scan findings include basal ganglia calcification and cortical atrophy. Cardiac abnormalities include pericardial disease, myocardial dysfunction, and dysrhythmias.

VI. **Diagnosis.** Diagnosis is based on suspicion of infection based on epidemiological risk or clinical presentation, and confirmation by different virologic assays in infants <18 months old or serologic tests if the infant is >18 months old.

  A. **All other causes of immunodeficiency must be excluded.** These include both primary and secondary immunodeficiency states. Primary immunodeficiency diseases include DiGeorge or Wiskott-Aldrich syndromes, ataxia-telangiectasia, agammaglobulinemia, severe combined immunodeficiency, and neutrophil function abnormality. Secondary immunodeficiency states include those caused by immunosuppressive therapy, starvation, and lymphoreticular cancer.

  B. **Laboratory studies**

    1. **HIV serology.** Antibodies against HIV-1 are found in all infants born to mothers with HIV infection because of transplacental passage of immunoglobulin G. HIV serology (enzyme-linked immunosorbent assay [ELISA] or Western blot) should not be used to diagnose HIV infection in infants <18 months of age.

    2. **Virologic assays.** (HIV-1 DNA and RNA polymerase chain reaction [PCR].) These are considered the gold standard for diagnosis of HIV in infants and children <18 months. With the use of these tests, HIV infection may be diagnosed as early as the first day after birth in some infants and by 1 month of age in most infected infants. The **HIV-1 DNA PCR** assay is the preferred diagnostic tool. Amplification of proviral DNA allows detection of cells that harbor quiescent provirus as well as cells with actively replicating virus. Approximately 30% of infants with perinatal HIV infection have a positive DNA PCR in samples obtained by 48 hours of age. A positive result identifies infants who were infected in utero. The test routinely can detect 1–10 DNA copies. The test will be positive in 93 and 99% of all infected infants by 2 weeks and 1 month of age, respectively. **HIV-1 RNA PCR** assays detect plasma (cell-free) viral RNA by PCR amplification. These assays are available as either "standard" or "ultrasensitive," and the lower limit of detection when using the ultrasensitive assays is in the range of 50–75 HIV-1 copies per milliliter of plasma. The reported sensitivity for RNA assays range from 25 to 50% within the first few days of life to 100% by 6–12 weeks of

age. HIV-1 RNA assays are commonly used for quantifying the amount of virus present as one predictor of disease progression. They are used in follow-up testing of patients during treatment for HIV-1 infection. The first test result should be confirmed as soon as possible by a repeat virologic test on a second specimen because false-positive results can occur with both RNA and DNA assays. Zidovudine (ZDV) prophylaxis does not appear to alter the diagnostic sensitivity of either HIV DNA PCR or RNA assays. It is also established that HIV DNA PCR remains positive even in infected individuals receiving therapeutic HAART.

Virologic assays should be performed within the first 48 hours after birth, at 14–21 days, between 1 and 2 months, and at 4–6 months of age. Cord blood should not be used because of the possibility of contamination with maternal blood. A positive virologic test confirmed at 2 weeks of age warrants a change in the recommended ZDV prophylactic monotherapy. HIV infection can be *presumptively* excluded in non–breast-fed infants with 2 or more negative virologic tests, with 1 test obtained at ≥14 days of age and 1 obtained at ≥4 weeks of age; or 1 negative virologic test obtained at ≥8 weeks of age; or 1 negative HIV antibody test obtained at ≥6 months of age. PCP prophylaxis is recommended for infants with indeterminate HIV infection status starting at 4–6 weeks of age until they are determined to be HIV uninfected or presumptively uninfected. *Definitive* exclusion of HIV infection in a non–breast-fed infant is based on 2 or more negative virologic tests, with 1 obtained at ≥1 month of age and one at ≥4 months of age; or 2 negative HIV antibody tests from separate specimens obtained at ≥6 months of age (in the absence of hypogammaglobulinemia). For both *presumptive* and *definitive* exclusion of HIV infection, the child must have no other laboratory (eg, no positive virologic test results or low CD4 count/percentage) or clinical evidence of HIV infection and not be breast-feeding. Many experts confirm the absence of HIV infection in infants with negative virologic tests by performing an antibody test at 12–18 months of age to document seroreversion to HIV antibody–negative status. The p_{24} antigen assay is less sensitive than DNA or RNA PCR and is generally not recommended. Viral HIV-1 culture is labor intensive and poses a significant biohazard risk. It is largely supplanted by DNA and RNA PCR virologic assays.

3. **Rapid tests.** A number of rapid tests for detection of HIV antibodies in blood, urine, or oral fluid have been licensed in the United States (**www.fda.gov/cber/products/testkits.htm**). These tests are comparable with enzyme immunoassays (EIAs) in both sensitivity (99.3–100%) and specificity (98.6–100%). As with routine EIAs, confirmation of positive results is necessary, but confirmation of a negative result is not. The rapid tests are valuable as a screening tool for pregnant women with no or limited prenatal care or for infants with unknown maternal HIV status. They have the potential to reduce MTCT, with immediate provision of antiretroviral prophylaxis and formula feeding to prevent postnatal transmission. They should be available in all hospitals providing delivery services in the United States. In 2012, a home HIV test received U.S. Food and Drug Administration (FDA) approval.

4. **Surrogate markers for disease.** Immunologic abnormalities found in HIV-infected infants include hypergammaglobulinemia, a low $CD4^+$ T-lymphocyte count, or a decreased $CD4^+$ percentage.

C. **Presence of a "marker" disease that indicates cellular immunodeficiency.** Marker diseases include candidiasis, cryptococcosis, *Mycobacterium avium* infection, Epstein-Barr virus infection, PCP, strongyloidiasis, and Kaposi sarcoma. Cytomegalovirus (CMV) infection and toxoplasmosis are included if toxoplasmosis occurs >1 month after birth and CMV infection presents >6 months after birth.

VII. **Management.** Isolation precautions for all infectious diseases, including maternal and neonatal precautions, breast-feeding, and visiting issues, can be found in Appendix F.

A. **Prevention.** MTCT can take place in utero, during labor, at delivery, and postnatally through breast-feeding. Before the widespread use of MTCT interventions (described later), transmission rates in the United States ranged from 16 to 30%. More recently, MTCT has dropped below 1–2%.

   1. **Identification of HIV infection in pregnant women and newborns.** A prerequisite for the application of successful MTCT interventions is identifying mothers who are HIV positive. The CDC issued revised guidelines in 2006 regarding HIV testing in pregnant women. The guidelines recommended that HIV screening be included in the routine panel of prenatal screening tests for **all pregnant women**. HIV screening is recommended after the patient is notified that testing will be performed unless the patient declines (opt-out screening). **Separate written consent for HIV testing should not be required**, and a general consent for medical care should be considered sufficient to encompass consent for HIV testing. Repeat screening in the third trimester is recommended in certain jurisdictions with elevated rates of HIV infection among pregnant women. The AAP and American College of Obstetricians and Gynecologists (ACOG) issued a recommendation similar to the CDC with all organizations supporting routine testing and the opt-out strategy. Most guidelines now state that health care providers have a responsibility not only to offer, but also to recommend, antenatal HIV testing. The benefits of antenatal HIV testing extend beyond the potential to reduce vertical transmission risk and include the opportunity to evaluate the infected woman's health status, to initiate HAART if required, and to allow the woman to reduce the risk of transmitting HIV to her sexual partner. For a **newborn infant whose mother's HIV infection status is unknown**, the newborn infant's physician should perform rapid HIV antibody testing on the mother or the infant (with appropriate consent). Test results should be reported to the physician as soon as possible to allow effective ARD prophylaxis, ideally within 12 hours. In some states, rapid testing of the neonate is required by law if the mother has refused to be tested.

   2. **Antiretroviral prophylaxis and treatment.** Antiretroviral drugs (ARDs) are prescribed to HIV-infected pregnant women to treat their own disease and to decrease MTCT of HIV. For optimal prevention of perinatal HIV transmission, combined antepartum, intrapartum, and infant antiretroviral prophylaxis are recommended. The ACTG 076 trial published in 1994 showed that an intensive regimen of oral ZDV given prenatally, intrapartum, and postpartum decreased perinatal transmission risk by two-thirds when compared with placebo. Widespread implementation of trial regimen led to sharp decreases in perinatal HIV transmission. Furthermore, since the late 1990s, most HIV-infected women in the United States have been prescribed combination regimens, which further reduced the risk. Widespread use of HAART, which is usually composed of 3 antiretrovirals from 2 drug classes, has substantially reduced MTCT rates to below 1–2%. Antiretroviral therapy or prophylaxis should be recommended to all pregnant HIV-infected women regardless of plasma HIV RNA copy number or $CD4^+$ cell count. According to the 2007 Public Health Service Task Force recommendations, HAART should be considered the standard of care for all pregnant women with HIV infection, even those who do not require treatment for their own health. Regimens for prophylaxis against perinatal HIV transmission should include a 3-drug combination from 2 classes of antiretroviral drugs. The use of ZDV alone is *controversial* but may be considered for those women initiating prophylaxis with plasma HIV RNA levels <1000 copies/mL on no therapy. ZDV should be included in the antenatal antiretroviral regimen unless there is severe toxicity or documented resistance. ZDV rapidly crosses the placenta, providing protective drug levels for the fetus. Clinical trial data clearly demonstrate the efficacy and safety of ZDV in reducing the risk of perinatal HIV transmission. Lamivudine (3TC) is the preferred drug to be used in

combination with ZDV. Both drugs are usually given together (Combivir) as 1 pill twice daily. Lopinavir/ritonavir (LPV/r) is the preferred protease inhibitor with a favorable safety profile for the mother and the fetus. The details of what combination drugs to use in pregnancy are outlined by guidelines released by the U.S. Department of Health and Human Services. These guidelines are updated regularly and are available online at (http://aidsinfo.nih.gov/ContentFiles/PerinatalGL.pdf).

3. **Safety of antiretroviral drugs (ARDs) during pregnancy.** There are limited human safety data on the antenatal use of ARDs. Efavirenz is a category D drug and thus contraindicated in pregnancy. Women are at increased risk of nevirapine (NVP)-related hepatotoxicity. Lactic acidosis is a relatively uncommon side effect of nucleoside reverse-transcriptase inhibitor (NRTI) drugs. HAART in pregnancy may increase the risk of gestational diabetes, preeclampsia, and premature delivery. Although animal studies suggest an increased risk of malformations associated with the use of certain ARDs, to date there appears to be no increased risk of congenital malformations associated with HAART exposure in pregnancy according to a registry's data (**www.apregistry.com**). ZDV treatment in infants is associated with a transient anemia. In utero exposure to HAART was shown to result in mild but statistically significant hematologic abnormalities like neutropenia and thrombocytopenia.

4. **Mode of delivery.** Data from individual patient meta-analysis and a randomized controlled trial confirmed that cesarean section (CS) performed before labor and rupture of membranes reduces MTCT by 50–80%, independent of the use of antiretroviral therapy or ZDV prophylaxis. The ACOG and the Department of Health and Human Services (DHHS) Panel on Treatment of HIV Infected Pregnant Women and Prevention of Perinatal Transmission recommend early CS for HIV-infected women with plasma viral loads of more than 1000 copies/mL. Elective CS is associated with a higher rate of postpartum complications among HIV-infected women than vaginal delivery. The added benefit of elective CS on reducing risk of MTCT in women with low-plasma HIV RNA loads (<1000 copies/mL) is uncertain, and most experts now recommend that women in this category can be offered vaginal delivery. The use of invasive procedures in labor (eg, amniocentesis, fetal scalp electrodes, operative vaginal delivery, and episiotomy) should be avoided because of the potential risk for enhanced transmission.

5. **Postdelivery.** Amniotic fluid and blood should be cleaned thoroughly. The infant should be isolated with the same precautions as for hepatitis B (blood and secretion precautions). Zidovudine (ZDV) is used. See dose in Chapter 148. Among infants whose mothers did not receive any ARDs before onset of labor, the current recommendation for neonatal postexposure prophylaxis is a 2-drug regimen of ZDV for 6 weeks with 3 doses of nevirapine during the first week of life (at birth, 48 hours, and 96 hours of life) rather than ZDV alone. Serial virologic studies should be obtained as discussed previously. The HIV-infected mother may be coinfected with other pathogens that can be transmitted from mother to child, such as cytomegalovirus, herpes simplex virus, hepatitis B, hepatitis C, syphilis, toxoplasmosis, or tuberculosis. Infants born to mothers with such coinfections should undergo appropriate evaluations as indicated to rule out transmission of additional infectious agents. Breast-feeding must be discouraged. Both mother and infant should have prescriptions for the HIV drugs when they leave the hospital, and the infant should have an appointment for a postnatal visit at 2–4 weeks of age to monitor medication adherence, obtain virologic testing (HIV DNA PCR), and screen the infant for anemia from ZDV.

6. **Treatment of infected patients.** Management of HIV-1 infection is an area of medicine that is changing rapidly. Current treatment recommendations for HIV-1–infected children are available online (**http://aidsinfo.nih.gov**) and

are **continuously updated**. ARDs therapy is indicated for all HIV-1–infected infants <12 months of age as soon as infection is confirmed, irrespective of clinical symptoms, immune status, or viral load. The principal objectives of therapy are to suppress viral replication maximally, to restore and preserve immune function, to reduce HIV-associated morbidity and mortality, to minimize drug toxicity, to maintain normal growth and development, and to improve quality of life. Aggressive therapy is warranted in the youngest children who are at greatest risk of rapid disease progression. In general, combination ARDs therapy with at least 3 drugs is recommended. Drug regimens most often used include 2 nucleoside analogue reverse-transcriptase inhibitors (NRTIs) plus either a protease inhibitor or a nonnucleoside reverse-transcriptase inhibitor (NNRTI). ARDs resistance testing (viral genotyping) is recommended before starting treatment, because infected infants may acquire resistant virus from their mothers. Suppression of the virus to undetectable levels is the desired goal. Early diagnosis and aggressive treatment of opportunistic infections may prolong survival and should be strongly pursued.

- B. **General supportive care**
  1. **Intravenous immune globulin (IVIG).** HIV-infected infants who have recurrent, serious bacterial infections (like bacteremia, meningitis, or pneumonia) are appropriate candidates for routine IVIG prophylaxis (400 mg/kg/dose every 28 days). Trimethoprim-sulfamethoxazole prophylaxis may provide comparable protection.
  2. **Immunization**
     a. **Active immunization.** All routine infant immunizations should be given to HIV-1–exposed infants. If HIV-1 infection is confirmed, then guidelines for the HIV-1–infected child should be followed. Children with HIV-1 infection should be immunized as soon as is age appropriate with inactivated vaccines. Trivalent inactivated influenza vaccine (TIV) should be given annually. Additionally, live virus–containing measles-mumps-rubella (MMR) and varicella vaccines should be given to asymptomatic HIV-1–infected children and those with appropriate CD4 percentages (ie, CD4$^+$ T-lymphocyte count >15% in children). Rotavirus vaccine may be given to HIV-1–exposed and HIV-1–infected infants. Measles-mumps-rubella-varicella (MMRV) vaccine should not be administered to HIV-infected infants because of lack of safety data in this population. The immunologic response to these vaccines in HIV-1–infected children may be less robust and less persistent than in immunologically normal children. Members of households in which a child has HIV-1 infection can receive MMR vaccine. Yearly influenza immunization is recommended to all household members 6 months of age or older. Immunization with varicella vaccine of siblings and susceptible adult caregivers of patients with HIV-1 infection is encouraged.
     b. **Passive immunization.** HIV-1–infected children exposed to **measles** should receive intramuscular immune globulin (IG) prophylaxis regardless of immunization status. Additionally, children with HIV-1 infection who sustain wounds classified as **tetanus** prone should receive tetanus immune globulin regardless of immunization status. Finally, for **chickenpox** or shingles exposure, HIV-infected children without a history of previous chickenpox or varicella vaccination should receive varicella zoster immune globulin (VariZIG) or, if not available, IVIG within 10 days after exposure.
  3. **Nutrition.** Close nutritional monitoring should be part of the routine care of these children.
  4. *Pneumocystis jiroveci* **prophylaxis.** CDC guidelines state that all infants born to HIV-infected women receive prophylaxis for 1 year beginning at 4–6 weeks regardless of CD4$^+$ lymphocyte count. If HIV infection is excluded, then prophylaxis can be stopped. The drug of choice for this is trimethoprim-sulfamethoxazole. The need

for prophylaxis after 1 year can be determined by the degree of immunosuppression as determined by CD4$^+$ T-lymphocyte count.

5. **Other aspects of supportive care.** Neurodevelopmental supportive services include preschool early intervention programs and school-based developmental disability programs. Aggressive management and protocols for pharmacologic and nonpharmacologic pain management should be used.

VIII. **Prognosis.** In developed countries, 2 patterns of symptomatic infection have been recognized in children who are not treated. Some children become symptomatic quickly and die before 4 years of age, with a median age of death of 11 months (15–20%, termed *rapid progressors*). The majority (80–85%) of untreated children, on the other hand, have delayed onset of milder symptoms and survive beyond 5 years of age (termed *slow progressors*). Only a minority of patients remain asymptomatic by 8 years. Clinical and laboratory factors associated with poor prognosis include being born to mothers with low CD4$^+$ counts or high viral load (ie, >100,000 copies/mL), high virus copy number in the cord blood, and early manifestation of symptoms (opportunistic infections, encephalopathy, severe wasting, and hepatosplenomegaly). Use of **HAART** has substantially reduced both mortality and morbidity and improved quality of life in HIV-infected children. Children with HIV infection acquired through blood transfusion tend to have a prolonged asymptomatic period. In the United States, mortality in HIV-infected children has declined from 7.2 per 100 person years in 1993 to 0.8 per 100 person years in 2006. In resource-limited developing countries, before the use of ARDs, the prognosis is much worse with one study showing 89% of the infected children having died by 3 years of age, 10% having been in HIV disease category B or C, and only ~1% having remained without HIV symptoms. With availability of ARDs to some developing countries, the prognosis is significantly improving. Recent studies from South Africa showed that implementation of a national antiretroviral treatment program resulted in 1 year and 3 year mortality rates of 4.6 and 7.7%, respectively.

Selected References

American Academy of Pediatrics. Human immunodeficiency virus infection. In: Pickering LK, Baker CJ, Kimberlin DW, Long SS, eds. *Red Book: 2012 Report of the Committee on Infectious Diseases.* 29th ed. Elk Grove Village, IL: American Academy of Pediatrics; 2012:418–439.

Chasela CS, Hudgens MG, Jamieson DJ, et al. Maternal or infant antiretroviral drugs to reduce HIV-1 transmission. *N Engl J Med.* 2010;362:2271–2281.

Davies MA, Keiser O, Technau K, et al. Outcomes of the South African National Antiretroviral Treatment Programme for children: the IeDEA Southern Africa collaboration. *S Afr Med J.* 2009;99:730–737.

Joint United Nations Program on HIV/AIDS (UNAIDS). UNAIDS Report on Global AIDS Epidemic 2010. Geneva, Switzerland: UNAIDS, 2010. http://www.unaids.org/globalreport. Accessed July 2012.

Panel on Antiretroviral Therapy and Medical Management of HIV-Infected Children. Guidelines for the Use of Antiretroviral Agents in Pediatric HIV Infection. August 11, 2011:1–268. http://www.aidsinfo.nih.gov/contentfiles/lvguidelines/pediatricguidelines.pdf. Accessed July 2012.

Panel on Treatment of HIV-Infected Pregnant Women and Prevention of Perinatal Transmission. Recommendations for Use of Antiretroviral Drugs in Pregnant HIV-1-Infected Women for Maternal Health and Interventions to Reduce Perinatal HIV Transmission in the United States. May 24, 2010:1–117. http://aidsinfo.nih.gov/guidelines/html/3/perinatal-guidelines/0/. Accessed July 2012.

Phadke MA, Gadgil B, Bharucha KE, et al. Replacement-fed infants born to HIV-infected mothers in India have a high early postpartum rate of hospitalization. *J Nutr.* 2003;133:3153–3157.

Read JS; Committee on Pediatric AIDS, American Academy of Pediatrics. Diagnosis of HIV-1 infection in children younger than 18 months in the United States. *Pediatrics.* 2007;120:e1547–e1562.

Taha TE, Kumwenda J, Cole SR, et al. Postnatal HIV-1 transmission after cessation of infant extended antiretroviral prophylaxis and effect of maternal highly active antiretroviral therapy. *J Infect Dis.* 2009;200:1490–1497.

The European Mode of Delivery Collaboration. Elective caesarean section versus vaginal delivery in preventing vertical HIV-1 transmission: a randomized clinical trial. *Lancet.* 1999;353:1035–1039.

Thorne C, Newell ML. HIV. *Semin Fetal Neonatal Med.* 2007;12:174–181.

World Health Organization. Antiretroviral drugs for treating pregnant women and preventing HIV infection in infants: recommendations for a public health approach, 2010 Version. Geneva, Switzerland: WHO Press; 2010. http://www.who.int/hiv/pub/mtct/antiretroviral2010/en/index.html. Accessed July 2012.

98 Hydrocephalus and Ventriculomegaly

I. **Definition.** **Hydrocephalus** is the progressive enlargement of the ventricular system secondary to excessive cerebrospinal fluid (CSF) volume. It is caused by an imbalance between CSF production, absorption, and impaired CSF circulation. Hydrocephalus is associated with increased intracranial pressure (ICP) and an enlarging head.

Typically, an occipitofrontal head circumference of >2 standard deviations of normal is consistent with macrocephaly due to hydrocephalus. Occasionally, hydrocephalus can present with normal head size but with marked ventricular dilatation.

CSF is primarily produced in the choroid plexus that lines the ventricles (mostly by lateral ventricles in humans). Approximately 80% is choroid plexus in origin, and the remainder is contributed from substance of the brain and spinal cord. Cerebral fluid acts as a buffer between the brain and the skull. Normally secretion of CSF occurs at a rate of 0.3–0.4 mL/min (500 mL/d). Total volume of CSF ranges from 10 to 30 mL for preterm infants and 40 mL for full-term infants; 99% of CSF is water. Sodium is a major cation. Replacement occurs in every 4–6 hours.

The mean CSF opening pressure in neonates and preterm infants is typically lower (100 mmH$_2$O and 95 mmH$_2$O, respectively). CSF values for cell count, protein, and glucose concentrations vary with gestational age (GA) and postmenstrual age (PMA). CSF protein concentrations decrease with both advancing PMA and postnatal age. The white blood cell count is higher in the CSF of neonates as compared with older children.

CSF drains from lateral ventricles via the foramen of Monro into the third ventricle, via the aqueduct of Sylvius into the fourth ventricle, and then into the subarachnoid space via the foramina of Luschka and Magendie. CSF enters the venous circulation by way of the absorptive arachnoid villi that line the superior sagittal sinus. Disruption in this pathway can cause hydrocephalus. Two mechanisms exist to explain the pathologic accumulation of CSF:

A. **Noncommunicating (or obstructive) hydrocephalus.** This may be any blockage along the ventricular CSF pathway that keeps it from reaching the subarachnoid space or disrupts the normal resorptive function of the arachnoid villi. For example, blockage may be aqueductal stenosis, ventriculitis, or a clot following an extensive intraventricular hemorrhage resulting in noncommunicating hydrocephalus.

B. **Communicating (absorptive) hydrocephalus.** Results when CSF is able to pass through all the foramina, including the foramina at the base of the skull (cisterna magna), but is not absorbed into the venous drainage of the cerebral circulation because of the obliteration of the arachnoid villi, as in bacterial meningitis or following an extensive subarachnoid hemorrhage.

II. **Incidence.** The incidence of neonatal hydrocephalus alone is unknown. When included in the diagnosis of spina bifida, it occurs in 2–5 births per 1000.

III. **Pathophysiology**

A. **Congenital hydrocephalus (CH).** CH is a state of progressive ventricular enlargement that starts before birth and is apparent on the first day of life. CH is noncommunicating (obstructive) in presentation and results from developmental malformations of the brain that disturb CSF pathways. Most malformations occur between 6 and 17 weeks of gestation. CH is usually accompanied by other anomalies of the brain, namely holoprosencephaly or encephalocele. Fifty percent of CH cases presenting as fetal hydrocephalus are associated with myelomeningocele, Arnold-Chiari malformation, aqueduct stenosis, or Dandy-Walker malformation.

B. **Postinfectious hydrocephalus.** May be either communicating or noncommunicating. Bacterial meningitis (eg, group B *Streptococcus, Escherichia coli,* or *Listeria monocytogenes*) and subsequent arachnoiditis cause communicating hydrocephalus due to loss of the CSF absorptive sites. However, a ventriculitis leads to obstruction within the ventricular system, usually the floor of the third ventricle and within the aqueduct of Sylvius (tuberculosis, or toxoplasmosis). Indirectly related to the CSF circulatory disturbance can be the formation of postinfectious subdural effusion with ICP and subsequent hydrocephalus.

C. **Posthemorrhagic ventricular dilation (PVD) and posthemorrhagic hydrocephalus (PHH).** It is important to distinguish between PVD and PHH. Progression of ventricular enlargement and evidence of ICP are major factors. PVD follows more severe germinal matrix/intraventricular hemorrhage (GM/IVH) in nearly one-third of all cases and presents as asymmetric or symmetric dilation of the lateral ventricles.

1. **Posthemorrhagic ventricular dilation.** PVD may present early as an acute ventricular dilation within the first week of hemorrhage or develop slowly over ≥2 weeks. By definition, hydrocephalus must present with some signs of ICP. PVD does not present with signs of increased pressure; moreover, recognizing PVD and following it closely will reveal whether it is self-limiting and possibly self-resolving without intervention. It may simply represent ventriculomegaly due to disturbed CSF flow after hemorrhage. Hemorrhagic blood and clots may dissipate and allow resumption of CSF circulation.

2. **Posthemorrhagic hydrocephalus.** PHH may acutely complicate a massive IVH, but more typically evolves posthemorrhage and presents as either communicating or noncommunicating hydrocephalus with ICP. A helpful overview by Goddard-Feingold et al suggests the following outcomes of ventriculomegaly after GM/IVH:

   a. PVD that resolves, leaving normal ventricles.

   b. Transient PHH that resolves, leaving some residual, but a static ventriculomegaly, and may also be referred to as an arrested hydrocephalus.

   c. PHH that is progressive and requires intervention to maintain a stable ICP.

   d. Ventriculomegaly with cerebral atrophy and no ICP.

D. **Ventriculomegaly (VM).** VM is an enlargement of the cerebral ventricles. However, increased ventricular dimension can be due to increased intraventricular pressure (as in hydrocephalus) or the result of passive ventricular enlargement caused by brain atrophy. Early diagnosis of fetal ventriculomegaly and hydrocephalus remains a diagnostic dilemma. The incidence of congenital cerebral lateral VM ranges between 0.3 and 1.5 per 1000 births. Fetal VM can be caused by an abnormal turnover of CSF (obstructive and nonobstructive), agenesis of corpus callosum, neuronal migration disorders (lissencephaly, schizencephaly), neuronal proliferation disorders (megalencephaly, microcephaly), holoprosencephaly, and cerebral vascular abnormalities. VM is frequently associated with syndromes caused by chromosomal abnormalities. Clinical presentation and management of neonatal VM depends on the etiology, type of parenchymal malformation, and whether the VM is associated with increased CSF volume and pressure.

Ventriculomegaly that reflects cortical atrophy has been called hydrocephalus ex vacuo; the term is no longer used because the condition is not a true hydrocephalus. Ventriculomegaly with loss of periventricular white matter is a complication of periventricular hemorrhagic infarction (PVHI). It can present as either unilateral or bilateral and decidedly asymmetric. PVHI with loss of periventricular white matter may present as a large extended porencephalic cyst. Increasing ICP is not a factor in either ventriculomegaly with cortical atrophy or periventricular white matter loss.

Ventriculomegaly associated with hydrocephalus should not be confused with **hydranencephaly.** An infant with hydranencephaly has an absence of the cerebral hemispheres, but the midbrain and brainstem are relatively intact. It may be caused by herpes simplex cerebritis, congenital toxoplasmosis, or ischemic brain necrosis; however, in many cases, the cause is unknown. These infants may have normal or enlarged head size at birth, but progressive enlargement soon becomes apparent and readily transilluminates with a head lamp. See Table 98–1 for other causes of ventriculomegaly.

Table 98–1. **CAUSES OF HYDROCEPHALUS/VENTRICULOMEGALY**

Communicating
    Achondroplasia
    Basilar enlargement of subarachnoid space
    Choroid plexus papilloma
    Meningeal malignancy
    Meningitis
    Posthemorrhagic
Noncommunicating
    Aqueductal stenosis
        Infectious
        X-linked
    Chiari malformation
    Dandy-Walker malformation
    Klippel-Feil syndrome
    Mass lesions
        Abscess
        Hematoma
        Tumors of neurocutaneous disorders
        Vein of Galen malformation
        Walker–Warburg syndrome
    Hydranencephaly
        Holoprosencephaly
        Massive hydrocephalus
        Porencephaly

Adapted and reproduced, with permission, from Fenichel GM. *Clinical Pediatric Neurology.* 5th ed. Philadelphia, PA: Elsevier; 2005:354.

IV. **Risk factors.** Congenital malformations (eg, aqueductal stenosis), CNS hemorrhages, and infections are the more common risk factors for the development of hydrocephalus.

V. **Clinical presentation**

A. **Head circumference.** Daily head circumferences (HC) performed by a primary medical caregiver improve the reliability of the measurements. Normal head growth is 0.5–1 cm/wk. Abnormally increased head circumference remains a hallmark of clinical findings. Additionally, distended scalp veins, separating scalp sutures, a full or bulging fontanel, or cerebral bruit are signs of significantly increased ICP and PHH.

B. **Apnea.** Apnea with bradycardia in association with post GM/IVH monitoring is a strong clinical sign of increasing ICP.

C. **Bradycardia, hypertension, and widening of pulse pressure** are known as Cushing's triad and are signs of increased ICP.

D. **Gastrointestinal.** Feeding intolerance, with or without vomiting, is an association with PHH.

E. **Eye findings.** The "setting-sun sign" of the eyes shows increased appearance of sclera above the iris and is suggestive of increased ICP. It is an important but inconsistent sign in preterm and term infants.

F. **Behavioral state changes.** Irritability or lethargy not previously attributed to the infant's day-to-day behavior is noteworthy when seen with any of preceding signs.

G. **Seizures.** Seizures may develop, but are not of any particular presentation or of any specific electroencephalographic character.

VI. **Diagnosis**

A. **Antenatal diagnosis.** Fetal hydrocephalus may be detected by fetal ultrasound as early as 15–18 weeks' gestation. Amniocentesis is advisable to evaluate chromosomal abnormalities (trisomy 13 and 18), fetal sex (X-linked aqueductal stenosis), and α-fetoprotein levels. Maternal serology may establish an suspected intrauterine infection (toxoplasmosis, syphilis, or cytomegalovirus).

B. **Newborn physical examination.** Head growth of 2 cm/wk is a sign of progressive ventricular dilation.

1. Make a note of the parents' head sizes. Some parents may have a constitutionally large head size, and so might their infant. Normal HC for adult women is 54 ± 3 cm and for men is 55 ± 3 cm. No further evaluation of the infant is needed unless there are risk factors for an enlarging head or signs of increasing ICP.

2. Infants with X-linked aqueductal stenosis may have a characteristic flexion deformity of the thumb.

3. Infants with Dandy-Walker malformation have occipital cranial prominence.

4. Funduscopic evaluation may reveal chorioretinitis indicative of intrauterine infection.

C. **Cerebral bruit.** May be sign of arteriovenous malformation of the vein of Galen or increased ICP due to hydrocephalus or subdural hematoma.

D. **Cranial ultrasound (CUS).** The most important screening tool for premature infants at risk for ventriculomegaly or hydrocephalus (see Figure 11–4D, E, and F views). Ventricular dilation may precede clinical signs of hydrocephalus by days and weeks. Clearly, signs of increasing HC dictate a screening CUS. Likewise, infants with difficult labor and delivery, or those who may have needed resuscitation measures, are candidates for screening CUS. Ventricular size, change in shape, rate of posthemorrhagic ventricular dilation, and the clinical picture guide the management.

1. In our institution, initial CUS is obtained for every infant ≤32 weeks GA between days 10 and 14.

2. CUS can be considered sooner than 10 days under certain conditions (eg, infant with multiple clinical complications).

3. If initial CUS is normal, second CUS is obtained at 36 weeks' GA or at discharge, whichever comes sooner.

4. If initial CUS is abnormal, consider weekly CUS to monitor progression of hemorrhage and posthemorrhagic hydrocephalus. Continue weekly monitoring until the injury is stable.

E. **CT cranial scanning.** Remains useful for image studies in selected patients. It provides the following information:

1. Ventricular dilation identification

2. Determination of size of the cerebral mantle

3. Detection of associated CNS anomalies

4. Detection of parenchymal destruction (calcification or cyst)

5. Determination of a likely site of disturbance of CSF dynamics

F. **Magnetic resonance imaging (MRI).** MRI has become the most effective means of detailing brain injury, hypoxic ischemic events, hemorrhage, malformations, and ventriculomegaly. Fetal brain imaging with new ultrafast MRI studies negates the motion artifact of the fetus. Ultrafast MRI now lends itself to in utero imaging for congenital anomalies of the brain and fetal hydrocephalus. For infants with GM/IVH and at risk for PVHI, studies by MRI are more accurate at documenting parenchymal loss and the formation of porencephalic cysts. Disadvantages of MRI are poor identification of calcifications and requirement of sedation and transport.

VII. **Management**

A. **Fetal hydrocephalus**

1. If fetal pulmonary maturity can be assured, consider prompt cesarean delivery.

2. If the lungs are immature, there are 3 options:

   a. Immediate delivery with the risk of prematurity.

   b. Delayed delivery until the lungs are mature with the risk of persistently increasing ICP. Antenatal steroids can be administered for induction of lung maturity, with delivery of the infant as soon as lung maturity is established.

   c. Fetal surgery options of in utero ventricular drainage with ventriculoamniotic shunt or transabdominal external drainage.

3. **Consultation.** Ideal management calls for a team approach with the obstetrician, neonatologist, neurosurgeon, ultrasonographer, geneticist, ethicist, and family members.

B. **Congenital aqueductal stenosis or neural tube defects.** Decompress by prompt placement of a ventricular bypass shunt into an intracranial or extracranial compartment.

C. **Posthemorrhagic hydrocephalus**

1. **Mild hydrocephalus.** Usually arrests within 4 weeks of progressive ventricular dilation or returns to normal within the first few month of life.

2. **Temporizing measures**

   a. **Serial lumbar punctures (LPs).** May be instituted if there is communicating hydrocephalus. Removal of 10–15 mL/kg CSF is frequently necessary. Approximately two-thirds of infants undergo arrest with partial or total resolution, and one-third still require extracranial shunting of CSF. The resistive index (RI) is the systolic velocity—diastolic velocity/systolic velocity. It can be evaluated by measuring systolic and diastolic blood flow velocities using Doppler ultrasound. Because it is a measure of resistance to blood flow, high values indicate a decrease in cerebral perfusion caused by ischemic brain injury or increasing ICP. Measuring RI may guide management of PHH. A significant rise in RI (>30%) from the baseline can be considered as an indication for CSF removal.

   b. **Drainage, irrigation, and fibrinolytic therapy.** Advocated as another means of minimizing clot obstruction with improved outcomes of neurodevelopmental function at 2 years of age.

      c. **Drugs to decrease CSF production.** Acetazolamide may be administered with or without furosemide with limited clinical improvement. Complications include significant metabolic acidosis, hypercalciuria, and nephrocalcinosis.

      d. **Ventricular drainage.** This can be done by direct or tunneled external ventricular drain or by a subcutaneous ventricular catheter that drains to a reservoir or to subgaleal or supraclavicular spaces. This is indicated for infants who have not responded adequately to LP and who are not good candidates for placement of extracranial shunt. The incidence of infection with these devices is ~5%.

      e. **Ventriculostomy.** Of more recent development has been the success of a third ventricle ventriculostomy. It is an endoscopic procedure that creates a communication (stoma) from the floor of the third ventricle directly into the subarachnoid space at the level of the foramina of the cistern magna. It is a redirection of CSF and a preservation of the subarachnoid to venous pathway for CSF resorption. It has been particularly promising for obstructive PHH with occlusion of the aqueduct of Sylvius.

   3. **Surgical management.** The method of choice is placement of ventriculoperitoneal (VP) shunts. The outcome is better with "early" shunting. It remains *controversial* whether elevated CSF protein level increases the risk of shunt complications and whether shunting should be delayed in patients with a high CSF protein content. VP shunt placement is indicated in nearly all cases to facilitate control of occipital frontal circumference, improved head control, skin care, general nursing care, and patient comfort. VP shunt function depends on shunt valve integrity. The Holter valve was a standard device for almost 50 years, but its limitations included over-drainage of CSF, causing symptoms of headache and dizziness, and renewed obstruction because of collapse of the ventricles (the slit ventricle syndrome). Newer shunts combine programmable magnetic valves with added anti-siphon controls for protection against over-drainage when the patient is in the upright position. In our institution, VP shunts usually are placed when the patient reaches 2 kg of body weight.

   4. **Long-term complications of shunts.** Include scalp ulceration, infection (usually staphylococcal), arachnoiditis, occlusion, development or clinical worsening of an inguinal hernia or hydrocele, organ perforation (secondary to intraperitoneal contact of a catheter with a hollow viscus), blindness, endocarditis, and renal and heart failure. The age of <6 month appears to be a major risk factor for shunt infection in infants.

VIII. **Prognosis**

  A. **Outcomes have significantly improved with modern neurosurgical techniques for PHH.** Long-term survival now approaches 90% with functioning shunts in place.

  B. **Predictors of unfavorable outcome**

    1. Cerebral mantle with <1 cm before shunt placement.

    2. Regarding the cause of hydrocephalus, prognosis decreases in the following order: communicating hydrocephalus and myelomeningocele > aqueduct stenosis > Dandy-Walker malformation.

    3. Reduced size of the corpus callosum is associated with decreased nonverbal cognitive skills and motor abilities.

    4. Mean intelligence quotient is low compared with that of the general population.

    5. Accelerated pubertal development is noted in patients with meningocele or shunted hydrocephalus due to increased gonadotropin production.

    6. Visual problems, such as strabismus, visual field defects, visuospatial abnormalities, and optic atrophy with decreased acuity due to increased ICP, are common.

7. In preterm infants with PHH, poor long-term outcome is directly correlated with the severity of IVH, the presence of PVHI or cystic periventricular leukomalacia, the need for VP shunt, shunt infections, and a high number of shunts.

Selected References

Cohen AR. Disorders in head shape and size. In: Martin RJ, Fanaroff AA, Walsh MC, eds. *Fanaroff's & Martin's Neonatal-Perinatal Medicine: Diseases of the Fetus and Newborn.* 9th ed. Philadelphia, PA: Elsevier Mosby; 2010.

Foroughi M, Wong A, Steinbok P, Singhal A, Sargent MA, Cochrane DD. Third ventricular shape: a predictor of endoscopic third ventriculostomy success in pediatric patients. *J Neurosurg Pediatr.* 2011;7:389–396.

Gaglioti P, Oberto M, Todros T. The significance of fetal ventriculomegaly: etiology, short- and long-term outcomes. *Prenat Diagn.* 2009;29:381–388.

Hassanein SM, Moharram H, Monib AH, Ramy A, Ghany WA. Perinatal ventriculomegaly. *J Pediatr Neurol.* 2008;6:298–307.

Khalid HK, Magram G. Siphon regulatory devises: their role in the treatment of the hydrocephalus. *Neurosurg Focus.* 2007;22:E5–E14.

Kondageski C, Thompson D, Reynolds M, Hayward RD. Experience with the Strata valve in the management of shunt overdrainage. *J Neurosurg.* 2007;106(suppl):95–102.

Lacy M, Pyykkonen BA, Hunter SJ, et al. Intellectual functioning in children with early shunted post-hemorrhagic hydrocephalus. *Pediatr Neurosurg.* 2008;44:376–368.

Perlman J. *Neonatology: Questions and Controversies Series: Neurology.* 1st ed. Philadelphia, PA: Elsevier Saunders; 2008.

Rizvi S, Wood M. Ventriculo-subgaleal shunting for post haemorrhagic hydrocephalus in premature Infants. *Pediatr Neurosurg.* 2010;46:335–339.

Volpe JJ. *Neurology of the Newborn.* 5th ed. Philadelphia, PA: Elsevier Saunders; 2008.

Whitelaw A, Jary S, Kmita G, et al. Randomized trial of drainage, irrigation and fibrinolytic therapy for premature infants with post-hemorrhagic ventricular dilatation: developmental outcome at 2 years. *Pediatrics.* 2010;125:e852–e858.

99 Hyperbilirubinemia, Direct (Conjugated Hyperbilirubinemia)

Jaundice is the most common transitional finding in the newborn period, occurring in 60–70% of term and ~80% of preterm infants. An elevation of serum bilirubin concentration >2 mg/dL is found in virtually all newborns in the first several days of life. Jaundice becomes clinically apparent at serum bilirubin concentration of ≥5 mg/dL.

Bilirubin is the end product of the catabolism of heme derived primarily from the breakdown of red blood cell hemoglobin. The rate-limiting step in this production is the oxidation of heme to form a green pigment called biliverdin, a process controlled by the enzyme heme oxygenase. Each molecule of heme catabolized results in equimolar quantities of bilirubin and carbon monoxide. Other sources of heme include heme-containing proteins such as myoglobin, cytochromes, and nitric oxide synthase. Bilirubin exists in several forms in the blood but is predominantly bound to serum albumin; other compounds, such as drugs and metal ions, may compete with bilirubin for albumin binding sites. Elevated concentration of free unconjugated bilirubin can enter the central nervous system (CNS) and become toxic to neurons. The precise mechanism of toxicity is unknown.

Inside liver cells, unconjugated bilirubin is bound immediately to intracellular proteins, the most important one being ligandin. It is then converted into an excretable and soluble form through the process of conjugation that consists of the transfer of 1 or 2 glucuronic acid residues from uridine diphosphoglucuronic acid (UDPGA) to form a monoglucuronide or diglucuronide conjugate. Uridine diphosphoglucuronyl transferase (UDPGT) is the major enzyme involved in this process. Conjugation is impaired in newborns due to reduced UDPGT activity and a relatively low level of uridine diphosphoglucuronic acid. Conjugated bilirubin is water soluble and can be excreted in the urine, but most of it is rapidly excreted as bile into the intestine. Conjugated bilirubin is further metabolized by bacteria in the intestine and excreted in the feces.

Hyperbilirubinemia presents as either **unconjugated hyperbilirubinemia or conjugated hyperbilirubinemia.** The 2 forms involve different pathophysiologic causes with distinct potential complications. In contrast to unconjugated hyperbilirubinemia, which can be transient and physiologic in the newborn period, conjugated hyperbilirubinemia is always pathologic. **See Chapter 100 for a discussion of unconjugated hyperbilirubinemia.**

I. **Definition. Conjugated hyperbilirubinemia** is defined as a measure of direct reacting bilirubin of >1.0 mg/dL, if the total serum bilirubin (TSB) is ≤5.0 mg/dL, or more than 20% TSB. It is the biochemical marker of cholestasis and a sign of hepatobiliary dysfunction. Unlike physiologic unconjugated hyperbilirubinemia, typically known as "physiologic jaundice of the newborn," it is important to emphasize that **there is no physiologic conjugated hyperbilirubinemia.** Chapter 57 provides information for rapid "on-call" assessment and management.

II. **Incidence.** Conjugated hyperbilirubinemia affects ~1 in every 2500 infants and is much less common than unconjugated hyperbilirubinemia.

III. **Pathophysiology.** Normal bile production involves 2 main processes: bile acid uptake by the hepatocytes from the blood, and bile excretion into the biliary canaliculus. Bile uptake from the blood is an active process facilitated by 2 main receptors at the basolateral membranes, while bile secretion at the canalicular membrane is mediated largely by the bile salt export pump. In healthy newborns, the cellular processes that regulate bile flow are immature and do not function at the normal adult level, making them more susceptible to cholestasis.

IV. **Risk factors.** Well-known risk factors include congenital infections, sepsis, neonatal hepatitis, ABO incompatibility, trisomy 21, and the use of total parenteral nutrition (TPN).

V. **Clinical presentation.** Prolonged clinical jaundice is the main presenting complaint of conjugated hyperbilirubinemia, along with pale (acholic) stools and dark urine. The Cholestasis Guideline Committee recommends that any infant noted to be jaundiced at 2 weeks of age be evaluated for cholestasis. Breast-fed infants who have a normal history and physical examination and can reliably be monitored should be evaluated for cholestasis at 3 weeks of age, if jaundice is persistent. No single screening test can predict which infant will develop cholestasis.

The differential diagnosis of cholestasis is extensive. It can be classified based on the anatomic location of the pathologic process (extrahepatic vs intrahepatic causes), or it can be categorized into broad etiologic causes, such as infectious, familial, metabolic, toxic, chromosomal, vascular, and bile duct anomalies. Recent understanding in molecular genetics has pointed to new directions of investigations that resulted in identification of the molecular mechanisms of a subset of hepatobiliary diseases that often can lead to ongoing liver dysfunction. The most common differential diagnoses of neonatal cholestasis are listed in Table 99–1.

A. Specific diseases

1. **Biliary atresia.** The most common cause of cholestasis in term infants, it remains the single most common reason for liver transplantation in children. It is a progressive idiopathic inflammatory process that leads to chronic cholestasis and fibrosis of both the intrahepatic and extrahepatic bile ducts and subsequent biliary cirrhosis. It has a worldwide estimated incidence of 1 in 15,000 live births,

Table 99–1. CAUSES OF CONJUGATED HYPERBILIRUBINEMIA

Extrahepatic biliary disease
  Biliary atresia
  Choledochal cyst
  Bile duct stenosis
  Spontaneous perforation of the bile duct
  Cholelithiasis
  Neoplasms
Intrahepatic biliary disease
  Intrahepatic bile duct paucity (syndromic or nonsyndromic)
  Progressive intrahepatic cholestasis
  Inspissated bile
Hepatocellular disease
  Metabolic and genetic defects
    α_1-antitrypsin deficiency, cystic fibrosis, mitochondrial hepatopathies, Dubin-Johnson syndrome, Rotor syndrome, galactosemia, progressive familial intrahepatic cholestasis (Byler disease), hereditary fructose intolerance, tyrosinemia, recurrent cholestasis with lymphedema, cerebrohepatorenal syndrome (Zellweger syndrome), congenital erythropoietic porphyria, Niemann-Pick disease, Menkes' kinky hair syndrome
  Infections
    Viral: hepatitis B virus; non-A, non-B hepatitis virus; cytomegalovirus; herpes simplex virus; coxsackievirus; Epstein-Barr virus; adenovirus
    Bacterial: *Treponema pallidum*, *Escherichia coli*, group B *Streptococcus*, *Staphylococcus aureus*, *Listeria monocytogenes*; urinary tract infection caused by *E. coli* and other gram-negative organisms
    Other: *Toxoplasma gondii*
  Total parenteral nutrition
  Idiopathic neonatal hepatitis
  Neonatal hemochromatosis
Miscellaneous
  Shock
  Extracorporeal membrane oxygenation/extracorporeal life support (ECMO/ECLS)

with the highest incidence in Taiwan and French Polynesia (1 in 3000 live births). There are 2 distinct phenotypes identified: **the embryonic or fetal form** is less common, associated with an earlier onset of cholestasis and multiple congenital anomalies, and **the perinatal or acquired form**, occurring in 80% of cases, without associated congenital anomalies. In the perinatal or acquired form, infants are presumed to have a normal and patent biliary system at birth that subsequently undergoes progressive inflammation and fibro-obliteration due to a perinatal insult. It is critical to confirm or exclude the diagnosis of biliary atresia as the cause of conjugated hyperbilirubinemia by 45–60 days of age. Evidence suggests that early surgical intervention leads to a better outcome and prognosis.

2. Genetic intrahepatic cholestasis. There are multiple forms of genetic intrahepatic cholestasis, each with different clinical features and variable clinical presentation and prognosis. Some progressive familial forms (formerly called progressive familial intrahepatic cholestasis [PFIC]) are potentially fatal; the syndromic paucity of intrahepatic bile ducts (Alagille syndrome) tends to have a more favorable prognosis. The pathogenetic mechanisms of this group of disorders have been defined only partially, and the techniques of molecular genetics have only been recently applied. These disorders, although individually rare, are collectively common.

a. **Alagille syndrome.** A syndromic condition thought to be due to altered embryogenesis; it is also known as arteriohepatic dysplasia. It is a genetic disorder, transmitted as autosomal dominant inheritance with variable expression. Mutations in JAG1 (protein associated with Alagille syndrome) on chromosome 20p have been identified. Its major clinical features include a paucity of the intrahepatic bile ducts (chronic cholestasis), cardiovascular anomalies (peripheral pulmonic stenosis), skeletal abnormalities (butterfly vertebrae), ophthalmologic findings (posterior embryotoxon), and "typical facies" (facial shape of an inverted triangle, with broad forehead, deep-set eyes, mild hypertelorism, straight nose with flattened tip, prominent chin, and small, low-set, malformed ears). Although it may not be present in 20–40% of young infants, the abnormality of bile ducts is considered to be the most consistent finding in Alagille syndrome; repeat liver biopsies may be needed in patients with a clinically suspected diagnosis but not confirmed on initial histologic diagnosis. Long-term prognosis depends on severity and duration of cholestasis, severity of cardiovascular defect, and liver status as it relates to need for liver transplantation.

b. **Progressive familial intrahepatic cholestasis (PFIC).** A group of genetic disorders, with autosomal recessive inheritance and characterized by progressive intrahepatic cholestasis. The predominant mechanism for the intrahepatic cholestasis is altered canalicular transport. Currently, 3 types of PFIC are recognized:

   i. **PFIC-1.** Originally called Byler disease. It presents with conjugated hyperbilirubinemia early in life, typically within the first 3 months. Diarrhea, pancreatitis, and deficiency of fat-soluble vitamins are seen. Cirrhosis is seen by the first decade of life, and liver transplantation is usually needed by the second decade of life.

   ii. **PFIC-2.** Caused by bile salt export pump (BSEP) deficiency, resulting in altered bile acid transport. It has a presentation similar to PFIC-1 with no evidence of pancreatitis. Serum γ-glutamyl transpeptidase (γ-GTP) is not elevated despite cholestasis.

   iii. **PFIC-3.** Due to multidrug resistance protein 3 (MDR3) deficiency, resulting in altered phospholipid transport into the canaliculus. It is clinically similar to PFIC-1 and PFIC-2, except that PFIC-3 has an elevated level of γ-GTP.

3. **Inborn errors of metabolism.** (See Chapter 101.) In the neonatal period, several inborn metabolic disorders can result in hepatocellular injury that can give rise to a clinical syndrome of neonatal hepatitis. The most common metabolic disease that presents as cholestasis is α_1-**antitrypsin deficiency**. Metabolic diseases that can present with rather fulminant liver dysfunction include galactosemia, tyrosinemia, and hereditary fructose intolerance. Hereditary fructose intolerance does not present in the neonatal period unless the infant was exposed to a fructose-containing diet.

a. **Galactosemia.** An autosomal recessive disorder of galactose metabolism that is caused by deficiencies in one of 3 enzymes involved in the metabolism of galactose: galactose-1-phosphate uridyltransferase (GALT), galactokinase (GALK), and uridine diphosphate galactose-4-epimerase (GALE).

   Classic galactosemia is the most common and most severe and is caused by deficiency of the galactose-1-phosphate uridyltransferase (GALT) enzyme. It affects ~1 in 10,000 to 1 in 30,000 live births. Deficiency of the GALT enzyme results in accumulation of galactose-1-phosphate and other metabolites that are thought to be toxic to the liver and other organ systems. The gold standard of diagnosis is measurement of GALT activity in the erythrocytes. Clinical presentation is variable and nonspecific in the neonatal period (occurs after ingestion of galactose-containing formula) and includes vomiting, loose stools, prolonged jaundice, irritability, and poor weight gain. Continued ingestion of galactose results in multiorgan toxicity with hepatomegaly, worsening liver dysfunction, splenomegaly, renal dysfunction, and CNS involvement. These infants, while on lactose-containing formula, have galactose in the urine, resulting in a positive reducing substance in the urine (Clinitest reagent tablets) but negative urine dipstick test for glucose (glucose oxidase). A cataract may be detected on examination. **"Oil-drop" cataracts** are highly typical of galactosemia and may resolve with treatment if diagnosed early. Neonatal sepsis due to *Escherichia coli* and other gram-negative organisms is more frequent in galactosemic infants. The reason for this unique predisposition remains unclear. Treatment for galactosemia consists of immediate removal of galactose in the diet as soon as diagnosis is suspected. Liver disease usually improves, but long-term neurodevelopmental complications may develop later despite good dietary control.

Galactokinase deficiency (GALK) results in accumulation of galactose, galactitol, and galactonate and leads to early onset of juvenile bilateral cataract. Although uncommon, pseudotumor cerebri, mental retardation, hepatosplenomegaly, hypoglycemia, and seizures have been described in GALK-deficient patients.

The rarest and most poorly understood among the 3 types is **epimerase deficiency (GALE)**. Natural history of epimerase-deficiency galactosemia is limited due to the small number of patients reported to date. When a diet containing lactose is not removed immediately, infants typically present with generalized hypotonia, poor feeding, vomiting, weight loss, progressive cholestatic jaundice, hepatomegaly, liver dysfunction, aminoaciduria, and cataracts. Prompt removal of galactose from their diet resolves or prevents acute symptoms.

b. **Tyrosinemia.** Biochemical basis for this disorder is a defect in tyrosine metabolism due to lack of fumarylacetoacetate hydrolase. It is inherited as an autosomal recessive disorder that clinically presents with hepatocellular damage, renal tubular dysfunction, and neuropathy. One characteristic pattern of tyrosinemia is a very high α-fetoprotein. For those patients who survived infancy, they are at high risk of developing hepatocellular carcinoma.

c. **Zellweger or cerebrohepatorenal syndrome.** This is a peroxisomal disorder characterized by the absence of peroxisomes and deranged mitochondria. It is inherited as an autosomal recessive trait and presents in the neonatal period with cholestasis, hepatomegaly, profound hypotonia, and dysmorphic features. Diagnosis is confirmed by the presence of abnormal levels of very-long-chain fatty acid in the serum. Most infants die within 1 year. Survivors beyond 1 year of age have severe mental retardation and seizures.

d. **α_1-Antitrypsin deficiency.** The **most common inherited cause of neonatal hepatitis syndrome**, with an incidence of 1 in 1600 to 1 in 2000 live births in North American and European populations, α_1-antitrypsin is the most abundant proteinase inhibitor, and it acts by inhibiting destructive proteases. Clinical diagnosis is made by documenting low serum concentration of α_1-antitrypsin and identifying the phenotypic variant based on differences in isoelectric point (Pi), with M being normal and Z being most deficient. There are several phenotypes; however, the homozygous Pi (protease inhibitor) ZZ is the most likely associated with neonatal liver disease and adult emphysema. Despite carrying the same mutation, only 10–15% of newborns present clinically. Treatment is mostly supportive or liver transplantation if cirrhosis is progressive. Outcome is related to severity of neonatal liver disease; 50% of children are clinically normal by 10 years of age, 5–10% require liver transplantation, and in 20–30% of patients, cholestasis resolves with residual evidence of cirrhosis that may eventually require liver transplantation.

e. **Mitochondrial hepatopathies.** Usually presents as metabolic crises with associated multiorgan dysfunction. However, mitochondrial disorders can be organ specific with subtle clinical findings to frank liver failure with or without signs of other organ involvement. Infant presenting with features suggestive of liver dysfunction, such as lactic acidosis, hypoglycemia, cholestasis, and coagulopathy should be worked up for mitochondrial hepatopathies. A muscle tissue biopsy or direct enzyme assay of cultured skin fibroblasts may not reveal a diagnosis, especially if the dysfunction is primarily in the liver; 80–95% of patients with clinically suspected mitochondrial disease do not have a detectable pathogenic DNA mutation. Treatment is mainly supportive, and in some cases liver transplantation is necessary.

4. **Idiopathic neonatal hepatitis.** A diagnosis given to neonatal hepatitis with liver histology showing giant cell multinucleated hepatocytes where no known infectious or metabolic cause has been found. Diagnosis is one of exclusion. Management is mostly supportive. Overall prognosis is difficult to estimate but generally good for infants whose liver disease resolves in the first year.

5. **Infection**

   a. **Congenital infections.** (TORCH [*t*oxoplasmosis, *o*ther infections, *r*ubella, *c*ytomegalovirus, and *h*erpes simplex virus]) Congenitally acquired infections have a spectrum of manifestations but are usually asymptomatic. They share clinical similarities such as hepatosplenomegaly, jaundice, petechial rash, and intrauterine growth restriction. Liver dysfunction is a possible presentation with any of these viral agents, but it is most common with herpes simplex infection. Vertical transmission of hepatitis viruses (B and C) is generally asymptomatic, but clinical hepatitis, including hepatic failure, may develop later.

   b. **Bacterial infections.** Inflammation-induced cholestasis has been linked predominantly with gram-negative infections (particularly *E. coli*), although gram-positive infections can also lead to cholestasis. Recent studies point to lipopolysaccharide (LPS) or endotoxin and the subsequent release of cytokines during infections as the major factors in sepsis-associated cholestasis. Disproportionate elevation of serum bilirubin in comparison with serum transaminases should prompt a search for an underlying infection. Infection should be part of the differential diagnosis of new-onset or worsening jaundice in an infant. Urinary tract infection in particular has been reported to be associated with persistent hyperbilirubinemia (both indirect and direct).

6. **Total parenteral nutrition (TPN)-related cholestasis.** The frequency, not necessarily the severity, of cholestasis is partly a function of the degree of prematurity. Cholestasis develops in >50% of infants with birthweight of <1000 g and <10% of term infants after prolonged hyperalimentation. Of infants who require long-term TPN for intestinal failure, 40–60% develop TPN-related liver disease. Pathogenesis is unknown but thought to be multifactorial and directly related to prematurity, low birthweight, episodes of sepsis, and duration of TPN use. One of the most important contributing factors is lack of enteral feeding leading to decreased gut hormone secretion, reduction of bile flow, and biliary stasis. Even small oral feedings (continuous or bolus) during hyperalimentation may prevent TPN-related liver disease. The resumption of normal enteral feeds is associated with improvement of cholestasis in 1–3 months, with minimal or no residual fibrosis and normal hepatic function. Hepatic complications are potentially reversible if TPN is discontinued before significant liver damage has ensued. A single component of parenteral nutrition (PN) solution has not been definitely identified as the cause of cholestasis; however, more recent evidence suggests that soy bean lipid emulsion (predominantly omega-6 polyunsaturated

fatty acids [PUFAs]) contributes to hepatotoxicity. Studies have demonstrated the benefit of fish oil lipid emulsions (predominantly omega-3 fatty acids [FAs]) in reversing cholestasis and hepatic injury in patients with intestinal failure–associated liver disease.

7. **Inspissated bile.** The "inspissated bile syndrome" is the term traditionally used for conjugated hyperbilirubinemia resulting from severe jaundice associated with hemolysis due to Rh or ABO incompatibility, although a multifactorial cause cannot be entirely excluded. Intrahepatic cholestasis is found on liver biopsy, and cholestasis is probably related to direct hepatocellular damage produced by unconjugated hyperbilirubinemia. Prognosis is generally good.

VI. **Diagnosis.** Evaluation of cholestasis can be extensive; therefore, it should be individualized to establish a diagnosis efficiently and promptly. **Figure 57–1 provides a concise algorithm for an infant with conjugated hyperbilirubinemia.**

A. **Laboratory studies**

1. **Bilirubin levels (total and direct).** The most important initial investigation in a persistently jaundiced infant is determining the fractionated serum bilirubin levels. Presence of direct reacting bilirubin of >1.0 mg/dL, if TSB is ≤5.0 mg/dL, or more than 20% of TSB is consistent with conjugated hyperbilirubinemia.

2. **Liver enzymes.** Serum transaminases (alanine transaminase [ALT] and aspartate transaminase [AST]) are sensitive indicators of hepatocellular inflammation but are neither specific nor of any prognostic value. They may be helpful in monitoring the course of the disease. Alkaline phosphatase is nonspecific because it is found in the liver, kidney, and bone.

3. **Prothrombin time and partial thromboplastin time.** May be more reliable indicators of liver synthetic function.

4. **γ-Glutamyl transpeptidase (GGT).** An enzyme in the biliary epithelium. Elevated levels are a very sensitive marker of biliary obstruction or inflammation. A normal level makes biliary atresia an unlikely diagnosis. Normal levels of GGT in the presence of cholestasis indicate failure of bile excretion at the canalicular level and can be seen in progressive familial hepatic cholestasis.

5. **Complete blood count (CBC), C-reactive protein, blood and urine cultures.** Should be considered to screen for any clinical evidence of infection.

6. **Serum cholesterol, triglycerides, and albumin levels.** Triglyceride and cholesterol levels may aid in nutritional management and assessment of liver failure. Albumin is a long-term indicator of hepatic function.

7. **Ammonia levels.** Should be checked if liver failure is suspected.

8. **Serum glucose levels.** Should be checked if the infant appears ill. Metabolic disorders may present with hypoglycemia along with conjugated hyperbilirubinemia.

9. **Urine testing for reducing substances.** A simple screening test that should always be performed to screen for metabolic disease, especially for galactosemia. Galactose in the urine results in a positive reducing substance in the urine on a Clinitest reagent tablet but has a negative urine test for glucose (glucose oxidase).

10. **TORCH titers and urine cultures for cytomegalovirus (CMV).** The use of TORCH titers is less preferable; direct identification of viral infection or measurement of specific IgM antibodies should be done for rapid diagnosis. Polymerase chain reaction (PCR)-based diagnostic studies are extremely helpful and specific.

11. **Other tests.** More specific tests are indicated in the investigation of the specific causes of conjugated hyperbilirubinemia.

    a. **Urine organic acid and plasma amino acid.** Screens for inborn errors of metabolism as a cause of neonatal liver dysfunction. High concentrations of tyrosine and methionine, and their metabolic derivatives, are seen in the urine in cases of tyrosinemia.

b. **α₁-Antitrypsin serum level.** Decreased serum α_1-antitrypsin concentration and liver biopsy showing periodic acid–Schiff–positive cytoplasmic granules will reveal variable degrees of hepatic necrosis and fibrosis.

c. **Sweat test.** Done for confirmatory diagnosis of cystic fibrosis.

B. **Imaging studies**

1. **Chest radiograph.** Presence of cardiovascular or situs anomalies may be suggestive of biliary atresia. Skeletal abnormalities, such as butterfly vertebrae, may be consistent with a diagnosis of Alagille syndrome.

2. **Ultrasonography.** A simple and noninvasive test that should be done in all infants presenting with cholestasis after a 4-hour fast; a small or absent gallbladder is suggestive of biliary atresia, whereas the presence of a normal-looking gallbladder makes this diagnosis unlikely. Ultrasound is a sensitive method for recognizing other surgical causes of neonatal cholestasis, such as a choledochal cyst or structural abnormalities of the biliary tree.

3. **Hepatobiliary scanning.** Contrast agents are taken up by the liver and excreted into the bile; they are technetium labeled and provide a clear image of the biliary tree after intravenous injection. Serial images are taken for up to 24 hours or until gut activity is visualized. Nonvisualization of contrast material within the intestine in 24 hours is considered an abnormal finding indicative of biliary obstruction or hepatocellular dysfunction. Sensitivity of this test for biliary atresia is high, but specificity is low because patients without anatomic obstruction may not excrete the tracer. Neonatal hepatitis, hyperalimentation, and septo-optic dysplasia are reported causes of absent gastrointestinal contrast excretion and must be considered in the differential diagnosis. Administration of phenobarbital a few days prior to the study may improve the precision of the test.

4. **Endoscopic retrograde cholangiopancreatography.** Sensitivity and specificity are excellent. This procedure can be both diagnostic and therapeutic in cases of cholestasis caused by bile duct stones. It is technically demanding and currently has a limited role in the evaluation of cholestasis in neonates.

C. **Other studies**

1. **Percutaneous liver biopsy.** The single most definitive procedure in the evaluation of neonatal cholestasis; however, biopsy interpretation requires a pathologist with expertise in pediatric liver disease. If a liver biopsy is obtained early in the course of biliary atresia, findings may be indistinguishable from hepatitis. Evidence supports that liver biopsy can be performed safely in young infants; it is therefore recommended that liver biopsy be performed in infants with undiagnosed cholestasis.

2. **Magnetic resonance cholangiopancreatography (MRCP).** The few reports available to date regarding the use of MRCP in children are encouraging. The procedure requires deep sedation or general anesthesia. Based on current available data, this modality is not routinely recommended in the evaluation of cholestasis in neonates.

VII. **Management.** Rapid "on-call" assessment and management is discussed in Chapter 57.

A. **Medical management.** Few conditions causing neonatal cholestasis are treatable, and these conditions (ie, biliary atresia and choledochal cyst) need timely diagnosis and management. Medical treatment is mostly supportive and should be directed toward promoting growth and development and in treating the other complications of chronic cholestasis, such as pruritus, malabsorption, nutritional deficiencies, and portal hypertension. Management involves dietary manipulation and fat-soluble vitamin support.

1. **Special formula.** Elemental formula containing medium-chain triglycerides is preferable because it can be better absorbed regardless of luminal concentration of bile acids.

2. **Medium-chain triglycerides (MCTs).** Infants with cholestasis often require a diet that includes MCTs, which can be absorbed without the action of bile salts. Some formulas containing MCTs include Enfaport and Pregestimil. Breast-fed cholestatic infants should be given supplemental MCT.

3. **Vitamin supplementation.** Fat malabsorption interferes with maintenance of adequate levels of fat-soluble vitamins. Supplementation of vitamins A, D, E, and K is needed. Extra vitamin K supplementation may be necessary if a bleeding tendency develops.

4. **Dietary restrictions.** Removal of galactose and fructose from the diet may prevent the development of cirrhosis and other manifestations of galactosemia and hereditary fructose intolerance, respectively. Dietary restrictions may also be used to treat tyrosinemia but usually are less successful. Most other metabolic causes of cholestatic jaundice have no specific therapy.

B. **Pharmacologic management.** See Chapter 148 for drug dosages.

1. **Ursodiol (ursodeoxycholic acid [UDCA], Actigall).** A naturally occurring dihydroxy bile acid that appears to help cholestasis in 2 ways: substitution in the bile acid pool for more hydrophobic bile acids, and stimulation of bile flow. It was found to lower levels of aminotransferases in patients with viral hepatitis, and to lower biochemical markers and slow the progression of hepatic fibrosis in PFIC. Recommended dose is 20 mg/kg/d in divided doses. The only common side effect is diarrhea, which usually responds to dose reduction.

2. **Phenobarbital.** Mode of action is to enhance bile acid synthesis, increase bile flow, and induce hepatic microsomal enzymes. Recommended dose is 3–5 mg/kg/d. Use is limited by its behavioral and sedative side effects.

3. **Cholestyramine.** Binds bile acids in the intestinal lumen, thereby decreasing enterohepatic circulation of bile acids, which leads to increased fecal excretion and increased hepatic synthesis of bile acids from cholesterol, which may lower serum cholesterol levels. Side effects include binding of fat-soluble vitamins, metabolic acidosis, and constipation.

4. **Rifampin.** Effective in the management of pruritus due to cholestasis, but experience is very limited in neonates. Patients should be monitored for hepatotoxicity and idiosyncratic hypersensitivity reaction, such as renal failure, hemolytic anemia, and thrombocytopenia.

C. **Surgical management**

1. **Kasai procedure.** Surgical procedure such as Kasai portoenterostomy should be done to establish biliary drainage in patients diagnosed with biliary atresia. Optimal results are obtained if the procedure is done before 8 weeks of age. The most significant predictor of long-term outcome is resolution of jaundice. The procedure is used as a bridge to transplantation.

2. **Liver transplantation.** When end-stage liver disease is inevitable, liver transplantation is the last resort. Biliary atresia remains the most common indication for liver transplantation in the United States. Overall, the success of liver transplantation has improved significantly. A review of a single-center 9-year experience reports patient survival of 94 and 92% at 1 and 5 years, respectively. Long-term complications include immunosuppression, infection, renal failure, and growth retardation.

VIII. **Prognosis.** Based on individual etiologies (see Section V).

Selected References

American Academy of Pediatrics. Subcommittee on hyperbilirubinemia. Management of hyperbilirubinemia in the newborn infant 35 or more weeks of gestation. *Pediatrics.* 2004;114:297–316.

Balistreri WF, Bezerra JA. Intrahepatic cholestasis: summary of an American Association for the Study of Liver Diseases single-topic conference. *Hepatology.* 2005;42:222–235.

Balistreri WF, Bezerra JA. Whatever happened to "neonatal hepatitis"? *Clin Liver Dis.* 2006;10:27–53.

Bosch AM. Classical galactosemia revisited. *J Inherit Metab Dis.* 2006;29:516–525.

Cies JJ, Giamalis JN. Treatment of cholestatic pruritus in children. *Am J Health Syst Pharm.* 2007;64:1157–1162.

Darwish AA, Bourdeaux C, Kader HA, et al. Pediatric liver transplantation using left hepatic segments from living related donors: surgical experience in 100 recipients at Saint-Luc University Clinics. *Pediatr Transplant.* 2006;10:345–353.

De Bruyne R, Van Biervliet S, Vande Velde S, Van Winckel M. Clinical practice: neonatal cholestasis. *Europ J Pediatr.* 2011;170:279–284.

Fellman V, Kotarsky H. Mitochondrial hepatopathies in the newborn period. *Semin Fetal Neonatal Med.* 2011;16(4):222–228.

Kaplan M, Wong RJ, Sibley E, Stevenson DK. Neonatal jaundice and liver disease. In: Martin RJ, Fanaroff AA, Walsh MC, eds. *Fanaroff & Martin's Neonatal-Perinatal Medicine: Diseases of the Fetus and Infant.* 9th ed. St. Louis, MO: Mosby; 2011:1481–1490.

Mack CL. The pathogenesis of biliary atresia: evidence of a virus-induced autoimmune disease. *Semin Liver Dis.* 2007;27:233–242.

Madan A, MacMahon JFR, Stevenson DK. Neonatal hyperbilirubinemia. In: Tauesch HW, Ballard RA, Gleason CA, eds. *Avery's Diseases of the Newborn.* 8th ed. Philadelphia, PA: Elsevier Saunders; 2005:1226–1256.

Mayatepek E, Hoffmann B, Meissner T. Inborn error of carbohydrate metabolism. *Best Pract Res Clin Gastroenterol.* 2010;24:607–617.

Moseley RH. Sepsis and cholestasis. *Clin Liver Dis.* 2004;8:83–94.

Moyer V, Freese DK, Whitington PF, et al. Guideline for the evaluation of cholestatic jaundice in infants: recommendations of the North American Society for Pediatric Gastroenterology, Hepatology and Nutrition. *J Pediatr Gastroenterol Nutr.* 2004;39:115–128.

Sokol RJ, Mack C. Etiopathogenesis of biliary atresia. *Semin Liver Dis.* 2001;2:517–524.

Vanderhoof JA, Zach TI, Adrian TE. Gastrointestinal disease. In: MacDonald MG, Seshia MMK, Mullett MD, eds. *Avery's Neonatology: Pathophysiology and Management of the Newborn.* 6th ed. Philadelphia, PA: Lippincott Williams & Wilkins; 2005:940–964.

Venick RS, Calkins K. The impact of intravenous fish oil emulsions on pediatric intestinal failure-associated liver disease. *Curr Opin Organ Transplant.* 2011;16:306–311.

Venigalla S, Gourley GR. Neonatal cholestasis. *Semin Perinatol.* 2004;28:348–355.

Wong LJ, Scaglia F, Graham BH, Craigen WJ. Current molecular diagnostic algorithm for mitochondrial disorders. *Mol Genet Metab.* 2010;100(2):111–117.

Zinn AB. Inborn errors of metabolism. In: Martin RJ, Fanaroff AA, Walsh MC, eds. *Fanaroff & Martin's Neonatal-Perinatal Medicine: Diseases of the Fetus and Infant.* 9th ed. St. Louis, MO: Mosby; 2011:1621–1677.

100 Hyperbilirubinemia, Indirect (Unconjugated Hyperbilirubinemia)

I. **Definition.** When the rate of bilirubin production exceeds the rate of elimination, the end result is an increase in the total serum bilirubin (TSB), a clinical condition called hyperbilirubinemia. The accumulation of bilirubin (yellow-orange pigment) in the skin, sclera, and mucosa is called jaundice.

II. **Incidence.** Neonatal hyperbilirubinemia is a common problem. Approximately 60–70% of term and ~80% of preterm infants develop jaundice in the first week of life. Incidence is higher in populations living at higher altitudes. Incidence also varies with ethnicity. It is lower in African Americans and higher in East Asians, Greeks, and Native Americans.

III. **Pathophysiology**

A. **Physiologic jaundice.** In newborns, a progressive elevation of serum unconjugated bilirubin is almost universal during the first week of life. Although most of these infants are healthy and will not need therapy, they need to be monitored closely because severe unconjugated hyperbilirubinemia can be potentially toxic to the neurons. Physiologic ranges of TSB remain *controversial* because levels are affected by several factors, such as gestational age, birthweight, disease state, degree of hydration, nutritional status, and ethnic background. Data from recent studies suggest that the upper limits of TSB levels (95th percentile) found in diverse populations of normal newborn infants may be as high as 17–18 mg/dL. Studies published for predominantly term breast-fed infants suggest that a typical peak for TSB is ~8–9 mg/dL. Preterm infants have no established "physiologic" bilirubin guidelines.

1. **Exclusion criteria for diagnosis of physiologic jaundice**

   a. Jaundice appearing within the first 24 hours of life.

   b. TSB level >95th percentile for age in hours based on a nomogram for hour-specific serum bilirubin concentration (Figure 100–1).

   c. Bilirubin level increasing at a rate >0.2 mg/dL/h or >5 mg/dL/d.

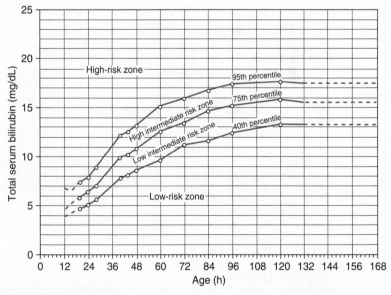

FIGURE 100–1. Nomogram for designation of risk in well newborns at ≥36 weeks' gestation with birthweight ≥2000 g or ≥35 weeks' gestation with birthweight ≥2500 g based on the hour-specific serum bilirubin values. (*Reproduced, with permission, from Bhutani VK, Johnson L, Sivieri EM. Predictive ability of a pre-discharge hour-specific serum bilirubin for subsequent significant hyperbilirubinemia in healthy term and near-term newborns. Pediatrics. 1999;103:6–14.*)

      d. Direct serum bilirubin level >1.5–2.0 mg/dL or >20% of the TSB.

      e. Jaundice persisting for >2 weeks in full-term infants.

  2. **Pathophysiologic mechanisms that predispose newborn infants to hyperbilirubinemia**

      a. **Increased bilirubin synthesis.** Increased synthesis due to larger red blood cell (RBC) mass, increased hemoglobin breakdown up to 2–3 times the adult rate (due to shorter life span of neonatal RBCs), and increased rate of RBC degradation in the bone marrow before release to the circulation.

      b. **Decreased binding and transport.** Decreased hepatic uptake of bilirubin from plasma due to decreased plasma albumin and liver transfer protein, ligandin.

      c. **Impaired conjugation and excretion.** Relatively reduced transferase (uridine diphosphate glucuronyl transferase [UDPGT]) activity in the newborn liver resulting in decreased mono- and diglucuronide bilirubin conjugates that can be excreted in the bile.

      d. **Enhanced enterohepatic circulation.** Conjugated bilirubin is unstable and can be hydrolyzed by the intestinal enzyme β-glucuronidase to its unconjugated form. Once hydrolyzed and unconjugated, bilirubin is readily absorbed through the intestinal mucosa. Sterility of intestinal mucosa prevents further formation of the more excretable products, urobilin and stercobilin.

B. **Breast-feeding and jaundice.** Most studies indicate that breast-feeding is a significant risk factor for hyperbilirubinemia. Jaundice associated with breast-feeding is divided into 2 types based on the age of onset: **Early-onset breast-feeding-associated jaundice** begins within the first week of life, with an incidence of 12.9% in infants having a bilirubin level >12 mg/dL; **late-onset breast milk jaundice** begins after the first week of life, with 2–4% of infants having a bilirubin level of >10 mg/dL at 3 weeks of age. Demographic, environmental, and genetic factors are involved in the development of hyperbilirubinemia in breast-fed neonates. A recent study has shown that breast-fed neonates who have 211 variants in the *UGT1A1*, are G6PD deficient, and are born by vaginal delivery are at higher risk for hyperbilirubinemia.

  1. **Breast-feeding–associated jaundice.** Caloric deprivation (ie, starvation and increased enterohepatic circulation) had been implicated as the cause of breast-feeding–associated jaundice. The exact mechanism is unclear but may involve shifts in bilirubin pools, less efficient conjugation, and enhanced bilirubin absorption in the intestines.

  2. **Breast milk (BM) jaundice.** Prolonged indirect hyperbilirubinemia, beyond the second to third week of life, has been reported to occur in as much as 10–30% of breast-fed infants and may persist up to 3 months of age. No single and exclusive cause has been identified as cause of BM jaundice. Some infants with prolonged BM jaundice have been found to have Gilbert syndrome. Although BM jaundice was considered by some experts as an extension of physiologic jaundice, kernicterus has been reported in apparently healthy term and late preterm infants, and so it cannot be considered totally benign. It has been shown that almost 50% of jaundice appearing between days 4 and 7 of life of exclusively breast-fed infants is related to BM intake.

C. **Pathologic unconjugated hyperbilirubinemia**

  1. **Disorders of production**

      a. **Hemolytic disease.** Results in the destruction of the RBCs and is the most common cause of pathologic hyperbilirubinemia in the newborn period. The process may begin in fetal life or immediately after birth depending on the etiology.

      b. **Blood group incompatibilities**

         i. **Rh (D-antigen) incompatibility** as well as other antigens in the Rh blood-group system (c, C, e, E, cc, and Ce) can cause

immune-mediated hemolytic disease. Alloimmunization occurs when as little as 0.1 mL of RBC from an Rh (D)-positive fetus crosses the placenta into the circulation of an Rh (D)-negative mother. The initial response in the maternal circulation is the production of immunoglobulin (Ig) M that does not cross the placenta and is then later followed by Ig G, which in subsequent pregnancies crosses the placenta and causes a hemolytic process that can begin in utero. The severe form of this process can result in erythroblastosis fetalis with hydrops.

ii. **ABO incompatibility.** Occurs in 3% of all infants. Antigens present on the surface of RBCs react with antibodies in the plasma of opposing blood types, resulting in ABO incompatibility with sensitization. Hemolytic disease related to blood groups is generally limited to group A or B infants born to group O mothers. Risk of recurrence of ABO hemolytic disease is reported to be as high as 88% in those infants with the same blood type as their index sibling. ABO incompatibility is somewhat protective of Rh sensitization because the fetal ABO-incompatible RBCs are rapidly destroyed in the maternal circulation, thereby decreasing the opportunity of Rh antigen to mount an immune response. (See Chapter 80.)

c. **Red cell enzyme deficiencies**

i. **Glucose-6-phosphate dehydrogenase deficiency (G6PD)** is the most common enzyme deficiency; known to affect millions of people. The major function of G6PD is in preventing oxidative damage of cells. The G6PD gene is located on the X chromosome. Prevalence of hyperbilirubinemia is twice that of general population in males who carry the defective gene and in homozygous females. Although it is more common in the African, Middle Eastern, southern European, and Asian populations, the ease of migration and intermarriage has transformed G6PD deficiency into a global problem. The rapid rise in TSB in infants with this enzyme deficiency may not be accompanied by evidence of a hemolytic process.

ii. **Pyruvate kinase deficiency** is inherited in an autosomal recessive manner and is most common in northern European descendants. It presents in the newborn period with jaundice, anemia, and reticulocytosis. This condition has to be considered in a newborn with a nonspherocytic and negative direct antiglobulin test (DAT) hemolytic anemia.

d. **Hemoglobinopathies.** As developmental differences in globin chain synthesis, these are responsible for the different clinical manifestations of α-chain and β-chain defects in the perinatal period. Although these conditions generally do not present in the newborn period, patients with deletion of 3 α-globin genes (hemoglobin H) are often born with hypochromic hemolytic anemia and are at risk for developing severe hyperbilirubinemia.

e. **Infection.** Infection, as sepsis, causes hyperbilirubinemia by increasing bilirubin concentrations via hemolysis, and it may impair conjugation, leading to decreased excretion of bilirubin. Both early- and late-onset jaundice are reported to be one of the more common clinical manifestations of urinary tract infection.

f. **Increased erythrocyte load**

i. **Blood sequestration.** Extravascular blood can result in increased bilirubin production due to breakdown of RBCs. The catabolism of 1 g of hemoglobin yields 35 mg of bilirubin. Occult hemorrhages, such as bruising, cephalohematomas, and intracranial bleeding, can cause significant hyperbilirubinemia.

ii. **Polycythemia.** Increased RBC mass is a known risk factor for hyperbilirubinemia due to an increase in the bilirubin load presented to the liver for conjugation and excretion.

     iii. Infants of diabetic mothers. Such infants have high erythropoietin levels that cause increased erythropoiesis, leading to polycythemia that contributes to hyperbilirubinemia.

2. **Disorders of bilirubin clearance**
   a. **Crigler-Najjar syndrome (CNS) type I.** Autosomal recessive disease characterized by almost complete absence of hepatic uridine diphosphate glycosyl transferase (UGT) activity. TSB is commonly >20 mg/dL. The diagnosis of CNS-I can usually be made by microassay of UGT activity or by measurement of menthol glucuronide in urine after oral menthol. Treatment consists of exchange transfusion soon after birth, followed by daily phototherapy for 12–24 hours and liver transplantation later on. The use of tin protoporphyrin may help decrease the bilirubin level temporarily and may shorten the need for daily phototherapy. Oral calcium supplementation makes phototherapy more efficient. TSB is unresponsive to phenobarbital therapy.
   b. **Crigler-Najjar syndrome type II.** Also known Arias disease, it is more common than CNS-I and is typically benign. CNS-II can occur as an autosomal recessive and dominant inheritance. It is caused by a single base pair mutation leading to decreased but not totally absent enzyme activity. TSB rarely exceeds 20 mg/dL and is lowered by phenobarbital administration. A definitive diagnosis is made by identifying the genetic defect.

   For routine clinical practice, CNS-I and CNS-II can be differentiated by their response to phenobarbital therapy and bile analysis. In CNS-I, bile is totally devoid of bilirubin conjugates, whereas bilirubin monoconjugates are present in CNS-II, and some diconjugates may be detectable after phenobarbital treatment.
   c. **Gilbert syndrome.** Characterized by mild, lifelong, unconjugated hyperbilirubinemia in the absence of hemolysis or evidence of liver disease. Autosomal dominant and recessive patterns of inheritance have been suggested. Hepatic glucuronidating activity is 30% of normal, resulting in an increased proportion of monoglucuronide. Studies have shown that neonates who carry the genetic marker for Gilbert syndrome have a more rapid rise and duration of neonatal jaundice. It is important to remember that Gilbert syndrome is a condition with no consequences for adults, but it can put a neonate at significant risk for hyperbilirubinemia and the potential for complications of bilirubin encephalopathy.
   d. **Lucey-Driscoll syndrome.** Also known as transient familial neonatal hyperbilirubinemia, it is associated with TSB concentrations that usually reach ≥20 mg/dL. The sera of affected neonates and their mothers are found to contain a high concentration of an unidentified UGT inhibitor when tested in vitro.
3. **Metabolic and endocrine disorders**
   a. **Galactosemia.** Jaundice may be one of the presenting signs; however, infants with significant hyperbilirubinemia due to galactosemia typically have other presenting signs and symptoms such as poor feeding, vomiting, and lethargy. Hyperbilirubinemia during the first week of life is almost always unconjugated, and then it becomes mostly conjugated during the second week, reflective of developing liver disease.
   b. **Hypothyroidism.** Prolonged jaundice is found in up to 10% of newborns diagnosed with hypothyroidism. It is due to deficient activity of UGT. Early-onset hyperbilirubinemia has been reported as the only presenting sign of congenital hypothyroidism. Treatment with thyroid hormone improves hyperbilirubinemia.
4. **Increased enterohepatic recirculation of bilirubin**
   a. Conditions that cause gastrointestinal obstruction (eg, pyloric stenosis, duodenal atresia, annular pancreas) or a decrease in gastrointestinal motility may result in exaggerated jaundice due to increased enterohepatic

recirculation of bilirubin. Blood swallowed during delivery and decreased caloric intake may also be contributing factors.

    b. **Breast-feeding jaundice**

        i. **Breast-feeding–associated jaundice.** Thought to be primarily due to poor breast-feeding practices and poor enteral intake leading to a state of relative starvation and delayed meconium passage with increased enterohepatic circulation of bilirubin.

        ii. **Breast milk jaundice.** Increased intestinal absorption of bilirubin facilitated by enzyme β-glucuronidase appears to be the explanation for increased jaundice in breast-fed infants.

    5. **Substances affecting binding of bilirubin to albumin.** Certain drugs occupy bilirubin-binding sites on albumin and increase the amount of free unconjugated bilirubin that can cross the blood–brain barrier. Drugs in which this effect may be significant include aspirin and sulfonamides. Chloral hydrate competes for hepatic glucuronidation with bilirubin and thus increases serum unconjugated bilirubin. Common drugs used in the neonates such as penicillin and gentamicin also compete with bilirubin for albumin-binding sites.

IV. **Risk factors.** Sepsis, acidosis, lethargy, asphyxia, temperature instability, G6PD deficiency, hemolytic disease (ABO or G6PD deficiency), borderline prematurity (35–38 weeks), exclusive breast-feeding, East Asian ethnicity, cephalohematoma or significant bruising, male sex, Native American infants, maternal diabetes, family history of neonatal jaundice, and use of oxytocin in labor.

V. **Clinical presentation**

  A. **Clinical assessment**

    1. **Monitor for jaundice.** All newborn infants should be monitored routinely for development of jaundice. Each nursery should have an established guideline for the routine assessment of jaundice. Jaundice is visible when the serum bilirubin level approaches 5–7 mg/dL. The yellow color is seen more easily in the "fingerprint" area than in the surrounding skin. Progression is cephalocaudal, so that for a given bilirubin level, the face appears more yellow than the rest of the body.

    2. **History.** Family history of jaundice, anemia, splenectomy, or metabolic disorder is significant and may suggest underlying etiology for jaundice. Maternal history of infection or diabetes may increase the newborn's risk for jaundice. Breast-feeding and factors affecting normal gastrointestinal function in the newborn period increase the tendency for more severe jaundice.

    3. **Physical examination.** Areas of bleeding such as cephalhematoma, petechiae, or ecchymoses indicate blood extravasations. Hepatosplenomegaly may signify hemolytic disease, liver disease, or infection. Physical signs of prematurity, plethora with polycythemia, pallor with hemolytic disease, and large infants with maternal diabetes all can be associated with jaundice. Omphalitis, chorioretinitis, microcephaly, petechiae, and purpuric lesions suggest infectious causes of increased serum bilirubin.

    4. **Neurologic examination.** Severe hyperbilirubinemia can be toxic to the auditory pathways and to the central nervous system, which can result in hearing loss and encephalopathy. The appearance of subtle abnormal neurologic signs heralds the onset of early bilirubin encephalopathy. Clinical signs may include lethargy, poor feeding, vomiting, hypotonia, and seizures. The progression of neurologic changes parallels the stages of bilirubin encephalopathy from acute to chronic and irreversible changes.

VI. **Diagnosis**

  A. **Basic laboratory studies**

    1. **Total serum bilirubin**

        a. TSB level determination is indicated in all infants who develop jaundice in the first 24 hours of life. Jaundice appearing that early is almost always associated with a pathologic process.

b. Total bilirubin level and the direct fraction have to be obtained. Indirect bilirubin (also called the unconjugated fraction) is derived by subtracting the direct fraction from the TSB.

c. Indicated for all infants with progressive jaundice and/or prolonged jaundice.

d. During the first few days of life, all bilirubin levels should be interpreted based on the infant's age in hours.

2. **Blood type and Rh status in both mother and infant**

a. ABO and Rh incompatibility can be easily diagnosed by comparing infant and maternal blood types.

b. Cord blood can be sent for routine blood typing of the newborn infant.

3. **Direct antibody test (direct antiglobulin test [DAT]; also known as direct Coombs test)**

a. Detects antibodies bound to the surface of RBCs.

b. Usually positive in hemolytic disease as a result of isoimmunization.

c. Does not correlate with severity of jaundice.

d. Can be obtained from the cord blood.

4. **Complete blood count and differential**

a. Presence of anemia may be suggestive of a hemolytic process; polycythemia increases risk for exaggerated jaundice.

b. Evaluate RBC morphology; spherocytes suggest ABO incompatibility or hereditary spherocytosis.

c. Evaluate for indices suggestive of infection (eg, leukopenia, neutropenia, and thrombocytopenia).

5. **Reticulocytes**

a. Elevation suggests hemolytic disease.

b. Can also be elevated in cases of occult or overt hemorrhage.

6. **Other laboratory tests**

a. Urine should be tested for reducing substances (to rule out galactosemia if the infant is receiving a galactose-containing formula) and for infectious agents.

b. If hemolysis is present, in the absence of ABO or Rh incompatibility, further testing by hemoglobin electrophoresis, G6PD screening, or osmotic fragility testing may be required to diagnose RBC defects.

c. Prolonged jaundice (>2 weeks of life) may require additional tests for thyroid and liver function, blood and urine cultures, and metabolic screening workup, such as plasma amino acid and urine organic acid measurements.

7. **Measurement of serum albumin.** Bilirubin is mostly bound to albumin in the circulation; evidence suggests that neurotoxicity is caused by unbound bilirubin fraction. Therefore, **measurement of serum albumin** may help assess the fraction of unbound bilirubin in the circulation and thereby determine the need of an albumin infusion. It may be useful in the determination of exchange transfusion.

B. **Transcutaneous bilirubinometry (TcB).** A portable instrument that uses reflectance measurements on the skin to determine the amount of yellow color present in the skin. A multicenter evaluation showed that TcB measurement correlates well with laboratory TSB measurement. Accuracy is independent of race, birthweight, and gestational age, and postnatal age of the newborn. A TcB value of >13 mg/dL should be correlated with TSB. Any jaundice noticeable within the first 24 hours of life should be confirmed with serum bilirubin level.

C. **Expired carbon monoxide (CO) breath analyzer.** An equimolar amount of CO is produced for every molecule of bilirubin formed from the degradation of heme. Measurement of CO in end-tidal breath is an index of total bilirubin production (end-tidal CO corrected for ambient CO). This method can alert the attending physician to the presence of hemolysis irrespective of the timing of jaundice.

VII. **Management of infants ≥35 weeks' gestation.** Three methods of treatment are commonly used to decrease the level of unconjugated bilirubin: phototherapy, exchange transfusion, and pharmacologic therapy. The American Academy of Pediatrics (AAP) has published guidelines on risk designation and when to start phototherapy for infants ≥35 weeks' gestation. Preterm infants <35 weeks are excluded from these guidelines and are discussed on page 682. The authors suggest that each institution and its practicing physicians establish their criteria for phototherapy and exchange transfusion by gestational age, weight groups, postnatal age, and the infant's condition, consistent with current standard of pediatric practice. The "on-call" approaches to indirect hyperbilirubinemia are discussed in Chapter 58.

A. **Practice guidelines.** In 2004, the AAP put together evidence-based recommendations to reduce the incidence of severe hyperbilirubinemia and bilirubin-induced encephalopathy in infants ≥35 weeks' gestation. The recommendations include the following: to promote and support successful breast-feeding, to perform a systematic risk assessment for severe hyperbilirubinemia before discharge, to provide early and focused follow-up for the high-risk patient, and to initiate immediate therapeutic intervention when indicated.

B. **Phototherapy.** Reduces serum bilirubin level through photoisomerization and photooxidation of bilirubin to an excretable form.

1. **Indication.** Most infants with increasing jaundice are treated with phototherapy when it is believed that bilirubin levels could enter the toxic range (Figure 100–2).

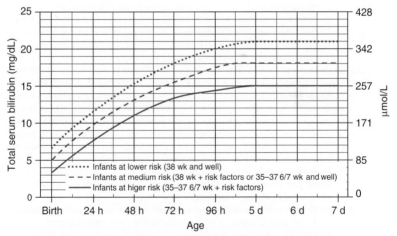

- Use total bilirubin. Do not subtract direct reacting or conjugated bilirubin.
- Risk factors–isoimmune hemolytic disease, G6PD deficiency, asphyxia, significant lethargy, temperature instability, sepsis, acidosis, or albumin <3.0 g/dL (if measured).
- For well infants 35–37 6/7 wk can adjust TSB levels for intervention around the medium risk line. It is an option to intervene at lower TSB levels for infants closer to 35 wks and at higher TSB levels for those closer to 37 6/7 wk.
- It is an option to provide conventional phototherapy in hospital or at home at TSB levels 2–3 mg/dL (35–50 mmol/L) below those shown, but home phototherapy should not be used in any infant with risk factors.

FIGURE 100–2. Guidelines for phototherapy in hospitalized infants of ≥35 weeks' gestation. TSB, total serum bilirubin. (*Reproduced, with permission, from the American Academy of Pediatrics, Subcommittee on Hyperbilirubinemia. Management of hyperbilirubinemia in the newborn infant 35 or more weeks of gestation. Pediatrics. 2004;114:297–316.*)

2. Factors influencing effective phototherapy
   a. Spectrum of light delivered. Researchers have shown that blue high-intensity light-emitting diodes (LEDs) are most effective in degrading bilirubin compared with conventional phototherapy devices.
   b. Energy output. Conventional phototherapy has an irradiance of 6–12 μW/cm^2/nm^{-1}. High-intensity phototherapy provides an irradiance of >25 μW/cm^2/nm^{-1}. The AAP defines intensive phototherapy as an irradiance of at least 30 μW/cm^2/nm^{-1}. Light intensity is a function of the distance from the light source; therefore, light source should be as close to the infant as possible (12–16 in).
   c. Surface area exposed. Maximize the skin exposure to the light source. Systems that provide light source under the infant and standard lighting above are recommended. To maximize exposure, infants should be naked in servo-controlled incubators.
3. Side effects. Phototherapy is relatively safe and easy to use. Minor side effects include rashes, dehydration, and ultraviolet light irradiation. No changes in growth, development, and infant behavior have been reported.
   a. Bronze baby syndrome (BBS). With conjugated hyperbilirubinemia, phototherapy causes photodestruction of copper porphyrins, causing urine and skin to become bronze in color. Clinical significance is unknown, and is generally regarded as harmless; however, recent report has indicated that BBS may pose an additional risk to development of kernicterus.
   b. Congenital erythropoietic porphyria. A rare disease in which phototherapy is contraindicated. Exposure to visible light of moderate to high intensity produces severe bullous lesions on exposed skin and may lead to death.
   c. Retinal effects. The retinal effects of phototherapy to the exposed infant's eyes are unknown; however, animal studies suggest that retinal degeneration may occur. Eye shields must be used. The infant's eyes should be covered with opaque patches for overhead lamp phototherapy.
C. Exchange transfusion. (See also Chapter 30.) Exchange transfusion is used when the risk of kernicterus for a particular infant is significant. A double-volume exchange replaces 85% of the circulating RBCs and decreases the bilirubin level to about half of the preexchange value. It appears that no specific level of bilirubin can be considered safe or dangerous for all infants because patient-to-patient variations exist for the permeability of the blood–brain barrier. Clinical practice parameters published by the AAP in July 2004 provide guidelines for exchange transfusions in healthy newborns ≥35 weeks of gestation (Figure 100–3).
   1. Exchange transfusion. Should be considered in the following circumstances: (Note: Direct or conjugated fraction should not be subtracted from the TSB when considering exchange transfusion)
      a. There is evidence of an ongoing hemolytic process and TSB level failed to decline by 1–2 mg/dL with 4–6 hours of intensive phototherapy.
      b. Rate of rise indicates that the level will reach 25 mg/dL within 48 hours.
      c. High concentration of TSB and early signs of bilirubin encephalopathy.
      d. Hemolysis causing anemia and hydrops fetalis.
   2. General guidelines for exchange transfusion
      a. Generally, type O Rh-negative blood is used for ABO or Rh incompatibility. If the infant is type A or B and the mother is of the same blood type, type-specific, Rh-negative donor blood can be used.
      b. Donor blood must always be crossmatched with maternal serum.
      c. Donor blood should be warmed to ~37°C.
      d. Use fresh blood that is no more than 4 days old.
      e. Consider calcium gluconate infusion during the course of the exchange transfusion because citrate (blood preservative) chelates calcium.
      f. Obtain parental consent.

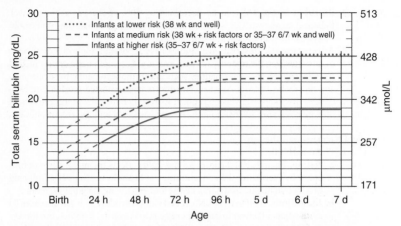

- The dashed lines for the first 24 h indicate uncertainty due to a wide range of clinical circumstances and a range of responses to phototherapy.
- Immediate exchange transfusion is recommended if infant shows signs of acute bilirubin encephalopathy (hypertonia, arching, retrocollis, opisthotonos, fever, high-pitched cry) or if TSB is 5 mg/dL (85 μmol/L) above these lines.
- Risk factors: isoimmune hemolytic disease, G6PD deficiency, asphyxia, significant lethargy, temperature instability, sepsis, acidosis.
- Measure serum albumin and calculate B/A ratio (see legend).
- Use total bilirubin. Do not subtract direct reacting or conjugated bilirubin.

Note that these suggested levels represent a consensus of most of the committee but are based on limited evidence, and the levels shown are approximations. During birth hospitalization, exchange transfusion is recommended if the TSB rises to these levels despite intensive phototherapy.

The following B/A ratios can be used together with but not in lieu of the TSB level as an additional factor in determining the need for exchange transfusion:

	B/A Ratio at Which Exchange Transfusion Should be Considered	
	Risk Category	TSB mol/L/Alb, mol/L
Infants 38 0/7 wk	8.0	0.94
Infants 35 0/7–36 6/7 wk and well or 38 0/7 wk if higher risk or isoimmune hemolytic disease or G6PD deficiency	7.2	0.84
Infants 35 0/7–37 6/7 wk if higher risk or isoimmune hemolytic disease or G6PD deficiency	6.8	0.80

If the TSB is at or approaching the exchange level, send blood for immediate type and crossmatch. Blood for exchange transfusion is modified whole blood (red cells and plasma) crossmatched against the mother and compatible with the infant.

FIGURE 100-3. Guidelines for exchange transfusion in infants ≥35 weeks' gestation. B/A, bilirubin/albumin ratio; G6PD, glucose-6-phosphate dehydrogenase deficiency; TSB, total serum bilirubin. (*Reproduced, with permission, from the American Academy of Pediatrics, Subcommittee on Hyperbilirubinemia. Management of hyperbilirubinemia in the newborn infant 35 or more weeks of gestation. Pediatrics. 2004;114:297–316.*)

3. **Bilirubin levels.** TSB can be decreased by 50% of the preexchange level. Rebound increase in TSB is expected after an exchange transfusion as bilirubin in tissues "migrates" back into circulation.

4. **Adverse events.** Observational studies have reported a high rate of adverse events; however, the majority of these events are asymptomatic, transient, and treatable laboratory abnormalities such as thrombocytopenia, hypocalcemia, and metabolic acidosis. More recent studies have reported mortality rates of 0.5–2%. Exchange transfusion is not risk-free; therefore, the procedure should only be done after intensive phototherapy has failed and the risk of bilirubin encephalopathy outweighs the risk of the procedure.

D. **Pharmacologic therapy**

1. **Phenobarbital**

   a. **Action.** Phenobarbital (dose: 2.5 mg/kg/d) affects the metabolism of bilirubin by increasing the concentration of ligandin in liver cells, inducing production of glucuronyl transferase and enhancing bilirubin excretion.

   b. **Indications.** Used to treat CNS-II and Gilbert syndrome. It can also be used as an adjunct therapy in cases of exaggerated neonatal jaundice, but it takes 3–7 days to become effective. Phenobarbital is not helpful in immediate treatment of unconjugated hyperbilirubinemia in the newborn period.

2. **Metalloporphyrins.** A synthetic heme analog, metalloporphyrin, inhibits heme oxygenase (HO), the rate-limiting enzyme in the catabolism of heme. By acting as a competitive inhibitor, the metalloporphyrin decreases the production of bilirubin. **Tin-mesoporphyrin (SnMP)** is a potent HO inhibitor that has been extensively studied. Strong evidence suggests that a single dose of SnMP reduces the need for phototherapy and exchange transfusion. A single intramuscular injection (6 mmol/kg) in patients with hemolytic disease results in a significant drop in TSB concentration, thereby avoiding the need for exchange transfusion. An immediate untoward effect noted was a non–dose-dependent transient erythema when used in conjunction with phototherapy; however, long-term safety of SnMP remains to be studied, and until then its use must be limited to infants who are at increased risk of developing bilirubin-induced neurotoxicity. It remains an unlicensed drug at this time and is available on an investigational or "compassionate" use basis.

3. **Albumin.** Administration of intravenous albumin may be helpful because an increased reserve of albumin provides more binding sites for free bilirubin and therefore reduces the unbound fraction that may be protective against bilirubin toxicity. An albumin level <3.0 g/dL can be considered as one risk factor for lowering the threshold for phototherapy (dose: 1 g/kg over 2 hours).

4. **Intravenous γ-globulin.** Works by blockage of Fc receptors in the neonatal reticuloendothelial system, thus competing with sensitized neonatal RBCs and preventing further hemolysis. It is recommended if the TSB is rising despite intensive phototherapy. Studies have shown that use of intravenous γ-globulin has decreased the use of exchange transfusion in hemolytic disease of the newborn.

VIII. **Management of infants <35 weeks' gestation.** Premature infants are at greater risk for developing severe hyperbilirubinemia and bilirubin-induced neurologic dysfunction because they are more likely to be sicker (common conditions such as respiratory distress, acidosis, sepsis, and hypoxia) and have lower serum albumin level than their near-term/term newborn counterparts. Because there has been no definitive evidence-based recommendation regarding what level of bilirubin necessitates treatment in premature infants, it is a common practice to use lower TSB levels to initiate phototherapy. Most recently, a consensus-based recommendation has been published that provides a gestational age–guided approach to the use of phototherapy and exchange transfusion in preterm infants. See Table 100–1. When using this table, follow these recommended guidelines: Measure the serum albumin level in all infants. Use the lower range of

Table 100–1. SUGGESTED PHOTOTHERAPY AND EXCHANGE TRANSFUSION CONCENSUS RECOMMENDATIONS IN PRETERM INFANTS <35 WEEKS' GESTATIONAL AGE

Gestational Age[a] (wk)	Begin Phototherapy (total serum bilirubin mg/dL)	Exchange Transfusion (total serum bilirubin mg/dL)
<26	Optional: start right after birth	N/A
<28 0/7	5–6	11–14
28 0/7–29 6/7	6–8	12–14
30 0/7–31 6/7	8–10	13–16
32 0/7–33 6/7	10–12	15–18
34 0/7–34 6/7	12–14	17–19

[a]Use postmenstrual age for phototherapy. Example, when an infant with 29 0/7 weeks' gestational age is 7 days old, use the TSB level for 30 0/7 weeks (see page 42 for postmenstrual vs gestational age determination).
Based on data from Maisels MJ, Watchko JF, Bhutani VK, Stevenson DK. An approach to the management of hyperbilirubinemia in the preterm infant less than 35 weeks of gestation. *J Perinatol.* 2012;32:660–664.

the listed TSB level for infants at greater risk for bilirubin toxicity, for example, these include but are not limited to:

A. Lower gestational age
B. Serum albumin levels <2.5 g/dL
C. Rapidly rising TSB levels, suggesting hemolytic disease
D. Clinically unstable (see page 405)

Recommendations for exchange transfusion apply to infants who are receiving appropriate intensive phototherapy but whose TSB continues to increase to the levels listed. For all infants, an exchange transfusion is recommended if the infant shows signs of acute bilirubin encephalopathy, such as hypertonia, arching, retrocollis, opisthotonus, or high-pitch cry (which rarely occur in very low birthweight infants).

IX. **Prognosis**

A. **General.** Unconjugated bilirubin in high concentration can cross the blood–brain barrier and can penetrate the brain cells, which may lead to neuronal dysfunction and death. The exact mechanism of bilirubin-induced neuronal cell injury is not completely understood; however, high concentrations of unconjugated bilirubin can have neurotoxic effects on cellular membranes and intracellular calcium homeostasis resulting in neuronal excitotoxicity and mitochondrial energy failure. The factors that determine toxicity of bilirubin in neurons of neonates is not completely understood. Specific bilirubin concentrations that put a preterm infant at risk for kernicterus have not been identified. The incidence of kernicterus in this group is unknown, and the relationship of serum bilirubin and neurodevelopmental outcome in the very low birthweight infant remains unclear.

B. **Encephalopathy**

1. **Transient.** Early bilirubin-induced neurologic dysfunction is transient and reversible. The auditory system serves as an objective window for looking at the central nervous system in cases of severe hyperbilirubinemia, and it can be used as an early predictor of bilirubin encephalopathy. Auditory brainstem responses show significant prolongation of latency of specific wavelengths. These changes may be reversed with either exchange transfusions or with spontaneous decrease in bilirubin levels. More recent data showed that TSB level of ≥22 mg/dL, Rh incompatibility, and early jaundice are independent predictors of abnormal development in babies with neonatal jaundice.

2. **Acute bilirubin encephalopathy.** A preventable neurologic sequela of untreated severe hyperbilirubinemia. It is an evolving encephalopathy that can progress in

3 clinical phases over several days. The major clinical features involve distur-bances in level of consciousness, tone and movement, and brainstem function, especially relating to feeding and crying. The severity of abnormalities appears to correlate with both the severity and duration of hyperbilirubinemia.

   a. Initial phase. Noted by lethargy, hypotonia, decreased movement, and poor suck. Clinical findings are nonspecific. A high index of suspicion is needed to recognize these signs as a signal of impending acute bilirubin encepha-lopathy. Prompt therapeutic intervention is critical to prevent deterioration and poor prognosis.

   b. Intermediate phase. This phase has cardinal signs of moderate stupor, irri-tability, and increased tone. Infant may exhibit backward arching of the neck (retrocollis) or of the back (opisthotonos). Fever has been reported to occur during this phase of the syndrome.

   c. Advanced phase. Characterized by deep stupor or coma, increased tone, inability to feed, and a shrill cry. Seizures may occur. This is an ominous stage of acute bilirubin encephalopathy suggesting irreversible central nervous system injury, and the later development of chronic bilirubin encephalopa-thy occurs in most infants.

3. **Chronic bilirubin encephalopathy.** A devastating and disabling neurologic disorder, also called **kernicterus,** and is characterized by a clinical tetrad:

   a. Choreoathetoid cerebral palsy
   b. High-frequency sensorineural hearing loss
   c. Palsy of vertical gaze
   d. Dental enamel hypoplasia

4. **Cognitive deficits.** These are unusual but can be severe. **Mortality rate can be as high as 10%. Kernicterus** is a pathologic diagnosis, describing the yellow discol-oration of the deep nuclei of the brain. Clinical terminology is **bilirubin encepha-lopathy.** Severity varies from mild to severe in children and adults. Mildly affected individuals remain highly functional; moderately affected individuals have more prominent dystonia and are likely to have athetoid movements. Severely affected individuals have speech difficulty and a more disabling dystonia to the point of not being ambulatory. This is a form of static encephalopathy, in which the degree of disability may change slightly overtime but only within limits and is never dra-matic. Brainstem regions that are typically affected by bilirubin encephalopathy are the following: globus pallidus, subthalamic nucleus, metabolic sector of the hippocampus, oculomotor nuclei, ventral cochlear nuclei, and the Purkinje cells of the cerebellar cortex. The pattern of involvement is similar across different ages of affected individuals. Bilirubin encephalopathy is not a reportable condition in the United States; therefore, its true prevalence is not known.

Selected References

Ahmed M, Mostafa S, Fisher G, Reynolds TM. Comparison between transcutaneous bili-rubinometry and total serum bilirubin measurements in preterm infants <35 weeks gestation. *Ann Clin Biochem.* 2010;47:72–77.

American Academy of Pediatrics; the American College of Obstetricians and Gynecolo-gists. Neonatal complications. In: *Guidelines for Perinatal Care.* 6th ed. Atlanta GA: ACOG; 2007:251–259.

American Academy of Pediatrics. Clinical practice guideline: management of hyperbili-rubinemia in the newborn infant 35 weeks or more weeks of gestation. *Pediatrics.* 2004;114:297–316.

Arun Babu T, Bhat BV, Joseph NM. Association between peak serum bilirubin and neu-rodevelopmental outcomes in term babies with hyperbilirubinemia. *Indian J Pediatr.* 2012;79:202–206.

Bertini G, Dani C, Fonda C, Zorzi C, Rubaltelli FF. Bronze baby syndrome and the risk of kernicterus. *Acta Paediatr.* 2005;94:968–971.

Chang PF, Lin TC, Liu K, et al. Risk of hyperbilirubinemia in breastfed infants. *J Pediatr.* 2011;159:561–565.

Elalfy MS, Elbarbary NS, Abaza HW. Intravenous immunoglobin (two-dose regimen) in the management of severe Rh hemolytic disease of newborn—a prospective randomized controlled trial. *Eur J Pediatr.* 2011;170:461–467.

Ghaemi S, Fesharaki RJ, Kelishadi R. Late onset jaundice and urinary tract infection in neonates. *Indian J Pediatr.* 2007;74:139–141.

Johnson L, Bhutani VK. The clinical syndrome of bilirubin-induced neurologic dysfunction. *Semin Perinatol.* 2011;35:101–113.

Kaplan M, et al. Neonatal jaundice and liver disease. In: Martin RJ, Fanaroff AA, Walsh MC, eds. *Fanaroff & Martin's Neonatal Perinatal Medicine: Diseases of the Fetus and Infant.* 9th ed. Philadelphia, PA: Mosby Elsevier; 2011:1443–1481.

Kappas A, Drummond GS, Munson DP, Marshall JR. Sn-Mesoporphyrin interdiction of severe hyperbilirubinemia in Jehovah witness newborns as an alternative to exchange transfusion. *Pediatrics.* 2001;108:1374–1377.

Keenan WJ, Novak KK, Sutherland JM, Bryla DA, Fetterly KL. Morbidity and mortality associated with exchange transfusion. *Pediatrics.* 1985;75:417–441.

Maisels MJ. Jaundice. In: MacDonald MG, Seshia MMK, Mullett MD, eds. *Avery's Neonatology: Pathophysiology & Management of the Newborn.* 6th ed. Philadelphia, PA: Lippincott Williams & Wilkins; 2005:768–846.

Maisels MJ, Watchko JF, Bhutani VK, Stevenson DK. An approach to the management of hyperbilirubinemia in the preterm infant less than 35 weeks of gestation. *J Perinatol.* 2012;32:660–664.

Murray NA, Roberts IA. Haemolytic disease of the newborn. *Arch Dis Child Fetal Neonatal Ed.* 2007;92:F83–F88.

Patra K, Storfer-Isser A, Siner B, Moore J, Hack M. Adverse events associated with neonatal exchange transfusion in the 1990s. *J Pediatr.* 2004;144:626–631.

Rubaltelli FF, Gourley GR, Loskamp N, et al. Transcutaneous bilirubin measurement: a multicenter evaluation of a new device. *Pediatrics.* 2001;107:1264–1271.

Shapiro SM, Bhutani VK, Johnson L. Hyperbilirubinemia and kernicterus. *Clin Perinatol.* 2006;33:387–410.

Sharma P, Chhangani NP, Meena KR, Jora R, Sharma N, Gupta BD. Brainstem evoked response audiometry (BAER) in neonates with hyperbilirubinemia. *Indian J Pediatr.* 2006;73:413–416.

Steiner LA, Gallagher PG. Erythrocyte disorder in the perinatal period. *Semin Perinatol.* 2007;31:254–261.

Stevenson DK, Wong RJ. Metalloporphyrins in management of neonatal hyperbilirubinemia. *Semin Fetal Neonatal Med.* 2010;15:164–168.

Volpe JJ. Bilirubin and brain injury. In: Volpe JJ, ed. *Neurology of the Newborn.* 5th ed. Philadelphia, PA: Saunders Elsevier; 2008:619–651.

Vreman HJ, Wong RJ, Stevenson DK, et al. Light emitting diodes: a novel light source for phototherapy. *Pediatr Res.* 1998;44:804–809.

Watchko JF. Hyperbilirubinemia and bilirubin toxicity in the late preterm infant. *Clin Perinatol.* 2006;33:839–852.

Watchko JF. Kernicterus and the molecular mechanisms of bilirubin-induced CNS injury in newborns. *Neuromolecular Med.* 2006;8:513–529.

Weng YH, Chiu YW. Clinical characteristics of G6PD deficiency in infants with marked hyperbilirubinemia. *J Pediatr Hematol Oncol.* 2010;32:11–14.

101 Inborn Errors of Metabolism with Acute Neonatal Onset

Inborn errors of metabolism (IEMs) are a group of disorders that are of great importance to physicians treating newborns. The immediate diagnosis and appropriate treatment of these conditions are often directly linked to the patient's outcome to the extremes of avoiding death or irreversible brain damage. Pediatricians may feel overwhelmed by the number and complexity of these disorders (Table 101–1) and the interpretation of laboratory tests needed to establish the diagnosis. This chapter, therefore, concentrates on the symptom patterns, laboratory tests and their interpretation, as well as the initial stabilization of the patient rather than discussing details of the specific biochemical and genetic defects or special treatment measures of IEMs. Usually, the patient's ongoing treatment is supervised by a geneticist specially trained in biochemical genetics.

I. **Classification**
   A. **Classification by time of onset.** Because of the nature of this manual, we concentrate here on metabolic disorders with onset in the neonatal period and early infancy. Be aware, however, that onset of a disease in later infancy or even in adolescence and adulthood does not exclude the diagnosis of an IEM. It is also important to realize that, even with comprehensive and well-organized neonatal screening programs, a number of IEMs present clinically before they are detected by screening tests or before the test result is available to the treating physicians. The use of **tandem mass spectrometry (TMS)** in newborn screening is now widespread. Due to the large amount of biochemical information obtained through tandem mass spectrometry analysis, physicians involved in newborn care now often encounter new issues regarding the follow-up evaluations and referrals of patients with a positive screening test.
   B. **Classification by clinical presentation.** Subdividing IEMs by clinical presentation may be the most useful approach to aid in establishing the correct diagnosis. Note that some **syndromes with dysmorphic features** are now known to be IEMs (eg, Smith-Lemli-Opitz syndrome or Zellweger syndrome [see Section IX.A and B]). Other classic examples of IEMs are discussed only briefly because they are clinically asymptomatic in the neonatal period (eg, phenylketonuria [PKU]). Note that some **skeletal dysplasias** and disorders affecting bone and cartilage formation (not discussed here) are, strictly speaking, also IEMs (eg, rhizomelic chondrodysplasia punctata and hypophosphatasia). The following classification system serves as the basis for the more detailed sections of this chapter. IEMs may present with the following:
      1. **Encephalopathy with or without metabolic acidosis**
      2. **Impairment of liver function**
      3. **Impairment of cardiac function**
      4. **Dysmorphic syndromes**
      5. **Less commonly, nonimmune hydrops fetalis**
   C. **Classification according to the biochemical basis of the disease.** A concept that divides IEMs according to their biochemical characteristics helps in understanding the pathogenesis of symptoms and different approaches to treatment but seems to be of less utility for those providing patient care.
II. **Incidence.** By some estimates, IEMs may account for as much as 20% of disease among full-term infants not known to have been born at risk. Cumulatively, an IEM may be present in >1 in 500 live births.
III. **Pathophysiology.** Metabolic processes are catalyzed by genetically encoded enzyme proteins. The classical mechanism of a metabolic defect is lack or deficiency of an

Table 101–1. **INBORN ERRORS OF METABOLISM PRESENTING IN THE NEONATAL PERIOD AND INFANCY**

Disorders of carbohydrate metabolism
  Galactosemia
  Fructose-1,6-bisphosphatase deficiency
  Glycogen storage disease (types IA, IB, II, III, and IV)
  Hereditary fructose intolerance
Disorders of amino acid metabolism
  Maple syrup urine disease
  Nonketotic hyperglycinemia
  Hereditary tyrosinemia
  Pyroglutamic acidemia (5-oxoprolinuria)
  Hyperornithinemia-hyperammonemia-homo citrullinemia syndrome
  Lysinuric protein intolerance
  Methylene tetrahydrofolate reductase deficiency
  Sulfite oxidase deficiency
Disorders of organic acid metabolism
  Methylmalonic acidemia
  Propionic acidemia
  Isovaleric acidemia
  Multiple carboxylase deficiency
  Glutaric acidemia type II (multiple acyl-CoA dehydrogenase deficiencies)
  HMG-CoA lyase deficiency
  3-Methylcrotonoyl-CoA carboxylase deficiency
  3-Hydroxyisobutyric aciduria
Disorders of pyruvate metabolism and the electron transport chain
  Pyruvate carboxylase deficiency
  Pyruvate dehydrogenase deficiency
  Electron transport chain defects
Disorders of the urea cycle
  Ornithine-transcarbamylase deficiency
  Carbamyl phosphate synthetase deficiency
  Transient hyperammonemia of the neonate
  Argininosuccinate synthetase deficiency (citrullinemia)
  Argininosuccinate lyase deficiency
  Arginase deficiency
  N-acetylglutamate synthetase deficiency
Lysosomal storage disorders
  GM_1 gangliosidosis type I (β-galactosidase deficiency)
  Gaucher disease (glucocerebrosidase deficiency)
  Niemann-Pick disease types A and B (sphingomyelinase deficiency)
  Wolman disease (acid lipase deficiency)
  Mucopolysaccharidosis type VII (β-glucuronidase deficiency)
  I-cell disease (mucolipidosis type II)
  Sialidosis type II (neuraminidase deficiency)
  Fucosidosis
Peroxisomal disorders
  Zellweger syndrome
  Neonatal adrenoleukodystrophy
  Single enzyme defects of the peroxisomal β-oxidation
  Rhizomelic chondrodysplasia punctata
  Infantile Refsum disease

(Continued)

Table 101–1. **INBORN ERRORS OF METABOLISM PRESENTING IN THE NEONATAL PERIOD AND INFANCY (*CONTINUED*)**

Miscellaneous disorders
Adrenogenital syndrome (21-hydroxylase and other deficiencies)
Disorders of bilirubin metabolism (Crigler-Najjar syndrome and others)
Pyridoxine-dependent seizures
α_1-Antitrypsin deficiency
Fatty acid oxidation disorders (short, medium, and long chain)
Cholesterol biosynthesis defects (Smith-Lemli-Opitz syndrome)
Congenital disorders of protein glycosylation (carbohydrate-deficient glycoprotein syndromes)
Neonatal hemochromatosis

CoA, coenzyme A; HMG, 3-hydroxy-3-methylglutaryl.

enzyme resulting in **substrate accumulation** and conversion of intermediary metabolites to products not usually present. In addition, end products of the normal pathway will be deficient. Symptoms may result from an increased level of the normal substrate (eg, in urea cycle disorders, the substrate ammonia is toxic and leads to cerebral edema, central nervous system [CNS] dysfunction, and eventually death). Additionally, a **lack of normal end products** of metabolism can lead to symptoms (eg, lack of cortisol in 21-hydroxylase deficiency [see Chapter 91]). The **alternative products may interfere with normal metabolic processes** (eg, accumulated propionyl-CoA may participate in reactions normally using acetyl-CoA in propionic acidemia). Finally, an **inability to degrade end products** of a metabolic pathway may lead to symptoms (eg, myocardial dysfunction in **glycogen storage disease** type II or hepatomegaly in glycogen storage disease type I). The time of clinical presentation often relates to the question of whether the symptoms are caused by metabolites that are able to prenatally transport across the placenta. These are usually of low molecular weight and, therefore, prenatally removed from the fetus and cleared by the maternal metabolism.

IV. **Risk factors. IEMs are genetic disorders.** Therefore, there are no definite behavioral or environmental risk factors for the presence of an inborn metabolic defect (although environment and especially nutrition may affect presentation). A history of relatives with mental retardation, protein avoidance, and, for many disorders, neonatal or childhood deaths or severe illness (liver disease, abnormal heart function, mental and physical decline, episodic illness) could be an indicator of increased risk. A history of protein avoidance, liver dysfunction/failure, or mental changes in pregnancy and labor may be seen in female carriers of X-linked inherited urea cycle defects. Presence of consanguinity and, for a number of inborn errors, ethnic background are also risk factors.

V. **Clinical presentation.** Although there are several specific situations (listed next) in which an IEM must be considered, the safest guideline for clinical practice is that **an IEM should be considered in any sick newborn.** The newborn has a "limited repertoire" of symptoms that are often nonspecific. The differential diagnosis of symptoms such as **poor feeding, lethargy, hypotonia, vomiting, hypothermia, seizures, and disturbances of breathing** is extensive. Although the diagnosis of sepsis is often at the top of the differential diagnosis list, it is important for a timely diagnosis and in the best interest of the patient to evaluate for other causes, including IEMs, at the same time that laboratory investigations are initiated to rule out sepsis. This can be accomplished with a relatively small number of laboratory tests readily available in most hospitals, as discussed in the following sections.

   A. An IEM must be strongly considered under the following circumstances:
      1. History of unexplained neonatal deaths in the family (prior siblings or male infants on the mother's side of the family).

2. Infants who are the offspring of consanguineous matings (because of the higher incidence of autosomal recessive conditions; autosomal recessive inheritance is common among IEMs).
3. Onset of signs and symptoms after a period of good health that may be as short as a few hours.
4. The infant may have had an uneventful perinatal and early newborn course. It is not uncommon for an infant with an IEM to have no significant perinatal history.
5. The introduction and progression of enteral feedings may be related to the symptoms.
6. Failure of usual therapies to alleviate the symptoms or inability to prove a suggested diagnosis such as sepsis, CNS hemorrhage, or other congenital or acquired conditions.
7. Progression of symptoms.
8. Although patients with an IEM might be born prematurely, they are typically full-term infants. An exception is the diagnosis of transient hyperammonemia of the neonate, a condition that typically affects preterm infants. Although this condition is briefly discussed in this chapter, the exact cause of the hyperammonemia in these patients remains unclear and may well be related to prematurity rather than being a typical IEM.

B. Signs and symptoms. Those seen in different IEMs are summarized in Table 101-2. Table 101-3 lists some of the conditions with which infants with IEMs have been misdiagnosed. Keep in mind that **symptoms may overlap** with

Table 101-2. SIGNS AND SYMPTOMS AND ASSOCIATED METABOLIC DISORDERS

Neurologic (hypotonia, lethargy, poor sucking, seizures, coma)
Glycogen storage disease, galactosemia, organic acidemias, hereditary fructose intolerance, maple syrup urine disease, urea cycle disorders, hyperglycinemia, pyridoxine dependency, peroxisomal disorders, congenital disorders of glycosylation, fatty acid oxidation disorders, and respiratory chain defects

Hepatomegaly/liver dysfunction
Lysosomal storage diseases, galactosemia, hereditary fructose intolerance, glycogen storage disease, tyrosinemia, α_1-antitrypsin deficiency, Gaucher disease, Niemann-Pick disease, Wolman disease, fatty acid oxidation defects, and respiratory chain defects

Hyperbilirubinemia
Galactosemia, hereditary fructose intolerance, tyrosinemia, α_1-antitrypsin deficiency, Crigler-Najjar syndrome, and other disorders of bilirubin metabolism

Nonimmune hydrops
Gaucher disease, Niemann-Pick disease, GM_1 gangliosidosis, congenital disorders of glycosylation

Cardiomegaly/cardiomyopathy
Glycogen storage disease type II, fatty acid oxidation defects, and respiratory chain defects

Macroglossia
GM_1 gangliosidosis, glycogen storage disease type II

Abnormal odor
Maple syrup urine disease (odor of maple syrup or burnt sugar)
Isovaleric acidemia, glutaric acidemia (odor of sweaty feet)
HMG-CoA lyase deficiency (odor of cat urine)

Abnormal hair
Argininosuccinic acidemia, lysinuric protein intolerance, Menkes kinky hair syndrome

Hypoglycemia
Galactosemia, hereditary fructose intolerance, tyrosinemia, maple syrup urine disease, glycogen storage disease, methylmalonic acidemia, propionic acidemia, fatty acid oxidation defects, and respiratory chain defects

(Continued)

Table 101–2. SIGNS AND SYMPTOMS AND ASSOCIATED METABOLIC DISORDERS (*CONTINUED*)

Ketosis
Organic acidemias, tyrosinemia, methylmalonic acidemia, maple syrup urine disease
Metabolic acidosis
Galactosemia, hereditary fructose intolerance, maple syrup urine disease, glycogen storage disease,
    organic acidemias
Hyperammonemia
Urea cycle defects, transient hyperammonemia of the neonate, organic acidurias, HMG-CoA lyase deficiency,
    fatty acid oxidation disorders
Neutropenia
Organic acidemias, especially methylmalonic acidemia and propionic acidemia; nonketotic hyperglycinemia,
    carbamyl phosphate synthetase deficiency
Thrombocytopenia
Organic acidemias, lysinuric protein intolerance
Dysmorphic features
Glutaric aciduria type II, 3-hydroxyisobutyric aciduria, Smith-Lemli-Opitz syndrome, peroxisomal disorders,
    congenital disorders of glycosylation
Renal cysts
Glutaric aciduria type II, peroxisomal disorders
Abnormalities of the eye (eg, glaucoma, retinopathy)
Galactosemia, lysosomal storage disorders, peroxisomal disorders
Abnormal fat distribution/inverted nipples
Congenital disorders of glycosylation
Epiphyseal stippling in radiograph
Peroxisomal disorders (Zellweger syndrome, neonatal adrenoleukodystrophy, rhizomelic chondrodysplasia
    punctata)

CoA, coenzyme A; HMG, 3-hydroxy-3-methylglutaryl.

frequent neonatal conditions; for example, a child with an IEM may have transient tachypnea of the newborn or be at risk for sepsis for unrelated reasons. Occasionally, two conditions may be present with a causative relationship. A typical example is the frequently quoted but still unexplained increased incidence of *Escherichia coli* sepsis in infants with galactosemia.

C. **Asymptomatic IEMs in the newborn.** Untreated PKU does not cause any symptoms in the newborn. It causes irreversible brain damage while the patient appears clinically well. Verify that newborn screening tests have been done and check results as soon as available. Early detection of PKU in the newborn allows a well-established treatment plan that prevents extreme mental retardation. (See Section XI.)

Table 101–3. MISDIAGNOSES OF METABOLIC DISEASE IN THE NEWBORN INFANT

Bacterial sepsis
Acute viral infection
Asphyxia
Gastrointestinal tract obstruction
Hepatic failure, hepatitis
Central nervous system catastrophe
Persistent pulmonary hypertension
Cardiomyopathy
Neuromuscular disorder

D. **To guide the clinician in the diagnostic workup, signs and symptoms are discussed further for 5 different major clinical presentations.** IEM presenting with encephalopathy, IEM presenting with liver disease, IEM presenting with impairment of cardiac function, IEM presenting as dysmorphic syndromes, and IEM presenting as nonimmune hydrops (see Sections VI to X). Flow diagrams in Figures 101–1 and 101–2 are designed to assist in the diagnostic workup. Details regarding the different **laboratory tests** are outlined in Section XII.

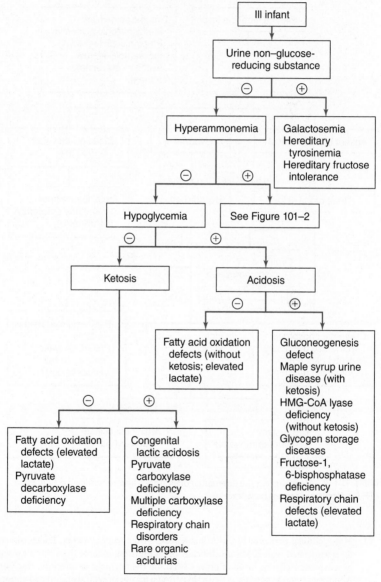

FIGURE 101–1. Algorithm for the diagnosis of metabolic disorders of acute onset (guideline only; for details, see text and references).

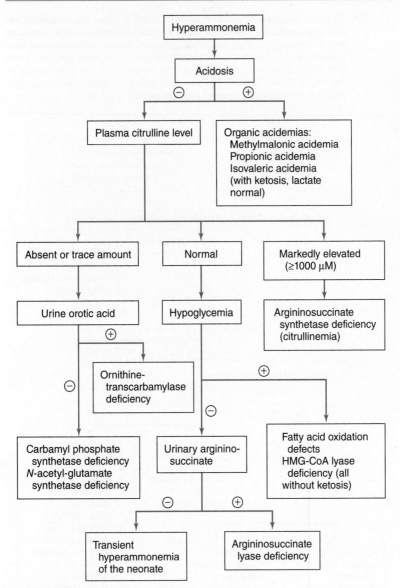

FIGURE 101–2. Algorithm for the differential diagnosis of hyperammonemia (guideline only; for details, see text and references).

VI. **Major clinical presentation: IEM presenting with encephalopathy.** Encephalopathies associated with IEMs are clinically often indistinguishable from those caused by a hypoxic-ischemic insult or other CNS insult (hemorrhage or infectious disease). **Abnormal tone** (hypotonia as well as hypertonia may be of central origin) and **abnormal movements and seizures** clearly indicate CNS involvement. Clinically, seizures may present as lip smacking, tongue thrusting, bicycling movements of the lower extremities, opisthotonos, tremors, or generalized tonic-clonic movements. In severe encephalopathy, burst suppression pattern may be seen on **electroencephalography (EEG) using conventional multilead EEG or bedside monitoring with amplitude-integrated enchalography (aEEG)**. Discontinuous patterns detected by aEEG may be seen with less severe encephalopathy.

A. Laboratory evaluation

  1. Acute evaluation. **In any patient with encephalopathy of any degree**, careful **evaluation of the acid-base status** is advisable. Some IEMs present with quite pronounced metabolic acidosis. In addition to an arterial or venous blood gas, the following tests (for details, see Section XII) should be performed as part of the **acute evaluation** of patients with encephalopathy:

      a. Arterial or venous blood gas

          i. When interpreting the venous or arterial blood gas of a newborn, the **alterations in respiratory status** that are so frequent in this patient group must be taken into careful consideration. An isolated respiratory acidosis is likely pulmonary, and a metabolic or mixed acidosis, especially shortly after delivery, may be related to perinatal events.

          ii. In case of a **severe and prolonged metabolic acidosis** without the presence of an underlying condition (such as septic or hypovolemic shock and malperfusion) explaining the finding, it is mandatory to evaluate whether **acidic metabolites** (eg, the excessive production of lactic acid) could be the cause of the imbalance. When considering compensatory mechanisms (eg, respiratory correction of a metabolic acidosis), remember that the resulting blood gas should reflect a mixed acid-base status.

          iii. Presence of an **isolated respiratory alkalosis** is suspicious for central disturbance of the respiratory pattern (hyperpnea), and **hyperammonemia** should be ruled out in this situation. Ammonia directly stimulates the respiratory center resulting in primary hyperventilation, which in turn leads to respiratory alkalosis.

      b. Serum electrolytes with calculation of the anion gap.

      c. Ammonia level.

      d. Lactate and pyruvate levels and ratio.

      e. Urine collection should be initiated and collected and the urine refrigerated or, ideally, frozen.

  2. Other causes of encephalopathy should be assessed by appropriate studies (eg, imaging studies, sepsis workup, lumbar puncture) as indicated and outlined in other sections of this manual. If cerebrospinal fluid (CSF) is obtained, it is advisable to freeze a sample for possible future testing (eg, ~1–2 mL for tests such as CSF amino acid analysis to rule out nonketotic hyperglycinemia [NKH]). If an IEM remains a diagnostic possibility after the initial evaluation, the analysis of plasma amino acids and urine organic acids should be arranged.

B. Differential diagnosis. Although the **differential diagnosis** of IEMs associated with encephalopathy is extensive, the following conditions are discussed in more detail because of either their frequency or clinical significance. (Items 1–4 are typically without severe metabolic acidosis at presentation; items 5 and 6 are typically associated with a severe metabolic acidosis.)

  1. Urea cycle defects (and transient hyperammonemia of the neonate)

      a. Clinical presentation. Presentation with hyperammonemia (not caused by liver dysfunction) with 3 major diagnostic possibilities:

          i. A primary defect of one of the enzymes of the urea cycle (that degrades ammonia produced in the metabolism of amino acids). The most common urea cycle defect is **ornithine-transcarbamylase (OTC) deficiency**, which is transmitted in an X-linked recessive fashion. Newborn patients, therefore, are usually male. **Female heterozygotes** can be symptomatic, depending on the X-chromosome inactivation pattern in the liver, but females usually present later in life. It is important to note that a mother heterozygous for OTC deficiency may develop symptoms (hyperammonemia) at the time of delivery because of the metabolic stresses of labor and delivery. The other urea cycle defects are inherited in an autosomal recessive fashion, with **carbamyl phosphate synthetase deficiency** being the second most common.

    ii. **An organic acidemia as an underlying cause** with secondary impairment of the urea cycle (see Section VI.B.5).

    iii. **Transient hyperammonemia of the neonate (THAN)**, a condition usually seen in premature infants. By anecdotal report, the frequency of THAN seems to have declined over the last few years.

  b. **Diagnosis.** Information regarding the diagnostic workup of patients with hyperammonemia is outlined in Figure 101–2. Quantitative measurement of plasma amino acids and orotic acid is necessary to establish the exact diagnosis. Urine organic acids should also be examined.

  c. **Treatment.** Initial treatment is similar, independent of the final diagnosis (see Section XIII.A). Immediate transfer to a facility able to perform hemodialysis is strongly advised when hyperammonemia is detected. The use of medication such as sodium phenyl acetate and butyrate should be supervised by a biochemical geneticist. In some defects (eg, argininosuccinate lyase deficiency), substitution of arginine (intravenous arginine hydrochloride) may alleviate symptoms; arginine becomes secondarily deficient as a metabolite of the cycle located after the deficient reaction. Long-term **protein restriction** is necessary (see Section XIII.B.1). Acute treatment of THAN is similar to that of inborn errors of the urea cycle, but deficiency of the metabolic pathway is temporary and normal protein intake is tolerated later in life.

  d. **Outcome.** Outcome (especially in regard to CNS damage) is much more favorable for THAN compared with the inherited urea cycle defects.

2. **Maple syrup urine disease (MSUD).** Accumulation of **branched-chain amino acids (leucine, isoleucine, and valine)** is secondary to a defect in the decarboxylase involved in the catabolism of these amino acids. 2-Keto metabolites of the 3 amino acids also accumulate. Leucine is the amino acid that has been implied to be the most neurotoxic.

  a. **Clinical presentation.** Presentation is commonly after the second week of life but may be as early as at 24 hours of age and, therefore, may precede the report of the **neonatal screening** test result. Typical symptoms are feeding intolerance, lethargy, signs of encephalopathy such as hypotonia or posturing, abnormal movements, or frank seizures (late in the course). **Typical odor** (maple syrup or "burnt sugar") may not be prominent, and metabolic acidosis is a late presentation of untreated MSUD.

  b. **Diagnosis.** Diagnosis is by quantitative amino acid analysis (elevated leucine, isoleucine, valine, and glycine) and detection of 2-keto metabolites in urine organic acid analysis. The 2, 4-dinitrophenylhydrazine (DNPH) test detects 2-keto acids and may be available at certain specialized laboratories.

  c. **Treatment.** Restrict all protein acutely while providing high amounts of glucose and fluid (see Section XIII.A). Later, provide formula low in leucine, valine, and isoleucine with restriction of natural protein. **Dialysis** may be needed as acute therapy if severe encephalopathy has developed. Some patients may show response to thiamine (see Section XIII.B.3).

3. **Nonketotic hyperglycinemia (NKH) (glycine encephalopathy)**

  a. **Clinical presentation.** A **typical presentation** for NKH is a patient suffering from a severe encephalopathy that is rapidly progressing and eventually results in respiratory arrest, but standard evaluation for IEMs and other causes of this presentation does not reveal any abnormalities (no acidosis, hypoglycemia, or hyperammonemia and no other organ system affected). **Pronounced and sustained "hiccoughs"** in an encephalopathic infant have been described as a typical observation in NKH.

b. Diagnosis. **Hyperglycinemia** in plasma is typical but may not be pronounced in young infants because of decreased renal reabsorption of this amino acid. In addition, other IEMs also result in increased blood glycine levels, such as MSUD (which is sometimes referred to as ketotic hyperglycinemia). This diagnostic situation is one of the few indications for **urine amino acids** to detect the high renal glycine excretion. A more specific diagnostic test is to determine the **CSF-to-plasma glycine ratio** because an elevation of glycine in the CSF is specific for NKH. A CSF-to-blood glycine ratio of >0.08 is considered abnormal (0.02–0.08 is uncertain; <0.02 is normal).

c. Treatment. Options remain limited at this point. Restoration of normal glycine levels in blood can be achieved through hydration or the use of sodium benzoate (see Section XIII.A.5), but the glycine accumulation in CSF remains unaffected. Several medications (dextromethorphan, diazepam, and even strychnine) have been used to try to affect the CNS symptomatology but have achieved only limited success.

d. Outcome. Patients may survive because the respiratory depression has the potential to improve, but severe brain damage is the rule. A few patients with a transient form of NKH have been reported.

4. **Peroxisomal disorders**

a. Clinical presentation. Defects of peroxisome biogenesis (eg, Zellweger syndrome and neonatal adrenoleukodystrophy) and some of the peroxisomal single enzyme defects (eg, multifunctional enzyme deficiency) present with encephalopathy in the neonatal period. Patients are **extremely floppy** as a result of severe central hypotonia and develop **seizures** (usually within the first week of life). Hepatomegaly, renal and hepatic cysts, and skeletal or retinal abnormalities may also be found.

b. Diagnosis. Most peroxisomal defects can be detected by analysis of **very long-chain fatty acids (VLCFAs)** (with carbon chains of 24 and more) in plasma. To fully exclude a peroxisomal defect, additional studies such as plasmalogen levels in red blood cells, phytanic acid, and others (see Section XII.C.8) are necessary.

5. Organic aciduria/acidemias (OAs). This group of IEMs is complex, and many clinicians feel overwhelmed by the biochemical details regarding these conditions. Relevant clinical information is as follows:

a. Clinical presentations. Many OAs present later in infancy. Three conditions commonly present in the neonatal period and are clinically nearly indistinguishable: **methylmalonic acidemia**, **propionic acidemia**, and **isovaleric acidemia**. Diagnostic landmarks are encephalopathy with severe acidosis, hyperammonemia, and seizures; an unusual **odor** (most noticeable in urine [see Table 101–2]) may be noted; **neutropenia** and **thrombocytopenia** may occur. More OAs are listed in Table 101–1.

b. Diagnosis. Analysis of plasma amino acids and urine organic acids is the appropriate **diagnostic evaluation** for OAs. Interpretation of these tests by an experienced biochemical geneticist familiar with the clinical presentation of the patient is strongly recommended.

c. Treatment. If this diagnosis is suspected, the following **treatment** should be initiated: hydration and glucose infusion (both at least 1.5 times the maintenance level), treatment of hyperammonemia (see Section XIII.A, and especially XIII.A.5), and careful correction of metabolic acidosis with bicarbonate while ensuring appropriate ventilation. Involvement of a geneticist in

      5. **Other common findings** include cataracts, hypotonia, and significant psycho-motor retardation.

  B. **Zellweger syndrome and other peroxisomal disorders.** Although Zellweger syndrome and **neonatal adrenoleukodystrophy** were initially described based on clinical characteristics, they are now known to be disorders of peroxisome biogenesis, as is **infantile Refsum disease.** These 3 conditions are all clinical phenotypes of defects in peroxisomal biogenesis and function (hence the term *Zellweger spectrum*). The diagnosis is established by measurement of VLCFAs and other biochemical parameters affected by peroxisomal dysfunction (see Section XII.C.8). Typical findings are as follows:

      1. **Dysmorphic features.** A high forehead, a wide and flat nasal bridge, epicanthal folds, and dysplastic ears; the fontanelles are wide open.

      2. **Severe hypotonia, seizures, and lack of psychomotor development.**

      3. **Hepatomegaly with fibrosis.**

      4. **Ocular abnormalities.** Corneal clouding, cataract, and retinal changes.

      5. **Punctate calcifications of the skeleton.**

      6. **Small renal cortical cysts.**

  C. **Pyruvate dehydrogenase (PDH) deficiency.** Patients with congenital lactic acidosis (LA) (see Section VI.B.6) resulting from PDH deficiency often display dysmorphic features, including a high and prominent forehead, a widened nasal bridge, a small anteverted nose, and dysmorphic and enlarged ears.

  D. **Congenital defects of glycosylation.** (See Section VI.C.9.) Dysmorphic features include broad nasal bridge, prominent jaw and forehead, large ears, and strabismus. **Unusual fat pads in the buttock area and inverted nipples** are believed to be characteristic findings.

X. **Major clinical presentation: IEM presenting as nonimmune hydrops.** Although the differential diagnosis of nonimmune hydrops is extensive and this condition is discussed in other sections of this manual, **2 groups** of **inherited disorders that can present with hydrops** are briefly mentioned here. *Note:* Congenital disorders of glycosylation rarely present with nonimmune hydrops fetalis (based on a small number of case reports).

  A. In **inherited hematologic conditions** (eg, glucose-6-phosphate dehydrogenase deficiency and pyruvate kinase deficiency), the hydrops is due to anemia and heart failure.

  B. **Genetic conditions with disturbed lysosomal function.** Cases of hydrops have been reported in **GM$_1$ gangliosidosis, Gaucher disease, Niemann-Pick disease**, and other genetic conditions with disturbed lysosomal function. Although the occurrence of hydrops in lysosomal disorders is well established, little has been published about the possible mechanism. The presence of **hepatomegaly, dysostosis multiplex**, and abnormal **vacuolated mononuclear cells** in the peripheral blood smear are diagnostic clues. Presence of a lysosomal storage disorder should be considered in any hydropic patient without established etiology, and involvement of a geneticist and consequent specific enzymatic assays using white blood cells or fibroblasts are both warranted.

XI. **Phenylketonuria.** Although PKU is an IEM of foremost interest because of its frequency and well-established treatment that prevents the extreme mental retardation characteristic of untreated PKU, it is not discussed in detail here because **untreated PKU does not cause symptoms in the neonate.** Even though the patient is clinically well, **irreversible brain damage** occurs as a result of accumulating phenylalanine and its metabolites. Therefore, patients benefit enormously from detection by neonatal screening for PKU.

  A. If an **abnormal neonatal screening** for PKU is reported, formula or breast milk must be discontinued and hydration provided (short-term enteral feedings with electrolyte solutions are feasible; intravenous therapy is usually not mandated). The patient should immediately (within hours) be referred to a geneticist for further evaluation (including differentiation between classic PKU and hyperphenylalaninemia), initiation of diet, and family education, training, and counseling.

B. Occasionally, the clinician takes care of a **child of a mother with PKU**; considering that this child is an obligate heterozygote for PKU combined with the high frequency of the PKU allele in the general population (1 in 20), this child has a 1 in 80 risk of being affected, and measurement of phenylalanine levels after enteral feedings are established is mandatory. Although institutional practices vary, many geneticists recommend early quantitative amino acid analysis rather than routine newborn screening in this scenario. Newborns of affected mothers with insufficient treatment manifest with **microcephaly, congenital heart disease,** and **mental deficiencies** (even if the infant is not homozygous for PKU).

XII. Diagnosis

A. Prenatal. The ability to diagnose IEMs prenatally has increased in recent years. Biochemical methods (eg, detection of metabolites in amniotic fluid and enzyme assays using cultured cells) as well as DNA analysis (mutation detection) are used. Diagnostic procedures routinely available are **chorionic villus sampling** and **amniocentesis.** In some centers, analysis of **fetal cells in maternal circulation** or **preimplantation testing of the embryo with in vitro fertilization** may also be offered. In some cases, in utero treatment can be achieved (eg, dietary control in maternal PKU or experimental therapies such as fetal stem cell treatment). Otherwise, appropriate therapies may be instituted immediately after delivery of the infant. Prenatal counseling is essential so that parents are well educated and able to make an informed decision regarding continuation of the pregnancy.

B. Postnatal. These postnatal tests are usually the initial tests done to evaluate for the possibility of a metabolic disorder while obtaining quick results and limiting the number of secondary tests that may be needed; considering that the limitation of the blood volume drawn is often a significant concern in neonates. Although some of these laboratory tests and their significance in aiding the diagnostic process have already been discussed, details regarding the specifics of these tests and their interpretations are briefly outlined here. Refer also to Table 101–4.

1. **Complete blood count (CBC) with differential, hemoglobin, and platelets.** Be aware that neutropenia (especially when accompanied by metabolic acidosis) not only is typically found in sepsis and poor perfusion but may be present in a patient with organic acidopathy (most common are propionic acidemia, methylmalonic acidemia, and isovaleric acidemia). Thrombocytopenia may be present. These IEMs are also accompanied by hyperammonemia; measurement of an ammonia level is mandatory in a newborn with acidosis, leukopenia, or thrombocytopenia with no established diagnosis.

2. **Blood gas.** Interpretation of the acid-base status is important in the differential diagnosis and has already been discussed (see Section VI.A.1a). IEMs must be especially considered in the scenario of a **severe metabolic acidosis** or **respiratory alkalosis** (note that although hyperventilation may be induced by the painful stimulus with a blood draw, a pure respiratory alkalosis should not easily be dismissed as artifact). Ammonia measurement is indicated in this situation to rule out an organic aciduria with secondary hyperammonemia or a urea cycle defect causing a respiratory alkalosis as a result of the direct stimulation of the respiratory center by ammonia with hyperventilation. Be aware that excess heparin in a blood gas specimen may mimic a metabolic acidosis. Those specimens that are not instantly processed should be stored in ice water.

3. **Electrolyte determination.** In addition to the interpretation of the different electrolyte components, the **anion gap** should be calculated. The concentration of negatively and positively charged electrolytes is compared: Add the sodium and potassium levels (in mEq/L), and subtract the sum of the chloride and bicarbonate concentrations. An excess of negatively charged ions (eg, lactate or metabolites found in an organic acidopathy) is suggested if the anion gap is

Table 101–4. LABORATORY FINDINGS SUGGESTIVE OF METABOLIC DISEASE

Variable	Galactosemia	Glycogen Storage Disease	Maple Syrup Urine Disease	Nonketotic Hyperglycinemia	Glutaric Acidemia Type II	Organic Acidemia	Disorders of Pyruvate Metabolism	Disorders of the Urea Cycle	Transient Hyperammonemia of the Newborn
Hypoglycemia	+	+	±	−	±	±	±	−	−
Metabolic acidosis with or without elevated anion gap	+	±	+	−	±	+	+	±	±
Respiratory alkalosis	−	−	−	−	−	−	−	+	±
Hyperammonemia	−	−	−	−	−	+	−	+	+
Urine ketones	−	±	+	−	−	+	±	−	−
Urine abnormal odor or color	−	−	+	−	+	+	−	−	−
Neutropenia or thrombocytopenia	−	−	−	−	−	+	−	−	−

Note: Guidelines only; for details, see text and references.

>17 mEq/L (consult with your local laboratory because cutoffs may vary some depending on assays and methods used). Be aware that in a hemolyzed specimen, potassium is released from cells that will distort the anion gap calculation (artificially increased). Disturbance of electrolytes is also found in other inherited conditions (eg, adrenogenital syndrome).

4. **Ammonia level.** Although the measurement of ammonia levels can be of foremost importance in making the diagnosis of an IEM, this test is unfortunately very susceptible to artifacts, resulting in a false elevation of ammonia levels. Several precautions must be strictly followed to avoid incorrect test results.

   a. The specimen must be placed on ice at the bedside.

   b. Timely transfer to the laboratory with instant preparation of the sample for analysis. If samples have to be stored, the blood must be centrifuged and the plasma maintained at −20°C. Without strict adherence to these precautionary measures, false elevation by as much as 60–100 mcg/dL may occur. Normal neonatal levels are up to 80 mcg/dL. IEMs typically result in levels in the hundreds and thousands. If a result is equivocal, a repeat measurement must be done quickly since the hyperammonemia in IEM most likely will be progressive.

5. **Liver function tests.** Transaminases (aspartate aminotransferase [**SGOT**] and alanine aminotransferase [**SGPT**]) are released from hepatocytes with cell damage. γ-Glutamyl transferase (**GGT**) is produced in the liver cell but also is present in bile ducts. It is a very sensitive indicator of liver dysfunction and/or cholestasis; it may be elevated even with fairly minor exposures to medications/toxins. **Conjugated bilirubin** and **alkaline phosphatase** are elevated with cholestasis. Cholesterol, albumin, and coagulation factor levels reflect the **synthetic function** of the liver. The **plasma amino acid pattern** is affected by liver dysfunction. **Ammonia** levels are increased in liver failure.

6. **Urine testing for ketones.** The presence of ketones in the urine of a neonate should always be considered abnormal. One of the IEMs that typically results in strongly positive testing is MSUD.

7. **Urine testing for reducing substances.** The main indication in the neonate is suspected galactosemia. It is important that a nonenzymatic assay is done. A negative test does not rule out the diagnosis. Even a few hours of galactose restriction may result in a negative test. Consider which enteral nutrition the patient is receiving. For example, soy formulas are often galactose-free, whereas breast milk is not (lactose ["milk sugar"] is a disaccharide of glucose and galactose).

8. **Lipid levels and profile.** Low cholesterol may be noted in patients with Smith-Lemli-Opitz syndrome. Hyperlipidemia may be present in some glycogen storage disorders.

C. **Laboratory testing more specific for IEMs.** Although some of the following tests might still be available through laboratories at many larger hospitals or through reference laboratories, we consider them to be a second line of more specific tests. The following tests are usually performed to further evaluate a specific diagnosis or abnormalities found on previous testing or to confirm a diagnosis that is clinically suspected.

   1. **Lactic acid level and lactate-to-pyruvate ratio.** Determination of lactate and pyruvate levels may be indicated in the evaluation of patients with severe metabolic acidosis. When excess lactate is present, the anion gap (see Section XII.B.3) is elevated. Lactic acid is best obtained from a central line or arterial specimen because even short stasis of blood (venous sampling using a tourniquet) may result in a significant increase in lactate. The lactate-to-pyruvate ratio is normal (15–20) in PDH deficiency and defects of gluconeogenesis (glycogen storage diseases) and elevated to >25 in pyruvate decarboxylase deficiency and mitochondrial defects of the respiratory/electron transport chain.

2. **Amino acid analysis.** Amino acid analysis must be quantitative to aid in the diagnosis of IEMs. Amino acid analysis of urine is usually not indicated in the evaluation of newborns. There are only a few indications for this test: to rule out cystinuria with renal calculi or to demonstrate a high renal glycine when NKH is suspected (see Section VI.B.3). **Plasma amino acid results** are best evaluated (in a sample obtained after a 4-hour fast) by concentrating on certain patterns of abnormalities rather than on single abnormal values that may be nutritional or artifacts (eg, taurine is often increased with delayed analysis of the sample). Discussion of the many diagnostic patterns of plasma amino acid abnormalities is beyond the scope of this manual. Interpretation of results by an experienced biochemical geneticist who is aware of the clinical presentation and nutritional status of the patient is strongly recommended.

   Plasma amino acid analysis not only is indicated in classic IEMs of amino acid metabolism (eg, MSUD or PKU) but also helps evaluate urea cycle defects because several metabolites of the urea cycle are chemically amino acids (eg, citrulline, arginine, and ornithine; see Figure 101–2). Conditions resulting in hyperammonemia often show elevated glutamine levels (glutamine synthesis incorporates ammonia).

   At least 1–2 mL of blood should be obtained. Laboratories usually request heparinized blood or samples without additives. Samples should be sent on ice. If analysis is to be deferred to a later time, serum or plasma should be separated and frozen.

3. **Urine organic acid analysis.** This complex analytic test is usually performed by laboratories specializing in biochemical genetics. In expert hands, this test can provide an enormous amount of information. Urine organic acid analysis helps establish the diagnosis of organic acidemias. The most common of this large group of disorders are methylmalonic acidemia, propionic acidemia, and isovaleric acidemia (see Section VI.B.5). Most laboratories request at least 5–10 mL of "fresh" urine. As soon as the specimen is collected, it should either be transported to the laboratory on ice or frozen at –20°C.

4. **Succinylacetone in urine.** This test is specific for hepatorenal tyrosinemia. A sample is collected and used to wet a filter paper (as used for the routine neonatal screening tests). After air drying, the sample can be forwarded to the testing laboratory by mail or courier services.

5. **Acyl carnitine profile.** Fatty acids that are metabolized in the mitochondria are conjugated with carnitine to facilitate their transport into the mitochondrion. The acyl carnitine profile determines the levels of fatty acid metabolites of different carbon length allowing for the recognition of diagnostic patterns for different fatty acid oxidation defects (note that VLCFAs with carbon chains of 24 carbons or more are metabolized in the peroxisome; see Section XII.C.8). Acyl carnitine profiles are now often evaluated as part of the newborn screening by tandem mass spectrometry; alternatively, specialized biochemical genetics laboratories perform the test. Dried whole-blood spot samples placed on filter paper cards are used. An additional test useful in patients with suspected fatty acid oxidation defect is the determination of **total and free carnitine plasma levels** (measured in heparinized blood).

6. **Tandem mass spectrometry (MS/MS).** MS/MS detects a large number of disorders of amino and organic acid metabolism as well as fatty acid oxidation defects. This makes it a valuable tool for newborn screening, and MS/MS is **now used routinely by many neonatal metabolic screening programs**; many laboratories also accept samples obtained beyond the neonatal period from infants presenting with symptoms suggestive of an inborn error of metabolism. Testing is easily done (blood spot samples mailed to laboratories) and usually quite cost-effective.

7. **Galactosemia testing.** To measure galactose-1-phosphate levels and GALT activity, whole blood is usually requested by the laboratory because the

metabolites and enzyme are localized in the erythrocytes. Blood must therefore be obtained before blood transfusions. An alternative in already transfused patients is to evaluate the heterozygous parents of the patient because heterozygote detection is possible with the enzymatic assay.

8. **Peroxisomal function tests.** Measurement of VLCFAs is done by gas chromatography. Normally, only trace amounts of fatty acids with carbon chains of 24 carbons or more are detectable. Measurement of VLCFAs, therefore, detects all peroxisomal disorders that affect the degradation of these compounds. Note that VLCFAs will be normal in a small subgroup of patients with peroxisomal defects (eg, rhizomelic chondrodysplasia punctata). Tests assessing other aspects of peroxisomal function (eg, plasmalogens, phytanic acid, or pipecolic acid measurements) may be necessary. Most of these analyses are done on plasma obtained from ethylenediaminetetraacetic acid (EDTA) blood. The red blood cell pellet of the sample should also be sent to the laboratory (separated) because plasmalogen levels are evaluated in red blood cells. Samples do not need to be frozen.

9. **Transferrin electrophoresis analysis.** A suspected diagnosis of carbohydrate-deficient glycoprotein syndromes (see Section VI.C.9) is first evaluated by electrophoresis analysis of a glycoprotein, usually transferrin. The measurement of transferrin levels is inappropriate as a diagnostic test for these conditions (levels usually are normal). Involvement of a geneticist is essential as electrophoresis patterns are not abnormal in all patients and further specialized testing may be indicated. If electrophoresis of a patient of <2 months of age is normal, repeat testing beyond 2 months of age is recommended.

10. **Muscle, liver, and skin biopsies.** In patients with lactic acidosis, **skeletal muscle biopsies** may be needed to establish diagnosis of a mitochondrial respiratory chain defect. Examination by electron microscopy, special stains, and enzyme essays may also be needed. Certain IEMs may require determination of enzyme activities in **cultured skin fibroblasts**. Glycogen storage disorders may require **liver biopsies** to establish the exact diagnosis.

11. **DNA analysis and sequencing.** Molecular defects are now known for many genetic conditions, including IEMs. Although diagnoses can usually be established through biochemical testing, analysis of **genomic or mitochondrial DNA** may be indicated in certain scenarios. Considering the complexity of these tests and the associated cost, DNA testing should usually be initiated and supervised by a geneticist. The discussion of specifics is beyond the scope of this manual. With the increasing use of array technologies, it is possible to detect segments of the genome with loss of heterozygosity; the patient is at higher risk for recessive disorders located in these areas. Whole exome and genome sequencing may become available for selected patients in the near future.

D. **Postmortem evaluation when an IEM is suspected.** If an IEM is suspected as a possible cause of death in a newborn or young infant, we recommend obtaining the following samples postmortem:

1. **Blood.** Blood should be collected. If no central access was established, a postmortem cardiac puncture may be necessary to obtain a sufficient volume of blood. Serum as well as plasma should be frozen. Also, keep the red blood cell pellets (not frozen). EDTA blood (nonseparated) and blood spots on filter paper should be kept to allow for later isolation of DNA.

2. **Urine.** Collect urine, if possible, and freeze it at $-20°C$. If no urine can be obtained but urine organic acid analysis is indicated, swabs of the bladder surface can be obtained on autopsy to attempt urine organic acid analysis.

3. **Skin.** A full-thickness sterile skin biopsy should be obtained (skin to be cleansed with alcohol, not iodine). Store in a sterile culture medium (if not available, serum from the patient may be used). Do not freeze the specimen, and transport it immediately to a tissue culture laboratory for fibroblast culture and storage.

4. **CSF.** If a lumbar puncture was not performed before death, a lumbar or ventricular puncture can be obtained postmortem. This procedure may be indicated to rule out infection or an IEM. In addition to obtaining cultures, we recommend freezing a 1- to 2-mL CSF specimen at −20°C.

5. **Percutaneous liver biopsy.** May be performed to obtain a specimen soon after death (freeze for enzyme analysis) or if the family did not consent to a full autopsy.

6. **Full autopsy and consultation with a geneticist (even postmortem).** May be helpful if an IEM is suspected. The geneticist may give special recommendations for postmortem specimens to be obtained on autopsy (eg, frozen or specially prepared samples rather than standard formalin processing). Genetic counseling may be indicated.

XIII. **Management.** For most IEMs, therapy is currently restricted to dietary measures and in some cases special medications and vitamin supplementation. In some metabolic disorders, **liver, bone marrow, or stem cell transplantation** may be an option.

A. **Acute care while awaiting results of diagnostic studies**

1. **Supportive care.** Following the standards of neonatal and intensive care, this includes securing an **airway**, supporting **respiration** and **circulation**, and establishing **intravenous access**. General measures may also include correction of the acid-base balance, electrolyte abnormalities, and **hydration** status. Assisted ventilation may be required in severely affected neonates, and aggressive **antibiotic therapy** is frequently indicated because of the overlap in symptomatology with bacterial disease.

2. **Nutritional measures.** An acutely ill newborn will receive nothing by mouth. For almost all IEMs, a **supply of sufficient glucose** to avoid a catabolic state is strongly indicated. Try to achieve a caloric intake of 80–100 kcal/kg/d. **Eliminate protein** acutely (24–48 hours) but not over prolonged periods because breakdown of endogenous protein may otherwise occur and may worsen the patient's clinical status. **Intravenous lipids may be contraindicated** in certain FAO defects.

3. **Hemodialysis or peritoneal dialysis.** May be needed to remove toxic metabolites and in cases in which acidosis is intractable. Exchange transfusions are not effective, and early transfer to a facility where hemodialysis is possible is mandatory in these situations (eg, hyperammonemia).

4. **Vitamin treatment.** Several IEMs have vitamin-responsive forms. Often, a combination of vitamin cofactors (vitamin B$_{12}$, biotin, riboflavin, thiamine, pyridoxine, and folate) is considered while specific test results are still outstanding. Give vitamins only after appropriate specimens have been obtained for full metabolic investigation and after consultation with a geneticist. **Carnitine substitution** may be indicated in some patients (eg, FAO defects or OAs). Carnitine (L-carnitine) may be given intravenously (IV) (30–50 mg/kg/d, some recommend giving a loading dose followed by divided doses; some patients may need higher doses) or carnitine orally (usually at higher doses than IV).

5. **Medications to treat hyperammonemia.** In patients with hyperammonemia, several medications can be used to provide an alternative pathway for ammonia excretion. These include **sodium phenyl acetate, sodium phenyl butyrate,** and **sodium benzoate.** A sodium phenyl acetate/sodium benzoate 10%/10% preparation is commercially available in the United States. Because of the intrinsic side effects, different indications, coordination with nutritional interventions, and frequent dosage adjustments necessary, the use of these medications should be initiated and supervised by an experienced biochemical geneticist.

6. **Other medications.** In tyrosinemia, NTBC (2-[2-nitro-4-trifluoromethylbenzoyl]-1,3-cyclohexanedione) may be used to prevent tyrosine degradation and production of succinylacetone.

B. **Long-term therapy**

1. **Diet.** One of the classic principles for the treatment of IEMs is the restriction of the substance leading to the accumulation of a toxic metabolite

(eg, phenylalanine in PKU). In some disorders (eg, urea cycle defects), the overall protein intake is restricted. Careful monitoring is necessary to avoid essential amino acid deficiencies.

2. **Provision of a deficient substance** is effective when the deficient product is readily available and can reach the appropriate tissue (eg, cortisol and mineralocorticoid in 21-hydroxylase deficiency). Carnitine replacement may be needed in organic acidurias because carnitine is lost through renal excretion of metabolites bound to carnitine. Patients with urea cycle defects (with the exception of arginase deficiency) require arginine (and/or citrulline in some defects) replacement due to decreased synthesis.

3. **Vitamin, cofactor, and other disease-specific therapy.** Large doses of specific cofactors may increase the activity of partially deficient enzymes: vitamin B_6 (homocystinuria), vitamin B_{12} (methylmalonic acidemia), biotin (multiple carboxylase deficiency), thiamine (MSUD), and riboflavin (glutaric acidemia II). A subgroup of patients with **PKU** may respond to commercially available **sapropterin dihydrochloride** with a reduction of phenylalanine levels. For a number of lysosomal storage disorders, **enzyme replacement** therapies are either commercially available or under clinical investigation.

4. **Supportive therapy** may help to reduce the morbidity associated with specific IEMs. **Splinting** may reduce deformities in mucopolysaccharidoses. **Splenectomy** may be indicated for thrombocytopenia associated with Gaucher disease.

5. **Long-term therapy.** Genetic disorders require lifelong nutritional, medical, and laboratory monitoring by a team of specialists in these disorders. Many times, intercurrent illnesses and stress may precipitate the recurrence of symptoms.

6. **Early intervention and special education programs** may be beneficial in those disorders characterized by intellectual impairment. Families may find a forum for their concerns and stresses, and resources for valuable information in **family support groups** such as the Genetic Alliance (www.geneticalliance.org), the National Organization for Rare Disorders (NORD; www.rarediseases.org), and numerous other disease- and syndrome-specific support groups.

7. **Liver, bone marrow, or stem cell transplantation** may be a treatment option in some IEMs.

XIV. **Prognosis.** Due to the great variety of inborn errors of metabolism, prognosis ranges from extremely favorable with normal development and life expectancy to severe physical and/or mental disability and death. In general, early diagnosis and, if available, treatment seem associated with more favorable outcomes.

XV. **Additional resources.** In order to assist the clinician with the care of newborns with inborn errors of metabolism, Table 101–5 provides a listing of useful resources.

Table 101–5. USEFUL RESOURCES FOR THE CLINICIAN IN THE EVALUATION, DIAGNOSIS, AND TREATMENT OF NEWBORNS WITH INBORN ERRORS OF METABOLISM

- **Genetics Home Reference** (ghr.nlm.nih.gov) maintained by the National Library of Medicine of the United States.
- **Multiple databases at the National Center for Biotechnology Information (NCBI)** (www.ncbi.nlm.org), which includes Online Mendelian Inheritance of Man (OMIM), GeneTests, and GeneReviews.
- **Information through support and family organizations**: Genetic Alliance (www.geneticalliance.org), the National Organization for Rare Disorders (NORD; www.rarediseases.org), and numerous other disease- and syndrome-specific support groups
- **Laboratory resources**:
  1. GeneTests (available via the National Center for Biotechnology Information (NCBI) at www.ncbi.nlm.org), a helpful resource to localize a laboratory for a specific genetic test.
  2. The American Association for Clinical Chemistry (www.aacc.org) publishes DORA (the Directory of Rare Analyses).
  3. Published test catalogs or websites of major regional referral laboratories are often also helpful resources.

Selected References

Blau N, Hoffman GF, Leonard J, Clarke JTR, eds. *Physician's Guide to the Treatment and Follow-Up of Metabolic Diseases*. Berlin: Springer; 2005.

Bosch AM. Classical galactosemia revisited. *J Inherit Metabol Dis*. 2006;29:516–525.

Christodoulou J, Wilcken B. Perimortem laboratory investigation of genetic metabolic disorders. *Semin Neonatol*. 2004;9:275–280.

Clarke JTR. *A Clinical Guide to Inherited Metabolic Diseases*. 3rd ed. Cambridge, UK: Cambridge University Press; 2006.

Dagli AI, Zori RT, Heese BA. Testing strategies for inborn errors of metabolism in the neonate. *NeoReviews*. 2008;9:e291–e298.

de Baulny HO, Benoist JF, Rigal O, Touati G, Rabier D, Saudubray JM. Methylmalonic and propionic acidemias: management and outcomes. *J Inherit Metal Dis*. 2005;28:415–423.

DiMauro S, Garone C. Metabolic disorders of fetal life: glycogenoses and mitochondrial defects of the mitochondrial respiratory chain. *Semin Fetal Neo Med*. 2011;16:181–189.

Enns GM. Inborn errors of metabolism masquerading as hypoxic-ischemic encephalopathy. *NeoReviews*. 2005;6:e549–e558.

Garganta CL, Smith WE. Metabolic evaluation of the sick neonate. *Semin Perinatol*. 2005;29:164–172.

Grünewald S. The clinical spectrum of phosphomannomutase 2 deficiency (CDG-Ia). *Biochim Biophys Acta*. 2009;1792:827–834.

Hicks JM, Young DS. *DORA 2005–2007. The Directory of Rare Analysis*. Washington, DC: American Association for Clinical Chemists; 2005.

Hoffmann GF, Zschocke J, Nyhan WL, eds. *Inherited Metabolic Diseases*. New York, NY: Springer; 2010.

Jaeken J, Matthijs G. Congenital disorders of glycosylation: a rapidly expanding disease family. *Annu Rev Genomics Hum Genet*. 2007;8:261–287.

Kahler SG. Metabolic disorders associated with neonatal hypoglycemia. *NeoReviews*. 2004;5:e377–e381.

Kambij M. Clinical approach to the diagnosis of inborn errors of metabolism. *Pediatr Clin N Am*. 2008;55:1113–1127.

Lehotay DC, Hall P, Lepage J, Eichhorst JC, Etter ML, Greenberg CR. LC-MS/MS progress in newborn screening. *Clin Biochem*. 2011;44:21–31.

Leonard JV, Morris AAM. Diagnosis and early management of inborn errors of metabolism presenting around the time of birth. *Acta Paediatr*. 2006;95:6–14.

Levy PA. Inborn errors of metabolism: part 1: overview. *Pediatr Rev*. 2009;30:131–138.

Levy PA. Inborn errors of metabolism: part 2: specific disorders. *Pediatr Rev*. 2009;30:e22–e28.

Liang JS, Lu JF. Peroxisomal disorders with infantile seizures. *Brain Develop*. 2011;33:777–782.

Malklova E, Albahari ZA. Screening and diagnosis of congenital disorders of glycosylation. *Clin Chim Acta*. 2007;385:6–20.

Marsden D, Larson C, Levy HL. Newborn screening for metabolic disorders. *J Pediatr*. 2006;148:577–584.

Mayatepek E, Hoffmann B, Meissner T. Inborn errors of carbohydrate metabolism. *Best Pract Res Clin Gastroenterol*. 2010;24:607–618.

National Organization for Rare Disorders (NORD). *NORD Resource Guide*. 5th ed. Danbury, CT: NORD; 2005.

Newborn Screening Authorizing Committee. Newborn screening expands: recommendations for pediatricians and medical homes—implications for the system. *Pediatrics*. 2008;121:192–217.

Noh GJ, Jane Tavyev Asher Y, Graham JM Jr. Clinical review of genetic epileptic encephalopathies. *Eur J Med Gen.* 2012;55(5):281–298. DOI:10.1016/j.ejmg.2011.12.010.

Nyhan WL, Barshop BA, Al-Aqeel AI. *Atlas of Inherited Metabolic Diseases.* 3rd ed. London: Hodder Arnold; 2012.

Patay Z. MR imaging workup of inborn errors of metabolism of early postnatal onset. *Magn Reson Imaging Clin N Am.* 2011;19:733–759.

Porter FD. Smith-Lemli-Opitz syndrome: pathogenesis, diagnosis and management. *Eur J Hum Genet.* 2008;16(5):535–451.

Saudubray JM. Inborn errors of metabolism (multiple articles). *Semin Neonatol.* 2002;7(1): 1–100.

Saudubray JM, Sedel F, Walter JH. Clinical approach to treatable inborn metabolic diseases: an introduction. *J Inherit Metab Dis.* 2006;29:261–274.

Saudubray JM, Walter JH, van den Berghe G, eds. *Inborn Metabolic Diseases: Diagnosis and Treatments.* 5th ed. Berlin: Springer; 2012.

Seashore MR, Seashore CJ. Newborn screening and the pediatric practitioner. *Sem Perinatol.* 2005;29:182–188.

Shimozawa N. Molecular and clinical aspects of peroxisomal diseases. *J Inherit Metab Dis.* 2007;30:193–197.

Staretz-Chacham O, Lang TC, LaMarca ME, Krasnewich D, Sidransky E. Lysosomal storage disorders in the newborn. *Pediatrics.* 2008;123:1191–1207.

Theda C. Use of amplitude integrated electroencephalography (aEEG) in patients with inborn errors of metabolism—a new tool for the metabolic geneticist. *Mol Genet Metabol.* 2010;100:S42–S48.

Valle D, Beaudet AL, Vogelstein B, et al. The online metabolic and molecular bases of inherited disease. New York, NY: McGraw-Hill. www.ommbid.com. Accessed February 2012.

Yu H, Patel SB. Recent insights into the Smith-Lemli-Opitz syndrome. *Clin Genet.* 2005;68: 383–391.

102 Infant of a Diabetic Mother

Maternal diabetic control is a key factor in determining fetal outcome for the infant of a diabetic mother (IDM). Data indicate that perinatal morbidity and mortality rates in the offspring of women with diabetes mellitus have improved with dietary management and insulin therapy. However, complications may still arise in the infant, including hypoglycemia, hypocalcemia, hypomagnesemia, perinatal asphyxia, respiratory distress syndrome (RDS), other respiratory illnesses, hypertrophic cardiomyopathy, hyperbilirubinemia, polycythemia, renal vein thrombosis, macrosomia, birth injuries, and congenital malformations. Because of better current understanding of the pathophysiology of diabetic pregnancies, these complications can be recognized and treated.

I. Classification
   A. **White's classification.** White's classification system is based on the age at onset, duration of the disorder, and complications. It is currently used to group women with diabetes during pregnancy and provide a method to compare groups of infants. The original table was revised (Table 102–1).
   B. **The Expert Committee on the Diagnosis and Classification of Diabetes Mellitus.** Table 102–2 presents the nomenclature of the Expert Committee for the classification diabetes mellitus.

Table 102–1. **WHITE'S MODIFIED CLASSIFICATION OF DIABETES IN PREGNANCY**

White's Class	Description
Gestational diabetes A1	Diet-controlled gestational diabetes[a] (fasting glucose <105 mg/dL 2 hours postprandial glucose <120 mg/dL)
Gestational diabetes A2	Insulin-treated gestational diabetes[a] (fasting glucose >105 mg/dL 2 hours postprandial glucose >120 mg/dL)
A	Abnormal GTT at any age or of any duration; treated only by diet therapy
B	Onset at age ≥20 years and duration <10 years
C	Onset at age 10–19 years or duration of 10–19 years
D	Onset before 10 years of age, duration >20 years, benign retinopathy, or hypertension (not pregnancy induced)
D1	Onset before age 10 years
D2	Duration >20 years
D3	Calcification of vessels of the leg (macrovascular disease), formerly called Class E
D4	Benign retinopathy (microvascular disease)
D5	Hypertension (not pregnancy induced)
R	Proliferative retinopathy or vitreous hemorrhage
F	Nephropathy with >500 mg/d proteinuria
RF	Criteria for both classes R and F
G	Many pregnancy failures
H	Evidence of arteriosclerotic heart disease
T	Prior renal transplantation

GTT, glucose tolerance test.
[a]Any degree of glucose intolerance with onset or first recognition during pregnancy.
Classes B through T require insulin treatment. Classes R, F, RF, H, and T have no onset or duration criterion, but usually occur with long-standing diabetes.
Modified and reproduced, with permission, from Brown FM, Hare JW. *Diabetes Complicating Pregnancy: The Joslin Clinic Method.* 2nd ed. New York: Wiley-Liss; 1995.

Table 102–2. **NOMENCLATURE OF THE EXPERT COMMITTEE ON THE DIAGNOSIS AND CLASSIFICATION OF DIABETES MELLITUS**

Class	Description
I. Type 1 diabetes	β-Cell destruction usually leading to absolute insulin deficiency (immune or idiopathic)
II. Type 2 diabetes	May range from predominantly insulin resistance with relative insulin deficiency to a predominantly secretory defect with insulin resistance
III. Other specific types	Genetic defects of β cell function, genetic defects in insulin action, diseases of exocrine pancreas, endocrinopathies, drug or chemical induced, infections, uncommon forms of immune-mediated diabetes, other genetic syndromes sometimes associated with diabetes
IV. Gestational diabetes mellitus	Any degree of glucose intolerance with onset or first recognition during pregnancy. A fasting plasma glucose of >126 mg/dL (7.0 mmol/L) or a casual glucose >200 mg/dL (11.1 mmol/L) meets the minimal criteria for the diagnosis of gestational diabetes. If the diagnosis is not clear, repeat on a subsequent day. If hyperglycemia is confirmed, no further testing needed. If the diagnosis is unclear, perform a 1- or 2-step oral glucose tolerance test.

Data from Diagnosis and Classification of Diabetes Mellitus. *Diabetes Care.* 2002;229:S43–S48.

II. **Incidence.** It is currently estimated that 2–3% of all pregnancies are complicated by diabetes and that 90% of these are women with gestational diabetes.

III. **Pathophysiology**

A. **Macrosomia.** This is the classic presentation of the infant of a poorly controlled diabetic mother (IDM). It is the result of biochemical events along the maternal hyperglycemia-fetal hyperinsulinemia pathway, as described by Pedersen. Macrosomia occurs in more than 25% of diabetic pregnancies and plays a role in both the birth injuries, including shoulder dystocia, brachial plexus injuries, subdural hemorrhage, cephalohematoma, and the increased rate of asphyxia seen in infants of diabetic mothers.

B. **Small for gestational age (SGA).** Mothers with renal, retinal, or cardiac diseases are more likely to have small for gestational age or premature infants, poor fetal outcome, fetal distress, or fetal death.

C. **Specific disorders frequently encountered in IDMs**

1. **Metabolic disorders**

   a. **Hypoglycemia.** Because an absolute definition of hypoglycemia as a specific value can not be given, the definition of hypoglycemia is based on treatment guidelines by the American Academy of Pediatrics (AAP). A blood glucose <40 or <45 mg/dL in a late preterm or term IDM, SGA, or large for gestational age infant depending on postnatal age and if the infant has symptoms, requires treatment. See Figure 62–1. It is present in up to 40% of IDMs, most commonly in macrosomic infants. It usually presents within 1–2 hours after delivery. According to Pedersen, at birth the transplacental glucose supply is terminated, and, because of high concentrations of plasma insulin, blood glucose levels fall. Mothers with well-controlled blood glucose levels have fewer infants with hypoglycemia. Hypoglycemia in SGA infants born to mothers with diabetic vascular disease is caused by decreased glycogen stores; it appears 6–12 hours after delivery.

   b. **Hypocalcemia.** Hypocalcemia has various definitions, but serum levels of <8 mg/dL in a term infant or <7 mg/dL in a preterm infant and ionized calcium levels of <4 mg/dL are considered hypocalcemic. The incidence is up to 50% of IDMs. The severity of hypocalcemia is related to the severity of maternal diabetes and involves decreased function of the parathyroid glands. Serum calcium levels are lowest at 24–72 hours of age.

   c. **Hypomagnesemia.** A serum magnesium level <1.52 mg/dL in any infant indicates hypomagnesemia. It is related to maternal hypomagnesemia and the severity of maternal diabetes.

2. **Cardiorespiratory disorders**

   a. **Perinatal asphyxia.** In a prospective study, 27% of IDMs, White's class B-R-T, suffered asphyxia. Nephropathy appearing in pregnancy, maternal hyperglycemia before delivery, and prematurity were significant risk factors.

   b. **Respiratory distress syndrome**

      i. **Incidence.** The incidence has decreased to only 3% of IDMs because of better management of diabetes during pregnancy. Most cases are the result of premature delivery, delayed maturation of pulmonary surfactant production, or delivery by elective cesarean section.

      ii. **Fetal lung maturity.** Pulmonary surfactant production in the IDM is deficient or delayed principally in class A, B, and C diabetics. Fetal hyperinsulinism may adversely affect the lung maturation process in the IDM by interfering with the incorporation of choline into lecithin. More recent evidence suggests that a change in insulin signaling leads to a decrease in the amount of surfactant production.

      iii. **Cesarean section.** Infants delivered by elective cesarean section are at risk for RDS because of lack of appropriate surfactant production and decreased prostaglandin production and increased pulmonary vascular resistance.

    c. **Other causes of respiratory distress**

      i. **Transient tachypnea of the newborn.** Occurs especially after elective cesarean section. This disorder may or may not require oxygen therapy and usually responds by 72 hours of age. (See Chapter 143.)

      ii. **Hypertrophic cardiomyopathy and septal hypertrophy.** Occurs in up to 25–75% of IDMs, although most are without signs of disease. It is currently not well understood how the combination of insulin and insulin-like growth factor-1 and high levels of glucose work together to produce the septal and cardiac hypertrophy seen in IDMs.

  3. **Hematologic disorders**

    a. **Hyperbilirubinemia.** Bilirubin production is apparently increased in the IDM secondary to prematurity, macrosomia, hypoglycemia, polycythemia, and delayed clearance.

    b. **Polycythemia and hyperviscosity.** The cause of polycythemia is unclear but may be related to increased levels of erythropoietin in the IDM, increased red blood cell production secondary to chronic intrauterine hypoxia in mothers with vascular disease, and intrauterine placental transfusion resulting from acute hypoxia during labor and delivery. (See Chapters 71 and 122.)

    c. **Renal venous thrombosis.** A rare complication most likely caused by hyperviscosity, hypotension, or disseminated intravascular coagulation. It is usually diagnosed by ultrasonography and may present with hematuria and an abdominal mass (see page 539).

  4. **Congenital malformations.** Congenital malformations occur more frequently in IDMs than in the general population. It is suspected that poor diabetic control in the first trimester is associated with a higher percentage of congenital malformations. Congenital malformations account for a significant portion of perinatal deaths and include cardiac defects (eg, transposition of the great vessels, ventricular septal defect, or atrial septal defect), renal defects (eg, agenesis), gastrointestinal tract defects (eg, small left colon syndrome or situs inversus), neurologic defects (eg, anencephaly or meningocele syndrome), skeletal defects (eg, hemivertebrae or caudal regression syndrome), unusual facies, and microphthalmos.

IV. **Risk factors.** The following factors or conditions may be associated with an increased risk for problems in IDMs.

  A. **Maternal class of diabetes**

    1. In gestational diabetes and class A diabetes controlled by diet alone, infants have few complications.

    2. Women with class A diabetes controlled with insulin and class B, C, and D diabetes are prone to deliver macrosomic infants if diabetes is inadequately controlled.

    3. Diabetic women with renal, retinal, cardiac, and vascular disease have the most severe fetal problems.

  B. **Hemoglobin A_{1C}.** To decrease perinatal morbidity and mortality rates, the diabetic woman should attempt to achieve good metabolic control before conception. Elevated hemoglobin A_{1C} levels during the first trimester appear to be associated with a higher incidence of congenital malformations.

  C. **Diabetic ketoacidosis.** Pregnant women with insulin-dependent diabetes are apt to develop diabetic ketoacidosis. The onset of this complication may be life-threatening for the mother and fetus or may lead to preterm delivery.

  D. **Preterm labor.** Premature onset of labor in a diabetic woman is a serious problem because of the increased likelihood of RDS in the fetus. Furthermore, sympathomimetic agents used to prevent preterm delivery may be associated with maternal hyperglycemia, hyperinsulinemia, and acidosis.

  E. **Immature fetal lung profile.** Diabetic women who present between 36 and 39 weeks' gestation may undergo amniocentesis to evaluate fetal lung maturity.

A mature lecithin–sphingomyelin ratio may not ensure normal respiratory function in the IDM. However, the presence of phosphatidylglycerol in the amniotic fluid is more apt to be associated with normal neonatal respiratory function (see also Chapter 1).

V. **Clinical presentation**

A. **At birth.** The infant may be large for gestational age or, if the mother has vascular disease, small for gestational age. The size of most infants is appropriate for gestational age; however, if macrosomia is present, birth trauma may occur.

B. **After birth.** Hypoglycemia can present as lethargy, poor feeding, apnea, or jitteriness in the first 6–12 hours after birth (AAP states IDMs can manifest hypoglycemia as early as 1 hour after birth and usually by 12 hours after birth). Jitteriness that occurs after 24 hours of age may be the result of hypocalcemia or hypomagnesemia. Signs of respiratory distress secondary to immature lungs can be noted on examination. Cardiac disease may be present as an enlarged cardiothymic shadow on a chest x-ray film or by physical evidence of heart failure. Gross congenital anomalies may be noted on physical examination.

VI. **Diagnosis**

A. **Laboratory studies.** The following tests must be closely monitored in the IDM.

1. **Serum glucose levels** should be checked at delivery and at 1/2, 1, 1 1/2, 2, 4, 8, 12, 24, 36, and 48 hours of age. AAP states to screen at-risk infants with a frequency and duration related to risk factors (for IDM, screen 0–12 hours). Glucose levels should be checked with bedside measurement tools. Readings <45 mg/dL at the bedside should be verified by serum glucose measurements.

2. **Serum calcium levels** should be obtained at 6, 24, and 48 hours of age. If serum calcium levels are low, serum magnesium levels should be obtained because they may also be low.

3. **Hematocrit** should be checked at birth and at 4 and 24 hours of age.

4. **Serum bilirubin levels** should be checked as indicated by physical examination.

5. **Other tests.** Arterial blood gas levels, complete blood cell counts, cultures, and Gram stains should be obtained as clinically indicated.

B. **Radiologic studies** are not necessary unless there is evidence of cardiac, respiratory, or skeletal problems.

C. **Electrocardiography and echocardiography** should be performed if hypertrophic cardiomyopathy or a cardiac malformation is suspected.

VII. **Management**

A. **Initial evaluation.** Upon delivery, the infant should be evaluated in the usual manner. In the nursery, blood glucose levels and the hematocrit should be obtained. The infant should be observed for jitteriness, tremors, convulsions, apnea, weak cry, and poor sucking. A physical examination should be performed, paying particular attention to the heart, kidneys, lungs, and extremities.

B. **Continuing evaluation.** Over the first several hours after delivery, the infant should be assessed for signs of respiratory distress. During the first 48 hours, observe for signs of jaundice and for renal, cardiac, neurologic, and gastrointestinal tract abnormalities.

C. **Metabolic management**

1. **Hypoglycemia.** See Chapter 62.

2. **Hypocalcemia**

a. **Calcium therapy.** Symptomatic infants should receive 10% calcium gluconate intravenously. The infusion should be given slowly to prevent cardiac arrhythmias, and the infant should be monitored for signs of extravasation. After the initial dose, a maintenance dose is given by continuous intravenous infusion. The hypocalcemia should respond in 3–4 days; until then, serum calcium levels should be monitored every 12 hours (see Chapter 85).

b. **Magnesium maintenance therapy.** Magnesium is usually added to intravenous fluids or given orally as magnesium sulfate 50%, 0.2 mL/kg/d (4 mEq/mL). See Chapter 148 for specific dosing information.

D. Management of cardiorespiratory problems
   1. **Perinatal asphyxia.** Close observation for fetal distress should continue throughout labor and delivery (see Chapter 119).
   2. **Respiratory distress syndrome.** Obtaining amniotic fluid for a fetal lung maturity profile is still an option and can decrease the incidence of hyaline membrane disease. However, some infants must be delivered even if the lung profile is immature.
   3. **Cardiomyopathy.** The treatment of choice is with propranolol (for dosage information, see Chapter 148). Digoxin is contraindicated because of possible ventricular outflow obstruction.
E. Hematologic therapy
   1. **Hyperbilirubinemia.** Frequent monitoring of serum bilirubin levels may be necessary. Phototherapy and exchange transfusion for infants with hyperbilirubinemia are discussed in Chapter 100.
   2. **Polycythemia.** See Chapter 71.
   3. **Renal venous thrombosis.** Treatment consists of fluid restriction and close monitoring of electrolytes and renal status. Supportive therapy is indicated to ensure adequate blood circulation. Nephrectomy is usually only a last resort in unilateral disease.
F. Management of morphologic and functional problems
   1. **Macrosomia and birth injury**
      a. **Fractures of the extremities** should be treated with immobilization.
      b. **Erb palsy** can be treated with range-of-motion exercises.
   2. **Congenital malformations.** If a gross malformation is discovered, a specialist should be consulted.

VIII. **Prognosis.** Less morbidity and mortality occur with adequate control during the diabetic pregnancy. Preconceptional counseling is used as an adjunct to preventive health care of the diabetic patient. The known pregnant diabetic is currently receiving better health care than before, but the challenge is early identification of women with biochemical abnormalities of gestational diabetes. The risk of subsequent diabetes in the infants of these women is at least 10 times greater than in the normal population.

Selected References

Committee on Fetus and Newborn. Postnatal glucose homeostasis in late-preterm and term infants. *Pediatrics.* 2011; 127:575–579. DOI:10.1542/peds.2010–3851.

Expert Committee on the Diagnosis and Classification of Diabetes Mellitus. Report. *Diabetes Care.* 2002;25(S5).

Frantz ID, Epstein MF. Fetal lung development in pregnancies complicated by diabetes. *Semin Perinatol.* 1978;2:347–352.

Hay WW. Care of the infant of the diabetic mother. *Curr Diab Rep.* 2012;12:4–15.

Key TC, Giuffrida R, Moore TR. Predictive value of early pregnancy glycohemoglobin in the insulin-treated diabetic patient. *Am J Obstet Gynecol.* 1987;156:1096–1100.

Landon MB, Catalano PM, Gabbe SG. Diabetes mellitus complicating pregnancy. In: Gabbe SG, Niebyl JR, Simpson JL, eds. *Obstetrics: Normal and Problem Pregnancies.* 5th ed. Philadelphia, PA: Churchill Livingstone; 2007:976–1010.

Mimouni F, Miodovnik M, Siddiqi TA, Khoury J, Tsang RC. Perinatal asphyxia in infants of insulin-dependent diabetic mothers. *J Pediatr.* 1988;113:345–353.

Pedersen J. *The Pregnant Diabetic and her Newborn.* 2ed ed. Baltimore, MD: Williams and Wilkins; 1977.

Rosenn B, Tsang RC. The effects of maternal diabetes on the fetus and neonate. *Ann Clin Lab Sci.* 1991;21:153–170.

Schaefer UM, Songster G, Xiang A, Berkowitz K, Buchanan TA, Kjos SL. Congenital malformations in offspring of women with hyperglycemia first detected during pregnancy. *Am J Obstet Gynecol.* 1997;177:1165–1171.

Smith BT, Giroud CJ, Robert M, Avery ME. Insulin antagonism of cortisol action on lecithin synthesis by cultured fetal lung cells. *J Pediatr.* 1975;87(Pt 1):953–955.

Stephenson MJ. Screening for gestational diabetes mellitus: a critical review. *J Fam Pract.* 1993;37:277–283.

Tsang RC, Brown DR, Steichen J. Diabetes and calcium disturbances in infants of diabetic mothers. In: Merkatz IR, Adam P, eds. *The Diabetic Pregnancy. A Perinatal Perspective.* New York, NY: Grune and Stratton; 1979:207–225.

White P. Diabetes mellitus in pregnancy. *Clin Perinatol.* 1974;1:331–347.

103 Infant of Substance-Abusing Mother

Existing studies on the neonatal effects of drug exposure in utero are subject to many confounding factors. Many studies have relied on the history obtained from the mother, which is notoriously inaccurate. In addition to recall bias, there is a considerable incentive to withhold information. Testing of urine for drugs of abuse does not reflect drug exposure throughout pregnancy and does not provide quantitative information. Many women who abuse drugs are multiple drug abusers and also drink alcohol and smoke cigarettes. It is thus difficult to isolate the effects of any one drug. Social and economic deprivation is common among drug abusers, and this factor not only confounds perinatal data but has a major effect on long-term studies of infant outcome.

I. **Definition.** An infant of a substance-abusing mother (ISAM) is one whose mother has taken drugs that may potentially cause neonatal withdrawal symptoms. The constellation of signs and symptoms associated with withdrawal is called the neonatal withdrawal syndrome. Table 103–1 lists the drugs associated with this syndrome.

II. **Incidence.** Maternal substance abuse has increased over the past decade. It is estimated that ~5–10% of deliveries nationwide are to women who have abused drugs (excluding alcohol) during pregnancy. The incidence is considerably higher in inner-city hospitals.

III. **Pathophysiology.** Drugs of abuse are of low molecular weight and usually water soluble and lipophilic. These features facilitate their transfer across the placenta and accumulation in the fetus and amniotic fluid. The half-life of drugs is usually prolonged in the fetus compared with an adult. Most drugs of abuse either bind to various central nervous system (CNS) receptors or affect the release and reuptake of various neurotransmitters. This may have a long-lasting trophic effect on developing dendritic structures. Drugs of abuse have also been suggested to alter in-utero or perinatal programming through either epigenetic or other factors. In addition, some drugs are directly toxic to fetal cells. The developing fetus may also be affected by the direct physiologic effects of a drug. Many of the fetal effects of cocaine, including its putative teratogenic effects, are thought to be due to its potent vasoconstrictive property.

Some drugs appear to have a partially beneficial effect. The incidence of respiratory distress syndrome (RDS) is decreased after maternal use of heroin and possibly also cocaine. These effects are probably a reflection of fetal stress rather than a direct maturational effect of these drugs. Particularly in the case of cocaine, the decreased incidence of RDS is more than offset by the considerable increase in preterm deliveries after its use. The major concern in ISAMs is the long-term outcome. The importance of direct and indirect effects of drugs on the developing CNS predominates, and the risks of drug abuse far outweigh the benefits. Pathophysiology of specific drugs are as follows:

Table 103–1. DRUGS CAUSING NEONATAL WITHDRAWAL SYNDROME

Opiates	Barbiturates	Miscellaneous
Codeine	Butalbital	Alcohol
Heroin	Phenobarbital	Amphetamine
Meperidine	Secobarbital	Chlordiazepoxide
Methadone		Clomipramine
Morphine		Cocaine
Pentazocine		Desmethylimipramine
Propoxyphene		Diazepam
		Diphenhydramine
		Ethchlorvynol
		Fluphenazine
		Glutethimide
		Hydroxyzine
		Imipramine
		Meprobamate
		Phencyclidine
		Selective serotonin reuptake inhibitors (SSRIs)

A. **Opiates.** Opiates bind to opiate receptors in the CNS; part of the clinical manifestations of narcotic withdrawal result from α_2-adrenergic supersensitivity (particularly in the locus ceruleus).

B. **Cocaine.** Cocaine prevents the reuptake of neurotransmitters (epinephrine, norepinephrine, dopamine, and serotonin) at nerve endings and causes a supersensitivity or exaggerated response to neurotransmitters at the effector organs. Cocaine is a CNS stimulant and a sympathetic activator with potent vasoconstrictive properties. It causes a decrease in uterine and placental blood flow with consequent fetal hypoxemia. It causes hypertension in the mother and the fetus with a reduction in fetal cerebral blood flow.

C. **Alcohol.** Ethanol is an anxiolytic-analgesic with a depressant effect on the CNS. Both ethanol and its metabolite, acetaldehyde, are toxic. Alcohol crosses the placenta and also impairs its function. The risk of affecting the fetus is related to alcohol dose, but there is a continuum of effects and no known safe limit.

IV. **Risk factors.** Associated with an increased incidence of drug abuse are the following:

A. **Maternal history**
1. Poor social and economic circumstances.
2. Poor antenatal care.
3. Teenage or unwed mothers.
4. Poor education.
5. Associated conditions include infectious diseases (hepatitis B, syphilis, and other sexually transmitted diseases/sexually transmitted infections), human immunodeficiency virus (HIV)-positive serology, multiple drug abuse, poor nutritional status, and anemia.

B. **Obstetric complications**
1. Premature delivery.
2. Premature rupture of membranes.
3. Chorioamnionitis.
4. Fetal distress.
5. Intrauterine growth restriction (IUGR).
6. With cocaine use, the following may be present (in addition to the conditions just mentioned):

Table 103–2. SIGNS AND SYMPTOMS OF NEONATAL ABSTINENCE

Hyperirritability
   Increased deep-tendon and primitive reflexes
   Hypertonus, hyperacusis
   Tremors
   High-pitched cry
Seizures
Wakefulness
Increased rooting reflex
Uncoordinated or ineffectual sucking and swallowing
Regurgitation and vomiting
Loose stools and diarrhea
Tachypnea, apnea
Yawning, hiccups
Sneezing, stuffy nose
Mottling
Fever
Failure to gain weight
Lacrimation

---

      a. Hypertension.
      b. Abruptio placentae.
      c. Cardiac. Arrhythmias, myocardial ischemia, and infarction.
      d. Cerebrovascular accident.
      e. Respiratory arrest.
      f. Fetal demise.
  V. **Clinical presentation.** Signs and symptoms of drug withdrawal are listed in Table 103–2. These signs essentially reflect CNS "irritability," altered neurobehavioral organization, and abnormal sympathetic activation. Although each drug may have its own effects, these signs and symptoms must be noted for every ISAM (because of multiple drug abuse); conversely, drug abuse should be suspected in infants exhibiting these signs and symptoms. Signs and symptoms for specific drugs are as follows:
    A. **Opiates.** Infants born to opiate-addicted mothers show an increased incidence of IUGR and perinatal distress. Even when these infants are not small for gestational age, they have lower weight and a smaller head circumference compared with drug-free infants.
      1. **Signs and symptoms of withdrawal occur in 60–90% of exposed infants.** The onset of symptoms may be minutes after delivery up to 1–2 weeks of age, but most infants exhibit signs by 2–3 days of life. The onset of withdrawal may be delayed beyond 2 weeks in infants exposed to methadone (parents should be appropriately informed).
      2. **The clinical course is variable, ranging from mild symptoms of brief duration to severe symptoms.** The clinical course may be protracted, with exacerbations or recurrence of symptoms after discharge. Restlessness, agitation, tremors, wakefulness, and feeding problems may persist for 3–6 months. There is a reduced incidence of both RDS and hyperbilirubinemia.
    B. **Cocaine**
      1. **Symptoms seen in neonates exposed to cocaine in utero.** Irritability, tremors, hypertonia, a high-pitched cry, hyperreflexia, frantic fist sucking, feeding problems, sneezing, tachypnea, and abnormal sleep patterns. A specific cocaine withdrawal syndrome has not been described. The symptoms just mentioned may be a reflection of cocaine intoxication rather than withdrawal, and after an

initial period of irritability and overactivity, a period of lethargy and decreased tone has been described.

2. *Controversial* cocaine associations
   a. In the neonate, the following have been described. Necrotizing enterocolitis, transient hypertension, and reduced cardiac output (on the first day of life), intracranial hemorrhages and infarcts, seizures, apneic spells, periodic breathing, abnormal electroencephalogram, abnormal brainstem auditory evoked potentials, abnormal response to hypoxia and carbon dioxide, and ileal perforation. These reports were mostly case reports or insufficiently controlled case series with numerous confounding factors. There are large case-control studies that have found no association between cocaine exposure and intraventricular hemorrhage. Despite earlier concerns, there does not appear to be an increased risk of sudden infant death syndrome (SIDS).
   b. Cocaine has been suggested as a teratogen. Its teratogenic potential is presumed to be due to its vascular effects, although direct toxicity on various cell lines may also play a role. Numerous CNS anomalies as well as cardiovascular abnormalities, limb reduction defects, intestinal atresias, and other malformations have been attributed to cocaine. However, most of these associations were derived from case reports, case series, or poorly controlled studies, and a detailed examination of the data does not substantiate most of these teratogenic associations. An exception appears to be an increased risk of genitourinary tract defects associated with cocaine exposure during gestation. Moreover, there does not appear to be a dysmorphism recognizable as a "cocaine syndrome." Cocaine is associated with an increased incidence of spontaneous abortion, stillbirth, abruptio placentae, premature labor, and IUGR.

C. Alcohol. Probably the foremost drug of abuse today. **The risk that an alcoholic woman will have a child with fetal alcohol syndrome (FAS) is ~35–40%.** However, even in the absence of FAS, and also with lower alcohol intakes, there is an increased risk of congenital anomalies and impaired intellect. It is estimated that alcohol is the major cause of congenital mental retardation today. **FAS consists of the following**:
   1. Prenatal or postnatal growth retardation, CNS involvement such as irritability in infancy or hyperactivity in childhood, developmental delay, hypotonia, or intellectual impairment.
   2. Facial dysmorphology. Microcephaly, microphthalmos, or short palpebral fissures, a poorly developed philtrum, a thin upper lip (vermilion border), and hypoplastic maxilla.
      Numerous congenital anomalies have been described after exposure to alcohol in utero both with and without full-blown FAS. CNS symptoms may appear within 24 hours after delivery and include tremors, irritability, hypertonicity, twitching, hyperventilation, hyperacusis, opisthotonos, and seizures. Symptoms may be severe but are usually of short duration. Abdominal distention and vomiting are less frequent than with most other drugs of abuse. In premature infants of women who were heavy alcohol users (>7 drinks/wk), there is an increased risk of both intracranial hemorrhage and white matter CNS damage.

D. Barbiturates. Symptoms and signs of withdrawal are similar to those observed in narcotic-exposed infants, but symptoms usually appear later. Most infants become symptomatic toward the end of the first week of life, although onset may be delayed up to 2 weeks. The duration of symptoms is usually 2–6 weeks.

E. Benzodiazepines. Symptoms are indistinguishable from those of narcotic withdrawal, including seizures. The onset of symptoms may be shortly after birth.

F. Phencyclidine (PCP). Symptoms usually begin within 24 hours of birth, and the infant may show signs of CNS "hyperirritability" as in narcotic withdrawal. Gastrointestinal symptoms of withdrawal are less common.

G. **Marijuana.** Studies have suggested a slightly shorter duration of gestation and somewhat reduced birthweight, but the extent of these differences was of no clinical importance. The drug may have some mild effect on a variety of newborn neurobehavioral traits.

H. **Selective serotonin reuptake inhibitors (SSRIs).** Symptoms, occurring in up to 30% of exposed infants, may include irritability, seizures, myoclonus, hyperreflexia, jitteriness, persistent crying, shivering, increased tone, feeding difficulties, tachypnea, and temperature instability. It may be difficult to make a clinical distinction between symptoms of withdrawal and those of a neonatal variant of the serotonin syndrome.

I. **Buprenorphine.** This drug, a partial μ-receptor opiate agonist, is being increasingly used as an alternative to methadone in the treatment of pregnant opiate users. Its short-term effects on the neonate are similar to that of methadone, although duration of symptoms appears to be decreased. Symptoms of withdrawal usually occur within the first 3 days of life.

VI. **Diagnosis**

A. **History.** Many, if not most, drug abusers withhold this information. Details of the extent, quantity, and duration of abuse are unreliable. However, the history is the simplest and most convenient means of diagnosis.

B. **Laboratory tests.** The most commonly used tests to detect drugs of abuse are immunoassays (enzymatic assays or radioimmunoassays). They are, however, subject to a low rate of false-negative and, because of cross-reactivity, false-positive testing. They are thus viewed as screening tests. When it is either medically or legally important, these tests should be supplemented by the more sensitive and specific chromatographic or mass spectrometric tests.

1. **Urine.** Easily obtained and is the most common substance used for drug testing. It reflects intake only in the last few days before delivery. Urine may be obtained from both the mother and the infant (in whom the substance may persist for a longer time).

   a. **False-negative immunoassays.** May be due to dilution (low specific gravity) or high sodium chloride content (detected by high specific gravity). Various adulterants may also affect detection; this is unlikely in the neonate but may occur in maternal urine.

   b. **False-positive immunoassays.** Although these depend on the specific assay used, the following have been reported:

      i. **Detected as morphine.** Codeine (found in many cold and cough medications and in analgesics). About 10% of codeine is metabolized to morphine in the liver. The consumption of baked goods containing poppy seeds (eg, bagels) can result in detectable amounts of morphine in the urine. These are "physiologic" false-positive results, but chromatography or mass spectrometry may determine the source by quantitative assays of other metabolites.

      ii. **Detected as amphetamines.** Ranitidine, chlorpromazine, ritodrine, phenylpropanolamine, ephedrine, pseudoephedrine, phenylephrine, phentermine, and phenmetrazine. Some of these (eg, pseudoephedrine) are found in many over-the-counter preparations.

2. **Meconium.** Easily obtained, and drugs may be found up to 3 days after delivery. It reflects drug use after the first trimester, has a lower rate of false negatives, is a more sensitive test than urine for detecting drug abuse, and reflects usage over a longer period than is detectable by urine testing. Its main disadvantage is that the specimen requires processing before testing and hence places an additional burden on the laboratory. The ability to detect drugs is reduced after formation of fed stools.

3. **Hair.** This is by far the **most sensitive test** available for detection of drug abuse. Hair grows at 1–2 cm/mo; hence maternal hair can be segmented and each

segment analyzed for drugs. Thus details of drug abuse throughout pregnancy may be obtained. There is a quantitative relationship between amounts of drug used and amounts incorporated in growing hair. Hair may be obtained from the mother or the infant (in whom it will reflect usage only during the last trimester). Hair may also be obtained from the infant a long time after delivery should symptoms occur that suggest in-utero drug exposure that was previously unsuspected. The test requires processing before assay, is more expensive, and is currently not as widely available as other test methods

    4. **Routine laboratory testing.** Routine laboratory tests are usually not required in ISAMs (other than tests to confirm the diagnosis). Laboratory tests are required to rule out other causes of particular signs and symptoms (eg, calcium and glucose for cases of jerky movements) or to follow up and manage some particular complication of drug abuse appropriately.

  C. **Other studies.** A **scoring system** has been devised for assessment of withdrawal signs. Commonly called the **Finnegan score**, after its originator, the score was devised for neonates exposed to opiates in utero. Its usefulness for assessing signs after exposure to other drugs or for guiding management in these cases has not been established, but it can be used as a guide. The scoring system is shown in Table 103–3. Other tools for assessing neonatal abstinence are the **Lipsitz tool, Neonatal Narcotic Withdrawal Index, and the Neonatal Withdrawal Inventory**, but these are less commonly used.

VII. Management. Manifestations of drug withdrawal in many infants resolve within a few days, and drug therapy is not required. Supportive care suffices in many, if not most, infants. It is not appropriate to treat prophylactically infants of drug-dependent mothers. The infant's withdrawal score should be assessed to monitor the progression of symptoms and the adequacy of treatment.

  A. **Supportive care**

    1. **Minimal stimulation.** Attempt to keep the infant in a darkened, quiet environment. Reduce other noxious stimuli.

    2. **Swaddling and positioning.** Use gentle swaddling with positioning that encourages flexion rather than extension.

    3. **Prevent excessive crying with a pacifier, cuddling, and so on.** Feedings should be on demand if possible, and treatment should be individualized based on the infant's level of tolerance.

  B. **General drug treatment.** *Warning:* **Naloxone (Narcan) may precipitate acute drug withdrawal in infants exposed to narcotics. It should not be used in infants born to mothers suspected of abusing opiates.**

    The general aim of treatment is to allow sleep and feeding patterns to be as close to normal as possible. When supportive care is insufficient to do this, or if symptoms are particularly severe, drugs are used. Indications for drug treatment are progressive irritability, continued feeding difficulty, and significant weight loss. A score >7 on the Finnegan score for 3 consecutive scorings (done every 4 hours during the first 2 days) may also be regarded as an indication for treatment. However, the Finnegan score should not be followed slavishly and treated as a definitive laboratory value. Many centers use the Finnegan score only every 12 hours and increase the frequency of its application if the infant's scores rapidly escalate. Drugs used for withdrawal are discussed next. Additional treatment may be required for some symptoms (eg, dehydration or convulsions). There have been very few clinical trials in this area, and drug therapy is based largely on anecdotal evidence and hence is variable. Cumulative reports suggest that drugs that act on the relevant receptors are superior to sedatives. When compared with opiates, phenobarbital, at doses required to suppress symptoms of withdrawal, may impair sucking in infants withdrawing from maternal opiates, and may require a more protracted duration of treatment.

    1. **Morphine.** A recent randomized trial comparing morphine with tincture of opium showed that infants treated with morphine required a somewhat longer

Table 103–3. **MODIFIED FINNEGAN'S SCORING SYSTEM FOR NEONATAL WITHDRAWAL**

Signs and symptoms are scored between feedings.

Cry:	High-pitched	2
	Continuous	3
Sleep hours after feed:	1 h	3
	2 h	2
	3 h	1
Moro reflex:	Hyperactive	2
	Marked	3
Tremors when disturbed:	Mild	2
	Marked	3
Tremors when undisturbed:	Mild	3
	Marked	4
Muscle tone increased:	Mild	3
	Marked	6
Convulsions:		8
Feedings:		
	Frantic sucking of fists	1
	Poor feeding ability	1
	Regurgitation	1
	Projectile vomiting	1
Stools:	Loose	2
	Watery	3
Fever:	100–101°F	2
	>101°F	2
Respiratory rate:	>60/min	1
	Retractions	2
Excoriations:	Nose	1
	Knees	1
	Toes	1
Frequent yawning:		1
Sneezing:		1
Nasal stuffiness:		1
Sweating:		1
Total scores per day		( )

Once an objective score has been attained, a dose for treatment can be decided on.

Reproduced, with permission. Initiated by Loretta Finnegan, MD, and modified by J. Yoon, MD. Initiated by Finnegan LP, Connaughton JF Jr, Kron RE, Emich JP. A scoring system for evaluation and treatment of neonatal abstinence syndrome: a new clinical and research tool. In: Morselli PL, Garattini S, Sereni F, eds. *Basic and Therapeutic Aspects of Perinatal Pharmacology.* New York, NY: Raven Press; 1975.

duration of treatment but had better weight gain. An appropriate schedule of treatment would be to start at a morphine dose of 0.04 mg/kg every 4 hours. Dosage may be increased every 4 hours at increments of 0.04 mg/kg until symptoms are under control (absent side effects). Once the symptoms are under control (eg, Finnegan score <8), treatment is maintained at that dosage for 72 hours and then weaning is commenced. Weaning is done by decreasing the daily dose by 10% every day, as long as symptoms do not relapse. If the infant becomes symptomatic during weaning, the dose is increased back to the last previous dose that had controlled the symptoms. There are no reports of any maximal dose of morphine used for withdrawal, but prudence suggests that infants be closely watched for side effects, and some centers recommend cardiorespiratory monitoring if morphine dosage exceeds 0.8 mg/kg/d. As mentioned, there is a paucity of controlled trials on this topic, and treatment schedules are highly variable between institutions. The schedule just suggested is within the range of common practice but is not carved in stone.

2. **Paregoric (camphorated opium tincture).** This has 0.4 mg/mL morphine equivalent and is thought to be more "physiologic" than nonnarcotic agents but is no longer recommended due to other constituents present in the preparation (eg, camphor, alcohol, benzoic acid).

3. **Opium tincture, also called tincture of opium.** This is similar to paregoric and has the advantage of fewer additives. It has a 10 mg/mL morphine equivalent and should be diluted to provide the same morphine dosage as in Section VII.B.1.

4. **Phenobarbital.** An adequate drug for controlling withdrawal from narcotics, especially those of irritability, fussiness, and hyperexcitability. It is not as effective as morphine for control of gastrointestinal symptoms. It is not suitable for dose titration because of its long half-life. It is mainly useful for treatment of withdrawal from nonnarcotic agents. The dosage is a 10–20 mg/kg loading dose, followed by 2–4 mg/kg/d maintenance. Once symptoms have been controlled for 1 week, decrease the daily dose by 25% every week.

5. **Chlorpromazine.** Quite effective in controlling symptoms of withdrawal from both narcotics and nonnarcotics. It has multiple untoward side effects (it reduces seizure threshold, cerebellar dysfunction, and hematologic problems) that make it **potentially undesirable** for use in neonates when alternatives can be used. The dosage is 3 mg/kg/d, divided into 3–6 doses per day.

6. **Clonidine.** This has been used for withdrawal from both narcotic and nonnarcotic agents. The dosage is 3–4 mcg/kg/d, divided into 4 doses per day.

7. **Diazepam.** This has been used to treat withdrawal from narcotics. One study showed a greater incidence of seizures after methadone withdrawal when infants were treated with diazepam rather than paregoric. When used to treat methadone withdrawal, it also impairs nutritive sucking more than methadone does alone. It may produce apnea when used with phenobarbital. It may be used for treatment of withdrawal from benzodiazepines and possibly also for the hyperexcitable phase after cocaine exposure. The dosage is 0.5–2 mg every 6–8 hours.

8. **Bupernorphine.** In a randomized trial, sublingual bupernorphine was found to reduce the duration of pharmacotherapy and length of stay in neonatal abstinence syndrome. Results are promising but further trials are required before its widespread use.

9. **Combination therapy (failure of monotherapy).** In one study, the combination of diluted tincture of opium (1:25 dilution of opium tincture to water) in combination with phenobarbital was superior to treatment with diluted tincture of opium alone. Patients given this combination spent less time with severe withdrawal and required less diluted tincture of opium, and duration of hospitalization was reduced by 48%. In another randomized trial, clonidine (1 mcg/kg/dose every 4 hours) when combined with tincture of opium was found to reduce duration of pharmacotherapy for neonatal abstinence.

C. **Long-term management.** If the infant is discharged after 4 days, an early appointment with the pediatrician should be arranged and the parents should be informed as to possible signs of delayed-onset withdrawal. Minor signs and symptoms of drug withdrawal may continue for a few months after discharge. This places a difficult infant in a difficult home situation. There are a few reports of an increased incidence of child abuse in these circumstances. Thus, frequent follow-up visits and close involvement of social services may be required.

D. **Breast-feeding.** The various drugs of abuse may be presumed to enter breast milk, and there have been case reports of intoxication in breast-fed infants whose mothers had continued to abuse drugs. Mothers on low-dose methadone have been allowed to breast-feed, but this required close supervision, and there was a constant concern that unsupervised weaning would precipitate withdrawal. A recent study demonstrated that concentration of methadone in breast milk, even at peak maternal plasma levels, was low in the perinatal period. The mothers had been receiving methadone doses of 76 $\pm$22 mg. The data support recommendations of breast-feeding for women on methadone maintenance. However, methadone-dependent women require special considerations and support and should also be counseled as to the unknown CNS effects of long-term exposure to small amounts of methadone present in breast milk. Similarly, there is no evidence that breast-feeding should not be discouraged in mothers who are receiving treatment with SSRIs. However, pending definitive evidence, caution suggests that breast-feeding might be discouraged in the particular case of fluoxetine use, due to its long elimination half-life and risk of accumulation.

VIII. **Prognosis.** During the first few years of life, infants exposed to drugs in utero may have various neurobehavioral problems. Prognosis is largely dependent on the drug used.

A. **Opiates.** There are increased risks of sudden infant death syndrome (SIDS) and strabismus. A substantial proportion of children demonstrate good catch-up growth by 1–2 years of age, although they may still be below the mean. There are limited data on long-term follow-up, but at 5–6 years of age these children appear to function within the normal range of mental and motor development. Some differences have been found in various behavioral, adaptive, and perceptual skills. At 9 years of age, there is a trend, in opiate-exposed children, to score lower than controls in some measures of language processing. Some children require special education classes. A positive and reinforcing environment can improve infant outcome significantly.

B. **Cocaine.** No major deficits in motor development have been found after gestational exposure to cocaine. By 1–6 years of age, there are no significant differences in weight, height, and head circumference between cocaine-exposed and nonexposed children. Gestational cocaine exposure may, however, be associated with long-term effects on behavior. Cocaine-exposed children exhibited more behavioral problems (both internalizing and externalizing) on follow-up to age 7 years, and these issues were related to degree of cocaine exposure during gestation. A long-term study found a 4.4-point decrease in IQ at 4.5–7 years of age after gestational exposure to cocaine. In addition, cocaine-exposed children are more likely to be referred for special education services at school when compared with unexposed children.

C. **Phencyclidine.** Very few studies have been done, but at 2 years of age these infants appear to have lower scores in fine motor, adaptive, and language areas of development. Although weight, length, and head circumference are somewhat reduced at birth, most children demonstrate adequate catch-up growth.

D. **Marijuana.** There is no definitive evidence of long-term dysfunction. Some scientific studies have found that infants born to women who used marijuana during their pregnancy display altered responses to visual stimulation, increased tremors, and a high-pitched cry, which may indicate problems with nervous system development. During preschool and early school years, marijuana-exposed children have been reported to have more behavioral problems and difficulties with sustained attention and memory than nonexposed children.

Selected References

Jansson LM, Velez M. Neonatal abstinence syndrome. *Curr Opin Pediatr.* 2012;24(2):252–258.

Rayburn WF. Maternal and fetal effects from substance use. *Clin Perinatol.* 2007;34:559–571.

Shankaran S, Lester BM, Das A, et al. Impact of maternal substance use during pregnancy on childhood outcome. *Semin Fetal Neonatal Med.* 2007;12:143–150.

Sie SD, Wennink JM, van Driel JJ, et al. Maternal use of SSRIs, SNRIs and NaSSAs: practical recommendations during pregnancy and lactation. *Arch Dis Child Fetal Neonatal Ed.* 2011 (Epub ahead of print).

104 Intracranial Hemorrhage

An **intracranial hemorrhage (ICH)** can occur in term and preterm infants. An **ICH occurring in term infants** tends to be subdural, subarachnoid, or subtentorial and is most related to birth trauma, hypoxic-ischemic events, coagulopathies (eg, thrombophilias or thrombocytopenia), and undetermined causes. The **most common ICH in preterm infants** is bleeding from the subependymal germinal matrix and may result in intraventricular or periventricular hemorrhage, either of which can potentially cause hemorrhagic infarctions of the white matter. This chapter reviews the following clinical conditions: subdural hemorrhage (SDH), epidural hemorrhage, subarachnoid hemorrhage (SAH), intracerebral parenchymal hemorrhage, intracerebellar parenchymal hemorrhage (ICPH), and germinal matrix and intraventricular hemorrhage (GM/IVH).

SUBDURAL HEMORRHAGE

I. **Definition.** A **subdural hemorrhage (SDH)** is an accumulation of blood between the dura and the arachnoid membrane and involves tears of bridging veins of the subdural compartment. The vascular structures most affected are superficial cerebral veins, infratentorial posterior fossa venous sinuses, the inferior sagittal sinus, and tentorial sinuses and veins (eg, vein of Galen). Blood may accumulate and cause acute symptoms of intracranial pressure (ICP) or reside as a hematoma that slowly evolves as a chronic subdural hematoma with increasing fluid accumulation and increasing ICP.

II. **Incidence.** A SDH is very common after birth: up to 50% of term asymptomatic infants may have SDH. It usually follows a traumatic delivery of a late preterm or term infant. Only on rare occasions does SDH become serious.

III. **Pathophysiology.** A SDH is typically related to traumatic birth events involving labor and delivery. Undue pressure on the skull and torsion may produce shear forces resulting in rupture of superficial cerebral bridging veins or tears in the dura or dural reflections (eg, either the falx cerebri or tentorium and associated venous sinuses). These events are usually found over the cerebrum or within the posterior fossa. Occasionally skull fractures accompany these findings. Timing of the onset of SDH and clinical findings may be acute or delayed. Clinical signs may be minimal to none with the SDH self-resolving, or subtle findings of slight irritability or a seemingly hyperalert state may foretell an underlying accumulating SDH with delayed onset of more serious neuropathic circumstances. Latent SDH can lead to a subdural hematoma and subdural effusion with increasing intracranial pressure.

IV. **Risk factors.** Include precipitous labor and delivery, instrumented deliveries utilizing forceps or vacuum-assist devices, a large for gestational age infant with cephalopelvic disproportion, and coagulopathies including familial thrombophilias and vitamin K deficiency.

V. **Clinical presentation.** Signs include lethargy alternating with irritability or asymmetric hypotonia of upper and lower extremities on the contralateral side of the SDH. More specific to SDH is impaired third cranial nerve function ipsilateral to the SDH. Focal seizures may present at any time and are much more likely to occur in low birthweight infants. Signs of increasing ICP may include a bulging fontanel, deviations of eye movements, and increasing occipital-frontal head circumference. Additional clinical signs can be decreased feeding, intermittent vomiting, and failure to thrive, all of which are more often related to late post-SDH neuropathic events.

VI. **Diagnosis**
   A. **Laboratory**
      1. **Hematocrit.** Unexplained anemia.
      2. **Total serum bilirubin.** Persistent newborn jaundice.
      3. **Cerebral spinal fluid (CSF) studies** are indicative but not diagnostic of SDH. Emphasis on ICH hemorrhage can be taken if a combination of CSF findings is seen: large numbers of red bloods cells (especially if crenated), xanthochromia, elevated protein content, and hypoglycorrhachia (ie, CSF glucose <50% of concomitant blood glucose).
   B. **Imaging studies**
      1. **Computed tomography (CT)** readily identifies most SDH.
      2. **Magnetic resonance imaging (MRI)** is best for detailing posterior fossa lesions and accumulations of blood or effusion.
      3. **Ultrasound (US)** does not readily lend itself to SDH identification, except for possible midline shifts.

VII. **Management.** Documentation of risk factors and appropriate cogent observation are the most important first clinical steps. Careful and repeated neurologic examinations will reveal neurologic signs that should be followed by laboratory and imaging studies.

VIII. **Prognosis.** The outcome of SDH ranges from early death to minimal or no disabling conditions. Much of the neurologic outcome of SDH depends on accompanying conditions soon after birth (eg, prematurity, birth asphyxia, shock, hypoxic-ischemic encephalopathy, or infection). Massive tentorial tears and hemorrhage dictate death or severe and long-term handicap. Infants with major SDH can have mortality rates upward of 45%. Conversely, in most cases SDH can be limited, produce few clinical signs, and have a good outcome. More than 50% of infants with minimal early clinical findings and later good outcomes have been largely found to have had small cerebral convexity SDH hemorrhages.

EPIDURAL HEMORRHAGE

An **epidural hemorrhage**, blood between the inner skull and dura, is extremely rare in newborns. It is usually caused by injury to the middle meningeal artery, which is less susceptible to injury because it moves freely. Causes include birth trauma or an infant being dropped at delivery. Diagnosis is by CT or MRI. Affected infants usually have a skull fracture and cephalhematoma, and treatment is supportive with possible surgical/needle aspiration.

SUBARACHNOID HEMORRHAGE

I. **Definition.** A **subarachnoid hemorrhage (SAH)** is an accumulation of blood between the arachnoid mater and the pia mater. The arachnoid mater is an avascular membrane situated below the dura mater and, together with the pia mater, constitutes what is known as the leptomeninges. Unlike adult SAH, which is arterial, infant SAH is venous in origin, coming from bridging veins within the subarachnoid space; however, on rare occasions it may be arterial, coming from leptomeningeal arteries of the subarachnoid space. SAH may be primary, coming from the vessels of the subarachnoid space, or secondary, occurring when the blood extends from existing intraventricular, cerebral, or cerebellar hemorrhages.

II. **Incidence.** A small SAH is commonly seen in preterm and term newborn infants. It is of limited significance unless other conditions are present, such as prematurity, coagulopathies, birth trauma, or asphyxia. Primary bleeding within the subarachnoid space is usually self-limited, and it is the second most common ICH seen in newborns.

III. **Pathophysiology.** Rupture of the small vessels of the subarachnoid space can be associated with trauma in term infants, or birth asphyxia in preterm infants, and is most often idiopathic and insignificant.

IV. **Risk factors.** See Pathophysiology.

V. **Clinical presentation.** In term infants, a SAH is mostly asymptomatic. Mild to intermittent irritability or lethargy may herald the onset of seizures on the second to third day of life.

VI. **Diagnosis**
   A. **Laboratory.** CSF findings in SAH mirror those already discussed for SDH.
   B. **Imaging studies.** CT and MRI studies establish the existence of primary SAH or identify other lesions that may be the source of secondary SAH.

VII. **Management.** Close observation and repeated neurologic examinations suffice for those infants at risk but without signs of SAH. Anticonvulsant medication and intravenous fluid therapy are needed if the infant has lethargy and/or seizure activity. Serum electrolyte and urine output monitoring for possible syndrome of inappropriate antidiuretic secretion is recommended if a significant amount of SAH has been identified. Regular sequential head circumference measurements will identify suspect cases of posthemorrhagic hydrocephalus. The latter is due to obliteration of CSF resorption sites by the organizing blood. Follow-up cranial imaging studies will also be needed.

VIII. **Prognosis.** A primary isolated SAH is mostly uncomplicated. Infants who have seizures that resolve before discharge from the hospital have an expected 90% uncomplicated outcome. Infants who develop long-term complications are mostly within those who had coexisting problems associated with birth trauma or perinatal asphyxia.

INTRACEREBRAL INTRAPARENCHYMAL HEMORRHAGE

I. **Definition.** An **intracerebral parenchymal hemorrhage** occurs deep within the brain tissue after venous infarction and is commonly referred to as **periventricular hemorrhagic infarction (PVHI).** Periventricular leukomalacia in preterm infants and porencephalic cysts in term infants are not uncommon complications of PVHI.

II. **Incidence.** The occurrence of PVHI may be as much as 10–15% among infants with ICH.

III. **Pathophysiology.** It is postulated that venous thrombosis and/or stasis causes PVHI through increased intravascular pressure that leads to rupture of parenchymal vessels; however, the exact mechanism remains unclear. Affected preterm infants have hemorrhagic venous infarction of subcortical and periventricular white matter, whereas affected term infants develop subcortical hemorrhage with infarction of overlying cortex.

IV. **Risk factors.** PVHI is seen most often after a perinatal hypoxic-ischemic event.

V. **Clinical presentation.** Clinical signs of PVHI follow those of severe neonatal encephalopathy and overlap with clinical signs as seen with SDH, SAH, or IVH.

VI. **Diagnosis**
   A. **CT** is most useful for detecting recent hemorrhage.
   B. **MRI** findings of hypodensities suggest evolving areas of brain injury.

C. **Cranial US** is particularly useful in identifying PVHI. An echodense lesion of periventricular white matter with an associated germinal matrix (GM) hemorrhage or IVH usually identifies coexisting PVHI. Whether the PVHI is unilateral or bilateral, it is always an asymmetric lesion.

VII. **Management.** PVHI requires observational and supportive care, much as severe SDH or SAH. If imaging studies suggest a midline shift, neurosurgical consultation should follow. Subsequent posthemorrhagic hydrocephalus (PHH) is always a threat, which also requires neurosurgical consultation.

VIII. **Prognosis.** Developmental studies of preterm infants with PVHI have shown that significant cognitive and/or motor delays complicate overall recovery in at least two-thirds of survivors. Careful follow-up is thus indicated in every case of PVHI.

INTRACEREBELLAR PARENCHYMAL HEMORRHAGE

I. **Definition.** An **intracerebellar parenchymal hemorrhage (ICPH)** is most often seen in preterm infants with complications of labor and delivery and for whom intense respiratory management is required. ICPH in term infants is almost always associated with birth trauma.

II. **Incidence.** Reports vary by gestational age. In neuropathologic reports, preterm infants <1500 g have an occurrence of 15–25%. A report using cranial US has defined the incidence as 2.8% in a population of <1500 g infants and an incidence of 8.7% for the smallest infants weighing <750 g. In another report using brain MRI in infants <34 weeks' gestation, the incidence was ~10%.

III. **Risk factors.** Traumatic delivery.

IV. **Pathogenesis.** Four mechanisms for intracerebellar parenchymal hemorrhage are possible:

A. **Primary hemorrhage** into either cerebellar hemisphere or into the vermis.

B. **Venous infarction.**

C. **Supratentorial IVH and SAH** is associated with reduction of preterm cerebellar growth, which may reflect concurrent cerebellar injury or direct effect of the blood on cerebellar development.

D. **Direct trauma to the posterior fossa with rupture of cerebellar bridging veins** or the occipital sinuses. This is seen primarily in term infants. Most ICPH is unilateral and focal with a predilection to the right cerebellar hemisphere.

V. **Clinical presentation.** An ICPH is unique in causing unexplained motor agitation, in addition to respiratory compromise, apnea, and breathing irregularities. Otherwise, the general symptoms of ICH are present as well.

VI. **Diagnosis.** CT and MRI have superior ability over US in diagnosing ICPH. However, US done via the mastoid fontanel can provide additional information.

VII. **Management.** All management modalities presented for other ICH patients apply to infants with confirmed or suspected ICPH. For infants at risk for ICPH, the added combination of shock and acidosis are closely related and warrant diagnostic efforts specific for ICPH.

VIII. **Prognosis.** Infants with ICPH usually require longer periods of mechanical ventilation. They will need close neurodevelopmental assessment, much as required with other types of ICH. In general, cerebellar hemorrhages seen only on MRI have much better prognosis than those detectable by US.

GERMINAL MATRIX AND INTRAVENTRICULAR HEMORRHAGE

I. **Definition.** IVH is the most common CNS complication of a preterm birth. The occurrence is greatly associated with the immaturity of the germinal matrix of the lateral ventricles. Acidosis, birth asphyxia, shock, blood pressure fluctuations, and hypoxia are common related problems.

The germinal matrix, located between the caudate nucleus and the ependymal lining of the lateral ventricle, is normally not seen on cranial US. When germinal matrix hemorrhage occurs, it becomes readily identified by US and is seen as subependymal bleeding originating between the groove of the thalamus and the head of the caudate nucleus. Bleeding may be confined to the germinal matrix or it may rupture into either lateral ventricle and thereby become a unilateral or bilateral GM/IVH.

By 36 weeks' postconceptional age, the germinal matrix has involuted in most infants, although some residual may persist. If IVH occurs in term infants, it originates most often in the choroid plexus; however, residual subependymal germinal matrix may also be a point of origin. Following IVH, further insult by venous thromboses may result in thalamic infarction.

II. **Incidence.** The overall occurrence of IVH in preterm infants <1500 g is ~13–15%. Rates vary by gestation, with the greatest risk of GM/IVH in preterm infants with birthweights <750 g. Because IVH is rarely seen in term infants, their incidence rates are exceptionally low and associated with birth-related injury or asphyxia. Curiously, 2–3% of seemingly normal term infants, when studied prospectively, have been noted to have asymptomatic IVH.

III. **Pathophysiology.** The germinal matrix is a marginally supported and highly vascularized area. The blood vessels (as arterioles, venules, or capillaries) in this area of immature cerebrum are especially prone to hypoxic-ischemic injury. The vessels are irregular, with large luminal areas, and readily rupture. The GM begins to involute after 34 weeks' postconceptional age, and thus the peculiar vulnerability and predilection for GM/IVH for preterm infants lessens, but is not totally removed. Late preterm infants (34–37 weeks' gestation) may have IVH that reflects those of early preterm infants. **Fluctuations in cerebral blood flow (CBF)** play an important role in the pathogenesis of GM/IVH because sick premature infants have **pressure-passive cerebral circulation.** A sudden rise or fall in systemic blood pressure can result in an increase in CBF with subsequent rupture of the germinal matrix vessels. Decreases in CBF can also result in ischemic injury to the GM vessels and surrounding tissues, making them prone to secondary rupture following reperfusion.

The unique deep venous anatomy at the level of the foramen of Monroe and the open communication between the GM vessels and the venous circulation contribute to the danger of abrupt or sharp fluctuations in cerebral venous pressure. Given this anatomic proximity, rupture through the GM subependymal layer results in entrance of blood into the lateral ventricles in nearly 80% of affected infants.

A. **Neuropathologic consequences of IVH**

1. **GM ventricular-subventricular zone contains the migrating cells of origin for the cerebral cortex.** It is the site of production of neurons and glial cells of the cerebral cortex and basal ganglia. GM destruction may result in impairment of myelination, brain growth, and subsequent cortical development. Moreover, in preterm infants, GM-IVH leads to reduction of cerebral perfusion in the first 2 weeks after the hemorrhage. The reduction was found to be most severe around day 5 and was irrespective of the IVH grade.

2. **Periventricular hemorrhagic infarction (PVHI)** is venous in origin, associated with severe and usually asymmetric IVH, and invariably occurs on the side with the larger amount of intraventricular blood. It is a distinct pathologic event following venous stasis; it is often mistakenly described as an "extension" of IVH, of which it is not. Moreover, PVHI is neuropathologically distinct from periventricular leukomalacia (PVL). See preceding discussion under PVHI.

3. **Posthemorrhagic hydrocephalus (PHH)** is more common in those infants with the highest grade of hemorrhage. It is most frequently attributable to obliterative arachnoiditis either over the convexities of the cerebral hemispheres with occlusion of the arachnoid villi or in the posterior fossa with obstruction

of outflow of the fourth ventricle. Rarely, aqueductal stenosis is caused by an acute clot or reactive gliosis.

4. **Periventricular leukomalacia (PVL)** is a frequent accompaniment of IVH but is not directly caused by IVH. PVL is an ischemic brain injury followed by necrosis of periventricular white matter adjacent to the lateral ventricles. It is usually a nonhemorrhagic event resulting from hypotension, apnea, and other hypoxic-ischemic events known to decrease CBF. Most PVL lesions are symmetrical in distribution.

IV. **Risk factors.** Prematurity and respiratory distress syndrome have remained as the most closely related clinical circumstances to GM/IVH. As mentioned earlier, the immature cerebral vascular structures of preterm infants are extremely vulnerable to volume and pressure changes and to hypoxic and acidotic changes. Secondarily, respiratory distress, and its attendant limitations for oxygenation, further attenuates the immature vasculature of the preterm brain. Birth asphyxia, pneumothorax, shock/hypotension, acidosis, hypothermia, and therapeutic volume and/or osmolar overloads all serve to multiply the risk for GM/IVH. Even procedures that we perceive as routine in the care of premature infants may also be contributory, such as tracheal suctioning, abdominal examination, and handling to reposition or to instill mydriatics for an eye examination.

Of growing importance for the understanding of preterm GM/IVH is the possible role of fetal and neonatal **inflammatory responses.** Chorioamnionitis and funisitis may be harbingers of postnatal cerebral vascular events leading up to GM/IVH. Fetal inflammatory responses and subsequent neonatal hypotension and sepsis are closely related processes to IVH. Mediators of an inflammatory response, such as cytokines, have vasoactive properties that may be the source of exaggerated blood pressure changes that overwhelm the pressure passive state of the germinal matrix.

V. **Clinical presentation.** The clinical presentation is diverse, and diagnosis requires neuroimaging for confirmation. Signs may mimic those of other ICH or common neonatal disorders such as metabolic disturbances, asphyxia, sepsis, or meningitis. IVH may be totally asymptomatic, or there may be subtle symptoms, for example, a bulging fontanel, a sudden drop in hematocrit, apnea, bradycardia, acidosis, seizures, changes in muscle tone, or changes in level of consciousness. A catastrophic syndrome may accompany an extensive IVH. It is characterized by a precipitous fall of hematocrit, a rapid onset of stupor or coma, respiratory failure, seizures, decerebrate posturing or a profound flaccid quadriparesis, and fixed pupils.

VI. **Diagnosis**

A. **Cranial US.** Cranial US (see Chapter 11 for imaging examples) is the procedure of choice for screening and diagnosis. CT and MRI are acceptable alternatives but are more expensive and require transport to the imaging service. They are valuable for a more definitive diagnosis or documentation of static brain injury before discharge from the hospital. Two systems for classifying GM/IVH have been advanced for clinical use. The older and most time honored has been that of Papile, based originally on CT but adapted for interpretation of cranial US. The second is the classification promulgated by Volpe, based also on cranial US. The utility of classification schema resides in the ability of clinicians to communicate degrees of severity and to have a source of information for comparison of lesions as well as having a means to follow progression or regression and recovery of the initial insult of IVH. **The GM/IVH classification by Papile** (updated in 2002) gives classes I to IV. Classes I and II are small hemorrhages. **Class I** is hemorrhage only seen in the GM. **Class II** shows hemorrhage from the GM extending into the lateral ventricles but without ventricular dilation. **Classes III and IV** are moderate to severe lateral ventricular hemorrhages, with the former resulting in acute ventricular dilation and the latter marked by extension into parenchymal hemorrhages.

IVH classification by Volpe offers a somewhat different perspective. His class I is confined to the GM with little or no IVH. Class II is an IVH seen on parasagittal view and extends into >50% of the lateral ventricles. Class III is IVH >50% on parasagittal view with distention of the lateral ventricles. Lastly, Volpe points out that a cranial US finding of any periventricular echo density is an obvious and more serious intracranial vascular insult, such as PVHI or PVL.

A cranial US is indicated for screening sick preterm infants for IVH from the first day of life and throughout the hospitalization. Typically a cranial US is done between day 1 and day 7, depending on clinical presentation and institutional protocols, keeping in mind that 50% of GM/IVH may occur on day 1, but 90% have occurred by day 4 of life. Of all GM/IVH identified by day 4 of life, 20–40% will progress to more extensive hemorrhage. Most clinicians obtain a final cranial US, CT, or MRI before discharge, or at 36 weeks' postconceptional age.

B. **Laboratory studies.** CSF initially shows elevated red and white blood cells, with elevated protein concentration. The degree of elevation of CSF protein correlates approximately with the severity of the hemorrhage. It is frequently difficult to distinguish IVH from a "traumatic tap." Within a few days after hemorrhage, the CSF becomes xanthochromic, with a decreased glucose concentration as in other forms of ICH. Often, the CSF shows a persistent increase in white blood cells and protein and a decreased glucose level, making it difficult to rule out meningitis.

VII. **Management**

A. **Prenatal prevention**

1. Avoidance of premature delivery.
2. Transportation in utero.
3. Data suggest that active preterm labor may be a risk factor for early IVH and there may be a protective role for cesarean delivery. However, Anderson et al showed that cesarean birth before the active phase of labor resulted in a lower frequency of severe IVH and less progression to severe IVH, although it did not affect the overall incidence of IVH. In a study by Durie et al, there was no correlation between mode of delivery and the incidence of IVH in very low birthweight infants who are presenting by the vertex.
4. **Antenatal steroid therapy.** Several large multicenter trials have shown a clear efficacy of antenatal steroids in reducing IVH. In one study the incidence of GM hemorrhage or IVH was 2- to 3-fold lower in infants whose mothers received a complete course of antenatal steroids compared with those whose mothers received no steroids or an incomplete course (<48 hours). Moreover, this beneficial effect appears to be independent of the improvement in respiratory status. The prevention of IVH may be a composite effect of enhanced vascular integrity, decreased respiratory distress, and possibly altered cytokine production. Blickstein and coworkers have reported that antenatal steroids (given between 24 and 32 weeks' gestation) as a completed course (48 hours) resulted in a 2.5 times lower incidence of GM/IVH (7.7% vs 19.4%) for singleton and multiple births.

B. **Postnatal prevention**

1. Avoid birth asphyxia.
2. Avoid large fluctuations in blood pressure.
3. Avoid rapid infusion of volume expanders or hypertonic solutions.
4. Use prompt but cautious cardiovascular support to prevent hypotension.
5. Correct acid-base abnormalities.
6. Correct abnormalities of coagulation.
7. Avoid poorly synchronized mechanical ventilation. Consider sedation and in difficult situations pharmacologic paralysis.
8. **Postnatal pharmacologic intervention with indomethacin.** Ment et al reported in 1994 that low-dose prophylactic indomethacin significantly lowered the incidence and severity of IVH but did not appear to be of benefit in the prevention or extension of early IVH. Subsequent reviews and reports over the ensuing years have not confirmed indomethacin prophylaxis for prevention of IVH, and the approach remains *controversial*. There are reports of reduced

cerebral blood flow after indomethacin as well as no difference in long-term neurologic outcome for treated versus nontreated infants. More recently, Ment et al have reported on long-term follow-up of school-age preterm infants, indicating improved vocabulary scores with a striking favorable sex response to indomethacin therapy for male subjects. In the same year, Miller et al reported less white matter injury after 3–6 doses of low-dose indomethacin therapy for infants of <28 weeks' gestation. Much of the controversy today surrounding low-dose prophylactic indomethacin therapy for the prevention or amelioration of GM/IVH involves the continuing concerns for indomethacin-related complications of necrotizing enterocolitis, spontaneous intestinal perforation, decreased renal function (albeit transient in most cases), and the threat of persistent pulmonary hypertension. Jones et al reported in a meta-analysis published in 2010 that there is no statistical difference in the incidence of IVH as a complication due to the use of either ibuprofen or indomethacin to treat patent ductus arteriosus.

C. **Management of acute hemorrhage**
1. **General supportive care** to maintain a normal blood volume and a stable acid-base status.
2. **Avoid fluctuations** of arterial and venous blood pressures.
3. **Follow-up serial imaging** (cranial US or CT) to detect progressive hydrocephalus (see Chapter 98).

VIII. **Prognosis**
A. **Short-term outcome of GM/IVH is directly related to birthweight, gestational age, and the ensuing severity of the hemorrhagic insult to the immature brain.** For the years 1995–1996, 1997–2002, and 2003–2007, very low birthweight infants in the National Institute of Child Health and Human Development (NICHD) Neonatal Research Network saw survival steady at 84–85%. Meanwhile, the occurrence of severe IVH remained unchanged at 12%. A broader view of the 1997–2002 infants weighing 501–1500 g reveals 15% mortality, 25% survival with short-term complications of bronchopulmonary dysplasia/chronic lung disease, severe IVH, and necrotizing enterocolitis, with ~60% survival for infants without the short-term complications; however, long-term outcomes remain in question.
B. **Long-term major neurologic sequelae of GM/IVH depend primarily on the extent of associated parenchymal injury, laterality, and any added effects of the short-term complications.** From the NICHD studies noted previously, long-term outcomes of seemingly normal extremely low birthweight infants at time of hospital discharge are worrisome. At 8–9 years of age, and in comparison with control term infants, studies now reveal strikingly lower IQ scores, greater learning problems, poor motor skills, markedly increased behavioral problems, and considerable hearing loss. Also, bilateral IVH has been proved to correlate with severe cerebral palsy and Mental Developmental Index <70 after 12 months of age, as opposed to unilateral IVH, in a multicenter retrospective study done by Maitre et al in 2009.

Selected References

Bassan H, Limperopoulos C, Visconti K, et al. Neurodevelopmental outcome in survivors of periventricular hemorrhagic infarction. *Pediatrics.* 2007;120:785–792.

Brouwer AJ, Groenendaal F, Koopman C, Nievelstein RJ, Han SK, de Vries LS. Intracranial hemorrhage in full-term newborns: a hospital based cohort study. *Neuroradiology.* 2010;52:567–576.

de Viers LS. Intracranial hemorrhage and vascular lesions. In: Martin RJ, Fanaroff AA, Walsh MC, eds. *Fanaroff & Martin's Neonatal-Perinatal Medicine: Diseases of the Fetus and Infant.* 9th ed. St. Louis, MO: Elsevier Mosby; 2011:936–952.

Durie DE, Sciscione AC, Hoffman MK, Mackley AB, Paul DA. Mode of delivery and outcomes in very low-birth weight infants in the vertex presentation. *Am J Perinatol.* 2011;28:195–200.

Ecury-Goossen GM, Dudink J, Lequin M, Feijen-Roon M, Horsch S, Govaert P. The clinical presentation of preterm cerebellar haemorrhage. *Eur J Pediatr.* 2010;169:1249–1253.

Kaukola T, Herva R, Perhomaa M, et al. Population cohort associating chorioamnionitis, cord, inflammatory cytokines and neurologic outcome in very preterm, extremely low birth weight infants. *Pediatr Res.* 2006;59:478–483.

Laughon M, Bose C, Allred E, et al. Factors associated with treatment for hypotension in extremely low gestational age newborns during the first postnatal week. *Pediatrics.* 2007;119:273–280.

Levene MI, de Vries LS. Hypoxia-ischemic encephalopathy: pathophysiology, assessment tools, and management. In: Martin RJ, Fanaroff AA, Walsh MC, eds. *Fanaroff & Martin's Neonatal-Perinatal Medicine: Diseases of the Fetus and Infant.* 9th ed. St. Louis, MO: Elsevier Mosby; 2011:952–976.

Maitre NL, Marshall DD, Price WA, et al. Neurodevelopmental outcome of infants with unilateral or bilateral periventricular hemorrhagic infarction. *Pediatrics.* 2009;124:e1153–e1160.

Ment LR, Peterson BS, Meltzer JA, et al. A functional magnetic resonance imaging study of the long term influences of early indomethacin exposure on language processing in the brains of prematurely born children. *Pediatrics.* 2006;118:961–970.

Mohamed AM, Aly H. Transport of premature infants is associated with increased risk for intraventricular hemorrhage. *Arch Dis Child Fetal Neonatal Ed.* 2010;95:F403–F407.

Stoll BJ, Hansen NI, Bell EF, et al. Neonatal outcomes of extremely preterm infants from the NICHD neonatal research network. *Pediatrics.* 2010;126:443–456.

Tam EW, Rosenbluth G, Rogers EE, et al. Cerebellar hemorrhage on magnetic resonance imaging in preterm newborns associated with abnormal neurologic outcome. *J Pediatr.* 2011;158:245–250.

Verhagen EA, Ter Horst HJ, Keating P, Martijn A, Van Braeckel KN, Bos AF. Cerebral oxygenation in preterm infants with germinal matrix-intraventricular hemorrhages. *Stroke.* 2010;41:2901–2907.

Volpe JJ. Intracranial hemorrhage. *Neurology of the Newborn.* 5th ed. Philadelphia, PA: Saunders; 2008:481–588.

Whitby EH, Griffiths PD, Rutter S, et al. Frequency and natural history of subdural haemorrhages in babies and relation to obstetric factors. *Lancet.* 2004;363:846–851.

Yang JYK, Chan AK, Callen DJ, Paes BA. Neonatal cerebral sinovenous thrombosis: sifting the evidence for a diagnostic plan and treatment strategy. *Pediatrics.* 2010;126:e693–e700.

105 Intrauterine Growth Restriction (Small for Gestational Age)

I. **Definition.** The terms **intrauterine growth restriction (IUGR)** and **small for gestational age (SGA)** are sometimes used interchangeably. Although related, they are not synonymous. SGA describes an infant whose weight is lower than population norms or lower than a predetermined cutoff weight. Most commonly, **SGA infants** are defined as having a birthweight below the 10th percentile for gestational age or >2 standard deviations below the mean for gestational age. In contrast, **IUGR infants have not attained optimal intrauterine growth.**

The **ponderal index**, arrived at by the following formula, can be used to identify infants whose soft tissue mass is below normal for the stage of skeletal development. A ponderal index <10th percentile may be used to identify IUGR infants. Thus, all IUGR infants may not be SGA, and all SGA infants may not be small as a result of a growth-restrictive process.

$$\text{Ponderal index} = \frac{\text{Birthweight} \times 100}{\text{Crown} - \text{heel length}^3}$$

A. **Symmetric IUGR.** (HC = Ht = Wt, all <10%) The head circumference (HC), length (Ht), and weight (Wt) are all proportionally reduced for gestational age. Symmetric IUGR is due to either decreased growth potential of the fetus (congenital infection or genetic disorder) or extrinsic conditions that are active early in pregnancy.

B. **Asymmetric IUGR.** (HC = Ht < Wt, all <10%) Fetal weight is reduced out of proportion to length and head circumference. The head circumference and length are closer to the expected percentiles for gestational age than is the weight. In these infants, brain growth is usually spared. The usual causes are uteroplacental insufficiency, maternal malnutrition, or extrinsic conditions appearing late in pregnancy.

C. **More recently, fetal growth restriction (FGR)** is being used to denote impaired fetal growth based on **healthy fetal growth standards.** An individual baby's growth potential is determined by both maternal and fetal factors. Recent attempts have been made to develop individualized growth charts taking into account maternal physiological characteristics such as race, ethnicity, parity, height, and so on, as well as fetal characteristics like gender.

   Term optimal weight (TOW) is defined as the optimal weight based on fetal weight curves of healthy infants born at term. For an individual pregnancy, fetal growth can be combined with TOW to show the **gestation-related optimal growth (GROW)** curve. GROW charts adjusted for maternal height, weight, parity, and ethnicity are available at www.gestation.net.

   Estimation of fetal growth velocity with serial measurements may be useful to identify FGR. For example, a fetus with weight >10th percentile may be growth restricted if fetal growth velocity declines. FGR may be early or late, comparable to symmetric and asymmetric IUGR.

   Early FGR is difficult to identify (by measuring crown-rump length), as often the timing of conception is not known. However, slow growth velocity between the first and second trimesters can identify infants at risk for perinatal death before 34 weeks' gestation. The onset of FGR before 34 weeks is associated with sequential changes on Doppler studies that parallel worsening placental function. Typically, umbilical artery Doppler changes precede biophysical profile parameters. Late FGR after 34 weeks' gestational age is more difficult to identify and has less characteristic Doppler changes.

II. **Incidence.** About 3–10% (up to 15%) of all pregnancies are associated with IUGR, and 20% of stillborn infants are growth retarded. The perinatal mortality rate is 5–20 times higher for growth-retarded fetuses, and serious short- or long-term morbidity is noted in half of the affected surviving infants. IUGR is estimated to be the predominant cause for low birthweight in developing countries. It is estimated that a third of infants with birthweights <2500 g are in fact growth retarded and not premature. Term infants with birthweights <3rd percentile have a higher morbidity and a 10 times higher mortality than appropriate for gestational age infants. In the United States, uteroplacental insufficiency is the leading cause of IUGR. An estimated 10% of cases are secondary to congenital infection. Chromosomal and other genetic disorders are reported in 5–15% of IUGR infants.

III. **Pathophysiology.** Fetal growth is influenced by fetal, maternal, and placental factors.
   A. **Fetal factors**
      1. **Genetic.** Approximately 20% of birthweight variability in a given population is determined by fetal genotype. Genetic determinants of fetal growth have their greatest impact in early gestation during the period of rapid cell development. Racial and ethnic backgrounds influence size at birth irrespective of socioeconomic status. Males weigh an average of 150–200 g more than females at birth. This weight increase occurs late in gestation. Birth order affects fetal size; infants born to primiparous women weigh less than subsequent siblings.
      2. **Chromosome anomalies.** Chromosomal deletions or imbalances result in diminished fetal growth. Nearly 20% of fetal growth restriction is due to chromosomal aberration.
      3. **Congenital malformations.** Anencephaly, gastrointestinal atresia, Potter syndrome, and pancreatic agenesis are examples of congenital anomalies associated with IUGR. Frequency of IUGR increases as the number of congenital defects increases.
      4. **Cardiovascular anomalies.** (With the possible exception of transposition of the great vessels and tetralogy of Fallot.) Abnormal hemodynamics are thought to be the basis of IUGR.
      5. **Congenital infection.** TORCH infections (*t*oxoplasmosis, *o*ther, *r*ubella, *c*ytomegalovirus, and *h*erpes simplex virus) are often associated with IUGR and account for ~5% of IUGR fetuses. The incidence of IUGR is highest when infection occurs in the first trimester. The clinical findings in different congenital infections are nonspecific and overlap considerably. Cytomegalovirus and rubella are associated with severe IUGR. Rubella causes damage during organogenesis and results in a decreased number of cells, whereas cytomegalovirus infection results in cytolysis and localized necrosis within the fetus.
      6. **Inborn errors of metabolism.** Transient neonatal diabetes, galactosemia, and phenylketonuria are other disorders associated with IUGR. Single-gene defects associated with impaired insulin secretion or action are associated with impaired fetal growth (see Chapter 101).
   B. **Maternal factors** (Table 105–1)
      1. **Reduced uteroplacental blood flow.** Maternal disorders such as preeclampsia-eclampsia, chronic renal vascular disease, and chronic hypertensive vascular disease often result in decreased uteroplacental blood flow and associated IUGR. Impaired delivery of oxygen and other essential nutrients is thought to limit organ growth and musculoskeletal maturation. Risk of placental thrombi is increased in conditions of inherited thrombophilias.
      2. **Maternal malnutrition.** The major risk factors for IUGR include small maternal size (height and prepregnancy weight) and minimal maternal weight gain. Low body mass index, defined as (weight [kg]/height [m^2])/100, is a major predictor of IUGR. Maternal malnutrition leads to deficient substrate supply to the fetus. Total caloric consumption rather than protein or fat consumption appears to be the principal nutritional influence on birthweight. A balanced protein energy supplementation during pregnancy decreases the risk of IUGR birth.
      3. **Multiple pregnancies.** Impaired growth results from failure to provide optimal nutrition for more than 1 fetus in utero. There is a progressive decrease in weight of singletons, twins, and triplets. In parabiotic twins, the smaller twin has decreased nutrient delivery secondary to abnormal placental blood flow resulting from arteriovenous communication in the chorionic plate.
      4. **Maternal substance use.** See also Chapter 103.
         a. **Cigarettes and alcohol.** Chronic abuse of cigarettes or alcohol is demonstrably associated with IUGR. The effects of alcohol and tobacco seem to be dose dependent, with IUGR becoming more serious and predictable with heavy abuse.

Table 105–1. **MATERNAL FACTORS IN INTRAUTERINE GROWTH RESTRICTION**

Pregnancy-induced hypertension (>140/90 mm Hg)
Weight gain (<0.9 kg every 4 weeks)
Uterus fundus growth lag (<4 cm for gestational age)
Cyanotic heart disease
Heavy smoking
Residing at high altitude
Substance abuse and drugs
Short stature
Low socioeconomic class
Anemia (hematocrit <30%)
Asthma
Prepregnancy weight (<50 kg)
Prior history of IUGR
Chronic hypertension, diabetes mellitus
Collagen vascular disorders such as lupus
Renal disease
Severe maternal malnutrition
Multiple pregnancy
Low maternal age
Preeclampsia
Inherited thrombophilias
Previous growth restricted baby

      b. **Heroin.** Maternal heroin addiction is also often associated with IUGR.

      c. **Cocaine.** Cocaine use in pregnancy is associated with increased rates of IUGR. The IUGR may be mediated by placental insufficiency or direct toxic effect on the fetus.

      d. **Others.** Other drugs and chemical agents causing IUGR include known teratogens, antimetabolites, and therapeutic agents such as trimethadione, warfarin, and phenytoin. Each of these agents causes characteristic malformation syndromes. Repeated use of antenatal steroids and lithium use are also associated with low birthweight.

   5. **Maternal hypoxemia.** Hypoxemia is seen in mothers with hemoglobinopathies, especially sickle cell disease, and they often have IUGR infants. Infants born at high altitudes tend to have lower mean birthweights for gestational age.

   6. **Other maternal factors.** Maternal short stature, young maternal age, short interpregnancy interval, uterine anomalies, low socioeconomic class, primiparous, grand multiparous, and low prepregnancy weight are associated with subnormal birthweight. Maternal hyperhomocysteinemia is also associated with low birthweight.

   7. **DNA damage.** Measured by micronucleus (MN) formation, may play a role. MNs are formed by the lagging chromosomal fragments during anaphase in both mitosis and meiosis. Increased MN count in maternal lymphocytes at 20 weeks' gestation is associated with increased risk of IUGR and preeclampsia.

 C. **Placental factors**

   1. **Placental insufficiency.** In the first and second trimesters, fetal growth is determined mostly by inherent fetal growth potential. By the third trimester, placental factors (ie, an adequate supply of nutrients) assume major importance for fetal growth. When the duration of pregnancy exceeds the nurturing capacity

of the placenta, placental insufficiency results with subsequent impaired fetal growth. This phenomenon occurs mostly in post-term gestations but may occur at any time during gestation.

2. **Uteroplacental insufficiency (UPI).** Seen in almost 70% of infants with IUGR. Impaired oxygen extraction and nutrient delivery (glucose and amino acids) lead to fetal hypoglycemia and hypoxia. The latter is associated with decrease in cell size and number, lighter brain weight, and lower DNA content. Small placental volume and a reduction in terminal villi are seen in IUGR placentas.

3. **Placenta structural abnormalities.** Various anatomic factors, such as multiple infarcts, aberrant cord insertions, umbilical vascular thrombosis, and hemangiomas, are described in IUGR placentas. IUGR is twice as common with a 2-vessel-cord pregnancy as compared with 3-vessel-cord pregnancies. Premature placental separation may reduce the surface area exchange, resulting in impaired fetal growth. An adverse intrauterine environment is apt to affect both placental and fetal development, hence IUGR infants usually have small placentas.

4. **IUGR fetuses.** These fetuses have downregulation of placental amino acid and lipoprotein lipase transporters Na^+/K^+ ATPase and Na^+/H^+ exchanger, leading to lower plasma amino acid levels and decreased fatty acid transfer. Genetic imprinting may also play a role (eg, alterations of the placenta-specific gene IGF-2 in knockout mice has produced IUGR fetuses).

5. **Fetal endocrine responses.** Include alterations in the hypothalamic-pituitary axis, resulting in elevated corticotropin-releasing hormone, adrenocorticotropic hormone, and cortisol with a decrease in insulin-like growth factor-1 (IGF-1). Thyroid-stimulating hormone is high, but thyroxine and triiodothyronine are low, as are serum vitamin D and osteocalcin. High cortisol levels are associated with decreased postnatal catch-up growth and delayed neurodevelopmental outcomes.

6. **Fetal response to placental dysfunction.** Different for early FGR and late FGR. In early FGR, decrease in umbilical venous flow and decreased fetal cardiac return to the placenta (due to increased resistance) precede clinical FGR. Fetal events include increased ductal shunting to the heart, decreased hepatic flow, downregulation of glucose-insulin-IGF, and decreased hepatic glycogen stores. With increasing villous obliteration, middle cerebral artery Doppler changes precede changes in the biophysical profile (BPP) with the loss of fetal heart rate reactivity, breathing, and loss of body movements. BPP changes also correlate with fetal acidosis. A decrease in amniotic fluid occurs in 20–30% of FGR that is independent of Doppler changes and correlates with fetal cardiac decompensation. Doppler changes usually progress over 4–6 weeks.

7. **Others.** Placental mosaicism, wherein the placental cytogenetics are different from the fetal cytogenetics, may account for ~15% of IUGR. Fibrin deposition in the decidua basalis, the intervillous space, and mesenchymal dysplasia are associated with an increased risk for placental thrombosis and IUGR.

IV. **Risk factors.** Related to fetal, maternal, or placental pathophysiologic factors (see previous text) (Table 105–2).

V. **Clinical presentation.** The maternal history will raise the index of suspicion regarding suboptimal fetal growth. The infant will have a reduced birthweight for gestational age. Using growth charts and the Ballard score can help assess gestational age, and intrauterine and postnatal growth. See Figures 5–1, 5–3 through 5–5.

VI. **Diagnosis**

A. **Establishing gestational age.** Determining the correct gestational age is imperative. The last menstrual period, size of the uterus, time of quickening (fluttering movements in the abdomen caused by fetal activity, appreciated by the mother for the first time), and early ultrasound measurements are used to determine gestational age. (See Chapter 5.)

Table 105–2. **PLACENTAL FACTORS IN INTRAUTERINE GROWTH RESTRICTION**

Two-vessel cord
Abruptio placentae, placental hematoma, placenta previa, chronic abruption
Hemangioma
Single umbilical artery
Infarction
Aberrant cord insertion
Umbilical vessel thrombosis
Circumvallate placentation
Confined placental mosaicism
Massive perivillous fibrin deposition (immune mediated)
Chronic villitis of unknown etiology (VUE)
Placental mesenchymal dysplasia

B. **Fetal assessment**
   1. **Clinical diagnosis.** Manual estimations of weight, serial measurements for fundus height, and maternal estimates of fetal activity are simple clinical measures.
   2. **Ultrasonography.** Because of its reliability to date pregnancy and to detect impaired fetal growth by anthropomorphic measurements and fetal anomalies, ultrasonography currently offers the greatest promise for diagnosis. The following anthropomorphic measurements are used in combination to predict growth impairment with a high degree of accuracy.
      a. **Biparietal diameter (BPD).** When serial measurements of BPD are less than optimal, 50–80% of infants have subnormal birthweights.
      b. **Abdominal circumference.** The liver is the first organ to suffer the effects of growth retardation due to redistribution of ductus venosus blood flow to the heart and a decrease in glycogen deposition in the liver. Reduced growth of the abdominal circumference (<5 mm/wk) is the earliest sign of asymmetric growth retardation and diminished glycogen storage. Abdominal circumference <10th percentile for age is suggestive of growth retardation.
      c. **Ratio of head circumference to abdominal circumference.** This ratio normally changes as pregnancy progresses. In the second trimester, the head circumference is greater than the abdominal circumference. At about 32–36 weeks' gestation, the ratio is 1:1, and after 36 weeks the abdominal measurements become larger. Persistence of a head-to-abdomen ratio <1 late in gestation is predictive of **asymmetric IUGR**.
      d. **Femur length.** Femur length appears to correlate well with crown-heel length and provides an early and reproducible measurement of length. Serial measurements of femur length are as effective as head measurements for detecting symmetric IUGR.
      e. **Placental morphology and amniotic fluid assessment.** May help in distinguishing a constitutionally small fetus from a growth-retarded fetus. For example, placental aging with oligohydramnios suggests IUGR and fetal jeopardy, whereas normal placental morphology with a normal amount of amniotic fluid suggests a constitutionally small fetus.
      f. **Placental volume measurements.** May be helpful in predicting subsequent fetal growth. Placental weight and/or volume is decreased before fetal growth decreases. IUGR with decreased placental size is more likely to be associated with fetal acidosis. Placental volume correlates with placental flow indices.
   3. **Doppler measurements.** In both maternal and various fetal vascular beds are increasingly used to detect, monitor, and optimize time of delivery in IUGR infants. Doppler studies are more helpful in diagnosing moderate to severe IUGR than mild IUGR. The various groups of vessels used are as follows:

a. **Uterine artery (UtA) flow abnormalities.** Used to predict IUGR as early as 12–14 weeks. A persistent abnormality at 23–24 weeks has a ~75% sensitivity in predicting early FGR.

b. **Umbilical artery (UA) flow abnormalities.** Used to evaluate placental insufficiency, particularly in high-risk pregnancies. Normally, the UA resistance declines with pregnancy. Increased pulsatility index (PI), decreased end-diastolic velocity (EDV), and absent or reversed EDV (AREDV) occur with worsening fetal compromise. AREDV is associated with 20–68% mortality. Decreased EDV is seen when 30% placental flow is attenuated, and ARDEV is noted when 60–70% placental flow is affected. Absent EDV and AREDV are associated with a 4.0- and 10.6-fold increased risk of mortality, respectively, compared to those with normal Doppler.

c. **Fetal cerebral arterial flow.** Usually studied in the middle cerebral artery as a pulsatility index (MCA PI) and middle cerebral artery peak systolic velocity (MCA PSV). With worsening IUGR, MCA PSV increases. Abnormal MCA PI precedes MCA PSV changes. Changes in MCA PI are not as consistent in predicting mortality, although decreased MCA resistance is associated with worse perinatal outcomes.

d. **Doppler venous flow studies** of the vena cava, umbilical vein (UV), and ductus venosus (DV) provide information about fetal cardiovascular and respiratory responses. Decreased venous blood flow in the UV and an abnormal deep or retrograde "a" wave in DV are suggestive of ventricular decompensation. Changes in venous flow are usually late and represent more severe decompensation. Absent or reversed DV flow correlates with acidosis and is associated with 63–100% mortality.

e. **Aortic isthmus (AoI).** Absolute flow velocities are decreased in growth-restricted fetuses. Retrograde flow in the AoI correlates strongly with adverse perinatal outcome.

4. **Biophysical profile (BPP).** Used for noninvasive fetal monitoring.

5. **Cardiotocography (CTG).** Used more commonly in Europe to assess timing of delivery for situations wherein significant fetal acidosis is suspected.

6. **Placental magnetic resonance imaging (MRI).** This can assess severity of FGR on the basis of decreased placental volume and changes in placental thickness-to-volume ratio. Fetal demise can also be predicted by abnormal signal intensity.

7. **Compensated versus decompensated fetus.** Persistence of UPI results in fetal adaptation to maintain adequate cerebral oxygenation and growth.

a. **UPI results in increased placental vascular resistance and fetal hypoxemia by reducing umbilical blood flow.** The fetus responds by redistribution of blood to the brain (brain sparing) by cerebral vasodilatation, mesenteric vasoconstriction, preferential shunting through the foramen ovale, increased fractional extraction of oxygen (O_2), polycythemia, and a relative decrease in fetal O_2 consumption. Fetal growth velocity and weight gain are decreased. Nonstress test (NST), BPP, and CTG are normal. Decreased or absent diastolic flow in the umbilical artery and increased diastolic component in the MCA are seen. The fetus is hypoxemic but does not have cerebral hypoxemia at this stage.

b. **With worsening fetal compromise.** There is cerebral hypoxemia and acidemia associated with no fetal weight gain, oligohydramnios, decreased fetal heart rate variability, and abnormal NST, CTG, and BPP. Umbilical arteries show **absence or reversal of end-diastolic flow (AREDV).** Deep "a" wave is seen in the ductus venosus, suggestive of ventricular dysfunction. With severe acidosis, MCA PI and MCA PSV decrease, suggesting imminent collapse of the fetus.

c. **Acute fetal decompensation.** AREDV in umbilical arteries (UAs) in early-onset FGR babies can be present up to 1 week before acute decompensation.

Table 105–3. SEQUENTIAL CHANGES OF DOPPLER STUDIES IN DECOMPENSATING FETAL GROWTH RESTRICTION

Initial changes	Decreased amniotic fluid index
	Increased uterine artery resistance with EDV
Early changes	Decreased MCA resistance (brain sparing)
(in 50% 2–3 weeks before nonreactive FHR)	Absent uterine artery EDV
Late changes	Increased resistance in DV-reversed EDV in uterine artery
(~6 days before nonreactive FHR)	
Very late changes	Reversed flow in DV and pulsatile flow in umbilical vein
(in 70%, 24 hours before changes in BPP)	

BPP, biophysical profile; DV, ductus venosus; EDV, end-diastolic flow; FHR, fetal heart rate; MCA, middle cerebral artery.

Approximately 40% of fetus with acidosis have AREDV pattern. MCA vasodilation with abnormal PI may be present for up to 2 weeks before acute deterioration in 50–80% of infants. MCA vasodilation may be independently associated with abnormal outcomes in late-onset FGR. Oligohydramnios develops in 20–30% of IUGR infants about 1 week before acute deterioration (Table 105–3).

C. **Neonatal assessment**

1. **Reduced birthweight for gestational age.** This is the simplest method of diagnosing IUGR. However, this method tends to misdiagnose constitutionally small infants.

2. **Physical appearance.** When infants with congenital malformation syndromes and infections are excluded, the remaining groups of IUGR infants have a characteristic physical appearance. These infants in general are thin with loose, peeling skin because of loss of subcutaneous tissue, a scaphoid abdomen, and a disproportionately large head.

3. **Appropriate growth charts should be used.** Several standardized growth charts are available to assess intrauterine and postnatal growth. See Lubchenco and Olsen charts (Chapter 5). Additional growth charts for infants based on Centers for Disease Control and Prevention (CDC) and World Health Organization (WHO) data from birth to 36 months can be found at the CDC website: http://www.cdc.gov/growthcharts/.

4. **Ponderal index** <10th percentile helps identify neonates with IUGR, especially those with birthweight <2500 g.

5. **Ballard score.** Gestational age can also be assessed by means of the Ballard scoring system. This examination is accurate within 2 weeks of gestation in infants weighing <999 g at birth and is most accurate at 30–42 hours of age. (See Chapter 5.)

D. **Observe for the following complications:**

1. **Hypoxia**

   a. **Perinatal asphyxia.** IUGR infants frequently have birth asphyxia because they tolerate the stress of labor poorly. IUGR accounts for a large proportion of stillborn infants with hypoxia in utero.

   b. **Persistent pulmonary hypertension.** Many IUGR infants are subjected to chronic intrauterine hypoxia, which results in abnormal thickening of the smooth muscles of the small pulmonary arterioles. This in turn reduces pulmonary blood flow and results in varying degrees of pulmonary artery hypertension. IUGR infants are particularly at risk for persistent pulmonary hypertension.

   c. **Respiratory distress syndrome.** Several reports suggest accelerated fetal pulmonary maturation in association with IUGR secondary to chronic intrauterine stress. Hyaline membrane disease is less frequently seen in IUGR because these infants tend to manifest advanced pulmonary maturity secondary to chronic intrauterine stress.

   d. **Meconium aspiration.** Post-term IUGR infants are particularly at risk for meconium aspiration.

   e. **Patent ductus arteriosus (PDA).** Conflicting data suggest that hemodynamically significant PDA may be bigger and occur earlier in IUGR infants than in appropriate for gestational age (AGA) infants, but spontaneous closure of PDA is more frequent in IUGR infants <1000 g birthweight. IUGR infants with PDA are at greater risk for pulmonary hemorrhage, intraventricular hemorrhage (IVH), necrotizing enterocolitis (NEC), and renal failure.

2. **Hypothermia.** Thermoregulation is compromised in IUGR infants because of diminished subcutaneous fat insulation. Infants with IUGR secondary to fetal malnutrition late in gestation tend to be thin as a result of loss of subcutaneous fat.

3. **Metabolic**

   a. **Hypoglycemia.** Carbohydrate metabolism is seriously disturbed, and IUGR infants are highly susceptible to hypoglycemia as a consequence of diminished glycogen reserves and decreased capacity for gluconeogenesis. Oxidation of free fatty acids and triglycerides is reduced in IUGR infants, which limits alternate fuel sources. Hyperinsulinism, excess sensitivity to insulin, and deficient catecholamine release during hypoglycemia suggest abnormality of counterregulatory hormone mechanisms during periods of hypoglycemia in IUGR infants. Hypothermia may potentiate the problem of hypoglycemia.

   b. **Hyperglycemia.** Very low birthweight infants have low insulin secretion, resulting in hyperglycemia.

   c. **Hypocalcemia.** Hypocalcemia may occur in asphyxiated IUGR infants.

   d. **Liver disease.** IUGR infants are at greater risk for developing cholestasis associated with parenteral nutrition. There is also an increased risk of non–fatty liver disease in children born SGA.

   e. **Other.** Hypertriglyceridemia, increased sympathetic tone, and reduced concentrations of IGF-1 have been associated with increased aortic intimal thickness in IUGR infants.

4. **Hematologic disorders.** Hyperviscosity and polycythemia may result from increased erythropoietin levels secondary to fetal hypoxia associated with IUGR. Thrombocytopenia, neutropenia, and altered coagulation profile are also seen in IUGR infants. Polycythemia may also contribute to hypoglycemia and lead to cerebral injury. There is an increased number of nucleated red cells secondary to extramedullary hematopoiesis. Persistent elevated nucleated red cell counts are associated with worse prognosis.

5. **Altered immunity.** IUGR infants have decreased immunoglobulin G (IgG) levels. In addition, the thymus is reduced in size by 50%, and peripheral blood lymphocytes are decreased. Reduction in total white cell count, neutrophils, monocyte and lymphocyte subpopulations, and thrombocytopenia may occur, and selective suppression of helper and cytotoxic T cells can be seen.

6. **Others.** IUGR infants are at increased risk of developing NEC, particularly when associated with an absent or reversed end-diastolic flow on an umbilical artery Doppler. Preterm IUGR infants are also at increased risk of pulmonary hemorrhage, chronic lung disease, more severe IVH, and renal failure.

VII. **Management.** Antenatal diagnosis is the key to proper management of IUGR.

   A. **History of risk factors.** The presence of maternal risk factors should alert the obstetrician to the likelihood of fetal growth retardation. Ultrasonography confirms the diagnosis. Correctable causes of impaired fetal growth warrant immediate attention.

   B. **Delivery and resuscitation.** The optimal timing for delivery of IUGR infants is still debated, but Doppler measurements provide an important tool for monitoring fetal well-being. IUGR infants have a 2- to 3-fold increased risk of preterm delivery when fetal growth standards are used for diagnosis. IUGR infants delivered before 28–30 weeks have worse outcomes. Outcomes are more favorable with cesarean delivery. Delivery is usually undertaken when the lungs are mature or when biophysical data obtained by monitoring reveal fetal distress. Labor is particularly stressful to IUGR fetuses. Skilled resuscitation should be available because perinatal depression is common.

 C. **Prevention of heat loss.** Meticulous care should be taken to conserve body heat (see Chapter 7).

 D. **Hypoglycemia.** Close monitoring of blood glucose levels is essential for all IUGR infants. Hypoglycemia should be treated promptly with parenteral dextrose and early feeding (see Chapter 62).

 E. **Hematologic disorders.** A central hematocrit reading should be obtained to detect polycythemia.

 F. **Congenital infection.** IUGR infants should be examined for congenital malformations or signs of congenital infections. Many intrauterine infections are clinically silent, and screening for these should be done routinely in IUGR infants.

 G. **Genetic anomalies.** Screening for genetic anomalies should be done as indicated by the physical examination.

VIII. **Prognosis.** Mortality increases with decreasing gestational age when IUGR is also present. Mortality decreases by 48% for each week that the fetus remains in utero before 30 weeks' gestation. **Neurodevelopmental morbidities are seen 5–10 times more often in IUGR infants compared with AGA infants.** Neurodevelopmental outcome depends not only on the cause of IUGR but also on the adverse events in the neonatal course (eg, perinatal depression or hypoglycemia). Many studies reveal evidence of minimal brain dysfunction, including hyperactivity, short attention span, and learning problems. Preterm IUGR infants also show alterations in early neurobehavioral functions like attention-interaction capacity and cognitive and memory dysfunction that persist. Increased risk of cerebral palsy, a wide spectrum of learning disabilities, mental retardation, pervasive developmental disorders, and neuropsychiatric disorders are seen in later years. The risk of morbidities is higher in term IUGR infants. IUGR infants who have normal Doppler studies have better outcomes than those with abnormal antenatal Doppler studies. Even mild FGR increases the risk of mortality and long-term development.

 A. **Symmetric versus asymmetric IUGR.** Infants with symmetric IUGR caused by decreased growth potential generally have a poor outcome, whereas those with asymmetric IUGR in which brain growth is spared usually have a better outcome. Smaller head circumference is associated with cognitive, psychomotor, and behavioral delays that persist into adolescence. Neuroimaging studies using MRI and ultrasound show that preterm IUGR infants have a high incidence of white matter loss and reduced myelination in the internal capsule associated with decreased cortical gray matter volume by as much as 28%. The total brain volume is also reduced by 10% when compared with AGA infants, particularly in the hippocampal, parietal, and parieto-occipital areas.

 B. **Preterm IUGR.** These infants have a higher incidence of abnormalities than the general population because they are subjected to the risks of prematurity in addition to the risks of IUGR. Outcomes are significantly poorer for children whose brain growth failure occurred before 26 weeks' gestation. Gestational age may be a more important predictor of developmental outcomes than FGR, particularly before 32–34 weeks.

 C. **Chromosomal disorders.** IUGR infants with major chromosomal disorders have a 100% incidence of disability.

 D. **Congenital infections.** Infants with congenital rubella or cytomegalovirus infection with microcephaly have a poor outcome, with a disability rate >50%.

 E. **Learning ability.** The school performance of IUGR infants is significantly influenced by social class; children from higher social classes score better on achievement tests.

 F. **Adult disorders.** Epidemiologic evidence indicates that obesity, insulin-resistant diabetes, hypertension, and cardiovascular diseases are more common among adults who were IUGR at birth.

G. **Risk for recurrence of IUGR in subsequent pregnancies.** Depends on the underlying condition. The presence of previous fetal growth retardation, preeclampsia, abruption, infarction, and acquired or inherited thrombophilias increase the risk of fetal growth retardation in the subsequent pregnancies. Placental pathologic examination should be attempted in all IUGR infants as the risk of FGR in subsequent pregnancy is very high (eg, risk of recurrence is 50–100% with fibrin deposition). In selected cases, folic acid, aspirin, and supplementation with L-arginine to improve placental blood flow may improve outcomes.

H. **FGR and stillbirth.** FGR is an important predictor of unexplained stillbirths. Greater than 50% of fetuses without congenital anomalies are IUGR. Maternal obesity increases the risk of concomitant FGR and stillbirth.

Selected References

Barker DJP. Fetal and infant origin of adult disease. *Brit Med J.* 1993;301:1111.

Baschat A. Fetal growth restriction—from observation to intervention. *J Perinatal Med.* 2010;38:239–246.

Baschat A. Neurodevelopment following fetal growth restriction and its relationship with antepartum parameters of placental dysfunction. *Ultrasound Obstet Gynecol.* 2011;37:501–514.

Battaglia FC, Lubchenco LO. A practical classification of newborn infants by weight and gestational age. *J Pediatr.* 1967;17:159.

Del Rio M, Martínez JM, Figueras F, et al. Doppler assessment of the aortic isthmus and perinatal outcome in preterm fetuses with severe intrauterine growth restriction. *Ultrasound Obstet Gynecol.* 2008;31:41–47.

Gardosi J. Intrauterine growth restriction: new standards for assessing adverse outcome. *Best Pract Res Clin Obstet Gynecol.* 2009;23:741–749.

Gardosi J. Intrauterine growth restriction: new concepts in antenatal surveillance, diagnosis, and management. *Am J Obstet Gynecol.* 2011; 204(4):288–300. DOI:10.1016/j/ajog.2010.08.055.

Kinzler W, Kaminsky L. Fetal growth restriction and subsequent pregnancy risks. *Semin Perinatol.* 2007;31:126–134.

Kleigman RM. Intrauterine growth retardation. In: Martin RJ, Fanaroff AA, Walsh MC, eds. *Fanaroff & Martin's Neonatal-Perinatal Medicine: Diseases of the Fetus and Newborn.* 9th ed. St. Louis, MO: Elsevier Mosby; 2011.

Mari G, Hanif F, Kruger M, Cosmi E, Santolaya-Forgas J, Treadwell MC. Middle cerebral artery peak systolic velocity: a new Doppler parameter in the assessment of growth restricted fetuses. *Ultrasound Obstet Gynecol.* 2007;29:310–316.

Mari G, Hanif F, Treadwell MC, Kruger M. Gestational age at delivery and Doppler waveforms in the very preterm intrauterine growth-restricted fetuses as predictors of perinatal mortality. *J Ultrasound Med.* 2007;26:555–559.

Odibo A, Zhong Y, Longtine M, et al. First-trimester serum analytes, biophysical tests and the association with pathological morphometry in the placenta of pregnancies with preeclampsia and fetal growth restriction. *Placenta.* 2011;32:e333–e338.

Sibley CP, Turner MA, Cetin I, et al. Placental phenotypes of intrauterine growth. *Pediatr Res.* 2005;58:827–832.

Skilton MR, Evans N, Griffiths KA, Harmer JA, Celermajer DS. Aortic wall thickness in newborns with intrauterine growth restriction. *Lancet.* 2005;365:1484–1486.

Urban G, Vergani P, Ghidini A, et al. State of the art: non-invasive ultrasound assessment of the utero-placental circulation. *Semin Perinatol.* 2007;31:232–239.

Yigiter A, Kavak ZN, Durukan B, et al. Placental volume and vascularization flow indices by 3D power Doppler US using VOCAL technique and correlation with IGF-1, free beta-hCG, PAPP-A, and uterine artery Doppler at 11-14 weeks of pregnancy. *J Perinat Med.* 2011;39:137–141.

106 Lyme Disease

I. **Definition.** Lyme disease was first reported in 1977, following an unusual cluster of adults and children with oligoarticular arthritis in a certain neighborhood of Lyme, Connecticut. Subsequently, a multisystem disease was described and attributed to the spirochete *Borrelia burgdorferi*. Lyme disease manifests as a spectrum of skin, musculoskeletal, cardiac, and neurologic findings. It is a vector-borne disease following the bite of an Ixodes tick—usually the black-legged *Ixodes scapularis*, commonly known as the deer tick. The species Ixodes includes additional subspecies (eg, *I. pacificus, I. dammini, and I. ricinus*) that contribute to a worldwide distribution of the disease and is known to be endemic in North and South America, Europe, Asia, Africa, and Australia. **Prenatal exposure to *B. burgdorferi* and the development of gestational borreliosis can result in maternal Lyme disease with placentitis and transplacental infection of the fetus and newborn.**

II. **Incidence.** In 2009, more than 38,000 cases of Lyme disease were reported to the Centers for Disease Control and Prevention. In the United States, 44 continental states reported cases of Lyme disease, with an incidence of 12.71 in 100,000 nationwide. No specific data for the number of pregnancy-related Lyme disease is available. Estimates for active infection after exposure to a deer-tick bite are only 1–3%. Presumably the number of infected pregnant women in the United States is small.

III. **Pathophysiology**

   A. **Transmission.** The Ixodes tick lives a 2-year life cycle consisting of 3 life stages: larval, nymph, and adult. The preferred reservoirs for the larval and nymph tick are the white-footed field mouse and for the adult tick it is the white-tailed deer. The larval stage emerges from eggs in early summer and feeds on previously infected mice from which they acquire the *B. burgdorferi* spirochete. The infected nymph stage emerges the next spring and is the most likely source of human infection because the activity of the feeding nymph corresponds to the outdoor activity of humans in spring and summer. The adult tick may infect before laying eggs in summer and dying soon after.

   B. **Human spirochetemia.** Following the tick bite, the incubation period of the spirochetes is 1–32 days with a median of 11 days, followed by the first clinical signs of disease. The disease is characterized by "early" and "late" manifestations. Early disease is in 2 stages. Spirochete dissemination is presumed to be facilitated by the surface of the organism binding to human plasminogen and subsequently binding to integrins, matrix glycosaminoglycans, and extracellular matrix proteins. These complexes may explain the propensity of the spirochetes to localize to collagen fibrils in the extracellular matrices of the heart, nervous system, and bone joints. Late Lyme disease occurs months to a year or more after dissemination.

   C. **Placentitis and transplacental disease.** Before 1990, a number of case reports had confirmed the transplacental passage of *B. burgdorferi* by way of identification of spirochetes in placental tissues, umbilical vessels, and fetal brain, heart, spleen, kidneys, bone marrow, liver, and adrenal glands. In 1989, MacDonald reported finding 13 cases of transplacental transmission of *B. burgdorferi* by way of fetal tissue cultures or immune serology.

   D. **Newborn disease secondary to *B. burgdorferi* remains undefined.** A number of reviews have documented fetal demise, stillbirths, preterm births, and newborns with hyperbilirubinemia, petechial rashes, respiratory distress, and various birth defects, all thought to be related to gestational borreliosis. The most frequently studied newborn condition has been a variety of congenital heart defects, but none have been confirmed as a clinical syndrome unique to infants of mothers with documented gestational borreliosis.

IV. **Risk factors.** Maternal Lyme disease is a result of exposure to deer ticks in known endemic areas of the United States or other endemic areas of the world. Once an expectant mother presents with a history of outdoor exposure or has dogs or cats in the home, a known tick embedment, or cutaneous lesions consistent with early disease, **prompt antibiotic therapy lessens the risk for transplacental transmission of spirochetes.** There are no other known predilections to Lyme disease related to pregnancy.

V. **Clinical presentation**

   A. **Maternal**

   1. **Early localized.** The cutaneous stage begins with a papule at the site of the tick bite, becoming an annular erythematous migrating rash (also known as erythema migrans) with central clearing. Rash may last 3–4 weeks and is nonpruritic and painless. The early stage is often accompanied by low-grade fever, evanescent arthralgias, myalgia, fatigue, headache, and neck muscle stiffness.

   2. **Early disseminated.** This is most often characterized by multiple erythema migrans, several weeks after the tick bite. This stage is accompanied by worsening fatigue, severe malaise, and migratory musculoskeletal pain. Systemic disease affecting target organs becomes more apparent, namely as mono- or pauciarticular arthritis, and cardiac manifestations, such as heart block. Nervous system involvement can include lymphocytic meningitis or cranial nerve palsies.

   3. **Late Lyme disease.** Months after exposure to disease, arthralgias and pauciarticular arthritis persist and recur. The knees are the most often affected joint with marked swelling, but with pain that is less than that of rheumatoid-type arthritis. On rare occasions, chronic neurologic conditions of encephalopathy, peripheral neuropathy, demyelination, or dementia have been reported.

   B. **Neonatal**

   1. **No specific clinical presentation of Lyme disease in the newborn or neonatal period has been described.** Of importance is the maternal history of disease and whether or not she has been adequately treated. Placental pathology in suspect cases may offer information that would prompt testing and perhaps treatment for at-risk neonates.

   2. **Congenital Lyme disease as a clinical entity has been reviewed and found not to be substantive.** In particular, congenital heart defects have been reviewed in large follow-up studies of mothers with positive *B. burgdorferi* serology. Williams et al reported in 1999 a cohort study of >5000 cord blood serologic surveys within a highly endemic area for Lyme disease (New York State). They did not find any correlation of congenital heart defects or other major or minor malformations attributable to positive maternal or cord blood serology. In 2001, Elliott et al reported a search of the world literature for teratogenic effects of gestational Lyme disease. They concluded that no effect was found, and any otherwise adverse pregnancy outcome was of low risk in the face of adequately treated gestational borreliosis. More recently, Walsh et al searched the worldwide literature for obstetric associations to Lyme disease with these conclusions:

      a. **Women who are seropositive at conception** have no increased incidence of adverse pregnancy.

      b. **Women who develop a confirmed diagnosis** of Lyme disease in pregnancy should receive appropriate antimicrobial treatment.

      c. **Women with Lyme disease in pregnancy** and who have been appropriately treated have shown no association with specific adverse fetal outcomes.

VI. **Diagnosis.** Laboratory testing for Lyme disease should follow if careful history taking and physical examination strongly suggest active disease.

   A. **Early localized disease.** Diagnosis is made largely on clinical grounds (history of exposure, rash, and symptoms). Serologic tests are not recommended secondary to late development of antibodies to *B. burgdorferi*.

B. **Early disseminated disease.** Dissemination of the disease is diagnosed clinically as described earlier. If rash is not present, serologic studies should be obtained.
   1. Enzyme immunoassay (EIA).
   2. Immunofluorescent-antibody assay (IFA).
   3. If both tests are negative, no further testing is needed, and clinical reevaluation for other conditions is indicated. Screening tests are known to have high false-positive rates.
   4. If either is positive, it should be followed by:
      a. **Western immunoblot standardized for antibodies to** *B. burgdorferi.* Subsequently, positive Western blot assays should include specific immunoglobulin G (IgG) and immunoglobulin M. If the Western blot assays are negative, the false-positive EIA or IFA testing suggests other spirochetal diseases, that is, syphilis, leptospirosis, an intercurrent viral disease (eg, Epstein–Barr), or an autoimmune condition such as lupus erythematosus.
      b. **Late disease.** If late disease is suspected, only a positive IgG immunoblot is needed.

VII. **Management**
   A. **Maternal**
      1. **Early localized disease.** *Note:* Doxycycline is the drug of choice for Lyme disease, *except* in pregnancy or in children <8 years of age.
         a. **Amoxicillin**
         b. **Cefuroxime axetil (alternative)**
      2. **Early disseminated or late disease**
         a. **Oral antibiotic therapy** is considered adequate.
         b. **Parenteral antibiotics** for a maximum of 4 weeks are only indicated in patients with symptoms of increased intracranial pressure and pleocytosis in cerebral spinal fluid. Routine lumbar puncture is not recommended.
   B. **Newborn**
      1. **Treat if infant is thought to be symptomatic at birth** especially if mother is confirmed with Lyme disease but has not been adequately or appropriately treated. Consider ceftriaxone, cefotaxime, or penicillin. Obtain infectious disease consultation before starting treatment.
      2. **If the infant is asymptomatic at birth** given low risk for active disease, current recommendations do not call for empirical treatment, especially if the mother was appropriately treated during pregnancy. Placental pathology may offer information helpful in the decision to treat or not; consultation with an infectious disease specialist is recommended.
      3. **Lyme disease is *not* a contraindication for breast-feeding.** No evidence is known for the passage of *B. burgdorferi* to the infant through breast-feeding.

VIII. **Prognosis.** Prompt diagnosis and antibiotic therapy are essential. One report has revealed that 25% of infants had adverse outcomes, 15% were sick or had an abnormality, 8% resulted in fetal death, and 2% resulted in neonatal death. Antibiotic therapy resulted in only 15% with adverse outcomes. Long-term follow-up is important for recurrence of the disease.

Selected References

American Academy of Pediatrics. Lyme disease. In: Pickering LK, Baker CJ, Kimberlin DW, Long SS, eds. *Red Book: 2009 Report of the Committee on Infectious Diseases.* 29th ed. Elk Grove Village, IL: American Academy of Pediatrics; 2012:474–479.

Centers for Disease Control and Prevention. Lyme Disease—United States 2003–2005. *Morb Mortal Wkly Rep.* 2007;56:573–576.

Centers for Disease Control and Prevention. Summary of Notifiable Diseases—United States, 2009. *Morb Mortal Wkly Rep.* 2011;58:1–100.

Elliott DJ, Eppes SC, Klein JD. Teratogen update: Lyme disease. *Teratology.* 2001;64:276–281.

Gibbs RS, et al. Maternal and fetal infectious disorders. In: Creasy RK, Resnik R, Iams JD, eds. *Maternal-Fetal Medicine: Principles and Practice.* 5th ed. Philadelphia, PA: Elsevier Saunders; 2004:758–760.

Mylonas I. Borreliosis during pregnancy: a risk for the unborn child? *Vector Borne Zooonotic Dis.* 2011;11:891–898.

Shapiro ED, Gerber MA. Lyme disease. In: Remington JS, Klein JO, Wilson CB, Nizet V, Maldonado Y, eds. *Infectious Diseases of the Fetus and Newborn Infant.* 6th ed. Philadelphia, PA: Elsevier Saunders; 2006:485–497.

Walsh CA, Mayer EW, Baxi LV. Lyme disease in pregnancy: case report and review of the literature. *Obstet Gynecol Surv.* 2007;62:41–50.

107 Magnesium Disorders (Hypomagnesemia, Hypermagnesemia)

As noted in Chapter 85, abnormalities of magnesium (Mg^{+2}) and calcium (Ca^{+2}) metabolism are commonly seen in the neonatal intensive care unit. Calcium disturbances may be mirrored by magnesium, as in hypocalcemia with hypomagnesemia or hypercalcemia with hypermagnesemia. Infants of diabetic mothers (IDMs) and infants with intrauterine growth restriction (IUGR) may present with hypocalcemia, hypomagnesemia, or both. Abnormalities in serum values for Ca^{+2} and Mg^{+2} are of concern in any infant and warrant further investigation.

I. **Hypomagnesemia**

   A. **Definition.** Normal serum levels for Mg^{+2} are typically 0.6–1.0 mmol/L (1.6–2.4 mg/dL). Hypomagnesemia is usually seen as any value <0.66 mmol/L (1.6 mg/dL); however, clinical signs do not manifest until levels drop below 0.5 mmol/L (1.2 mg/dL).

   B. **Incidence.** True overall incidence in neonates is not well documented and remains to be determined; however, neonates appear to be more predisposed than other groups of patients, and the most frequent occurrence tends to follow that of those infants with hypocalcemia.

   C. **Pathophysiology.** Mg^{+2} is a key trace element for maintaining skeletal integrity, and it acts as a catalyst for intracellular enzymes for adenosine triphosphate (ATP) activation in skeletal and myocardial contractility. It has an important role in different processes related to cell physiology, hormonal and metabolic pathways, nerve conduction, and blood coagulation. It is also integral to protein synthesis, vitamin D metabolism, parathyroid function, and calcium homeostasis.

   D. **Risk factors**

      1. Hypocalcemia
      2. Preterm and late-preterm infants
      3. Inadequate intake of magnesium
      4. Infant of diabetic mother (IDM), reflecting maternal Mg^{+2} deficiency secondary to gestational diabetes
      5. IUGR, especially if mother had preeclampsia
      6. Inherited renal wasting (eg, Gitelman syndrome, Na^+-K-ATPase mutation, others)
      7. Hypoparathyroidism
      8. Associated hypocalciuria and nephrocalcinosis
      9. Magnesuria secondary to furosemide or gentamicin
      10. Citrated blood exchange transfusions

   E. **Clinical presentation**

      1. Similar to hypocalcemia (see Chapter 85, Section I.E) (eg, jitteriness, apnea, feeding intolerance), and may also present as seizures.

   2. Clinical signs may be masked as hypocalcemia. If symptoms persist after adequate calcium gluconate therapy, hypomagnesemia should be considered.

F. **Diagnosis.** Laboratory testing to establish serum levels.

   1. **Serum magnesium level.** Normal values are 0.6–1.0 mmol/L (1.6–2.4 mg/dL), although it may vary minimally with gestational age. Twin gestation, multiple births, or vaginal delivery may result in lower levels of Mg^{+2}. It is important to note that most methods to assess Mg^{+2} levels measure total Mg^{+2} concentration, while only free Mg^{+2} is biologically active and almost 30% is inactive bound to albumin.

   2. **Total and ionized calcium levels.** Usually hypomagnesemia is associated with hypocalcemia, and hypercalcemia may inhibit magnesium reabsorption in the distal loop of Henle and cause hypomagnesemia.

G. **Prevention.** Adequate intake of magnesium should be assured in parenteral and enteral nutrition to prevent hypomagnesemia (recommend 8–15 mg/kg/d).

H. **Management.** **Acute hypomagnesemia should be treated with intravenous magnesium sulfate** (see Chapter 148 for specific dosing guidelines). Infusion must be monitored closely for cardiac arrhythmias and hypotension. Maintenance Mg^{+2} can be by parenteral nutrition solutions or by oral feeds with 5-fold dilution of Mg^{+2} salt solution. Mg^{+2} infusion should be used cautiously if patient has impaired renal function due to its accumulated toxicity.

I. **Prognosis.** Hypomagnesemia generally has good outcome if diagnosed promptly and treated adequately. The exception is a clinical presentation that includes hypomagnesemia-induced seizures with follow-up studies suggesting ≥20% incidence of neurologic abnormalities.

II. **Hypermagnesemia**

A. **Definition.** Reference levels of serum magnesium signifying hypermagnesemia vary from >1.15 mmol/L (2.3 mg/dL) to >1.5 mmol/L (3.0 mg/dL).

B. **Incidence.** Largely unknown, however, it occurs more frequently in infants whose mothers have been treated with magnesium sulfate. Otherwise, it occurs rarely in healthy newborns. There have been 5 trials over the past decade, which included a total of 6145 patients, to study the effects of magnesium sulfate as neuroprotection to reduce the incidence of cerebral palsy in neonates. Two published meta-analyses analyzed these trials and concluded that there is enough evidence to support the use of magnesium sulfate for reducing cerebral palsy. The American College of Obstetrics and Gynecology and Australian national guidelines have recommended the prenatal administration of magnesium sulfate as neuroprotection for preterm infants. This new trend of magnesium sulfate use may increase the incidence of hypermagnesemia in preterm infants being admitted to neonatal units.

C. **Pathophysiology.** Increased serum Mg^{+2} levels depress the central nervous system, impair electrical conduction, and decrease skeletal muscle contractility. Antenatal magnesium sulfate administration to mothers before preterm delivery may have a neuroprotective role and decreased incidence of cerebral palsy in infants. Magnesium may serve as an N-methyl-D-aspartate (NMDA) receptor antagonist, membrane stabilizer, vasodilator, and anticonvulsive. Mg^{+2} also has anticonvulsive properties (by blocking neuromuscular transmission and decreasing the amount of acetylcholine liberated at the end plate by the motor nerve impulse) that may contribute to diminish extension of brain damage. Mg^{+2} may reduce vascular instability, prevent hypoxic damage, and mitigate cytokine or excitatory amino acid damage, all of which threaten the vulnerable preterm brain.

D. **Risk factors**

   1. **Increased maternal serum levels** following magnesium sulfate therapy for pregnancy-related hypertension, preeclampsia, and neonatal neuroprotection before preterm delivery.

   2. **Excessive magnesium sulfate administration** to an infant with hypomagnesemia (iatrogenic medication error) or following administration of Mg^{+2}-containing antacids, especially if dehydrated. Excess magnesium in total parenteral nutrition (TPN) is a cause.

E. **Clinical presentation.** Severity of symptoms and signs of hypermagnesemia may not correlate with serum Mg^{+2} levels. Symptoms may mimic hypercalcemia.
   1. Hypotonia, hypotension, hyporeflexia, seizures
   2. Respiratory depression, hypoventilation, apnea
   3. Bradycardia, hypotension, cardiac arrest with toxic Mg^{+2} levels (ie, >7.5 mmol/L)
   4. Poor suck, feeding intolerance, decreased gastrointestinal motility, increased gastric aspirates, abdominal distention, and delayed meconium passage
   5. Meconium plug syndrome, intestinal perforation
   6. Urinary retention
F. **Diagnosis**
   1. **Laboratory studies**
      a. **Serum magnesium.** Normal levels are 0.6–1.0 mmol/L (1.6–2.4 mg/dL).
      b. **Serum calcium.** Always determine both total and ionized calcium levels with Mg^{+2} abnormalities.
   2. **Electrocardiogram.** May reveal a prolonged PR interval, increased QRS interval, prolonged QT interval, and AV block.
G. **Management**
   1. **Identify and remove the source of excess magnesium** (ie, TPN, antacids).
   2. **Urinary excretion** is the only mechanism for decreasing serum Mg^{+2} levels.
   3. **Maintain IV hydration** if the patient is symptomatic.
   4. **Furosemide diuresis** may facilitate Mg excretion, but close monitoring of electrolytes is needed and its effect is not well studied.
   5. **Monitor serum electrolytes,** urine output, and acid-base status.
   6. **With acute signs such as seizures or electrocardiogram (ECG) changes,** give IV calcium gluconate in doses as for hypocalcemia (page 578).
   7. **Avoid aminoglycosides** as they may potentiate the neuromuscular manifestations of hypermagnesemia.
   8. **Respiratory support** may be needed in severely affected infants (hypoventilation, apnea).
   9. **Exchange transfusion** has been used. Dialysis is uncommon in neonates.
H. **Prognosis** is good following treatment, especially if normal renal function has been preserved. In general, antenatal use of magnesium sulfate is very safe in the postnatal period. It has been successfully used in multiple trials, but in 1 recent study, increased mortality in neonates has been reported with the use of magnesium sulfate administration for neuroprotection.

Selected References

Basu SK, Chickajajur V, Lopez V, Bhutada A, Pagala M, Rastogi S. Immediate clinical outcome in preterm infants receiving antenatal magnesium for neuroprotection. *J Perinat Med.* 2011;40(2):185–189.

Doyle LW, Crowther CA, Middleton P, Marret S, Rouse D. Magnesium sulphate for women at risk of preterm birth for neuroprotection of the fetus. *Cochrane Database Syst Rev.* 2009;(1):CD004661.

Rigo J, Mohamed MW, De Curtis M. Disorders of calcium, phosphorus and magnesium metabolism. In: Martin RJ, Fanaroff AA, Walsh MC, eds. *Fanaroff & Martin's Neonatal-Perinatal Medicine: Diseases of the Fetus and Infant.* 9th ed. Philadelphia, PA: Elsevier Mosby; 2011:1523–1555.

Schulpis KH, Karakonstantakis T, Vlachos GD, et al. Maternal-neonatal magnesium and zinc serum concentrations after vaginal delivery. *Scand J Clin Lab Invest.* 2010;70(7):465–469.

VII. **Management**
  A. **Prenatal management.** The key to management of meconium aspiration lies in prevention of fetal distress during the prenatal period.
    1. **Identification of high-risk pregnancies.** The approach to prevention begins with recognition of predisposing maternal factors that may cause uteroplacental insufficiency and subsequent fetal hypoxia during labor. In pregnancies that continue past the due date, induction as early as 41 weeks may help prevent meconium aspiration. (Risk of MAS is highest in those infants with gestational age >41 weeks).
    2. **Monitoring.** During labor, careful observation and fetal monitoring should be performed. Any signs of fetal distress (eg, appearance of meconium-stained fluid, loss of beat-to-beat variability, fetal tachycardia, or deceleration patterns) warrant assessment of fetal well-being by scrutiny of fetal heart tracings and fetal scalp pH. If the assessment identifies a compromised fetus, corrective measures should be undertaken or the infant should be delivered in a timely manner.
    3. **Amnioinfusion.** In mothers with moderate or thick MSAF, amnioinfusion is effective in reducing the occurrence of variable fetal heart rate decelerations by relieving umbilical cord compression during labor. However, its efficiency in altering the risk or severity of meconium aspiration has not been well demonstrated except in settings with limited perinatal surveillance. In this setting, amnioinfusion is associated with substantial improvements in perinatal outcomes.
  B. **Delivery room management.** Chapter 3 discusses the delivery room management of the meconium-stained infant. The appropriate intervention in an infant born through meconium-stained fluid depends on whether the infant is "vigorous," as demonstrated by spontaneous respirations, a heart rate >100 beats/min, spontaneous movements, or extremities in a flexion position. For those vigorous infants, routine care only should be provided regardless of the meconium consistency. Those infants who are depressed or who show signs of airway obstruction from thick MSAF should be intubated as quickly as feasible and the endotracheal tube connected to a meconium trap aspirator attached to wall suction at a pressure of 100 mm Hg. Positive pressure ventilation should be avoided, if possible, until tracheal suctioning is accomplished.
  C. **Management of the newborn with meconium aspiration.** Infants with meconium below the vocal cords are at risk for pulmonary hypertension, air leak syndromes, and pneumonitis and must be observed closely for signs of respiratory distress.
    1. **General management.** Infants who have aspirated meconium and require resuscitation often develop metabolic abnormalities such as hypoxia, acidosis, hypoglycemia, and hypocalcemia. Because these patients may have suffered perinatal asphyxia, surveillance for any end-organ damage is essential.
      a. **Maintain a neutral thermal environment.**
      b. **Minimal handling protocol to avoid agitation.**
      c. **Maintain adequate blood pressure and perfusion.** Volume expansion may be necessary with normal saline or packed red blood cells if warranted. Vasopressor support such as dopamine may be necessary.
      d. **Correct any metabolic abnormalities** such as hypoglycemia, hypocalcemia, or metabolic acidosis.
      e. **Sedation** may be needed in infants on mechanical ventilation.
    2. **Respiratory management**
      a. **Pulmonary toilet.** If suctioning the trachea does not result in clearing of secretions, it may be advisable to leave an endotracheal tube in place in symptomatic infants for pulmonary toilet. Chest physiotherapy every 30 minutes to 1 hour, as tolerated, will aid in clearing the airway (*controversial*). Chest physiotherapy is contraindicated in labile infants when associated PPHN is suspected.
      b. **Arterial blood gas levels.** On admission to the neonatal intensive care unit, arterial blood gas measurements to assess ventilatory compromise and supplemental oxygen requirements should be obtained. If the patient requires >0.4

FIO_2 or demonstrates pronounced lability, an arterial catheter for frequent sampling should be inserted.

c. **Oxygen monitoring.** A pulse oximeter provides important information regarding the severity of the infant's respiratory status and also assists in preventing hypoxemia. Comparing oxygen saturation values from a pulse oximeter on the right arm to those placed on the lower extremities may help identify those infants with right-to-left ductal shunting secondary to MAS-associated pulmonary hypertension.

d. **Chest radiograph.** A chest radiograph should be obtained after delivery if the infant is in distress. It may also help determine which patients will experience respiratory distress. However, radiographs often poorly correlate with the clinical presentation.

e. **Antibiotic coverage.** Although meconium is sterile, it inhibits the normally bacteriostatic quality of amniotic fluid. MAS alone is not an indication for antibiotic therapy. However, because it is difficult to differentiate meconium aspiration from pneumonia radiographically, infants with infiltrates on a chest radiograph should be started on broad-spectrum antibiotics (ampicillin and gentamicin; for dosages, see Chapter 148) after appropriate cultures have been obtained.

f. **Supplemental oxygen.** A major goal is to prevent episodes of alveolar hypoxia leading to hypoxic pulmonary vasoconstriction and the development of PPHN. For that purpose, supplemental oxygen is provided "generously," to maintain the arterial oxygen tension at least in the range of 80–90 mm Hg. Some clinicians may elect to maintain Pao_2 at a higher level because the risk of retinopathy should be negligible among full-term infants. The same goal of preventing alveolar hypoxia requires cautious weaning from oxygen therapy. Many of the patients are very labile, and weaning from oxygen should be made slowly, sometimes at a pace of 1% at a time. The prevention of alveolar hypoxia includes a high index of suspicion for the diagnosis of air leak as well as efforts to minimize handling of the child.

g. **Continuous positive airway pressure (CPAP).** This can be used to improve oxygenation if the FIO_2 exceeds 40–50%. If hyperinflation is present, use CPAP cautiously since it can make air trapping worse.

h. **Mechanical ventilation.** Patients with severe disease who are in impending respiratory failure with hypercapnia and persistent hypoxemia require mechanical ventilation.

 i. **Specific ventilatory strategies.** Ventilation must be tailored to the individual patient. Volume-targeted ventilation may decrease lung over-distension. The use of relatively short inspiratory time may further limit potential air trapping. Modes of ventilation that allow the infant to regulate the frequency and degree of mechanical assistance (assist/control or pressure support ventilation) may be preferable. Infants with MAS typically require higher pressures and faster rates than those with respiratory distress syndrome.

 ii. **Pulmonary complications.** With the development of atelectasis, air trapping, and decreased lung compliance, high mean airway pressures may be required in a patient who is at risk for air leak. For any unexplained deterioration of clinical status, the possibility of a **pneumothorax** or **pneumomediastinum** should be considered and appropriate evaluation undertaken. The approach to ventilation must be directed at preventing hypoxemia and providing adequate ventilation at the lowest mean airway pressure possible to reduce the risk of catastrophic air leak.

 iii. **High-frequency ventilation (HFV).** Randomized controlled trials supporting the use of HFV specifically for MAS are lacking. Other prospective studies have demonstrated that HFV can be an effective modality. Both high-frequency jet ventilation and high-frequency oscillatory ventilation are efficacious in infants in whom adequate ventilation cannot be maintained on conventional ventilation without using excessive ventilatory pressures. HFV has also been used to maximize the beneficial effects of inhaled nitric oxide (see Chapter 8).

iv. **Heliox ventilation.** In a limited study, the use of heliox was associated with improved oxygenation but failed to demonstrate significant improvement in other outcomes, including oxygenation index, survival, or degree of respiratory support, beyond the reduction in F_{IO_2}

i. **Surfactant.** A number of randomized controlled trials have shown that infants with severe MAS who require mechanical ventilation and have radiologic evidence of parenchymal lung disease are likely to benefit from early surfactant therapy. Doses may exceed those used for preterm infants with respiratory distress syndrome. Because of the potential for concomitant pulmonary hypertension, close observation is required to prevent the consequences of transient airway obstruction that may develop during the tracheal instillation of surfactant. Surfactant lavage has been shown to decrease the overall oxygen requirement. Current clinical trials have failed to demonstrate a statistically significant impact on other outcome measures but did demonstrate a trend toward improved survival. Surfactant lavage has also been shown to decrease systemic proinflammatory cytokines that normally accompany MAS.

j. **Inhaled nitric oxide.** Pulmonary hypertension commonly affects infants with severe MAS. This can be effectively treated by inhaled nitric oxide (see Chapter 120). In an update of an earlier Cochrane System Review, data suggest that in settings without access to nitric oxide or HFV, sildenafil has been shown to be effective in reducing PVR and improving oxygenation and decreasing mortality.

k. **Extracorporeal membrane oxygenation/extracorporeal life support (ECMO/ECLS).** The use of inhaled nitric oxide and surfactant therapy has decreased the number of infants who go on to require ECMO/ECLS. Compared with other population subsets that require ECMO/ECLS, infants with meconium aspiration have a high survival rate (93–100%). (See Chapter 18.)

l. **Steroids.** Although some animal data and limited human trials suggest a potential benefit, there are not sufficient data to warrant the use of steroids. Some human trials suggest that steroid therapy for MAS may be harmful. Until sufficient data are available, steroids should not be employed as a therapeutic measure for MAS.

3. **Persistent pulmonary hypertension.** Meconium aspiration is the most common respiratory disorder associated with PPHN. It occurred in ~40% of cases. (See Chapter 120.)

D. **Prognosis.** Complications are common and associated with significant mortality. New modalities of therapy such as administration of exogenous surfactant, HFV, inhaled nitric oxide, and ECMO/ECLS have reduced the mortality to <5%. In patients surviving severe meconium aspiration, bronchopulmonary dysplasia/chronic lung disease may result from prolonged mechanical ventilation. MAS is associated with neurodevelopmental sequela, including global developmental delay, cerebral palsy, and autism, and therefore warrants long-term follow-up.

Selected References

Beligere N, Rao R. Neurodevelopmental outcome of infants with meconium aspiration syndrome: report of a study and literature review. *J Perinatol.* 2008;28:s93–s101.

Dargaville PA, Copnell B, Mills JF, et al. Randomized controlled trial of lung lavage with dilute surfactant for meconium aspiration syndrome. *J Pediatr.* 2011;158:383–389.

De Luca D, Minucci A, Tripodi D, et al. Role of distinct phospholipases A2 and their modulators in meconium aspiration syndrome in human neonates. *Intensive Care Med.* 2011;37:1158–1165.

Gardener H, Spiegelman D, Buka SL. Perinatal and neonatal risk factors for autism: a comprehensive meta-analysis. *Pediatrics.* 2011;128:344–355.

Hernderson-Smart DJ, De Paoli AG, Clark RH, Bhuta T. High frequency oscillatory ventilation versus conventional ventilation for infants with severe pulmonary dysfunction born at or near term. *Cochrane Database Syst Rev.* 2009;CD002974.

Hofmeyr GJ, Xu H. Amnioinfusion for meconium-stained liquor in labour. *Cochrane Database Syst Rev.* 2010;CD000014.

Raghavendran K, Willson D, Notter RH. Surfactant therapy for acute lung injury and acute respiratory distress syndrome. *Crit Care Clin.* 2011;27:525–559.

Shah PS, Ohlsson A. Sildenafil for pulmonary hypertension in neonates. *Cochrane Database Syst Rev.* 2011;CD005494.

Szczapa T, Gadzinowski J. Use of heliox in the management of neonates with meconium aspiration syndrome. *Neonatology.* 2011;100:265–270.

109 Meningitis

I. **Definition.** Neonatal meningitis is an infection of the meninges and central nervous system (CNS) in the first month of life. This is the most common time of life for meningitis to occur.

II. **Incidence.** The incidence is ~0.16–0.45 per 1000 live births in developed countries. The incidence may be higher in underdeveloped countries.

III. **Pathophysiology.** In most cases, infection occurs because of hematogenous seeding of the meninges and CNS. In cases of CNS or spinal anomalies (eg, myelomeningocele), there may be direct inoculation by flora on the skin or in the environment. Neonatal meningitis is often accompanied by **ventriculitis**, which makes resolution of infection more difficult. There is also a predilection for vasculitis, which may lead to hemorrhage, thrombosis, and infarction. Subdural effusions and brain abscess may also complicate the course.

Most organisms implicated in neonatal sepsis also cause neonatal meningitis. Some have a definite predilection for CNS infection. **Group B *Streptococcus* (GBS)** (especially type III) and the **gram-negative rods** (especially *Escherichia coli* with K1 antigen) are the **most common causative agents**. Galactosemia should be considered if *E. coli* is the causative agent in late-onset meningitis. Other causative organisms include *Listeria monocytogenes* (serotype IVb), other streptococci (enterococci, *Streptococcus pneumoniae*), other gram-negative enteric bacilli (*Klebsiella, Enterobacter,* and *Serratia* spp), and rarely *Neisseria meningitides.* In the very low birthweight infant, coagulase-negative staphylococci need to be considered as causative organisms in bacterial meningitis.

With CNS anomalies involving open defects or indwelling devices (eg, ventriculoperitoneal shunts), staphylococcal disease (*Staphylococcus aureus* and *Staphylococcus epidermidis*) is more common, as is disease caused by other skin flora, including streptococci and diphtheroids. Many unusual organisms, including *Ureaplasma*, fungi, and anaerobes, have been described in case reports of neonatal meningitis.

IV. **Risk factors.** Premature infants with sepsis have a much higher incidence (up to 3-fold) than term infants of CNS infection. The characteristics of some bacteria make them more virulent, especially for neonates (eg, capsular polysaccharide of GBS type III, *E. coli* K1, and *L. monocytogenes* serotype IVb all contain sialic acid in high concentrations). Infants with CNS defects necessitating ventriculoperitoneal shunt procedures also are at increased risk.

V. **Clinical presentation.** The clinical presentation is usually nonspecific and indistinguishable from those caused by sepsis. Meningitis must be excluded in any infant being evaluated for sepsis or infection. Signs and symptoms of meningitis include temperature instability (the most common), lethargy, irritability, poor tone, seizures, feeding intolerance, vomiting, respiratory distress, apnea, or cyanotic episodes. Seizures, often focal, can be the presenting manifestation in up to 50% of the cases. Late manifestations of meningitis include a bulging anterior fontanelle and coma. Syndrome of inappropriate antidiuretic hormone may accompany meningitis.

VI. **Diagnosis**

A. **Laboratory studies.** The clinical presentation of bacterial meningitis in the neonate is nonspecific; therefore, neonates with suspected bacterial meningitis should undergo a full sepsis evaluation including a complete blood count with differential, blood culture, urine culture (if >3–5 days), and lumbar puncture (LP) to examine cerebrospinal fluid (CSF) for Gram stain, culture, protein, glucose, and cell count. CSF examination is critical in the investigation of possible meningitis and the only way to confirm the diagnosis. Approximately 15–50% of all infants with positive CSF cultures for bacteria have negative blood cultures. The technique for obtaining CSF fluid and CSF normal values are discussed in Chapter 35.

1. **Culture.** A **CSF culture is the gold standard** for the diagnosis of bacterial meningitis. It may be positive in association with a normal or minimally abnormal CSF analysis.

2. **CSF pleocytosis** is variable. There are usually more cells with gram-negative rods than with GBS disease. Normal values range from 0 to 35 white blood cells (WBCs), some of which may be polymorphonuclear cells. Traumatic LP (>500 red cells/mm^3) occur in up to 40% of the attempts, and adjustment of CSF white cells down to account for increased red cells does not improve diagnostic utility of the CSF examination. Reactive pleocytosis may be seen secondary to CNS hemorrhage.

3. **Gram-stained smear** can be helpful in making a more rapid definitive diagnosis and identifying the initial classification of the causative agent.

4. **Decreased CSF glucose.** CSF glucose level must be compared with serum glucose level. Normal CSF values are one-half to two-thirds of serum values. Typically, neonates with meningitis have CSF glucose level <20–30 mg/dL.

5. **CSF protein** is usually elevated (>100–150 mg/dL), although normal values for infants, especially premature infants, may be much higher than in later life, and the test may be confounded by the presence of blood in the specimen.

B. **Imaging studies** are recommended to detect the complications of meningitis, especially when the clinical course is complicated. Infection with certain microorganisms such as *Citrobacter koseri* and *Enterobacter sakazakii* predispose for the development of brain abscesses. The most useful and noninvasive method of imaging is ultrasonography, which provides information regarding ventricular size, inflammation (echogenic strands), and the presence of hemorrhage. Computed tomography (CT) or magnetic resonance imaging (MRI) are useful in detecting cerebral abscesses and later in the treatment course in identifying areas of encephalomalacia that may dictate prolonged therapy.

VII. **Management.** General supportive measures like ventilation/oxygenation, cardiovascular support, intravenous dextrose, and anticonvulsant therapy are considered essential components of managing the neonate with bacterial meningitis. Isolation precautions for all infectious diseases, including maternal and neonatal precautions, breast-feeding, and visiting issues, can be found in Appendix F.

A. **Drug therapy.** For drug dosages and other pharmacologic information, see Chapter 148. (*Note:* Dosages for ampicillin, nafcillin, and penicillin G are **doubled** when treating meningitis.)

1. **Empirical therapy.** Optimal antibiotic selection depends on culture and sensitivity testing of the causative organisms. **Ampicillin** and **gentamicin** are usually started as empirical therapy for suspected early sepsis. If meningitis is suspected, **cefotaxime** should be added. For hospitalized infants with late-onset presentation, empiric therapy consists of **vancomycin** (cover gram-positive organisms, especially coagulase-negative staphylococci) and **gentamicin** with the addition of **cefotaxime** when CSF findings suggest meningitis (extended coverage of gram-negative rods). Lastly, for the infant <60 days who is coming from home to the emergency department, the empiric therapy consists of **ampicillin** and **cefotaxime**.

2. **Gram-positive meningitis (GBS and *Listeria*).** **Penicillin or ampicillin** is the drug of choice. These infections usually respond well to treatment for 14 days of therapy.

3. **Staphylococcal disease.** Because of the increased prevalence of methicillin-resistant staphylococci both in the nosocomial setting and in the community, **vancomycin** should be substituted for penicillin or ampicillin as initial coverage.

4. **Gram-negative meningitis.** Most clinicians would use **ampicillin plus cefotaxime plus** an **aminoglycoside** as initial therapy. Further therapy is dictated by sensitivity results. "Double" gram-negative coverage is maintained for 10 days after sterility of CSF. Subsequently, cefotaxime can be continued alone to complete 21 days of therapy. There is an emerging problem with multidrug-resistant enteric microorganisms (especially *Klebsiella pneumoniae*); for this situation, the drug of choice is **meropenem**. (See Chapter 148.) Studies have shown no advantage for intrathecal or intraventricular gentamicin.

5. **Repeat lumbar puncture 48 hours into antibiotic therapy** is recommended to document CSF sterilization. Persistence of infection may indicate a focus, such as obstructive ventriculitis, subdural empyema, or multiple small-vessel thrombi. Infants with repeat positive CSF cultures after initiation of appropriate antibiotics are at risk for complications as well as a poor outcome. In general, ~3 days are required to sterilize the CSF in infants with gram-negative meningitis, whereas in gram-positive meningitis, sterilization usually occurs within 36–48 hours. Follow-up CSF examination is recommended until sterility is documented. External ventricular drainage may be indicated in certain cases complicated by ventriculitis. Treatment should continue until 14 days after cultures are negative or for 21 days, whichever is longer.

6. **Adjunctive therapy.** Contrary to childhood meningitis, dexamethasone does not seem to improve the outcome of neonatal meningitis. Other therapies focusing on enhancing the immune system in the newborn, such as hematopoietic growth factors or intravenous immune globulins, do not seem to help either.

B. **Supportive measures and monitoring for complications.** Head circumference should be measured daily, and neurologic examination should be performed frequently. Imaging studies (especially MRI) are helpful for prognosis and guiding the length of therapy. Hearing and vision evaluation should be done in all neonates who develop meningitis. All of them should undergo long-term neurodevelopmental follow-up.

VIII. **Prognosis.** The **mortality rate** has decreased over the past 15 years to 3–13%, compared with 25–30% from earlier decades. There is a higher incidence (20–50%) of neurodevelopmental sequelae in survivors, and this figure has not changed over the years. Factors predictive of death or serious sequelae include preterm birth, neutropenia, seizures persisting more than 72 hours after hospitalization, focal neurologic deficits, initial inotropic support, delayed sterilization of the CSF, and parenchymal lesions (abscess, thrombi, infarcts, and encephalomalacia) on neuroimaging studies.

Selected References

Ansong AK, Smith PB, Benjamin DK, et al. Group B streptococcal meningitis: cerebrospinal fluid parameters in the era of intrapartum antibiotic prophylaxis. *Early Hum Dev.* 2009;85:S5–S7.

Doctor BA, Newman N, Minich NM, Taylor HG, Fanaroff AA, Hack M. Clinical outcomes of neonatal meningitis in very-low birth-weight infants. *Clin Pediatr.* 2001;40:473–480.

Gaschignard J, Levy C, Romain O, et al. Neonatal bacterial meningitis: 444 cases in 7 years. *Pediatr Infect Dis J.* 2011;30(3):212–217.

Greenberg RG, Benjamin DK Jr, Cohen-Wolkowiez M, et al. Repeat lumbar punctures in infants with meningitis in the neonatal intensive care unit. *J Perinatol.* 2011;31(6): 425–429.

Greenberg RG, Smith PB, Cotten CM, Moody MA, Clark RH, Benjamin DK Jr. Traumatic lumbar punctures in neonates: test performance of the cerebrospinal fluid white blood cell count. *Pediatr Infect Dis J.* 2008;27:1047–1051.

Heath PT, Nik Yusoff NK, Baker CJ. Neonatal meningitis. *Arch Dis Child Fetal Neonatal Ed.* 2003;88:F173–F178.

Malbon K, Mohan R, Nicholl R. Should a neonate with possible late onset infection always have a lumbar puncture? *Arch Dis Child.* 2006;91:75–76.

Philip AG. Neonatal meningitis in the new millennium. *NeoReviews.* 2003;4:e73–e80.

Smith PB, Cotten CM, Garges HP, et al. Comparison of neonatal gram-negative rod and gram-positive cocci meningitis. *J Perinatol.* 2006;26:111–114.

110 Methicillin-Resistant *Staphylococcus aureus* Infections

I. **Definition.** Infection with methicillin-resistant *Staphylococcus aureus* (**MRSA**) (**clustered gram-positive cocci**) causes a variety of localized and invasive suppurative infections and toxin-mediated syndromes such as toxic shock syndrome and scalded skin syndrome. MRSA infections used to be limited to health care facilities (HC-MRSA) and were strictly nosocomial; however, a significant increase in community-acquired MRSA (CA-MRSA) has been seen in the last decade. The separation between HC-MRSA and CA-MRSA is becoming less distinct, as CA-MRSA is becoming more virulent and causing significantly more health care–associated infections.

II. **Incidence.** The methicillin-sensitive *Staphylococcus aureus* normally colonizes the nose, umbilicus, and the groin area by 1 week of age, with a colonization rate of 20–90%. Maternal anogenital colonization with MRSA ranges from 0.5% to 10.4%, with little risk for early-onset disease in the newborn. There are several documented outbreaks of invasive CA-MRSA that developed in healthy newborn infants discharged from normal newborn nurseries as well as neonatal intensive care units (NICUs). The majority of MRSA infections in the NICU are of late onset. According to neonatal data reported from National Nosocomial Infections Surveillance System for the years 1995–2004, MRSA accounted for 23% of all hospital-associated *S. aureus* infections. The incidence of MRSA infections per 100,000 patient-days increased by 308% during the study period from 0.7 in 1995 to 3.1 in 2004. The NICU colonization rate is variable; one study showed a rate of 10.4%, with a mean time to acquire MRSA of 17 days.

III. **Pathophysiology.** If the newborn infant is exposed to MRSA, whether from the community or the hospital, then he or she will be colonized with more virulent strains that are more likely to cause invasive disease. MRSA has specific virulence factors that make it more invasive than methicillin-sensitive *S. aureus*. These include staphylococcal chromosome cassette (SCC) *mecA*, Panton-Valentine leukocidin (PVL), and staphylococcal enterotoxins. The SCC *mecA* has the genes that encode antibiotic resistance. PVL genes lead to the production of cytotoxins that form pores in the cellular membrane and cause tissue necrosis and cell lysis.

IV. **Risk factors.** Include overcrowding, inconsistent hand washing, invasive procedures (eg, central lines, endotracheal intubations, nasogastric tubes), low birthweight, the practice of kangaroo (skin-to-skin) mother care, a high MRSA colonization rate, and prolonged hospital stay.

V. **Clinical presentations.** Invasive MRSA disease is likely to be preceded by colonization (skin, umbilicus, and nasopharynx). The source of the bacteria could be a health care worker, another patient, equipment, or a family member.

A. **Bloodstream infections.** These are usually catheter related. Common clinical signs are nonspecific and include apnea or hypoxia, fever, elevated C-reactive protein, and leukocytosis. The infant needs to be examined repeatedly and meticulously for subtle clues of focal infection (eg, phlebitis, pustulosis).

B. **Septic arthritis and osteomyelitis.** *Staphylococcus aureus* is the primary cause of septic arthritis and osteomyelitis in the neonate. Symptoms are nonspecific, such as poor feeding or increased irritability. Signs include soft tissue swelling and erythema.

C. **Endocarditis.** Neonates with congenital heart disease and percutaneous central catheters are at a higher risk for endocarditis.

D. **Skin and soft tissue infections.** *Staphylococcus aureus* is the most common pathogen causing pustulosis and cellulitis in the neonate. MRSA has virulence factors that contribute to the pathogen's ability to damage the neonatal skin that is already compromised.

E. **Conjunctivitis.** See Chapter 53.

F. **Pneumonia.** Pneumonia can be primary or associated with ventilator therapy. The course is frequently complicated by alveolar necrosis, pneumatocele formation, and pleural empyema.

G. **Surgical site infections.**

VI. **Diagnosis.** The **gold standard for diagnosing a bloodstream infection is a positive blood culture.** Diagnosing arthritis and osteomyelitis can be challenging. In addition to a blood culture, the workup should include a joint aspirate, bone culture (if surgical debridement is done), radiography, and possibly magnetic resonance imaging. Echocardiography (to diagnose endocarditis) is strongly recommended in infants with >1 positive blood culture. For skin and soft tissue infections, incision and drainage, with subsequent Gram stain and culture of aspirated fluid, is recommended. Real-time polymerase chain reaction (PCR) has been used recently for active surveillance of MRSA in the NICU; however, studies have shown PCR to have low reproducibility, low positive predictive value, and high false-positive rate. Therefore, PCR should not be used for screening MRSA in the NICU.

VII. **Management**

A. **Eradication of colonization.** Adult intensive care unit studies demonstrated that eradication of MRSA colonization using a combination of 5 days of intranasal mupirocin and 3 daily chlorhexidine baths resulted in reducing MRSA infections. There are no studies in neonates showing similar efficacy; however, mupirocin has been used effectively in controlling outbreaks of MRSA in NICU populations.

B. **Antibiotic therapy.** The Infectious Diseases Society of America issued guidelines for the management of invasive MRSA infections in adults and children including infants ≤30 days of age. Vancomycin is the first-line therapy for MRSA, and many NICUs with endemic MRSA use vancomycin as an empirical therapy for late-onset sepsis while awaiting culture results. In cases of vancomycin intermediate

S. aureus (VISA) or vancomycin allergy, linezolid and clindamycin have been used effectively. Treatment duration depends on the specific infection. For **skin and soft tissue infections** and **bacteremia**, a 7- to 10-day course is generally appropriate. In cases of **endocarditis** and **osteomyelitis**, 6–8 weeks of treatment is necessary. In patients with **extensive disease with persistently positive blood cultures** despite therapeutic doses of vancomycin, both rifampin and gentamicin can be used for synergy. Mupirocin may be adequate for mild cases of localized neonatal pustulosis in the well-appearing full-term infant.

VIII. Prevention

   A. **Hand hygiene.** The Centers for Disease Control and Prevention recommends using an alcohol-based hand sanitizer before touching patients, after touching patients, after removing gloves, and after touching the patient care environment and equipment due to the ability of MRSA to survive on inanimate objects. Alcohol-based hand sanitizers improve compliance with hand hygiene policies as well as improve the skin integrity of health care workers.

   B. **Controlling outbreaks.** During an outbreak, many measures are instituted concurrently. In 2006, Gerber et al released a consensus statement from the Chicago Department of Public Health on the management of outbreaks of MRSA in a NICU. Their recommendations included an alcohol-based rub for hand hygiene, isolation and cohorting of MRSA-colonized infants, and regular neonatal surveillance cultures (Table 110–1). They also emphasized the use of molecular typing as an integral part of control because it can determine the ongoing transmission of a particular clone. They did not make a recommendation for decolonization with mupirocin; this intervention was left to the discretion of the primary clinical care team because the efficacy of this strategy is uncertain. Passive protection of neonates by using the monoclonal antibody tefibazumab, which binds to the surface-expressed adhesion protein clumping factor A, has not proven to be efficacious.

Table 110–1. GUIDELINES FOR OUTBREAKS OF METHICILLIN-RESISTANT *STAPHYLOCOCCUS AUREUS* IN THE NICU

Recommendation Type, Rating Category[a]	Consensus Recommendation
Hand hygiene	
IA	A waterless, alcohol-based hand hygiene product should be made available and easily accessible; soap and water should be used if hands are visibly soiled.
IA	Monitoring of hand hygiene is a key component in preventing MRSA transmission in the NICU. Direct observations of hand hygiene practices on a regular basis, or consistent enforcement of proper hand hygiene (eg, use of a unit guard, providing feedback), contribute to increased rates of compliance.
Cohorting and isolation	
IA	MRSA-positive infants should be placed under contact precautions and cohorted (placed in a designated room or area), as should the supplies used in the care of these infants.
IA	Gloves and gowns should be worn when caring for or visiting infants known or suspected to be MRSA positive.
IA	Masks should be worn for aerosol-generating procedures, such as suctioning. The environment in the area of the infant should be kept clean and neat at all times.

(Continued)

Table 110–1. GUIDELINES FOR OUTBREAKS OF METHICILLIN-RESISTANT *STAPHYLOCOCCUS AUREUS* IN THE NICU (*CONTINUED*)

Recommendation Type, Rating Category[a]	Consensus Recommendation
NR/UI	Disposal of infant supplies used in the care of the MRSA-positive cohort should be decided by the institution's infection control experts.
IA	Whenever possible, nurses should be cohorted (designated exclusively) for care of MRSA-positive infants. Other HCWs should also be cohorted to the maximum extent allowed by the institution's resources.
II	If cohorting of nurses is not possible, nurses should care for the non-cohorted patients before working with the cohorted neonates, when feasible.
II	The number of people (including HCWs and visitors) who enter a room or area designated for MRSA-positive infants should be limited to the minimum possible.
II	Cohorting of infants should be maintained until the last infected or colonized infant has been discharged from the NICU.

Neonatal surveillance cultures

IB	Infants in the NICU should be screened periodically to detect MRSA colonization. The frequency of screening should increase (eg, to once per week) when clusters of colonization are detected; after evidence suggests a halt in transmission, it may decrease to a lower frequency (eg, to once per month) until the investigation is over.
IA	Although cultures of swab specimens from multiple body sites, including nares, throat, rectum, and umbilicus, have been used to detect MRSA colonization, culture of nasal or nasopharyngeal specimens alone is sufficiently sensitive to detect MRSA colonization in neonates.

Screening of HCWs

IB	Screening of HCWs in response to a cluster of MRSA colonization or infection in the NICU should be performed only to corroborate or refute epidemiologic data that link an HCW to transmission.

Decolonization

IB	Mupirocin may be used for decolonization of neonates and/or HCWs if deemed necessary by the affected institution (off-label use).

Environmental cultures

IA	Environmental cultures should be performed in response to a cluster of MRSA colonization or infection in the NICU only to corroborate or refute epidemiologic data that link an environmental source to transmission.

Molecular analysis

IA	When investigating an outbreak, molecular analysis with pulsed-field gel electrophoresis or a comparable molecular epidemiologic tool should be performed to assess the relatedness of strains found in NICU patients, HCWs, and the environment.
IB	If the hospital cannot perform genotyping in-house, then the isolates should be sent to a suitable laboratory for molecular analysis.

(*Continued*)

Table 110–1. **GUIDELINES FOR OUTBREAKS OF METHICILLIN-RESISTANT *STAPHYLOCOCCUS AUREUS* IN THE NICU (*CONTINUED*)**

Recommendation Type, Rating Category[a]	Consensus Recommendation
Communication	
II	Open communication between regional NICUs is essential to prevent spread between NICUs at different institutions, particularly when an infant is transferred from one NICU to another.
II	In the intake of a transferred patient, the receiving facility should be able to determine whether the infant has been screened previously for MRSA, and if so, the date, specimen source, and result of the culture.
II	In the intake of a transferred patient, the receiving facility should be able to determine whether the transferring institution currently knows of any MRSA-positive infants in its NICU.
IB	The receiving facility should consider isolation and screening of any infant transferred from another NICU, regardless of the transferring institution's MRSA status.
II	Standardized instruction sheets describing methods to prevent transmission of MRSA should be developed as a resource for parents and visitors of infants in NICUs in which MRSA has been detected.
Regulation	
IA	Overcrowding increases the likelihood of MRSA transmission in the NICU; institutions should adhere to all appropriate licensing requirements.
IA	Agency HCWs should be oriented to and monitored periodically for compliance with the institution's infection control and hand hygiene procedures.
II	Logs of shifts worked by agency HCWs should be updated frequently to ensure that, in the case of an epidemiologic investigation, transmission links to these staff may be evaluated.
IC	Hospitals must comply with all local and state regulations regarding the reporting of MRSA in NICUs.
Hospital and public health collaboration	
II	Hospital officials should collaborate with state and local public health officials to conduct surveillance for MRSA in NICUs, facilitate interinstitutional communication and coordination of prevention activities, and provide laboratory support to allow detection of shared MRSA clones among NICUs in multiple institutions.

MRSA, methicillin-resistant *Staphylococcus aureus*; NICU, neonatal intensive care unit; HCW, health care worker.

[a] Rating categories are defined as follows. **IA:** Strongly recommended for implementation and strongly supported by well-designed experimental, clinical, or epidemiologic studies. **IB:** Strongly recommended for implementation and supported by some experimental, clinical, or epidemiologic studies and a strong theoretical rationale. **IC:** Required by state or federal regulations, rules, or standards. **II:** Suggested for implementation and supported by suggestive clinical or epidemiologic studies or a theoretical rationale. **NR/UI:** No recommendation or unresolved issue for which evidence is insufficient or no consensus regarding efficacy exists. Definitions from Boyce et al.

Reproduced with permission from Gerber SI, Jones RC, Scott MV, et al. Management of outbreaks of methicillin-resistant *Staphylococcus aureus* infection in the neonatal intensive care unit: a consensus statement. *Infect Control Hosp Epidemiol.* 2006;27:139–145.

Selected References

American Academy of Pediatrics. Staphylococcal infections. In: Pickering LK, Baker CJ, Kimberlin DW, Long SS, eds. *Red Book: 2012 Report of the Committee on Infectious Diseases.* 29th ed. Elk Grove Village, IL: American Academy of Pediatrics; 2012:656–657.

Andrews WW, Schelonka R, Waites K, Stamm A, Cliver SP, Moser S. Genital tract methicillin-resistant *Staphylococcus aureus:* risk of vertical transmission in pregnant women. *Obstet Gynecol.* 2008;111:113–118.

Beigi RH. Clinical implications of methicillin-resistant *Staphylococcus aureus* in pregnancy. *Curr Opin Obstet Gynecol.* 2011;23:82–86.

Carey AJ, Duchon J, Della-Latta P, Saiman L. The epidemiology of methicillin-susceptible and methicillin-resistant *Staphylococcus aureus* in a neonatal intensive care unit, 2000-2007. *J Perinatol.* 2010;30:135–139.

Carey AJ, Long SS. *Staphylococcus aureus*: a continuously evolving and formidable pathogen in the neonatal intensive care unit. *Clin Perinatol.* 2010;37:535–546.

Centers for Disease Control and Prevention (CDC). Community-associated methicillin-resistant *Staphylococcus aureus* infection among healthy newborns—Chicago and Los Angeles County, 2004. *MMWR Morb Mortal Wkly Rep.* 2006;55:329–332.

Fortunov RM, Hulten KG, Allen CH, et al. Nasal *Staphylococcus aureus* colonization among mothers of term and late preterm previously healthy neonates with community-acquired *Staphylococcus aureus* infections. *Pediatr Infect Dis J.* 2011;30:74–76.

Gerber SI, Jones RC, Scott MV, et al. Management of outbreaks of methicillin-resistant *Staphylococcus aureus* infection in the neonatal intensive care unit: a consensus statement. *Infect Control Hosp Epidemiol.* 2006;27:139–145.

Lessa FC, Edwards JR, Fridkin SK, Tenover FC, Horan TC, Gorwitz RJ. Trends in incidence of late-onset methicillin-resistant *Staphylococcus aureus* infection in neonatal intensive care units: data from the National Nosocomial Infections Surveillance System, 1995-2004. *Pediatr Infect Dis J.* 2009;28:577–581.

Liu C, Bayer A, Cosgrove SE, et al. Clinical practice guidelines by the Infectious Diseases Society of America for the treatment of methicillin-resistant *Staphylococcus aureus* infections in adults and children. *Clin Infect Dis.* 2011;52:e18–e55.

Maraqa NF, Aigbivbalu L, Masnita-Iusan C, et al. Prevalence of and risk factors for methicillin-resistant *Staphylococcus aureus* colonization and infection among infants at a level III neonatal intensive care unit. *Am J Infect Control.* 2011;39:35–41.

Sarda V, Molloy A, Kadkol S, Janda WM, Hershow R, McGuinn M. Active surveillance for methicillin-resistant *Staphylococcus aureus* in the neonatal intensive care unit. *Infect Control Hosp Epidemiol.* 2009;30:854–860.

Vergnano S, Menson E, Smith Z, et al. Characteristics of invasive *Staphylococcus aureus* in United Kingdom Neonatal Units. *Pediatr Infect Dis J.* 2011;30:850–854.

111 Multiple Gestation

I. **Definition.** A multiple gestation occurs when more than one fetus is carried during a pregnancy.

II. **Incidence.** In 2008, the overall rate of twin births was 32.6 in 1000 live births, and the rate of triplet births was 147.6 in 100,000 live births. The incidence of multiple gestation pregnancies is probably underestimated. Fewer than half of twin pregnancies diagnosed by ultrasonography during the first trimester are delivered as twins, a phenomenon that has been termed **vanishing twin**. Two gestational sacs can be identified with ultrasonography by 6 weeks' gestation. In addition, routine screening for maternal α-fetoprotein (AFP) may identify pregnancies with multiple gestations at an early gestational age. Between 1980 and 2004, the twinning rate climbed 70% (18.9–32.2/100 live births). The rate was stable between 2004 and 2007 but climbed 1% between 2007 and 2008. The rate of triplet births escalated more rapidly, increasing 400% during the 1980s and 1990s with a peak in 1998. Since 1998 there has been a steady reduction in triplet and other higher order multiple births. About a third of twins in the United States are monozygotic. The incidence of monozygotic twinning is constant at 3–5 per 1000 pregnancies, whereas the rate for dizygotic twinning varies from 4–50 per 1000 pregnancies.

III. **Pathophysiology.** Placental classification and determination of zygosity are important in the pathophysiology of twins.

   A. **Classification.** Placental examination affords a unique opportunity to identify two-thirds to three-fourths of monozygotic twins at birth.

      1. **Twin placentation is classified according to the placental disk** (single, fused, or separate), number of chorions (monochorionic or dichorionic), and number of amnions (monoamniotic or diamniotic) (Figure 111–1).

      2. **Heterosexual (assuredly dizygotic) twins** always have a dichorionic placenta.

      3. **Monochorionic twins** are always of the same sex. All monochorionic twins are believed to be monozygotic. In 70% of monozygotic twin pregnancies, the placentas are monochorionic, and the possibility exists for commingling of the fetal circulations. Less than 1% of twin pregnancies are monoamniotic.

   B. **Placental complications.** Twin gestations are associated with an increased frequency of anomalies of the placenta and adnexa, for example, a single umbilical artery or velamentous or marginal cord insertion (6–9 times more common with twin gestation). The cord is more susceptible to trauma from twisting. The vessels near the insertion are often unprotected by Wharton jelly and are especially prone to thrombosis when compression or twisting occurs. Intrapartum fetal distress from cord compression and fetal hemorrhage from associated vasa previa are potential problems with velamentous insertion of the cord.

   C. **Determination of zygosity.** The most efficient way to identify zygosity is as follows:

      1. **Gender examination.** Male-female pairs are dizygotic. The dichorionic placenta may be separate or fused.

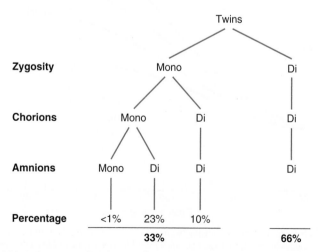

FIGURE 111–1. Percentage distribution of twins according to placental type. Mono, monoamniotic; Di, diamniotic.

2. **Placental examination.** Twins with a monochorionic placenta (monoamniotic or diamniotic) are monozygotic. Care should be taken not to confuse apposed fused placentas for a single chorion. If doubt exists on a gross inspection of the dividing membranes, a transverse section should be studied. The zygosity of twins of the same sex with dichorionic membranes cannot be immediately known. Genetic studies are needed (eg, blood typing, human leukocyte antigen typing, DNA markers, and chromosome marking) to determine zygosity.

IV. **Risk factors.** Use of assisted reproductive technology is a major risk factor for multiple births. The incidence of dizygotic twinning increases with a family history of twins, maternal age (peak at 35–39 years), previous twin gestation, increasing parity, maternal height, fecundity, social class, frequency of coitus, and exposure to exogenous gonadotropins, clomiphene, or in vitro fertilization. The risk of twinning decreases with undernourishment. Ethnic background (African Americans > Caucasians > Asians) is a preconception risk factor for naturally conceived multiple gestation births.

V. **Clinical presentation.** Twins are more likely to have prematurity, intrauterine growth restriction, congenital anomalies, and twin-twin transfusion.

A. **Prematurity and uteroplacental insufficiency.** The major contributors to perinatal complications. In 2008, 1% of singletons, 10% of twins, and 36% of triplets had birthweights of <1500 g.

B. **Intrauterine growth restriction (IUGR).** The incidence of low birthweight in twins is ~50–60%, a figure that is 5–7 times higher than the incidence of low birthweight in singletons. In general, the more fetuses in a gestation, the smaller their weight for gestational age (Figure 111–2). Twins tend to grow at normal rates up to about 30–34 weeks'

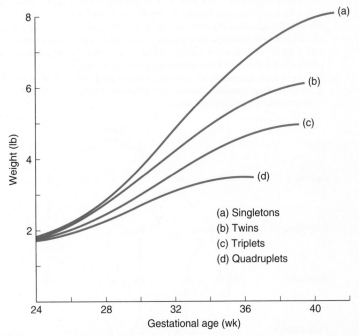

FIGURE 111–2. Growth curve showing the mean weights of infants from single and multiple pregnancies by gestational age. (*Modified from McKeown T, Record RG. Observations of foetal growth in multiple pregnancy in man.* J Endocrinol. *1952;8:386.* Reproduced, with permission, from the Society for Endocrinology.)

gestation when they reach a combined weight of 4 kg. Thereafter, they grow more slowly. Two-thirds of twins show some signs of growth restriction at birth.

C. **Uteroplacental insufficiency.** The incidence of acute and chronic uteroplacental insufficiency is increased in multiple gestations. Five-minute Apgar scores of 0–3 are reported for 5–10% of twin gestations. These low scores may relate to acute stresses of labor, cord prolapse (1–5%), or trauma during delivery superimposed on chronic uteroplacental insufficiency.

D. **Congenital anomalies.** Birth defects are 2 to 3 times more common in monozygotic twins than in singletons or dizygotic twins, who have a 2–3% incidence of major defects diagnosed at birth. Three mechanisms are postulated for the increased frequency of structural defects in monozygotic twins: deformations caused by intrauterine space constraint, disruption of normal blood flow secondary to placental vascular anastomoses, and defects in morphogenesis. Such defects are usually discordant in monozygotic twins; however, in purely genetic conditions (eg, chromosomal abnormalities or single-gene defects), concordance would be the rule. Twins conceived by in vitro fertilization have twice the risk of major congenital anomalies compared with twins conceived naturally.

1. **Anomalies unique to multiple pregnancies.** Certain anomalies, such as conjoined twins and acardia, are unique to multiple pregnancies.

2. **Deformations.** Twins are more likely to suffer from intrauterine crowding and restriction of movement, leading to synostosis, torticollis, facial palsy, positional foot defects, and other defects.

3. **Vascular disruptions.** Disruptions related to monozygotic vascular shunts may result in birth defects. Acardia occurs from an artery-to-artery placental shunt, in which reverse flow leads to the development of an amorphous recipient twin. In utero death of a co-twin may result in a thromboembolic phenomenon, including disseminated intravascular coagulation, cutis aplasia, porencephaly or hydranencephaly, limb reduction defects, intestinal atresias, or gastroschisis.

E. **Twin-twin transfusion syndrome**

1. **Vascular anastomoses.** Almost all monochorionic placentas demonstrate vascular anastomoses, whereas dichorionic placentas rarely do. Vascular anastomoses may be superficial direct communications easily visible on inspection between arteries (most common) or veins (uncommon), deep connections from arteries to veins via villi, or combinations of superficial and deep connections.

2. **Incidence.** Despite the high frequency of vascular anastomosis in monochorionic placentation, the twin-twin transfusion syndrome is relatively uncommon (~15% of monochorionic gestations).

3. **Clinical manifestations.** Clinically, the twin-twin transfusion syndrome is diagnosed when twins have a hemoglobin difference of >5 g/dL and is due to artery-to-vein anastomoses.

   a. **The donor twin** tends to be pale and have a low birthweight, oligohydramnios, anemia, hypoglycemia, decreased organ mass, hypovolemia, and amnion nodosum. Donor twins often require volume expansion, red blood cell transfusion, or both.

   b. **The recipient twin** is frequently plethoric and has a high birthweight, polyhydramnios, polycythemia or hyperviscosity, increased organ mass, hypervolemia, and hyperbilirubinemia. Recipient twins often require partial exchange transfusion.

   c. **Infants born with twin-twin transfusion syndrome** have an increased risk of being diagnosed with antenatally acquired severe cerebral lesions and are at an increased risk of neurodevelopmental sequelae, even when treatment is initiated antenatally. Antenatal treatment with fetoscopic selective laser coagulation may reduce the risk of death or long-term impairment.

   d. **Very low birthweight infants** who are multiple births may have an increased risk of mortality and intraventricular hemorrhage compared with singletons.

VI. **Diagnosis.** Multiple gestation is usually diagnosed prenatally by ultrasound as early as 5 weeks (can see gestational sacs) and by an increased AFP (in twin pregnancies, the average AFP is double that found in a singleton pregnancy).

VII. **Management**

A. **Site of delivery.** When a complicated twin gestation has been identified, delivery should ideally be conducted at a high-risk perinatal center with experienced pediatric delivery teams in attendance.

B. **Physical examination.** Infants should be examined for evidence of intrauterine growth restriction, congenital anomalies, and twin-twin transfusion syndrome. Central hematocrits should be obtained in both infants. When one of the infants has a congenital anomaly, the other twin is at increased risk for complications. In particular, death of one fetus puts the others at risk for fetal disseminated intravascular coagulation.

C. **Complications in newborn period.** The second-born twin is more likely to develop respiratory distress syndrome, bronchopulmonary dysplasia, and die.

D. **Co-bedding of multiples** (*controversial*). Coincident with the rise in multiple births has been an interest in co-bedding of multiples. Although co-bedding multiples has become common practice, the safety or the benefit of this practice has not been definitively established.

E. **Economic considerations.** It has been estimated that the care of assisted reproductive-related preterm infants born in the United States is approximately $1 billion annually.

F. **Risks beyond the neonatal period**

1. **Catch-up growth.** In monozygotic twins, birthweight differences may be as much as 20%, but the lighter twin has a remarkable ability to make up intrauterine growth deficits.

2. **Social problems.** Parents of multiple births may have an increased level of stress and may respond differently to their children compared with singletons. Counseling for parents of twins may be invaluable.

VIII. **Prognosis.** Although perinatal mortality rates for singleton pregnancies have continued to fall during the last decade, there has been little change in mortality rates for multiple pregnancies.

A. **Twins.** The perinatal death rate for twins is 9 times the rate for first-born singletons and 11 times the rate for second-born singletons.

1. **Monoamniotic twins.** Monoamniotic twins have the highest mortality rate among the different types of twins, largely because of cord entanglement.

2. **Monozygotic twins.** Monozygotic twins have a perinatal mortality and morbidity rate that is 2 to 3 times that of dizygotic twins. Diamniotic monochorionic twins have a mortality rate of 25%, and dichorionic twins have a mortality rate of 8.9%.

3. **Fetal death in twins.** When the cause of death is intrinsic to one dichorionic fetus and does not threaten the other fetus, complications are rare. Hazardous intrauterine environments threaten both twins, whether monochorionic or dichorionic. With monochorionic placentas, the incidence of major complications or death in the surviving twin is ~50%.

B. **Triplets.** The neonatal mortality rate for triplets is 18.8%, and the perinatal mortality rate is 25.5%. The risk of death or neurodevelopmental impairment has been shown to be increased in extremely low birthweight triplets and other higher-order multiples compared to singletons (adjusted odds 1.7, 95% confidence intervals 1.3–2.2).

Selected References

Bromer JG, Ata B, Seli M, Lockwood CJ, Seli E. Preterm deliveries that result from multiple pregnancies associated with assisted reproductive technologies in the USA: a cost analysis. *Curr Opin Obstet Gynecol.* 2011;23:168–173.

Hayes EJ, Paul D, Ness A, Mackley A, Berghella V. Very-low-birthweight neonates: do outcomes differ in multiple compared with singleton gestations? *Am J Perinatol.* 2007;24:373–376.

Lopriore E, Middeldorp JM, Sueters M, Oepkes D, Vandenbussche FP, Walther FJ. Long-term neurodevelopmental outcome in twin-to-twin transfusion syndrome treated with fetoscopic laser surgery. *Am J Obstet Gynecol.* 2007;196:231.e1–231.e4.

Lopriore E, van Wezel-Meijler G, Middeldorp JM, Sueters M, Vandenbussche FP, Walther FJ. Incidence, origin, and character of cerebral injury in twin-to-twin transfusion syndrome treated with fetoscopic laser surgery. *Am J Obstet Gynecol.* 2006;194:1215–1220.

Martin JA, Hamilton BE, Sutton PD, Ventura SJ, Mathews TJ, Osterman MJ. Births: final data for 2008. *Natl Vital Stat Rep.* 2010;59:1–72.

Salomon LJ, Ortqvist L, Aegerter P, et al. Long-term developmental follow-up of infants who participated in a randomized clinical trial of amniocentesis vs laser photocoagulation for the treatment of twin-twin transfusion syndrome. *Am J Obstet Gynecol.* 2010;203:e1–e7.

Shinwell ES, Blickstein I, Lusky A, Reichman B. Effect of birth order on neonatal morbidity and mortality among very low birthweight twins: a population based study. *Arch Dis Child Fetal Neonatal Ed.* 2004;89:F145–F148.

Tomashek KM, Wallman C; Committee on Fetus and Newborn, American Academy of Pediatrics. Cobedding twins and higher-order multiples in a hospital setting. *Pediatrics.* 2007;120:1359–1366.

Wadhawan R, Oh W, Vohr BR, et al. Neurodevolopmental outcomes of triplets or higher order extremely low birth weight infants. *Pediatrics.* 2011;127:e654–e660.

112 Myasthenia Gravis (Transient Neonatal)

I. **Definition. Myasthenia gravis** is a neuromuscular disorder affecting synaptic transmission at the motor end plate. It is characterized by abnormal muscle fatigability and can be either genetic or acquired. Infants born with the genetic form of the disease (very rare) are born to healthy mothers and suffer permanent disability. **Transient neonatal myasthenia gravis (TNMG)** is an acquired form of the disease that occurs only in infants born to mothers with myasthenia gravis and is the predominant type and is discussed here.

II. **Incidence.** The incidence of myasthenia gravis varies from 9 to 21 cases per million. **TNMG** is a rare disorder affecting 10–15% of infants born to mothers with myasthenia gravis. There is no race or sex preference. There is no correlation between disease severity in the mother and the clinical outcome of the infant. The risk of disease in a sibling is significantly higher than that of a first born.

III. **Pathophysiology**

   A. **Anti-acetylcholine receptor antibodies.** A total of 75–80% of mothers with myasthenia gravis have anti-acetylcholine receptor (anti-AChR) antibodies. These antibodies cause nicotinic acetylcholine receptor loss by accelerating their degradation, blocking acetylcholine binding, and inducing the lysis of the postsynaptic membrane through induction of the complement system. TNMG is caused by the passive transfer of these maternal antibodies to the fetus. The antibodies can be directed against the fetal acetylcholine receptor (present until 33 weeks' gestation) or the adult receptor. Higher maternal antibody titers directed against the fetal versus the adult acetylcholine receptor has been shown to increase the risk and severity of TNMG.

   B. **Anti–muscle-specific kinase antibodies.** Although anti-AChR antibody–mediated TNMG is the most common cause of the disease, there have been case reports of infants developing TNMG as a result of anti–muscle-specific kinase (anti-MuSK) antibodies. There is some suggestion that this form of TNMG may be more difficult to treat with anticholinesterase agents.

IV. **Risk factors.** See Sections II and III.

V. **Clinical presentation**

A. **Antenatal.** Although rare, neonatal weakness can present in utero, and mothers may comment on reduced fetal movements. Polyhydramnios can be present as a result of poor fetal swallowing. Arthrogryposis multiplex congenita can also rarely occur as a result of decreased fetal movement.

B. **Postnatal.** In 67% of patients symptoms are present within a few hours after birth, and 78% of patients will have symptoms within 24 hours of life. Infants whose mothers have been taking anticholinesterase agents tend to present later than infants whose mothers have not been treated. There have been no known cases with symptoms presenting after day 3 of life. **The majority of patients present with hypotonia and inadequate suck.** Many will have a weak cry, facial diparesis, lack of facial expression, feeding difficulties, and mild respiratory distress. Ptosis and ophthalmoparesis can be present although this is less common. Deep tendon reflexes should still be present.

VI. **Diagnosis.** The key to making the diagnosis is a history of myasthenia gravis in the mother with a symptomatic infant. The diagnosis is confirmed with the use of pharmacologic challenge tests.

A. **Anticholinesterase agents.** To confirm the diagnosis of TNMG, the infant should show a symptomatic improvement after the administration of an anticholinesterase agent. When evaluating the patient, improvement should be defined as the reversal of definite neurologic impairments (usually sucking or swallowing difficulties) or a decrease in ventilatory requirements. Observing for changes in hypotonia or spontaneous motor activity is not as accurate, particularly in premature infants, infants with hypoxic ischemic encephalopathy, or those with intraventricular hemorrhage. When administering these drugs, atropine may be required to help manage the muscarinic side effects (ie, diarrhea and tracheal secretions).

1. **Neostigmine methylsulfate.** Most commonly used diagnostic agent. Consists of a single, 0.15 mg/kg dose administered intramuscularly (IM) or subcutaneously (SC). In a positive test, neurologic improvement is seen 10–15 minutes after administration and persists for 1–3 hours. Muscarinic side effects, in particular, tracheal secretions, can be problematic. False-negative results have been reported.

2. **Edrophonium chloride (Enlon).** Administer 0.15 mg/kg IM or SC or 0.1 mg/kg intravenously (IV). Positive effects are seen within 3 minutes (IV) or 3–5 minutes (IM or SC) and last for 10–15 minutes. Muscarinic side effects are not as severe. Can rarely cause respiratory arrest (especially in larger doses). False-negative results are known, particularly in premature infants.

B. **Repetitive nerve stimulation.** Used rarely for diagnosis when pharmacologic testing has yielded equivocal results. May be useful in patients with prematurity or intrapartum asphyxia where the response to an anticholinesterase inhibitor is questionable and also as a quantitative assessment of neuromuscular function. In the test, the amplitude of the fifth evoked muscle action potential is compared with the first both before and after an anticholinesterase agent is administered. The test is considered positive when the fifth action potential is noted to be decreased by at least 10% and restored to normal after anticholinesterase treatment.

VII. **Management**

A. **Supportive care.** The management of TNMG focuses mainly on supportive care. In 20% of patients, symptoms are mild, requiring only small, frequent oral feeding and close observation. These patients are usually discharged from hospital after 1 week. The majority of patients, however, will present with moderate/severe symptoms, many of whom will require gavage feeds and ventilatory support.

B. **Anticholinesterase treatment.** In addition to supportive care, affected infants can benefit from anticholinesterase treatment. Neostigmine methylsulfate 0.05 mg/kg IM or SC administered 20 minutes before feeding or 0.5 mg/kg NG administered 30 minutes before feeding is the treatment of choice. Doses may be titrated gradually until sucking and swallowing are reestablished. As the dose is increased, careful monitoring for side effects (eg, diarrhea, increased secretions, muscle fasciculations) must occur. As symptoms improve, the dose can be decreased. When symptoms are no longer present and/or when repetitive nerve stimulation is normal, the medication can slowly be discontinued. For the patients presenting with moderate/severe symptoms, 50% will require anticholinesterase treatment for 1–2 weeks, 30% will require treatment for 3–4 weeks, and 20% will need more than 5 weeks of therapy.

C. **Intravenous immunoglobulin (IVIG).** IVIG has been used with some benefit in those few infants who have anti-MuSK–mediated TNMG and are resistant to anticholinesterase therapy.

D. **Plasmapheresis.** In mothers with a history of previous children with TNMG, plasmapheresis during pregnancy may help to reduce symptoms in subsequent infants.

VIII. **Prognosis.** Although TNMG can be life-threatening if not identified and treated promptly, for the majority of infants it is a transient illness with no lasting effects. Symptoms last for an average of 18 days (5 days to 4 weeks), and full recovery is seen in 90% of patients by 2 months of age. The remaining 10% of patients recover by 4 months. There have been reports of more prolonged illness; however, these are usually associated in the more atypical cases and in infants with arthrogryposis. Permanent facial diparesis has also rarely been reported.

Selected References

Ahlsten G, Lefvert AK, Osterman PO, Stålberg E, Säfwenberg J. Follow-up study of muscle function in children of mothers with myasthenia gravis during pregnancy. *J Child Neurol.* 1992;7:264–269.

Angelini C. Diagnosis and management of autoimmune myasthenia gravis. *Clin Drug Invest.* 2011;31:1–14.

Eynard B. Antibodies in myasthenia gravis. *Rev Neurol (Paris).* 2009;165:137–143.

O'Carroll P, Bertorini TE, Jacob G, Mitchell CW, Graff J. Transient neonatal myasthenia gravis in a baby born to a mother with new-onset anti-MuSK mediated myasthenia gravis. *J Clin Neuromuscul Dis.* 2009;11:69–71.

Oskoui M, Jacobson L, Chung WK, et al. Fetal acetylcholine receptor inactivation syndrome and maternal myasthenia gravis. *Neurology.* 2008;71:2010–2012.

Papzian O. Transient neonatal myasthenia gravis. *J Child Neurol.* 1992;7:135–141.

113 Necrotizing Enterocolitis

I. **Definition. Necrotizing enterocolitis (NEC)** is an ischemic and inflammatory necrosis of the bowel primarily affecting premature neonates after the initiation of enteral feeding.

II. **Incidence.** NEC is predominantly a disorder of preterm infants, with an incidence of 6–10% in infants weighing <1500 g, with the highest incidence in the most premature infants. NEC can also occur in term infants, many of whom have preexisting medical conditions.

III. **Pathophysiology.** Multifactorial theory has been suggested in which several risk factors, including prematurity, formula feeds, ischemia, and bacterial colonization, interact to initiate mucosal damage via a final common pathway involving activation of an inflammatory cascade. Mucosal damage results in invasion of the bowel walls by gas-producing bacteria, resulting in intramural gas accumulation (pneumatosis intestinalis). This sequence of events may then progress to transmural necrosis or gangrene of the bowel wall and finally to perforation and peritonitis.

IV. **Risk factors**

  A. **Prematurity.** There is an inverse relationship between gestational age and risk for developing NEC. While most preterm infants develop NEC at postmenstrual age (PMA) of 30–32 weeks, various factors resulting from premature birth places them at increased risk for NEC. These may involve immature mucosal barrier, mucosal enzymes, and various gastrointestinal (GI) hormones. Premature infants may have an imbalance between pro- and anti-inflammatory factors and thus have increased activation of inflammatory mediators and decreased inactivation of specific mediators like platelet activating factor (PAF), which has been linked to NEC. Abnormal toll-like receptor 4 (TLR 4) signaling in the premature intestine and increased activation of nuclear factor-κB may play a role in the pathogenesis of NEC. An inability to effectively regulate the intestinal microcirculation and differences in bacterial colonization may also make preterm infants more susceptible to NEC.

  B. **Microbial colonization.** NEC has not been shown to occur in germ-free animals. While bacterial and viral pathogens including *Escherichia coli*, *Klebsiella* spp, *Clostridium* spp, *Staphylococcus epidermidis*, rotavirus, and enterovirus have been implicated, no single organism has been consistently associated with NEC. Blood cultures are positive in only 20–30% of cases. While colonization by normal gut flora supports the intestinal mucosa through toll-like receptors, pathological bacteria induce inflammation and apoptosis by signaling pathways such as nuclear factor-κB. The growth of these noncommensal bacteria may also result in endotoxin release, leading to mucosal damage.

  C. **Enteral feedings.** NEC is rare in unfed infants, and 90–95% infants with NEC have received at least 1 enteral feed. Enteral feeding provides necessary substrate for proliferation of enteric pathogens. Hyperosmolar formula/medications may alter mucosal permeability and cause mucosal damage. Short-chain fatty acids produced as a result of colonic fermentation (due to deficient lactase activity in premature infants) may add to the damage.
      Breast milk significantly lowers risk of NEC. It has the benefit of providing immunoprotective as well as local growth-promoting factors not available with commercially prepared formulas. Early initiation of small-volume feeds with human milk for a few days followed by slow advancement of feeds (about 20 cc/kg/d) has been shown to decrease the incidence of NEC. This can be effectively accomplished by using weight-based feeding guidelines.

  D. **Circulatory instability.** During periods of circulatory stress, blood is diverted away from the splanchnic circulation (diving reflex). The resulting intestinal ischemia followed by reperfusion may lead to bowel damage. Imbalance between vascular dilator and constrictor molecules leading to defective splanchnic blood flow autoregulation in newborns may contribute to the injury. Infants with NEC have been shown by Doppler flow to have higher flow resistance in the superior mesenteric artery on the first day of life. A diminished blood supply to the gut in infants exposed to maternal cocaine may also increase the risk for NEC.

  E. **Maternal cigarette smoking.** A recent study has found an association between maternal cigarette smoking and development of NEC in the infant. The underlying mechanism may be the effect of maternal smoking or nicotine on blood vessel development in the fetal gastrointestinal tract.

  F. **Congenital heart disease.** Infants with hypoplastic left heart or univentricular heart disease with or without arch obstruction, truncus arteriosus or aortopulmonary window, congestive heart failure and infants who have had systemic-to-pulmonary shunts placed are at increased risk for NEC. Infants with symptomatic patent ductus arteriosus are also at higher risk for NEC. A common feature of many of these conditions is decreased mesenteric perfusion from diastolic steal. Hypoxemia from cardiac failure or cardiac procedures may add to this risk.

G. **Polycythemia and hyperviscosity syndromes.** These increase the risk for NEC by diminished perfusion and intestinal ischemia in watershed areas of the GI tract.

H. **Blood transfusion.** A significant association between red blood cell transfusion and NEC has been reported in recent retrospective studies with about 25–35% cases of NEC occurring within 48 hours of packed red blood cell (PRBC) transfusions. The pathogenic mechanism is uncertain but the following mechanisms have been proposed:

   1. **Immunologic mechanism.** Transfusion-related gut injury (TRAGI) may be similar to the transfusion-related lung injury (TRALI) described in adults with immunologically mediated damage to the gut. Impaired maturation of T cells or priming of neutrophils from prior transfusions may play a role.

   2. **Anemia.** Transfusions are given for symptomatic anemia. Anemia may impair the oxygen-carrying capacity of blood, leading to reduced oxygen delivery to the intestine resulting in injury. In 1 retrospective case-control study, NEC cases had lower hematocrit (Hct), and each one-point decrease in nadir Hct was associated with a 10% increase in the odds of NEC. Thus, withholding treatment of severe anemia may increase the risk for NEC. The critical Hct level where the risk of NEC from anemia outweighs the risk of blood transfusion has yet to be determined.

   3. **Storage effects.** Stored erythrocytes have depleted nitric oxide levels and could act as nitric oxide sink in the microcirculation predisposing to vasoconstriction and ischemic insult. The 3 mechanisms described previously may not be mutually exclusive and may all play a role in the pathogenesis of NEC. **Feeding prior to, during, and after PRBC transfusion remains *controversial*.** One institutional experience with withholding feeds prior and during PRBC transfusion showed a significant reduction in the incidence of NEC in their neonatal intensive care unit (NICU). Although many centers have instituted different feed-holding policies with blood transfusions, more prospective research is needed before uniform recommendations can be made.

V. **Clinical presentation.** While term infants who develop NEC often have underlying illnesses predisposing to NEC and are often diagnosed in the first week of life, most premature infants who develop NEC are between 14 and 20 days of age or 30–32 weeks' postmenstrual age. The early clinical presentation may include feeding intolerance, increased gastric residuals, and blood in stools. Specific abdominal signs include abdominal distension, tenderness, abdominal skin discoloration, emesis, and bilious drainage from nasogastric tube. Nonspecific signs include symptoms and signs of neonatal sepsis including increased apnea/bradycardia episodes, temperature instability, hypotension, and circulatory shock.

The clinical course of NEC is variable. While about 30% may have a mild presentation that responds to medical treatment, about 7% may have a fulminant course with rapid progression to NEC totalis, septic shock, severe metabolic acidosis, and death. **The modified Bell's staging criteria** is often used to classify NEC according to clinical and radiographic presentations.

A. **Stage I: suspected NEC**
   1. **Systemic signs.** Nonspecific, including apnea, bradycardia, lethargy, and temperature instability.
   2. **Intestinal findings.** Feeding intolerance, recurrent gastric residuals, and abdominal distension.
   3. **Radiographic findings.** Normal or nonspecific.

    B. **Stage II: proven NEC**
      1. **Systemic signs.** Include Stage I signs plus abdominal tenderness and thrombocytopenia.
      2. **Intestinal findings.** Prominent abdominal distension, tenderness, bowel wall edema, absent bowel sounds, and gross bloody stools.
      3. **Radiographic findings.** Pneumatosis with or without portal venous gas.
    C. **Stage III: advanced NEC**
      1. **Systemic signs.** Respiratory and metabolic acidosis, respiratory failure, hypotension, decreased urine output, shock, neutropenia, and disseminated intravascular coagulation (DIC).
      2. **Intestinal findings.** Tense, discolored abdomen with spreading abdominal wall edema, induration, and discoloration.
      3. **Radiographic findings.** Pneumoperitoneum (see Figure 11–22).
VI. **Diagnosis** A high index of suspicion must be maintained for any infant with a combination of risk factors enumerated under Section IV.
    A. **Clinical diagnosis.** NEC is a tentative diagnosis in any infant presenting with the triad of feeding intolerance, abdominal distension, and grossly bloody stools. Alternatively, the earliest signs may be identical to those of neonatal sepsis.
    B. **Laboratory studies.** The following studies should be performed and repeated as necessary:
      1. **Complete blood count (CBC) with differential and platelets.** The white blood cell (WBC) count may be normal but is frequently either elevated with increased left shift or low (leucopenia). Thrombocytopenia is often seen.
      2. **C-reactive protein (CRP)** correlates with the inflammatory response. Since initial CRP may be normal, serial CRP levels done at 12- to 24-hour intervals are more useful.
      3. **Blood culture** for aerobes, anaerobes, and fungi (*Candida* spp).
      4. **Stool cultures** for rotavirus and enteroviruses.
      5. **Electrolyte panel.** Electrolyte imbalance, including hypo- and hypernatremia, as well as hyperkalemia, are common.
      6. **Arterial blood gas measurements.** Metabolic or combined acidosis may be seen.
      7. **Coagulation studies** include prothrombin time (PT), partial thromboplastin time (PTT), fibrinogen, and fibrin degradation products (D-dimer). A rise in PT, PTT, and fibrinogen degradation products indicates DIC, a frequent finding in infants with severe NEC.
    C. **Imaging and other studies**
      1. **Flat plate radiograph of the abdomen**
        a. **Supportive for NEC.** Abnormal bowel gas pattern, ileus, fixed sentinel loop of bowel, or areas suspicious for pneumatosis intestinalis.
        b. **Confirmatory for NEC.** Pneumatosis intestinalis and intrahepatic portal venous gas (in the absence of umbilical venous catheter). (See Figures 11–23 and 11–24.)
      2. **Lateral decubitus and cross-table lateral studies of the abdomen.** Presence of free air is indicative of intestinal perforation. Serial radiographic studies of the abdomen should be obtained every 6–8 hours in the presence of pneumatosis intestinalis or portal venous gas to look for pneumoperitoneum as they are at risk for perforation within 48–72 hours. Serial radiographs may be discontinued with clinical improvement after 48–72 hours.
      3. **Abdominal sonography.** May be useful in the presence of nonspecific clinical and radiologic findings or in infants with NEC not responding to medical management. Ultrasound can detect intermittent gas bubbles in the liver parenchyma and the portal venous system that are not detected on abdominal radiograph. Free gas and focal fluid collections can also be viewed by sonography. Color Doppler ultrasound (US) is useful in detecting bowel necrosis and perfusion.

4. **Mesenteric oxygen saturation.** Recent studies have shown the possibility of using near-infrared spectroscopy (NIRS) to detect mesenteric oxygen saturations. This provides hope of early detection and real-time noninvasive monitoring for decreased bowel perfusion in infants who have NEC. This technique is still experimental.

VII. **Management.** The main principle of management for confirmed NEC is to treat it as an acute abdomen with impending or septic peritonitis. The goal is to prevent progression of disease, intestinal perforation, and shock. If NEC occurs in epidemic clusters, cases need to be isolated.

A. **Medical management**

1. **Nil per os (NPO)** to allow gastrointestinal rest for 7–14 days (shorter course for Stage I NEC). Total parenteral nutrition (TPN) to provide basic nutritional needs.

2. **Gastric decompression** with large-bore orogastric tube (Replogle) at low intermittent or continuous suctioning.

3. **Close monitoring** of vital signs and abdominal circumference.

4. **Monitoring for gastrointestinal bleeding.** Check all gastric aspirates and stools for blood.

5. **Respiratory support.** Provide optimal respiratory support to maintain acceptable blood gas parameters. Progressive abdominal distension causing loss of lung volume may increase need for positive-pressure ventilation.

6. **Circulatory support.** There may be excessive third spacing of fluid, which requires effective volume replacement. Inotropic support may be needed to maintain normal blood pressure.

7. **Strict fluid intake and output monitoring.** Try to maintain urine output of 1–3 cc/kg/h. Fluid replacement to correct third space losses. Removal of potassium from IV fluids in the presence of hyperkalemia or anuria.

8. **Laboratory monitoring.** Check CBC and electrolyte panel every 12–24 hours until stable. Obtain blood and urine culture prior to starting antibiotics.

9. **Antibiotic therapy.** Treat with parenteral antibiotics for 10–14 days. Antibiotic regimen should cover pathogens that can cause late-onset sepsis in premature infants. Add anaerobic coverage if bowel necrosis or perforation is suspected. Reasonable antibiotic regimens include

    a. **Vancomycin, gentamicin, and clindamycin (or metronidazole).**

    b. **Vancomycin and piperacillin/tazobactam.**

    c. **Vancomycin, gentamicin, and piperacillin/tazobactam.**

    d. **Term infants may be treated with ampicillin, gentamicin, and clindamycin.**

10. **Monitoring for DIC.** Infants in Stage II and III may develop DIC and require fresh frozen plasma and cryoprecipitate. Packed red blood cell transfusions and platelet transfusions may also be needed.

11. **Imaging studies.** Obtain an abdominal flat plate with lateral decubitus of cross-table lateral studies every 6–8 hours in the acute stage (usually the first 24–48 hours) to detect bowel perforation.

12. **Surgical consultation** is needed for confirmed NEC Stage II and III, especially when the condition is rapidly progressing or there is evidence of GI perforation.

B. **Surgical management.** A pneumoperitoneum is an absolute indication for surgical intervention. Relative indications for surgery include portal venous gas, abdominal wall edema and cellulitis (indicating peritonitis), fixed dilated intestinal segment by x-ray (sentinel loop), tender abdominal mass, and clinical deterioration refractory to medical management.

1. **Exploratory laparotomy.** This involves examining the bowel and resecting the necrotic segments. A portion of viable bowel is used to create an enterostomy and mucous fistula. Reanastomosis takes place after 8–12 weeks. If NEC only involves a short segment of bowel or limited resection, primary anastomosis is

used by some surgeons, avoiding complications associated with ileostomy and need for second surgery for reanastomosis. In situations of widespread areas of intestinal necrosis, abdomen may be closed after placement of a drain and reexplored later. A poor prognosis is associated with severe short-bowel syndrome, and foregoing further treatment may be considered.

2. **Peritoneal drainage (PD) placement.** A small transverse incision is made at McBurney's point. Abdominal layers are bluntly dissected and a Penrose drain is threaded into the abdomen and secured.

Two multi-center trials have shown use of PD and laparotomy in infants with bowel perforation to have similar mortality, need for total parenteral nutrition, and length of hospital stay. There has been concern for the requirement of delayed laparotomy in infants managed with PD. This has varied from 38% in the study by Moss et al and 74% in that by Rees et al, without affecting survival. PD is a relatively simple procedure and can be done with local anesthesia at the bedside. Hence, it is often used as a temporizing procedure in critically sick infants. However, this too has been questioned by Rees et al, and they have shown lack of improvement in physiologic measurements following PD. Currently, the optimal surgical management for infants with bowel perforation remains ***controversial*** and needs further study.

VIII. **Prevention**

A. **Human milk** has been shown to prevent NEC. While mother's own milk is ideal, a meta-analysis of 5 randomized clinical trials of donor human milk versus formula suggests that human milk was beneficial and formula-fed infants had a 2.5 times increased risk of NEC. Another study showed that the risk of NEC decreased by a factor of 0.8 for each 10% increase in the proportion of human milk intake. The rate of NEC was also shown to be lower in infants receiving human milk fortifier compared to those receiving bovine milk–based fortifier.

B. **Use of feeding protocol with initial period of trophic feeds** followed by gradual advancement of feeds has been shown to decrease the incidence of NEC. A cautious approach to feeds in high-risk infants with circulatory compromise, congenital heart disease, or those receiving a blood transfusion is recommended.

C. **Probiotics.** There has been recent work promoting use of probiotics to decrease the risk for NEC in preterm infants. Probiotics may prevent NEC by promoting colonization of the gut with beneficial organisms, preventing colonization by pathogens, improving the maturity and function of gut mucosal barrier and modulation of the immune system. A meta-analysis of 11 published trials on use of probiotics showed a 30% reduction in the incidence of NEC with no significant adverse effects. However, additional studies regarding the safety of specific probiotic preparations, dosage, duration, and practicality of administration in this fragile population are awaited before routine treatment with probiotics can be recommended. Probiotics have not been approved by the U.S. Food and Drug Administration.

D. **Prebiotics, or nutrients that enhance the growth of beneficial microbes,** have been proposed as a preventive strategy. These include oligosaccharides, inulin, galactose, fructose, lactose, and others. While prebiotics enhance the proliferation of endogenous flora, their efficacy in prevention of NEC is unclear.

E. **Avoidance of prolonged empiric antibiotic use.** These alter the gut flora, promoting growth of pathogens, and should be avoided in premature infants. This is supported by a retrospective study that showed that extremely low birthweight infants receiving initial antibiotic course of >5 days had an increased risk of NEC or death.

IX. **Complications**

A. **Recurrence of NEC** may occur in about 5% of cases.

B. **Colonic strictures** may occur in 10–20% cases and present with recurrent abdominal distension and persisting feeding intolerance. Contrast radiographic studies are usually diagnostic.

    C. **Short bowel syndrome** may develop in infants undergoing extensive resection of bowel. The traditional limits of intestinal length for successful survival are at least 20 cm of viable small bowel remaining with an intact ileocecal valve, or 40 cm viable remaining small bowel with loss of ileocecal valve. Intestinal transplantation, with variable outcome, remains an option for some of these infants.

    D. **Parenteral nutrition–associated liver disease** occurs more frequently in infants with surgical therapy for NEC.

X. **Prognosis**

    A. **Infants with NEC** have an overall mortality of 12.5%. NEC with perforation is associated with mortality of 20–40%.

    B. **Infants with surgical NEC** are at risk for significant growth delay and adverse neurodevelopmental outcomes.

Selected References

Blau J, Calo JM, Dozor D, Sutton M, Alpan G, La Gamma EF. Transfusion-related acute gut injury: necrotizing enterocolitis in very low birth weight neonates after packed red blood cell transfusion. *J Pediatr.* 2011;158:403–409.

Christensen RD, Gordon PV, Besner GE. Can we cut the incidence of necrotizing enterocolitis I half—today? *Fetal Pediatr Pathol.* 2010;29:185–198.

Deshpande G, Rao S, Patole S, Bulsara M. Updated meta-analysis of probiotics for preventing necrotizing enterocolitis in preterm neonates. *Pediatrics.* 2010;125:921–930.

Downard CD, Grant SN, Maki AC, et al. Maternal cigarette smoking and the development of necrotizing enterocolitis. *Pediatrics.* 2012;130:78–82.

Duro D, Mitchell PD, Kalish LA, et al. Risk factors for parenteral nutrition-associated liver disease following surgical therapy for necrotizing enterocolitis. *J Pediatr Gastroenterol Nutr.* 2011;52:595–600.

El-Dib M, Narang S, Lee E, Massaro AN, Aly H. Red blood cell transfusions, feeding and necrotizing enterocolitis. *J Perinatol.* 2011;31:183–187.

Lambert DK, Christensen RD, Baer VL, et al. Fulminant necrotizing enterocolitis in a multi-hospital healthcare system. *J Perinatol.* 2011(Epub ahead of print).

Martin CR, Dammann O, Allred EN, et al. Neurodevelopment of extremely preterm infants who had necrotizing enterocolitis with or without late bacteremia. *J Pediatr.* 2010;157:751–756.

Moss LR, Dimmit RA, Henry MCW, et al. A meta-analysis of peritoneal drainage versus laparotomy for perforated necrotizing enterocolitis. *J Ped Surg.* 2001;36:1210–1213.

Mukherjee D, Zhang Y, Chang DC, Vricella LA, Brenner JI, Abdullah F. Outcome analysis of necrotizing enterocolitis within 11,958 neonates undergoing cardiac surgical procedures. *Arch Surg.* 2010;145:389–392.

Neu J, Walker WA. Necrotizing enterocolitis. *N Engl J Med.* 2011;364:255–264.

Rees CM, Eaton S, Kiely EM, Wade AM, McHugh K, Pierro A. Peritoneal drainage or laparotomy for neonatal bowel perforation? A randomized controlled trial. *Ann Surg.* 2008; 248:44–51.

Singh R, Visintainer PF, Frantz ID 3rd, et al. Association of necrotizing enterocolitis with anemia and packed red blood cell transfusions in preterm infants. *J Perinatol.* 2011;31:176–182.

Sullivan S, Schanler RJ, Kim JH, et al. An exclusively human milk-based diet is associated with a lower rate of necrotizing enterocolitis than a diet of human milk and bovine milk-based products. *J Pediatr.* 2010;156:562–567.

Zabaneh RN, Cleary JP, Lieber CA. Mesenteric oxygen saturations in premature twins with and without necrotizing enterocolitis. *Pediatr Crit Care Med.* 2010 (Epub ahead of print).

114 Neural Tube Defects

I. **Definitions. Neural tube defects (NTDs)** are malformations of the developing brain and spinal cord. In normal development, the closure of the neural tube occurs over a 4- to 6-day period with completion around the 29th day postconception, often before a woman has realized that she is pregnant. Most current hypotheses consider NTDs to be defects from failure of a neural tube closure rather than the reopening of a previously closed tube. Most likely, the closure starts at several distinct sites rather than being one continuous process. The nomenclature for NTDs is not standardized and is thus often confusing. Frequently used terms are as follows:

A. **Anencephaly.** The defective closure of the upper or rostral end of the anterior neural tube. Hemorrhagic and degenerated neural tissue is exposed through an uncovered cranial opening extending from the lamina terminalis to the foramen magnum. Infants with anencephaly have a typical appearance with prominent eyes when viewed face on. **Craniorachischisis totalis** (a neural platelike structure without skeletal or dermal covering resulting from complete failure of neural tube closure) and **myeloschisis** or **rachischisis** (in which the spinal cord is exposed posteriorly without skeletal or dermal covering because of failure of posterior neural tube closure) are other, less frequent open lesions.

B. **Encephalocele.** Herniation of brain tissue outside the cranial cavity resulting from a mesodermal defect occurring at or shortly after anterior neural tube closure; usually a closed lesion. Approximately 80% of encephaloceles occur in the occipital region.

C. **Myelomeningocele.** Often also referred to as **spina bifida** (protrusion of the spinal cord into a sac on the back through a deficient axial skeleton with variable dermal covering). Considering that, strictly speaking, "spina bifida" only describes the bony defect, the term **spinal dysraphism** is considered more accurate by some. More than 80% of defects in this category occur in the lumbar region, and ~80% are not covered by skin. In contrast to myelomeningoceles, **meningoceles** (closed lesions involving the meninges only) usually do not result in neurologic deficits.

D. **Spina bifida occulta and occult spinal dysraphism.** Disorders of the caudal neural tube that are covered by skin (skin dimples or only very small skin lesions are present). These dysraphic disturbances range from cystic dilation of the central canal (**myelocystocele**), over bifida spinal cords with or without a separating bony, cartilaginous, or fibrous septum (**diastematomyelia** or **diplomyelia**), to a **tethered cord with a dermal sinus** or other visible changes such as hair tufts, lipomas, or hemangiomas. The term *spina bifida occulta* is used incorrectly when it is applied to an incomplete ossification of the posterior vertebral arch, a frequent and insignificant finding that is neither clinically nor genetically related to NTDs.

II. **Incidence.** Ninety-five percent of children with NTDs are born to couples with no family history of such defects.

A. **Statistics related to NTDs are to be interpreted with caution** and in the context of population, location, and time because occurrence of NTDs is affected by many epidemiologic and medical factors (see later sections).

B. **The overall worldwide incidence** has been quoted as ~1 in 1000 live births. More recently, frequency has been given as ~0.2 per 1000 live births.

C. **Spina bifida occulta, myelomeningocele, and anencephaly** are the more frequently encountered NTDs.

D. **At early embryonic stages, the incidence of NTDs is as high as 2.5%;** many abort spontaneously.

E. **The Centers for Disease Control and Prevention (CDC) reports that ~1500 infants with spina bifida are born in the United States per year.** The prevalence of neural tube defects (spina bifida and anencephaly) is decreasing (data include more than half of the U.S. states): prevalence was 7.92 per 10,000 for 1996 (year of birth) and decreased during the years after introduction of mandatory fortification to a prevalence of 4.61 per 10,000 in 2006 (year of birth).

F. **Medical costs are significant.** For 2009, the medical costs for an infant with spina bifida in the United States are estimated at more than $50,000; even later in life, the costs of health care are estimated to be 3–6 times higher for a person with a neural tube defect as compared with a person without such defect.

G. **Countries that have implemented mandatory fortification programs have reported a 30–50% reduction in incidence.** For the United States, a 19% reduction in the birth prevalence of NTDs was reported after the introduction of folic acid fortification of the U.S. food supply.

H. Geographic variation, sex, race, and social class
   1. The incidence is higher in females versus males.
   2. **The risk is approximately doubled for infants born to Hispanic women compared with white women.** The risk seems lower in Ashkenazi Jews than in whites of European descent.
   3. **Some populations with frequent consanguineous matings have an increased risk.**
   4. **The risk for African Americans and Asians is lowest.** But the incidence in northern China is higher: 5–6 in 1000 births.
   5. **The risk is increased in infants of particularly young or particularly older mothers of lower socioeconomic class.** This increase may be related to nutritional factors and/or lower compliance with the recommendations for vitamin and folate supplementation.

III. **Pathophysiology.** The causes of NTDs seem to be multifactorial in most cases of anencephaly, encephalocele, myelomeningocele, and meningocele. Interactions between genetic and environmental factors result in disturbance of normal development. Recognized causes or contributing factors include the following:
   A. **Nutritional and vitamin deficiencies.** Main concern: folic acid deficiency; other deficiencies linked to NTDs: vitamin B_{12} and zinc.
   B. **Chromosome abnormalities.** Include trisomies 13 and 18, triploidy, unbalanced translocations, and ring chromosomes.
   C. **Genetic syndromes.** NTDs have been observed as part of a variety of syndromes, some with Mendelian inheritance patterns. A typical example is **Meckel-Gruber syndrome** (autosomal recessive), which presents with encephalocele, microcephaly, polydactyly, cystic dysplastic kidneys, and other anomalies of the urogenital system. Genetic references and databases list >50 syndromes associated with NTDs in the differential diagnosis. Recent advances into the understanding of neurodevelopment emphasize the importance of intact primary cilia and signaling pathways for normal development.
   D. **Teratogens. Nitrates** (cured meat, blighted potatoes, salicylates, and hard water), **antifolates** (aminopterin, methotrexate, phenytoin, phenobarbital, primidone, carbamazepine, and valproic acid), **thalidomide**, and **abnormal glucose homeostasis in diabetic mothers** have all been implicated as causes of neural tube defects. The role of other potential causes of NTD remains *controversial*; a potential interference with normal neurodevelopment has been discussed for a variety of exposures, including (but not limited to) **lead, glycol, clomiphene, hazardous waste**, and **maternal hyperthermia**.
   E. **Other causes.** An overall increase in birth defects has been reported in infants of teenage mothers (<20 years old) compared with those mothers in the 25- to 29-year age range. The relative risk of nervous system defects in infants of teen mothers is 3.4 times that for children of 25- to 29-year-old mothers. Although a low body mass index does not increase the risk for NTDs, obesity does. The parents' ages are not related to the occurrence of NTDs per se; the risk for twins seems higher (a 2- to 5-fold increase).

IV. Risk factors
A. The occurrence of NTDs appears higher in the following:
1. **Women with insulin-dependent diabetes mellitus** (the risk appears to be influenced by the level of control).
2. **Women with seizure disorders** who are being treated with valproic acid or carbamazepine.
3. **Women with a family history of NTDs.**
B. The recurrence risk is as follows:
1. **Two to three percent with 1 affected sibling.** Some types of NTDs may be folic acid resistant, and even with folic acid treatment, a residual risk of ~1% remains.
2. **Approximately 4–6% with 2 affected siblings.** Higher if other associated findings suggest a syndrome/condition with possible Mendelian inheritance.
V. **Clinical presentation.** Clinical presentations of the most severe NTDs are the obvious cranial defect in anencephaly and open spinal defects of the thoracic and/or lumbar spine with open spinal NTDs, both with exposure of neural tissue. NTDs with an intact skin cover may show an obvious mass (eg, an occipital encephalocele) or be more subtle. Subtle findings include bulging of the skin cover over the occipital or spinal defect, small openings sometimes missed on initial examination, dimples, or hair patches. See Section I for definitions and description of the different NTDs.
VI. Diagnosis
A. **Prenatal screen using maternal serum α-fetoprotein (AFP) at 14–16 weeks'** gestation. Elevated levels (>2.5 multiples of the mean, which are adjusted to gestational age) are indicative of open NTDs at a sensitivity of 90–100%, a specificity of 96%, and a negative predictive value of 99–100% but a low positive predictive value.
B. **Prenatal diagnosis.** Documentation of an elevated maternal serum AFP is followed by:
1. **Genetic counseling.** The patient should receive counseling on the risk of NTDs and other conditions with elevated AFP (gastroschisis or other conditions leading to fetal skin defects) in her fetus. Causes of possible false-positive results (imprecise dates or twin pregnancies) need to be investigated. Options regarding further evaluation (see later) are to be discussed, and nondirective counseling regarding treatment options should be provided.
2. **Detailed fetal ultrasonography with anomaly screening.** In skilled hands, a detailed ultrasonogram (now often enhanced by 3-dimensional images) can be extremely sensitive and specific for detection of NTDs. Sonographic determination of the level of the lesion is useful in predicting the ambulatory potential of fetuses with NTDs. Ultrasonography is also done to rule out other major congenital defects and is now often aided by fetal magnetic resonance imaging (MRI).
3. **Measurement of the amniotic fluid AFP and acetylcholinesterase.** Amniocentesis is usually done between 16 and 18 weeks' gestation, although it can technically be done as early as 14 weeks' gestation. If indicated, a karyotype can also be obtained. The detection rate for anencephaly and open spina bifida is 100% when results of amniotic fluid acetylcholinesterase and AFP are combined, with a false-positive rate of only 0.04%.
VII. Management
A. Prevention of NTDs
1. The British Medical Research Council (MRC) demonstrated in 1991 that high-dose folate (4 mg/d) reduced the recurrence risk of NTDs by 72%.
2. Based on results from the MRC, the U.S. National Institute of Child Health and Human Development (NICHD), CDC, U.S. Preventative Services Task Force, and American Academy of Pediatrics (AAP) published recommendations regarding folic acid intake for women of childbearing age. The **American Academy of Pediatrics Committee on Genetics** gives the following recommendations in their policy statement from 1999 (reaffirmed in 2007):

    a. **All women of childbearing age who are capable of becoming pregnant should consume 0.4 mg of folic acid daily.** The committee encourages food fortification. In the absence of optimal fortification, supplementation is encouraged. Use of a multivitamin with 0.4 mg of folic acid is quoted as the most convenient, inexpensive, and direct way to meet the recommended dosage.

    b. **Women with a previous pregnancy resulting in a fetus affected by an NTD should consume 4 mg of folic acid.** High levels of folic acid intake should not be achieved by use of over-the-counter multivitamin preparations. The higher-level folic acid intake is also recommended for certain other high-risk persons.

    c. **Folic acid should ideally be taken before conception and at least through the first few months of gestation.** See the AAP Policy Statement for further details of the recommendations.

  3. Sources of folic acid

    a. **Dietary.** The average U.S. diet used to contain about 0.2 mg of folate, which is less bioavailable than folic acid. Folate intake of 0.4 mg/d can be achieved through careful selection of folate-rich foods (spinach and other leafy green vegetables, dried beans, peas, liver, and citrus fruits). **Since January 1998, enriched grains (including flour, bread, rolls, cornmeal, pasta, and rice) in the United States are fortified with folic acid by order of the U.S. Food and Drug Administration.** Some countries have opted against food fortification due to concerns about adverse effects (masking of vitamin B_{12} deficiency, potential promotion of tumor growth) and issues relating to freedom of choice.

    b. **Supplementation.** Folic acid is available over the counter and by prescription. Prenatal vitamins typically contain 0.8 or 1 mg of folic acid. A survey by the March of Dimes revealed that only 27% of nonpregnant women 18–45 years of age took a vitamin preparation containing folic acid in 2001. Awareness of the U.S. Public Health Service recommendation regarding folic acid did more than double from 1995–2002 (from 15 to 32%) for the same group. Multiple sources are available to provide educational material: March of Dimes (www.marchofdimes.com), CDC (www.cdc.gov), AAP (www.aap.org), and American College of Obstetrics and Gynecology (www.acog.org).

  4. Current epidemiologic and biochemical evidence suggests that NTDs are not primarily due to folate insufficiency but rather arise from changes in the metabolism of folate and possibly vitamin B_{12} in predisposed women. The mechanisms may also involve homocysteine metabolism. Polymorphisms of methylene tetrahydrofolate reductase and other genes encoding proteins involved in folate metabolism may be associated with an increased frequency of NTDs. Due to the homocysteine-lowering effect of folic acid, **supplementation may also reduce the risk for cardiovascular disease**. Some studies suggest that **folate and vitamin supplementation may also reduce the risk for other birth defects** (including congenital heart defects, orofacial clefts, urinary tract and limb defects, or even occurrence of trisomy 21). Other reports suggest an inverse association between folate intake and breast cancer, childhood neuroblastoma, and acute lymphoblastic leukemia. Promotion of tumor growth and the obscuring of vitamin B_{12} deficiency have been discussed as **potential adverse effects** of folate supplementation.

B. **Specific management**

  1. Anencephaly

    a. **Approximately 75% of anencephalic infants are stillborn.** Most live-born infants with anencephaly die within the first 2 weeks of birth.

    b. **Considering the lethality of anencephaly, usually only supportive care is given.** This includes warmth, comfort, and enteral nutrition. Support services for the family, including social work and genetic and general counseling, are essential. There are some ethically *controversial* issues regarding the extent of care and other issues (eg, organ donation), and it may be advisable to involve other support systems (eg, ethics committees, support groups, or religious guidance—if desired by the family). For family support or other resources, see Section VII.B.3h.

2. **Encephalocele**
   a. **Physical examination and initial management.** In addition to the general principles of neonatal resuscitation, an especially careful physical examination is indicated. Look for **associated malformations.** As mentioned in Section III.C, some genetic reference texts and databases list >50 syndromes associated with NTDs. We recommend that the child be given nothing by mouth until the **consultations** by subspecialties such as neurosurgery are obtained and a treatment plan has been formulated. **Imaging studies** (ultrasonography, computed tomography, and MRI) should be arranged. Genetic evaluation and testing should be initiated early, considering the turnaround time of many tests that may be ordered (eg, karyotype and others).
   b. **Neurosurgical intervention.** May be indicated to prevent ulceration and infection, except in those cases with massive lesions and marked microcephaly. The encephalocele and its contents are often excised because the brain tissue within is frequently infarcted and distorted. Surgery may be deferred, depending on the size, skin coverage, and location. **Ventriculoperitoneal (VP) shunt** placement may be required because as many as 50% of cases have secondary hydrocephalus.
   c. **Counseling and long-term outcome.** A multidisciplinary approach is necessary to counsel the family regarding recurrence risk, long-term outcome, and follow-up. For family support and other resources, see Section VII.B.3h. The degree of **deficits** is determined mainly by the extent of herniation and location; one or both cerebral hemispheres, the cerebellum, and even the brainstem can be involved. **Visual deficits** are common with occipital encephaloceles. **Motor and intellectual deficits** are found in ~50% of patients.

3. **Myelomeningocele.** Traditionally, postnatal surgery and management by a multidisciplinary team is the treatment for myelomeningocele. After the publication of the Management of Myelomeningocele Study (MOMS) in 2011, a review of this approach might need to be considered. The study found that prenatal surgery for myelomeningocele reduced the need for placement of a cerebrospinal fluid shunt and improved motor outcomes at 30 months but was associated with maternal and fetal risks. After birth, a multidisciplinary team approach, including the primary care physician, geneticist, genetic counselor, neonatologist, urologist, neurosurgeon, orthopedic surgeon, and social worker, is necessary.
   a. **Physical examination.** A physical examination should include careful evaluation for other malformations (see Section III.C). In addition, special efforts should be made to correlate motor, sensory, and sphincter function and reflexes to the functional level of lesion (Table 114–1). Voluntary muscle movements are difficult to elicit in newborns with myelomeningocele and therefore are not helpful during initial evaluation. Furthermore, motor examination may be distorted initially by reversible spinal cord dysfunction above the level of the actual defect induced by exposure of the open cord.
      i. **Extent of neurologic dysfunction** tends to correlate with the level of the spinal cord lesion.
      ii. **Paraplegia** typically below the level of the defect.

    iii. **The presence of the anal wink and anal sphincter tone** suggests functioning sacral spinal segments and is prognostically important. In one study, 90% of patients with a positive anocutaneous reflex were determined to be "dry" on a regimen of intermittent catheterization as opposed to 50% of those with a negative reflex.

  b. **Initial management.** In addition to following the general principles of neonatal resuscitation and newborn care, appropriate management of the spinal lesion is essential.

    i. There are institutional differences in the specifics of how to cover the lesion, and provision of a **sterile cover** can be achieved by several means. Some surgeons request that the infant be placed in a sterile plastic bag; others prefer application of plastic wrap to cover the lesion. Many recommend avoiding contact with gauze or other material that could adhere to the tissue and result in mechanical damage when removed. It is advisable to try to keep the defective area moist while avoiding bacterial contamination. If tolerated, the patient should be positioned on the side. Fecal contamination should be avoided, which sometimes is easier with methods covering the site only rather than placement of the infant's complete lower body in a plastic bag.

    ii. Be aware that a high rate of **latex allergies** are reported in patients with NTDs. All patients with myelodysplasia should be considered at risk for anaphylaxis and other allergic complications. **Latex avoidance** is practiced as a preventive protocol. One study showed that after 6 years of a latex-free environment, the prevalence of latex sensitization fell from 26.7% to 4.5% of children with spina bifida. A resource regarding issues relating to latex allergy is the website of the American Latex Allergy Association (www.latexallergyresources.org).

    iii. In most centers, patients are started on antibiotics and given nothing by mouth.

    iv. Arrange for **imaging studies** to evaluate for hydrocephalus or other malformations detected or suspected on physical examination.

  c. **Surgical management.** Usually closure of the back lesion is done within 48 hours to prevent infection and further loss of function.

  d. **Hydrocephalus.** Common and often **noncommunicative** secondary to associated **Arnold-Chiari malformation** of the foramen magnum and upper cervical canal (usually type II) with resultant downward displacement of the medulla, pons, and cerebellum and obstruction of cerebrospinal fluid flow.

    i. **The risk of hydrocephalus** is 95% for infants with thoracolumbar, lumbar, and lumbosacral lesions and 63% for those with occipital, cervical, thoracic, or sacral lesions.

    ii. **In some cases, hydrocephalus may not be evident** until after closure of the myelomeningocele, and placement of a **VP shunt** may be required at a later date.

    iii. **Aggressive treatment with early VP shunt placement may improve cognitive function.**

    iv. **Serial ultrasound scans are necessary to monitor the degree of hydrocephalus** because ventricular dilation may occur without rapid head growth or signs of increased intracranial pressure. The hydrocephalus often becomes clinically overt 2–3 weeks after birth.

    v. **Despite treatment of the myelomeningocele and hydrocephalus,** some infants may still succumb to death from complications or associated anomalies.

  e. **Urinary tract dysfunction.** One of the major causes of morbidity and mortality after the first year of life.

    i. **More than 85% of myelomeningoceles located above S2 are associated with neurogenic bladder dysfunction, urinary incontinence, and ureteral reflux.** Poor bladder emptying immediately after NTD closure may be temporary ("spinal shock") and improvement of bladder function may be observed up to 6 weeks after repair.

    ii. **Without proper management, hydronephrosis** may develop, with progressive scarring and destruction of the kidneys.

    iii. **Renal ultrasonography and a voiding cystourethrogram** may identify patients who may benefit from anticholinergic medication, clean and intermittent catheterization, prophylactic antibiotics, or early surgical intervention.

    iv. **Other associated renal anomalies** may be present in patients with NTDs, including renal agenesis, horseshoe kidneys, and ureteral duplications.

f. Orthopedic issues

    i. **With impairment of lower extremity innervation, the risk of atrophy is high.**

    ii. **Deformities of the foot, knee, hip, and spine** are common as a result of muscle imbalance, abnormal in utero positioning, or teratologic factors.

    iii. **Hip dislocation or subluxation** may occur and is usually evident within the first year of life; common in patients with midlumbar myelomeningocele.

    iv. **Treatment of orthopedic abnormalities** should be instituted as soon as there is sufficient healing of the back wound.

    v. **Physical therapists** assist with proper positioning of the extremities to minimize contractures and to maximize function.

g. Outcome of aggressive therapy

    i. **The overall mortality rate** is now <15% by 3–7 years of age; 1-year survival of infants with spina bifida has been reported as high as 87.2%. In multivariable analysis, factors associated with increased mortality were low birthweight and high lesions.

    ii. **Infants with sacral lesions** have essentially no mortality.

    iii. **The outcome in regard to the highest potential for ambulation** depends largely on the level of the original lesion (see Table 114–1) and is modified by the orthopedic treatment and potential complications (see Section VII.B.3f).

    iv. **A significant percentage of children with lumbar myelomeningocele score within the normal range on intelligence and achievement tests.** Deficits, possibly progressive, for performance IQ, arithmetic achievement, and visuomotor integration have been reported; reading and spelling may be less affected.

    v. **An IQ >80** is found in essentially all patients with lesions below S1; ~50% of survivors with thoracolumbar lesions have IQ >80.

    vi. **Cognitive function** is improved in the presence of favorable socioeconomic and environmental factors.

h. Family support groups, educational material and other resources. Educational material and information regarding existing support groups may be found at the following sites: March of Dimes (www.marchofdimes.com); Spina Bifida Association of America (www.spinabifidaassociation.org); International Federation for Spina Bifida and Hydrocephalus (based in Europe; www.ifglobal.org); National Institute of Neurological Disorders and Stroke (www.ninds.nih.gov). For information about latex allergy and its prevention, see American Latex Allergy Association (www.latexallergyresources.org).

4. Spina bifida occulta

    a. Neonatal features. The presence of spina bifida occulta is suggested by overlying abnormal collections of hair, hemangiomas, pigmented macules,

Table 114–1. CORRELATION OF THE LEVEL OF MYELOMENINGOCELE WITH LEVELS OF CUTANEOUS SENSATION, SPHINCTER FUNCTION, REFLEXES, AND POTENTIAL FOR AMBULATION

Level of Lesion	Innervation	Cutaneous Sensation (Pinprick)	Sphincter Function	Reflexes	Ambulation Potential
Thoracolumbar	T12–L2	Groin (L1) Anterior upper thigh (L2)	—	—	Full braces Wheelchair bound
Lumbar	L3–L4	Anterior lower thigh and knee (L3) Medial leg (L4)	—	Knee jerk	May ambulate with braces and crutches
Lumbosacral	L5–S1	Lateral leg and medial foot (L5) Sole of foot (S1)	—	Ankle jerk	May ambulate with or without short leg braces
Sacral	S2–S4	Posterior leg and thigh (S2) Medial buttock (S4) Middle of buttock (S3)	Bladder and rectal function	Anal wink	May ambulate without braces

aplasia cutis congenita, skin tags, subcutaneous masses, cutaneous dimples, or tracts, usually in the lumbosacral area.

b. **If undetected in the neonatal period,** clinical presentation later in infancy may include delay in development of sphincter control, delay in walking, development of a foot deformity, and/or recurrent meningitis. Sudden symptoms may represent vascular insufficiency produced by tension on a **tethered cord**, angulation of the cord around fibrous or related structures, or cord compression from a tumor or cyst.

c. **Diagnosis**

   i. **Ultrasonography** is useful for screening. Note that the acoustic window used to diagnose a tethered cord closes at 3–6 months.

   ii. **Magnetic resonance imaging** provides superior anatomic details. An advantage of an MRI is the lack of exposure to radiation; contrast is usually not needed.

d. **Early surgical correction** may be necessary to avoid the onset of symptoms. A timely surgical release of a tethered cord or decompression of the spinal cord in patients developing symptoms may completely or partially reverse recently acquired deficits.

VIII. **Prognosis.** See individual topics in management section.

Selected References

Adzick NS, Thom EA, Spong CY, et al. A randomized trial of prenatal versus postnatal repair of myelomeningocele. *N Engl J Med.* 2011;364:993–1004.

American Academy of Pediatrics, Committee on Genetics. Folic acid for the prevention of neural tube defects. *Pediatrics.* 1999;104:325–327.

Boulet SL, Yang Q, Mai C, et al. Trends in the postfortification prevalence of spina bifida and anencephaly in the United States. *Birth Defect Res A Clin Mol Teratol.* 2008:82:527–532.

Brand MC. Examining the newborn with an open spinal dysraphism. *Adv Neonatal Care.* 2006;6:181–196.

Burke R, Liptak GS; Council on Children with Disabilities. Providing a primary care medical home for children and youth with spina bifida. *Pediatrics.* 2011;128:e1645–e1657.

Dias MS. Neurosurgical management of myelomeningocele (spina bifida). *Pediatr Rev.* 2005;26:50.

Fletcher JM, Brei TJ, eds. *Spina Bifida: A Multidisciplinary Perspective.* Developmental Disability Research Reviews, Vol 16, Issue 1. Hoboken, NJ: Wiley Periodicals; 2010.

Lipak GS, Dosa NP. Myelomeningocele. *Pediatr Rev.* 2010;31:443.

Logan CV, Abdel-Hamed Z, Johnson CA. Molecular genetics and pathogenic mechanisms for the severe ciliopathies: insights into neurodevelopment and pathogenesis of neural tube defects. *Mol Neurobiol.* 2011;43:12–26.

Medical Research Council Vitamin Study Research Group. Prevention of neural tube defects: results of the Medical Research Council Vitamin Study. *Lancet.* 1991;338:131.

Oppenheimer SG, ed. *Neural Tube Defects.* New York, NY: Informa Health Care; 2007.

Swanson ME, Sandler A, eds. *Spina Bifida: Health and Development Across the Life Course (multiple articles).* Pediatric Clinics of North America, Vol 57, No 4. Philadelphia, PA: Elsevier Saunders; 2010.

Thompson DNP. Postnatal management and outcomes for neural tube defects including spina bifida and encephaloceles. *Prenat Diagn.* 2009;29:412.

Wyszynski DF, ed. *Neural Tube Defects: From Origin to Treatment.* New York, NY: Oxford University Press; 2005.

115 Orthopedic and Musculoskeletal Problems

Orthopedic problems are common in neonates. The problems can be isolated deformities or part of a generalized disorder. Usually these deformities are obvious, but a comprehensive musculoskeletal examination is the key for diagnosis of associated generalized disorders. This chapter provides an overview of the common problems encountered in the neonatal intensive care unit. **Many images of these neonatal orthopedic and musculoskeletal conditions, designated by [⟳], can be found online by visiting www.neonatologybook.com and clicking on the image tab.**

I. **Spine problems**
   A. **Scoliosis**
      1. **Definition.** Scoliosis is a lateral deviation of the spine that is >10 degrees and typically includes the rotation and sagittal deformity. Scoliosis is classified into several types including idiopathic, congenital, and neuromuscular.
         a. **Infantile idiopathic scoliosis** is more common in boys and in Europe than North America. It is an uncommon scoliosis and thought to be related to infant positioning. Most children are diagnosed within the first 6 months of life and have left-sided thoracic curves. Plagiocephaly is a common association. The natural history is *controversial*, but these curves can improve spontaneously. Radiographic measures described by Mehta have been used to predict the likelihood of progression. Neuro-axis abnormalities have been noted in over 20% of these children, and a magnetic resonance image (MRI) of the spine is recommended for children with curves measuring 20 degrees

or more. Casting and bracing have been successful treatment modalities in this condition. Occasionally surgical treatment is required, and the instrumentation is typically a growing rod.

b. **Congenital scoliosis** is caused by anomalies in the growing vertebra. The etiology is unknown, but studies have indicated that carbon monoxide exposure may be a factor, and recent genetic studies suggest a possible congenital basis. The neuro-axis, vertebral column, and organ systems develop at similar periods in utero. Neuro-axis abnormalities can occur in up to a third of these children, 20% will have a genitourinary abnormality, and 20% will have a cardiac abnormality. The classification consists of 2 basic abnormalities: defects of vertebral formation and defects of vertebral segmentation. The hemivertebrae is an example of a defect in formation, while defects of segmentation include block vertebra and unilateral bars (this is where 1 side of 2 vertebrae are connected, leading to a growth tether).

Progression of the deformity is typically due to unbalanced growth and can be highly variable. A hemivertebrae with normal growth caudally and cranially can progress significantly. The unilateral bar is the most common cause of congenital scoliosis and can result in significant deformity, particularly if there are hemivertebrae associated.

2. **Treatment.** Bracing is usually not a successful treatment regimen. Surgical management may be indicated for progressive curves. It may consist of vertebral resection and spine realignment or fusion to prevent further progression.

B. **Spina bifida** [☼]
   1. **Definition.** This group of disorders is characterized by congenital malformation of the spinal cord and vertebral column. Whereas the etiology of spina bifida is unknown, inadequate maternal intake of folic acid, gestational diabetes, and history of previously affected siblings with the same partner are contributory factors. There are 2 types:
      a. **Spina bifida occulta** is a defective formation of the posterior elements with intact skin and normal meninges and spinal cord.
      b. **Spina bifida cystica** is open skin with abnormal meninges and spinal cord. Spina bifida cystica is further subdivided into 3 types:
         i. **Meningocele.** The meningeal cyst herniates through a defect of the posterior elements of the spine but without the spinal cord or roots.
         ii. **Myelocele.** All the neural tissues are exposed without overlying tissues.
         iii. **Myelomeningocele.** This is the most common type (90%). The spinal cord and the nerve roots protrude outside the spinal canal through a defect in the posterior arch along with the meninges (dura, arachnoid). Other abnormalities of the spinal cord often occur with the myelomeningocele, including duplication of the cord (**diplomyelia**) and vertebral bony anomalies, such as defects in segmentation and failure of fusion of vertebral bodies, which cause congenital scoliosis, kyphosis, and kyphoscoliosis.
   2. **Diagnosis.** The diagnosis can be made prenatally by elevated maternal serum α-fetoprotein or by ultrasound, or postnatally by the presence of the lesion in the neonate's back. **A tuft of hair over the neonate's lumbosacral spine or skin dimple may be a sign of underlying anomalies.** Associated conditions are hydrocephalus, Arnold-Chiari malformation, congenital spinal deformity, and tethered cord syndrome. Ambulation is usually lost in upper thoracic or high lumbar lesions and is often preserved in lower lumbar and sacral lesions.
   3. **Treatment.** Surgical repair is usually indicated within 48 hours after birth. If hydrocephalus is present, a shunt is required.

C. **Torticollis**
   1. **Definition.** A lateral tilt of the neck and head typically due to a tight sternocleidomastoid muscle. The head and neck tilt toward the involved side, and the chin is turned toward the contralateral side. The most common causes are

       a. **Congenital muscular torticollis.** [✿] Fibrosis of the sternomastoid muscle, which may be due to a localized compartment syndrome or uterine packing problems.

       b. **Vertebral anomalies.** Klippel-Feil syndrome (congenital anomalies of the cervical spine) or congenital occipitocervical anomalies.

   2. **Diagnosis.** The diagnosis can be made with the observation of the typical deformity as well as palpation of a tight sternocleidomastoid muscle. A palpable mass in the muscle may appear in the postnatal period and resolve later on. Examination of the neonate for other congenital anomalies (developmental dysplasia of hip [DDH], metatarsus adductus) is essential. Radiographs of the cervical spine should be done to rule out any vertebral anomalies when there is no response to stretching exercises of the sternomastoid. Complications include plagiocephaly with facial asymmetry and restriction of neck movement.

   3. **Treatment.** Stretching exercises are successful in 90% of the cases. Surgical correction may be considered in resistant cases after 1 year of age.

II. **Upper limb and hand anomalies**

  A. **Radial club hand**

    1. **Definition.** Radial club hand is a longitudinal partial or complete deficiency of the radius. The typical deformity is radial deviation of the wrist and hand with or without thumb hypoplasia. The ulna is usually short and deformed. It may be associated with thrombocytopenia (TAR [thrombocytopenia with absent radius] syndrome), Fanconi anemia, Holt-Oram syndrome, Nager syndrome, VATER/VACTERL (*v*ertebral defects, *a*nal atresia, *t*racheoesophageal fistula, and *r*adial or *r*enal dysplasia/*v*ertebral defects, *a*nal atresia, *c*ardiac malformations, *t*racheo esophageal fistula, *r*enal dysplasia, and *l*imb abnormalities) syndrome, and other skeletal and cardiac abnormalities.

    2. **Treatment.** Splinting, stretching, physical therapy, and surgery.

  B. **Below-elbow amputation (congenital amputation)**

    1. **Definition.** Below-elbow amputation is a transverse deficiency resulting in the complete absence of the forearm just below the elbow. It is the most common form of congenital amputation (1 in 20,000 newborns has a transverse forearm deficiency). The hand or its remnants can be attached to the proximal forearm. Commonly, it is unilateral with no genetic basis or known cause.

    2. **Treatment.** There is no treatment required, although prosthesis fitting may be useful.

  C. **Polydactyly**

    1. **Definition.** Polydactyly is duplication of 1 or more fingers. It is most common among African Americans. It may be associated with Ellis-van Creveld syndrome or chromosomal anomalies.

      a. **Ulnar polydactyly, postaxial type.** [✿] It may affect the little finger. It has an autosomal dominant inheritance with variable penetration.

      b. **Central polydactyly.** It affects the central 3 fingers (central polydactyly). It typically has autosomal dominant inheritance.

      c. **Thumb polydactyly, preaxial type.** [✿] It affects the thumb.

    2. **Treatment.** Surgical reconstruction is often indicated.

  D. **Macrodactyly**

    1. **Definition.** Macrodactyly is an abnormal enlargement of the digits due to an osseous and/or soft tissue enlargement. Generalized enlargement may be due to a complex vascular malformation or neurofibromatosis. Klippel-Trenaunay-Weber syndrome (triad of port-wine stain, varicose veins, and bony and soft tissue hypertrophy involving an extremity) or Proteus syndrome are rare syndromes associated with macrodactyly. There are 2 varieties of macrodactyly: one presents as a large digit at birth, which grows at a normal growth rate, and in the other, the digit is normal at birth and then grows at a faster rate subsequently.

    2. **Treatment.** Surgical reconstruction is usually indicated.

E. **Syndactyly**
   1. **Definition.** Syndactyly [✿] is congenital webbing between the fingers. The fusion may be complete if it extends to the fingertips or complex if it involves the bony elements of the adjacent digits. It may be an isolated anomaly or associated with chromosomal or genetic disorders (eg, trisomies 21, 13, 18; Silver syndrome; Prader-Willi syndrome; or focal dermal hypoplasia). It is more common in boys, often with bilateral involvement. Also, it is more common in the ring and middle fingers than the index and thumb.
   2. **Treatment.** Surgical reconstruction is often indicated in the first year of life to allow for development of hand function.

III. **Hip disorders**
   A. **Developmental dysplasia of the hip (DDH).** [✿] (See also Chapter 6.) A wide spectrum of hip abnormalities ranging from hip instability to frank dislocation. In certain cultures newborn cradling may be an etiologic factor in DDH (eg, American Indians' use of the cradleboard with the hip extended and adducted). Hip examinations usually demonstrate hip instability. The following tests are used for clinical screening of the neonates:
      1. **Ortolani test** (reduction test for the dislocated hip). [✿] The child should be positioned supine with both the knees and hips flexed 90 degrees. The test is then performed with one hand stabilizing the pelvis and the other hand with the thumb over the hip adductors and the index finger over the greater trochanter. The hip is slowly abducted, so the dislocated femoral head slips toward the acetabulum, creating reduction (audible and palpable). The positive Ortolani test is a sign of dislocated hip.
      2. **Barlow test** (provocative test for the dislocatable hip). [✿] The child is positioned as for the **Ortolani test.** The hip is mildly adducted and pressure is applied posteriorly. If the femoral head slips over the posterior rim of the acetabulum and slides back again into the acetabulum when the pressure is released, this is considered Barlow positive, which means the hip is dislocatable.
      3. **Hip ultrasound examination** is indicated for screening of high-risk neonates (Table 115–1), although some clinical communities do ultrasound screening of all children. **Pavlik harness** is the treatment of choice for neonates with dislocated hips (positive Ortolani test). In the majority of Barlow-positive neonates, the hips stabilize in the postnatal period. Neonates with a positive Barlow test should have a repeat clinical and ultrasound examination after 4 weeks. If the hip is not stable at that time, a Pavlik harness should be used. Surgical treatment is rarely indicated in the postnatal period [✿].

IV. **Lower extremity disorders**
   A. **Proximal focal femoral deficiency (PFFD)** [✿]
      1. **Definition.** PFFD is a congenital anomaly of the proximal femur and pelvis resulting in a short femur and hip deformity. There is no known genetic etiology. The femoral segment is short, abducted, flexed, and externally rotated. There may be genu valgum and anterior cruciate ligament deficiency of the knee joint. The deformity is bilateral in 15% of cases. Fibular hemimelia may be associated with PFFD.

Table 115–1. RISK FACTORS FOR DEVELOPMENTAL DYSPLASIA OF THE HIP

Breech presentation
Female gender
First-born infant
Family history of DDH
Second infant of identical twin if the other had DDH (34% risk), nonidentical twin (3% risk)

DDH, developmental dysplasia of the hip.

2. **Treatment.** Either reconstruction (limb lengthening and realignment) or amputation.

B. **Fibular hemimelia [✿]**

1. **Definition.** This is characterized by congenital complete or partial absence of the fibula. There is no known genetic etiology. The tibia is short with a valgus and procurvatum deformity. There is often a skin dimple at the apex of the deformity. Fibular hemimelia is frequently associated with foot deformities with or without deletion of the lateral foot rays. Equinovalgus foot deformity is the most common associated foot deformity.

2. **Treatment.** Depends on the foot deformity and degree of limb length discrepancy (LLD). The surgical options are limb reconstruction (lengthening and realignment) or amputation of the deformed foot and fitting of a prosthesis.

C. **Tibial hemimelia [✿]**

1. **Definition.** This is a congenital partial or complete absence of the tibia. The infant usually presents with a short extremity with a rigid equinovarus, supinated foot deformity. [✿] Preaxial polydactyly is a relatively common associated anomaly. Other congenital anomalies may be associated with tibial hemimelia, such as congenital cardiac anomalies and or spine deformities. It is one of the few congenital limb deformities that have a genetic etiology and is seen with syndromes associated with ectrodactyly (cleft hand and foot deformity).

2. **Treatment.** The surgical options are either reconstruction or knee disarticulation.

D. **Posteromedial bowing of the tibia**

1. **Definition.** This is a benign condition characterized by a posteromedial bowing of the tibia. It is associated with a calcaneovalgus foot deformity and LLD. The condition should be differentiated from anterolateral bowing of the tibia (associated with congenital pseudarthrosis of the tibia and neurofibromatosis) and from fibular hemimelia.

2. **Treatment.** The natural history is complete resolution of the tibial deformity, although LLD may be significant.

E. **Hyperextension deformity of the knee (congenital knee dislocation)**

1. **Definition.** It is a rare deformity and varies from a simple hyperextension of the knee to a frank anterior dislocation of the tibia on the femur. It is seen as an isolated deformity and may be associated with other conditions (eg, Larsen syndrome). There is a loss of ability to flex the knee actively or passively. Radiographs are helpful to make the diagnosis and to differentiate simple hyperextension deformities from congenital knee dislocation.

2. **Treatment.** Mild cases respond to serial manipulation and casting. Surgery may be required in severe cases.

V. **Foot disorders.** Foot disorders are common and require careful assessment for proper diagnosis. Examples of common foot disorders are noted in the following text and in Table 115–2.

A. **Syndactyly**

1. **Definition.** Syndactyly is congenital webbing between toes. There are usually no functional problems associated with foot syndactyly. The fusion may be complete if it extends to the toenails or complex if it involves the bony elements of the adjacent digits. It may be associated with polydactyly.

2. **Treatment.** Surgical release is rarely indicated for foot syndactyly.

B. **Cleft foot [✿]**

1. **Definition.** Cleft foot is due to an absence of the central 2 or 3 rays of the foot. The cone-shaped cleft of the forefoot tapers proximally. Autosomal inheritance is common in bilateral cases and uncommon in unilateral cases. In bilateral cases, the hand may be affected as well.

2. **Treatment.** Surgery may be indicated to improve shoe fitting.

tenderness over the clavicle, loss of motion of the affected arm, an asymmetric Moro reflex, and pseudo paralysis. **The radiograph is diagnostic with the fracture at the junction between the middle and outer thirds.** The condition should be differentiated from a humerus fracture or brachial plexus injury. Prognosis is very benign.

    2. **Treatment.** Treatment is immobilization with pinning of the sleeve of the shirt to the chest of the neonate's clothes for 7–10 days.

B. **Humeral and femoral fractures**

    1. **Definition.** These fractures are less common than the clavicle fracture. **Both are associated with prolonged labor, extension of the injured extremity during breech presentation, rapid extraction of the infant during fetal distress, and forceps delivery.** The fracture usually occurs through the diaphysis (femur; less commonly the humerus) or through the growth plate (proximal or distal humerus, distal femur). The neonate usually has pain, limitation of movements, pseudo paralysis, tenderness, and crepitus at the fractured ends. Periarticular fractures can be easily overlooked. The diagnosis is made by radiograph.

    2. **Treatment.** Immobilization of the limb with splints for 3 weeks is satisfactory, and the prognosis is excellent. There is a remarkable remodeling potential and rarely residual shortening or angulation.

C. **Brachial plexus injuries**

    1. **Definition.** Stretching of the cervical nerve roots during delivery results in brachial plexus injuries. **The condition is usually associated with oversized neonates with a vertex presentation and shoulder dystocia, or after a breech presentation.** The fifth and sixth cervical nerve roots are commonly affected and result in **Erb palsy.** The arm is adducted and internally rotated with elbow extension and forearm pronation with normal hand function. The extremity sensation is intact, and the Moro reflex and biceps reflex are usually absent in the affected limb. If the lower cervical and first thoracic roots are affected, it is called **Klumpke paralysis.** There is a loss of grasp response of the hand with forearm paralysis, and both are poor prognostic signs. Examination of the other extremities is essential to exclude neonatal quadriplegia. Occasionally it may be bilateral, especially with breech deliveries. Full muscle testing is essential 48 hours after delivery. **Horner syndrome is usually present on the affected side.** Recovery may occur within 48 hours, but it may take up to 6 months. Imaging studies include plain radiograph, computed tomographic myelography, and MRI. Nerve conduction studies may be helpful to differentiate between root avulsion versus neurapraxia. For upper plexus injuries, the biceps function is a marker of spontaneous recovery. A preserved biceps function has a better prognosis. The prognosis depends on the type of injury to nerve roots (neurapraxia, axonotmesis, or neurotmesis) and the extent of nerve involvement and degree of recovery after initial palsy.

    2. **Treatment.** Surgery is rarely indicated in neonates. Surgical options include a microsurgical repair, tendon transfers to replace the weak muscles, or humeral osteotomy to correct the residual deformities in untreated cases.

VIII. **Orthopedic infections (osteomyelitis).** [✿] Prematurity, skin infections, and a complicated delivery are known risk factors for osteomyelitis. Hematogenous spread is the most common route of spread. The organisms may gain access to the circulation through venous or umbilical catheters, intravenous feeding lines, or invasive monitoring. The infection usually starts in the metaphysis of long bones. Because the nutrient vessels cross the growth plate to supply the epiphysis, septic thrombophlebitis of these vessels can lead to a growth plate injury and growth disturbances later in life. The thin cortex and periosteum of the neonate's bones are poor barriers for infection spread, allowing an infection to be easily spread to the adjacent tissues. When the metaphysis of long tubular bones is intracapsular, these infections usually result in septic arthritis (hip joint, shoulder joints). The osteomyelitis in premature infants or severely ill full-term infants tends to be multifocal with or without septic arthritis (usually 2 or 3 sites). **The most common organism is _Staphylococcus aureus_; the least common organism is group B streptococci, although other organisms may be isolated.** Diagnosis may be difficult due to a lack of symptoms and signs, especially in mild cases, but limitation of movements or pseudo paralysis and/or local swelling should be taken seriously. Less common presentations are pain on passive motion and abnormal posture of the limb. Once the sepsis is suspected, joint or bone aspiration is indicated to confirm the diagnosis. Laboratory tests include a complete blood count, erythrocyte sedimentation rate, C-reactive protein, and blood culture. Other diagnostic tools include a plain radiograph (usually normal or might only show a soft tissue swelling), ultrasound, bone scan, or MRI. Surgical drainage is indicated when an abscess is formed. The common sites are hip, shoulder, and knee joints. It is considered a surgical emergency to avoid the long-term results of infection.

Selected References

Bevan WP, Hall JG, Bamshad M, Staheli LT, Jaffe KM, Song K. Arthrogryposis multiplex congenita (amyoplasia): an orthopaedic perspective. _J Pediatr Orthop._ 2007;27(5):594–600.

Bora FW. _The Pediatric Upper Extremity: Diagnosis and Management._ Philadelphia, PA: Saunders; 1986.

Bowen JR, Neto AK. _Developmental Dysplasia of the Hip._ Towson, MD: Data Trace Publishing; 2006.

Fegin RD, Cherry JD. _Textbook of Pediatrics: Infectious Diseases._ 5th ed. Philadelphia, PA: Saunders; 2004.

Herring JA. _Tachdjian's Pediatric Orthopaedics._ Philadelphia, PA: Saunders; 2008.

Knudsen CJ, Hoffman EB. Neonatal osteomyelitis. _J Bone Joint Surg Br._ 1990;72(5):846–851.

Mehta MH. The rib-vertebra angle in the early diagnosis between resolving and progressive infantile scoliosis. _J Bone Joint Surg._ 1972; 54-B(2):230–243.

Mok PM, Reilly BJ, Ash JM. Osteomyelitis in the neonate. Clinical aspects and the role of radiography and scintigraphy in diagnosis and management. _Radiology._ 1982;145(3):677–682.

Morrissy RT, Weinstein S. _Lovell and Winter's Pediatric Orthopaedics._ 6th ed. Philadelphia, PA: Lippincott Williams & Wilkins; 2005.

Shenaq SM, Bullocks JM, Dhillon G, Lee RT, Laurent JP. Management of infant brachial plexus injuries. _Clin Plastic Surg._ 2005;32:79–98.

116 Osteopenia of Prematurity

I. **Definition.** Prematurity affects bone mineralization and bone growth—thus the entity known as **osteopenia of prematurity**; however, some authors use the term "**rickets of prematurity**." Normal bone is formed by the deposition of minerals, predominantly calcium (Ca^{+2}) and phosphorus (P), onto an organic matrix (osteoid) secreted by the osteoblasts. Osteoclasts play an important role in bone resorption and remodeling. Although osteopenia and rickets result in decreased bone mineralization and may have similar clinical findings, they are not identical processes and thus the term "rickets of prematurity" is not used in this chapter. Osteopenia of prematurity is principally a result of inadequate calcium intake to meet bone growth demands. Rickets, however, is principally due to vitamin D deficiency, but vitamin D supplementation alone will not resolve either osteopenia or rickets. Both disease processes involve the utilization of calcium, phosphorous, and vitamin D.

A. **Osteopenia.** Refers to a decrease in the amount of organic bone matrix (osteoid) due to a decrease in the thickness or number of trabeculae and/or decreased thickness of the bone cortex. These can be due to either insufficient deposition or increased resorption of the organic bone matrix.

B. **Osteomalacia.** Refers to the lack of mineralization of the organic bone matrix resulting in accumulation of nonmineralized osteoid and softening of bones. When involving the growth plate, it results in **rickets**. Bone density and bone mineral content (BMC) are both decreased.

C. **Osteoporosis.** Refers to a decrease in bone mineral density <2.5 standard deviations from the norm (adults). There is no accepted definition of osteoporosis in infants.

II. **Incidence.** Due to improvements in nutritional management such as initiation of early feedings, changes in nutritional formulas, and other clinical practices such as initiation of early parenteral nutrition, the current incidence of osteopenia is difficult to estimate. It is now more commonly seen in extreme prematurity and preterm infants with chronic illnesses such as bronchopulmonary dysplasia/chronic lung disease and necrotizing enterocolitis.

Previously, osteopenia has been reported in 23% of very low birthweight infants (VLBW) and in 55–60% of extremely low birthweight infants <1000 g. It was more commonly reported in breast-fed (40%) compared with formula-fed (16%) infants. Fractures have been reported in up to 10% of VLBW infants but are likely to be less common now.

III. **Pathophysiology.** Intrauterine bone formation occurs either as endochondral ossification (axial and appendicular skeleton) with the deposition of an osteoid matrix with a cartilaginous core or as membranous without the cartilaginous precursors (skull, maxilla, mandible). Several vitamins (A, C, D), cytokines, minerals (calcium), and hormones (thyroid hormone, growth hormone, parathyroid hormone related peptide) play important roles in fetal bone growth. The placenta is essential to fetal nutrient and mineral accretion.

A. **An increase in trabecular thickness and bone volume occurs faster in utero compared with ex utero.** After birth, bone growth is secondary to cyclical bone formation and resorption. In the first year, bone growth occurs by increases in length and diameter but with a decrease in cortical thickness; however, there is an overall 3-fold increase in bone strength. This adaptation occurs earlier in preterm infants than in term infants. Mineral retention is affected more than linear growth, contributing to a reduction in bone density following preterm birth. In preterm infants, the bone mineral content remains lower at term-equivalent than for full-term infants.

B. **Approximately 99% of body Ca^{+2} and 80% of P is in the skeleton at a term birth, and nearly 80% of this transfer occurs between 25 weeks' gestation and term.** Fetal accretion rate for Ca^{+2} and P cannot be met ex utero. Furthermore, inadequate intake (Ca^{+2} and P) in the face of increased growth demands results in nutrient deficiency.

C. **Vitamin D hydroxylation.** This is fully functional at 24 weeks' gestation, and preterm infants can form 1,25 dihydroxy vitamin D.

D. **Genetics and bone disease.** In adults and in VLBW infants, osteoporosis is associated with polymorphisms involving VDR, ER, and COLIA1 genes. In VLBW infants, homozygous allelic variants of ERα genotype with low number of thymidine-adenine repeat [(TA)n] were correlated with high urinary pyridinoline crosslink levels (indicating increased bone resorption) and with the development of metabolic bone disease. The locus interaction between VDR and COLIA1 was found to be protective in the development of bone disease.

IV. **Risk factors**

A. **Fetal and neonatal causes**

1. **Prematurity and birthweight.** Preterm birth results in Ca^{+2} and P deficiency. The frequency of osteopenia is inversely related to gestational age and

birthweight. Both conditions predispose these infants to mineral deficiencies in the face of increased nutritional and growth requirements.

2. **Feeding practices.** Delayed enteral feeding, prolonged use of parenteral nutrition, use of unfortified human milk, enteral feeding restrictions, and malabsorption states can result in mineral deficiencies.

3. **Human milk** is low in P, and donor milk content is even lower compared with preterm maternal milk. Prolonged use can result in low serum phosphate levels and decreased incorporation into the organic bone matrix. Unfortified human milk cannot match the mineral accretion that can be achieved across the placenta.

4. **Drugs.** Corticosteroids, furosemide, and methylxanthines are commonly used in preterm infants and cause mobilization of Ca^{+2} from the bone, resulting in decreased bone mineral content.

5. **Lack of mechanical stimulation.** Bone growth requires mechanical stimulation that is interrupted by preterm birth, illness, sedation, and paralysis. Neurologically impaired infants with spina bifida or arthrogryposis have limited mobility and poor bone growth.

6. **Vitamin D.** Preterm infants can absorb vitamin D and convert 25-OH to 1,25-dihydroxy vitamin D. Vitamin D is also converted to 1,25-dihydrocholecalciferol in the placenta, which is important in the transfer of phosphate to the fetus. Postnatal vitamin D deficiency may occur in breast-fed infants without fortification due to low levels (25–50 IU/L) in breast milk. Other causes of vitamin D deficiency in preterm infants include the following:
   a. Renal (osteodystrophy) disorders.
   b. **Drugs** such as phenytoin and phenobarbital increase vitamin D metabolism.
   c. **Pseudo–vitamin D deficiency** (absence of 1-α hydroxylase enzyme that converts 25 [OH] to 1,25 dihydroxy vitamin D or type I, or tissue resistance to 1,25 dihydroxy vitamin D or type II).

7. **Aluminum contamination of parenteral nutrition.**

8. **Malabsorption of vitamin D and Ca^{+2}** can occur in infants with prolonged cholestasis and short gut syndrome.

B. **Maternal factors**

1. **Maternal deficiency of vitamin D** results in low fetal levels. Maternal vitamin D deficiency in Europe, particularly in the winter, is associated with a low total BMC and a decreased intrauterine long bone growth. Maternal vitamin D status may also influence head circumference (at 3–6 months) and bone mineral content at 9 years of age.

2. **Maternal smoking, thin body habitus,** low Ca^{+2} intake, and increased physical activity in the third trimester result in a decreased BMC in the fetus.

3. **Exposure to high doses of magnesium** in utero, preeclampsia, chorioamnionitis, and placental infections are associated with osteopenia.

4. **Higher incidence of postnatal rickets** is seen in infants with intrauterine growth restriction (chronic damage to the placenta may alter phosphate transport).

5. **Increased maternal parity and boys** have higher incidence.

6. **Placental hormones** including estrogen and parathyroid hormone (PTH) and PTH-related protein also play a role.

V. **Clinical presentation.** Clinically, osteopenia manifests between 6 and 12 weeks of age and is usually asymptomatic; however, severe manifestations may include the following:

A. **Severe manifestations**

1. **Poor weight gain and growth failure.**

2. **Rickets-like findings** may include growth retardation, frontal bossing, craniotabes, prominence of the costochondral junction (rachitic rosary), and epiphyseal widening.

3. **Fractures** may manifest as pain on handling.
4. **Respiratory difficulties** or failure to wean off ventilator support due to poor chest wall compliance.

B. **Consequences of osteopenia.** Osteopenia can result in myopia of prematurity due to alterations in the shape of the skull. In childhood, infants remain thinner and shorter with a decreased total BMC and density. Increased urinary calcium excretion has also been reported.

VI. **Diagnosis**

A. **Radiographs.** Most commonly, osteopenia is recognized on radiographs, which are often subjective. Objective changes are not seen until a 20–40% decrease in bone mineralization occurs. Thin "washed-out" bones, cupping, fraying, and rarefaction of the end of long bones may occur. Subperiosteal new bone formation and fractures may also be visible. Serial radiographs in 3–4 weeks may be useful for follow-up.

B. **Biochemical markers of bone turnover**

1. **Markers of bone activity**

   a. **Calcium levels** may remain normal until late in the course.

   b. **Phosphorous.** Serum phosphate levels are low (<3 mg/dL). Low phosphate levels have low sensitivity but high specificity. Low levels of inorganic phosphate (P_i) <1.8 mmol/L with elevated alkaline phosphatase may be more specific for diagnosing inadequate intake.

   c. **Alkaline phosphatase (ALP).** Serum ALP is the sum of 3 isoforms (liver, intestine, and bone). The bone isoform contributes to the largest proportion (90%). ALP in infants can be up to 5 times the normal adult values. Elevated levels can be due to both osteoblastic and osteoclastic activity. The use of bone-specific isoform has not been found to improve sensitivity for predicting the development of osteopenia.

      i. **Elevated levels of ALP** can be seen with normal growth, healing rickets, fractures, or with copper deficiency.

      ii. **Low levels of ALP** are seen with zinc deficiency, severe malnutrition, and congenital hypophosphatasia.

      iii. **ALP is also negatively correlated with phosphate levels;** high levels (>1200 units/L) have been associated with short stature in childhood.

      iv. **Isolated elevation in ALP** without Ca^{+2} and P may occur with transient hyperphosphatasemia of infancy.

   d. **C-terminal procollagen peptide or propeptide of type I collagen** correlates with collagen turnover and bone formation in premature infants.

   e. **1,25 Dihydroxy vitamin D levels** are elevated with osteopenia.

   f. **Routine serum vitamin D and PTH levels** are not needed.

   g. **Osteocalcin (marker for osteoblastic activity)** may be elevated.

   h. **Osteoprotegerin (osteoclastogenesis inhibitory factor)** inhibits osteoclast activation and differentiation and its overexpression causes severe osteopetrosis. However, levels do not correlate with metabolic bone disease.

2. **Markers of bone resorption**

   a. **Urinary calcium and phosphorous.** Extreme prematurity is associated with a low phosphate threshold and an increased excretion even with low serum phosphate levels. High tubular resorption of phosphate suggests inadequate intake. Urinary calcium excretion >1.2 mmol/L and an inorganic phosphorus at >0.4 mmol/L suggest a high bone mineral accretion.

   b. **Cross-linked carboxy-terminal telopeptide of type I collagen,** urinary pyridinium crosslink products, cross-linked N-telopeptides of type I collagen, and pyridinoline cross-links of collagen are markers for bone resorption but are in limited clinical use.

C. **Ultrasound.** Quantitative ultrasound, using broadband ultrasound measurement, speed of sound (SOS), or bone transmission time, has been used. However, SOS cannot be used as surrogate for dual-energy x-ray absorptiometry (DXA).

1. **Advantages.** Ultrasound offers several advantages, including easy accessibility and lack of exposure to ionizing radiation. It uses peripheral sites such as the calcaneus and tibia. It measures both qualitative and quantitative bone properties, such as bone mineralization and cortical thickness, respectively, in addition to bone mass (osteopenia), elasticity, and microarchitecture.

2. **Speed of sound is most commonly used.** The SOS decreases in preterm infants from birth to term (corrected age) and is suggestive of decreased BMC. Inverse correlation between tibial SOS at birth and serum ALP has also been noted. Higher calcium intake my inversely affect the decline in SOS noted after preterm birth.

   D. **Dual-energy x-ray absorptiometry (DEXA).** DEXA is the gold standard used to assess both bone size and bone mineral status and can predict risk of fractures in newborn infants. However, limitations in its use and interpretation of data preclude wide clinical application.

VII. **Management**

   A. **Feeding and nutritional practices.** Establishment of early enteral feeding, decreasing length of parenteral nutrition, fortification of human milk, and using specialized preterm formula can limit osteopenia. Postdischarge use of specially designed preterm or transitional formulas (see also Chapter 10 on nutrition) and human milk fortification promotes mineralization. Ca^{+2} and P supplementation to achieve adequate *retention* levels range from 60 to 90 mg/kg/d of phosphate (provide 100–160 mg/kg/d to ensure adequate bioavailability). Care should be taken to avoid adding them directly to milk to prevent precipitation. Adequate vitamin D intake is also essential.

   B. **Vitamin D.** Vitamin D sufficiency in mothers is important to prevent deficiency in the fetus. Requirements have been reported to vary between 150 and 1000 IU/d of vitamin D.

   C. **Stimulation.** Mechanical stimulation by passive exercises to improve bone mineralization has yielded conflicting outcomes. Improved BMC, bone length, and bone area have been reported in individual studies. Current evidence does not justify the standard use of physical activity programs in preterm infants.

   D. **Minimize use of furosemide and corticosteroids.** The use of thiazide diuretics, although of theoretical advantage, has not been shown to prevent osteopenia.

   E. **Malabsorption.** Infants at risk of cholestasis and malabsorption may benefit from additional supplementation with fat-soluble vitamins and use of a specialized formula to facilitate fat absorption.

VIII. **Prognosis.** Osteopenia of prematurity appears to be decreasing with improved prevention and treatment practices. BMC remains 25–70% lower at term in the extremely premature infants. Catch-up mineralization occurs by 6 months of age. Long-term follow-up suggests that bone growth and adult height may also be impacted in these infants.

Selected References

Atkinson SA, Tsang RC. Calcium, magnesium, phosphorous, and vitamin D. In: Tsang RC, Uauy R, Koletzlo B, Zlotkin SH, eds. *Nutrition of the Preterm Infant: Scientific Basis and Practical Guidelines.* 2nd ed. Cincinnati, OH: Digital Education Publishing; 2005:245–275.

Chen HL, Lee CL, Tseng HI, Yang SN, Yang RC, Jao HC. Assisted exercise improves bone strength in very low birthweight infants by bone quantitative ultrasound. *J Pediatr Child Health.* 2010;46:653–659.

Funke S, Morava E, Czakó M, Vida G, Ertl T, Kosztolnyi G. Influence of genetic polymorphisms on bone disease of preterm infants. *Pediatr Res.* 2006;60:607–612.

Harrison CM, Johnson K, McKechnie E. Osteopenia of prematurity: a national survey and review of practice. *Acta Pediatr.* 2008;97:407–413.

McDevitt H, Ahmed SF. Quantitative ultrasound assessment of bone health in the neonate. *Neonatology.* 2007;91:2–11.

Pereira-da-Silva L, Costa A, Pereira L, et al. Early calcium and phosphorous intake by parenteral nutrition prevents short-term bone strength decline in preterm infants. *J Pediatr Gastroenterol Nutr.* 2011;52:203–209.

Rack B, Lochmüller EM, Janni W, et al. Ultrasound for the assessment of bone quality in preterm and term infants. *J Perinatol.* 2012;32:218–226.

Rigo J, Pieltain C, Salle B, Senterre J. Enteral calcium, phosphate and vitamin D requirements and mineralization in preterm infants. *Acta Pediatr.* 2007;96:969–974.

Schulzke SM, Trachsel D, Patole SK. Physical activity programs for promoting bone mineralization and growth in preterm infants. *Cochrane Database Syst Rev.* 2007;2:CD005387.

Tomlinson C, McDevitt H, Ahmed SF, White MP. Longitudinal changes in bone health as assessed by the speed of sound in very low birth weight preterm infants. *J Pediatr.* 2006;148:450–455.

117 Parvovirus B19 Infection

I. **Definition.** Human parvovirus B19 (PB19) is a small, single-stranded, nonenveloped DNA virus.

II. **Incidence.** Infection with PB19 is common worldwide. Infection occurs mostly among school-aged children where the major manifestation is **erythema infectiosum** (fifth disease). The prevalence of immunoglobulin G (IgG) antibodies directed against PB19 ranges from 15 to 60% in children 6–19 years old. About 35–45% of women of childbearing age do not possess protective IgG antibodies against PB19 and therefore are susceptible to primary infection. The incidence of acute PB19 infection in pregnancy is 3.3–3.8%. Annual seroconversion rates in pregnant women in the United States range from 1 to 1.5%.

III. **Pathophysiology.** The only known natural host cell of PB19 is the human erythroid progenitor cell. PB19 is a potent inhibitor of hematopoiesis. The cellular receptor for PB19 is globoside or P-antigen, which is found on erythrocyte progenitor cells, synovium, placental tissue, fetal myocardium, and endothelial cells. The B19-associated red blood cell aplasia is related to caspase-10–mediated apoptosis of erythrocyte precursors. Infection with PB19 is usually acquired through respiratory droplets, but the virus can also be transmitted by blood or blood products and vertically from mother to fetus. In children and adults, viremia develops 2 days after exposure and reaches its peak at ~1 week. During the phase of viral replication and shedding, the patient is generally asymptomatic. When the typical rash (characterized by a "slapped cheek" appearance on the face and a "lace-like" erythematous rash on the trunk and extremities) or arthralgias develop, the patient is no longer infectious to others. Symptoms during pregnancy are nonspecific and include a flulike syndrome with a low-grade fever, sore throat, generalized malaise, and headache. Pregnant women rarely develop the characteristic "slapped cheek." The fetus may become infected during the maternal viremic stage. Because of active erythropoiesis in the fetus with a shortened red-cell life span, marked fetal anemia, high-output cardiac failure, and fetal hydrops may develop. Myocarditis, and less often fetal hepatic infection, may contribute to fetal cardiac failure. Teratogenicity from PB19 has been described in case reports; also, one recent study found high prevalence of trisomy in pregnancy loss ascribable to PB19/erythrovirus infection. Despite that, PB19 is considered nonteratogenic based on large epidemiologic studies.

IV. **Risk factors.** The risk of acquiring PB19 infection during pregnancy is highest in schoolteachers, day care workers, and women who have school-aged children at home.

V. **Clinical presentation**

A. **During pregnancy.** The mother may report a history of exposure to a child with **erythema infectiosum**. More commonly, the mother does not recall such exposure and the diagnosis is made based on ultrasound findings. Fortunately, most maternal infections are associated with normal pregnancy outcomes. The overall risk of adverse outcomes after primary infection is probably <10% despite transplacental transmission rate of 33–50%. Adverse outcomes include the following:

1. **Fetal death.** Infection in the first trimester may result in fetal loss or miscarriage. A large prospective study of PB19 infection in pregnant women reported fetal death in 6.3% of pregnancies (up to 10.2% in other smaller studies). All deaths were limited to PB19 infections diagnosed in the first half of pregnancy (13% for first trimester infections, 9% for infections diagnosed between 13 and 20 weeks of gestation). Fetal death in the third trimester is exceedingly rare (<1%) and those fetuses (stillborn) are usually nonhydropic.

2. **Nonimmune hydrops fetalis.** The observed risk of PB19-induced hydrops fetalis is ~4% after maternal infection throughout pregnancy, with a maximum of ~10% when infection occurs between 9 and 20 weeks' gestation. The median interval between diagnosis of maternal infection and hydrops is 3 weeks. Hydrops can progress rapidly to fetal death (days to weeks) or can resolve spontaneously with an apparently normal infant at delivery. The spontaneous resolution is estimated at 34%. Severe thrombocytopenia can develop in 37% of parvovirus-infected fetuses with hydrops. This can lead to significant blood loss and exsanguination at the time of periumbilical blood sampling (PUBS) or other fetal procedures; for this reason, the platelet count should be determined and platelets should be available for transfusion if needed.

B. **Neonatal period.** The newborn infant may present with anemia and thrombocytopenia, especially if maternal infection occurred in the third trimester. Few cases of encephalopathy, meningitis, and severe central nervous system abnormalities following intrauterine PB19 infection have been reported.

VI. **Diagnosis**

A. **Laboratory studies**

1. **Serologic tests. PB19 IgG and IgM antibodies are first ordered when PB19 infection is suspected.** PB19-specific IgM antibodies become detectable in maternal serum within 7–10 days after infection, sharply peak at 10–14 days, and then rapidly decrease within 2 or 3 months. IgG antibodies rise considerably more slowly and reach a plateau at 4 weeks after infection. Measurement of maternal IgM is highly sensitive and specific. However, at the time of clinically overt hydrops fetalis, IgM levels may already have become low or (rarely) even undetectable. In contrast to maternal testing, serologic examination of fetal and neonatal blood samples is highly unreliable.

2. **Polymerase chain reaction (PCR)** to detect PB19 DNA is extremely sensitive. This method is especially useful in patients lacking an adequate antibody-mediated immune response, in immunocompromised or immunosuppressed individuals, and in fetuses. Using standard procedures, detection of PB19-specific IgM in fetal blood has a sensitivity of 29% compared with almost 100% for PCR. However, low viral DNA levels may persist for years after acute infection, and therefore low-positive PCR results do not prove recent infection.

B. **Ultrasound and Doppler velocimetry** are very useful noninvasive measures to monitor the pregnant woman who is exposed to PB19. Ultrasound is used to monitor for hydrops and fluid accumulation in fetal body cavities. **Doppler velocimetry is used to detect blood flow pattern in the fetal middle cerebral artery (MCA).** An increase in the MCA peak systolic velocity (MCA-PSV) is a very sensitive measure of fetal anemia.

VII. **Management.** Isolation precautions for all infectious diseases, including maternal and neonatal precautions, breast-feeding, and visiting issues, can be found in Appendix F.

    A. **Monitoring of the exposed pregnant woman.** Women who have been exposed or symptomatic should be assessed by determining their PB19 IgG and IgM status. Blood PCR is recommended when the fetus is hydropic. If the woman is immune to PB19 (IgG positive, IgM negative), she can be reassured that recent exposure will not result in adverse consequences in her pregnancy. If there is no immunity to the virus and seroconversion has not taken place after 2 weeks, the woman is not infected but remains at risk. If the woman has been infected with PB19 (IgM positive), the fetus should be monitored for the development of hydrops fetalis by ultrasound examination and Doppler assessment of MCA-PSV, preferably weekly until 8–10 weeks postexposure.

    B. **Intrauterine blood transfusion (IUT).** If the fetus subsequently develops hydrops and/or anemia (increase in MCA-PSV), PUBS and IUT (PUBS-IUT) should be considered. PUBS-IUT is an invasive procedure and carries a complication rate of 2–5% but can be lifesaving. It should be considered only for fetuses that are symptomatic. In most cases, one transfusion is sufficient for fetal recovery. When preparing for fetal transfusion, both packed red blood cells (PRBCs) and platelets must be available because some fetuses have severe thrombocytopenia in addition to anemia. Platelet transfusion may help if the fetus develops a hemorrhagic complication secondary to the procedure.

    C. **Packed red blood cell (PRBC) transfusion.** PRBC transfusion may be indicated for the symptomatic anemic newborn patient.

    D. **Intravenous immune globulin (IVIG).** IVIG has been used to treat acute B19 infection in immunodeficient adults and human immunodeficiency virus (HIV)-infected children with aplastic crisis. However, there is only 1 case report on its use during pregnancy. Given these limited data, the use of IVIG cannot be recommended.

    E. **Antiviral agents.** No antiviral agents are effective against PB19.

VIII. **Prognosis.** Mortality with parvovirus-related fetal hydrops is better than the generally reported mortality for nonimmune fetal hydrops (50–98%). With treatment, the long-term prognosis is good. Apparently, there is no increase in the frequency of developmental delays in children with exposure in utero to PB19.

Selected References

American Academy of Pediatrics. Parvovirus B19. In: Pickering LK, Baker CJ, Kimberlin DW, Long SS, eds. *Red Book: 2012 Report of the Committee on Infectious Diseases.* 29th ed. Elk Grove Village, IL: American Academy of Pediatrics; 2012:539–541.

Bonvicini F, Puccetti C, Salfi NC, et al. Gestational and fetal outcomes in B19 maternal infection: a problem of diagnosis. *J Clin Microbiol.* 2011(Epub ahead of print).

Brkic S, Bogavac MA, Simin N, Hrnjakovic-Cvetkovic I, Milosevic V, Maric D. Unusual high rate of asymptomatic maternal parvovirus B19 infection associated with severe fetal outcome. *J Maternal Fetal Neonatal Med.* 2011;24:647–649.

Carlsen K, Beck BL, Bagger PV, Christensen LS, Donders GG. Pregnancy loss ascribable to parvovirus B19/erythrovirus is associated with a high prevalence of trisomy. *Gynecol Obstet Invest.* 2010;70:328–334.

de Haan TR, van den Akker ES, Porcelijn L, Oepkes D, Kroes AC, Walther FJ. Thrombocytopenia in hydropic fetuses with parvovirus B19 infection: incidence, treatment and correlation with fetal B19 viral load. *BJOG.* 2008;115:76–81.

Enders M, Klingel K, Weidner A, et al. Risk of fetal hydrops and non-hydropic late intrauterine fetal death after gestational parvovirus B19 infection. *J Clin Virol.* 2010;49:163–168.

Riipinen A, Väisänen E, Nuutila M, et al. Parvovirus B19 infection in fetal deaths. *Clin Infect Dis.* 2008;47:1519–1525.

Sarfraz AA, Samuelsen SO, Bruu AL, Jenum PA, Eskild A. Maternal human parvovirus B19 infection and the risk of fetal death and low birth weight: a case-control study within 35940 pregnant women. *BJOG*. 2009;116:1492–1498.

Simms RA, Liebling RE, Patel RR, et al. Management and outcome of pregnancies with parvovirus B19 infection over seven years in a tertiary fetal medicine unit. *Fetal Diagn Ther*. 2009;25:373–378.

118 Patent Ductus Arteriosus

I. **Definition.** The ductus arteriosus is a large vessel that connects the main pulmonary trunk (or proximal left pulmonary artery) with the descending aorta, some 5–10 mm distal to the origin of the left subclavian artery. In the fetus, it serves to shunt blood away from the lungs and is essential (closure in utero may lead to fetal demise or pulmonary hypertension). In full-term healthy newborns, functional closure of the ductus occurs rapidly after birth. Final functional closure occurs in almost half of full-term infants by 24 hours of age, in 90% by 48 hours, and in all by 96 hours after birth. **Patent ductus arteriosus (PDA) refers to the failure of the closure process and continued patency of this fetal channel.**

II. **Incidence.** The incidence varies according to means of diagnosis (eg, clinical signs vs echocardiography).

   A. **Factors associated with increased incidence of PDA**
      1. **Prematurity.** The incidence is inversely related to gestational age. PDA is found in ~45% of infants <1750 g; in infants weighing <1000 g, the incidence is closer to 80%.
      2. **Respiratory distress syndrome (RDS) and surfactant treatment.** The presence of RDS is associated with an increased incidence of a PDA, and this is correlated with the severity of RDS. After surfactant treatment, there is an increased risk of a clinically symptomatic PDA; moreover, surfactant may lead to an earlier clinical presentation of a PDA.
      3. **Fluid administration.** An increased intravenous fluid load in the first few days of life is associated with an increased incidence of PDA.
      4. **Asphyxia.**
      5. **Congenital syndromes.** PDA is present in 60–70% of infants with congenital rubella syndrome. Trisomy 13, trisomy 18, Rubinstein-Taybi syndrome, and XXXXX (Penta X) syndrome are associated with an increased incidence of PDA.
      6. **High altitude.** Infants born at a high altitude have an increased incidence of PDA.
      7. **Congenital heart disease.** A PDA may occur as part of a congenital heart disease (eg, coarctation, pulmonary atresia with intact septum, transposition of the great vessels, or total anomalous pulmonary venous return).

   B. **Factors associated with a decreased incidence of PDA**
      1. **Antenatal steroid administration**
      2. **Intrauterine growth restriction**
      3. **Prolonged rupture of membranes**

III. **Pathophysiology.** In the fetus, the ductus is essential to divert blood flow from the high-resistance pulmonary circulation to the descending aorta. After birth, functional closure of the ductus occurs within hours (but up to 3–4 days). The patency of the ductus depends on the balance between the various constricting effects (eg, of oxygen) and the relaxing effects of various substances (most importantly: prostaglandin E's). The effects of oxygen and prostaglandins vary at different gestational ages. Oxygen has less of a constricting effect with decreasing gestational age. However, the sensitivity of the ductus to the relaxing effects of prostaglandin E_2 is greatest in immature animals (and decreases with advancing gestational age). In term infants, responsiveness is lost shortly after birth, but this does not occur in the immature ductus. Indomethacin constricts the immature ductus more than it does in the close-to-term ductus.

The magnitude and direction of the ductus shunt are related to the vessel size (diameter and length), the pressure difference between the aorta and the pulmonary artery, and the ratio between the systemic and pulmonary vascular resistances. The clinical features associated with a left-to-right ductal shunt depend on the magnitude of the shunt and the ability of the infant to handle the extra volume load. Left ventricular output is increased by the extra volume return. The increase in pulmonary venous return causes an increase in ventricular diastolic volume (preload). Left ventricular dilation will result, with an increase in left ventricular end-diastolic pressure and a secondary increase in left atrial pressure. This may eventually result in left heart failure with pulmonary edema. Eventually, these changes may lead to right ventricular failure. With a PDA, there is also a redistribution of systemic blood flow secondary to retrograde aortic flow (ductal steal, or "run off"). Renal and mesenteric blood flows are thus reduced, as is cerebral blood flow.

IV. **Risk factors.** See Section II.

V. **Clinical presentation.** The initial presentation may be at birth but is usually on days 1–4 of life. The cardiopulmonary signs and symptoms are as follows:

A. **Heart murmur.** The murmur is usually systolic and heard best in the second or third intercostal space at the left sternal border. The murmur may also be continuous and sometimes heard only intermittently. Frequently, it may be necessary to disconnect the infant from mechanical ventilation to appreciate the murmur.

B. **Hyperactive precordium.** The increased left ventricular stroke volume may result in a hyperactive precordium.

C. **Bounding peripheral pulses and increased pulse pressure.** The increased stroke volume with diastolic runoff through the PDA may lead to these signs.

D. **Hypotension.** A PDA is associated with a decreased mean arterial blood pressure. In some infants (particularly those of extremely low birthweight), hypotension may be the earliest clinical manifestation of a PDA, sometimes without a murmur (ie, the "silent" PDA).

E. **Respiratory deterioration.** Respiratory deterioration after an initial improvement in a small premature infant with RDS should arouse suspicion of a PDA. The deterioration may be gradual (days) or brisk (hours) but is usually not sudden (as in pneumothorax). PDA may similarly complicate the respiratory course of chronic lung disease.

F. **Other signs.** These may include tachypnea, crackles, or apneic spells. If the PDA is untreated, the left-to-right shunt may lead to heart failure with frank pulmonary edema and hepatomegaly.

VI. **Diagnosis**

A. **Echocardiography.** Two-dimensional echocardiography combined with Doppler ultrasonography is by far the most sensitive means of diagnosing a PDA. The ductus can be directly visualized, and the direction of flow may be demonstrated. In addition, echocardiography can assess the secondary effects of the PDA (eg, left atrial and ventricular size) and contractility. The echocardiogram will also rule out alternative or additional cardiac diagnoses.

B. **Imaging studies.** On initial presentation, the chest film may be unremarkable, especially if the PDA has occurred against a background of preexisting RDS. Later, pulmonary plethora and increased interstitial fluid may be noted with subsequent florid pulmonary edema. True cardiomegaly is usually a later sign.

VII. **Management**

A. **Ventilatory support.** Respiratory distress secondary to a PDA may require intubation and mechanical ventilation. If the infant is already ventilated, the PDA may lead to increased ventilatory requirements. These should be determined by blood gases. Increasing positive end-expiratory pressure is helpful in controlling pulmonary edema.

B. **Fluid restriction.** Decreasing fluid intake as far as possible decreases the PDA shunt as well as the accumulation of fluid in the lungs. Increased fluid intake in the first few weeks of life is associated with an increased risk of patency of the ductus in premature infants with RDS.

C. **Increasing hematocrit (Hct).** Increasing the Hct above 40–45% will decrease the left-to-right shunt. Frequently, an increase in Hct abates some of the signs of the PDA (eg, the murmur may disappear).

D. **Indomethacin.** A prostaglandin synthetase inhibitor that has proved to be effective in promoting ductal closure. Its effectiveness is limited to premature infants and also decreases with increasing postnatal age; thus it has limited efficacy beyond 3–4 weeks of age, even in premature infants. There are essentially 3 approaches to administering indomethacin for ductal closure in premature infants: **prophylactic, early symptomatic, and late symptomatic.** *Note:* There are minor variations in dosage regimens, and what follows are guidelines. Pharmacologic information on indomethacin can be found in Chapter 148.

1. **Prophylactic indomethacin.** A dose of 0.1 mg/kg/dose is given intravenously (infused over 20 minutes) every 24 hours from the first day of life for 6 days. In this regimen, indomethacin is given prophylactically to all infants <1250 g birthweight who have received surfactant for RDS (before any clinical signs suggestive of PDA). It would also be appropriate to limit this regimen to infants with RDS who are <1000 g birthweight. Clinical trials have shown that this treatment is safe and effective in reducing the incidence of symptomatic PDA in these infants. The major drawback is that up to 40% of these infants probably would never have had a symptomatic PDA and hence did not require treatment.

2. **Early symptomatic indomethacin.** Infants are given indomethacin, 0.2 mg/kg intravenously (infused over 20 minutes). Second and third doses are given 12 and 36 hours after the first dose. The second and third doses are 0.1 mg/kg/dose if the infant is <1250 g birthweight and <7 days old. If the infant is either >7 days old or >1250 g, the second and third doses are also 0.2 mg/kg/dose. Indomethacin is given if there is any clinical sign of a PDA (eg, a murmur) and before there are signs of overt failure. This is usually on days 2–4 of life.

3. **Late symptomatic indomethacin.** Infants are given indomethacin when signs of congestive failure appear (usually at 7–10 days). Dosage is as described in Section VII.D.2. The problem with this approach is that if indomethacin fails to constrict the ductus significantly, there is less opportunity for a second trial of indomethacin, and the infant is more likely to require surgery.

4. **Ductus reopening and indomethacin failure.** In 20–30% of infants, the ductus reopens after the first course of indomethacin. In such cases, a second course of indomethacin may be worthwhile because a significant proportion of these infants have their PDA closed with this course. The ductus is more likely to reopen in infants of very low gestational age and in those who had received a greater amount of fluids previously. Infection and necrotizing enterocolitis (NEC) are also risk factors for ductus reopening (and may be contraindications for indomethacin).

5. **Complications of indomethacin**

   a. **Renal effects.** Indomethacin causes a transient decrease in the glomerular filtration rate and urine output. In such cases, fluid intake should be reduced to correct for the decreased urine output, which should improve with time (usually within 24 hours).

   b. **Gastrointestinal bleeding.** Stools may be heme-positive after indomethacin. This is transient and usually of no clinical significance. Indomethacin is a mesenteric vasoconstrictor, but the PDA itself also decreases mesenteric blood flow. In most trials of indomethacin, there was no increased incidence of NEC.

   c. **Spontaneous intestinal perforation.** Indomethacin exposure has been associated with spontaneous intestinal perforation, especially when the drug was given early or when given together with postnatal corticosteroids. Caution is warranted, although none of the randomized trials comparing indomethacin with placebo have shown this finding.

   d. **Platelet function.** Indomethacin impairs platelet function for 7–9 days regardless of platelet number. In the various trials of indomethacin, there is no increased incidence of intraventricular hemorrhage (IVH) associated with the drug, and there is no evidence that it extends the degree of pre-existing IVH. Nevertheless, it may be unwise to impose additional platelet dysfunction in infants who are also significantly thrombocytopenic.

6. Indomethacin contraindications
   a. **Serum creatinine >1.7 mg/dL.**
   b. **Frank renal or gastrointestinal bleeding or generalized coagulopathy.**
   c. **Necrotizing enterocolitis (NEC).**
   d. **Sepsis.** All anti-inflammatory drugs should be withheld if there is sepsis. Indomethacin may be given once sepsis is controlled.

E. **Ibuprofen.** Another nonselective cyclooxygenase inhibitor that closes the ductus in animals. Clinical studies have shown that ibuprofen is as effective as indomethacin for the treatment of PDA in preterm infants. It has an advantage in that it does not reduce mesenteric and renal blood flow as much as indomethacin and is associated with fewer renal side effects. Urine output is higher and serum creatinine is lower in infants treated with ibuprofen compared with those treated with indomethacin. However, in trials comparing indomethacin with ibuprofen, no differences were found in incidence of significant clinical side effects (eg, NEC, renal failure, IVH). Choice of one drug over the other is largely a matter of institutional preference and may be often based on physiologic rather than clinical considerations. The dose used is an initial dose of 10 mg/kg followed by 2 doses of 5 mg/kg each after 24 and 48 hours if treatment is given in the first week of life. Due to change in pharmacokinetics, dosages of 18 mg/kg, 9 mg/kg, and 9 mg/kg at 24-hour intervals have been recommended when given in the second week of life.

F. **Surgery.** Surgery should be performed in patients with a hemodynamically significant PDA in whom medical treatment has failed or in whom there is a contraindication to the use of indomethacin. Surgical mortality is low (<1%). However, recent observational studies have suggested that surgical ligation is associated with an increased risk of chronic lung disease and neurodevelopmental/neurosensory impairment in extremely premature infants. It is not clear whether this association is causal or whether the need for ligation served as a marker for a higher-risk subgroup of patients.

G. **PDA in the full-term infant.** PDA accounts for ~10% of all congenital heart disease in full-term infants. The PDA in a full-term infant is structurally different, which may explain why it does not respond appropriately to the various stimuli for closure. Indomethacin is usually ineffective. The infant should be monitored carefully, and surgical ligation should be considered at the earliest signs of significant congestion. Even without signs of failure, the PDA should be ligated before 1 year of age to prevent endocarditis and pulmonary hypertension.

H. **Should the ductus be treated?** (*Controversial*) The issues of when and, in fact, whether at all, to treat the PDA in the preterm infant is a matter of ongoing controversy. There is no doubt that there is an association between the PDA and various morbidities of the premature infant. However, there is a debate whether this relation is a causal one and hence whether treatment is likely to be of benefit.

Numerous controlled trials have failed to show clinical benefit to the pharmacologic closure of the symptomatic PDA in terms of duration of mechanical ventilation, incidence of bronchopulmonary dysplasia/chronic lung disease, NEC, retinopathy of prematurity, or length of hospitalization. Early pharmacologic closure is, unsurprisingly, associated with a decreased need for later surgical ligation (and hence surgical morbidities). Meta-analyses have confirmed these findings. The only beneficial effect of very early prophylactic treatment with indomethacin appears to be a reduction in the incidence of severe pulmonary hemorrhage and of severe IVH, and even this does not necessarily translate into improved long-term neurodevelopmental outcome. Moreover, indomethacin's ability to reduce the incidence of severe IVH is independent of its effect on the PDA, and this effect has not been observed with ibuprofen. A differing overview and analysis of the clinical trials carried out to date has suggested, however, that exposure to a symptomatic PDA for ≥6 days is associated with a prolonged need for supplemental oxygen or mechanical ventilation. Also, studies in premature baboons have shown diminished alveolar development and impaired pulmonary mechanics in animals exposed to a moderate PDA for 14 days. The impaired alveolarization and pulmonary mechanics were attenuated by pharmacologic closure of the PDA (but not by surgical ligation). It is thus possible that the adverse effects of the ductus would be primarily seen in those infants destined to have either a PDA with a sizable shunt and/or prolonged exposure to significant ductal patency. Thus only a subgroup of neonates may require treatment. Various attempts to identify such a select subgroup of high-risk neonates who might benefit from treatment have been made using a variety of clinical and echocardiographic criteria or biochemical ones (eg, B-type natriuretic peptide). However, no outcome-based controlled trials have been done to demonstrate improved outcomes with selective treatment based on these criteria.

    I. **Feeding infants with PDA (or on treatment)** *(controversial).* Given the physiologic effects of the PDA, and medications used to treat it, on intestinal blood flow, there is no consensus regarding whether feedings should be withheld or continued in the presence of a PDA or during its treatment. Data are lacking, and there is wide variability in clinical practice.

VIII. **Prognosis.** Prognosis is excellent in those infants who only have a PDA. Studies show that premature infants <30 weeks have a spontaneous closure of the PDA 72% of the time. Conservative treatment (with medication) has a closure rate of ~94%.

Selected References

Benitz WE. Patent ductus arteriosus: to treat or not to treat. *Arch Dis Child Fetal Neonatal Ed.* 2012;97:F80–F82.

Benitz WE. Treatment of persistent patent ductus arteriosus in preterm infants: time to accept the null hypothesis? *J Perinatol.* 2010;30:241–252.

Chorne N, Leonard C, Piecuch R, Clyman RI. Patent ductus arteriosus and its treatment as risk factors for neonatal and neurodevelopmental morbidity. *Pediatrics.* 2007;119: 1165–1174.

Hamrick SEG, Hansmann G. Patent ductus arteriosus of the preterm infant. *Pediatrics.* 2010;125:1020–1030.

Johnston PG, Gillam-Krakauer M, Fuller MP, Reese J. Evidence-based use of indomethacin and ibuprofen in the neonatal intensive care unit. *Clin Perinatol.* 2012;39:111–136.

Noori S. Patent ductus arteriosus in the preterm infant: to treat or not to treat? *J Perinatol.* 2010;30:S31–S37.

119 Perinatal Asphyxia

I. **Definition**
   A. **Perinatal asphyxia** is a condition of impaired blood gas exchange that, if persistent, leads to progressive hypoxemia and hypercapnia. **Hypoxic-ischemic encephalopathy (HIE)**, which is a subset of **neonatal encephalopathy (NE)**, can result from perinatal asphyxia.
   B. **Neonatal encephalopathy (NE)** is clinically defined as a disturbance in neurologic function demonstrated by difficulty in maintaining respirations, hypotonia, altered level of consciousness, depressed or absent primitive reflexes, seizures, and poor feeding. NE does not imply HIE. NE may represent a metabolic disorder, infection, drug exposure, or neonatal stroke, but it is the preferred terminology to describe a depressed newborn from any cause at the time of birth.
   C. In order for an **acute intrapartum hypoxic event** to be considered a cause of cerebral palsy (CP), the American Academy of Pediatrics (AAP) and the American College of Obstetrics and Gynecology (ACOG) define 4 essential criteria that must be met:
      1. Evidence of a metabolic acidosis in fetal umbilical cord arterial blood obtained at delivery (pH <7 and base deficit ≥12 mmol/L).
      2. Early onset of severe or moderate neonatal encephalopathy in infants born at 34 or more weeks of gestation.
      3. CP of the spastic quadriplegic or dyskinetic type.
      4. Exclusion of other identifiable etiologies, such as trauma, coagulation disorders, infectious conditions, or genetic disorders.
   D. Criteria that collectively suggest an acute intrapartum hypoxic event (within 0–48 hours to labor and delivery) but are individually nonspecific to asphyxial insults:
      1. A sentinel hypoxic event occurring immediately before or during labor
      2. A sudden and sustained fetal bradycardia or the absence of fetal heart rate variability in the presence of persistent, late, or variable decelerations, usually after a hypoxic sentinel event when the pattern was previously normal
      3. Apgar scores of 0–3 beyond 5 minutes
      4. Onset of multisystem involvement within 72 hours of birth
      5. Early imaging showing evidence of acute nonfocal cerebral abnormality
II. **Incidence.** Data regarding perinatal asphyxia rates from 2001 indicate a prevalence rate of 25 per 1000 term live births and 73 per 1000 preterm live births, with 15 and 50% moderate to severe cases, respectively. The overall incidence of NE attributable to perinatal asphyxia was ~1.6 per 10,000 live births in the absence of preconception or antepartum abnormalities. European data indicate an overall CP rate of 2.08 per 1000 live births for the period 1980–1990, with increased rates seen in infants with birthweight <1500 g. While earlier studies showed a stable rate of CP between the 1950s and 1990s, more recent data indicate a decline in the prevalence of CP for preterm infants born after 1980, possibly reflecting improved perinatal care. Only 8–17% of CP in term infants is associated with adverse perinatal events suggestive of asphyxia; the cause of ≥90% of cases remains unknown.
III. **Pathophysiology**
   A. **Hypoxic-ischemic injury.** The asphyxial event results in cerebral ischemia, which precipitates an immediate drop in cellular high-energy phosphate levels, termed **primary energy failure**. Glutamate, an excitatory amino acid, is also released in substantial amounts due to cellular depolarization. *N*-methyl-D-aspartate (NMDA) receptors are subsequently overstimulated by glutamate and result in increased intracellular calcium and necrotic cell death. Cerebral blood flow is

restored in the **reperfusion period** with normalization of cellular energy levels within 2–3 hours after the insult. A **latent phase** follows and lasts 6–15 hours, during which oxidative metabolism returns to baseline, but secondary inflammation and cellular apoptosis are initiated. Without intervention, the latent phase can progress to **secondary energy** failure, which is characterized by cellular excitotoxicity, oxidative damage, and neuronal death within 3 days. The severity of the insult determines the extent of brain injury. Neurodevelopmental outcomes have specifically been correlated with the degree of secondary energy failure. Current neuroprotective therapies are therefore designed to intervene within the latent phase and before the onset of secondary energy failure.

B. **Adaptive responses of the fetus or newborn to asphyxia.** The fetus and neonate are much more resistant to asphyxia than adults. In response to asphyxia, the mature fetus redistributes blood flow to the heart, brain, and adrenals to ensure adequate oxygen and substrate delivery to these vital organs.

  1. **Impairment of cerebrovascular autoregulation.** Results from direct cellular injury and cellular necrosis from prolonged acidosis and hypercarbia.

  2. **Majority of neuronal disintegration.** Occurs after termination of the asphyxial insult because of persistence of abnormal energy metabolism and low adenosine triphosphate (ATP) levels (primary energy failure).

  3. **Major circulatory changes during asphyxia (reperfusion phase):**

    a. **Loss of cerebrovascular autoregulation** under conditions of hypercapnia, hypoxemia, or acidosis, cerebral blood flow (CBF) becomes "pressure passive," leaving the infant at risk for cerebral ischemia with systemic hypotension and cerebral hemorrhage with systemic hypertension.

    b. **Increase in cerebral blood flow** (occurs in phase of secondary energy failure) secondary to redistribution of cardiac output, initial systemic hypertension, loss of cerebrovascular autoregulation, and local accumulation of vasodilator factors (H^+, K^+, adenosine, and prostaglandins).

    c. **In prolonged asphyxia,** there is a decrease in cardiac output, hypotension, and a corresponding fall in CBF. In general, brain injury occurs only when the asphyxia is severe enough to impair CBF.

    d. **The postasphyxia newborn** is in a persistent state of vasoparalysis and cerebral hyperemia, whose severity is correlated with the severity of the asphyxial insult. Cerebrovascular hemorrhage may occur on reperfusion of the ischemic areas of the brain. However, when there has been prolonged and severe asphyxia, local tissue recirculation may not be restored because of collapsed capillaries in the presence of severe cytotoxic edema.

C. **Neurophysiology**

  1. **Cerebral edema** is a consequence of extensive cerebral necrosis rather than a cause of ischemic cerebral injury.

  2. **Regional central nervous system (CNS)** vulnerability changes with postconceptional age (PCA) and as the infant matures.

    a. **Periventricular white matter** is most severely affected in infants <34 weeks' PCA. The "watershed" areas between the anterior and middle cerebral arteries and between the middle and posterior cerebral arteries are predominantly involved in term infants.

    b. **Areas of brain injury in profound asphyxia** correlate temporally and topographically with the progression of myelination and of metabolic activity within the brain at the time of the injury. White matter, therefore, is more susceptible to hypoxic injury.

    c. **The topography of brain injury** observed in vivo corresponds closely to the topography of glutamate receptors.

    d. **When cerebral blood flow is increased** in response to asphyxia, regional differences exist such that there is relatively more blood flow to the brainstem than to higher cerebral structures.

D. **Neuropathology.** Experimental models in animal studies have been used extensively in the study of human asphyxia to establish the basic physiology of the CNS injury. Findings in humans include the following:

1. **Cortical edema,** with flattening of cerebral convolutions, is followed by cortical necrosis until finally a healing phase results in gradual cortical atrophy, and may result in microcephaly.

2. **Selective neuronal necrosis** is the most common type of injury observed in neonatal HIE. The pathogenesis most likely involves hypoperfusion and reperfusion with injury promulgated by glutamate.

3. **Other findings** in infants include status marmoratus, a marbled histopathological appearance caused by hypermyelination of the basal ganglia and thalamus, and parasagittal cerebral injury (bilateral and usually symmetric) with the parieto-occipital regions affected more often than regions anteriorly.

4. **Periventricular leukomalacia (PVL)** is hypoxic-ischemic necrosis of periventricular white matter resulting from cerebral hypoperfusion and the vulnerability of the oligodendrocyte within the white matter to free radicals, excitotoxin neurotransmitters, and cytokines. Injury to the periventricular white matter is the most significant problem contributing to long-term neurologic deficit in the premature infant, although it does occur in sick full-term infants as well. The incidence of PVL increases with the length of survival and the severity of postnatal cardiorespiratory disturbances. PVL involving the pyramidal tracts usually results in spastic diplegic or quadriplegic CP. Visual perception deficits may result from involvement of the optic radiation.

5. **Porencephaly, hydrocephalus, hydranencephaly, and multicystic encephalomalacia** may follow focal and multifocal ischemic cortical necrosis, PVL, or intraparenchymal hemorrhage.

6. **Brainstem damage** is seen in the most severe cases of hypoxic-ischemic brain injury and results in permanent respiratory impairment.

IV. **Risk factors.** Perinatal asphyxia can occur in the antepartum, intrapartum, or postnatal period.

A. **Antepartum risk factors** such as maternal trauma, maternal hypotension, and uterine hemorrhage account for 20% of HIE cases.

B. **About 70% of cases are estimated to occur in the intrapartum period** due to factors (sentinel events) such as placental abruption, umbilical cord prolapse, uterine rupture, and conditions associated with placental vascular insufficiency (maternal diabetes, intrauterine growth restriction, preeclampsia, and multiple gestation).

C. **Postnatal risk factors,** which account for 10% of HIE cases, are due to cardiorespiratory failure and congenital heart disease.

V. **Clinical presentation.** Perinatal asphyxia can result in CNS injury alone (16% of cases), CNS and other end-organ damage (46%), isolated non-CNS organ injury (16%), or no end-organ damage (22%).

A. **CNS injury in severe cases of HIE manifest with variable clinical signs that evolve over time:**

1. **Birth–12 hours.** Deep stupor or coma, respiratory failure or periodic breathing, diffuse hypotonia, intact pupillary and oculomotor responses, and subtle or focal clonic seizures by 6–12 hours in term infants. Preterm infants can present with generalized tonic seizures.

2. **12–24 hours.** The level of alertness can appear to improve in less critical cases of brain injury. However, severe seizures, marked jitteriness, and apnea also present at this time. Term infants can present with weakness of the proximal upper limbs, while preterm infants have lower extremity weakness.

3. **24–72 hours.** The consciousness level worsens leading to deep stupor and coma, leading to respiratory failure. Pupillary and oculomotor disturbance are now present due to brainstem involvement. Death due to HIE most often

occurs at this time with a median time of 2 days. Preterm infants who die at this time often have severe intraventricular hemorrhage (IVH) and periventricular hemorrhagic infarction.

4. **After 72 hours.** Mild to moderate stupor may persist, but the overall level of alertness improves. Diffuse hypotonia may persist or hypertonia can become evident. Feeding difficulties become obvious due to abnormal sucking, swallowing, and tongue movements.

B. **Non-CNS multi-organ dysfunction can present as follows:**

1. **Renal.** Acute tubular necrosis can present with hematuria or renal insufficiency or failure.

2. **Pulmonary.** Respiratory failure and meconium aspiration are due to fetal distress and persistent pulmonary hypertension.

3. **Cardiac.** Myocardial dysfunction and congestive heart failure may result in arrhythmias and hypotension.

4. **Hepatic.** Abnormal liver enzymes, elevated serum bilirubin, and decreased coagulation factors secondary to hepatic dysfunction.

5. **Hematologic.** Thrombocytopenia due to bone marrow suppression and decreased platelet survival add to the coagulopathy.

6. **Gastrointestinal.** Paralytic ileus or necrotizing enterocolitis (NEC) are due to decreased end-organ perfusion.

7. **Metabolic.** Acidosis (elevated lactate), hypoglycemia (hyperinsulinism), hypocalcemia (increased phosphate load, correction of metabolic acidosis), and hyponatremia/syndrome of inappropriate antidiuretic hormone secretion (SIADH).

VI. **Diagnosis**

A. **Maternal data**

1. **History.** A thorough maternal history (prior pregnancy loss, thyroid disease, fever, drug use, infection) and family history (thromboembolic disorders, seizure disorder) can help identify causes of NE other than HIEs.

2. **Fetal heart rate (FHR) patterns.** The following FHR tracings may serve as antepartum indictors of uteroplacental insufficiency or fetal compromise. Reactive FHR and subsequent prolonged FHR deceleration is suggestive of a sudden catastrophic event (pattern of acute asphyxia). A reactive FHR, which, during labor, becomes nonreactive, is associated with rising FHR baseline and repetitive late decelerations (pattern of intrapartum asphyxia). A persistent nonreactive FHR tracing with a fixed baseline rate, from admission until delivery, is suggestive of prior neurologic injury. This FHR pattern is often associated with reduced fetal movement, old passage of meconium, oligohydramnios, and abnormal fetal pulmonary vasculature (persistent pulmonary hypertension). FHR patterns are not always specific and have a substantial false-positive rate.

3. **Umbilical cord blood gases.** Umbilical cord gases provide objective evidence regarding the intrapartum metabolic status of the fetus. An arterial cord pH <7 and base deficit ≥12 mmol/L are consistent with fetal metabolic acidosis. Neonatal morbidity increases as umbilical arterial pH falls below 7.0. The metabolic component (base deficit and bicarbonate) is more important than the respiratory component (Pco_2). Isolated respiratory acidosis is not typically associated with neonatal complications. The precise value that is required to define damaging acidemia is not known. A pH <7.0 realistically represents clinically significant acidosis. Acidemia alone does not establish that hypoxic injury has occurred. Umbilical artery Po_2 levels are not predictive of adverse neonatal outcome.

4. **Placental pathology.** Important information regarding the etiology of NE may be gleaned from abnormalities seen on the maternal or fetal side of the placenta. Pathological umbilical cord lesions, such as velamentous or marginal cord insertion or cord hematoma or tears, may indicate a disruption in the fetal vascular supply. Chorioamnionitis and funisitis may indicate an

infectious etiology of NE, while fetal thrombotic vasculopathy can point to a genetic coagulopathic disorder.

B. Neonatal data

1. **Apgar scores.** While the previous AAP/ACOG definition of perinatal asphyxia mandated an Apgar score of ≤3 at 5 minutes, it is not part of the updated criteria. The most recent AAP/ACOG policy statement concludes that while a low 5-minute Apgar score may be associated with neonatal mortality, low 1- and 5-minute Apgar scores are not definite markers of an asphyxial event. An infant with an Apgar score of 0–3 at 5 minutes, improving to ≥4 by 10 minutes, has >99% chance of not having CP at 7 years of age; 75% of children who develop CP have normal Apgar scores at birth.

2. **Physical examination.** Findings determine grading of HIE severity based on the Sarnat scale.

   a. **Stage 1 (mild).** Hyperalertness, normal muscle tone, weak suck, low threshold Moro, mydriasis, and absence of seizures.

   b. **Stage 2 (moderate).** Lethargic or obtunded, mild hypotonia, weak or absent suck, weak Moro, miosis, and focal or multifocal seizures.

   c. **Stage 3 (severe).** Stupor, flaccid muscle tone, intermittent decerebration, absent suck, absent Moro, and poor pupillary light response.

3. **Laboratory studies.** Complete blood count with differential, blood culture, serum electrolytes, blood urea nitrogen, creatinine, cardiac enzymes, liver enzymes, a coagulation panel, and blood gases should be obtained at time of admission and serially monitored as indicated.

4. **Imaging other than cranium.** An echocardiogram can be obtained to evaluate cardiac ventricular function. A renal and hepatic ultrasound may provide further information regarding end-organ damage.

5. **Conventional electroencephalogram (cEEG).** Multiple neonatal cEEG classification systems, with varying criteria, exist focusing on the following variables:

   a. **Amplitude.** Described as isoelectric (maximally depressed or flat), low voltage, or mild voltage suppression.

   b. **Symmetry.** Classified as mildly, moderately, or severely abnormal.

   c. **Continuity.** Categorized as burst suppression pattern, which has the worst prognosis; persistent discontinuity (moderately or severely abnormal); or mild discontinuity (mildly abnormal).

   d. **Sleep-wake state.** The presence of sleep-wake cycling (SWC), as expected in a normal EEG, may be poorly defined or absent in a neonate affected by HIE with the time from birth to onset of normal SWC predictive of outcome.

   e. **Frequency.** Background frequency or pattern may be described as diffuse delta pattern (moderately or severely abnormal), poorly developed background rhythms (moderately abnormal), mild disturbance in background rhythm (mildly abnormal), and presence of seizures (moderate or severely abnormal).

6. **Amplitude-integrated EEG (aEEG).** This mode of monitoring utilizes a bedside cerebral function monitor, which records and amplitude integrates a single-channel EEG from biparietal electrodes. aEEG has the advantage over cEEG of not requiring extensive formal training for interpretation. A meta-analysis has shown aEEG to be useful in predicting long-term neurodevelopmental outcomes in term infants with HIE. The appearance of SWC in the aEEG within the first 36 hours is indicative of a good prognosis. The following classification scheme is suggested to describe the aEEG findings (see Figure 16–1):

   a. **Continuous normal voltage.** Continuous activity with lower (minimum) amplitude around (5 to) 7–10 μV and maximum amplitude of 10–25 (to 50) μV.

b. **Discontinuous normal voltage.** Discontinuous background with minimum amplitude variable, but below 5 μV, and maximum amplitude above 10 μV.

c. **Burst suppression.** Discontinuous background with minimum amplitude without variability at 0–1 (2) μV and bursts with amplitude >25 μV.

d. **Continuous extremely low voltage.** Continuous background pattern of very low voltage (around or below 5 μV).

e. **Inactive, flat trace.** Primarily inactive (isoelectric tracing) background below 5 μV.

7. **MRI of the brain.** It is important to note that HIE infants with a normal MRI may still be at risk for neurodevelopmental dysfunction. Diffusion tensor magnetic resonance imaging (MRI) (vs T1- and T2-weighted MRI) may be more accurate at demarcating areas of brain injury due to the presence of cerebral edema in the first 48–72 hours.

   More than the severity of injury, the pattern of brain involvement identified by MRI correlates with neurodevelopmental outcomes for infants with HIE:

   a. **Watershed predominant pattern.** Involves the vascular watershed in white matter. Involvement of the cortical gray matter can be seen in severe HIE. This pattern results from partial prolonged asphyxia and is associated with cognitive impairment.

   b. **Basal ganglia/thalamus predominant pattern.** Affects the deep gray nuclei and perirolandic cortex. The total cortex can be involved in severe HIE. This pattern results from acute profound asphyxia and is associated with severe cognitive and motor deficiencies.

8. **Magnetic resonance spectroscopy (MRS).** Used to assess the concentration of cerebral metabolites, thereby providing information regarding the biochemical changes in the brain secondary to HIE. Specifically a high ratio of N-acetylaspartate to choline and a low ratio of lactate to choline are predictive of better neurodevelopment outcomes.

9. **Diffusion weighted imaging (DWI) and diffusion tensor imaging (DTI).** Provide important information regarding the directionality and magnitude of water diffusion in the brain. The apparent diffusion coefficient (ADC) reflects the rate of diffusion and is reduced rapidly after an ischemic insult. A low ADC translates into a high-intensity signal on diffusion imaging. While restricted diffusion has the highest sensitivity for early detection, it can lead to underestimation of injury if obtained within the first 24 hours. The diffusion abnormalities peak at 3–5 days and then normalize.

VII. **Management.** The management of infants with HIE begins with the identification of perinatal patients at high risk for asphyxia and optimal resuscitation in the delivery room. As many cases of perinatal asphyxia are unanticipated and unpreventable, clinical care mostly focuses on providing supportive care to prevent further exacerbation of injury and specific neuroprotective therapies targeted at the therapeutic window prior to the onset of irreversible secondary energy failure. The ethical and medicolegal aspects of care also need to be considered.

A. **Supportive care**

1. **Resuscitation.** The 2011 Neonatal Resuscitation Program guidelines (Kattwinkel et al, 2010) recommend initiating resuscitation with room air or blended oxygen with a targeted preductal SpO_2 of 60–65% by 1 minute of life and 80–85% by 5 minutes of life in all term and preterm infants. There are no current guidelines specific to neonates with HIE. While resuscitation with 100% O_2 more rapidly restores CBF and perfusion in animal studies, hyperoxia should be avoided, as oxidative damage from oxygen-free radicals can further exacerbate hypoxic-ischemic brain injury.

2. **Ventilation.** Assisted ventilation may be required to maintain PcO_2 within the physiologic range. While hypercarbia exacerbates cerebral intracellular acidosis

and impairs cerebrovascular autoregulation, hypocarbia ($Paco_2$ <20–25 mm Hg) decreases CBF and is associated with PVL in preterm infants and late-onset sensorineural hearing loss in full-term infants.

3. **Perfusion.** Arterial blood pressure should be maintained in the normotensive range for gestational age and weight. Due to the loss of cerebrovascular autoregulation, volume expanders and inotropic support should be used cautiously in order to avoid rapid shifts between systemic hypotension and hypertension.

4. **Acid-base status.** The base deficit is thought to increase in the first 30 minutes of life due to an initial washout effect secondary to improved perfusion and transient increase in lactic acid levels. However, acidosis normalizes in the majority of infants by 4 hours of life, regardless of bicarbonate therapy. The rate of recovery from acidosis is reflective of HIE severity but not duration, and is not predictive of outcomes. Sodium bicarbonate therapy is not recommended as it causes a concomitant rise in intracellular Pco_2 levels, negating any changes in pH, and is associated with increased rates of intraventricular hemorrhage and mortality. One must consider an inborn error of metabolism if the degree of acidosis seems out of proportion to history and presentation and if the metabolic acidosis persists despite vigorous therapy.

5. **Fluid status.** Initial fluid restriction is recommended as HIE infants are predisposed to a fluid overload state from renal failure secondary to acute tubular necrosis (ATN) and SIADH. The avoidance of volume overload helps avert cerebral edema. A single dose of theophylline (8 mg/kg) may be considered within the first hour to increase glomerular filtration by blocking adenosine-mediated renal vasoconstriction.

6. **Blood glucose.** Initial hypoglycemia (<40 mg/dL) in the context of HIE amplifies the risk of progression from moderate to severe encephalopathy. Timely and frequent monitoring of blood glucose levels is therefore essential.

7. **Seizures.** Seizure activity is both a consequence and determinant of brain injury. A Cochrane review showed no reduction in death, neurodevelopmental disability, or combined outcome with the prophylactic use of anticonvulsant therapy. Phenobarbital therapy is recommended as the first-line agent for prolonged or frequent clinical seizures. The use of prophylactic phenobarbital in conjunction with hypothermia has shown a reduction in clinical seizures but not neurodevelopmental outcome. Phenobarbital levels in asphyxiated infants should be carefully monitored because hepatic and renal dysfunction, as well as hypothermia, can increase the drug's half-life and plasma concentration.

B. **Neuroprotective strategies**

1. **Hypothermia.** (See Chapter 39.) Therapeutic hypothermia attenuates secondary energy failure by decreasing cerebral metabolism, inflammation, excitotoxicity, oxidative damage, and cellular apoptosis. Hypothermia is now emerging as standard of care for perinatal asphyxia. Early identification of neonates with perinatal asphyxia and their timely referral to tertiary care centers for hypothermia therapy is therefore crucial. Hypothermia protocols and recommended temperature regulation prior to admission (such as passive cooling or active cooling on transport) are institution specific and must be clarified with the accepting facility at the time of referral. To date, 3 large multicenter trials of cerebral hypothermia for HIE, initiated within 6 hours of birth and continued for 72 hours, have been completed. In a recent review (Wu, 2011), direct comparisons of selective head cooling and whole body cooling are lacking, but both appear to have similar safety and effectiveness. Whole body cooling is preferred in most centers in the United States due to ease of administration and easier access to the scalp for EEG monitoring.

    a. **The "Cool Cap" trial** utilized selective head cooling with mild systemic hypothermia (34–35°C) and an aEEG screen as part of entrance criteria.

In a subset of patients with less severe aEEG findings, an improvement in survival without severe neurodevelopmental disability was demonstrated.

b. **The National Institute of Child Health and Human Development (NICHD) trial** subjected infants to whole body cooling with moderate systemic hypothermia (33.5°C) without any aEEG entrance criteria. They demonstrated a reduction in the combined endpoint of death or moderate or severe disability.

c. **The Total Body Hypothermia for Neonatal Encephalopathy (TOBY) trial** also cooled infants to a body temperate of 33.5°C but used aEEG entrance criteria. Cooling did not reduce the combined rate of death or severe disability, but improved neurodevelopmental outcomes were seen among survivors.

d. **Selective head cooling (SHC)** increases the temperature gradient across the brain from the central to peripheral regions. This is in contrast to whole body cooling, which maintains a uniform temperature gradient across the brain. In a systematic review of 13 studies (Shah, 2010), systemic hypothermia, but not SHC, was associated with a reduction in outcomes of cognitive delay, psychomotor delay, and cerebral palsy. The reduction in mortality or neurodevelopmental disability among survivors was similar between both modes of cooling. There are no clinically significant adverse effects from therapeutic hypothermia, and the mode of cooling does not have any differential impact on multiorgan system dysfunction in asphyxiated infants.

2. **Pharmacotherapy.** While investigation of potentially neuroprotective drugs is ongoing, these drugs are not in wide clinical use. Antioxidant enzymes such as superoxide dismutase and catalase were effective when given in animals prior to brain injury. Free-radical inhibitors such as allopurinol were effective in asphyxiated infants when given soon after resuscitation. Deferoxamine, a free-radical inhibitor, was beneficial when given during the reperfusion phase of injury in animal studies. Magnesium, an N-methyl-D-aspartate (NMDA) glutamate receptor antagonist, may have a beneficial effect on preventing cerebral palsy, based on retrospective clinical data, but neonatal animal studies are equivocal. While the prophylactic use of calcium channel blockers, such as flunarizine, was beneficial in animal studies, their use in infants is currently contraindicated due to adverse cardiovascular effects. Erythropoietin has been shown to improve outcomes for term infants with mild to moderate HIE by modulating neuronal injury and promoting neural regeneration.

C. **Ethics.** Most cases of perinatal asphyxia are unanticipated and families are often unprepared to deal with the complexities of HIE. Direct and timely communication between the medical team and the neonate's family is therefore essential to foster shared decision making with difficult medical and emotional decisions such as discontinuation of life support. A multidisciplinary team approach is essential, as severely depressed infants may have multiple complex medical needs (see also Chapter 21). A neurological consult is helpful to provide parents with important prognostic information based on the infant's neurological assessment. A palliative care consult may offer families support while optimizing the quality of the life for the infant.

The use of therapeutic hypothermia has also raised some important ethical issues. The concern that hypothermia therapy would simply increase the survival rate of severely disabled infants but not actual neurologic outcomes was addressed by the deliberate use of a compound primary outcome of death or survival without disability in the research design. Another concern regarding whether hypothermia therapy would hinder discussion regarding the withdrawal of care in profoundly affected infants was not found to be valid in the 3 major cooling trials.

D. **Medicolegal aspects**

1. **Obstetric care.** Fetal status must be assessed with electronic fetal monitoring at the time of maternal admission to identify and categorize risk for intrapartum fetal distress. A reactive fetal heart rate (FHR) pattern is a reliable sign of fetal well-being, while a nonreactive pattern indicates a higher probability of intrapartum fetal distress and adverse fetal outcome. The early recognition of fetal heart rate patterns that are associated with brain-damaged infants and timely intervention may potentially alleviate brain injury. It is important to note, however, that FHR patterns may actually be reflective of preexisting or underlying neurological impairment that existed prior to the perinatal period. Also, only cerebral palsy of the spastic quadriplegic type is thought to have perinatal asphyxia as an etiological component. Caution must therefore be used in identifying a specific event as the cause for an adverse outcome, as the baseline fetal brain status is often unknown. One cannot state with a reasonable degree of medical certainty that CP in a given child was due to intrapartum asphyxia merely because the physician can find no other explanation.

2. **Neonatal care.** Many cases of perinatal asphyxia are unanticipated, and an experienced resuscitation team may not always be readily available. In an anticipated high-risk birth, clear communication between members of the obstetric and neonatal teams prior to delivery is imperative. The resuscitation team must be thoroughly prepared for the potential for vigorous resuscitation per current AAP Neonatal Resuscitation Program guidelines. Careful attention must be paid to avoiding hypoglycemia, hypotension, and hypocarbia in the postresuscitation stabilization period. Early referral for evaluation for hypothermia therapy is crucial, as transport and admission to the tertiary center is ideally achieved within 6 hours after birth. Documentation of the resuscitation and stabilization process as well as informed consent for transport is an important part of the medical record. Informed consent for hypothermia is institution specific.

VIII. **Prognosis.** The presence of neonatal encephalopathy is considered an essential etiologic link between perinatal events and permanent brain damage. Mild cases of neonatal HIE have a favorable outcome, while severe cases have a high rate of mortality and neurodevelopmental disability. Predictions of outcome can be categorized by the following time points:

A. **0–6 hours after birth.** One model used the following 3 factors: chest compression >1 minute, onset of respiration after age 20 minutes, and base deficit >16 mmol/L to predict outcome in patients with moderate or severe HIE. Severe adverse outcome rates were 46% with none of the 3 predictors, 64% with any 1 predictor, 76% with any 2 predictors, and 93% with all 3 predictors present. Abnormal aEEG tracings also have predictive value for death or moderate to severe disability.

B. **6–72 hours after birth.** The clinical examination focusing on the Sarnat stages of encephalopathy, presence of seizures, spontaneous activity, and brainstem function are all predictive of outcome.

The following findings on MRI and MRS are predictive of a poor outcome: absence of normal hyperintensity in the posterior limb of internal capsule, a watershed or basal ganglia/thalamus predominant pattern, a high lactate/choline ratio or a low N-acetylaspartate/choline ratio. Abnormalities seen on diffusion tensor imaging do not correlate with long-term outcome. Amplitude-integrated EEG findings of burst suppression or discontinuous background are predictive of death or severe disability.

C. **Prior to discharge.** A normal neurological examination at 1 week of age is highly correlated with a normal outcome. Establishment of oral feedings is a good prognostic indicator. Lesions on neuroimaging may evolve or become more apparent as cerebral edema resolves.

D. **Postdischarge follow-up.** Microcephaly at 3 months of age or an abnormal neurologic examination at 12 months of age predict poor neurodevelopmental outcome at 5 years of age. A decrease in head circumference (HC) ratios (actual HC/ mean HC for age × 100%) of >3.1% between birth and 4 months of age is highly predictive of the eventual development of microcephaly before 18 months of age. Suboptimal rate of head growth associated with moderate cerebral white matter changes on MRI may be a better predictor of poor neurodevelopmental outcome.

Selected References

American Academy of Pediatrics Committee on Fetus and Newborn; American College of Obstetricians and Gynecologists Committee on Obstetric Practice. The Apgar score. *Pediatrics.* 2006;117:1444–1447.

Chau V, Poskitt KJ, Miller SP. Advanced neuroimaging techniques for the term newborn with encephalopathy. *Pediatr Neurol.* 2009;40:181–188.

Evans DJ, Levene MI, Tsakmakis M. Anticonvulsants for preventing mortality and morbidity in full term newborns with perinatal asphyxia. *Cochrane Database Syst Rev.* 2007;3:CD001240. DOI:10.1002/14651858.CD001240.pub2.

Kattwinkel J, Perlman JM, Aziz K, et al. Neonatal resuscitation: 2010 American Heart Association guidelines for cardiopulmonary resuscitation and emergency cardiovascular care. *Pediatrics.* 2010;126:e1400–e1413.

Menkes JH, Sarnat HB. Perinatal asphyxia and trauma. In: Menkes JH, Sarnat HB, Maria, BL, eds. *Child Neurology.* 7th ed. Philadelphia, PA: Lippincott Williams & Wilkins; 2006:367–432.

Perlman JM. General supportive management of the term infant with neonatal encephalopathy following intrapartum hypoxia-ischemia. In: Perlman JM, ed. *Neurology: Neonatology Questions and Controversies.* Philadelphia, PA: Saunders Elsevier; 2008:79–87.

Perlman M, Shah PS. Hypoxic-ischemic encephalopathy: challenges in outcome and prediction. *J Pediatr.* 2011;158(suppl 2):e51–e54.

Sarkar S, Barks JD, Bhagat I, Donn SM. Effects of therapeutic hypothermia on multiorgan dysfunction in asphyxiated newborns: whole-body cooling versus selective head cooling. *J Perinatol.* 2009;29:558–563.

Shah PS. Hypothermia: a systematic review and meta-analysis of clinical trials. *Semin Fetal Neonatal Med.* 2010;15:238–246.

The American College of Obstetricians and Gynecologists Committee on Obstetric Practice. Umbilical cord blood gas and acid-base analysis. *Obstet Gynecol.* 2006;108:1319–1322.

Volpe JJ. Hypoxic-ischemic encephalopathy. In: Volpe JJ, ed. *Neurology of the Newborn.* 5th ed. Philadelphia, PA: Saunders Elsevier; 2008:245–480.

Walsh BH, Murray DM, Boylan GB. The use of conventional EEG for the assessment of hypoxic ischaemic encephalopathy in the newborn: a review. *Clin Neurophysiol.* 2011;122(7):1284–1294. DOI:10.1016/j.clinph.2011.03.032.

Wintermark P, Boyd T, Gregas MC, Labrecque M, Hansen A. Placental pathology in asphyxiated newborns meeting the criteria for therapeutic hypothermia. *Am J Obstet Gynecol.* 2010;203:579.e1–e9.

Wu Y. Clinical features, diagnosis, and treatment of neonatal encephalopathy. Up to Date 2011. http://www.uptodate.com. Accessed November, 2011.

Wyatt JS. Ethics and hypothermia treatment. *Semin Fetal Neonatal Med.* 2010;15:299–304.

120 Persistent Pulmonary Hypertension of the Newborn

I. **Definition.** **Persistent pulmonary hypertension of the newborn (PPHN)** is a condition characterized by marked pulmonary hypertension resulting from elevated pulmonary vascular resistance (PVR) and altered pulmonary vasoreactivity, leading to right-to-left extrapulmonary shunting of blood across the foramen ovale and the ductus arteriosus, if it is patent. It is associated with a wide array of cardiopulmonary disorders that may also cause intrapulmonary shunting. When this disorder is of unknown cause and is the primary cause of cardiopulmonary distress, it is often called "idiopathic PPHN" or persistent fetal circulation.

II. **Incidence.** 2–6 per 1000 live births.

III. **Pathophysiology.** PPHN may be the result of underdevelopment of the lung together with its vascular bed (eg, congenital diaphragmatic hernia and hypoplastic lungs), maladaptation of the pulmonary vascular bed to the transition occurring around the time of birth (eg, various conditions of perinatal stress, hemorrhage, aspiration, hypoxia, and hypoglycemia), and maldevelopment of the pulmonary vascular bed in utero from a known or unknown cause. It is convenient to think in terms of this basic pathologic classification. However, the clinical manifestations of PPHN are often not attributable to a single physiologic or structural entity, and many disorders exhibit more than one underlying pathology. Often, even when there is evidence of perinatal or postnatal stress (eg, meconium aspiration), the underlying cause of PPHN had been secondary to an in utero process of some duration.

Preacinar arteries are already present in the lungs by 16 weeks' gestation; thereafter, respiratory units are added with further growth of the appropriate arteries. Muscularization, differentiation, and growth of the peripheral pulmonary arteries are influenced by numerous trophic factors (eg, fibroblast growth factors) and by changes that occur in the connective tissue matrix. The lungs of infants with PPHN contain many undilated precapillary arteries, and pulmonary arterial medial thickness is increased. There may be extension of muscle in small and peripheral arteries that are normally nonmuscular. After a few days, there is already evidence of structural remodeling with connective tissue deposition.

In the fetus, PVR is high, and only 5–10% of the combined cardiac output flows into the lungs, with most of the right ventricular output crossing the ductus arteriosus to the aorta. After birth, with expansion of the lungs, there is a sharp drop in PVR and pulmonary blood flow increases ~10-fold. The factors responsible for maintaining high PVR in the fetus and for effecting the acute reduction in PVR that occurs after birth are incompletely understood. Fetal and neonatal pulmonary vascular tone is modulated through a balance between vasoconstrictive and vasodilatory stimuli. Vasoconstrictive stimuli include various products of arachidonic acid metabolism (eg, thromboxane) and the endothelins (ETs). The hemodynamic effect of the ETs are mediated by at least 2 receptors; ET-A and ET-B. The fetal lung also produces a number of cyclooxygenase (COX)–dependent metabolites that function as pulmonary vasodilators (eg, PGI_2, PGE_1, and PGE_2). It has also become clear that the endothelium (and its interaction with vascular smooth muscle cells) plays a crucial role in regulating pulmonary vascular tone. Nitric oxide (NO), a potent vasodilator, is synthesized from L-arginine by endothelial nitric oxide synthase (eNOS). NO stimulates soluble guanylate cyclase (sGC), which produces cGMP and causes vasodilation. cGMP, in turn, is hydrolyzed by cyclic nucleotide phosphodiesterases (PDEs), and manipulation of these control the intensity and duration of cGMP action. Various isoenzymes of PDE have been identified, and inhibition of PDE-5 (by, eg, sildenafil) causes pulmonary vasodilation.

In summary, for successful pulmonary circulatory transition to occur, various mechanical, physiologic, and biochemical factors, which maintain high fetal PVR, must be eliminated or reversed. Major events are the replacement of the fluid-filled lung of the fetus with the air-filled postnatal lung, the increase in oxygen tension, and the increase in pulmonary blood flow (which increases shear stress and thereby increases NO). At the same time, changes occur in the synthesis and release of various biochemical modulators of vascular tone, and there are interactions between the mechanical and biochemical events surrounding birth. Disturbances in this cascade of events may lead to PPHN. At the same time, manipulation of these pathways enables us to treat it.

IV. **Risk factors.** The following factors or conditions may be associated with PPHN:

A. **Lung disease.** Meconium aspiration, respiratory distress syndrome (RDS), pneumonia, pulmonary hypoplasia, cystic lung disease (including congenital cystic adenomatoid malformation and congenital lobar emphysema), diaphragmatic hernia, and congenital alveolar capillary dysplasia.

B. **Systemic disorders.** Polycythemia, hypoglycemia, hypoxia, acidosis, hypocalcemia, hypothermia, and sepsis.

C. **Congenital heart disease.** Particularly, total anomalous venous return, hypoplastic left heart syndrome, transient tricuspid insufficiency (transient myocardial ischemia), coarctation of the aorta, critical aortic stenosis, endocardial cushion defects, Ebstein anomaly, transposition of the great arteries, endocardial fibroelastosis, and cerebral venous malformations.

D. **Perinatal factors.** Asphyxia, perinatal hypoxia, and maternal ingestion of aspirin or indomethacin.

E. **Miscellaneous.** Central nervous system disorders, neuromuscular disease, and upper airway obstruction. Although still contentious, some observational studies have suggested that the use of selective serotonin reuptake inhibitors during the last half of pregnancy may be associated with PPHN in the newborn.

V. **Clinical presentation.** The primary finding is respiratory distress with cyanosis (confirmed by demonstrating hypoxemia). This may occur despite adequate ventilation. Other clinical findings are highly variable and depend on the severity, stage, and other associated disorders (particularly pulmonary and cardiac diseases).

A. **Respiratory.** Initial respiratory symptoms may be limited to tachypnea, and onset may be at birth or within 4–8 hours of age. In addition, in an infant with pulmonary disease, PPHN should be suspected as a complicating factor when there is marked lability in oxygenation. These infants may have significant decreases in pulse oximetry readings with routine nursing care or minor stress (eg, movement or noise). Furthermore, a minor decrease in inspired oxygen concentration may lead to a surprisingly large decrease in arterial oxygenation (eg, the $AaDO_2$ gradient changes more rapidly and is more labile than that seen in the normal course of progression of uncomplicated RDS or other pulmonary disease).

B. **Cardiac signs.** Physical findings may include a prominent right ventricular impulse, a single second heart sound, and a murmur of tricuspid insufficiency. In extreme cases, there may be hepatomegaly and signs of heart failure.

C. **Imaging.** The chest film may show either cardiomegaly or a normal-sized heart. If there is no associated pulmonary disease, the film may show normal or diminished pulmonary vascularity. If there is also a parenchymal lung disorder, the degree of hypoxemia may be out of proportion to the radiographic measure of severity of the pulmonary disease.

VI. **Diagnosis. PPHN is essentially a diagnosis of exclusion.**

A. **Differential oximeter readings.** In the presence of right-to-left shunting of blood via the PDA, the Pao_2 in preductal blood (eg, from the right radial artery) is higher than that in the postductal blood (obtained from left radial, umbilical, or tibial arteries). Hence simultaneous preductal and postductal monitoring of oxygen saturation is a useful indicator of right-to-left shunting at the ductal level. However, it is important to note that PPHN cannot be excluded if no difference is found because the right-to-left shunting may be predominantly at the atrial level (or the ductus may not be patent at all). A difference >5% between preductal and postductal oxygen saturations is considered indicative of a right-to-left ductal shunt. A difference >10–15 mm Hg between preductal and postductal Pao_2 is also considered suggestive of a right-to-left ductal shunt. Preductal and postductal oxygenation should be assessed simultaneously.

B. **Hyperventilation test.** PPHN should be considered if marked improvement in oxygenation (>30 mm Hg increase in Pao_2) is noted on hyperventilating the infant (lowering $Paco_2$ and increasing pH). When a "critical" pH value is reached (often ~7.55 or greater), PVR decreases, there is less right-to-left shunting, and Pao_2 increases. This test may differentiate PPHN from cyanotic congenital heart disease. Little or no response is expected in infants with the latter diagnoses. It has been suggested that infants subjected to this test should be hyperventilated for 10 minutes. Prolonged hyperventilation is not recommended, however, particularly in premature infants (see later discussion).

C. **Imaging.** Clear lung fields or only minor disease in the face of severe hypoxemia is strongly suggestive of PPHN, if cyanotic congenital heart disease has been ruled out. In an infant with significant pulmonary parenchymal disease, a chest film is of little help in diagnosing PPHN (although it is indicated for other reasons). In an infant with rapidly worsening oxygenation, the major value of a chest film is in the exclusion of alternative diagnosis (eg, pneumothorax or pneumopericardium).

D. **Echocardiography.** Often essential in distinguishing cyanotic congenital heart disease from PPHN because the latter is frequently a diagnosis of exclusion. Furthermore, whereas all the other previously mentioned signs and tests are suggestive, echocardiography (together with Doppler studies) can provide confirmatory evidence that is often diagnostic. The first question that needs to be answered is whether the heart is structurally normal. Then the pulmonary artery pressure can be assessed indirectly by measuring the velocity of the tricuspid regurgitant jet when present. A flattened interventricular septum, or one that is bowing into the left ventricle, also supports the diagnosis of PPHN. Similarly, information about right-to-left shunting at the atrial and ductal levels support the diagnosis of PPHN. Echocardiography can also be used to assess ventricular output and contractility (both of which may be depressed in infants with PPHN).

VII. **Management**

A. **Prevention.** Adequate resuscitation and support from birth may presumably prevent or ameliorate, to some degree, PPHN when it may occur superimposed on a preexisting condition. An example is adequate and timely ventilation of an asphyxiated infant with appropriate attention to temperature control.

B. **General management.** Infants with PPHN clearly require careful and intensive monitoring. Fluid management is important because hypovolemia aggravates the right-to-left shunt. However, once normovolemia can be assumed, there is no known benefit to be gained from repeated administration of either colloids or crystalloids. Normal serum glucose and calcium should be maintained because hypoglycemia and hypocalcemia aggravate PPHN. Temperature control is also crucial. Significant acidosis should be avoided. It is useful to use 2 pulse oximeters: 1 preductal and 1 postductal.

C. **Minimal handling.** Because infants with PPHN are extremely labile with significant deterioration after seemingly "minor" stimuli, this aspect of care deserves special mention. Endotracheal tube suctioning, in particular, should be performed only if indicated and not as a matter of routine. Noise level and physical manipulation should be kept to a minimum.

D. **Mechanical ventilation.** Often needed to ensure adequate oxygenation and should first be attempted using "conventional" ventilation. The goal is to maintain adequate and stable oxygenation using the lowest possible mean airway pressures. The lowest possible positive end-expiratory pressure should also be sought. However, atelectasis should be avoided because it may aggravate pulmonary hypertension and also impair effective delivery of inhaled nitric oxide (iNO) to the lungs. Hyperventilation should be avoided, and as a guide, arterial PCO_2 values should be kept >30 mm Hg if possible; levels of 40–50 mm Hg, or even higher, are also acceptable if there is no associated compromise in oxygenation. Initially, it would be wise to ventilate with 100% inspired oxygen concentration. Weaning should be gradual and in small steps. In those infants who cannot be adequately oxygenated with conventional ventilation, high-frequency oscillatory ventilation (HFOV) should be considered early. In the presence of parenchymal lung disease, infants treated with HFOV combined with iNO were less likely to be referred for extracorporeal membrane oxygenation/extracorporeal life support (ECMO/ECLS) than those treated with either therapy alone.

E. **Surfactant.** In infants with RDS, administration of surfactant is associated with a fall in PVR. Surfactant may also be of benefit in various other pulmonary disorders (eg, meconium aspiration), although it is unknown whether its actions in these is related to a reduction in PVR. There is evidence for surfactant deficiency in some patients with PPHN.

F. **Pressor agents.** Some infants with PPHN have reduced cardiac output. In addition, increasing systemic blood pressure reduces the right-to-left shunt. Hence at least normal blood pressure should be maintained, and some recommend maintaining blood pressure of ≥40 mm Hg. **Dopamine is the most commonly used drug for this purpose.** Dobutamine has the disadvantage, in this context, that, although it may improve cardiac output, it has less of a pressor effect than dopamine. **Milrinone,** a type 3 phosphodiesterase inhibitor, is also sometimes employed to improve cardiac output. Milrinone reduces pulmonary hypertension in experimental animal models, and 2 small case series have reported on its beneficial effects in neonates with PPHN. However, the use of milrinone has been associated with occasional cases of systemic hypotension in adults and of higher heart rates in neonates. Hence more data are needed before widespread use of milrinone can be recommended.

G. **Sedation.** The lability of these infants has been mentioned previously, and hence sedation is commonly used. Pentobarbital (1–5 mg/kg) or midazolam (0.1 mg/kg) is frequently used, and analgesia with morphine (0.05–0.2 mg/kg) is also used.

H. **Inhaled nitric oxide (iNO).** See also Chapters 8 and 148.

1. **Background.** Controlled clinical trials have shown that nitric oxide (NO), when given by inhalation, reduces PVR and improves oxygenation and outcomes in a significant proportion of term and near-term neonates with PPHN. The administration of iNO to infants with PPHN reduces the number requiring ECMO/ECLS without increasing morbidity at 2 years of age. In another large multicenter trial, iNO was demonstrated to reduce both the need for ECMO/ECLS and the incidence of bronchopulmonary dysplasia (BPD)/chronic lung disease (CLD). Oxygenation can also improve during iNO therapy via mechanisms additional to its effect of reducing extrapulmonary right-to-left shunting. iNO can also improve oxygenation by redirecting blood from poorly aerated or diseased lung regions to better aerated distal air spaces (which are better exposed to the inhaled drug), thereby improving ventilation-perfusion mismatching. Although the benefits of iNO have been demonstrated in full- and near-term neonates with pulmonary hypertension, iNO treatment of preterm infants is more *controversial*. In preterm neonates, the hope was that iNO would decrease the incidence of BPD/CLD and, possibly, mitigate other morbidities. However, results of clinical trials have been conflicted, and respiratory distress in premature infants is regarded as a *controversial* indication for which further studies are necessary.

2. **Physiology.** NO is a colorless gas with a half-life of seconds. Exogenous iNO diffuses from alveoli to pulmonary vascular smooth muscle and produces vasodilation. Excess NO diffuses into the bloodstream, where it is rapidly inactivated by binding to hemoglobin and subsequent metabolism to nitrates and nitrites. This rapid inactivation thereby limits its action to the pulmonary vasculature. Dosage of iNO is measured as ppm (parts per million) of gas.

3. **Toxicity.** NO reacts with oxygen to form other oxides of nitrogen and, in particular, NO_2 (nitrogen dioxide). The latter may produce toxic effects and hence must be removed from the respiratory circuit (which can be done by using an adsorbent). When NO combines with hemoglobin, it forms methemoglobin, and this is also of potential concern. In the several large trials that have been completed, methemoglobinemia has not been a significant complication at NO doses <20 ppm. The rate of accumulation of methemoglobin depends on both the dose and duration of NO administration. Even when using doses >20 ppm, clinically significant methemoglobinemia does not appear to be a frequent complication. NO inhibits platelet adhesion to endothelium. Hence another potential complication is the prolongation of bleeding time described at NO doses of 30–300 ppm. NO may also have an adverse effect on surfactant function, but this appears to require much higher doses than those relevant in clinical applications. On the contrary, low-dose NO also has antioxidant effects, and these may be potentially beneficial. Because of these potential complications, when administering NO, NO_2 levels should be monitored. Also, blood methemoglobin concentration should be measured. Follow-up studies in infants receiving iNO have not shown any adverse effects.

4. **Dosage and administration.** Available evidence supports the use of doses of iNO beginning at 20 ppm. Among infants with a positive response to iNO, the response time is rapid. There is no agreement, however, about the duration of treatment and criteria for discontinuation; these vary and often reflect institutional preferences. Thus some recommend weaning once arterial Po_2 is >50 mm Hg; others suggest an oxygenation index <10 as an indications for weaning. Moreover, no evidence suggests the superiority of one weaning regimen over another. However, some observations are available to assist in weaning considerations. One point is, however, beyond contention: weaning should be done under careful and intensive monitoring of each step. Particular note should be made of the observation that sudden discontinuation of iNO can be associated with "rebound" pulmonary hypertension (see Section VII.H.4b).

   a. **Initial dose.** Start treatment with iNO at 20 ppm. Little is to be gained by administering higher doses because, at most, only a few patients will respond to these higher doses after not having responded to a dose of 20 ppm. Higher doses may significantly increase the rate of methemoglobinemia. Also, initial treatment with subtherapeutic low-dose iNO may diminish the subsequent response to iNO at 20 ppm. Among infants with a positive response to iNO, the response time is rapid.

   b. **Weaning.** Wean inspired oxygen concentration until F_{IO_2} <0.6. Then start weaning iNO concentrations in steps of 5 ppm until iNO is 5 ppm. Weaning may be initiated as early as 4–6 hours after starting treatment, or later, and should be attempted at least once per day, but may be done as frequently as every 30 minutes. Hemodynamic stability and adequate oxygenation should be monitored closely 30–60 minutes after each weaning step. Significant deterioration should be an indication of reversing the previous weaning step. Once iNO is at 5 ppm, weaning should be continued at a slower pace, in steps of 1 ppm, until iNO is 1 ppm. Once the patient has demonstrated stability at iNO of 1 ppm for a few hours, iNO may be discontinued. Some decline in oxygen saturation should be anticipated, and an increase of 10–20% in required inspired oxygen concentration may be considered reasonable when discontinuing iNO and need not be an indication for reinstating therapy. However, if an FIO_2 >0.75 is required to maintain adequate oxygenation, the patient may benefit from being placed back on iNO. *Caution:* Although there are various weaning regimens of iNO, evidence suggests that iNO should be discontinued from a dose of 1 ppm and not from a higher one. The rate of success is higher when discontinuation is done from a dose of 1 ppm than from 5 ppm or higher. Moreover, the phenomenon of rebound pulmonary hypertension should be kept in mind after discontinuation of iNO. Sudden discontinuation of iNO can be associated with "rebound" pulmonary hypertension, and this rebound can be severe and may occur even in infants who had initially failed to respond to iNO treatment when it was initiated. We should emphasize that this protocol is merely a suggestion and is compatible with data derived from trials and experience with the use of iNO. Many other regimens would be just as reasonable.

5. **Failure to respond to iNO or the need for prolonged administration.** Patients not responding to iNO or those in whom iNO cannot be weaned after 5 days of treatment merit a reevaluation. Effective therapy requires adequate lung inflation, and an infant who fails to respond should be evaluated by chest radiograph for airway obstruction and atelectasis. Lung volume recruitment strategies may be required, as may surfactant treatment in appropriate circumstances. Pressor support or volume administration may be required because impaired cardiac output may render iNO treatment ineffective. An echocardiogram is warranted to rule out cardiac anomalies that may have been missed and to assess cardiac function. Consideration should be directed toward lung diseases that respond poorly to iNO, such as alveolar-capillary dysplasia or those associated with pulmonary hypoplasia. Fewer than 35% of infants with congenital diaphragmatic hernia respond to iNO or survive without ECMO/ECLS.

I. **Sildenafil.** The phosphodiesterase PDE5 is abundantly expressed in lung tissue and degrades cGMP. Sildenafil, a PDE5 inhibitor, prolongs the half-life of cGMP and would be expected to enhance the actions of both endogenous and exogenous nitric oxide. A few small randomized trials in infants have shown its effectiveness in treating pulmonary hypertension. Additional reports are in the form of case series. It has been successful in treating pulmonary hypertension in infants after cardiac surgery, and case series have shown it to be useful in attenuating the rebound pulmonary hypertension after withdrawal of iNO. In some patients sildenafil may confer benefit additional to that obtained by iNO alone. In some units, sildenafil is given prophylactically before the final step in weaning off iNO. Patients treated with sildenafil have not shown an increased propensity for systemic hypotension. Concern has been raised about possible adverse effects of this drug in those infants at risk for retinopathy of prematurity, although the putative association has been questioned. Larger trials will be required to address issues of risk and benefits. Although an intravenous (IV) preparation is available, the drug is mostly given enterally. Reported dosages vary and range from 1–3 mg/kg every 6 hours.

J. **Prostacyclin.** Prostacyclin (PGI_2) is a short-acting, potent vasodilator of both the pulmonary and systemic circulations. The greatest experience of its use is as a continuous IV infusion of epoprostenol. Trials in adults and older children with pulmonary hypertension have shown an improvement in symptoms and mortality. However, epoprostenol treatment is associated with various limitations. The drug has a very short half-life and requires continuous infusion. There are special storage requirements, and side effects include systemic hypotension. The data in neonates is sparse and consists of a few case reports of the drug's successful use in this patient population. Reported dosages have varied between 4 ng/kg/min to 40 ng/kg/min IV, and it is suggested that a low starting dose be initiated, with increasing dosage rate being titrated according to response. Higher doses are associated with increased risk of systemic hypotension, and blood pressure should be monitored.

K. **Inhaled/nebulized PGI$_2$ (Iloprost).** This is a stable PGI$_2$ analogue with a longer half-life, and it acts by stimulating adenyl cyclase and increasing cAMP. It is gaining wider acceptance owing to its selective pulmonary vasodilation without decreasing systemic blood pressure. Randomized trials in adults have shown its effectiveness and safety, but the pediatric and neonatal literature consists of a few case series and case reports. The use of inhaled prostacyclin was reported in 4 neonates with PPHN refractory to iNO. All 4 infants showed a rapid improvement. One neonate subsequently deteriorated and was found to have alveolar-capillary dysplasia. No systemic vascular effects were noted. Dosage varies between reports but is mostly in the range of 0.25–2 mcg/kg per inhalation with inhalations being given over 5–10 minutes every 2–8 hours.

L. **Bosentan.** ET-1 is a potent vasoconstrictor and is increased in newborns with PPHN. Bosentan is an endothelin receptor antagonist that improves hemodynamics and quality of life in adults with pulmonary hypertension. Up to 10% of patients are affected by liver toxicity. Bosentan improved hemodynamics in a study of its use in pediatric patients with pulmonary hypertension. Its use also enabled a reduction of the epoprostenol dose. There is, however, little information on the use of bosentan in neonates with PPHN and the literature consists mostly of case reports. Bosentan is sometimes used anecdotally for refractory pulmonary hypertension in infants with congenital diaphragmatic hernia, severe BPD/CLD, and congenital heart diseases. There are no systematic data on its use and safety in neonates, either as a single therapy or as an adjunct in combination therapy. Reported dosage is 1–2 mg/kg twice per day.

M. **Paralyzing agents.** The use of these agents is *controversial*. Their use has been advocated in infants who have not responded to sedation and are still labile or who appear to "fight" the ventilator. In a retrospective survey, the use of paralysis was associated with increased mortality, although a causal relation cannot be inferred. Pancuronium is the drug most commonly used, although it may increase PVR to some extent and worsen ventilation-perfusion mismatch. Vecuronium (0.1 mg/kg) has also been used.

N. **Alkalinization.** In the past, it had been noted that hyperventilation, with the resulting hypocapnia, improved oxygenation secondary to pulmonary vasodilation. Subsequently, it was shown, in animal studies, that the beneficial effect of hypocapnia was actually a result of the increased pH rather than of the low Paco$_2$ values achieved. Furthermore, follow-up of infants with PPHN had suggested that hypocapnia was related to poor neurodevelopmental outcome (especially sensorineural hearing loss). Hypocapnia is known to reduce cerebral blood flow. The use of alkalinization is *controversial*, and there are no adequately controlled trials on its use to alleviate PPHN. If alkalinization is employed, it may be advisable to increase pH using an infusion of sodium bicarbonate (0.5–1 mEq/kg/h) if possible. Serum sodium should be monitored to avoid hypernatremia. Improvement in oxygenation has been anecdotally reported with arterial pH 7.50–7.55 (sometimes levels as high as 7.65 are required).

O. **Magnesium sulfate.** Magnesium causes vasodilation by antagonizing calcium ion entry into smooth muscle cells. A few small observational studies have suggested that MgSO$_4$ may effectively treat PPHN, but the evidence is conflicting, and there is some risk of systemic hypotension. The dose reported is a loading dosage of 200 mg/kg followed by an infusion of 20–150 mg/kg/h (the drug is given IV). Two small trials in neonates with PPHN have shown that sildenafil and iNO are each superior to IV MgSO$_4$.

P. **Adenosine.** Adenosine causes vasodilation by stimulation of adenosine receptors on endothelial cells and release of endothelial NO. A small randomized trial reported the effectiveness of adenosine infusion (25–50 mcg/kg/min) in treating PPHN in term babies. Subsequently a few further cases have been published. Despite initial favorable data, the drug has not attracted attention, and its use awaits further clinical trials.

Q. ECMO/ECLS. (See Chapter 18.) ECMO/ECLS may be indicated for term or near-term infants with PPHN who fail to respond to conventional therapy and who meet ECMO/ECLS entry criteria. The survival rate with ECMO/ECLS is reportedly >80%, although only the most severely afflicted infants are referred for this treatment.

VIII. **Pulmonary hypertension in BPD/CLD.** A significant number of cases of BPD/CLD exhibit pulmonary hypertension (PH). The pulmonary circulation in BPD/CLD exhibits elevated pulmonary vascular resistance and increased vasoreactivity, vascular remodeling, and decreased and disrupted growth. The disruption in angiogenesis also impairs alveolarization, and, furthermore, there is formation of bronchial and other systemic-to-pulmonary collateral vessels. The presence of PH complicating the course of BPD/CLD is associated with significantly increased mortality and morbidity. The rationale for aggressively diagnosing and treating PH complicating BPD/CLD is the hope that it would affect the increased mortality. Which patients with BPD/CLD should be screened for the presence of PH? There are no data to indicate an optimal approach, but a few guidelines have been suggested. Patients still requiring ventilatory assistance or significant supplemental oxygen at 36 weeks' postconceptional age might benefit from an echocardiographic evaluation. Furthermore, infants with severe respiratory disease that fails to improve, those with respiratory disease out of proportion to the expected course or radiologic findings, those with recurrent and persistent cyanotic spells or respiratory deteriorations, and those with repeated need for diuretic administration might also benefit of screening for PH. Screening for PH in patients with BPD/CLD may require serial interval echocardiograms. The echocardiographic evaluation of PH is far from perfect, and certain patients may require cardiac catheterization for diagnosis of PH and to assess its severity and response to treatment. The therapeutic options most commonly used are iNO, sildenafil, and bosentan. However, treatment of PH should always occur in a context whereby attempts have been made to optimize ventilatory support and complicating factors (eg, reflux and aspirations) have been considered and treated, if necessary.

IX. **Prognosis.** The overall survival rate is >70–75%. There is, however, a marked difference in survival and long-term outcome according to the cause of the PPHN. More than 80% of term or near-term neonates with PPHN are expected to have an essentially normal neurodevelopmental outcome. Abnormal long-term outcome in PPHN survivors (and a high incidence of sensorineural hearing loss) has been reported to correlate with duration of hyperventilation. However, the relationship may not be causal because prolonged hyperventilation may simply be a marker for the severity of PPHN and hypoxic insult. Survivors of idiopathic PPHN usually have no residual lung or heart disease. Very low birthweight infants with PPHN accompanying severe RDS have a much higher rate of mortality, and there are few data on the long-term outcome of the survivors.

Selected References

Gao Y, Raj JU. Regulation of pulmonary circulation in the fetus and newborn. *Physiol Rev.* 2010;90:1291–1335.

Kelly LK, Porta NF, Goodman DM, Carroll CL, Steinhorn RH. Inhaled prostacyclin for term infants with persistent pulmonary hypertension refractory to inhaled nitric oxide. *J Pediatr.* 2002;141:830–832.

Mourani PM, Abman SH. Pulmonary hypertension in bronchopulmonary dysplasia. *Prog Pediatr Cardiol.* 2009;27:43–48.

Mulligan C, Beghetti M. Inhaled Iloprost for the control of acute pulmonary hypertension in children. A systemic review. *Pediatr Crit Care Med.* 2012;13:472–480.

Rao S, Bartle D, Patole S. Current and future therapeutic options for persistent pulmonary hypertension in the newborn. *Expert Rev Cardiovasc Ther.* 2010;8:845–862.

Steinhorn RH. Neonatal pulmonary hypertension. *Pediatr Crit Care Med.* 2010;11(suppl):S79–S84.

121 Pertussis

I. **Definition.** Pertussis is an infection caused by the gram-negative bacteria *Bordetella pertussis*. In children it often presents with respiratory symptoms, including the classic whooping cough, but in neonates it tends to have an atypical and more severe presentation.

II. **Incidence.** The overall incidence of pertussis has been increasing in recent years, with the highest incidence seen in infants <6 months of age in the United States. There are an estimated 300,000 deaths due to pertussis worldwide each year, mostly affecting young infants. The incidence of pertussis in pregnant women is thought to be similar to that of the general population.

III. **Pathophysiology.** Transmission of *Bordetella pertussis* occurs through the respiratory route via close contact with respiratory secretions or aerosolized droplets. The parents of infants are estimated to be the source of infection in 25% of cases, and household members are thought to be the source in about 80% of cases. *Bordetella pertussis* produces multiple toxins including the pertussis toxin, which inhibits neutrophil migration to the lungs, and tracheal cytotoxin, which damages cilia in the respiratory epithelium via a nitric oxide synthase (NOS)-dependent pathway. The lymphocytosis seen in cases of pertussis is attributed to the potent mitogen, lymphocytosis-promoting factor. The aggregation of leukocytes in the pulmonary circulation is thought to cause the refractory pulmonary hypertension seen in severe cases of neonatal pertussis.

IV. **Risk factors.** Infants <6 months of age are at highest risk for severe pertussis and complications or death from pertussis, especially if they are unvaccinated. Other risk factors include preterm (<37 weeks' gestation) and low birthweight infants. Infection during pregnancy does not appear to increase either maternal or fetal morbidity.

V. **Clinical presentation.** The 3 phases of classic pertussis, namely catarrhal (1–2 weeks), paroxysmal (2–6 weeks), and convalescent (2–6 weeks), are not typically observed in infants. Neonatal cases tend to present with paroxysmal cough, gagging, bradycardia, gasping, apnea, and cyanotic spells, but not fever and tachypnea. They do not have the characteristic "whoop" due to lack of prolonged inspiratory effort at the end of a paroxysm. Infants <6 months of age tend to have a shorter catarrhal and longer convalescent phase. The following complications may be observed in neonates and young infants with pertussis:

A. **Secondary infections.** Pertussis can be complicated by secondary infections such as pneumonia (22–25% of cases), meningoencephalitis, and otitis media.

B. **Ophthalmologic complications.** The forceful coughing paroxysms characteristic of pertussis can also result in ophthalmologic complications such as subconjunctival, scleral, and rarely retinal hemorrhages.

C. **Central nervous system manifestations.** Intraventricular and subarachnoid hemorrhages may result from increased intracranial pressure secondary to the Valsalva effect of paroxysmal coughing. Seizures (2–4% of cases) are attributed to hypoxemia from apnea or relentless coughing, but may also be due to hyponatremia secondary to pneumonia-induced syndrome of inappropriate antidiuretic hormone secretion. Encephalopathy is estimated to occur in 0.5–1% of cases and usually occurs during the paroxysmal stage. It can present with fever, convulsions, focal neurological signs including blindness and deafness, pareses and plegias, and altered mental state progressing to coma. Pertussis encephalopathy is fatal in one-third of patients and leads to neurodevelopmental delay in another third of patients.

D. **Respiratory complications.** Infants with pertussis are at increased risk for severe pulmonary hypertension due to pulmonary vasoconstriction from hypoxia and acidosis secondary to recurrent prolonged apnea, as well as restriction of pulmonary blood flow from leukocyte thrombi. Neonates with pertussis have a greater need for mechanical ventilation due to frequent apnea, respiratory compromise during paroxysms of coughing, and pulmonary hypertension.

E. **Miscellaneous.** The increased intrathoracic and intra-abdominal pressures associated with paroxysmal coughing can result in other physical sequelae such as epistaxis, upper body petechiae, pneumothorax, and umbilical and inguinal hernias. Post-tussive emesis can lead to alkalosis, dehydration, and malnutrition.

VI. **Diagnosis.** Pertussis should be differentiated from other infectious causes of respiratory distress in neonates. Adenoviral infections can produce apnea and intractable coughing but usually present with fever, lethargy, maculopapular rash, pharyngitis, conjunctivitis, and coagulopathy. *Mycoplasma pneumoniae* can present with protracted cough and pneumonia. *Chlamydia trachomatis* infections may present with conjunctivitis, nasal congestion, pneumonia, and a staccato cough in afebrile patients. Respiratory syncytial virus (RSV) can present with apnea and lower respiratory tract infection. Pertussis and RSV, as coexisting infections, is not infrequent.

A. **Laboratory studies**

   1. **Complete blood count (CBC) with differential.** Leukocytosis (white blood cell count of $\geq$20,000 cells/mm^3) with lymphocytosis ($\geq$50% lymphocytes) is suggestive of pertussis.

   2. **Bacterial culture.** The gold standard for diagnosis is bacterial culture of a nasopharyngeal specimen placed in a special transport medium (Regan-Lowe). While this method is 100% specific, false-negative cultures can occur if the specimen is obtained within or later than the third week of illness, or in pretreated or vaccinated patients.

   3. **Polymerase chain reaction (PCR).** Testing for pertussis by PCR has increased sensitivity over bacterial culture, especially in later stages of the disease and in pretreated individuals. False-positive PCR results have been noted and appear to be related to an absence of standardized procedures and laboratory variability.

B. **Imaging studies**

   1. **Chest radiograph.** Infants with uncomplicated pertussis usually have normal findings. Radiographic evidence of pneumonia may be seen in severe or complicated cases.

VII. **Management**

A. **Antimicrobial therapy.** Macrolide antibiotics alleviate disease severity if given during the initial catarrhal stage. Treatment in later phases is still recommended to reduce the risk of contagion. Due to an association between orally administered erythromycin and infantile hypertrophic pyloric stenosis, azithromycin (10 mg/kg/d in a single dose daily for 5 days) is the current drug of choice for treatment or prophylaxis of pertussis in infants <1 month of age.

B. **Supportive care.** Infants <3 months of age should be hospitalized with close monitoring of respiratory, hydration, and nutrition status.

C. **Respiratory support**

   1. **Mechanical ventilation.** Intubation and mechanical ventilation are often necessary due to frequent apnea or respiratory failure.

   2. **Airway therapies.** Bronchodilators, inhaled steroids, and cough suppressants are not routinely recommended.

   3. **Inhaled nitric oxide (iNO).** Pulmonary hypertension resulting from pertussis is thought to be refractory to iNO, because vasodilator therapy does not address the issue of leukocyte thrombi in the pulmonary vasculature. Current literature suggests caution in the use of iNO in the setting of pertussis; it is thought that tracheal cytotoxin induces NOS via generation of the cytokine interleukin (IL)-1, leading to increased levels of endogenous NO production that then diffuses to ciliated cells and causes the specific ciliated-cell cytopathology characteristic of *B. pertussis* infection.

4. **Double volume exchange transfusion.** Early consideration prior to the onset of hypotension and shock is suggested to alleviate the hyperleukocytosis contributing to severe cases of pulmonary hypertension, hypoxia, and cardiac failure. See Chapter 30.

5. **Extracorporeal membrane oxygenation/extracorporeal life support (ECMO/ECLS).** ECMO/ECLS should be considered for neonates with refractory respiratory failure and pulmonary hypertension. Survival after ECMO/ECLS is estimated at 20–30%, with a high neutrophil count at presentation and multiorgan dysfunction suggestive of a poor prognosis. The low survival rate has led to speculation that different pathophysiologic mechanisms are at play in pertussis other than those seen in neonatal persistent pulmonary hypertension. See Chapter 18.

D. **Prevention/control measures**

1. **Isolation.** Standard precaution is recommended for the entire course of illness. Droplet precaution is recommended for 5 days after initiation of effective therapy.

2. **Chemoprophylaxis.** Early chemoprophylaxis is recommended for all household contacts and other close contacts. Due to limited efficacy, late chemoprophylaxis (after 21 days) is only recommended for high-risk contacts (pregnant women and young infants or their contacts).

3. **Immunizations.** Six doses of pertussis vaccine (at 2, 4, and 6 months; 15–18 months; 4–6 years; 11 years) are recommended universally. Preterm birth is not a contraindication to the pertussis vaccine. See Appendix E.

4. **Newborn exposure.** Due to an increasing occurrence of outbreaks of pertussis (eg, California in 2011), immunization of pregnant women in either the second or third trimester has been endorsed by the American Congress of Obstetricians and Gynecologists and the Centers for Disease Control and Prevention (CDC). The intention is to prevent maternal pertussis from occurring in the immediate postpartum period should exposure occur, or in the event of exposure subsequently in the newborn and infant periods prior to routine immunizations beginning at 2 months of age. Secondarily, some passive transfer of maternal antibodies may protect the newborn. Additionally, the CDC, American Academy of Pediatrics, and American College of Obstetricians and Gynecologists advocate "cocooning" of newborns by providing postpartum immunization of all close family contacts and any family contacts that may have exposure to children 1 year of age or younger (the most actively infected population identified in recent outbreaks). Finally, immunization of newborn infants in the immediate postnatal period has been suggested as a possible consideration based on recent evidence of greater newborn immunocompetence than previously known. To date, no U.S.-based organizational approval has been established to support such a recommendation. However, in the face of a proximal community outbreak of pertussis, early infant immunization schedules at 6 weeks of age may be undertaken instead of 2 months (CDC, 2011).

VIII. **Prognosis.** Neonates with pertussis have demonstrated a need for longer hospitalization when compared to those with nonpertussis respiratory illnesses. A case fatality rate of 1% is reported for infants <2 months of age.

Selected References

American Academy of Pediatrics. Pertussis (whooping cough). In: Pickering LK, Baker CJ, Kimberlin DW, Long SS, eds. *Red Book 2012 Report of the Committee on Infectious Diseases.* Elk Grove Village, IL: American Academy of Pediatrics; 2012:553–566.

Castagnini LA, Munoz FM. Clinical characteristics and outcomes of neonatal pertussis: a comparative study. *J Pediatr.* 2010;156:498–500.

Centers for Disease Control and Prevention. Prevention of pertussis, tetanus, and diphtheria among pregnant and postpartum women and their infants: recommendations of the advisory committee on immunization practices. *MMWR.* 2011;60:1424–1426.

Flak TA, Heiss LN, Engle JT, Goldman WE. Synergistic epithelial responses to endotoxin and a naturally occurring muramyl peptide. *Infect Immun.* 2000;68:1235–1242.

Kirimanjeswara GS, Agosto LM, Kennett MJ, Bjornstad ON, Harvill ET. Pertussis toxin inhibits neutrophil recruitment to delay antibody-mediated clearance of *Bordetella pertussis. J Clin Invest.* 2005;115:3594–3601.

Long SS. Pertussis. In: Behrman RE, Kliegman RM, Jenson HB, eds. *Nelson Textbook of Pediatrics.* 17th ed. Philadelphia, PA: Elsevier; 2004:908–912.

Murphy TV, Slade BA, Broder KR, et al. Prevention of pertussis, tetanus, and diphtheria among pregnant and postpartum women and their infants. Recommendations of the Advisory Committee on Immunization Practices (ACIP). *MMWR Recomm Rep.* 2008;57:1–47, 51.

Paddock CD, Sanden GN, Cherry JD, et al. Pathology and pathogenesis of fatal *Bordetella pertussis* infection in infants. *Clin Infect Dis.* 2008;47:328–338.

Pooboni S, Roberts N, Westrope C, et al. Extracorporeal life support in pertussis. *Pediatr Pulmonol.* 2003;36:310–315.

Romano MJ, Weber MD, Weisse ME, Siu BL. Pertussis pneumonia, hypoxemia, hyperleukocytosis, and pulmonary hypertension: improvement in oxygenation after a double volume exchange transfusion. *Pediatrics.* 2004;114:e264–e266.

Wendelboe AM, Njamkepo E, Bourillon A, et al. Transmission of *Bordetella pertussis* to young infants. *Pediatr Infect Dis J.* 2007;26:293–299.

122 Polycythemia and Hyperviscosity

I. **Definitions.** Polycythemia is an increased total red blood cell (RBC) mass. Polycythemic hyperviscosity is an increased viscosity of the blood resulting from, or associated with, increased numbers of RBCs.

   A. **Polycythemia of the newborn.** Defined as a central venous hematocrit >65%. The clinical significance of this value results from the curvilinear relationship between the circulating RBC volume (hematocrit) and whole-blood viscosity. Above a hematocrit of 65%, blood viscosity, as measured in vitro, rises exponentially.

   B. **Hyperviscosity.** Defined as a viscosity >14 cP at a shear rate of 11.5/s measured by a viscometer. Serum viscosity is reported as centipoises [cP]. Hyperviscosity is the cause of clinical symptoms in infants presumed to be symptomatic from polycythemia. Many polycythemic infants are also hyperviscous, but this is not invariably the case. **The terms polycythemia and hyperviscosity are not interchangeable.**

II. **Incidence**

   A. **Polycythemia.** Polycythemia occurs in 2–4% of the general newborn population. Half of these patients are symptomatic, although it is not at all certain whether their symptoms are caused by polycythemia.

   B. **Hyperviscosity.** Hyperviscosity without polycythemia occurs in 1% of normal (nonpolycythemic) newborns. In infants with a hematocrit of 60–64%, a fourth have hyperviscosity.

III. **Pathophysiology.** Clinical signs attributed to hyperviscosity may result from the regional effects of hyperviscosity, including tissue hypoxia, acidosis, and hypoglycemia, and from the formation of microthrombi within the microcirculation. An important caveat, however, is that the same clinical signs may result from coexisting perinatal circumstances in the presence or absence of hyperviscosity. Potentially affected organs include the central nervous system, the kidneys and adrenal glands, the cardiopulmonary system, and the gastrointestinal tract. Blood viscosity depends on the interaction of frictional forces in whole blood. These forces are defined as **shear stress** (refers to frictional forces within a fluid) and **shear rate** (a measure of blood flow velocity). The shear rate in the aorta is 230/s and only 11.5/s in the small arterioles and venules. As the viscosity increases, such as in the microcirculation, blood with a high hematocrit may virtually cease flowing. The frictional forces identified within whole blood and their relative contributions to hyperviscosity in the newborn include the following:

A. **Hematocrit.** An increase in the hematocrit is the most important single factor contributing to hyperviscosity in the neonate. An increased hematocrit results from either an absolute increase in circulating RBC volume or a decrease in plasma volume.

B. **Plasma viscosity.** A direct linear relationship exists between plasma viscosity and the concentration of plasma proteins, particularly those of high molecular weight, such as fibrinogen. Term infants and, to a greater degree, preterm infants have low plasma fibrinogen levels compared with adults. Consequently, except for the rare case of primary hyperfibrinogenemia, plasma viscosity does not contribute to an increased whole-blood viscosity in the neonate. Under normal conditions, low plasma fibrinogen levels and, correspondingly, low plasma viscosity actually may protect the microcirculation of the neonate by facilitating perfusion and contributing to low whole-blood viscosity.

C. **RBC aggregation.** Occurs only in areas of low blood flow and is usually limited to the venous microcirculation. Because fibrinogen levels are typically low in term and preterm infants, RBC aggregation does not contribute significantly to whole-blood viscosity in newborn infants. There is some concern that the use of adult fresh-frozen plasma for partial exchange transfusion in neonates might critically alter the concentration of fibrinogen and paradoxically raise whole-blood viscosity within the microcirculation.

D. **Deformability of RBC membrane.** There are apparently no differences among term infants, preterm infants, and adults in terms of the membrane deformability of erythrocytes. RBC deformability is increased in preterm neonates as compared with term neonates and in term neonates as compared with adults. The increase in deformability is presumed to reduce blood viscosity and to reduce the likelihood that polycythemia will cause hyperviscosity. Because infants of diabetic mothers are thought to have RBCs with reduced deformability, hyperviscosity may be more likely at polycythemic hematocrits than in unaffected neonate.

IV. **Risk factors**
   A. **Conditions that alter incidence**
      1. **Altitude.** There is an absolute increase in RBC mass as part of physiologic adaptation to high altitude.
      2. **Neonatal age.** The normal pattern of fluid shifts during the first 6 hours of life is away from the intravascular compartment. The period of maximum physiologic increase in the hematocrit occurs at 2–4 hours of age.
      3. **Obstetric factors.** A delay in cord clamping beyond 30 seconds or stripping of the umbilical cord, if that is the prevailing practice, results in a higher incidence of polycythemia.
      4. **High-risk delivery.** A high-risk delivery is associated with an increased incidence of polycythemia, particularly if precipitous or uncontrolled.
   B. **Perinatal processes**
      1. **Enhanced fetal erythropoiesis.** Elevated erythropoietin levels result from a direct stimulus, usually related to fetal hypoxia, or from an altered regulation of erythropoietin production.
         a. Placental insufficiency
            i. **Maternal hypertensive disease (preeclampsia/eclampsia) or primary renovascular disease**

        ii. **Abruptio placentae** (chronic recurrent)
      iii. **Postmaturity**
      iv. **Cyanotic congenital heart disease**
       v. **Intrauterine growth restriction (IUGR)**
      vi. **Maternal cigarette smoking**
   b. **Endocrine disorders.** Increased oxygen consumption is the suggested mechanism by which hyperinsulinism or hyperthyroxinemia creates fetal hypoxemia and stimulates erythropoietin production.
       i. **Infant of a diabetic mother** (>40% incidence of polycythemia)
      ii. **Infant of a mother with gestational diabetes** (>30% incidence of polycythemia)
      iii. **Congenital thyrotoxicosis**
      iv. **Congenital adrenal hyperplasia**
       v. **Beckwith-Wiedemann syndrome** (secondary hyperinsulinism)
   c. **Genetic trisomies.** Trisomies 13, 18, and 21.
2. **Hypertransfusion.** Conditions that enhance placental transfusion at birth may create hypervolemic normocythemia, which evolves into hypervolemic polycythemia as the normal pattern of fluid shift occurs. A larger transfusion may create hypervolemic polycythemia at birth, with signs present in the infant. Conditions associated with hypertransfusion include the following:
   a. **Delay in cord clamping.** Placental vessels contain up to a third of the fetal blood volume, half of which is returned to the infant within 1 minute after birth. The risks associated with delayed cord clamping are probably negligible compared with the benefits that are in the term infant: reduction in the rate of iron deficiency in the first 2 years of life and in the sick preterm, decreased need for blood transfusions, inotrope support, and intraventricular hemorrhage. Representative blood volumes for term infants with a variable delay in cord clamping are as follows:
       i. 15-second delay, 75–78 mL/kg.
      ii. 60-second delay, 80–87 mL/kg.
      iii. 120-second delay, 83–93 mL/kg.
   b. **Gravity.** Positioning the infant below the placental bed (>10 cm below the placenta) enhances placental transfusion via the umbilical vein. Elevation of the infant >50 cm above the placenta prevents placental transfusion.
   c. **Maternal use of medications.** Drugs that enhance uterine contractility—specifically oxytocin—do not significantly alter the gravitational effects on placental transfusion during the first 15 seconds after birth. With further delay in clamping of the cord, however, blood flow toward the infant accelerates to a maximum at 1 minute of age.
   d. **Cesarean delivery.** In cesarean delivery, there is usually a lower degree of placental transfusion if the cord is clamped early because of the absence of active uterine contractions in most cases and because of gravitational effects.
   e. **Twin–twin transfusion.** Interfetal transfusion (**parabiosis syndrome**) is observed in monochorionic twin pregnancy with an incidence of 15%. The recipient twin, on the venous side of the anastomosis, becomes polycythemic, and the donor, on the arterial side, becomes anemic. Simultaneous venous hematocrits obtained after delivery differ by >12–15%, and both twins have a high risk of intrauterine or neonatal death and increased neurologic morbidity.
   f. **Maternal-fetal transfusion.** Approximately 10–80% of normal newborn infants receive a small volume of maternal blood at the time of delivery. The "reverse" Kleihauer-Betke acid elution technique documents maternal RBC "ghosts" on a neonatal blood smear. With large transfusions, the test is positive for several days. Because various conditions may lead to

a false-negative test result, new and more accurate flow cytometry techniques can be used when the index of suspicion for **maternal-fetal** transfusions is elevated.

g. **Intrapartum asphyxia.** Prolonged fetal distress enhances the net umbilical blood flow toward the infant until cord clamping occurs, and acidosis may encourage capillary leak, reduced plasma volume, and decreased red blood cell deformability.

V. **Clinical presentation.** Clinical signs observed in polycythemia are nonspecific and reflect the regional effects of hyperviscosity within a given microcirculation. The conditions listed next may occur independently of polycythemia or hyperviscosity and must be considered in the differential diagnosis.

A. **Central nervous system.** There may be an altered state of consciousness, including lethargy and decreased activity, hyperirritability, proximal muscle hypotonia, vasomotor instability, and vomiting. Seizures, thromboses, and cerebral infarction are extraordinarily rare.

B. **Cardiopulmonary system.** Respiratory distress and tachycardia may be present. Congestive heart failure with cardiomegaly may be seen but is rarely clinically prominent. Pulmonary hypertension may occur but is not usually severe unless other predisposing factors are present.

C. **Gastrointestinal tract.** Feeding intolerance occurs occasionally. Necrotizing enterocolitis has been reported but rarely without other factors (eg, IUGR), which casts doubt on the primary cause.

D. **Genitourinary tract.** Oliguria, acute renal failure/acute kidney injury, renal vein thrombosis, or priapism may occur.

E. **Metabolic disorders.** Hypoglycemia, hypocalcemia, or hypomagnesemia may be seen.

F. **Hematologic disorders.** There may be hyperbilirubinemia, thrombocytopenia, or reticulocytosis (with enhanced erythropoiesis only).

VI. **Diagnosis**

A. **Venous (not capillary) hematocrit.** Polycythemia is present when the central venous hematocrit is ≥65%.

B. **The following screening studies may be used:**
   1. A cord blood hematocrit >56% suggests polycythemia.
   2. A warmed capillary hematocrit ≥65% suggests polycythemia.

VII. **Management.** (See also Chapter 71). Clinical management of the polycythemic infant is more expectant now than a decade ago. Studies and reviews have created much doubt about any long-term benefits of partial exchange transfusion (PET). Consequently, PET should probably be performed only on infants in whom significant morbidity is in question.

A. **Asymptomatic infants.** Only expectant observation is required for virtually all asymptomatic infants. The possible exception is an infant with a central venous hematocrit of >75%, but even in this group the risks of central catheter insertion probably outweigh the benefits of PET.

B. **Symptomatic infants.** When the central venous hematocrit is ≥65%, PET with normal saline may ameliorate acute signs of polycythemia or hyperviscosity. Whether treatment of a self-limited problem justifies the risks of central catheter insertion and an exchange procedure is debatable, however. For the procedure for partial exchange transfusion, see Chapter 30.

VIII. **Prognosis.** The long-term outcome of infants with polycythemia or hyperviscosity and response to PET is as follows:

A. A causal relationship exists between PET and an increase in gastrointestinal tract disorders and necrotizing enterocolitis.

B. Older randomized controlled prospective studies of polycythemic and hyperviscous infants indicate that PET may reduce but not eliminate the risk of neurologic sequelae. More recent data suggest that no benefits accrue from PET.

C. Infants with "asymptomatic" polycythemia have an increased risk for neurologic sequelae, but normocythemic controls with the same perinatal histories have a similarly increased risk.

Selected References

Dempsey EM, Barrington K. Short and long term outcomes following partial exchange transfusion in the polycythaemic newborn: a systematic review. *Arch Dis Child Fetal Neonatal Ed.* 2006;91:F2–F6.

Dempsey EM, Barrington K. Crystalloid or colloid for partial exchange transfusion in neonatal polycythemia: a systematic review and meta-analysis. *Acta Paediatr.* 2005;94:1650–1655.

Mercer JS, Vohr BR, McGrath MM, Padbury JF, Wallach M, Oh W. Delayed cord clamping in very preterm infants reduces the incidence of intraventricular hemorrhage and late-onset sepsis: a randomized, controlled trial. *Pediatrics.* 2006;117:1235–1242.

Morag I, Strauss T, Lubin D, Schushan-Eisen I, Kenet G, Kuint J. Restrictive management of neonatal polycythemia. *Am J Perinatol.* 2011;28:677–682.

Oh W. Timing of umbilical cord clamping at birth in full-term infants. *JAMA.* 2007;11:1257–1258.

Rosenkrantz TS. Polycythemia and hyperviscosity in the newborn. *Semin Thromb Hemost.* 2003:29:515–527.

Seng YC, Rajadurai VS. Twin-twin transfusion syndrome: a five year review. *Arch Dis Child Fetal Neonatal Ed.* 2000;83:F168–F170.

---

123 Renal Failure, Acute (Acute Kidney Injury)

I. **Definition.** The term acute renal failure (ARF) has now been replaced with the term acute kidney injury (AKI), and is now used to encompass mild renal dysfunction to complete anuric kidney failure. In neonates, ARF/AKI is defined as a serum creatinine >1.5 mg/dL (132.6 μmol/L), regardless of age or urine output, with normal maternal renal function. ARF/AKI can be **anuric** (absence of urinary output by 24–48 hours of age), **oliguric** (urine output of <1.0 mL/kg), or **nonoliguric** (>1.0 mL/kg). ARF/AKI can present with normal urinary output (seen in asphyxiated neonates). Normal urine output is ~1–3 mL/kg/h with almost all infants voiding within 24 hours of birth. See Table 68–1, page 467.

II. **Incidence.** In some studies, as many as 24% of neonatal intensive care unit (NICU)-admitted neonates have some degree of renal failure. Prerenal is the most common type in the neonate, which may be identified in up to 85% of cases. Renal incidence is 6–8% and postrenal 3–5%.

III. **Pathophysiology.** The normal newborn kidney has poor concentrating ability (maximum specific gravity 1.025). Renal injury leads to problems with volume overload, hyperkalemia, acidosis, hyperphosphatemia, and hypocalcemia. Postnatally ARF/AKI is traditionally divided into 3 categories:

A. **Prerenal failure** is due to decreased renal blood flow/perfusion, which leads to a decreased renal function in a normal kidney. Any condition that causes inadequate renal perfusion can cause prerenal ARF/AKI. Common causes include hemorrhage, dehydration, septic shock, congestive heart failure, patent ductus arteriosus (PDA), and necrotizing enterocolitis (NEC). Other causes include respiratory distress syndrome (RDS), hypoxia, congenital heart disease, hypoalbuminemia, perinatal asphyxia, extracorporeal membrane oxygenation/ extracorporeal life support (ECMO/ECLS), and hypotension. Medications in neonates that can decrease renal blood flow include indomethacin, ibuprofen, angiotensin-converting enzyme (ACE) inhibitors, and phenylephrine eye drops. Maternal use of nonsteroidal anti-inflammatory drugs (NSAIDs), ACE inhibitors, or cyclooxygenase (COX)-2 inhibitors can also decrease renal blood flow.

B. **Intrinsic renal failure refers to structural damage** to the kidneys, which causes renal tubular dysfunction. It includes acute tubular necrosis, congenital anomalies, vascular lesions, and infections/toxins. **Acute tubular necrosis (ATN)** is the most common cause, and it can be caused by prolonged poor renal perfusion, ischemia or hypoxia, sepsis, cardiac surgery (blood product transfusions), or nephrotoxins (aminoglycosides, NSAIDs, amphotericin B, contrast agents, or acyclovir). Other causes include **congenital anomalies** (eg, bilateral renal agenesis, polycystic kidney disease, congenital nephrotic syndrome of the Finnish type, renal hypoplasia/dysplasia), **vascular lesions** (bilateral renal vein/artery thrombosis, cortical necrosis, disseminated intravascular coagulation [DIC]), **infections** (congenital: syphilis, toxoplasmosis; candidiasis, pyelonephritis), **exogenous toxins** (uric acid nephropathy, myoglobinuria, hemoglobinuria).

C. **Postrenal/obstructive.** All of the causes involve obstruction of urinary outflow after the urine has been produced by the kidneys. The most common cause in males is posterior urethral valves. Other causes include urethral strictures, meatal stenosis, bilateral uteropelvic/vesical junction obstruction, neurogenic bladder, large ureteroceles, blocked urinary drainage catheters, megaureter, and prune belly syndrome. Rare causes in neonates include extrinsic tumor compression of the bladder or ureters (sacrococcygeal teratoma) or intrinsic obstruction (nephrolithiasis, bilateral fungal bezoar).

IV. **Risk factors.** Include dehydration, sepsis, asphyxia, administration of nephrotoxic drugs, prematurity, very low birthweight infants, congenital heart disease undergoing cardiopulmonary bypass, and ECMO/ECLS. Maternal diabetes may increase the risk for renal vein thrombosis and subsequent renal insufficiency.

V. **Clinical presentation**

A. **Decreased or absent urine output.** Low or absent urine output is usually the presenting problem. Virtually all infants void by 24 hours after birth (see Chapter 68).

B. **Family history.** History of urinary tract disease in other family members; history of oligohydramnios, which frequently accompanies urinary outflow obstruction or severe renal dysplasia or agenesis; and maternal diabetes should be obtained.

C. **Physical examination**

1. **Abdominal mass** may be due to a distended bladder, polycystic kidneys, hydronephrosis, or tumors
2. **Potter facies** is associated with renal agenesis
3. **Meningomyelocele** is associated with neurogenic bladder
4. **Pulmonary hypoplasia** is due to severe oligohydramnios in utero
5. **Urinary ascites** may be seen with posterior urethral valves and severe upper urinary tract obstruction
6. **Prune belly syndrome.** Hypoplasia of the abdominal wall musculature, cryptorchidism, and dilated upper urinary tracts

VI. **Diagnosis**

A. **Urethral catheterization.** Use a 5F or 8F feeding tube to measure volume of retained urine of monitor output (see Chapter 26).

B. **Laboratory studies**

1. **Blood urea nitrogen (BUN) and creatinine**

a. **BUN.** 15–20 mg/dL suggests dehydration or renal insufficiency.

b. **Creatinine.** Normal serum creatinine values are 0.8–1.0 mg/dL at 1 day, 0.7–0.8 mg/dL at 3 days, and <0.6 mg/dL by 7 days of life. Higher values suggest renal disease except in low birthweight infants, in whom a creatinine

Table 123–1. **URINARY INDICES IN THE NEONATE USED IN THE EVALUATION OF ACUTE RENAL FAILURE/ACUTE KIDNEY INJURY**

Urinary Indices	Prerenal	Intrinsic
Urine osmolality (mosmol/kg water)	>400	<400
Urine sodium (mEq/L)	31 ±19	63 ±35
Urine/plasma creatinine ratio	29 ±16	10 ±4
Fractional excretion of sodium (FeNa) (%)	<2.5	>2.5
Renal failure index (RFI)	<3.0	>3.0

level of <1.6 mg/dL is considered normal. (Rule of thumb: If the creatinine doubles, then 50% of the renal function has been lost.)

2. **Urinary indices.** (Table 123–1) A spot urine osmolality, serum and spot urine sodium, and serum and urine creatinine are used to calculate the fractional excretion of sodium (FeNa) and the renal failure index (RFI). These indices are of limited value if measured while the effects of diuretics, such as furosemide, are present.

$$FENa = \frac{\text{Urine Na} \times \text{Plasma Cr}}{\text{Urine Cr} \times \text{Plasma Na}} \times 100$$

$$RFI = \frac{\text{Urine Na} \times \text{Serum Cr}}{\text{Urine Cr}}$$

3. **Complete blood count (CBC) and platelet count.** May reveal thrombocytopenia, which is seen with sepsis or renal vein thrombosis.
4. **Serum potassium.** May be increased with renal insufficiency.
5. **Urinalysis.** May reveal hematuria (associated with renal vein thrombosis, tumors, or DIC) or pyuria, suggesting urinary tract infection.
6. **Biomarkers**
   a. **Serum and urinary cystatic C levels.** Used to calculate glomerular filtration rate
   b. **Plasma and urinary neutrophil gelatinase–associated lipocalin (NGAL) levels.**
   c. **Serum and urinary interleukin (IL)-18 levels.**
   d. **Urinary albumin-to-creatinine ratio (ACR).**
C. **Diagnostic fluid challenge.** If the patient does not have clinical volume overload or congestive failure, give a fluid challenge. Administer normal saline or colloid solution, 5–10 mL/kg as an intravenous bolus, and repeat once as needed. If there is no response, give furosemide, 1 mg/kg IV. If there is still no increase in urine output, obstruction above the level of the bladder must be ruled out by ultrasound examination. If there is no evidence of obstruction, and the patient does not respond to these maneuvers, the most likely cause of anuria or oliguria is intrinsic renal failure.
D. **Imaging studies**
   1. **Abdominal ultrasonography.** May identify hydronephrosis, dilated ureters, abdominal masses, a distended bladder, or renal vein thrombosis.
   2. **Abdominal radiograph studies.** May show spina bifida or an absent sacrum, which may be associated with a neurogenic bladder. Displaced bowel loops suggest the presence of a space-occupying mass.
   3. **Radionuclide scanning.** May be used to assess function of renal parenchymal, but is less accurate in neonates due to immature kidneys.

VII. **Management.** See also Chapter 68.
  A. **General management**
  1. **Replace insensible fluid losses** (preterm, 50–70 mL/kg/d; term, 30 mL/kg/d) plus fluid output (urine and gastrointestinal tract).
  2. **Keep strict intake and output and frequent weights.**
  3. **Monitor serum sodium and potassium levels** frequently, and replace losses cautiously as needed. Hyperkalemia may be lethal.
  4. **Restrict protein** to <2 g/kg/d, and ensure adequate nonprotein caloric intake. Breast milk or formulas such as Similac PM 60/40 are frequently used for infants with renal failure.
  5. **Hyperphosphatemia and hypocalcemia frequently coexist,** and phosphate binders such as aluminum hydroxide, 50–150 mg/kg/d orally, should be used to normalize phosphate. Once phosphate is normalized, calcium (with or without vitamin D supplementation) is usually needed.
  6. **For tetany or convulsions,** acute intravenous calcium replacement with 10% calcium gluconate, 40 mg/kg, or 10% calcium chloride will increase the serum calcium 1 mg/dL. Monitor ionized calcium.
  7. **Metabolic acidosis may require chronic oral bicarbonate supplementation.** Blood pressure should be monitored serially because these infants are always at risk for chronic hypertension. Intravenous bicarbonate therapy should be given if the pH is <7.25 or the serum bicarbonate (HCO_3) is <12 mEq.

  $$HCO_3 \text{ deficit} = (24 - \text{observed}) \, 0.5 \times \text{body weight (kg)}$$

  B. **Definitive management**
  1. **Prerenal failure.** Treated by providing volume to increase and restore renal perfusion and to treat the underlying cause.
  2. **Postrenal failure.** Acute management involves bypassing the obstruction with a bladder catheter or by percutaneous nephrostomy drainage, depending on the level of the obstruction. Operative intervention with surgical repair may be indicated to relieve obstruction. Urinary tract infection prophylaxis may be indicated. Consult with pediatric urology.
  3. **Intrinsic renal disease.** Stop or adjust doses of any nephrotoxic medications if possible. Supportive therapy is indicated (see previous text). Diuretics (furosemide, 1–2 mg/kg/dose) may increase urine output and aid in fluid management, but studies show that it does not improve the course of kidney injury. Low-dose dopamine can increase renal perfusion. (**Note:** No studies in neonates are reported, but studies in adults have shown it does not improve survival.) Observe for hyponatremia, hyperkalemia, hyperphosphatemia, hypocalcemia, and metabolic acidosis as they can occur frequently in intrinsic renal disease. Follow blood pressure as hypertension can occur (more common in renal artery/venous thrombosis). Renal feeding formulas that have a low renal solute and phosphorus should be considered. Pediatric nephrology should be consulted.
  4. **Renal replacement therapy (peritoneal dialysis, hemodialysis, hemofiltration with or without dialysis).** This is used if other measures fail. If recovery of renal function is expected or if renal transplantation is considered an option when the child is older, **peritoneal dialysis** is **the treatment most commonly used in the neonate**.

VIII. **Prognosis.** The prognosis from ARF/AKI depends on the underlying cause or the extent of damage. If renal disease is caused by toxins or acute tubular necrosis, renal function may recover to some extent with time. Chronic renal failure may ensue as neonates with ARF/AKI are at increased risk. Mortality and morbidity are increased in newborns with multiorgan failure. Factors that increase mortality include hypotension, need for mechanical ventilation, dialysis, use of vasopressors, hemodynamic instability, and multiorgan failure. Follow-up with monitoring of urine, renal function, and blood pressure is necessary.

Selected References

Askenazi D, Koralkar R, Levitan EB, et al. Baseline values of candidate urine acute kidney injury (AKI) biomarkers vary by gestational age in premature infants. *Pediatr Res.* 2011;70:302–306.

Askenazi DJ, Ambalavanan N, Goldstein SL. Acute kidney injury in critically ill newborns: what do we know? What do we need to learn? *Pediatr Nephrol.* 2009;24:265–274.

Askenazi DJ, Ambalavanan N, Hamilton K, et al. Acute kidney injury and renal replacement therapy independently predict mortality in neonatal and pediatric noncardiac patients on extracorporeal membrane oxygenation. *Pediatr Crit Care Med.* 2011;12:e1–e6.

Askenazi DJ, Montesanti A, Hunley H, et al. Urine biomarkers predict acute kidney injury and mortality in very low birth weight infants. *J Pediatr.* 2011;159:907–912;e1.

Blinder JJ, Goldstein SL, Lee VV, et al. Congenital heart surgery in infants: effects of acute kidney injury on outcomes. *J Thorac Cardiovasc Surg.* 2012;143:368–374.

Chua AN, Sarwal MMl. Acute renal failure management in the neonate. *NeoReviews* 2005;6;e369–e376.

Gadepalli SK, Selewski DT, Drongowski RA, Mychaliska GB. Acute kidney injury in congenital diaphragmatic hernia requiring extracorporeal life support: an insidious problem. *J Pediatr Surg.* 2011;46:630–635.

Goldstein SL. Advances in pediatric renal replacement therapy for acute kidney injury. *Semin Dial.* 2011;24:187–191.

Jetton GJ, Askenazi DJ. Update on acute kidney injury in the neonate. *Curr Opin Pediatr.* 2012 (Epub ahead of print).

Koralkar R, Ambalavanan N, Levitan EB, McGwin G, Goldstein S, Askenazi D. Acute kidney injury reduces survival in very low birth weight infants. *Pediatr Res.* 2011;69:354–358.

Krawczeski CD, Woo JG, Wang Y, Bennett MR, Ma Q, Devarajan P. Neutrophil gelatinase-associated lipocalin concentrations predict development of acute kidney injury in neonates and children after cardiopulmonary bypass. *J Pediatr.* 2011;158: 1009–1015;e1.

124 Respiratory Distress Syndrome

I. **Definition. Respiratory distress syndrome (RDS) was previously called hyaline membrane disease.** The Vermont Oxford Network definition for RDS requires that babies have:
   A. **An arterial oxygen tension (Pao_2) <50 mm Hg and central cyanosis** in room air, a requirement for supplemental oxygen to maintain Pao_2>50 mm Hg, or a requirement for supplemental oxygen to maintain a pulse oximeter saturation over 85 %.
   B. **A characteristic chest radiographic appearance** (uniform reticulogranular pattern to lung fields with or without low lung volumes and air bronchogram) within the first 24 hours of life. The clinical course of the disease varies with the size of the infant, severity of disease, use of surfactant replacement therapy, presence of infection, degree of shunting of blood through the patent ductus arteriosus (PDA), and whether or not assisted ventilation was initiated.
II. **Incidence.** Incidence of RDS is ~91% at 23–25 weeks' gestation, 88% at 26–27 weeks' gestation, 74 % at 28–29 weeks' gestation, and 52% at 30–31 weeks' gestation. The incidence and severity of RDS are expected to decrease after the increase in use

of antenatal steroids in recent years. After the introduction of exogenous surfactant, the survival from RDS is at >90%. During the surfactant era, RDS accounts for <6% of all neonatal deaths.

III. **Pathophysiology.** Surfactant deficiency is the primary cause of RDS, often complicated by an overly compliant chest wall. Both factors lead to progressive atelectasis and failure to develop an effective functional residual capacity (FRC). Surfactant is a surface-active material produced by airway epithelial cells called type II pneumocytes. This cell line differentiates, and surfactant synthesis begins at 24–28 weeks' gestation. Type II cells are sensitive to and decreased by asphyxial insults in the perinatal period. The maturation of this cell line is delayed in the presence of fetal hyperinsulinemia. The maturity of type II cells is enhanced by the administration of antenatal corticosteroids and by chronic intrauterine stress such as pregnancy-induced hypertension, intrauterine growth restriction, and twin gestation. Surfactant, composed chiefly of phospholipid (75%) and protein (10%), is produced and stored in the characteristic lamellar bodies of type II pneumocytes. This lipoprotein is released into the airways, where it functions to decrease surface tension and maintain alveolar expansion at physiologic pressures.

A. **Lack of surfactant.** In the absence of surfactant, the small airspaces collapse; each expiration results in progressive atelectasis. Exudative proteinaceous material and epithelial debris, resulting from progressive cellular damage, collect in the airway and directly decrease total lung capacity. In pathologic specimens, this material stains typically as eosinophilic hyaline membranes lining the alveolar spaces and extending into small airways.

B. **Presence of an overly compliant chest wall.** In the presence of a chest wall with weak structural support secondary to prematurity, the large negative pressures generated to open the collapsed airways cause retraction and deformation of the chest wall instead of inflation of the poorly compliant lungs.

C. **Decreased intrathoracic pressure.** The infant with RDS who is <30 weeks' gestational age often has immediate respiratory failure because of an inability to generate the intrathoracic pressure necessary to inflate the lungs without surfactant.

D. **Shunting.** The presence or absence of a cardiovascular shunt through a PDA or foramen ovale, or both, may change the presentation or course of the disease process. Shortly after birth, the predominant shunting is right to left across the foramen ovale into the left atrium, which may result in venous admixture and worsening hypoxemia. After 18–24 hours, left-to-right shunting through the PDA may become predominant as a result of falling pulmonary vascular resistance, leading to pulmonary edema and impaired alveolar gas exchange. Unfortunately, this usually occurs when the infant is starting to recover from RDS and can be aggravated by surfactant replacement therapy.

IV. **Risk factors.** Table 124–1 lists factors that increase or decrease the risk of RDS.

Table 124–1. **RISK FACTORS THAT INCREASE OR DECREASE THE RISK OF RESPIRATORY DISTRESS SYNDROME**

Increased Risk	Decreased Risk
Prematurity	Prolonged rupture of membranes
Male sex	Female sex
Familial predisposition	Vaginal delivery
Cesarean delivery without labor	Narcotic/cocaine use
Perinatal asphyxia	Corticosteroids
Multiple gestation	Thyroid hormone
Maternal diabetes	Tocolytic agents

V. **Clinical presentation**
   A. **History.** The infant is often preterm or has a history of asphyxia in the perinatal period. Infants have some respiratory difficulty at birth, which becomes progressively more severe. The classic worsening of the atelectasis seen on chest radiograph and increasing oxygen requirement for these infants have been greatly modified by the availability of exogenous surfactant therapy and effective mechanical ventilatory support.
   B. **Physical examination.** The infant with RDS exhibits tachypnea, grunting, nasal flaring, and retractions of the chest wall. The infant may have cyanosis in room air. Grunting occurs when the infant partially closes the vocal cords to prolong expiration and develop or maintain some FRC. This mechanism actually improves alveolar ventilation. The retractions occur and increase as the infant is forced to develop high transpulmonary pressure to reinflate atelectatic air spaces.
VI. **Diagnosis**
   A. **Chest radiograph.** An anteroposterior chest radiograph should be obtained for all infants with respiratory distress of any duration. The typical radiographic finding of RDS is a uniform reticulogranular pattern, referred to as a ground-glass appearance, accompanied by peripheral air bronchograms (see Figure 11–13). During the clinical course, sequential radiographs may reveal air leaks secondary to mechanical ventilatory intervention as well as the onset of changes compatible with bronchopulmonary dysplasia/chronic lung disease (BPD/CLD) (see Figure 11–17).
   B. **Laboratory studies**
      1. **Blood gas sampling.** Essential in the management of RDS. Usually, intermittent arterial sampling is performed. Although there is no consensus, most neonatologists agree that arterial oxygen tensions of 50–70 mm Hg and arterial carbon dioxide tensions of 45–60 mm Hg are acceptable. Most would maintain the pH at or above 7.25 and the arterial oxygen saturation at 85–93%. In addition, continuous transcutaneous oxygen and carbon dioxide monitors or oxygen saturation monitors, or both, are proving valuable in the minute-to-minute monitoring of these infants.
      2. **Sepsis workup.** A partial sepsis workup, including complete blood cell count and blood culture, should be considered for each infant with a diagnosis of RDS because early-onset sepsis (eg, infection with group B *Streptococcus*) can be indistinguishable from RDS on clinical grounds alone.
      3. **Serum glucose levels.** May be high or low initially and must be monitored closely to assess the adequacy of dextrose infusion. Hypoglycemia alone can lead to tachypnea and respiratory distress.
      4. **Serum electrolyte levels and calcium.** Should be monitored every 12–24 hours for management of parenteral fluids. Hypocalcemia can contribute to more respiratory symptoms and is common in sick, nonfed, preterm, or asphyxiated infants.
   C. **Echocardiography.** A valuable diagnostic tool in the evaluation of an infant with hypoxemia and respiratory distress. It is used to confirm the diagnosis of PDA as well as to document response to therapy. Significant congenital heart disease can be excluded by this technique as well.
VII. **Management**
   A. **Prevention**
      1. **Antenatal corticosteroids.** Treatment with antenatal corticosteroids is associated with an overall reduction in neonatal death, RDS, intraventricular hemorrhage (IVH), necrotizing enterocolitis (NEC), respiratory support, intensive care admissions, and systemic infections in the first 48 hours of life. A single course of antenatal steroids is recommended between 24 and 34 weeks of gestation to all women at risk of preterm delivery within 7 days. A single course should be administered to women with premature rupture of membranes before 32 weeks of gestation to reduce the risks of RDS, perinatal mortality, and

other morbidities. The efficacy of corticosteroid use at 32–33 completed weeks for preterm prelabor rupture of membranes is unclear based on current evidence, but treatment may be beneficial, especially if pulmonary immaturity is documented. Antenatal corticosteroids should be considered for threatened preterm birth at 22–23 weeks of gestation. Antenatal corticosteroid exposure reduced improved survival of extremely preterm infants. Antenatal treatment with corticosteroids at 34–36 weeks of pregnancy has not reduced the risk of respiratory morbidity in neonates. The optimal treatment to delivery interval is >24 and <7 days after the start of steroid treatment. A second course should be considered if the risk from RDS is felt to outweigh the uncertainty about possible long-term adverse effects. The recommended glucocorticoid regimen consists of the administration to the mother of two 12-mg doses of betamethasone given intramuscularly 24 hours apart. Dexamethasone is not recommended because of increased risk for cystic periventricular leukomalacia among very premature infants exposed to the drug prenatally.

2. **Preventive measures.** Several preventive measures may improve the survival of infants at risk for RDS and include **antenatal ultrasonography** for more accurate assessment of gestational age and fetal well-being, **continuous fetal monitoring** to document fetal well-being during labor or to signal the need for intervention when fetal distress is discovered, **tocolytic agents** that prevent and treat preterm labor, and **assessment of fetal lung maturity** before delivery (lecithin-to-sphingomyelin ratio and phosphatidylglycerol; or amniotic fluid lamellar bodies, see Chapter 1) to prevent iatrogenic prematurity.

B. **Surfactant replacement.** (See also Chapter 8.) Now considered a standard of care in the treatment of intubated infants with RDS. Since the late 1980s, >30 randomized clinical trials involving >6000 infants have been conducted. Systematic reviews of these trials demonstrate that surfactant, whether used prophylactically in the delivery room or in the treatment of established disease, leads to a significant decrease in the risk of pneumothorax and the risk of death. These benefits were observed in both the trials of natural surfactant extracts and synthetic surfactants. Prophylactic surfactant replacement to prevent RDS in infants born at <31 weeks' gestation has reduced the risk of death or BPD/CLD but may result in some infants being intubated and receiving treatment unnecessarily. A recent consensus statement recommends surfactant prophylaxis (within 15 minutes of birth) to almost all infants <26 weeks' gestation. Prophylaxis should also be administered to all preterm infants with RDS who require delivery-room intubation for stabilization. Early rescue surfactant should be administered to preterm babies with an evidence of RDS. The effect of surfactant therapy is better the earlier in the course of RDS it is given. A second, sometimes a third dose of surfactant should be administered in cases with ongoing evidence of RDS (ie, persistent need of mechanical ventilation and oxygen supplementation).

Natural (derived from animal lungs) surfactant preparations are better than synthetic (protein-free) at reducing pulmonary air leaks. Natural surfactants are therefore the treatment of choice. Trials comparing natural bovine surfactants, given prophylactically or as rescue therapy, have shown similar outcomes. Trials comparing bovine and porcine-derived surfactants have shown a more rapid improvement in oxygenation in the latter. A better survival has been demonstrated in a meta-analysis comparing a 200-mg/kg dose of poractant alfa with 100 mg/kg of beractant, or 100 mg/kg poractant alfa, for rescue treatment of moderate to severe RDS. Poractant alfa treatment for RDS was in a retrospective study associated with a significantly reduced likelihood of death, when compared with calfactant, and a trend toward reduced mortality when compared with beractant.

Mechanical ventilation can be avoided by using the INSURE (Intubate-Surfactant-Extubate to CPAP [continuous positive airway pressure]) technique when surfactant is administered. This has reduced need for mechanical ventilation and development of BPD/CLD in randomized trials. Immediate (or early) extubation to noninvasive respiratory support (CPAP or nasal intermittent positive ventilation) following surfactant administration should be considered in otherwise stabile infants.

Currently, long-term follow-up studies have not shown significant differences between surfactant-treated patients and nontreated control groups with regard to PDA, IVH, retinopathy of prematurity, NEC, and BPD/CLD. Evidence exists that the length of stay on mechanical ventilation and total ventilator days have been reduced with the use of surfactant at all gestational age levels, even with the increase of extremely low birthweight infants. A dramatic fall in deaths from RDS began in 1991. This probably reflected the introduction of surfactant replacement therapy. In long-term follow-up studies, no adverse effects attributable to surfactant therapy have been identified.

C. **Respiratory support**
   1. **Endotracheal intubation and mechanical ventilation.** Mainstays of therapy for infants with RDS in whom apnea or hypoxemia with respiratory acidosis develops. Mechanical ventilation (MV) modes include conventional, such as intermittent positive pressure ventilation (IPPV), and high-frequency oscillatory ventilation (HFOV). Ventilators with the capacity to synchronize respiratory effort may generate less inadvertent airway pressure and lessen barotrauma. Ventilator settings should be adjusted frequently to maintain the lowest possible pressures and inspired oxygen concentrations in an attempt to minimize damage to parenchymal tissue. HFOV may be beneficial as a rescue therapy in infants with respiratory failure on IPPV. Rescue HFOV reduces pulmonary air leaks but is associated with an increased risk of IVH. Insufficient evidence exists to recommend the routine use of HFOV instead of conventional ventilation for preterm infants with lung disease. Hypocapnia is associated with increased risks of BPD/CLD and periventricular leukomalacia and should therefore be avoided. To minimize duration of MV, weaning from MV should be started as soon as satisfactory gas exchange is achieved. Caffeine should be routinely used for very preterm neonates with RDS to augment extubation.
   2. **Continuous positive airway pressure (CPAP) and nasal synchronized intermittent mandatory ventilation (SIMV).** Nasal CPAP (NCPAP) or nasopharyngeal CPAP (NPCPAP) can be used early to delay or prevent the need for endotracheal intubation and mechanical ventilation. CPAP treatment is recommended to be started from birth in all infants at risk of RDS, as those born at <30 weeks' gestation. In this way some infants with RDS can be managed without surfactant replacement. By not using surfactant, however, the risk of pneumothorax is increased. Use of NCPAP or NPCPAP on extubation after mechanical ventilation decreases the chance of reintubation, when at least 5 cm H_2O pressure is applied. **Nasal SIMV** is a potentially useful way of augmenting NCPAP. The ability to synchronize the ventilator breaths with the infant's own respiratory cycle has made this mode of ventilation feasible. In 3 trials, nasal SIMV has reduced the incidence of symptoms of extubation failure when compared with NCPAP. Short binasal prongs should be used instead of a single prong.
   3. **Humidified high-flow nasal cannula system.** This has been introduced to neonatal respiratory care as a way to provide positive distending pressure, even comparable to NCPAP, to a neonate with respiratory distress. It aims to maximize patient tolerance by using heated, humidified gas flow (≥ 1 L/min). Studies comparing high-flow nasal cannula with nasal SIMV for RDS are going on.
   4. **Complications.** Pulmonary air leaks, such as pneumothorax, pneumomediastinum, pneumopericardium, and pulmonary interstitial emphysema, may occur (see Chapter 81). Chronic complications include respiratory problems such as BPD/CLD (see Chapter 84) and tracheal stenosis.

D. **Fluid and nutritional support.** In the very ill infant, it is possible to maintain nutritional support with parenteral nutrition for an extended period. Full parenteral nutrition and minimal enteral feeding can be initiated on the first day of life. Careful fluid balance should, however, be maintained. The specific needs of preterm and term infants are becoming better understood, and the nutrient preparations available reflect this understanding (see Chapters 9 and 10).

E. **Antibiotic therapy.** Antibiotics that cover the most common neonatal infections are usually begun initially.

F. **Sedation.** Commonly used to control ventilation in these sick infants. **Morphine, fentanyl,** or **lorazepam** may be used for analgesia as well as sedation, but there is significant controversy surrounding such treatment. Reported advantages of treatment include improved ventilator synchrony and pulmonary function. Decreased adverse long-term neurologic sequelae have been suggested. Neuroendocrine responses to mechanical ventilation are alleviated by opioid treatment, which may be beneficial in the long term. However, clinicians should consider adverse effects of medication, especially opioids, including hypotension with morphine and chest wall rigidity with fentanyl. Tolerance, dependence, and withdrawal occur. In addition, pharmacologic treatment does not decrease adverse sequelae, at least in the short term. The most significant gaps in knowledge include the inability to assess chronic pain in this population and the long-term effects of treatment. Minimal handling to avoid pain is an important means to decrease need for pain management in ventilated infants. Muscle paralysis with **pancuronium** for infants with RDS remains *controversial*. Sedation might be indicated for infants who "fight" the ventilator and exhale during the inspiratory cycle of MV. This respiratory pattern may increase the likelihood of complication such as air leak and therefore should be avoided. Sedation of infants with fluctuating cerebral blood flow velocity theoretically decreases the risk of IVH. (See also Chapter 76.)

VIII. **Outcome.** Although the survival of infants with RDS has improved greatly, the survival with or without respiratory and neurologic sequelae is highly dependent on birthweight and gestational age. Major morbidity (BPD/CLD, NEC, and severe IVH) and poor postnatal growth remain high for the smallest infants.

Selected References

Committee on Obstetric Practice. Antenatal corticosteroid therapy for fetal maturation. *Obstet Gynecol.* 2011;117:422.

Davis P, Lemyre B, de Paoli AG. Nasal intermittent positive pressure ventilation (NIPPV) versus nasal continuous positive airway pressure (NCPAP) for preterm neonates after extubation. *Cochrane Database Syst Rev.* 2001;CD002272.

Davis PG, Henderson-Smart DJ. Nasal continuous airway pressure immediately after extubation for preventing morbidity in preterm infants. *Cochrane Database Syst Rev.* 2003;CD000143.

EuroNeoStat Annual Report for Very Low Gestational Age Infants 2006.The ENS Project: Barakaldo, Spain.

Greenough A, Milner AD, Dimitriou G. Synchronized mechanical ventilation for respiratory support in newborn infants. *Cochrane Database Syst Rev.* 2001;CD000456.

Hall RW, Boyle E, Young T. Do ventilated neonates require pain management? *Semin Perinatol.* 2007;31:289–297.

Henderson-Smart DJ, Cools F, Bhuta T, Offringa M. Elective high frequency oscillatory ventilation versus conventional ventilation for acute pulmonary dysfunction in preterm infants. *Cochrane Database Syst Rev.* 2007;CD000104.

Lampland A, Plumm B, Meyers PA, Worwa CT, Mammel MC. Observational study of humidified high-flow nasal cannula compared with nasal continuous positive airway pressure. *J Pediatr.* 2009;154:177–182.

Miller MJ, Fanaroff AA, Martin RJ. Respiratory disorders in preterm and term infants. In: Fanaroff AA, Martin RJ, eds. *Neonatal-Perinatal Medicine: Diseases of the Fetus and Infant.* 7th ed. St. Louis, MO: Mosby; 2002.

Mori R, Kusuda S, Fujimura M; Neonatal Research Network Japan. Antenatal corticosteroids promote survival of extremely preterm infants born at 22 to 23 weeks of gestation. *J Pediatr.* 2011;159:110.e1–114.e1.

Morley CJ, Davis PG, Doyle LW, et al. Nasal CPAP or intubation at birth for very preterm infants. *N Engl J Med.* 2008;358:700–708.

Ramanathan R, Bhatia JJ, Sekar K, Ernst FR. Mortality in preterm infants with respiratory distress syndrome treated with poractant alfa, calfactant or beractant: a retrospective study. *J Perinatol* (Epub ahead of print on September 1, 2011).

Roberts D. Antenatal corticosteroids in late preterm infants. *BMJ.* 2011;342:d1614.

Roberts D, Dalziel S. Antenatal corticosteroids for accelerating fetal lung maturation for women at risk of preterm birth. *Cochrane Database Syst Rev.* 2006;CD004454.

Soll RF, Morley CJ. Prophylactic versus selective use of surfactant for preventing morbidity and mortality in preterm infants. *Cochrane Database Syst Rev.* 2001;2:CD000510.

Stevens TP, Harrington EW, Blennow M, Soll RF. Early surfactant administration with brief ventilation vs. selective surfactant and continued mechanical ventilation for preterm infants with or at risk for respiratory distress syndrome. *Cochrane Database Syst Rev.* 2007;CD003063.

Sweet D, Carnielli V, Greisen G, et al. European consensus guidelines on the management of neonatal respiratory distress syndrome in preterm infants: 2010 update. *Neonatology.* 2010;97:402–417.

125 Respiratory Syncytial Virus

I. **Definition.** Respiratory syncytial virus (RSV) is a large, enveloped RNA paramyxovirus. Two major strains (groups A and B) have been identified and often circulate concurrently.

II. **Incidence.** Almost all children are infected at least once by 2 years of age. Humans are the only source of infection. Initial infection occurs most commonly during the child's first year. Reinfection throughout life is common. In the United States, RSV usually occurs in annual epidemics during winter and early spring (predominantly November through March). Communities in the southern United States, particularly some communities in the state of Florida, tend to experience the earliest onset of RSV activity (as early as July). RSV is the most common cause of acute lower respiratory tract infection (ALRI) in children <1 year of age. RSV is associated with up to 120,000 pediatric hospitalizations (1–3% of children in the first 12 months of life) each year in the United States. Approximately 400 deaths are attributed to RSV annually. Globally, an estimated 3.4 million new episodes of severe RSV ALRI necessitating hospital admission occur in children <5 years, of whom up to 200,000 die as a complication of infection. Also, RSV is a common cause of nosocomial infection. It can persist on environmental surfaces for several hours and for a half-hour or more on hands. Infection among hospital personnel and others may occur by hand-to-eye or hand-to-nasal epithelium self-inoculation with contaminated secretions.

III. **Pathophysiology.** The disease is generally limited to the respiratory tract. The inoculation of the virus occurs in the upper respiratory tract. The virus replicates in the nasopharynx and spreads to the small bronchiolar epithelium, sparing the basal cells. Subsequently, the virus extends to the type 1 and 2 alveolar pneumocytes in lung, presumably by cell-to-cell spread or via aspiration of secretions. In infants, the disease manifests itself as bronchiolitis or pneumonia. In very rare cases, RSV may be recovered from extrapulmonary tissues, such as liver, spinal, or pericardial fluid. Up to 20% of children with RSV bronchiolitis may be **coinfected** with another respiratory tract virus, such as human metapneumovirus or rhinovirus.

IV. **Risk factors.** Risk factors include infants <6 months of age, premature infants born <35 weeks' gestation, infants born with lung disease, infants <2 years of age with heart disease, infants with school-aged siblings, infants who attend day care, family history of asthma, regular exposure to secondhand smoke or air pollution, multiple birth babies, peak RSV season (fall to end of spring), being male, immunocompromised patients (eg, severe combined immunodeficiency, leukemia, or undergoing organ transplant), <1 month or no breast-feeding, and others sharing the bedroom with the infant. High altitude increases the risk of RSV hospitalization. **Risk factors for more severe or fatal RSV disease** include a premature infant, an infant with complex congenital heart disease (CHD), especially those that cause cyanosis or pulmonary hypertension; an infant with bronchopulmonary dysplasia (chronic lung disease [CLD]); and an infant with immunodeficiency with lymphopenia or receiving therapy that causes immune suppression.

V. **Clinical presentation.** RSV usually begins in the nasopharynx with coryza and congestion. During the first 2–5 days, it may progress to the lower respiratory tract with development of cough, dyspnea, and wheezing. RSV is the most common cause of bronchiolitis and pneumonia in infants <2 years old. Lethargy, irritability, and poor feeding are commonly present in young infants. **Apnea** may be the presenting symptom in ~20% of infants hospitalized with RSV and may be the cause of sudden, unexpected death. Most previously healthy infants infected with RSV do not require hospitalization. RSV infection may predispose to reactive airway disease and recurrent wheezing during the first decade of life; the association between RSV bronchiolitis early in life and subsequent asthma remains poorly understood.

VI. **Diagnosis**
   A. **Enzyme-linked immunosorbent assay (ELISA) and direct fluorescent antibody (DFA) tests** utilize antigen capture technology that can be performed in <30 minutes on nasal wash or tracheal aspirate. Their sensitivity and specificity exceed 80–90% (in comparison with culture). False-positive test results are more likely to occur when the incidence of disease is low. Viral isolation from nasopharyngeal secretions in cell culture requires 1–5 days (shell vial techniques can produce results within 24–48 hours). Reverse transcriptase–polymerase chain reaction (**RT-PCR**) is an alternative to culture for confirming the result of rapid antigen detection assay (which is rarely needed). Culture and PCR may be needed to confirm rapid antigen detection initially to mark the start of the RSV season. Diagnostic serology is not helpful in infants because of the passive transplacental transfer of maternal antibody.
   B. **Chest radiograph** usually reveals infiltrates or hyperinflation.
   C. **Blood gas analysis** may show hypoxemia and occasionally hypercarbia. Development of hypercarbia is an ominous sign of impending respiratory failure.

VII. **Management.** Isolation precautions for all infectious diseases, including maternal and neonatal precautions, breast-feeding, and visiting issues, can be found in Appendix F.
   A. **Immunization**
      1. **Passive**
         a. **Palivizumab (Synagis)** provides passive immunity. It is a humanized RSV monoclonal antibody administered intramuscularly (15 mg/kg) monthly during RSV season. It is well tolerated with infrequent or minimal side effects. According to the American Academy of Pediatrics guidelines, palivizumab should be considered for:

  i. **Infants and children <2 years with chronic lung disease** who have required medical therapy (supplemental oxygen, bronchodilator, diuretic, or corticosteroid therapy) for CLD within 6 months before the anticipated start of the RSV season. These infants and young children should receive a maximum of 5 doses. Patients with the most severe CLD who continue to require medical therapy may benefit from prophylaxis during a second RSV season. Consultation with an infectious disease specialist is recommended.

 ii. **Infants born before 32 weeks' gestation (31 weeks, 6 days or less).** Infants born at 28 weeks of gestation or earlier may benefit from prophylaxis during the RSV season, whenever that occurs during the first 12 months of life. Infants born at 29–32 weeks of gestation may benefit most from prophylaxis if <6 months of age at the start of the RSV season. Once an infant qualifies for initiation of prophylaxis at the start of the RSV season, administration should continue throughout the season and not stop at the point an infant reaches either 6 months or 12 months of age. A maximum of 5 monthly doses is recommended for infants in this category.

iii. **Infants born at 32 to <35 weeks' gestation (defined as 32 weeks, 0 days through 34 weeks, 6 days).** Prophylaxis may be considered for those infants who are born <3 months before the onset or during the RSV season and for whom at least 1 of 2 risk factors is present. **Risk factors include attendance at child care** (defined as a home or facility where care is provided for any number of infants or young toddlers in the child care facility), **or presence of a sibling <5 years of age** who lives permanently in the same household. Multiple births <1 year of age do not qualify as fulfilling this risk factor. Infants in this gestational age category should receive prophylaxis only until they reach 3 months of age and should receive a maximum of 3 monthly doses. Many of them will receive only 1 or 2 doses until they reach 3 months of age.

 iv. **Children who are ≤24 months of age with hemodynamically significant congenital heart disease.** Decisions regarding prophylaxis should be made on the basis of the degree of physiologic cardiovascular compromise. Children who are most likely to benefit include infants who are receiving medication to control congestive heart failure, infants with moderate to severe pulmonary hypertension, and infants with cyanotic heart disease. Because a mean decrease in palivizumab serum concentration of 58% was observed after cardiopulmonary bypass, for children who still require prophylaxis, a postoperative dose of palivizumab (15 mg/kg) should be considered as soon as the patient is medically stable. Infants and children with hemodynamically insignificant heart disease (eg, secundum atrial septal defect, small ventricular septal defect, pulmonic stenosis, uncomplicated aortic stenosis, mild coarctation of the aorta, and patent ductus arteriosus) are not at increased risk for RSV and generally should not receive immunoprophylaxis.

  v. **Infants with congenital abnormalities of the airway or neuromuscular disease.** Immunoprophylaxis may be considered for infants who have either significant congenital abnormalities of the airway or a neuromuscular condition that compromises handling of respiratory tract secretions. Infants and young children in this category should receive a maximum of 5 doses of palivizumab during the first year of life.

b. **Motavizumab** is another, more potent RSV-neutralizing antibody that is being considered for RSV prevention (not yet U.S. Food and Drug Administration approved).

2. **Active.** Several promising candidate RSV vaccines are currently in development both at the preclinical and early clinical stage.

B. **Ribavirin** has in vitro antiviral activity against RSV, but ribavirin aerosol treatment for RSV is not recommended routinely.

C. **Surfactant** two small, randomized studies showed that surfactant therapy improves gas exchange and shortens mechanical ventilation days and intensive care unit stay in infants with severe RSV-induced respiratory failure.

D. **β-Adrenergic agents** may be tried (once) for wheezing associated with RSV bronchiolitis. Repeated doses should be continued only in the small number of infants who demonstrate a well-documented improvement in respiratory function soon after the first dose.

E. **Antibiotics, theophylline, and corticosteroids** have not been shown to be helpful in the treatment of RSV.

F. **Isolation.** Contact precautions are recommended for the duration of the illness. RSV present in secretions remains viable for up to 6 hours on countertops. Gowns, gloves, and scrupulous hand-washing practices are required. Patients with RSV infection should be cared for in a single room or placed in a cohort.

VIII. **Prognosis.** The prognosis is generally excellent; however, infants with underlying cardiac or pulmonary conditions can have an increased risk of complications. In prematurely born infants with CLD who are hospitalized because of RSV in the first 2 years of life, there is a reduced airway caliber at school age. Even in normal infants, RSV infection in the first 3 years of life predisposes them to recurrent wheezing up to 11 years of age. Palivizumab prophylaxis given to premature infants in the first year of life has protective effect on physician-diagnosed recurrent wheezing through the ages of 2–5 years, especially in those children with no family history of asthma or atopy.

Selected References

American Academy of Pediatrics. Respiratory syncytial virus. In: Pickering LK, Baker CJ, Kimberlin DW, Long SS, eds. *Red Book: 2012 Report of the Committee on Infectious Diseases.* 28th ed. Elk Grove Village, IL: American Academy of Pediatrics; 2012:609–618.

Barreira ER, Precioso AR, Bousso A. Pulmonary surfactant in respiratory syncytial virus bronchiolitis: the role in pathogenesis and clinical implications. *Pediatr Pulmonol.* 2011;46:415–420.

Carbonell-Estrany X, Simões EA, Dagan R, et al. Motavizumab for prophylaxis of respiratory syncytial virus in high-risk children: a noninferiority trial. *Pediatrics.* 2010;125:e35–e51.

García CG, Bhore R, Soriano-Fallas A, et al. Risk factors in children hospitalized with RSV bronchiolitis versus non-RSV bronchiolitis. *Pediatrics.* 2010;126:e1453–e1460.

Greenough A, Alexander J, Boit P, et al. School age outcome of respiratory syncytial virus hospitalization of prematurely born infants. *Thorax.* 2009;64:490–495.

Hall CB, Weinberg GA, Iwane MK, et al. The burden of respiratory syncytial virus infection in young children. *N Engl J Med.* 2009;360:588–598.

Nair H, Nokes DJ, Gessner BD, et al. Global burden of acute lower respiratory infections due to respiratory syncytial virus in young children: a systematic review and meta-analysis. *Lancet.* 2010;375(9725):1545–1555.

Ralston S, Hill V. Incidence of apnea in infants hospitalized with respiratory syncytial virus bronchiolitis: a systematic review. *J Pediatr.* 2009;155(5):728–733.

Schmidt AC. Progress in respiratory virus vaccine development. *Semin Respir Crit Care Med.* 2011;32:527–540.

Simões EA, Carbonell-Estrany X, Rieger CH, et al. The effect of respiratory syncytial virus on subsequent recurrent wheezing in atopic and nonatopic children. *J Allergy Clin Immunol.* 2010;126:256–262.

126   Retinopathy of Prematurity

I. **Definitions**
   A. **Retinopathy of prematurity (ROP).** A disorder of the developing retinal vasculature resulting from interruption of normal progression of newly forming retinal vessels. Vasoconstriction and obliteration of the advancing capillary bed are followed in succession by neovascularization extending into the vitreous, retinal edema, retinal hemorrhages, fibrosis, and traction on, and eventual detachment of, the retina. In most cases, the process is reversed before fibrosis occurs. **Advanced stages may lead to blindness.**
   B. **Retrolental fibroplasia (RLF).** As originally described, the condition was seen only in its most advanced form, after extensive fibrosis and scarring had already occurred behind the lens. It was, therefore, termed *retrolental fibroplasia*. It is now understood that recognizable changes occur in the developing vasculature before end-stage fibrosis occurs, making this condition a true retinopathy. Because it is found chiefly in premature infants, it is called *retinopathy of prematurity*.
   C. **Cicatricial ROP.** The term *cicatricial ROP* refers to fibrotic disease.
II. **Incidence.** ROP represents ~20% of blindness in preschool children in the United States. Of particular concern are the increasing numbers of survivors weighing <1000 g, who have the highest incidence of ROP. The U.S. National Institutes of Health (NIH) sponsored the Cryotherapy for Retinopathy of Prematurity (CRYO-ROP) study in 1986–1987, which showed that 65.8% of infants weighing <1251 g developed ROP of any stage. Two percent of infants weighing 1000–1250 g developed threshold stage III+ disease eligible for treatment, whereas 15.5% of infants weighing <750 g did so. **Threshold disease occurred at a median postconceptional age of 36–37 weeks, regardless of gestational age at birth or chronologic age.** A study of earlier treatment, the ETROP (Early Treatment for Retinopathy of Prematurity) study, carried out in 2002, showed little difference in the overall incidence of the disorder and time of onset from the earlier CRYO-ROP study. The International NO-ROP Group, however, published data in 2005 suggesting that severe ROP in larger infants is an emerging worldwide issue. Care and survival of these premature infants is improving, whereas specialized treatment for ROP is not yet as prevalent.
III. **Pathophysiology**
   A. **Historical perspective.** RLF was first described by Terry in the 1940s and was associated with the use of oxygen in newborn infants by Patz in 1984. The **first epidemic**, estimated to be responsible for 30% of cases of blindness in preschool children by the end of the 1940s, occurred during a period of relatively liberal oxygen administration. After this association was recognized, oxygen use in nurseries was curtailed. Although the incidence of RLF fell, mortality rates in newborn infants increased. In the 1960s, improved oxygen monitoring techniques made possible the cautious reintroduction of oxygen into the nursery. Despite improved oxygen monitoring, however, a **second epidemic** of RLF (ROP) appeared in the late 1970s and is associated with the increased survival of very low birthweight infants.
   B. **Normal embryology of the eye.** In the normally developing retina, there are no retinal vessels until about 16 weeks' gestation. Until then, oxygen diffuses from the underlying choroidal circulation. At 16 weeks, in response to a stimulus (experimental evidence suggests relative hypoxia stimulating the release of angiogenic factors as the retina thickens), cells derived from mesenchyme traveling in the nerve fiber layer emanate from the optic nerve head. These cells are the precursors of the retinal vascular system. A fine capillary network advances through the retina to the ora serrata, or retinal edge. More mature vessels form behind this advancing

network. Vascularization on the nasal side of the ora serrata is complete at ~8 months' gestation, whereas that on the temporal side is ordinarily complete at term. Regulation of this process involves various factors including vascular endothelial growth factor (VEGF) and insulin-like growth factor 1 (IGF-1) working in combination. Once the retinal vasculature is completely vascularized, it is no longer susceptible to insults of the type that lead to ROP.

C. **Causes**
1. There appear to be 2 phases in the development of ROP. Clinical and experimental evidence lead to the following general concepts.
   a. **Early vasoconstriction and obliteration of the capillary network** occurs in response to high oxygen concentrations noted experimentally or another vascular insult. Concentrations of IGF-1 are low in the very low birthweight infant in the early postnatal period as maternal levels are no longer available. Experimental evidence in the mouse model suggests that low IGF-1 contributes to the lack of retinal blood vessel formation in early ROP.
   b. **Vasoproliferation** follows the period of high oxygen exposure or insult, in response to angiogenic factors such as VEGF released by the hypoxic retina. Recent data suggest that VEGF only leads to angiogenesis in the presence of adequate tissue concentrations of IGF-1. When endogenous IGF-1 levels rise in the maturing at-risk premature infant, vasoproliferation is triggered in the presence of VEGF. Considerable evidence has been developed to support this hypothesis. Phelps and Rosenbaum studied kittens made hyperoxic and then allowed to recover in room air (21% oxygen) or 13% oxygen. Those recovering in the hypoxic environment had worse retinopathy than those recovering in room air, suggesting that retinal hypoxia plays a role. VEGF is a known product of the hypoxic retina. Using a mouse model, Smith et al have shown that IGF-1 is an important factor in VEGF action and the development of ROP. Further research will surely elucidate other modulators of this process.

IV. **Risk factors.** The association of ROP with oxygen alone is not so clear. Transient hyperoxemia alone is not sufficient. Many other factors, such as extreme prematurity, apnea, sepsis, hyper- and hypocapnia, intraventricular hemorrhage, anemia, exchange transfusion, hypoxia, lactic acidosis, and possibly erythropoietin, which is angiogenic, have been implicated. Experimental studies have focused chiefly on the role of oxygen. Oxygen monitoring is an important part of the care of the premature infant, although **extreme prematurity is known to be the significant risk factor**. Recent data from Hellström et al have shown that postnatal weight gain also significantly affects the development of ROP.

V. **Clinical presentation.** Several methods of classification of ROP have been used. With development of the **International Classification of ROP**, there is general agreement on the staging of active disease.
A. **Stage I.** A thin demarcation line develops between the vascularized region of the retina and the avascular zone.
B. **Stage II.** This line develops into a ridge protruding into the vitreous.
C. **Stage III.** Extraretinal fibrovascular proliferation occurs with the ridge. Neovascular tufts may be found just posterior to the ridge (Figure 126–1).
D. **Stage IV.** Fibrosis and scarring occur as the neovascularization extends into the vitreous. Traction occurs on the retina, resulting in partial retinal detachment.
E. **Stage V.** Complete retinal detachment.
F. **Plus disease (eg, stage III+).** This may occur when vessels posterior to the ridge become dilated and tortuous. **Plus disease has become a primary factor in treatment decisions.**
G. **Pre-plus disease.** Dilation and tortuosity of posterior pole vessels in zone 1; less severe than plus disease.

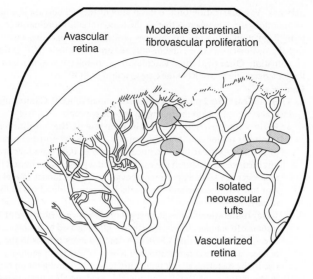

FIGURE 126–1. Schematic drawing of moderate stage III retinopathy of prematurity. Optic nerve head is shown at the bottom, and periphery of the retina is at the top. (*Reproduced, with permission, from Garner A. International classification of retinopathy of prematurity. Pediatrics. 1984;74:127.*)

    H. **Aggressive posterior ROP (AP-ROP).** Rapidly progressive ROP primarily zone I. **Requires immediate treatment.**
        The retina is divided into circumferential **zones I, II, and III** to designate how far from the back of the retina (the posterior pole) disease is present. The most severe disease is any stage with plus disease close to the posterior pole, in zone I. The least severe is disease in the peripheral retina, zone III. No treatment is necessary for peripheral zone III disease, as it regresses spontaneously.
  VI. **Diagnosis. Ophthalmoscopic examination** by an experienced examiner usually confirms the diagnosis. **Binocular indirect ophthalmoscopy (BIO)** is generally used. Assessment of newer digital camera technology in the multicenter PhotoROP study demonstrated 100% sensitivity in detecting ROP requiring treatment. However, it does not permit adequate assessment of ROP in the retinal periphery. BIO must be employed to determine when screening can be discontinued. A 2006 joint statement by the American Academy of Pediatrics (AAP), American Association for Pediatric Ophthalmology and Strabismus, and American Academy of Ophthalmology provided updated recommendations for ROP screening examinations in premature infants. These recommendations are evolving and may change as longer-term ROP outcomes are recognized. AAP pain management recommendations from 2006, reaffirmed in 2010, state that retinal examinations are painful, and pain relief measures should be used. They further state that a reasonable approach would be to administer local anesthetic eye drops and oral sucrose.
    A. Infants weighing ≤1500 g or ≤30 weeks' gestation and those weighing >1500 g with an unstable clinical course should have dilated eye examinations starting at 4–6 weeks of age or 31–33 weeks' postmenstrual age. Examinations should continue every 2–3 weeks until retinal maturity is reached, if no disease is present.
    B. Infants with ROP or very immature vessels should be examined every 1–2 weeks until vessels are mature or the risk of threshold disease has passed. Those at greatest risk should be examined every week.

VII. **Management**
   A. **Circumferential cryopexy.** Proven to be an effective treatment for progressive (stage III+) disease in an attempt to prevent further progression by destroying cells that may be releasing angiogenic factors. Results of the large collaborative NIH-sponsored trial indicate that cryopexy carried out at stage III+ can reduce the incidence of severe visual impairment by ~50% if performed within 72 hours of detecting threshold disease. Although myopia is a common feature of ROP, 10-year follow-up shows significant improvement in visual acuity of treated versus control eyes. It is imperative that an ophthalmologist skilled in cryopexy perform the procedure.
   B. **Laser photocoagulation.** Data suggest that this technique is equally effective yet safer than cryopexy, and it has become **the treatment of choice.** In 1994, the Laser ROP Study Group was formed to carry out a meta-analysis of 4 laser-ROP trials. Treatment was based on the same criteria used in the CRYO-ROP trial. Recognizing the limitations of a meta-analysis, the study group concluded that laser therapy is at least as effective as cryotherapy for ROP, despite a small risk of cataract formation. Ten-year follow-up of a small group of patients suggests better outcomes with laser photocoagulation. More recently, the ETROP study (2002) demonstrated improved outcomes with treatment at any stage when plus disease is present. AAP pain recommendations from 2006, reaffirmed in 2010, state that retinal surgery should be considered major surgery, and effective opiate-based pain relief should be provided while monitoring the infant with an appropriate pain assessment scale.
   C. **Oxygen for treatment of ROP.** In an attempt to reduce angiogenic factors from the hypoxic retina and the progression of ROP from prethreshold to threshold (III+) levels, oxygen therapy was attempted in a large collaborative trial, the Supplemental Therapeutic Oxygen for Prethreshold Retinopathy of Prematurity (STOP-ROP) study. Oxygen saturations were targeted at 96–99% in the treatment group and 89–94% in the conventional group once prethreshold ROP was diagnosed. No significant difference was seen in the rate of progression to threshold disease between the 2 groups, although there was a significant increase in bronchopulmonary dysplasia/chronic lung disease in the high-saturation group. The appropriate saturation ranges remain *controversial* and under study, although most neonatal intensive care units keep infants <1250 g at saturations <95% when in supplemental oxygen. Multicenter, randomized trials of reduced oxygen saturation therapy are currently being undertaken in several countries. Randomization is to oxygen saturations of 85–89% or 91–95% with similar study designs to allow a planned meta-analysis of the trials when completed.
   D. **Additional experimental therapies.** Therapies that show promise include suppression of VEGF with anti-VEGF therapy and **dietary supplementation of omega-3 polyunsaturated fatty acids (PUFA).** The balance of omega-3 and omega-6 PUFAs in the retina affects cell survival. Studies in the mouse model have shown a protective effect of omega-3 supplementation. **Anti-VEGF therapy has moved from animal studies to human clinical trials.** Mintz-Hittner et al recently published their results for the BEAT-ROP collaborative trial in which infants with stage 3+ ROP were randomly assigned to intravitreal bevacizumab monotherapy versus laser therapy. A significant benefit for zone 1 ROP (the most difficult to treat conventionally) was demonstrated. Outcomes were short, and safety could not be assessed due to the small size of the trial. Further study has been recommended.
   E. **Vitamin E.** The administration of pharmacologic doses of vitamin E for ROP has been studied with no proof of clear benefit. Reported side effects include sepsis, necrotizing enterocolitis, and intraventricular hemorrhage. Even so, maintenance of normal serum vitamin E levels is a prudent management objective. (For doses, see Chapter 148.)
   F. **Decreased lighting intensity.** A prospective, randomized, multicenter trial of 409 premature infants weighing <1251 g and 31 weeks' gestation concluded that a reduction in ambient light exposure does not alter the incidence of ROP.

G. **Retinal reattachment.** Stage IV disease has been treated by attempts at retinal reattachment without significant success to date. Reattachment of late retinal detachments in childhood has met with more success.

H. **Vitrectomy.** This has not substantially improved the outcome in cicatricial disease.

I. **Follow-up eye examinations.** Advocated every 1–2 years for infants with fully regressed ROP and every 6–12 months for those with cicatricial ROP. Premature infants are at risk for myopia even in the absence of ROP and should have an eye examination by 6 months of age.

VIII. **Prognosis.** Ninety percent of cases of stage I and stage II disease regress spontaneously. Current information suggests that ~50% of cases of stage III+ disease regress spontaneously. Of those that do progress to stage III+, the incidence of unfavorable structural outcomes can be reduced by ~50% and unfavorable visual outcomes by ~30% if circumferential cryopexy is carried out by a skilled ophthalmologist. Laser photocoagulation appears equally and possibly more effective than cryopexy. Sequelae of regressed disease such as myopia, strabismus, amblyopia, glaucoma, and late detachment require regular follow-up.

Selected References

American Academy of Pediatrics, Section on Ophthalmology; American Academy of Ophthalmology; American Association for Pediatric Ophthalmology and Strabismus. Screening examination of premature infants for retinopathy of prematurity [erratum appears in *Pediatrics.* 2006;118:1324]. *Pediatrics.* 2006;117:572–576.

American Academy of Pediatrics and American College of Obstetrics and Gynecology. Neonatal complications. In: Lockwood C, Lemons J, eds. *Guidelines for Perinatal Care.* 6th ed. Atlanta, GA: ACOG; 2007:262–264.

American Academy of Pediatrics, Committee of Fetus and Newborn and Section on Surgery, Section on Anesthesiology and Pain Medicine, Canadian Paediatric Society and Fetus and Newborn Committee. Prevention and management of pain in the neonate: an update. *Pediatrics.* 2006;118;2231–2241. Reaffirmed. *Pediatrics.* 2010;126;404.

Cryotherapy for Retinopathy of Prematurity Cooperative Group. Multicenter trial of cryotherapy for retinopathy of prematurity: ophthalmological outcomes at 10 years. *Arch Ophthalmol.* 2001;119:1110.

Early Treatment for Retinopathy of Prematurity Cooperative Group. The incidence and course of retinopathy of prematurity: findings from the Early Treatment for Retinopathy of Prematurity study. *Pediatrics.* 2005;116:15–23.

Fleck BW, McIntosh N. Retinopathy of prematurity: recent developments. *NeoReviews.* 2009;10: 20–30.

Heidary G, Löfqvist C, Mantagos IS, et al. Retinopathy of prematurity: clinical insights from molecular studies. *NeoReviews.* 2009:10;550–557.

International Committee for the Classification of Retinopathy of Prematurity. The international classification of retinopathy of prematurity revisited. *Arch Ophthalmol.* 2005;123:991–999.

Mintz-Hittner HA, Kennedy KA, Chuang AZ; BEAT-ROP Cooperative Group. Efficacy of intravitreal bevacizumab for stage 3+ retinopathy of prematurity. *N Eng J Med.* 2011;364:603–615.

Phelps DL. Retinopathy of prematurity: history, classification and pathophysiology. *NeoReviews.* 2001;2:153.

STOP-ROP Multicenter Study Group. Supplemental therapeutic oxygen for prethreshold retinopathy of prematurity (STOP-ROP), a randomized, controlled trial: I. Primary outcomes. *Pediatrics.* 2000;105:295.

127 Rh Incompatibility

I. **Definition.** Isoimmune hemolytic anemia of variable severity may result when Rh incompatibility develops between an Rh-negative mother previously sensitized to the Rh (D) antigen and her Rh-positive fetus. The onset of clinical disease begins in utero as the result of active placental transfer of maternal immunoglobulin (Ig)G-Rh antibody. It is manifested as a partially compensated, moderate to severe hemolytic anemia at birth, with unconjugated hyperbilirubinemia developing in the early neonatal period.

II. **Incidence.** Historically, Rh hemolytic disease of the newborn accounted for up to a third of symptomatic cases seen and was associated with detectable antibody in ~15% of Rh-incompatible mothers. **The use of Rh immunoglobulin (RhoGAM) prophylaxis has reduced the incidence of Rh sensitization to <1% of Rh-incompatible pregnancies.** Other alloimmune antibodies have become relatively more important as a cause of hemolysis. Anti-c, Kell (K and k), Duffy (Fya), Kidd (Jka and Jkb), MNS (M, N, S, and s), and less commonly anti-C and anti-E may cause severe hemolytic disease of the newborn. This cannot be prevented by the use of D antigen–specific Rh immunoglobulin.

III. **Pathophysiology.** Initial exposure of the mother to the Rh antigen occurs most often during parturition, miscarriage, abortion, and ectopic pregnancy. Invasive investigative procedures such as amniocentesis, chorionic villus sampling, and fetal blood sampling also increase the risk of fetal transplacental hemorrhage and alloimmunization. Recognition of the antigen by the immune system ensues after initial exposure, and reexposure to the Rh antigen induces a maternal anamnestic response and elevation of specific IgG-Rh antibody. Active placental transport of this antibody and immune attachment to the Rh-antigenic sites on the fetal erythrocyte are followed by extravascular hemolysis of erythrocytes within the fetal liver and spleen. The rate of the hemolytic process is proportionate in part to the levels of the maternal antibody titer but is more accurately reflected in the antepartum period by elevation of the amniotic fluid bilirubin concentration and in the postpartum period by the rate of rise of unconjugated bilirubin. In contrast to ABO incompatibility, the greater antigenicity and density of the Rh-antigen loci on the fetal erythrocyte facilitates progressive, rapid clearance of fetal erythrocytes from the circulation. A demonstrable phase of spherocytosis will be absent. Compensatory reticulocytosis and shortening of the erythrocyte generation time, if unable to match the often high rate of hemolysis in utero, results in anemia in the newborn infant and a risk of multiple systemic complications.

IV. **Risk factors**

A. **Birth order.** The firstborn infant is at minimum risk (<1%) unless sensitization has occurred previously. Once sensitization has occurred, subsequent pregnancies are at a progressive risk for fetal disease.

B. **Fetomaternal hemorrhage.** The volume of fetal erythrocytes entering the maternal circulation correlates with the risk of sensitization. The risk is ~8% with each pregnancy but ranges from 3 to 65%, depending on the volume of fetal blood (3% with 0.1 mL compared with 22% with >0.1 mL) that passes into the maternal circulation.

C. **ABO incompatibility.** Coexistent incompatibility for either the A or B blood group antigen reduces the risk of maternal Rh sensitization to 1.5–3.0%. Rapid immune clearance of these fetal erythrocytes after their entry into the maternal circulation exerts a partial protective effect. It confers no protection once sensitization has occurred.

D. **Obstetric factors.** Cesarean delivery or trauma to the placental bed during the third stage of labor increases the risk of significant fetomaternal transfusion and subsequent maternal sensitization.

E. **Gender.** Male infants are reported to have an increased risk of more severe disease than females, although the basis for this observation is unclear.

F. **Ethnicity.** Approximately 15% of whites are Rh negative compared with 7% of blacks and almost 0% in Asiatic Chinese and Japanese. The risk to the fetus varies accordingly.

G. **Maternal immune response.** A significant proportion of Rh-negative mothers (10–50%) fail to develop specific IgG-Rh antibody despite repeated exposure to Rh antigen.

V. **Clinical presentation**

A. **Symptoms and signs**

1. **Jaundice.** Unconjugated hyperbilirubinemia is the most common presenting neonatal sign of Rh disease, usually appearing within the first 24 hours of life.

2. **Anemia.** Low cord blood hemoglobin at birth reflects the relative severity of the hemolytic process in utero and is present in ~50% of cases.

3. **Hepatosplenomegaly.** Enlargement of the liver and spleen is seen in severe hemolysis, sometimes occurring in association with ascites, with an increased risk for splenic rupture.

4. **Hydrops fetalis.** Severe Rh disease has a historical association with hydrops fetalis and at one time was its most common cause. Clinical features in the fetus include progressive hypoalbuminemia with ascites, pleural effusion, or both; severe chronic anemia with secondary hypoxemia; and cardiac failure. There is an increased risk of late fetal death, stillbirth, and intolerance of active labor. The neonate frequently has generalized edema, notably of the scalp, which can be detected by antepartum ultrasonography, cardiopulmonary distress often involving pulmonary edema and severe surfactant deficiency, congestive heart failure, hypotension and peripheral perfusion defects, cardiac rhythm distur-bances, and severe anemia with secondary hypoxemia and metabolic acidosis. Currently, nonimmune conditions are more commonly associated with hydrops fetalis. Secondary involvement of other organ systems may result in hypoglycemia or thrombocytopenic purpura.

VI. **Diagnosis.** Obligatory screening in an infant with unconjugated hyperbilirubinemia includes the following studies:

A. **Blood type and Rh type (mother and infant).** These studies establish the likeli-hood of Rh incompatibility and exclude the diagnosis if the infant is Rh negative, with one exception (see direct antiglobulin test [direct Coombs test], Section VI.C).

B. **Reticulocyte count.** Elevated reticulocyte levels, adjusted for the degree of anemia and gestational age in preterm infants, reflect the degree of compensation and support a diagnosis of an ongoing hemolytic process. Normal values are 4–5% for term infants and 6–10% for preterm infants (30–36 weeks' gestational age). In symptomatic Rh disease, expected values are 10–40%.

C. **Direct antiglobulin test (direct Coombs test).** A strongly positive direct Coombs test indicates that fetal red blood cells (RBCs) are coated with anti-bodies and is diagnostic of Rh incompatibility in the presence of the appropriate setup and an elevated reticulocyte count. If Rh immunoglobulin was given at 28 weeks' gestation, subsequent passive transfer of antibody will result in a false-positive direct Coombs test without associated reticulocytosis. Very rarely, a strongly positive direct Coombs test is associated with a falsely Rh-negative infant when all fetal RBC Rh-antigenic sites are covered by a high titer of maternal antibodies.

D. **Blood smear.** Polychromasia and normoblastosis proportionate to the reticulocyte count are typically present. Spherocytes are not usually present. The nucleated RBC count is often >10 per 100 white blood cells.

E. **Bilirubin levels.** Progressive elevation of unconjugated bilirubin on serial testing provides an index of the severity of the hemolytic process. An elevated direct fraction is most likely to be secondary to a laboratory artifact in the first 3 days of life and should not be subtracted from the total bilirubin when making management decisions. In the most severely affected infants, particularly those who are hydropic, the intense extramedullary erythropoiesis may cause hepatocellular dysfunction and biliary canalicular obstruction with significant elevated direct bilirubin by 5–6 days of age.

F. **Bilirubin-binding capacity tests.** Correlation between measurements of serum albumin, free bilirubin, bilirubin saturation index, and reserve binding capacity and outcome has been variable. The role of these values in directing the management of patients remains unclear.

G. **Glucose and blood gas levels.** These should be monitored closely.

H. **Supplementary laboratory studies.** Supportive diagnostic studies may be required when the basis of the hemolytic process remains unclear.

1. **Direct Coombs test in the mother.** This study should be negative in Rh disease. This test can be positive in the presence of maternal autoimmune hemolytic disease, particularly collagen vascular disease.

2. **Indirect antiglobulin titer (indirect Coombs test).** This test detects the presence of antibodies in the maternal serum. Rh-positive RBCs are incubated with the serum being tested for the presence of anti-D. If present, the RBCs now coated with anti-D are agglutinated by an antihuman globulin serum reflecting a positive indirect antiglobulin (Coombs) test result. The reciprocal of the highest dilution of maternal serum that produces agglutination is the indirect antiglobulin titer.

3. **Carbon monoxide (CO).** The severity of Rh disease may be determined by measurement of endogenous CO production. When heme is catabolized to bilirubin, CO is produced in equimolar amounts. Hemoglobin binds the CO to form carboxyhemoglobin (CO Hb) and then is finally excreted in the breath. CO Hb levels are increased in neonates with hemolysis. CO Hb levels >1.4% have been correlated with an increased need for exchange transfusion.

VII. **Management**

A. **Antepartum treatment.** Verification of the Rh-negative status at the first prenatal visit may be obtained by the following measures:

1. **Maternal antibody titer.** Once an IgG-Rh antibody has been identified, it is important to determine the titer. Serial antibody titer determinations are required every 1–4 weeks (depending on the gestational age) during pregnancy. Invasive fetal testing becomes indicated when the titer is above a critical level, usually between 1:8 and 1:16. A negative antibody screen (indirect Coombs test) signifies absence of sensitization. This test should be repeated at 28–34 weeks' gestation.

2. **RhoGAM.** Current obstetric guidelines suggest giving immunoprophylaxis at 28 weeks' gestation in the absence of sensitization.

3. **Amniocentesis.** If maternal antibody titers indicate a risk of fetal death (usual range, 1:16–1:32), amniocentesis should be performed to assess fetal Rh genotype and assess severity. Fetal Rh-genotype determination can also be made from fetal cell free DNA found in maternal plasma. To reasonably predict the risk of moderate to severe fetal disease, serial determinations of amniotic fluid bilirubin levels present photometrically at 450 nm are plotted on standard graphs according to gestational age (known as the **Liley curve**). Readings falling into very high zone II or zone III indicate that hydrops will develop within 7–10 days. Zone I indicates no fetal hemolytic disease or no anemia.

4. **Ultrasonography.** As a screening study in pregnancies at risk, serial fetal ultrasound examinations allow detection of scalp edema, ascites, or other signs of developing hydrops fetalis. Peak systolic middle cerebral artery

velocity can reliably detect moderate and severe fetal anemia and thus reduce the need for more invasive diagnostic procedures such as amniocentesis and cordocentesis.

5. **Intrauterine transfusion.** Based on the studies just mentioned, intrauterine transfusion may be indicated because of possible fetal demise or the presence of fetal hydrops. This procedure must be performed by an experienced team. The goal is maintenance of effective erythrocyte mass within the fetal circulation and maintenance of the pregnancy until there is a reasonable chance for successful extrauterine survival of the infant.

6. **Glucocorticoids.** If premature delivery is anticipated, glucocorticoids should be given to accelerate fetal lung maturation and reduce the risk of intraventricular hemorrhage.

7. **Reduction of maternal antibody level.** Intensive maternal plasma exchange and high-dose intravenous immunoglobulins (IVIGs) have been reported of value in the severely alloimmunized pregnant woman to reduce circulating maternal antibodies levels by >50%.

B. **Postpartum treatment**

1. **Resuscitation.** Moderately to severely anemic infants with or without hydropic features are at risk for high-output cardiac failure, hypoxemia secondary to decreased oxygen-carrying capacity or surfactant deficiency, and hypoglycemia. These infants may require immediate single-volume exchange blood transfusion at delivery to improve oxygen-carrying capacity, mechanical support of ventilation, and an extended period of monitoring for hypoglycemia.

2. **Cord blood studies.** A cord blood bilirubin level >4 mg/dL, a cord hemoglobin <12 g/dL, or both usually suggests moderate to severe disease. The cord blood is used for these and initial screening studies, including blood typing, Rh typing, and Coombs test.

3. **Serial unconjugated bilirubin studies.** Determination of the rate of increase in unconjugated bilirubin levels provides an index of the severity of the hemolytic process and the need for exchange transfusion. Commonly used guidelines include a rise of >0.5 mg/dL/h or >5 mg/dL over 24 hours within the first 2 days of life or projection of a serum level that will exceed a predetermined "exchange level" for a given infant (usually 20 mg/dL in term infants).

4. **Phototherapy.** In severe Rh hemolytic disease, phototherapy is used only as an adjunct to exchange transfusion. Phototherapy decreases bilirubin levels and reduces the number of total exchange transfusions required. See Chapters 58 and 100 for phototherapy details.

5. **Exchange transfusion.** (For the procedure, see Chapter 30.) Exchange transfusion is indicated if the unconjugated bilirubin level is likely to reach a predetermined "exchange level" for that patient. Optimally, exchange transfusion is done well before this exchange level is reached to minimize the risk of entry of unconjugated bilirubin into the central nervous system. Consideration should be given to irradiation of blood before the transfusion is given, particularly in preterm infants or infants expected to require multiple transfusions, to reduce the risk of graft-versus-host disease. The process removes 70–90% of the fetal red cells, but only 25% of the total bilirubin because most of the bilirubin is in the extravascular space. A rapid rebound of serum bilirubin is common after reequilibration, and thus additional exchange transfusions may be required.

6. **Heme oxygenase inhibitors (stannsoporfin).** Tin (Sn) porphyrin can decrease the production of bilirubin and reduce the need for exchange transfusion and duration of phototherapy. It is an inhibitor of heme oxygenase, which is the enzyme that allows the production of bilirubin from heme. The dose of stannsoporfin is 6 μmol/kg IM as a single dose given within 24 hours of birth with severe hemolytic disease, and it is available via compassionate use protocol.

7. **IVIG.** By blocking neonatal reticuloendothelial Fc receptors, and thus decreasing hemolysis of the antibody-coated RBCs, high-dose IVIG (1 g/kg over 4 hours) reduces serum bilirubin levels and the need for blood exchange transfusion with ABO or Rh hemolytic diseases. (See Chapters 80 and 127.) Caution should be used when considering treatment with IVIG, as there are emerging reports of increased incidence of NEC in term and late-preterm infants with hemolytic disease of the newborn and isoimmune neonatal thrombocytopenia who were treated with IVIG.

C. **RhoGAM prophylaxis.** Most cases of incompatibility involve the D antigen. RhoGAM given at 28 weeks' gestation, within 72 hours of suspected Rh-antigen exposure, or both reduces the risk of sensitization to <1%; the recommended dosage (300 mcg) should be well in excess of the amount of Rh antigen transfused (300 mcg for every 25 mL of fetal blood in maternal circulation). The amount of fetal blood entering the maternal circulation may be estimated using the Kleihauer-Betke acid elution technique (page 562) during the immediate postpartum period.

No treatment equivalent to RhoGAM is available for maternal Rh sensitization to non-D antigens, notably C and E antigens. These antigens, however, are significantly less antigenic than the D antigen, clinical manifestations of incompatibility are frequently milder, and the risk of severe disease is considerably less.

D. **Hydrops fetalis.** Skilled resuscitation and anticipation of selective systemic complications may prevent early neonatal death.

1. **Isovolumetric partial exchange transfusion with type O Rh-negative packed erythrocytes.** Raises the hematocrit and improves the oxygen-carrying capacity (see Chapter 30).
2. **Central arterial and venous catheterization.** May be performed to provide the following measures:
   a. **Isovolumetric exchange transfusion**
   b. **Monitoring of arterial blood gas levels** and central venous and systemic blood pressures
   c. **Monitoring of fluid and electrolyte balance,** particularly renal and hepatic function, calcium-to-phosphorus ratio, and serum albumin levels, as well as appropriate hematologic studies and serum bilirubin levels
3. **Positive-pressure mechanical ventilation.** This measure may include increased levels of positive end-expiratory pressure, if pulmonary edema is present, as a means of stabilizing alveolar ventilation. Treatment with exogenous surfactant may be considered in particular when the infant is judged to be not fully mature.
4. **Therapeutic thoracentesis or paracentesis.** May be performed to remove fluid that may further compromise respiratory effort. Excessive removal of ascitic fluid may lead to systemic hypotension. (See Chapters 27 and 37.)
5. **Volume expanders.** May be necessary, in addition to erythrocytes, to improve peripheral perfusion defects. This should be done with caution because most hydropic infants are hypotensive or poorly perfused because of hypoxic heart failure rather than hypovolemia, or both.
6. **Drug treatment.** May include diuretics such as furosemide for pulmonary edema and pressor agents such as dopamine (for dosing, see Chapter 148). In the case of cardiac rhythm disturbances, appropriate drugs may be used if indicated.
7. **Electrocardiography or echocardiography.** May be needed to determine whether cardiac abnormalities are present.

VIII. **Prognosis.** Prenatal mortality for infants at risk of anti-D Rh isoimmunization is currently ~1.5% and has decreased significantly over the past 2 decades. Antenatal immune prophylaxis and improved management techniques, including amniotic fluid spectrophotometry, intrauterine transfusion, and advances in neonatal intensive care, have been largely responsible for this reduction. Isolated cases of severe isoimmunization still occur because of isoimmunization by other than anti-D antibody or failure to receive immune prophylaxis and may exhibit the full spectrum of disease, including an increased risk of stillbirths and early neonatal morbidity and mortality.

Selected References

Abrams ME, Meredith KS, Kinnard P, Clark RH. Hydrops fetalis: a retrospective review of cases reported to a large national database and identification of risk factors associated with death. *Pediatrics.* 2007;120(1):84–89.

Figueras-Aloy J, Rodríguez-Miguélez JM, Iriondo-Sanz M, Salvia-Roiges MD, Botet-Mussons F, Carbonell-Estrany X. Intravenous immunoglobulin and necrotizing enterocolitis in newborns with hemolytic disease. *Pediatrics.* 2010;125;139–144.

Moise KJ Jr. Management of rhesus alloimmunization in pregnancy. *Obstet Gynecol.* 2008;112(1):164–176.

Wagle S, Deshpande PG. Hemolytic disease of the newborn. http://emedicine.medscape.com/article/974349-overview. Last updated May 18, 2011. Accessed September 21, 2011.

128 Rubella

I. **Definition.** Rubella is a viral infection capable of causing chronic intrauterine infection and damage to the developing fetus. Rubella is classified as a member of the togavirus family.

II. **Incidence.** Rubella vaccination has virtually eliminated the majority of cases of congenital rubella syndrome (CRS) in the developed world. In the United States, between 2000 and 2005, only 4 cases of CRS have been reported, and only 1 was a child whose mother had been born in the United States. Rubella remains prevalent in developing countries and in nonvaccinated immigrant populations.

III. **Pathophysiology.** Rubella virus is an RNA virus that typically has an epidemic seasonal pattern of increased frequency in the spring. In developing countries with no vaccination programs, epidemics have occurred at 4- to 7-year intervals, with major pandemics every 10–30 years. Humans are the only known hosts, with an incubation period of ~18 days after contact. Virus is spread by respiratory secretions and also from stool, urine, and cervical secretions. A live virus vaccine has been available since 1969. In places with no vaccination, 15–20% of women of childbearing age are susceptible to rubella. Recent serologic surveys indicate that ~10% of the U.S.-born population >5 years of age is susceptible to rubella. There is a high incidence of subclinical infections. Maternal viremia is a prerequisite for placental infection, which may or may not spread to the fetus. Most cases occur after primary disease, although a few cases have been described after reinfection.

The fetal infection rate varies according to the timing of maternal infection during pregnancy. If infection occurs at 1–12 weeks and is associated with maternal rash, there is an 81% risk of fetal infection; at 13–16 weeks, 54%; at 17–22 weeks, 36%; at 23–30 weeks, 30%; there is a rise to 60% at 31–36 weeks; and 100% in the last month of pregnancy. No correlation exists between the severity of maternal rubella and teratogenicity. However, the incidence of fetal effects is greater the earlier in gestation that infection occurs, especially at 1–12 weeks, when 85% of infected fetuses will have congenital defects. Infection during weeks 13–16 results in 35% of fetuses having congenital defects; infection at later gestational ages rarely causes deafness or congenital malformations. The virus sets up chronic infection in the placenta and fetus. Placental or fetal infection may lead to resorption of the fetus, spontaneous abortion, stillbirth, fetal infection with multisystem disease, congenital anomalies, or unapparent infection.

Spontaneous abortion may occur in up to 20% of cases when rubella occurs in the first 8 weeks of pregnancy.

The disease involves angiopathy as well as cytolytic changes. Other viral effects include chromosome breakage, decreased cell multiplication time, induction of programmed cell death (apoptosis), and mitotic arrest in certain cell types. There is little inflammatory reaction.

IV. **Risk factors.** Women of childbearing age who are rubella nonimmune or foreign born are at risk. Laboratory confirmation of rubella infection is required because a clinical diagnosis is unreliable. Rubella is indistinguishable clinically from other infections that present with a rash, such as parvovirus B19, measles, human herpesvirus (HHV-6, HHV-7), enterovirus, and group A *Streptococcus* infections.

V. **Clinical presentation.** Congenital rubella infection has a wide spectrum of presentations, ranging from asymptomatic infection to acute disseminated infection to deficits not evident at birth.

   A. **Systemic transient manifestations** include low birthweight, hepatosplenomegaly, meningoencephalitis, thrombocytopenia, with or without purpura, and bony radiolucencies. These are probably a consequence of extensive virus infection and usually resolve spontaneously within days or weeks. Infants with these abnormalities usually fail to thrive during infancy.

   B. **Systemic permanent manifestations** include heart defects (eg, patent ductus arteriosus [PDA], pulmonary artery stenosis, pulmonary arterial hypoplasia), eye defects (eg, cataracts, iris hypoplasia, microphthalmos, retinopathy), central nervous system (CNS) problems (eg, mental retardation, psychomotor retardation, speech defects/language delay), microcephaly, and sensorineural or central auditory deafness (unilateral or bilateral). More than half of those children infected during the first 8 weeks of gestation have heart defects; **branch pulmonary artery stenosis** (78%) and **PDA** (62%) are the most common. Of the eye defects, a **"salt and pepper"** retinopathy is the most common. A **cataract** occurs in approximately a third of all cases of CRS, and in approximately half of these, they are bilateral. **Deafness** is a major disabling abnormality and may occur alone.

   C. **Developmental and late-onset abnormalities.** Rubella is a progressive disease due to the persistence of the viral infection and the defective immune response to the virus. Existing manifestations, such as deafness and CNS disease, may progress, and some abnormalities may not be detected until the second year of life or later. These include hearing, developmental and eye defects, diabetes mellitus (DM), thyroid disorders, behavioral and educational difficulties, and progressive panencephalitis. Insulin-dependent DM is the most frequent endocrine abnormality, occurring in ~20% of cases.

VI. **Diagnosis.** Timely diagnosis of congenital rubella infection is important both for management of the individual patient and for prevention of secondary infection because these infants may remain infectious for 1 year. The diagnosis may be suspected clinically, but needs to be confirmed with laboratory tests. The Centers for Disease Control and Prevention (CDC) has published an elaborate case definition for congenital rubella infection that is updated regularly (www.cdc.gov/osels/ph_surveillance/nndss/casedef/rubellasc_current.htm). Cases of CRS are classified as suspected, probable, confirmed, or infection only, depending on clinical findings and laboratory criteria for diagnosis.

   A. **CDC case definition**

      1. **Suspected.** **An infant who has 1 or more of the following findings (but does not meet the criteria for a confirmed or probable case):** cataracts or congenital glaucoma, congenital heart disease (most commonly PDA or peripheral pulmonary artery stenosis), hearing impairment, pigmentary retinopathy, purpura, hepatosplenomegaly, jaundice, microcephaly, developmental delay, meningoencephalitis, or radiolucent bone disease.

      2. **Probable.** **An infant who has at least 2 of the following findings (but does not have laboratory confirmation of rubella infection or a more**

plausible etiology): either cataracts or congenital glaucoma or both (count as 1), congenital heart disease (most commonly PDA or peripheral pulmonary artery stenosis), hearing impairment, or pigmentary retinopathy.

OR

An infant who has at least 1 or more of the following (but does not have laboratory confirmation or an alternative more plausible etiology etiology): either cataracts or congenital glaucoma or both (counts as 1), congenital heart disease (PDA or peripheral pulmonary artery stenosis), hearing impairment, or pigmentary retinopathy

AND

1 or more of the following of the following: purpura, hepatosplenomegaly, microcephaly, developmental delay, meningoencephalitis, or radiolucent bone disease.

3. Confirmed. **An infant with at least 1 symptom (listed previously) that is clinically consistent with congenital rubella syndrome and laboratory evidence of congenital rubella infection as demonstrated by:** isolation of rubella virus, or detection of rubella-specific immunoglobulin M (IgM) antibody, or infant rubella antibody level that persists at a higher level and for a longer period than expected from passive transfer of maternal antibody (ie, rubella titer that does not drop at the expected rate of a 2-fold decline per month), or a specimen that is polymerase chain reaction (PCR) positive for rubella virus.

4. Infection only. **An infant with laboratory evidence of infection but with no clinical symptoms or signs.** Laboratory evidence is documented by isolation of rubella virus or detection of rubella-specific IgM antibody or infant rubella antibody level that persists at a higher level and longer than expected from passive transfer of maternal antibody (eg, rubella titer that does not drop at the expected rate of a 2-fold decline per month), or a specimen that is PCR positive for rubella virus. **If any signs or symptoms are identified later such as hearing loss, then the diagnosis is reclassified as confirmed.**

B. **Laboratory studies**

1. **Open cultures.** The virus can be cultured for up to 1 year despite measurable antibody titer. The best specimens for viral recovery are from nasopharyngeal swabs, conjunctival scrapings, urine, and cerebrospinal fluid (CSF; in decreasing order of usefulness).

2. **Serologic studies.** These are the mainstay of rubella diagnosis. CRS is diagnosed by the detection of rubella-specific IgM in a serum or oral fluid taken before 3 months of age. IgM testing is less reliable after 3 months of age as levels of specific IgM decline. However, if sensitive assays are used, specific IgM may be detected in 85% of symptomatic infants at 3–6 months and >30% at 6–12 months of age. A negative result by IgM-capture enzyme immunosorbent assay in the first 3 months of age virtually excludes congenital infection. It is also possible to make a diagnosis by demonstrating persistence of rubella IgG in sera taken between 6 and 12 months of age. It is no longer possible to make a serologic diagnosis of congenital rubella after rubella vaccination. Testing of oral-fluid samples as an alternative to serum has been used and standardized. It offers many advantages for surveillance of CRS in developing countries. Serologic tests for detection of rubella-specific IgM in oral-fluid samples are accurate.

3. **Rubella virus PCR.** CRS may also be diagnosed by detection of viral RNA by nested reverse-transcriptase PCR (RT-PCR) in nasopharyngeal swabs, urine, oral fluid, CSF, lens aspirate, and EDTA-blood.

4. **CSF examination.** This may reveal encephalitis with an increased protein and cell count.

C. **Imaging studies.** Long-bone films may show metaphyseal radiolucencies that correlate with metaphyseal osteoporosis.

VII. **Management.** Cases of CRS (suspected or confirmed) in the US should be reported to the CDC through local and state health departments. All newborns who fail hearing screening should undergo evaluation for rubella (measurement of rubella-specific IgM antibodies) and other intrauterine infections. There is no specific treatment for rubella. Long-term follow-up is needed secondary to late-onset symptoms. Prevention consists of vaccination of the susceptible population (especially young children). Vaccine should not be given to pregnant women. Pregnancy should be avoided for 28 days after vaccination. Inadvertent vaccination of pregnant women does not cause CRS, although there is a 3% chance of congenital infection. Passive immunization does not prevent fetal infection when maternal infection occurs. Children with congenital rubella should be considered contagious until they are at least 1 year of age, unless 2 cultures of clinical specimens (nasopharyngeal and urine cultures) obtained 1 month apart are negative for rubella virus after 3 months of age. Rubella vaccine virus can be isolated from breast milk in lactating women who have received the vaccine. However, breast-feeding is not a contraindication to vaccination because no evidence indicates that the vaccine virus is in any way harmful to the infant.

VIII. **Prognosis.** Infection in the first or second trimester can cause growth restriction and deafness. Consequences of congenital rubella may present later (inguinal hernia, motor and mental retardation, hearing and communication disorders, and microcephaly).

Selected References

American Academy of Pediatrics. Rubella. In: Pickering LK, Baker CJ, Kimberlin DW, Long SS, eds. *Red Book: 2012 Report of the Committee on Infectious Diseases.* 29th ed. Elk Grove Village, IL: American Academy of Pediatrics; 2012:629–634.

Best JM. Rubella. *Semin Fetal Neonatal Med.* 2007;12:182–192.

Centers for Disease Control and Prevention. Rubella. In: Atkinson W, ed. *Epidemiology and Prevention of Vaccine-Preventable Diseases. The Pink Book.* 12th ed. Washington DC: Public Health Foundation; 2011;275–290.

Harlor AD, Bower C; Committee on Practice and Ambulatory Medicine; Section on Otolaryngology-Head and Neck Surgery. Hearing assessment in infants and children: recommendations beyond neonatal screening. *Pediatrics.* 2009;124:1252–1263.

Morice A, Ulloa-Gutierrez R, Avila-Agüero ML. Congenital rubella syndrome: progress and future challenges. *Expert Rev Vaccines.* 2009;8:323–331.

Oster ME, Riehle-Colarusso T, Correa A. An update on cardiovascular malformations in congenital rubella syndrome. *Birth Defects Res A Clin Mol Teratol.* 2010;88:1–8.

Plotkin SA, Reef SE, Cooper LZ, Alford CA, Jr. Rubella. In: Remington JS, Klein JO, Wilson CB, Nizet V, Maldonado Y, eds. *Infectious Diseases of the Fetus and Newborn Infant.* 7th ed. Philadelphia, PA: Elsevier Saunders; 2011:861–898.

Reef SE, Strebel P, Dabbagh A, Gacic-Dobo M, Cochi S. Progress toward control of rubella and prevention of congenital rubella syndrome: worldwide, 2009. *J Infect Dis.* 2011; 204(suppl 1):S24–S27.

129 Seizures

I. **Definition.** A seizure is defined clinically as a paroxysmal alteration in neurologic function (ie, behavioral, motor, or autonomic function).

II. **Incidence.** Neonatal seizures are relatively common and occur in 0.15–1.5% of all neonates.

III. **Pathophysiology.** The neurons within the central nervous system (CNS) undergo depolarization as a result of inward migration of sodium. Repolarization occurs via efflux of potassium. A seizure occurs when there is excessive depolarization, resulting in excessive synchronous electrical discharge. Volpe (2001) proposed the following 4 possible reasons for excessive depolarization: failure of the sodium-potassium pump because of a disturbance in energy production, a relative excess of excitatory versus inhibitory neurotransmitter, a relative deficiency of inhibitory versus excitatory neurotransmitter, and alteration in the neuronal membrane, causing inhibition of sodium movement. The basic mechanisms of neonatal seizures, however, are unknown.

IV. **Etiology.** There are numerous causes of neonatal seizures, but relatively few account for most cases (Table 129–1). Therefore, only common causes of seizures are discussed here.

    A. **Perinatal asphyxia** is the most common cause of neonatal seizures. These occur within the first 24 hours of life in most cases and may progress to overt status epilepticus. In premature infants, seizures are of the generalized tonic type, whereas in full-term infants they are of the multifocal clonic type. Accompanying subtle seizures are usually present in both types.

    B. **Intracranial hemorrhage,** whether subarachnoid, periventricular, or intraventricular, may occur as a result of hypoxic insults that can lead to neonatal seizures. Subdural hemorrhage, usually a result of trauma, can cause seizures.

        1. **In primary subarachnoid hemorrhage,** convulsions often occur on the second postnatal day, and the infant appears quite well during the interictal period.

Table 129–1. CAUSES OF NEONATAL SEIZURES

Perinatal asphyxia
Intracranial hemorrhage
   Subarachnoid hemorrhage
   Periventricular or intraventricular hemorrhage
   Subdural hemorrhage
Metabolic abnormalities
   Hypoglycemia
   Hypocalcemia
   Electrolyte disturbances: hyponatremia and hypernatremia
   Amino acid disorders
   Pyridoxine dependency
Congenital malformations
Infections
   Meningitis
   Encephalitis
   Syphilis, cytomegalovirus infections, toxoplasmosis, herpes simplex
   Cerebral abscess
Drug withdrawal
Toxin exposure (particularly local anesthetics)
Miscellaneous disorders
   Zellweger syndrome
   Tuberous sclerosis
   Benign familial neonatal seizures
   Benign idiopathic neonatal seizures ("fifth-day fits")
   Early myoclonic encephalopathy (EME)
   Early infantile epileptic encephalopathy (Ohtahara syndrome)
   Benign neonatal sleep myoclonus
   Hyperekplexia ("startle disease")
   Congenital hypothyroidism

2. **Periventricular or intraventricular hemorrhage** arising from the subependymal germinal matrix is accompanied by subtle seizures, decerebrate posturing, or generalized tonic seizures, depending on the severity of the hemorrhage.

3. **Subdural hemorrhage** over the cerebral convexities leads to focal seizures and focal cerebral signs.

C. **Metabolic disturbances**

1. **Hypoglycemia** is frequently seen in infants with intrauterine growth retardation and in infants of diabetic mothers (IDMs). The duration of hypoglycemia and the time lapse before initiation of treatment determine the occurrence of seizures. Seizures are less frequent in IDMs, perhaps because of the short duration of hypoglycemia.

2. **Hypocalcemia** has been noted in low birthweight infants, IDMs, asphyxiated infants, infants with DiGeorge syndrome, and infants born to mothers with hyperparathyroidism. Hypomagnesemia is a frequent accompanying problem.

3. **Hyponatremia** occurs because of improper fluid management or as a result of the syndrome of inappropriate antidiuretic hormone (SIADH).

4. **Hypernatremia** is seen with dehydration as a result of inadequate intake in breast-fed infants, excessive use of sodium bicarbonate, or incorrect dilution of concentrated formula.

5. **Other metabolic disorders**

   a. **Pyridoxine dependency.** Leads to seizures resistant to anticonvulsants. Infants with this disorder experience intrauterine convulsions and are born with meconium staining. They resemble asphyxiated infants.

   b. **Amino acid disorders.** Seizures in infants with amino acid disturbances are invariably accompanied by other neurologic manifestations. Hyperammonemia and acidosis are commonly present in amino acid disorders.

D. **Infections.** Intracranial infection secondary to bacterial or nonbacterial agents may be acquired by the neonate in utero, during delivery, or in the immediate perinatal period.

1. **Bacterial infection.** Meningitis resulting from **group B *Streptococcus*,** *Escherichia coli,* or *Listeria monocytogenes* infection is accompanied by seizures during the first week of life.

2. **Nonbacterial infection.** Nonbacterial causes such as toxoplasmosis and infection with herpes simplex, cytomegalovirus, rubella, and coxsackie B viruses lead to intracranial infection and seizures.

E. **Drug withdrawal.** Three categories of drugs used by the mother lead to passive addiction and drug withdrawal (sometimes accompanied by seizures) in the infant. These are **analgesics** such as heroin, methadone, and propoxyphene (Darvon); **sedative hypnotics** such as secobarbital; and **alcohol.** Current studies revealed that antidepressant exposure was associated with an increased risk for infant seizures, especially selective serotonin reuptake inhibitor (SSRI) exposure.

F. **Toxins.** Inadvertent injection of local anesthetics into the fetus at the time of delivery (paracervical, pudendal, or saddle block anesthesia) may cause generalized tonic-clonic seizures. Mothers often notice the absence of pain relief during delivery.

V. **Risk factors.** In a large study (2.3 million births) from California, the following risk factors were identified for seizures in the newborn during the birth admission: prematurity, birthweight <2500 g, delivery at ≥42 weeks, maternal diabetes mellitus, maternal age ≥40 years, nulliparity, intrapartum fever/infection (chorioamnionitis), and catastrophic delivery (placental abruption, uterine rupture, and cord prolapse).

VI. **Clinical presentation.** It is important to understand that **seizures in the neonate are different from those seen in older children.** The differences are perhaps due to the neuroanatomic and neurophysiologic developmental status of the newborn infant. In the neonatal brain, glial proliferation, neuronal migration, establishment of axonal and dendritic contacts, and myelin deposition are incomplete. Clinical seizures may occur without any electrographic correlation and vice versa (electroclinical dissociation). **Four types of seizures,** based on clinical presentation, are recognized: **subtle, clonic, tonic, and myoclonic.**

A. **Subtle seizures** are not clearly clonic, tonic, or myoclonic and are more common in premature than in full-term infants. Subtle seizures are more commonly associated with an electroencephalographic seizure in premature infants than in full-term infants. They consist of tonic horizontal deviation of the eyes with or without jerking; eyelid blinking or fluttering; sucking, smacking, or drooling; "swimming," "rowing," or "pedaling" movements; and apneic spells. Apnea as a manifestation of seizures is usually accompanied or preceded by other subtle manifestations. In premature infants, apnea is less likely to be a manifestation of seizures.

B. **Clonic seizures** are more common in full-term infants than in premature infants and commonly associated with an electroencephalographic seizure. There are 2 types of clonic seizures:
1. **Focal seizures.** Well-localized, rhythmic, slow jerking movements involving the face and upper or lower extremities on one side of the body or the neck or trunk on one side of the body. Infants are usually not unconscious during or after the seizures.
2. **Multifocal seizures.** Several body parts seize in a sequential, nonjacksonian fashion (eg, left arm jerking followed by right leg jerking).

C. **Tonic seizures** occur primarily in premature infants. Two types of tonic seizures are seen.
1. **Focal seizures.** Sustained posturing of a limb, asymmetric posturing of the trunk or neck, or both. These are commonly associated with an electroencephalographic seizure.
2. **Generalized seizures.** Most commonly, these occur with a tonic extension of both upper and lower extremities (as in decerebrate posturing) but may also present with tonic flexion of the upper extremities with extension of the lower extremities (as in decorticate posturing). It is uncommon to see electroencephalographic seizure disorders.

D. **Myoclonic seizures** are seen in both full-term and premature infants and are characterized by single or multiple synchronous jerks. Three types of myoclonic seizures are seen.
1. **Focal seizures.** Typically involve the flexor muscles of an upper extremity and are not commonly associated with electroencephalographic seizure activity.
2. **Multifocal seizures.** Exhibit asynchronous twitching of several parts of the body and are not commonly associated with electroencephalographic seizure activity.
3. **Generalized seizures.** Present with bilateral jerks of flexion of the upper and sometimes the lower extremities. They are more commonly associated with electroencephalographic seizure activity.

   Note: It is important to distinguish **jitteriness** from **seizures.** Jitteriness is accompanied by neither abnormal gaze nor eye movements, nor by autonomic changes. It is highly stimulus sensitive; tremor is the dominant movement, and it can be stopped by gentle flexion.

VII. **Diagnosis**
A. **History.** Although it is often difficult to obtain a thorough history in infants transported to tertiary care facilities from other hospitals, the physician must make a concerted effort to elicit pertinent historical data.
1. **Family history.** A positive family history of neonatal seizures is usually obtained in cases of metabolic errors and benign familial neonatal convulsions.
2. **Maternal drug history.** This is critical in cases of narcotic withdrawal syndrome.
3. **Delivery.** Details of the delivery provide information regarding maternal analgesia, the mode and nature of delivery, the fetal intrapartum status, and the resuscitative measures used. Information regarding maternal infections during pregnancy points toward an infectious basis for seizures in an infant.

B. **Physical examination**
  1. **Physical examination.** A thorough general physical examination (including measurement of head circumference and careful attention to any dysmorphic features) should precede a well-planned neurologic examination. Determine the following:
     a. **Gestational age**
     b. **Blood pressure**
     c. **Presence of skin lesions**
     d. **Presence of hepatosplenomegaly**
  2. **Neurologic evaluation.** A neurologic evaluation should include assessment of the level of alertness, cranial nerves, motor function, primary neonatal reflexes, and sensory function. Some of the specific features to look for are the size and "feel" of the fontanelle, retinal hemorrhages, chorioretinitis, pupillary size and reaction to light, extraocular movements, changes in muscle tone, and status of primary reflexes.
  3. **Notation of the seizure pattern.** When seizures are observed, they should be described in detail, including the site of onset, spread, nature, duration, and level of consciousness. Recognition of subtle seizures requires special attention.
C. **Laboratory studies.** In selecting and prioritizing laboratory tests, use the information obtained by history taking and physical examination and look for common and treatable causes.
  1. **Complete blood count (CBC) and differential.** To rule out infection and polycythemia.
  2. **Serum chemistries.** Estimations of serum glucose, calcium, sodium, blood urea nitrogen, and magnesium and blood gas levels must be performed. They may reveal the abnormality causing the seizures.
  3. **Spinal fluid examination.** Evaluation of the cerebrospinal fluid (CSF) is essential because the consequences of delayed treatment or nontreatment of bacterial meningitis are grave. CSF polymerase chain reaction (PCR) should be performed for herpes simplex virus if suspected. A low CSF glucose and normal blood glucose indicates meningitis or glucose transporter defect. Likewise, a low CSF glycine despite normal blood amino acids suggests hyperglycinemia, and elevated CSF lactate suggests a mitochondrial disorder.
  4. **Metabolic disorders.** (See also Chapter 101.) With a family history of neonatal convulsions, a peculiar odor about the infant, milk intolerance, acidosis, alkalosis, or seizures not responsive to anticonvulsants, other metabolic causes should be investigated.
     a. **Blood ammonia levels** should be checked.
     b. **Amino acids** should be measured in urine and plasma. The urine should be tested for reducing substances.
        i. **Urea cycle disorders.** Respiratory alkalosis is seen as a result of direct stimulation of the respiratory center by ammonia.
        ii. **Maple syrup urine disease.** With 2,4-dinitrophenylhydrazine (2,4-DNPH) testing of urine, a fluffy yellow precipitate is seen in cases of maple syrup urine disease.
D. **Imaging and other studies**
  1. **Ultrasonography of the head.** Performed to rule out intraventricular hemorrhage (IVH) or periventricular hemorrhage.
  2. **Computed tomography (CT) scanning of the head.** Provides detailed information regarding intracranial disease. CT scanning is helpful in looking for evidence of infarction, hemorrhage, calcification, and cerebral malformations. Experience with this technique suggests that valuable information is obtained in term infants with seizures, especially when seizures are asymmetric. Be mindful of heavy dose of radiation and avoid repeating unless it is essential.

3. **Magnetic resonance imaging (MRI).** MRI is the study of choice and can detect congenital abnormalities of brain such as lissencephaly, pachygyria, and polymicrogyria, along with IVH with infarct and hypoxic ischemic encephalopathy (HIE). A cranial MRI is the most sensitive test to determine the etiology of seizures in the neonate. It is difficult to do in an unstable infant and is a test that requires a lot of time.

4. **Electroencephalography.** Electroencephalograms (EEGs) obtained during a seizure are abnormal. Interictal EEGs may be normal. However, an order to obtain an ictal EEG should not delay other diagnostic and therapeutic steps. The diagnostic value of an EEG is greater when it is obtained in the first few days because diagnostic patterns indicative of unfavorable prognosis disappear thereafter. Electroencephalography is valuable in confirming the presence of seizures when manifestations are subtle or when neuromuscular paralyzing agents have been given, and in defining the interictal background features. EEGs are of prognostic significance in full-term infants with recognized seizures. For proper interpretation of EEGs, it is important to know the clinical status of the infant (including the sleep state) and any medications given. Video EEG monitoring can be done when infrequent seizures occur. Although continuous EEG monitoring with **amplitude-integrated electroencephalography (aEEG)** has improved seizure detection and is useful in full-term infants with hypoxia-ischemia, conventional full-array continuous video EEG remains the gold standard.

VIII. **Management.** Because repeated seizures may lead to brain injury, **urgent treatment is indicated. The method of treatment depends on the cause.** Neurologic consultation is recommended. Optimal treatment for neonatal seizures is *controversial* and highly variable between centers, especially concerning the use of anticonvulsants.

A. **Hypoglycemia.** Hypoglycemic infants with seizures should receive 10% dextrose in water, 2–4 mL/kg intravenously (IV), followed by 6–8 mg/kg/min by continuous infusion. (See Chapter 62.)

B. **Hypocalcemia.** Treated with slow IV infusion of calcium gluconate (for dosage and other information, see Chapter 85). If serum magnesium levels are low (<1.52 mEq/L), magnesium sulfate should be given. (See Chapter 107.)

C. **Anticonvulsant therapy.** Conventional anticonvulsant treatment is used when no underlying metabolic cause is found. Loading doses of phenobarbital and phenytoin control 85% of neonatal seizures.

1. **Phenobarbital** is usually given first (for dosage and other pharmacologic information, see Chapter 148). A recent review of treatment in 31 U.S. pediatric hospitals verified that most treated infants received phenobarbital. Worldwide, phenobarbital continues to be the initial drug of choice. Neither gestational age nor birthweight seem to influence the loading or maintenance dose of phenobarbital. When phenobarbital alone fails to control seizures, another agent is used. Gilman et al (1989) found that sequentially administered phenobarbital controlled seizures in term and preterm newborns in 77% of cases. If seizures are not controlled at a serum phenobarbital level of 40 mcg/mL, administer a second agent (eg, phenytoin [Dilantin]).

2. **Phenytoin (Dilantin)** is usually used next by many practitioners. Fosphenytoin may be a preferred form. (For dosage and other pharmacologic information, see Chapter 148.)

3. **If seizures still persist, then the third medication usually given is a benzodiazepine.**

   a. **Diazepam** has been used as single or repeated doses. Because of its very rapid brain clearance, it is more effective if given by continuous infusion of 0.3 mg/kg/h. It is falling out of favor because of rapid brain clearance, risk of circulatory failure when used with phenobarbital, narrow therapeutic/toxicity window, and greater depressant effect.

    b. Lorazepam, given IV, can be repeated 4 to 6 times in a 24-hour period. It is advantageous to use over diazepam because it causes less sedation and respiratory depression and has a less rapid brain clearance. It has been quite effective and safe. Some centers use lorazepam as a second-line drug in place of phenytoin. (For dosage and other pharmacologic information, see Chapter 148.)

  4. **If seizures are still present, then 3 disorders need to be ruled out before more medications are given:**

    a. Pyridoxine-dependent seizures. A trial of pyridoxine (vitamin B_6), 50–100 mg, given IV with EEG monitoring is now recommended. With pyridoxine dependency, the seizures stop quickly after the medication is given. The administration should be continued, as stoppage leads to recurrence of seizures, requiring reinstitution. Some institutions wait to give this after 3 medications have been given and failed; some try this after 2 medications have been given.

    b. Folinic acid–responsive seizures (rare). Obtain CSF neurotransmitter studies. Then folinic acid is given at 2.5 mg twice daily (up to 4 mg/kg/d initially) in 2 doses. After 24 hours of treatment, seizures may stop. Folinic acid can be given for 48 hours as a trial.

    c. DeVivo syndrome (glucose transporter deficiency). Treatment is a ketogenic diet.

  5. **If seizures still persist, the following drugs may be used depending on institutional preference:**

    a. High-dose phenobarbital. >30 mg/kg to achieve serum level >60 mcg/mL was effective in one review.

    b. Midazolam. IV: 0.2 mg/kg, then 0.1–0.4 mg/kg/h. It is also given intranasally.

    c. Pentobarbital. IV: 10 mg/kg, then 1 mg/kg/h.

    d. Thiopental. IV: 10 mg/kg, then 2–4 mg/kg/h.

    e. Clonazepam. Oral: 0.1 mg/kg in 2–3 doses. IV: 0.1 mg/kg, then 0.1–0.5 mg/kg/d.

    f. Valproic acid. Oral: 10–25 mg/kg, then 20 mg/kg/d in 3 doses. Same dose for IV use.

    g. Chlormethiazole (not available in the United States). IV: initial infusion rate of 0.08 mg/kg/min.

    h. Paraldehyde. Given rectally (IV preparation no longer available in the United States); used as a last effort.

    i. Lidocaine. IV: 2 mg/kg, then 6 mg/kg/h with cardiac monitoring. New infusion doses are used to decrease cardiac arrhythmias. Not recommended in infants who have been treated with phenytoin or who have congenital heart disease.

    j. Levetiracetam. IV: 10 mg/kg/d divided twice daily; increase dosage by 10 mg/kg over 3 days to 30 mg/kg/d. Oral: 10–30 mg/kg/d in 2 doses.

    k. Topiramate. Oral: 3 mg/kg/d.

    l. Lamotrigine. Oral: 12.5 mg in 2 doses.

    m. Carbamazepine. Oral: 10 mg/kg, then 15–20 mg/kg/d in 2 doses.

    n. Vigabatrin. Oral: 50 mg/kg/d in 2 doses up to 200 mg/kg/d.

    o. Zonisamide. Oral: 2.5 mg/kg/d.

  6. **Duration of anticonvulsant therapy.** The optimal duration of anticonvulsant therapy has not been established. Although some clinicians recommend continuation of phenobarbital for a prolonged period, others recommend stopping it after seizures have been absent for 2 weeks. Anticonvulsants may have to be continued when seizures are due to abnormality of the brain.

D. Therapeutic hypothermia. The incidence of seizures in neonates receiving therapeutic hypothermia for HIE is high. In a prospective study of term neonates undergoing whole-body hypothermia for HIE for 72 hours (followed by 24 hours of normothermia), electrographic seizures were noted in 65% (17 of 26) patients. These were entirely nonconvulsive in 47% (8 of 17), status epilepticus occurred in 23% (4 of 17); the seizure onset was in the first 48 hours in 76% (13 of 17). An earlier study of selective head cooling for HIE (Sarnat stage 2 and 3) revealed that seizures were almost universal. In therapeutic hypothermia for hypoxic-ischemic encephalopathy, seizures (clinical and electroclinical) are frequent. These are treated with phenobarbital and fosphenytoin. Midazolam or levetiracetam are used if the former 2 fail to control seizures. Anticonvulsants are not given prophylactically.

IX. **Prognosis.** The etiology of the seizure is critical in deciding the outcome and prognosis. Recent evidence suggests that neonatal seizures impair normal brain development. In infants with transient or metabolic disorders that can be corrected, the outcome is usually favorable. In infants with CNS infections, hypoxic-ischemic encephalopathy, or brain malformations, the outcome is not as favorable. The type of seizure can also dictate outcome. In one study, pure clonic seizures without facial involvement in term infants suggested favorable outcome, whereas generalized myoclonic seizures in preterm infants were associated with mortality. Prognosis is usually better for term infants than preterm infants. In one study of 34,615 infants, 90 were noted to have seizures by strict clinical classification. Of the 90 children, 27% of survivors had epilepsy, 25% had cerebral palsy, 20% had mental retardation, and 27% had a learning disorder. Poor prognosis was associated with severe encephalopathy, complicated IVH, infections in preterm neonates, abnormal interictal EEG, cerebral dysgenesis, and the use of multiple drugs to treat the seizures. Attempts have been made to develop a scoring system to predict outcomes since the 1980s. Recently, by scoring for birthweight, Apgar score at 1 minute, neurologic examination at seizure onset, head ultrasound, efficacy of anticonvulsant therapy, and presence of neonatal status epilepticus, a composite score was computed. The score ranged from 0 to 12 and a cutoff score of ≥4 provided greatest sensitivity and specificity for predicting neurodevelopmental outcome at 2 years. A simple scoring system used numerically scored and visually graded (independently) analysis of the EEG background. Higher score correlated with increasing incidence of mortality, neurodevelopmental impairment, cerebral palsy, vision and hearing impairment, and epilepsy.

Selected References

Blume HK, Garrison MM, Christakis DA. Neonatal seizures: treatment and treatment variability in 31 United States pediatric hospitals. *J Child Neurol.* 2009;24(2):148–154.

Gilman JT, Gal P, Duchowny MS, Weaver RL, Ransom JL. Rapid sequential phenobarbital treatment of neonatal seizures. *Pediatrics.* 1989;83:674.

Glass HC, Pham TN, Danielsen B, Towner D, Glidden D, Wu YW. Antenatal and intrapartum risk factors for seizures in term newborns: a population-based study, California 1998–2002. *J Pediatr.* 2009;154(1):24–28.

Nagarajan L, Palumbo L, Ghosh S. Neurodevelopmental outcomes in neonates with seizures: a numerical score of background encephalography to help prognosticate. *J Child Neurol.* 2010;25(8):961–968.

Pisani F, Sisti L, Seri S. A scoring system for early prognostic assessment after neonatal seizures. *Pediatrics* 2009;124(4):e580–e587.

Riviello JJ. Pharmacology review: drug therapy for neonatal seizures: part 2. *NeoReviews.* 2004;5:e262–e268.

Ronen GM, Buckley D, Penney S, Streiner DL. Long-term prognosis in children with neonatal seizures: a population-based study. *Neurology.* 2007;69(19):1812–1813.

Seshia SS, Huntsman RJ, Lowry NJ, Seshia M, Yager JY, Sankaran K. Neonatal seizures: diagnosis and management. *Zhongguo Dang Dai Er Ke Za Zhi.* 2011;13(2):81–100 (*Chin J Contemp Pediatr*).

Sutsko RP, Braziuniene I, Saslow JG, et al. Intractable neonatal seizures: an unusual presentation of congenital hypothyroidism. *J Pediatr Endocrinol Metab.* 2009;22(10):961–963.

Volpe JJ. Neonatal seizures. *Neurology of the Newborn.* 4th ed. Philadelphia, PA:WB Saunders Co; 2001:178–214.

Volpe JJ. *Neurology of the Newborn.* 5th ed. Philadelphia, PA: Saunders Elsevier; 2008.

Wusthoff CJ, Dlugos DJ, Gutierrez-Colina A, et al. Electrographic seizures during therapeutic hypothermia for neonatal hypoxic-ischemic encephalopathy. *J Child Neurol.* 2011;26(6):724–728.

130 Sepsis

I. **Definition.** Neonatal sepsis is a clinical syndrome of systemic illness accompanied by bacteremia occurring in the first month of life.

II. **Incidence.** The overall incidence of primary sepsis is 1–5 per 1000 live births. The incidence is much higher for very low birthweight (VLBW) infants (birthweight <1500 g), with early-onset sepsis rate of 2% and late-onset nosocomial sepsis rate of 36% according to data from the National Institute of Child Health and Human Development Neonatal Research Network (NICHD-NRN). The mortality rate is high (13–25%); higher rates are seen in premature infants and in those with early fulminant disease.

III. **Pathophysiology.** Neonatal sepsis can be classified into 2 relatively distinct syndromes based on the age of presentation: early-onset and late-onset sepsis.

A. **Early-onset sepsis (EOS).** Presents in the first 3–5 days of life and is usually a multisystem fulminant illness with prominent respiratory symptoms. Typically, the infant has acquired the organism during the antepartum or intrapartum period from the maternal genital tract. Several infectious agents, notably treponemes, viruses, *Listeria*, and probably *Candida*, can be acquired transplacentally via hematogenous routes. Acquisition of other organisms is associated with the birth process. With rupture of membranes, vaginal flora or various bacterial pathogens may ascend to reach the amniotic fluid and the fetus. Chorioamnionitis develops, leading to fetal colonization and infection. Aspiration of infected amniotic fluid by the fetus or neonate may play a role in the resultant respiratory symptoms. Finally, the infant may be exposed to vaginal flora as it passes through the birth canal. The primary sites of colonization tend to be the skin, nasopharynx, oropharynx, conjunctiva, and umbilical cord. Trauma to these mucosal surfaces may lead to infection. Early-onset disease is characterized by a sudden onset and fulminant course that can progress rapidly to septic shock and death.

B. **Late-onset sepsis (LOS).** May occur as early as 5 days of age. LOS is usually more insidious but it can be fulminant at times. It is usually not associated with early obstetric complications. In addition to bacteremia, these infants may have an identifiable focus, most often meningitis in addition to sepsis. Bacteria responsible for LOS and meningitis include those acquired after birth from the maternal genital tract (vertical transmission) as well as organisms acquired after birth from human contact or from contaminated equipment/environment (nosocomial). Therefore, horizontal transmission appears to play a significant role in late-onset disease. The reasons for the delay in development of clinical illness, the predilection for central nervous system (CNS) disease, and the less severe systemic and cardiorespiratory symptoms are unclear. Transplacental transfer of maternal antibodies to the mother's own vaginal flora may play a role in determining which exposed infants become infected, especially in the case of group B streptococcal infections. In case of nosocomial spread, the pathogenesis is related to the underlying illness and debilitation of the infant, the flora in the neonatal intensive care (NICU) environment, and invasive monitoring and other techniques used in the NICU. Breaks in the natural barrier function of the skin and intestine allow opportunistic organisms to invade and overwhelm the neonate. Infants, especially the premature, have an increased susceptibility to infection because of underlying illnesses and immature immune defenses that are less efficient at localizing and clearing bacterial invasion.

C. **Microbiology.** The principal pathogens involved in EOS have tended to change with time. Before 1965, *Staphylococcus aureus* and *Escherichia coli* used to be the most commonly isolated organisms. In the late 1960s, group B *Streptococcus* (GBS) emerged as the most common microorganism. Currently, most centers continue to report GBS as the most common microorganism, even though the incidence has decreased considerably after the widespread adoption of universal antenatal screening for GBS colonization at 35–37 weeks' gestation and intrapartum prophylaxis with penicillin or ampicillin for colonized women. The incidence of EOS secondary to GBS decreased from 1.7 per 1000 live births in 1993 to 0.28 per 1000 in 2008 (>80% reduction). The second most common bacteria are gram-negative enteric organisms, especially *E. coli*. An increase in the incidence of *E. coli* has been noted in EOS in VLBW infants to the extent that *E. coli* is currently the predominant microorganism in this group of patients. This increase was noted in late 1990s and early 2000s and appears to be stabilizing. Recent data from NICHD-NRN suggest that widespread use of intrapartum antibiotic prophylaxis to reduce vertical transmission of GBS has not resulted in a further increase in non-GBS EOS among the larger cohort of infants of all birthweights or among VLBW infants beyond what was noted previously. GBS and *E. coli* account for two-thirds of all cases of EOS. Other pathogens causing EOS include *Listeria monocytogenes, Staphylococcus,* enterococci, anaerobes, *Haemophilus influenzae,* and *Streptococcus pneumoniae.* The pathogens that cause LOS or nosocomial sepsis tend to vary in each nursery; however, coagulase-negative staphylococci (CoNS), especially *Staphylococcus epidermidis,* are the most predominant. Other microorganisms causing LOS include Gram-negative rods (including *Pseudomonas, Klebsiella, Serratia,* and *Proteus*), *S. aureus,* GBS, and fungal microorganisms.

IV. **Risk factors**

A. **Prematurity and low birthweight.** Prematurity (<37 weeks' gestation) is the single most significant factor correlated with sepsis. The risk increases in proportion to the decrease in birthweight and gestational age.

B. **Rupture of membranes (ROM) ≥18 hours.** The risk for proven sepsis increases 10-fold.

C. **Maternal peripartum infection.** Infections such as **chorioamnionitis,** urinary tract infection (UTI) especially **GBS bacteriuria, rectovaginal colonization with GBS,** and perineal colonization with *E. coli* are well-recognized risk factors for EOS. **Chorioamnionitis** is a major risk factor for neonatal sepsis. The essential criterion for the clinical diagnosis of chorioamnionitis is **maternal fever.** Other criteria are relatively insensitive. When defining intra-amniotic infection (chorioamnionitis) for clinical research studies, the diagnosis is typically based on the presence of maternal fever of >38°C (100.4°F) and at least 2 of the following criteria: **maternal leukocytosis** (>15,000 cells/mm³), **maternal tachycardia** (>100 beats/min), **fetal tachycardia** (>160 beats/min), **uterine tenderness,** and/or **foul odor of the amniotic fluid.**

D. **Previous delivery of a neonate with GBS disease.**

E. **Fetal and intrapartum distress.** Infants who had intrapartum fetal tachycardia, meconium-stained amniotic fluid, were born by traumatic delivery, or were severely depressed at birth and required intubation and resuscitation are either infected in utero or at significant risk for EOS.

F. **Multiple gestation.**

G. **Invasive procedures.** Invasive monitoring (fetal scalp electrodes), intravascular catheterization (percutaneously inserted central catheters [PICC] and umbilical catheters), and respiratory (endotracheal intubation) or metabolic support (total parenteral nutrition) are important risk factors for LOS. Continuous positive airway pressure has been associated with an increased risk of Gram-negative infections in VLBW infants.

H. **Metabolic factors.** Hypoxia, acidosis, inherited metabolic disorders (eg, galactosemia predisposing to *E. coli* sepsis), and immune defects (eg, asplenia) are factors that predispose as well as increase the severity of sepsis.

I. **Other factors.** Males are 4 times more affected than females, and the possibility of a sex-linked genetic basis for host susceptibility is postulated. Bottle-feeding (as opposed to breast-feeding) may predispose to infection. Persons of black African descent have been found to have an independent risk factor for GBS sepsis (both EOS and LOS). Reasons for the disproportionately high disease burden among black populations cannot be fully explained by prematurity or socioeconomic status. NICU staff and family members are often vectors for the spread of microorganisms, primarily as a result of improper or lack of hand washing.

V. **Clinical presentation.** Because the initial diagnosis of sepsis is, by necessity, a clinical one, it is crucial to begin treatment before the results of cultures are available. Clinical signs and symptoms of sepsis are nonspecific, and the differential diagnosis is broad. Some signs are subtle or insidious, and therefore a high index of suspicion is required to identify and evaluate infected neonates. Clinical signs and symptoms most often mentioned include the following:

A. **Temperature irregularity.** Hypothermia is more common than fever as a presenting sign for bacterial sepsis in premature infants. Hyperthermia is more common in full-term infants beyond the first 24 hours of life and if viral agents (eg, herpes) are involved.

B. **Change in behavior.** Lethargy, irritability, or change in tone.

C. **Skin.** Poor peripheral perfusion, cyanosis, mottling, pallor, petechiae, rashes, sclerema, or jaundice singularly or in combinations are known signs of sepsis.

D. **Feeding problems.** Feeding intolerance, vomiting, diarrhea, or abdominal distention with or without visible bowel loops.

E. **Cardiopulmonary.** Tachypnea, respiratory distress (grunting, flaring, and retractions), apnea within the first 24 hours of birth or of new onset (especially after 1 week of age), tachycardia, and hypotension singularly or in combinations should suggest sepsis. Hypotension tends to be a late sign.

Reduced variability and transient decelerations in heart rate (HR) may be present in the hours to days before diagnosis of LOS. These **abnormal HR characteristics (HRC)** in response to systemic infection and inflammation have been characterized mathematically, and the resulting **HRC index** can be computed in real time and displayed continuously at the bedside. Preliminary studies suggest that monitoring the HRC index in high-risk premature infants may result in improved outcomes and decreased mortality (through early warning with diagnosing early sepsis and prompt treatment with antibiotics).

F. **Metabolic.** Metabolic findings include hypoglycemia, hyperglycemia, or metabolic acidosis.

G. **Focal infections.** These may precede or accompany LOS. Look for cellulitis, impetigo, soft tissue abscesses, omphalitis, conjunctivitis, otitis media, meningitis, or osteomyelitis.

VI. **Diagnosis**

A. **Differential diagnosis.** Because signs and symptoms of neonatal sepsis are nonspecific, noninfectious etiologies need to be considered. If the infant is presenting with respiratory symptoms, respiratory distress syndrome, transient tachypnea of the newborn, meconium aspiration, and aspiration pneumonia are considered. If the infant is showing CNS symptoms, then intracranial hemorrhage, drug withdrawal, and inborn errors of metabolism are considered. Patients with feeding intolerance and bloody stool may have necrotizing enterocolitis, gastrointestinal perforation, or obstruction. Some nonbacterial infections such as disseminated herpes simplex virus can be indistinguishable from bacterial sepsis and should be considered in the differential diagnosis, especially if the infant has fever.

B. Laboratory studies

1. Cultures. Blood and other normally sterile body fluids (urine, spinal fluid, and tracheal aspirate) should be obtained for culture. Body surface cultures are not recommended.

   a. Blood cultures. Computer-assisted automated blood culture systems identify up to 94–96% of all microorganisms by 48 hours of incubation. Results may vary because of a number of factors, including maternal antibiotics administered before birth, organisms that are difficult to grow and isolate (ie, anaerobes), and sampling error with small sample volumes (the minimum volume for blood culture is 1 mL). One blood culture is typically obtained in cases of EOS and 2 blood cultures (1 from PICC and 1 peripheral) in cases of LOS. In many clinical situations, infants are treated for "presumed" sepsis despite negative cultures, with apparent clinical benefit (see Chapter 73). Positive bacterial cultures confirm the diagnosis of sepsis.

   b. Lumbar puncture (LP). Some *controversy* currently exists regarding whether an LP is needed in asymptomatic newborns being worked up for early-onset presumptive sepsis. Many institutions perform LPs only on infants who are clinically ill, infants who have CNS symptoms such as apnea or seizures, or in cases of documented positive blood cultures or if the decision is made to extend antibiotics beyond 48–72 hours for presumptive clinical sepsis. This practice is consistent with a recent report from the American Academy of Pediatrics (AAP) Committee on the Fetus and the Newborn that LP should be part of the routine evaluation for LOS. Meningitis is likely to happen without sepsis in VLBW infants, and therefore LP should be considered strongly in this group.

   c. Urine cultures. In neonates <24 hours of age, a sterile urine specimen is not necessary, given that the occurrence of UTIs is exceedingly rare in this age group. If indicated, urine for culture must be obtained by either a suprapubic tap (see Chapter 25) or catheterized specimen (see Chapter 26). Bag urine samples should not be used to diagnose UTI.

   d. Tracheal cultures. Should be obtained in intubated neonates with a clinical picture suggestive of pneumonia; if the mother developed chorioamnionitis with overwhelming EOS of the newborn; or when the quality and volume of tracheal secretions change substantially. Tracheal aspirates done after several days of intubation are of limited value.

2. Gram stain of various fluids. Gram staining is especially helpful for the study of cerebrospinal fluid (CSF). Gram-stained smears and cultures of amniotic fluid are helpful in diagnosing chorioamnionitis. A Gram stain of fluid obtained from the endotracheal tube can alert one of an inflammatory process.

3. Other laboratory tests

   a. Complete blood count with differential. These values alone are very nonspecific. There are reference values for total white blood cell (WBC) count, and absolute neutrophil counts are a function of postnatal age in hours (see Chapter 73, particularly Tables 73–1 and 73–2). Neutropenia may be a significant finding with an ominous prognosis when associated with sepsis. However, neutropenia has been described commonly as an incidental finding in otherwise healthy growing VLBW infants. The presence of immature forms is more specific but still rather insensitive. Ratios of bands to segmented forms >0.3 and of bands to total polymorphonuclear cells >0.1 have good predictive value, if present. The diagnostic yield of WBC count improves when testing is done after 4 hours of age. A variety of conditions other than sepsis can alter neutrophil counts and ratios, including maternal hypertension and fever, neonatal asphyxia, maternal intrapartum oxytocin, hypoglycemia, stressful labor, meconium aspiration syndrome, pneumothorax, and even prolonged crying. Serial WBC counts obtained several hours apart may be helpful in establishing a trend.

    b. Decreased platelet count. This is usually a late sign and very nonspecific.

    c. Acute-phase reactants (APRs). A complex multifunctional group comprising complement components, coagulation proteins, protease inhibitors, C-reactive protein (CRP), and others that rise in concentration in the serum in response to inflammation. The inflammation may be secondary to infection, trauma, or other processes of cellular destruction. An elevated APR does not distinguish between infectious and noninfectious causes of inflammation. Except for CRP, most of APRs are not commercially available for routine testing.

        i. CRP is an APR that increases the most in the presence of inflammation caused by infection or tissue injury. The highest concentrations of CRP are reported in patients with bacterial infections, whereas moderate elevations typify chronic inflammatory conditions. Synthesis of acute-phase proteins by hepatocytes is modulated by cytokines. Interleukin-1β (IL-1β), IL-6, IL-8, and tumor necrosis factor (TNF) are the most important regulators of CRP synthesis. CRP secretion starts within 4–6 hours after the inflammatory stimulus and peaks at ~36–48 hours. The biologic half-life of CRP is 19 hours, with a 50% reduction daily after the acute-phase stimulus resolves. Serial CRP measurements demonstrate high sensitivity and negative predictive value but low specificity for infection. A single normal value cannot rule out infection because the sampling may have preceded the rise in CRP. Serial determinations, therefore, are recommended. CRP elevations in noninfected neonates have been seen with fetal hypoxia, respiratory distress syndrome (RDS), meconium aspiration, after trauma/surgery, and after immunizations. A false-positive rate of 8% has been found in healthy neonates. Nonetheless, CRP is a valuable adjunct in the diagnosis of sepsis (ruling it out when serial CRPs are low), monitoring the response to treatment as well as guiding duration of treatment.

        ii. Cytokines IL-6, IL-8, and TNF are produced primarily by activated monocytes and macrophages and are major mediators of the systemic response to infection. Studies have shown that combining cytokines with CRP may be better than using CRP alone. IL-6, IL-8, and procalcitonin may be better than CRP in the diagnosis and follow-up of neonatal sepsis secondary to **coagulase-negative staphylococci (CoNS).**

        iii. Procalcitonin (PCT) is a propeptide of calcitonin that increases markedly with sepsis. It may not be useful to screen for early sepsis because it normally rises in the first 48 hours of life. However, PCT appears to be a sensitive marker for LOS and may be superior to CRP. PCT became commercially available recently.

        iv. Neutrophil surface antigen CD11 and CD64 are promising markers of early infection that correlate well with CRP but peak earlier.

C. Imaging and other studies

    1. Chest radiograph. A chest radiograph should be obtained in cases with respiratory symptoms, although it is often impossible to distinguish GBS or *Listeria* pneumonia from uncomplicated RDS. One distinguishing feature is the presence of pleural effusion, which occurs in 67% of cases of pneumonia.

2. **Urinary tract imaging.** Imaging with renal ultrasound examination, renal scan, and possibly voiding cystourethrogram should be considered when UTI accompanies sepsis.

D. **Other studies.** Examination of the placenta and fetal membranes may disclose evidence of chorioamnionitis and thus an increased potential for neonatal infection.

VII. **Management.** Isolation precautions for all infectious diseases, including maternal and neonatal precautions, breast-feeding, and visiting issues, can be found in Appendix F. (See Chapter 73 for AAP recommendations for management of neonates with suspected or proven early-onset bacterial sepsis.)

A. **Prevention**

1. **GBS prophylaxis.** Because of the widespread use of intrapartum antibiotic prophylaxis, EOS secondary to GBS has been reduced by 80%. Approximately 10–30% of pregnant women are colonized with GBS in the vaginal or rectal area. Consensus guidelines regarding management of GBS were published by the Centers for Disease Control and Prevention in 1996 and were later revised in 2002 and in 2010. These guidelines are supported by the AAP and the American College of Obstetricians and Gynecologists. The guidelines recommended that all pregnant women should be screened at 35–37 weeks' gestation for vaginal and rectal GBS colonization. At the time of labor or rupture of membranes, intrapartum chemoprophylaxis should be given to all pregnant women identified as GBS carriers. Women with GBS isolated from the urine (>10,000 colony-forming U/mL) during their current pregnancy should receive intrapartum chemoprophylaxis because such women usually are heavily colonized with GBS and are at increased risk of delivering an infant with EOS. Women who have previously given birth to an infant with invasive GBS disease should receive intrapartum chemoprophylaxis as well. Penicillin is the drug of choice, but ampicillin is an acceptable alternative. Cefazolin, and less commonly vancomycin, may be used for penicillin-allergic women. The risk-based approach is no longer acceptable except for circumstances in which screening results are not available before labor and delivery. In these circumstances, intrapartum antibiotic prophylaxis should be given to women <37 weeks' gestation, those with ROM ≥18 hours, and women who have a fever ≥38° C (100.4° F). The new guidelines recognize the availability of commercial nucleic acid amplification tests (NAAT) such as polymerase chain reaction for rapid detection of GBS. If available, NAAT intrapartum rectovaginal testing can be performed on women with unknown GBS status and no intrapartum GBS risk factors. Antibiotic prophylaxis should be given if the NAAT testing returns positive or an intrapartum risk factor develops regardless of NAAT results. In addition, the guidelines specifically addressed threatened preterm labor (PTL) and preterm premature rupture of membranes (pPROM) with detailed algorithms. Briefly, women with threatened PTL or pPROM should be screened for GBS colonization on admission unless a GBS culture was obtained within the preceding 5 weeks. In both of these situations, women should receive GBS prophylaxis (typically for 48 hours) unless the screening results are negative. The new recommendations also provided clarification on optimal GBS culturing methods. Finally, the guidelines provided specific recommendations for management of neonates born to mothers who are GBS colonized, have risk factors for sepsis, or were exposed to chorioamnionitis (Figure 130–1).

2. **Prevention of nosocomial sepsis in premature infants in NICU.** A subset of nosocomial sepsis is central line–associated bloodstream infections (CLABSIs). Although primary prevention of CLABSI relies on minimizing the use of central lines, novel technologies such as antiseptic and antimicrobial impregnated catheters in addition to meticulous care during PICC insertion and maintenance are key factors in preventing CLABSIs. **Hand hygiene** is the single most important strategy for avoiding transmission of contagions in the NICU. Fresh

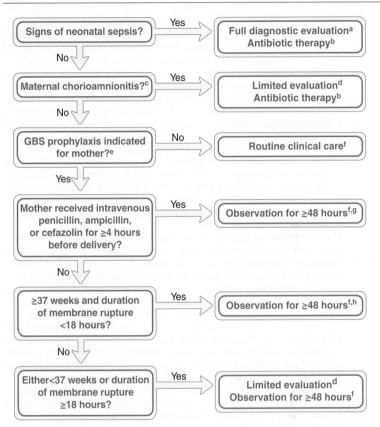

a Full diagnostic evaluation includes a blood culture, a complete blood count (CBC) including white blood cell differential and platelet counts, chest radiograph (if respiratory abnormalities are present), and lumbar puncture (if patient is stable enough to tolerate procedure and sepsis is suspected).

b Antibiotic therapy should be directed toward the most common causes of neonatal sepsis, including intravenous ampicillin for GBS and coverage for other organisms (including *Escherichia coli* and other gram-negative pathogens) and should take into account local antibiotic resistance patterns.

c Consultation with obstetric providers is important to determine the level of clinical suspicion for chorioamnionitis. Chorioamnionitis is diagnosed clinically and some of the signs are nonspecific.

d Limited evaluation includes blood culture (at birth) and CBC with differential and platelets (at birth and/or at 6–12 hours of life).

e Refer to Table 3 in *MMWR* Nov 19, 2010, Vol 59, No RR-10.

f If signs of sepsis develop, a full diagnostic evaluation should be conducted and antibiotic therapy initiated.

g If ≥37 weeks' gestation, observation may occur at home after 24 hours if other discharge criteria have been met, access to medical care is readily available, and a person who is able to comply fully with instructions for home observation will be present. If any of these conditions is not met, the infant should be observed in the hospital for at least 48 hours and until discharge criteria are achieved.

h Some experts recommend a CBC with differential and platelets at age 6–12 hours.

FIGURE 130–1. Centers for Disease Control and Prevention algorithm for secondary prevention of early-onset group B *Streptococcus* (GBS) sepsis among newborns including exposure to chorioamnionitis and other risk factors. (*Reproduced from Centers for Disease Control and Prevention. Prevention of perinatal group B streptococcal disease: revised guidelines from CDC, 2010. MMWR. 2010;59:22.*)

maternal milk contains a number of substances responsible for innate immune and humoral responses against pathogens; therefore, promotion of **breast-feeding** is a key step in the prevention of NICU infections. Medical stewardship of antibiotics, steroids, and H_2 blockers is mandatory; indiscriminate use of these agents has been associated with increased nosocomial sepsis. Enhancement of the enteric microbiome composition with the possible use of **probiotics** may restore gut immune function and help prevent necrotizing enterocolitis and sepsis. Use of bioactive substances with known anti-infective properties such as **lactoferrin** may be helpful. A recently published multicenter study conducted in Italy showed that oral bovine lactoferrin was beneficial in preventing LOS in VLBW infants during their stay in NICU, regardless of the type of nutrition. Finally, specific and targeted pharmacologic prophylactic interventions have been used with some success. For example, specific antifungal prophylaxis with fluconazole has been associated with 85% reduction in invasive fungal infection. However, the use of pagibaximab, a recombinant monoclonal antibody targeting staphylococcal species, does not appear to offer protection against gram-positive CLABSIs in NICU.

B. **Empiric antibiotic therapy.** Treatment is most often begun before a definite causative agent is identified. For EOS, it usually consists of **ampicillin** and **gentamicin**. This empirical regimen covers the most commonly encountered microorganism; namely GBS and *E. coli*, and has proved to be efficacious over the years. In nosocomial sepsis, the flora of the NICU must be considered; however, staphylococcal coverage with **vancomycin plus an aminoglycoside** such as gentamicin or amikacin is usually begun. Third-generation cephalosporins should be avoided as an empirical therapy for EOS or nosocomial sepsis because they are associated with increased risk for antibiotic resistance and invasive fungal infections. The empirical treatment for suspected LOS in a neonate admitted from the community is ampicillin and gentamicin; cefotaxime can be added only when there is a concern for meningitis. Dosages are presented in Chapter 148.

C. **Continuing therapy.** Based on culture and sensitivity results, clinical course, and other serial laboratory studies (eg, CRP). Monitoring for antibiotic toxicity is important, as well as monitoring levels of aminoglycosides and vancomycin. When GBS is documented as the causative agent, penicillin G is the drug of choice; however, an aminoglycoside is often added because of documented synergism in vitro.

D. **Complications and supportive therapy**
1. **Respiratory.** Ensure adequate oxygenation with blood gas monitoring, and initiate oxygen therapy or ventilator support if needed.
2. **Cardiovascular.** Support blood pressure and perfusion to prevent shock. Use volume expanders such as normal saline, and monitor the intake and output of fluids. Inotropes such as dopamine or dobutamine may be needed (see Chapter 65).
3. **Hematologic**
   a. **Disseminated intravascular coagulation (DIC).** With DIC, one may observe generalized bleeding at puncture sites, the gastrointestinal tract, or CNS. In the skin, large-vessel thrombosis may cause gangrene. Laboratory parameters consistent with DIC include thrombocytopenia, increased prothrombin time, and increased partial thromboplastin time. There is an increase in fibrin split products or D-dimers. Treatment options include fresh-frozen plasma, 10 mL/kg; vitamin K (see Chapter 148); platelet infusion; and possible exchange transfusion (see Chapter 30).
   b. **Neutropenia.** Multiple factors contribute to the increased susceptibility of neonates to infection, including developmental quantitative and qualitative neutrophil defects. Colony-stimulating factors (CSFs) comprise a group of cytokines that are central to the hematopoiesis of blood cells, as well as to the maintenance of homeostasis and overall immune competence.

Granulocyte CSF (G-CSF) and granulocyte-macrophage-CSF (GM-CSF) have been used in neonates with established sepsis associated with neutropenia, in neutropenic infants without sepsis, and prophylactically in neonates at risk for sepsis. Limited data suggest that CSFs administration may reduce mortality when systemic infection is accompanied by severe neutropenia. A recent randomized control trial that enrolled 280 small for gestational age extremely preterm infants and used early GM-CSF prophylactically showed no reduction in sepsis or improvement in survival in the treated group. Intravenous immunoglobulin does not appear useful either as a prophylactic or as an adjunct to antibiotic therapy in serious neonatal infection.

4. **Central nervous system.** Implement seizure control measures using phenobarbital, and monitor for the syndrome of inappropriate antidiuretic hormone (decreased urine output, hyponatremia, decreased serum osmolarity, and increased urine specific gravity and osmolarity).

5. **Metabolic.** Monitor for and treat hypoglycemia or hyperglycemia. Metabolic acidosis may accompany sepsis and is treated with bicarbonate and fluid replacement.

E. **Future developments.** Intensive research continues in the development of vaccines (especially for GBS) as well as synthetic monoclonal antibodies to the specific pathogens causing neonatal sepsis (ie, antistaphylococcal antibodies). Research is also ongoing into blocking some of the body's own inflammatory mediators that result in significant tissue injury, including endotoxin inhibitors, cytokine inhibitors, nitric oxide synthetase inhibitors, and neutrophil adhesion inhibitors. Finally, recent trials are showing probiotics and lactoferrin to be promising agents in the prevention of LOS and necrotizing enterocolitis.

VIII. **Prognosis.** With early diagnosis and treatment, most infants will recover and not have any long-term problems. However, the mortality rate is still significant. For early-onset disease, the mortality rate is 5–10%, and for late-onset disease, the rate is 2–6%. For VLBW infants with early-onset disease, the fatality rate is higher (16% based on recent report from NICHD NRN). *E. coli* sepsis is associated with higher mortality compared with GBS.

Selected References

Arnon S, Litmanovitz I. Diagnostic tests in neonatal sepsis. *Curr Opin Infect Dis.* 2008;21: 223–227.

Auriti C, Fiscarelli E, Ronchetti MP, et al. Procalcitonin in detecting neonatal nosocomial sepsis. *Arch Dis Child Fetal Neonatal Ed.* 2012;97:F368–F370.

Benitz WE. Adjunct laboratory tests in the diagnosis of early-onset neonatal sepsis. *Clin Perinatol.* 2010;37:421–438.

Carr R, Brocklehurst P, Doré CJ, Modi N. Granulocyte-macrophage colony stimulating factor administered as prophylaxis for reduction of sepsis in extremely preterm, small for gestational age neonates (the PROGRAMS trial): a single-blind, multicentre, randomised controlled trial. *Lancet.* 2009;373:226–233.

Centers for Disease Control and Prevention. Prevention of perinatal group B streptococcal disease: revised guidelines from CDC, 2010. *MMWR Recomm Rep.* 2010;59:1–36.

Cohen-Wolkowiez M, Benjamin DK Jr, Capparelli E. Immunotherapy in neonatal sepsis: advances in treatment and prophylaxis. *Curr Opin Pediatr.* 2009;21:177–181.

Cohen-Wolkowiez M, Moran C, Benjamin DK, et al. Early and late onset sepsis in late preterm infants. *Pediatr Infect Dis J.* 2009;28:1052–1056.

Dilli D, Oğuz SS, Dilmen U, Köker MY, Kızılgün M. Predictive values of neutrophil CD64 expression compared with interleukin-6 and C-reactive protein in early diagnosis of neonatal sepsis. *J Clin Lab Anal.* 2010;24:363–370.

Fairchild KD, O'Shea TM. Heart rate characteristics: physiomarkers for detection of late-onset neonatal sepsis. *Clin Perinatol.* 2010;37:581–598.

Kuhn P, Dheu C, Bolender C, et al. Incidence and distribution of pathogens in early-onset neonatal sepsis in the era of antenatal antibiotics. *Paediatr Perinat Epidemiol.* 2010;24: 479–487.

Manzoni P, Mostert M, Stronati M. Lactoferrin for prevention of neonatal infections. *Curr Opin Infect Dis.* 2011;24:177–182.

Manzoni P, Rizzollo S, Decembrino L, et al. Recent advances in prevention of sepsis in the premature neonates in NICU. *Early Hum Dev.* 2011;87:S31–S33.

Moorman JR, Carlo WA, Kattwinkel J, et al. Mortality reduction by heart rate characteristic monitoring in very low birth weight neonates: a randomized trial. *J Pediatr.* 2011;159:900–906.e1.

Muller-Pebody B, Johnson AP, Heath PT, et al. Empirical treatment of neonatal sepsis: are the current guidelines adequate. *Arch Dis Child Fetal Neonatal Ed.* 2011;96:F4–F8.

Newman TB, Puopolo KM, Wi S, Draper D, Escobar GJ. Interpreting complete blood counts soon after birth in newborns at risk for sepsis. *Pediatrics.* 2010;126:903–909.

Nizet V, Klein JO. Bacterial sepsis and meningitis. In: Remington JS, Klein JO, Wilson CB, Nizet V, Maldonado Y, eds. *Infectious Diseases of the Fetus and Newborn Infant.* 7th ed. Philadelphia, PA: Elsevier Saunders; 2011:222–275.

Polin RA; the Committee on Fetus and Newborn. Management of neonates with suspected or proven early-onset bacterial sepsis. *Pediatrics.* 2012;129:1006–1015.

Stoll BJ, Hansen NI, Bell EF, et al. Neonatal outcomes of extremely preterm infants from the NICHD Neonatal Research Network. *Pediatrics.* 2010;126:443–456.

Stoll BJ, Hansen NI, Sánchez PJ, et al. Early onset neonatal sepsis: the burden of group B streptococcal and E. coli disease continues. *Pediatrics.* 2011;127:817–826.

van den Hoogen A, Gerards LJ, Verboon-Maciolek MA, Fleer A, Krediet TG. Long-term trends in the epidemiology of neonatal sepsis and antibiotic susceptibility of causative agents. *Neonatology.* 2010;97:22–28.

Vouloumanou EK, Plessa E, Karageorgopoulos DE, Mantadakis E, Falagas ME. Serum procalcitonin as a diagnostic marker for neonatal sepsis: a systematic review and meta-analysis. *Intensive Care Med.* 2011;37:747–762.

Weinberg GA, D'Angio CT. Laboratory aids for diagnosis of neonatal sepsis. In: Remington JS, Klein JO, Wilson CB, Nizet V, Maldonado Y, eds. *Infectious Diseases of the Fetus and Newborn Infant.* Philadelphia, PA: Elsevier Saunders; 2011:1144–1160.

131 Spontaneous Intestinal Perforation

I. **Definition.** A **spontaneous intestinal perforation (SIP)** is a single intestinal perforation typically involving the antimesenteric border of distal ileum, which usually occurs without a defined prodrome in extremely premature infants in the first 1–2 weeks of life. These infants usually have not been fed (or have received minimum feeds). At the area of perforation, focal hemorrhagic necrosis with well-defined margins is observed in contrast to ischemic and coagulative necrosis seen in necrotizing enterocolitis (NEC). The bowel proximal and distal to the perforation appears normal.

II. **Incidence.** Five percent in extremely low birthweight infants.

III. **Risk factors.** Prematurity, maternal chorioamnionitis, outborn status (requiring transport to the neonatal intensive care unit [NICU]), and male gender have been linked with occurrence of SIP. Early administration of glucocorticoids (both dexamethasone and hydrocortisone) has been associated with development of SIP. Similarly, early use of indomethacin (first 3 days) has been associated with SIP. The risk is greater when there is combined exposure to indomethacin and either elevated endogenous cortisol levels or administration of exogenous glucocorticoids in the first 3 days of life.

IV. **Pathogenesis.** SIP histopathology is associated with robust mucosa, with or without submucosal hemorrhage, and segmental/focal necrosis or absence of muscularis externa. These findings are not consistent with an ischemic insult. While some cases of SIP (especially in larger infants) can be associated with congenital deficits in the muscularis layer of the bowel, theories have been developed for the unique association of SIP with perinatal stress and postnatal early steroids and indomethacin exposure. The following sequence of events has been proposed: Steroids promote mucosal growth at the expense of bowel wall integrity with thinning of the submucosal layer. Indomethacin, in combination with steroids, causes a transient ileus due to depletion of nitric oxide synthase. Swallowing of air and return of bowel motility at about 7 days' age leads to increased intraluminal pressure in the bowel leading to bowel perforation.

V. **Presentation.** These infants usually present at **about 7–10 days of life** (range of 0–15 days). They have not been fed or are receiving minimal feeds and present with sudden deterioration with abdominal distension, bluish discoloration over abdomen, hypotension, and metabolic acidosis.

VI. **Diagnosis.** SIP is suspected when low birthweight infants present with the symptoms and signs described in Section V.

    A. **Clinical diagnosis.** This is based on sudden presentation with abdominal distension and bluish discoloration of abdominal wall, often associated with hypotension and clinical deterioration. Three features are helpful in distinguishing SIP from NEC with perforation:

      1. **Early presentation** usually in the first week of life

      2. **Physical findings** of abdominal distension and bluish discoloration of abdominal wall, occasionally extending to the groin and to the scrotum in male infants

      3. **Free air with absence of pneumatosis or portal venous gas** on abdominal radiograph

    B. **Laboratory studies**

      1. **Complete blood count (CBC) with differential.** May have elevated or low white blood cell count. May also have low platelet count. Elevated percentage of bands may be present.

      2. **Disseminated intravascular coagulation (DIC) panel.** Prothrombin time (PT), partial thromboplastin time (PTT), fibrinogen degradation products, and fibrinogen level need to be corrected if abnormal and infant needs surgical intervention.

      3. **Blood culture.** Candida and *Staphylococcus epidermidis* have been associated with SIP. These organisms colonize the gastrointestinal tract of unfed or minimally fed infants and may be released after the bowel perforation.

      4. **Electrolyte panel.**

      5. **Blood gas.** May have respiratory and/or metabolic acidosis.

    C. **Imaging and other studies**

      1. **Flat plate radiograph of the abdomen.** There may be a gasless abdomen or ileus. Free air may be seen.

      2. **Lateral decubitus and cross-table lateral studies of the abdomen.** Presence of free air is indicative of intestinal perforation.

VII. **Management**

    A. **Medical management**

1. **NPO** to allow gastrointestinal rest for 7–14 days. Total parenteral nutrition to provide basic nutritional needs.
2. **Gastric decompression** with large-bore orogastric tube (Replogle) at low intermittent or continuous suctioning.
3. **Close monitoring** of vital signs and abdominal circumference.
4. **Respiratory support.** Provide optimal respiratory support to maintain acceptable blood gas parameters.
5. **Circulatory support.** There may be third spacing of fluid, which requires effective volume replacement. Ionotropic support may be needed to maintain normal blood pressure.
6. **Strict fluid intake and output monitoring.** Try to maintain urine output of 1–3 cc/kg/h. Provide fluid replacement to correct third-space losses.
7. **Antibiotic therapy.** Treat with parenteral antibiotics for 7–10 days. Antibiotic regimen to cover pathogens including *S. epidermidis* and Candida, along with effective gram-positive, gram-negative, and anaerobic coverage. See doses in Chapter 148. Recommendations are to **start fluconazole** and one of the following antibiotic regimens:
   a. **Vancomycin, gentamicin, and clindamycin (or metronidazole)**
   b. **Vancomycin and Zosyn (piperacillin/tazobactam)**
   c. **Vancomycin, gentamicin, and Zosyn**

B. **Surgical management.** The optimal surgical management continues to be *controversial*. The prospective randomized trials by Moss et al and Rees et al included infants with SIP, and both studies showed similar clinical outcomes using the 2 surgical techniques. The concern, expressed more in the latter study, was the high number of infants requiring secondary laparotomies for failure of clinical improvement or latter development of bowel obstruction. Peritoneal drain is an attractive option for very unstable low birthweight infants since it can be done with relative ease at the bedside using local anesthesia. In one retrospective study, infants with elevated percent band count and hypotension requiring vasopressor support were at higher risk for secondary laparotomy, and this subset may thus benefit from primary laparotomy.

1. **Laparotomy with primary repair.** An abdominal incision is made and the bowel is explored. The segment of the bowel with perforation is resected and followed by end-to-end anastomosis of the bowel loops, or creation of an ileostomy and distal mucous fistula. Reanastomosis is usually undertaken after 8–12 weeks.
2. **Peritoneal drain placement.** After making a small transverse incision in the abdomen, a Penrose drain is placed. The drain is removed when there is no meconium or intestinal drainage. After return of bowel function, feeds are started or a contrast enema is done to ensure patency of the distal ileum and colon.
3. **Laparoscopy with mini-laparotomy.** This is a procedure recently described in which a diagnostic laparoscopy is done at the bedside. The diagnosis is confirmed and the site of perforation is localized. The affected bowel loop is then either exteriorized or primarily repaired.

VIII. **Prognosis.** Lower morbidity and mortality as well as neurodevelopmental impairment, as compared to intestinal perforation following necrotizing enterocolitis. Long-term survival of infants with SIP is 64–90% with improved medical and surgical care in the NICU. However, infants who develop SIP do have higher risk for periventricular leukomalacia and retinopathy of prematurity when compared with infants of similar gestational age without SIP.

IX. **Prevention.** Caution regarding early use of indocin (within first week of life), especially in infants who may be stressed with endogenously elevated cortisol levels. Avoid combined use of indocin and hydrocortisone in preterm infants. Close monitoring of extremely low birthweight infants for any signs of SIP.

Selected References

Ahmad I, Davis KF, Emil S, Uy C, Sills J. Risk factors for spontaneous intestinal perforation in extremely low birth weight infants. *Open Pediatr Med J.* 2008;2:11–15.

Attridge JT, Clark R, Walker MW, Gordon PV. New insights into spontaneous intestinal perforation using a national data set: (1) SIP is associated with early indomethacin exposure. *J Perinatol.* 2006;26:93–99.

Emil A, Davis K, Ahmad I, Strauss A. Factors associated with definitive peritoneal drainage for spontaneous intestinal perforation in extremely low birth weight neonates. *Eur J Pediatr Surg.* 2008;18(2):80–85.

Gordon PV. Understanding intestinal vulnerability to perforation in the extremely low birth weight infant. *Pediatr Res.* 2009;65:138–144.

Moss RL, Dimmitt RA, Barnhart DC, et al. Laparotomy versus peritoneal drainage for necrotizing enterocolitis and perforation. *N Engl J Med.* 2006;354:2225–2234.

Nah SA, Tan HL, Tamba RP, Aziz DA, Azzam N. Laparoscopic localization and microlaparotomy for focal isolated perforation in necrotizing enterocolitis: an alternative approach to a challenging problem. *J Pediatr Surg.* 2011;46:424–427.

Rees CM, Eaton S, Khoo AK, Kiely EM; Members of NET Trial Group, Pierro A. Peritoneal drainage does not stabilize low birth weight infants with perforated bowel: data from NET Trial. *J Pediatr Surg.* 2010;45:324–329.

Rees CM, Eaton S, Kiely EM, Wade AM, McHugh K, Pierro A. Peritoneal drainage or laparotomy for neonatal bowel perforation? A randomized controlled trial. *Ann Surg.* 2008;248:44–51.

132 Surgical Diseases of the Newborn: Abdominal Masses

GASTROINTESTINAL MASSES

Gastrointestinal masses are palpable abdominal masses that arise from the gastrointestinal tract are unusual and tend to be cystic, smooth walled, and mobile (depending on size). Causes include intestinal duplications and mesenteric cyst. Malignancy is rare.

HEPATIC MASSES

Hepatomegaly results from a variety of conditions. When physical examination and ultrasonography suggest a discrete mass, magnetic resonance imaging (MRI) or computed tomography (CT) should be performed. These studies are often diagnostic and aid in surgical planning. Lesions include the following:

I. Hepatic cysts. Congenital, solitary, nonparasitic liver cysts are rare in newborns.
II. Solid, benign tumors
   A. Hamartomas commonly have a cystic component. They are characterized by fine internal septations without calcifications. Surgical removal and cyst marsupialization are options.
   B. Hemangioendotheliomas are the most common benign, solid hepatic tumors in children. They are often asymptomatic, but may present with high output heart failure, anemia, thrombocytopenia, and coagulopathy (Kasabach-Merritt syndrome).

Hepatic transaminases and α-fetoprotein are usually normal. Diagnosis can be made by contrast CT scan or MRI. Typically, lesions begin to regress at ~1 year of age. Treatment is reserved for symptomatic lesions. Options include interferon, systemic corticosteroids, or vincristine. Surgical resection, embolization, and liver transplantation have been described for select lesions.

III. **Malignant tumors.** Hepatoblastoma is the most common liver cancer in neonates. Serum α-fetoprotein is usually elevated. Although surgical resection remains the key to achieving a cure, new chemotherapeutic protocols (cisplatin and doxorubicin) have improved the formerly dismal prognosis for infants with this tumor. Hepatic transplantation for unresectable lesions is associated with improved outcomes.

OVARIAN MASSES

A **simple ovarian cyst** is a frequent cause of a palpable abdominal mass in the female neonate. It presents as a relatively mobile, smooth-walled abdominal mass. It is not associated with cancer, and excision with preservation of any ovarian tissue is curative. Smaller lesions (≤5 cm) may be followed with serial ultrasounds over the first year of life as long as they regress. Larger lesions may benefit from percutaneous aspiration to decrease risk of ovarian torsion.

RENAL MASSES

(See also Chapters 136 and 137.) In most clinical series, the majority of neonatal abdominal masses arise from the kidney. They may be unilateral or bilateral, solid or cystic. After physical examination, ultrasonography should be obtained to define whether the mass is solid or cystic, to determine the presence or absence of normal kidneys, and to assess for other intraabdominal abnormalities. In selected instances, additional procedures such as renal scan, CT, retrograde pyelography, venography, and arteriography may be needed to define the pathology and plan appropriate therapy.

I. **Multicystic dysplastic kidney.** Most common renal cystic disease of the newborn. It is usually unilateral. Ultrasonography can define the nature of the disorder, and CT/nuclear renal scans are useful in assessing the remainder of the urinary system. Nephrectomy may be warranted.

II. **Hydronephrosis.** Urinary obstruction, depending on location, can cause unilateral or bilateral flank and abdominal masses. Treatment is by correction of the obstructing lesion or by proximal decompression. A kidney rendered nonfunctional by back pressure is usually best removed. Obstructive uropathy may be suitable for in utero intervention. Decompressing the obstructed fetal urinary system may improve the postnatal status and increase survival.

III. **Infantile polycystic kidney disease.** Also known as autosomal recessive polycystic kidney disease. This entity involves both kidneys and carries a grim prognosis.

IV. **Renal vein thrombosis.** Typically presents within the first 3 days of life with hematuria and ≥1 flank masses. Maternal diabetes and dehydration are risk factors. Conservative management is generally recommended.

V. **Wilms tumor.** See Chapter 136.

Selected References

Albanese CT, ed. Abdominal masses in the newborn. *Semin Pediatr Surg.* 2000;9:107.

Holcomb GW, Murphy JP, eds. *Ashcraft's Pediatric Surgery.* 5th ed. Philadelphia, PA: Saunders Elsevier; 2010.

Leclair MD, El-Ghoneimi A, Audry G, et al; French Pediatric Urology Study Group: The outcome of prenatally diagnosed renal tumors. *J Urol.* 2005;173:186–189.

133 Surgical Diseases of the Newborn: Abdominal Wall Defects

GASTROSCHISIS

I. **Definition.** A gastroschisis is a centrally located, full-thickness abdominal wall defect with 2 distinct anatomic features.

   A. **The extruded intestine is never covered by a protective sac.**

   B. **The umbilical cord is an intact structure** at the level of the abdominal skin, just to the left of the defect. Typically, the abdominal wall opening is 2–4 cm in diameter, and the solid organs (liver and spleen) reside in the peritoneal cavity.

II. **Pathophysiology.** Exposure to irritating amniotic fluid renders the intestines edematous, indurated, and foreshortened. Appropriate peristalsis and effective intestinal absorption are significantly delayed, usually by several weeks. Associated congenital anomalies are rare.

III. **Clinical presentation.** The infant is born with varying amounts of intestine extruding through the defect. An inflammatory peel is often found on the intestines. Up to 10% of neonates with gastroschisis will have an associated intestinal atresia.

IV. **Diagnosis.** Although readily apparent in most cases, gastroschisis must be differentiated from ruptured omphalocele. Increasingly, prenatal ultrasonography identifies gastroschisis.

V. **Management**

   A. **General considerations.** Infants with gastroschisis should be delivered at a neonatal center capable of providing definitive care. Both vaginal and cesarean deliveries have been shown to be safe and should be left to the obstetrician's discretion.

   B. **Specific measures**

      1. **Fluid resuscitation.** Venous access should be obtained promptly and aggressive fluid resuscitation should be initiated to combat the large evaporative fluid losses from the exposed bowel.

      2. **Temperature regulation.** Immediate attention should be directed toward maintenance of normal body temperature. The tremendous intestinal surface area exposed to the environment puts these infants at great risk for hypothermia.

      3. **Protective covering/position.** To prevent evaporative heat loss, the bowel should be covered with a moist, clean dressing. The abdomen should be wrapped in layers of cellophane, or the baby's abdomen, bowel, and legs should be placed in a plastic bag. The newborn should be laid on its side to prevent "kinking" the intestine's vascular pedicle while awaiting surgical intervention.

      4. **Nasogastric/orogastric decompression.** This is helpful.

      5. **Broad-spectrum antibiotic coverage.** Appropriate given the unavoidable contamination.

      6. **Total parenteral nutrition.** Delayed bowel function should be expected, and appropriate intravenous nutritional support must be provided.

      7. **Surgical correction.** As soon as the infant's condition permits, operative correction should be undertaken. In some babies, reduction of the herniated intestine and primary closure of the abdominal wall can be performed. Others require placing the intestines in a protective silo with subsequent staged reduction. Central venous access is usually part of the surgical intervention.

OMPHALOCELE

I. **Definition.** An omphalocele is a herniation of abdominal contents into the base of the umbilical cord. The gross appearance of omphalocele differs from that of gastroschisis in 2 important respects:

A. The malpositioned abdominal contents are covered by a protective membrane (unless antenatal rupture has occurred).

B. Elements of the umbilical stalk course individually over the sac and come together to form a normal-appearing umbilical cord.

II. **Associated anomalies.** Significant congenital anomalies occur in 50% of infants with omphalocele. Chromosomal abnormalities, cardiac defects, and congenital diaphragmatic hernia are common.

III. **Clinical presentation.** The size of the omphalocele varies. Typically, smaller defects contain intestine only. Large or giant omphaloceles (<5 cm) may also contain liver and spleen. The peritoneal cavity may be small because growth has proceeded without the solid organs in proper position.

IV. **Diagnosis.** The anomaly is usually apparent. A ruptured omphalocele may be confused with a gastroschisis, but infants with omphalocele do not possess an intact umbilical cord at the level of the abdominal wall. Careful studies to identify associated congenital anomalies should be performed.

V. **Management.** Reduction, even when staged over a lengthy period, may be difficult to achieve. Infants fall into 2 treatment groups:

A. **Ruptured sac.** A ruptured omphalocele resembles a gastroschisis. Care of the unprotected intestines is as described for gastroschisis (see previous text). Emergent surgical intervention is necessary.

B. **Intact sac.** An intact omphalocele is a less urgent surgical problem. The omphalocele sac conserves heat, prevents evaporative loss, allows effective peristalsis, and must be protected. Timing of surgery is determined by the size of the defect, gestational age, and presence of other congenital anomalies. Primary closure can be attempted in neonates with small defects. The application of various topical agents has been described to allow gradual epithelialization of the sac. Staged reduction with a compressive dressing to encourage growth of the abdominal cavity may be appropriate.

INGUINAL HERNIA AND HYDROCELE

I. **Definition.** Persistence of a patent processus vaginalis (related to testicular descent) is responsible for inguinal hernias and hydroceles in the neonate.

A. **Inguinal hernia.** The opening of the processus at the inguinal ring is large enough to allow abdominal viscera to extrude through the defect with increased intra-abdominal pressure.

B. **Hydrocele.** The patent processus is too narrow to permit egress of intestine. Peritoneal fluid leaves the abdominal cavity and accumulates in the processus vaginalis. Hydroceles are classified as communicating, if the processus remains patent, and noncommunicating, if the processus obliterates.

II. **Diagnosis**

A. **Inguinal hernias** tend to present as bulges at the pubic tubercle that continue along the inguinal canal. Less commonly, they descend into the scrotum.

B. **Hydroceles** are typically are found in the scrotum, transilluminate, and are not reducible.

III. **Management**

A. **Inguinal hernias** carry a 5–15% risk of incarceration during the first year of life. Usually, they are repaired surgically when the infant's general medical condition permits.

B. **Hydroceles** frequently resolve without intervention because the processus vaginalis continues to obliterate after birth. Hydroceles that persist beyond 6–12 months should be repaired.

UMBILICAL HERNIA

I. **Definition.** An umbilical hernia is a skin-covered fascial defect at the umbilicus that allows protrusion of intra-abdominal contents.

II. **Diagnosis.** Physical examination establishes the diagnosis.

III. **Management.** During infancy, surgical intervention for an umbilical hernia is rarely warranted. Complications such as incarceration and skin breakdown are exceedingly rare. The natural history is one of gradual closure of the umbilical fascial defect, often leading to complete resolution. Surgical correction should be considered if the defect persists after the second birthday.

Selected References

Holcomb III GW, Murphy JP, eds. *Ashcraft's Pediatric Surgery.* 5th ed. Philadelphia, PA: Elsevier Saunders; 2010.

Ledbetter DJ. Gastroschisis and omphalocele. *Surg Clin North Am.* 2006;86(2):249–260.

O'Neill JA, Grosfeld JL, Fonkalsrud EW, Coran AG, Caldamone AA, eds. *Principles of Pediatric Surgery.* 2nd ed. St. Louis, MO: Mosby; 2004.

Snyder CL. Current management of umbilical abnormalities and related anomalies. *Semin Pediatr Surg.* 2007;16(1):41–49.

134 Surgical Diseases of the Newborn: Alimentary Tract Obstruction

ESOPHAGEAL ATRESIA WITH TRACHEOESOPHAGEAL FISTULA

I. **Definition. Type C tracheoesophageal (TE) fistula** is the most common type of esophageal atresia (85%). The esophagus ends blindly ~10–12 cm from the nares, and the distal esophagus communicates with the posterior trachea (distal tracheoesophageal fistula [TEF]). **Type A "pure" esophageal atresia** implies esophageal atresia without TEF (10% of cases). It has a similar presentation without the distal gastrointestinal air.

II. **Pathophysiology.** Because of the esophageal obstruction, the infant is unable to handle secretions, with subsequent "excess salivation" and aspiration of pharyngeal contents. Communication between the tracheobronchial tree and the distal fistula allows the crying newborn to greatly distend the stomach with air. This impairment of diaphragmatic excursion can promote basilar atelectasis and respiratory distress. Additionally, the distal TEF permits reflux of gastric secretions directly into the tracheobronchial tree, causing chemical pneumonitis or pneumonia.

III. **Clinical presentation.** Pregnancy can be complicated by polyhydramnios. Typically, the newborn is unable to manage oral secretions and requires frequent suctioning. Attempted feedings result in prompt regurgitation, coughing, choking, and cyanosis.

IV. **Diagnosis.** A nasogastric tube cannot be passed beyond 10–12 cm from the nares. Chest radiograph shows the tube ending in the region of the thoracic inlet. The upper pouch can be better visualized by insufflating 20–30 mL of air into the tube as the radiograph is being taken. Air in the gastrointestinal tract confirms presence of a distal fistula. The radiograph should also be examined for skeletal anomalies, pulmonary infiltrates, cardiac size and shape, and abdominal bowel gas patterns. Appropriate evaluation for VATER/VACTERL association is necessary.

V. **Management**

A. **Preoperative treatment** should focus on protecting the lungs by evacuating the proximal esophageal pouch with an indwelling Replogle tube or frequent suctioning. Placing the baby in an upright (45-degree) position lessens the likelihood of reflux of gastric contents up the distal esophagus into the trachea. Broad-spectrum antibiotics should be administered. An echocardiogram should be obtained to assess for cardiac and aortic arch anomalies.

B. **Surgical therapy.** The steps and timing of surgical therapy must be individualized to the baby's anatomy. Some surgeons perform preliminary gastrostomy to decompress the stomach and provide additional protection against reflux. Single-stage TEF ligation and esophageal anastomosis via thoracotomy or thoracoscopy is the preferred intervention if allowed by the neonate's clinical status.

C. **Type A esophageal atresia** is associated with a higher incidence of a long gap between the proximal and distal esophageal segments. Delayed surgical correction allows growth of the segments and permits primary anastomosis. Enteral nutrition is provided via gastrostomy.

DUODENAL OBSTRUCTION

I. **Definition.** Obstruction of the lumen of the duodenum may be complete, partial, pre- or postampullary, and caused by either intrinsic or extrinsic problems.

II. **Pathophysiology**

A. **Duodenal atresia** is a complete obstruction of the lumen, and duodenal stenosis is a partial obstruction. Frequently, it is associated with trisomy 21 (33%).

B. **Annular pancreas** is a congenital anomaly of pancreatic development in which pancreatic tissue encircles the descending duodenum. This results in either complete or partial duodenal obstruction.

C. **Malrotation** refers to various abnormalities of intestinal rotation and fixation that can cause complete or partial duodenal obstruction. Abnormal peritoneal attachments (Ladd bands) may extrinsically compress the duodenum. Volvulus occurs when the entire midgut twists on its vascular pedicle, the superior mesenteric artery. This results in duodenal obstruction, midgut ischemia, and eventual necrosis.

III. **Clinical presentation**

A. **General.** Neonates with duodenal obstruction typically present with bilious vomiting. Abdominal distention is not common. Polyhydramnios may be evident on prenatal examination.

B. **Duodenal atresia.** Down syndrome, esophageal atresia, and imperforate anus are associated with duodenal atresia. The emesis is nonbilious when the obstruction is proximal to the ampulla of Vater.

C. **Midgut volvulus.** Presents with bilious vomiting and evidence of intestinal ischemia (lethargy, acidosis, bloody stools, etc.). This occurs most frequently in the first few weeks of life. Previously, the baby may have been well or had only minor feeding difficulties. **This is a true surgical emergency.**

IV. **Diagnosis.** The exact cause of the obstruction may not be fully elucidated before laparotomy.

A. **Abdominal radiographic study.** The **"double bubble"** is the pathognomonic finding of complete duodenal obstruction. Only 2 abdominal lucencies are seen: 1 in the stomach and 1 in the first portion of duodenum. The remainder of the gastrointestinal (GI) tract is gasless.

B. **Radiologic contrast studies**

1. **Partial obstruction** probably requires an upper GI (UGI) series to identify the site of difficulty.

2. **Malrotation** is best evaluated by UGI study to identify the ligament of Treitz. Occasionally, contrast enema may be useful to document the position of the cecum. Malrotation with volvulus is an emergency, and imaging studies should not delay surgical intervention in a baby who is critically ill.

V. **Management**

A. **Duodenal atresia or annular pancreas.** In cases of atresia or annular pancreas, gastric decompression controls vomiting and allows for "elective" surgical correction.

B. **Malrotation. Malrotation mandates immediate surgical intervention** when identified because the viability of the intestine from the duodenum to the transverse colon may be at risk from midgut volvulus.

C. **Unknown proximal obstruction.** In cases in which the source of the obstruction is unclear, appropriate resuscitation and early surgical exploration are warranted to prove that the obstruction is not due to a lesion causing intestinal ischemia.

PROXIMAL INTESTINAL OBSTRUCTION

I. **Definition.** A proximal intestinal obstruction is an obstruction of the jejunum.
II. **Pathophysiology.** Jejunal obstruction typically results from segmental atresia of the bowel, usually as the result of an in utero vascular accident.
III. **Clinical presentation.** Infants with jejunal obstruction usually have bilious vomiting associated with minimal abdominal distention because only a few loops of intestine are involved in the obstructive process.
IV. **Diagnosis.** A plain **abdominal radiograph** reveals a few dilated small bowel loops with no distal gas. It may be difficult to distinguish between jejunal atresia and midgut volvulus by plain films alone. Small amounts of distal gas may indicate that a volvulus has occurred.
V. **Management.** Surgical correction is required. The dilated proximal bowel is usually resected or tapered. Outcome is determined by the remaining bowel length and other comorbidities.

DISTAL INTESTINAL OBSTRUCTION

I. **Definition.** The term **distal intestinal obstruction** denotes partial or complete obstruction of the distal portion of the GI tract. It may be either small bowel (ileum) or colon. It may be a physical obstruction (meconium disease or atresia) or a functional obstruction (small left colon syndrome or Hirschsprung disease). Differential diagnosis includes the following:
   A. **Jejunal/Ileal atresia** may be single or multiple. Usually, this is a complete obstruction.
   B. **Meconium ileus**
      1. **Uncomplicated (simple) obstruction of the terminal ileum** occurs by pellets of inspissated meconium. Meconium ileus is associated with cystic fibrosis (CF).
      2. **Complicated meconium ileus** implies compromise of bowel viability, either prenatally or postnatally, due to perforation, volvulus, or atresia.
   C. **Colonic atresia.**
   D. **Meconium plug syndrome.**
   E. **Hypoplastic left colon syndrome** is frequently found in babies of diabetic mothers.
   F. **Hirschsprung disease (congenital aganglionic megacolon).**
II. **Clinical presentation.** Neonates with obstructing lesions in the distal intestine have similar signs and symptoms. They typically have distended abdomens, failure to pass meconium, and bilious emesis.
III. **Diagnosis**
   A. **Abdominal radiographs.** These show multiple dilated loops of intestine. The site of obstruction (distal small bowel vs colon) cannot be determined on plain films.
   B. **Contrast radiologic studies.** The preferred diagnostic test is contrast enema. It may identify colonic atresia, outline microcolon (signifying complete distal small bowel obstruction), or suggest a transition zone (indicating Hirschsprung disease). The procedure can identify and treat meconium plug and hypoplastic left colon syndromes. If the test is normal, ileal atresia, meconium ileus, and Hirschsprung disease are possibilities.
   C. **Cystic fibrosis (CF) evaluation.** Newborn screening for immunoreactive trypsinogen (IRT) (done on all infants) is done as part of the newborn screening to rule out CF. If the level is high, further testing is done (blood tested to determine whether CF gene mutations are present or a repeat IRT is done), followed by sweat chloride.
   D. **Mucosal rectal biopsy for histologic detection of ganglion cells.** This is the appropriate test for Hirschsprung disease. Laparotomy is sometimes necessary to determine the exact nature of the problem in infants with normal results of barium enema.

IV. **Management.** See also Chapter 67.
  A. **Nonoperative management.** In cases of meconium plug and hypoplastic left colon, this is accomplished with stimulation and is "curative" by either water contrast enema(s) or rectal stimulation.
    1. **Passage of time and colonic stimulation by digital examination and rectal enemas** promote return of effective peristalsis.
    2. **Infants who achieve apparently normal bowel function** should be evaluated for Hirschsprung disease by rectal mucosa biopsy. A small percentage of patients with meconium plug syndrome are proven to have colonic aganglionosis.
    3. **Uncomplicated meconium ileus can often be treated by nonoperative means.** Repeated enemas with Hypaque or acetylcysteine (Mucomyst) may loosen the inspissated meconium in the terminal ileum and relieve the obstruction.
  B. **Surgical therapy.** Urgent surgical intervention is required for atresias, complicated meconium ileus, and whenever the diagnosis cannot be made by other means. Hirschsprung disease is always treated surgically. There are 3 accepted types of surgical intervention for Hirschsprung disease. Laparoscopic, open, and transanal procedures have been described:
    1. Staged repair with colostomy creation using ganglionic bowel in the neonatal period.
    2. One-stage pull-through procedure while the infant is in the neonatal intensive care unit.
    3. Delayed 1-stage repair when the infant has doubled his or her birthweight. Therapeutic irrigations/enemas are used to keep the distal colon decompressed.

IMPERFORATE ANUS

See also Chapter 67.
  I. **Definition.** An imperforate anus is the lack of an anal opening of proper location and size. There are 2 types: high and low.
    A. **High imperforate anus.** The rectum ends above the puborectalis sling, the main muscle responsible for maintaining fecal continence. There is never an associated fistula to the perineum. In males, there may be a fistula to the urinary tract. High imperforate anus is much more common in males.
    B. **Low imperforate anus.** The rectum has traversed the puborectalis sling in the correct position. Variants include anal stenosis, imperforate anus with perineal fistula, and imperforate anus without fistula.
  II. **Diagnosis.** Diagnosis is made by perineal inspection and calibration of any opening that drains meconium (eg, fifth digit probe, rectal thermometer, or soft feeding tube). All patients with imperforate anus should have radiographic studies of the lumbosacral spine and urinary tract because there is a high incidence of dysmorphism in these areas. Spinal ultrasound and magnetic resonance imaging are used to evaluate for tethered cord.
  III. **Management.** Neonatal surgical intervention consists of colostomy for high anomalies and perineal anoplasty or fistula dilation for low lesions. If the level is not known, colostomy creation is preferred to blind exploration of the perineum. If a colostomy is done, the distal limb can be studied with contrast enemas to ascertain the level at which the rectum ends and to determine whether a fistula exists.

NECROTIZING ENTEROCOLITIS

See also Chapter 113.
  I. **Definition.** In most centers, necrotizing enterocolitis (NEC) is the most common indication for abdominal operation in neonates. It is caused by a combination of mucosal injury, relative hypoxia, and infection of the intestinal wall.

II. **Diagnosis.** Radiographic diagnosis of "true" NEC requires the presence of pneumatosis intestinalis and/or portal venous air. Abdominal distention, bloody bowel movements, and feeding intolerance in a neonate who previously tolerated enteral feeds are all signs of NEC. Definitive diagnosis requires radiographic evidence or a pathologic specimen from the affected bowel.

III. **Management**

    A. **Nonoperative management.** Includes intestinal decompression with a Replogle-style nasogastric or orogastric tube, aggressive fluid resuscitation, broad-spectrum antibiotics (include anaerobic coverage), and inotropic support as necessary. Serial abdominal examinations, labs, and abdominal radiographs should be obtained. Early surgical consultation is encouraged.

    B. **Surgical therapy.** Abdominal exploration is usually reserved for infants with full-thickness necrosis of the intestine. Pneumoperitoneum indicates intestinal perforation and is best identified with a left lateral decubitus radiograph. Relative indications for surgery include abdominal wall erythema and a fixed abdominal mass. Delayed stricture formation complicates 15–25% of NEC cases and presents with signs of a bowel obstruction.

Selected References

Bianchi A. One stage neonatal reconstruction without stoma for Hirschsprung's disease. *Semin Pediatr Surg.* 1998;7:170.

Chwals WJ, Blakely ML, Cheng A, et al. Surgery-associated complications in necrotizing enterocolitis: a multi-institutional study. *J Pediatr Surg.* 2001;36:1722.

Grosfeld JL, O'Neill JA, Fonkalsrud EW, Coran AG, eds. *Pediatric Surgery.* 6th ed. St. Louis, MO: Mosby-Year Book; 2006.

Levitt MA, Peña A. Outcomes from the correction of anorectal malformations. *Curr Opin Pediatr.* 2005;17:394–401.

Moss RL, Dimmitt RA, Henry MC, Geraghty N, Efron B. A meta-analysis of peritoneal drainage versus laparotomy for perforated necrotizing enterocolitis. *J Pediatr Surg.* 2001;36:1210.

O'Neill JA, Grosfeld JL, Fonkalsrud EW, Coran AG, Caldmone AA, eds. *Principles of Pediatric Surgery.* 2nd ed. St. Louis, MO: Mosby; 2004.

135   Surgical Diseases of the Newborn: Diseases of the Airway, Tracheobronchial Tree, and Lungs

INTRINSIC ABNORMALITIES OF THE AIRWAY

I. **Definition.** Intrinsic abnormalities of the airway that cause partial obstruction of the airway fall into this category. Examples include laryngomalacia, vocal cord paralysis, subglottic web, and hemangioma.

II. **Pathophysiology.** Lesions result in partial obstruction of the airway and cause stridor and respiratory distress of varying severity.

    A. **Laryngomalacia** is due to delayed development of the supraglottic pharynx.

    B. **Congenital vocal cord paralysis** can be congenital or acquired (birth trauma, patent ductus arteriosus ligation) and unilateral or bilateral.

C. **Subglottic web** is a congenital short-segment obstruction that may be partial or complete.

D. **Hemangioma** can occur below the glottis, engorge, and obstruct with agitation.

III. **Clinical presentation.** This can vary from mild respiratory stridor to complete airway obstruction depending on pathology.

IV. **Diagnosis.** The diagnosis is established by airway endoscopy with careful visual inspection.

V. **Management.** Management is individualized. Some problems, such as laryngomalacia, will be outgrown and require only supportive care. Other lesions, such as subglottic webs and hemangiomas, may be amenable to endoscopic resection or laser therapy.

CHOANAL ATRESIA

I. **Definition.** Choanal atresia is a congenital blockage of the posterior nares caused by a persistence of a bony septum (90%) or a soft tissue membrane (10%).

II. **Pathophysiology.** True choanal atresia is complete and bilateral, and it is one cause of respiratory distress immediately after delivery. Neonates are obligate nose breathers and do not automatically breathe through the mouth. Unilateral defects may be well tolerated and often go unnoticed.

III. **Clinical presentation.** Respiratory distress resulting from partial or total upper airway obstruction is the mode of presentation.

IV. **Diagnosis.** Diagnosis is based on the **inability to pass a catheter into the nasopharynx via either side of the nose.**

V. **Management.** Making the baby cry will initiate mouth breathing and temporarily improves the respiratory status. Insertion of an oral airway maintains the ability to breathe until the atresia is surgically corrected. Definitive management requires resection of the soft tissue or bony septum in the nasopharynx.

PIERRE ROBIN SEQUENCE

I. **Definition.** This anomaly consists of mandibular hypoplasia (micrognathia) in association with cleft palate.

II. **Pathophysiology.** Airway obstruction is produced by posterior displacement of the tongue associated with the small size of the mandible.

III. **Clinical presentation.** Severity of symptoms varies, but most infants manifest a high degree of partial upper airway obstruction.

IV. **Management**
A. **Infants with mild involvement** can be cared for in the prone position and fed through a special Breck nipple. Over the next few weeks to months, the mandible grows and the degree of airway obstruction subsides.
B. **More severe cases** require nasopharyngeal tubes, mandibular distraction, or other procedures to hold the tongue in an anterior position. Tracheostomy is generally a last resort.

LARYNGOTRACHEAL ESOPHAGEAL CLEFT

I. **Definition.** A rare congenital anomaly in which there is an incomplete separation of the larynx (and sometimes the trachea) from the esophagus, resulting in a common channel of esophagus and airway. This communication may be short or may extend almost the entire length of the trachea.

II. **Pathophysiology.** The persistent communication between the larynx (and occasionally a significant portion of the trachea) and the esophagus results in recurring symptoms of aspiration and respiratory distress with feeding.

III. **Clinical presentation.** Respiratory distress during feeding is the presenting symptom.

IV. **Diagnosis.** Contrast swallow may suggest the anomaly, but endoscopy is essential to establish the diagnosis and delineate the extent of the defect.

V. **Management.** Laryngotracheal esophageal cleft is treated by surgical correction, which is difficult and often unsuccessful.

VASCULAR RING

I. **Definition.** A **vascular ring** denotes a variety of anomalies of the aortic arch and its branches that create a "ring" of vessels around the trachea and esophagus.

II. **Pathophysiology.** Partial obstruction of the trachea, the esophagus, or both may result from extrinsic compression by the encircling ring of vessels.

III. **Clinical presentation.** Dysphagia and/or stridor (respiratory insufficiency) are the modes of presentation. Airway compromise is rarely severe and usually presents as stridor.

IV. **Diagnosis.** Diagnosis is by barium swallow, which identifies extrinsic compression of the esophagus in the region of the aortic arch. Computed tomography (CT) and magnetic resonance imaging (MRI) are useful to further define the anatomy.

V. **Management.** Management consists of surgically dividing a portion of the constricting vascular ring. The surgical plan must be tailored to the specific type of anomaly.

TYPE E (OR H-TYPE) TRACHEOESOPHAGEAL FISTULA

I. **Definition.** This anomaly is an uncommon type of tracheoesophageal fistula (TEF), making up 5% of cases. Esophageal continuity is intact, but there is a fistulous communication between the posterior trachea and the anterior esophagus.

II. **Pathophysiology.** When the fistula is small, "silent" aspiration with resulting pneumonitis occurs during feedings. If the fistula is unusually large, coughing and choking may accompany each feeding.

III. **Clinical presentation.** Symptoms, as noted previously, depend on the size of the fistula. This TEF subtype frequently escapes diagnosis in the newborn period.

IV. **Diagnosis.** Barium swallow is the initial diagnostic study, but it sometimes fails to identify the fistula. The test's sensitivity can be increased with a "pull back" upper gastrointestinal (UGI) series. Here, a nasogastric tube placed in the distal esophagus is pulled out slowly while instilling water-soluble contrast. The most accurate procedure is bronchoscopy (often combined with esophagoscopy). This should allow discovery and perhaps cannulation of the fistula.

V. **Management.** Surgical correction is required. The approach (via the neck or chest) is determined by location of the fistula.

CONGENITAL LOBAR EMPHYSEMA

I. **Definition.** **Lobar emphysema** denotes hyperexpansion of the air spaces in a segment or lobe of the lung.

II. **Pathophysiology.** Inspired air is trapped in an enclosed space. As the entrapped air expands, the normal lung is increasingly compressed. Cystic problems are more common in the upper lobes.

III. **Clinical presentation.** Small cysts may cause few or no symptoms and are readily seen on radiograph. Giant cysts may cause significant respiratory distress, with mediastinal shift and compromise of the contralateral lung.

IV. **Diagnosis.** Usually, the cysts are easily seen on plain chest radiographs. However, the radiologic findings may be confused with tension pneumothorax. Chest CT is often useful.

V. **Management.** Therapeutic options include observation for small asymptomatic cysts, repositioning of the endotracheal tube to selectively ventilate the uninvolved lung for

6–12 hours, bronchoscopy for endobronchial lavage, and operative resection of the cyst with or without the lobe from which it arises.

CYSTIC ADENOMATOID MALFORMATION

I. **Definition.** The term **cystic adenomatoid malformation (CAM)** encompasses a spectrum of congenital pulmonary malformations involving varying degrees of cyst formation. They communicate with the normal tracheobronchial tree. There are 3 types (I, II, and III) depending on the size of the cysts within the malformation.

II. **Pathophysiology.** Severity of symptoms is related to the amount of lung involved and particularly to the degree to which the normal ipsilateral and contralateral lung is compressed.

III. **Clinical presentation.** Signs of respiratory insufficiency such as tachypnea and cyanosis are modes of presentation.

IV. **Diagnosis.** The characteristic pattern on chest radiograph is multiple discrete air bubbles, occasionally with air-fluid levels, involving a region of the lung. The radiographic appearance can mimic that of congenital diaphragmatic hernia (CDH).

V. **Management.** Treatment is surgical resection of the involved lobe of lung, allowing reexpansion of compressed normal pulmonary tissue. If small and without symptoms, the surgical management can wait until the infant is several months of age.

PULMONARY SEQUESTRATION

I. **Definition.** Pulmonary sequestration is masses of abnormal tissue with aberrant blood supply arising from a systemic and not a pulmonary source. They may be intralobar or extralobar. Intralobar sequestrations have abnormal connections to the tracheobronchial tree. Extralobar sequestrations have separate pleura and no connections to the tracheobronchial tree.

II. **Pathophysiology.** Sequestrations are usually not recognized in the neonate. Intralobar sequestrations are found after frequent recurrent infections. Extralobar sequestrations are usually not associated with infections.

III. **Clinical presentation.** Lung mass found with or without frequent recurrent infections.

IV. **Diagnosis.** Diagnosis is by chest radiograph and CT scan.

V. **Management.** Surgical resection is warranted. Aberrant blood supply may originate from below the diaphragm.

CONGENITAL DIAPHRAGMATIC HERNIA

I. **Definition.** A patent pleuroperitoneal canal through the foramen of Bochdalek is the most common defect in congenital diaphragmatic hernia (CDH) (95%). A central anterior defect of the diaphragm (Morgagni hernia) is less common and usually not associated with lung hypoplasia.

II. **Pathophysiology**

A. **Prenatal.** Abnormal communication between the peritoneal and pleural cavities allows herniation of intestine into the pleural space as the developing gastrointestinal (GI) tract returns from its extracoelomic phase at 10–12 weeks' gestation. Depending on the degree of pulmonary compression by herniated intestine, there may be marked diminution of bronchial branching, limited multiplication of alveoli, and persistence of muscular hypertrophy in pulmonary arterioles. These lung abnormalities are most notable on the same side as the CDH (usually the left); they are also present to some degree in the contralateral lung.

B. **Postnatal.** After delivery, the anatomic anomaly may contribute to the following pathologic conditions:

1. **Pulmonary parenchymal insufficiency.** Infants with CDH have an abnormally small functional lung mass. Some have so few conducting air passages

and developed alveoli—a condition known as **pulmonary parenchymal insufficiency**—that survival is unlikely.

2. **Pulmonary hypertension.** Infants with CDH are predisposed to persistent pulmonary hypertension of the newborn (PPHN), also known as persistent fetal circulation. In this condition, blood is shunted away from the lungs through the foramen ovale and patent ductus arteriosus (PDA). Shunting promotes acidosis and hypoxia, both of which are potent stimuli to additional pulmonary vasoconstriction. Thus, a vicious cycle of clinical deterioration is established.

III. **Clinical presentation.** Most infants with CDH exhibit significant respiratory distress within the first few hours of life.

IV. **Diagnosis.** Prenatal diagnosis can reliably be made by ultrasonography. Delivery should occur in a neonatal center with full resuscitation capability, including extracorporeal life support/extracorporeal membrane oxygenation (ECLS/ECMO). Afflicted infants tend to have scaphoid abdomens because a paucity of the GI tract is located in the abdomen. Auscultation reveals diminished breath sounds on the affected side. Diagnosis is established by a chest radiograph that reveals a bowel gas pattern in one hemithorax, with shift of mediastinal structures to the other side, and compromise of the contralateral lung.

V. **Management**

A. **Indwelling arterial catheter.** Blood gas levels should be monitored by an arterial catheter.

B. **Supportive care.** Intubation with positive-pressure ventilation should be initiated immediately. CDH lungs can be surfactant deficient, and replacement therapy may be helpful. Several different strategies for appropriate respiratory and metabolic support have been described. These include permissive hypercapnia with conventional ventilation, oscillator ventilation, and/or the addition of inhaled nitric oxide. All these therapies are aimed at providing maximal pulmonary vasodilatation with minimal secondary lung injury due to barotrauma.

C. **Nasogastric tube.** A nasogastric tube should be placed to lessen gaseous distention of the stomach and intestine. Care must be taken to make sure the tube remains functional and does not clog.

D. **Surgical correction.** This is done by reduction of intrathoracic intestine and closure of the diaphragmatic defect. Surgical intervention is an essential element of treatment, but it is not the key to survival. Most authorities favor a delayed approach, allowing the newborn to stabilize its hyperreactive pulmonary vascular bed and to improve pulmonary compliance. If indicated, ECMO/ECLS can be instituted, and repair of the hernia defect performed immediately after stabilization on ECMO/ECLS, when the infant is ready to wean from ECMO/ECLS, or after successful ECMO/ECLS decannulation.

E. **Extracorporeal life support/extracorporeal membrane oxygenation (ECLS/ECMO).** Used in the treatment of neonates with severe respiratory failure. Exposure of venous blood to the ECMO/ECLS circuit allows correction of Po_2 and Pco_2 abnormalities as the lungs recover from the trauma associated with positive-pressure ventilation (see Chapter 18).

VI. **Prognosis.** Mortality rates for infants with CDH are still in the range of 50%. This high rate has prompted a search for other modes of treatment in addition to the expensive, labor-intensive modality ECLS.

A. **Fetal surgery.** This has been performed successfully on a case study basis, with the idea that in utero intervention will lessen the risk for development of pulmonary hypoplasia, which may be incompatible with life after delivery. However, trials of fetal tracheal occlusion and complete fetal correction have been abandoned due to high mortality.

B. **Medications.** Another major area of research is the attempt to develop a pharmacologic agent to decrease pulmonary vascular resistance selectively. To date, early promising data on inhaled nitric oxide have been tempered with the realization that it does not reverse pulmonary hypertension. Sildenafil (0.5–1 mg/kg every 6 hours) is reported to lower pulmonary hypertension in neonates with PPHN.

Selected References

Dimmitt RA, Moss RL, Rhine WD, Benitz WE, Henry MC, Vanmeurs KP. Venoarterial versus venovenous extracorporeal membrane oxygenation in congenital diaphragmatic hernia: the extracorporeal life support organization registry, 1990–1999. *J Pediatr Surg.* 2001;36:1199.

Greenholz SK. Congenital diaphragmatic hernia: an overview. *Semin Pediatr Surg.* 1996;5:216.

Grosfeld JL, O'Neill JA, Coran AG, Fonkalsrud E, eds. *Pediatric Surgery.* 6th ed. St. Louis, MO: Mosby-Year Book; 2006.

Harting MT, Lally KP. Surgical management of neonates with congenital diaphragmatic hernia. *Semin Pediatr Surg.* 2007;16(2):109–114.

Logan JW, Rice HE, Goldberg RN, Cotten CM. Congenital diaphragmatic hernia: a systematic review and summary of best-evidence practice strategies. *J Perinatol.* 2007;27(9): 535–549.

Nuchtern JG, Harberg FJ. Congenital lung cysts. *Semin Pediatr Surg.* 1994;3:233.

O'Neill JA, Grosfeld J, Fonkalsrud E, Coran AG, Caldamone AA, eds. *Principles of Pediatric Surgery.* 2nd ed. St. Louis, MO: Mosby; 2004.

Skinner SC, Hirschl RB, Bartlett RH. Extracorporeal life support. *Semin Pediatr Surg.* 2006;15(4):242–250.

Wung JT, Sahni R, Moffitt ST, Lipsitz E, Stolar CJ. Congenital diaphragmatic hernia: survival treated with very delayed surgery, spontaneous respiration and no chest tube. *J Pediatr Surg.* 1995;30:406.

136 Surgical Diseases of the Newborn: Retroperitoneal Tumors

NEUROBLASTOMA

I. **Definition.** A neuroblastoma is a primitive malignant neoplasm that arises from neural crest tissue. Usually, it is located in the adrenal gland, but it can occur anywhere neural crest cells migrate. It is the most common extracranial solid malignancy of childhood. Incidence is ~1 per 100,000 children in the United States.

II. **Clinical presentation.** This tumor typically presents as a firm, fixed, irregular mass extending obliquely from the costal margin, occasionally across the midline, and into the lower abdomen.

III. **Diagnosis**

   A. **Laboratory studies.** A 24-hour urine collection should be analyzed for vanillylmandelic acid and other catecholamine metabolites. Elevated lactate dehydrogenase is associated with poor prognosis.

   B. **Imaging and other studies.** A plain abdominal radiograph may reveal calcifications within the tumor. Computed tomography (CT) typically shows extrinsic compression and inferolateral displacement of the kidney. Metastatic evaluation involves bone marrow aspiration and biopsy, bone scan, chest radiograph, and chest CT.

IV. **Management.** Treatment is based on stage. Complete surgical resection remains the best hope for cure unless the infant has type 4S disease, which is associated with spontaneous regression. Planned therapy should take into account this well-recognized but poorly understood fact. Advanced tumors require multimodality therapy with surgery, radiation, and chemotherapy, but this is uncommon in neonates.

MESOBLASTIC NEPHROMA

I. **Definition.** A mesoblastic nephroma is embryonic solid renal tissue that is not usually malignant.

II. **Clinical presentation.** A palpable mass is found on abdominal examination, or a solid kidney mass is seen on prenatal ultrasound.

III. **Diagnosis**
   A. **Physical examination.** The mass is found on examination in the newborn period or becomes apparent in first few months of life.
   B. **Imaging and other studies.** Ultrasonography is obtained when a solid mass is identified in the neonate.

IV. **Management**
   A. **Surgery.** Nephrectomy is indicated and includes lymph node sampling to assess for rare malignant degeneration.

WILMS TUMOR (NEPHROBLASTOMA)

I. **Definition.** A Wilms tumor is an embryonal renal neoplasm in which blastemic, stromal, and epithelial cell types are present. Renal involvement is usually unilateral but may be bilateral (5% of cases).

II. **Clinical presentation.** A palpable abdominal mass extending from beneath the costal margin is the usual mode of presentation.

III. **Risk factors.** Aniridia, hemihypertrophy, certain genitourinary anomalies, and a family history of nephroblastoma are well recognized.

IV. **Diagnosis**
   A. **Laboratory studies.** No tumor marker is available.
   B. **Imaging and other studies.** Ultrasonography is generally followed by CT, which reveals intrinsic distortion of the calyceal system of the involved kidney. The possibility of tumor thrombus in the renal vein and inferior vena cava should be evaluated by ultrasonography.

V. **Management.** Multimodality therapy combining surgery, radiation, and chemotherapy is the standard.
   A. **Unilateral renal involvement.** Radical nephrectomy with lymph node sampling is indicated. Surgical staging determines the need for radiotherapy and chemotherapy. Both are effective.
   B. **Bilateral renal involvement.** Treatment of bilateral tumors is highly individualized. Neoadjuvant therapy followed by nephron-sparing resection may be attempted.

TERATOMA

I. **Definition.** A teratoma is a neoplasm containing elements derived from all 3 germ cell layers: endoderm, mesoderm, and ectoderm. Neonatal teratomas are primarily sacrococcygeal in location. They may represent a type of abortive caudal twinning.

II. **Clinical presentation.** This tumor is usually grossly evident as a large external mass in the sacrococcygeal area. Occasionally, it may be presacral and retroperitoneal in location or may present as an abdominal mass.

III. **Diagnosis.** See Section II. Most sacrococcygeal teratomas are identified on prenatal ultrasound. Digital rectal examination of the presacral space is important. α-Fetoprotein levels should be assayed.

IV. **Management.** The incidence of malignant tumors increases with age. Prompt surgical excision is required.

Selected References

DeMarco RT, Casale AJ, Davis MM, Yerkes EB. Congenital neuroblastoma: a cystic retroperitoneal mass in a 34-week fetus. *J Urol.* 2001;166:2375.

Grosfeld JL, O'Neill JA, Fonkalsrud EW, Coran AG, eds. *Pediatric Surgery.* 6th ed. St. Louis, MO: Mosby-Year Book; 2006.

Maris JM, Hogarty MD, Bagatell R, Cohn SL. Neuroblastoma. *Lancet.* 2007;369:2106–2120.

O'Neill JA, Grosfeld JL, Fonkalsrud EW, Coran AG, Caldamone AA, eds. *Principles of Pediatric Surgery.* 2nd ed. St. Louis, MO: Mosby; 2004.

137 Surgical Diseases of the Newborn: Urologic Disorders

Renal masses are discussed in Chapter 136.

UNDESCENDED TESTIS (CRYPTORCHIDISM)

 I. **Definition.** Testicular descent can occur prior to birth or in the first 6 months of life, after which cryptorchidism or undescended testis occurs in up to 10% of premature infants and 0.8% of term infants.
 II. **Clinical presentation.** Testicles may be nonpalpable or located along the course of the inguinal canal, in the superior scrotum, retroscrotally, and in the perineum. The ipsilateral scrotum may be hypoplastic, and a hernia or hydrocele may also be present. Cryptorchidism may be associated with other anomalies such as disorders of sexual development (especially in the presence of hypospadias), prune-belly syndrome, bladder exstrophy, pituitary disorders, and multiple other syndromes.
 III. **Diagnosis.** Careful examination with a warm hand sweeping lateral to medial from the anterior superior iliac spine to the ipsilateral groin is the most effective method of distinguishing a palpable from a nonpalpable testis.
   A. **Palpable testes.** A palpable testis must be distinguished from hernia, hydrocele, nubbin, and a long, looping portion of vas or epididymis. Infants with a palpable undescended testis should be followed to ensure proper descent by 6 months of age.
   B. **Nonpalpable testes.** Imaging studies are not indicated to help identify nonpalpable testes. If testicles are nonpalpable at 3 months of age, referral to a pediatric urologist is needed. If both testes are nonpalpable, a disorder of sexual differentiation, including congenital adrenal hyperplasia in a genetic female, should be considered. The incidence of disorders of sexual differentiation in patients with hypospadias and bilateral nonpalpable testis is high and warrants a karyotype evaluation.
 IV. **Management.** Spontaneous descent is possible until 6 months of age, after which there is only a 1% likelihood of spontaneous decent. After 6 months of age, orchiopexy is indicated for malpositioned palpable testicles. For nonpalpable testes, laparoscopy is indicated to localize the testis or identify the characteristic blind-ending spermatic artery and vas deferens entering the internal ring.

SCROTAL AND TESTICULAR MASSES

 I. **Definition.** The differential diagnosis of an abnormal testicular examination in an infant includes the following:

A. **Hydrocele.** Fluid within the tunica vaginalis and/or along the spermatic cord. Hydroceles may have continuity with the peritoneal cavity via a patent processus vaginalis (communicating hydrocele), or be confined to the tunica vaginalis and spermatic cord distal to an obliterated processus vaginalis (noncommunicating hydrocele).

B. **Hernia (most commonly indirect inguinal).** Protrusion of intra-abdominal contents through a patent processus vaginalis lateral to the epigastric vessels along the spermatic cord.

C. **Testicular torsion.** Twisting of the spermatic cord with reduction or cessation of testicular blood flow.

D. **Testicular tumor.** Rare in newborns.

II. **Clinical presentation.** A noncommunicating hydrocele presents as a painless testicular enlargement that is not reducible and does not change in size. Hernias and communicating hydroceles both present as a bulge in the groin or testicular enlargement that changes size and is usually more prominent with increased intra-abdominal pressure. Hernias are usually painless; however, they may become painful if intraperitoneal contents become incarcerated. Scrotal discoloration and testicular induration with or without significant swelling is typical of perinatal testicular torsion. In the rare instance of a testicular tumor, a painless, firm mass can be palpated within the testicle or paratesticular soft tissue.

III. **Diagnosis.** Diagnosis is based on the history and physical examination. Ultrasound can quickly assess for torsion and evaluate for a potential mass.

IV. **Management.** Hernias and communicating hydroceles should be repaired when diagnosed. The majority of nonreducible hydroceles will spontaneously resolve within the first year of life and warrant observation. Perinatal torsion should be explored urgently in conjunction with a contralateral orchiopexy. Rare cases of scrotal masses should be managed via an inguinal orchiectomy.

HYPOSPADIAS

I. **Definition.** Hypospadias is defined by 3 components: altered development of the distal urethra, a dorsal hooded prepuce with lack of ventral prepuce, and ventral penile curvature. The megameatus variant is an isolated urethral defect with a normal complete foreskin and no curvature.

II. **Clinical presentation.** The defect is usually identified at birth with the classic findings of dorsal hooded foreskin, ventral curvature, and a proximally located urethral meatus. Megameatus may be identified during or after circumcision.

III. **Diagnosis.** Diagnosis is based on physical examination findings. Hypospadias is classified by the location of the urethral meatus and degree of curvature. About 10% of patients also have cryptorchidism, and up to half of these may have disorders of sexual development (see Chapter 91). Karyotyping should be performed on infants with proximal hypospadias and nonpalpable testes.

IV. **Management.** Preputial skin is used in surgical correction of hypospadias; therefore, newborn circumcision should not be performed if the defect is identified at birth. The need for repair and surgical approach is based on the severity of the defect and the cosmetic appearance of the phallus. Repair is an elective procedure, ideally performed between 6 and 18 months of age.

EPISPADIAS

I. **Definition.** Isolated epispadias is the least severe of the "exstrophic" embryologic malformations that results in incomplete development of the dorsal urethra.

II. **Clinical presentation.** In isolated epispadias, formation of the urethra is incomplete and the urethral plate is exposed dorsally. In males this results in dorsal curvature and incomplete fusion of the glans. Females present with a bifid clitoris and vagina that is positioned anteriorly. Involvement of the bladder neck is common, resulting in incontinence in both sexes.

III. **Diagnosis.** Diagnosis is based on physical examination. Voiding cystourethrography may be useful in defining urethral and bladder anatomy, but is not required.

IV. **Management.** Surgical correction of curvature and urethral reconstruction is performed between 6 and 18 months of age. Reconstruction of the bladder neck and restoration of continence mechanisms is delayed until 4–5 years of age.

CLASSIC BLADDER EXSTROPHY

I. **Definition.** Thought to be due to altered development of the cloacal membrane, classic bladder exstrophy is defined by incomplete formation of the anterior abdominal wall, bladder, and dorsal urethra.

II. **Clinical presentation.** The anomaly may be identified prenatally or at birth, and it occurs more commonly in males (3–6:1). The epispadias malformation described previously is present in addition to a large abdominal wall defect occupied by the bladder plate.

III. **Diagnosis.** Findings on prenatal ultrasound include lack of bladder filling, inferior umbilicus, widened pubic ramis, and lower abdominal mass. Physical examination findings include epispadias, external rotation of the pelvic bones, a wide pubic diastasis, anterior displacement of the anus, and a large abdominal wall defect with exposed bladder plate.

IV. **Management.** The bladder plate must be protected with a thin plastic covering or moist dressing. There has been debate within the pediatric urology community; however, today the majority of exstrophy patients undergo bladder closure, repair of the anterior abdominal wall, and restoration of pelvic anatomy within the first days of life. The epispadias defect is repaired either at that time or within the first year of life, with bladder neck reconstruction and repair of continence mechanisms being delayed until 4–5 years of age.

CLOACAL EXSTROPHY

I. **Definition.** The most severe presentation of "exstrophic" embryologic malformations, cloacal exstrophy is defined by the same features of bladder exstrophy in addition to altered hindgut development and the presence of an omphalocele.

II. **Clinical presentation.** Prenatal ultrasound (US) findings of absence of bladder, infraumbilical anterior midline abdominal wall defect, omphalocele, and myelomeningocele were present in over 50% of patients with exstrophy. At birth, the omphalocele extends superiorly while the open bladder plate is divided by hindgut structures, which often include a segment of intussuscepted ileum. Genital malformations are similar to those seen in exstrophy except are more severe, often with complete separation of the phallus or clitoris.

III. **Diagnosis.** In addition to the physical examination findings discussed previously, cloacal exstrophy is also associated with renal abnormalities, Müllerian fusion anomalies, intestinal anomalies, hip or limb defects, and neural tube defects.

IV. **Management.** As with classic exstrophy patients, the bladder plate should be protected with plastic wrap or a moist dressing. Imaging should include renal and spinal US and skeletal imaging. Reconstructive surgery consists of multiple staged procedures with the initial goal of closing the bladder plate in addition to repairing the omphalocele and any associated neural tube defects. Subsequent procedures are then needed to address the hindgut and genital malformations.

PRUNE-BELLY (EAGLE-BARRETT OR TRIAD) SYNDROME

I. **Definition.** The triad consists of deficient abdominal musculature, bilateral cryptorchidism, and dilation of the urinary tract in a male.

II. **Clinical presentation.** "Prune belly" refers to the classic appearance of abdominal wall wrinkling and bulging flanks caused by varying degrees of abdominal wall deficiency.

Presentation ranges from the most severe (category 1) disease associated with oligohydramnios, renal dysplasia, and pulmonary hypoplasia to category 3 with mild external features and stable renal function. The degree of renal dysplasia is the single most important factor in determining the severity of the disease.

III. Diagnosis. Clinical diagnosis is based on the classic appearance of the abdominal wall and associated genitourinary anomalies.

IV. Management. Initial management consists of antibiotic urinary tract infection (UTI) prophylaxis and assessment of renal function. The majority of patients will benefit from surgical repair of the abdominal wall defect and cryptorchidism. More invasive surgical decompression of the urinary tract and radical reconstruction is *controversial* and is reserved for those patients with recurrent febrile urinary tract infections or deteriorating renal function.

POSTERIOR URETHRAL VALVES

I. Definition. Posterior urethral valves (PUVs) are aberrant folds of tissue that extend from verumontanum to the external sphincter, creating a urethral obstruction.

II. Clinical presentation. The presentation of PUVs encompasses a wide spectrum, from mild bladder outlet obstruction to severe obstructive uropathy with renal insufficiency, oligohydramnios, and pulmonary hypoplasia. The majority of cases of PUVs present prenatally with bilateral hydroureteronephrosis and megacystis, with or without oligohydramnios.

III. Diagnosis. Voiding cystourethrogram (VCUG) is the gold standard for diagnosis and classically shows a thickened bladder wall, a dilated posterior urethra, and decreased urethral caliber beyond the verumontanum.

IV. Management. In cases diagnosed prenatally, in utero decompression of the bladder has been attempted with limited success. A randomized controlled trial (PLUTO trial), comparing intrauterine vesicoamniotic shunting and conservative care for fetal bladder outflow obstruction, showed an improvement in perinatal survival in those who underwent vesicoamniotic shunting in preliminary results. Postnatal treatment consists of placement of an indwelling catheter, initiating antibiotic prophylaxis, and elective cystoscopic ablation of the valves. Serial chemistries are needed to monitor renal function as maternal creatinine is cleared. However, decompression of the urinary tract will likely do little to improve renal function if significant renal dysplasia is present. Nadir serum creatinine of <0.8 in the first year of life suggests a better long-term renal prognosis.

HYDRONEPHROSIS (PRENATAL AND POSTNATAL)

I. Definition. Hydronephrosis is dilatation of the renal pelvis and calyces. Mild dilation of the renal pelvis is defined as an anteroposterior diameter of 5–10 mm between weeks 18 and 23 of gestation. Severe dilation is generally defined as an anteroposterior diameter >15 mm. Postnatally, hydronephrosis is classified as grade 1–4 based on the Society for Fetal Urology grading system.

II. Clinical presentation. Prenatal ultrasound will detect mild pelvic dilation in 2–5% of fetuses at 18–23 weeks; however, 80% will spontaneously resolve. Severe dilation, bilateral hydronephrosis, and oligohydramnios are all suggestive of a significant urinary tract obstruction. Vesicoureteral reflux (VUR) can cause hydronephrosis. With the common use of prenatal ultrasound, a large proportion of infants with significant VUR are now diagnosed long before they would present with UTI later in life.

III. Diagnosis. Prenatal hydronephrosis is most commonly diagnosed at routine prenatal ultrasound. Postnatal evaluation is as follows: Renal/bladder ultrasound may be performed 24–48 hours immediately after birth, especially if bladder outlet obstruction is suspected. Mild unilateral dilation that persists on postnatal ultrasound is followed with a repeat ultrasound at 3 months of age. All infants with severe unilateral or bilateral hydronephrosis should be started on antibiotic prophylaxis and evaluated with a VCUG under current guidelines.

IV. **Management.** Serial ultrasounds are used to document stabilization/improvement of mild to moderate dilation. Normal postnatal US precludes the need for additional studies. The differential diagnosis is broad, and specific surgical management will be dictated by the underlying pathology.

Selected References

Baker L, Grady R. Exstrophy and epispadias. In: Docimo SG, Canning DA, Khoury AE, eds. *The Kelalis-King-Belman Textbook of Clinical Pediatric Urology.* 5th ed. Andover, Hampshire: Thompson Publishing Services; 2007:99–1045.

Gearhart JP, Ben-Chaim J, Jeffs RD, Sanders RC. Criteria for the prenatal diagnosis of classic bladder exstrophy. *Obstet Gynecol.* 1995;85:961.

Hrebinko RL, Bellinger MF. The limited role of imaging techniques in managing children with undescended testes. *J Urol.* 1993;150(2 Pt 1):458–460.

Kaefer M, Diamond D, Hendren WH, et al. The incidence of intersexuality in children with cryptorchidism and hypospadias: stratification based on gonadal palpability and meatal position. *J Urol.* 1999;162:1003–1006; discussion 1006–1007.

Kolon T. Cryptorchidism. In: Docimo SG, Canning DA, Khoury AE, eds. *The Kelalis-King-Belman Textbook of Clinical Pediatric Urology.* 5th ed. Andover, Hampshire: Thompson Publishing Services; 2007:1295–1307.

Noh PH, Cooper CS, Winkler AC, Zderic SA, Snyder HM 3rd, Canning DA. Prognostic factors for long-term renal function in boys with the prune-belly syndrome. *J Urol.* 1999;162(4):1399–1401.

Morris R, Kilby M. The PLUTO trial: percutaneous shunting in lower urinary tract obstruction. *Am J Obstet Gynecol.* 2012;206(suppl):S14.

Pathak E, Lees C. Ultrasound structural fetal anomaly screening: an update. *Arch Dis Child Fetal Neonatal Ed.* 2009;94:F384–F390.

Sarhan OM, El-Ghoneimi AA, Helmy TE, Dawaba MS, Ghali AM, Ibrahiem el-HI. Posterior urethral valves: multivariate analysis of factors affecting the final renal outcome. *J Urol.* 2011;185(suppl 6):2491–2495.

Wenzler DL, Bloom DA, Park JM. What is the rate of spontaneous testicular descent in infants with cryptorchidism? *J Urol.* 2004;171(2):849–851.

138 Syphilis

I. **Definition.** Syphilis is a sexually transmitted infection caused by *Treponema pallidum*, which is a thin, motile spirochete that is extremely fastidious, surviving only briefly outside the host. According to the Centers for Disease Control and Prevention (CDC), a case of **congenital syphilis (CS)** is defined as illness in an infant from whom lesional, placental, umbilical cord, or autopsy material specimens demonstrated *T. pallidum* by dark-field microscopy, fluorescent antibody, or other specific stain; an infant whose mother had untreated or inadequately treated syphilis at delivery (ie, any nonpenicillin therapy or penicillin administered <30 days before delivery); or an infant or child who has a reactive treponemal test for syphilis and any of the following: **evidence of CS on physical examination, evidence of CS on radiographs of long bones, reactive cerebrospinal fluid (CSF) venereal disease research laboratory test (VDRL),** elevated CSF cell count or protein (without other causes) or a reactive fluorescent treponemal antibody absorbed–19S-immunoglobulin M (IgM) antibody test or IgM enzyme-linked immunosorbent assay. This definition includes infants who are stillborn to women with untreated syphilis.

II. Incidence. The incidence of CS parallels that of primary and secondary syphilis in the general population. The most recent incidence in the United States is 10.1 cases per 100,000 live births, which represented an increase of 23% between 2003 and 2008. Rates of infection remain disproportionately high in large urban areas and in the southern United States. Worldwide, syphilis continues to represent a serious public health problem with a recent increase in incidence documented in both the developed and underdeveloped world. The World Health Organization estimates that 1 million pregnancies are affected by syphilis worldwide. Of these, 460,000 will result in stillbirth, hydrops fetalis, abortion, or perinatal death; 270,000 will result in an infant born preterm or with low birthweight; and 270,000 will result in an infant with stigmata of CS. The rate of CS is increased among infants born to mothers with human immunodeficiency virus (HIV) infection.

III. Pathophysiology. Treponemes are able to cross the placenta at any time during pregnancy, thereby infecting the fetus. **Syphilis can cause stillbirth (30–40% of fetuses with CS are stillborn), preterm delivery, congenital infection, or neonatal death,** depending on the stage of maternal infection and duration of fetal infection before delivery. Untreated infection in the first and second trimesters often leads to significant fetal morbidity, whereas with third-trimester infection, many infants are asymptomatic. The most common cause of fetal death is placental infection associated with decreasing blood flow to the fetus, although direct fetal infection also plays a role. Infection can also be acquired by the neonate via contact with infectious lesions during passage through the birth canal. Kassowitz's law states that the risk of vertical transmission of syphilis from an infected, untreated mother decreases as maternal disease progresses. Thus transmission ranges from 70–90% in primary and secondary syphilis, to 40% for early latent syphilis, and to 8% for late latent disease. CS can cause placentomegaly and congenital hydrops. *T. pallidum* is not transferred in breast milk, but transmission may occur if the mother has an infectious lesion (eg, chancre) on her breast.

IV. Risk factors. At-risk group include infants whose mothers received no or inadequate treatment (dose was unknown, inadequate, or undocumented), the mother received a nonpenicillin treatment during pregnancy for syphilis, or the mother was treated within 28 days of the infant's birth. Infants of high-risk mothers (drug use, especially cocaine use; low socioeconomic levels; HIV infection; teen pregnancy; commercial sex work; and lack of prenatal care) are at increased risk for syphilis. **Lack of early prenatal care is the strongest predictor of CS.**

V. Clinical presentation. CS is a multiorgan infection that may cause neurologic or skeletal disabilities or death in the fetus or newborn. However, when mothers with syphilis are treated early in pregnancy, the disease is almost entirely preventable. Spirochetes can cross the placenta and infect the fetus from ~14 weeks' gestation, with the risk of fetal infection increasing with advancing gestation. Approximately two-thirds of liveborn neonates with CS are asymptomatic at birth but have low birthweight. Clinical manifestations after birth are arbitrarily divided into **early CS** (<2 years of age) and **late CS** (>2 years of age).

A. Early manifestations include nasal discharge (snuffles) and maculopapular or vesiculobullous rash that appears on the palms and soles. The rash may be associated with desquamation. Other early stigmata include fever, abnormal bone radiographs, hepatosplenomegaly, petechiae, lymphadenopathy, jaundice, pneumonia, osteochondritis, pseudoparalysis, hemolytic anemia, leukocytosis, thrombocytopenia, and central nervous system (CNS) involvement. Skin lesions and moist nasal secretions in infected babies are highly contagious. However, organisms rarely are found in lesions >24 hours after treatment has begun.

B. **Late manifestations** develop in untreated infants and are characterized by chronic granulomatous inflammation. The sites most often involved include bones and joints, teeth, eyes, and the nervous system. **Hutchinson triad** (blunted upper incisors, interstitial keratitis, and eighth nerve deafness) and saddle nose are distinct complications. Some of these consequences may not become apparent until many years after birth, such as interstitial keratitis (5–20 years of age) and eighth cranial nerve deafness (10–40 years of age). A poor response to antibiotic treatment is often noted.

VI. **Diagnosis.** Diagnosis relies on active surveillance and laboratory studies. Maternal testing during pregnancy to treat the mother and identify at-risk newborn is crucial. Most infants are asymptomatic at birth. Besides testing for syphilis, these infants should be tested for HIV infection as well.

A. **Laboratory studies.** Patients with congenital or acquired syphilis produce several different antibodies that can be tested in the laboratory. These are grouped as **nonspecific nontreponemal antibody (NTA) tests,** and **specific treponemal antibody (STA) tests.** NTA tests (including VDRL, rapid plasma reagin [RPR], and automated reagin test) are inexpensive, rapid, and convenient screening tests that may indicate disease activity. These tests measure antibody directed against lipoidal antigen from *T. pallidum*, antibody interaction with host tissues, or both. They are used as initial screening tests and quantitatively to monitor a patient's response to treatment and to detect reinfection and relapse. False-positive reactions can be secondary to autoimmune disease, intravenous drug addiction, aging, pregnancy, and many infections, such as hepatitis, mononucleosis, measles, and endocarditis. The interpretation of NTA and STA tests can be confounded by maternal immunoglobulin G antibodies that are passed transplacentally to the fetus.

1. **Nonspecific nontreponemal antibody (NTA) tests.** The 2 most often used of these nonspecific screening tests are **VDRL** and **RPR.** A titer of at least 2 dilutions (4-fold) higher in the infant than in the mother signifies probable active infection. Titers should be monitored and repeated every 2–3 months after therapy. A sustained 4-fold decrease in titer, equivalent to a change of 2 dilutions (eg, from 1:32 to 1:8), of the NTA test result after treatment usually demonstrates adequate therapy, whereas a sustained 4-fold increase in titer from 1:8 to 1:32 after treatment suggests reinfection or relapse. The NTA test titer usually decreases 4-fold within 6–12 months after therapy for primary or secondary syphilis and usually becomes nonreactive within 1 year. **VDRL (not RPR) should be used on CSF.** A normal test result is negative, and any positive test should be followed up with a specific treponemal test. When NTA tests are used to monitor treatment response, the same test (eg, VDRL or RPR) must be used throughout the follow-up period, preferably by the same laboratory, to ensure comparability of results.

2. **Specific treponemal antibody (STA) tests.** These tests verify a diagnosis of current or past infection and should be performed if NTA test results are positive. These antibody tests do not correlate with disease activity and are not quantified. They are useful for diagnosing a first episode of syphilis and for distinguishing a false-positive result of NTA tests. However, they have limited use for evaluating response to therapy and possible reinfections. Once the STA test is positive, it will stay positive for life. Also, STA tests are not 100% specific for syphilis; positive reactions variably occur in patients with other spirochetal diseases, such as yaws, pinta, leptospirosis, rat-bite fever, relapsing fever, and Lyme disease. NTA tests can be used to differentiate Lyme disease from syphilis, because the VDRL test is nonreactive in Lyme disease. Examples of STA tests include fluorescent treponemal antibody absorption (**FTA-ABS**), microhemagglutination test for antibodies to *T. pallidum* (**MHA-TP**), *T. pallidum* enzyme immunoassay (**TP-EIA**), and *T. pallidum* particle agglutination (**TP-PA**). *T. pallidum*-specific **IgM immunoblot** testing in the newborn is able to identify infants with CS with

high sensitivity; however, the test is not commercially available. Most recently, some clinical laboratories and blood banks have begun to screen samples using **TP-EIA**, rather than beginning with an NTA test; the reasons for this change in sequence of the screening relates to cost and manpower issues. However, this "reverse sequence screening" approach is associated with high rates of false-positive results, and in 2011 the CDC recommended against adopting it.

3. **Direct identification of T. *pallidum*.** Microscopic **dark-field examination** and **direct fluorescent antibody** staining can be performed on appropriate specimens to detect spirochetes and their antigens. Also, a polymerase chain reaction (**PCR**) test to detect spirochete DNA in clinical specimens has been developed but is not commercially available.

4. **Lumbar puncture.** CNS disease may be detected by examining CSF and finding positive serologic tests (VDRL or FTA-ABS), dark-field examination positive for spirochetes, positive syphilis PCR, elevated monocyte count, or elevated spinal fluid protein levels. VDRL is most commonly used, but some experts recommend the FTA-ABS test as well. FTA-ABS may be more sensitive but less specific than VDRL. Results from the VDRL test should be interpreted cautiously, because a negative result on a VDRL test of CSF does not exclude a diagnosis of neurosyphilis. Alternatively, a reactive VDRL test in the CSF of neonates can be the result of nontreponemal IgG antibodies that cross the blood–brain barrier. PCR testing of CSF may prove very useful for the diagnosis of CNS syphilis.

B. **Imaging studies.** Radiographic abnormalities may be noted in 65% of the cases. These manifestations noted on long bones include periostitis, osteitis, and sclerotic metaphyseal changes. Infants may also present with pseudoparalysis or pathologic fractures.

VII. **Management.** Isolation precautions for all infectious diseases, including maternal and neonatal precautions, breast-feeding, and visiting issues, can be found in Appendix F.

A. **Maternal testing during pregnancy.** CDC recommends serologic syphilis testing for all pregnant women at the first prenatal visit. As of 2003, syphilis screening of pregnant women during the first trimester or at the first prenatal care visit was required by law in 43 states and the District of Columbia. In communities and populations in which the risk for congenital syphilis is high, serologic testing and a sexual history also should be obtained at 28 weeks' gestation and at delivery. Any woman who delivers a stillborn infant after 20 weeks' gestation should be tested for syphilis. For women treated during pregnancy, follow-up serologic testing is necessary to assess the efficacy of therapy. The result of a positive NTA test (eg, VDRL) should be confirmed with STA test (eg, TP-PA). Rapid point-of-care pre-natal syphilis screening using immunochromographic strip is being considered for limited-resource countries.

B. **Evaluation and treatment of infants.** No newborn infant should be discharged from the hospital without determination of the mother's serologic status for syphilis at least once during pregnancy and also at delivery in communities and populations in which the risk for CS is high. Testing of umbilical cord blood or an infant serum sample is inadequate for screening, because these can be nonreactive if the mother's serologic test result is of low titer or she was infected late in pregnancy. All infants born to seropositive mothers require a careful examination and a quantitative NTA test. The test performed on the infant should be the same as that performed on the mother to enable comparison of titer results. **The diagnostic and therapeutic approach to infants being evaluated for CS is summarized in Figure 138–1.**

1. **Infants with proven or highly probable disease** (abnormal physical examination consistent with congenital syphilis, a serum quantitative NTA titer that is 4-fold higher than the mother's titer, or a positive dark-field or fluorescent antibody test of a body fluid). The recommended treatment according to the CDC

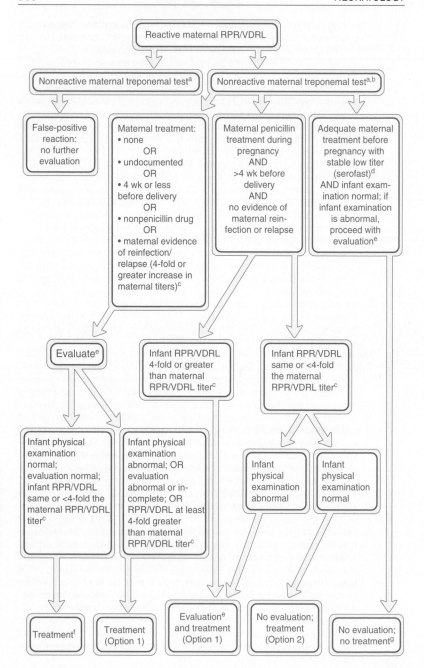

Reactive maternal RPR/VDRL

Nonreactive maternal treponemal test[a]

Nonreactive maternal treponemal test[a,b]

False-positive reaction: no further evaluation

Maternal treatment:
• none
  OR
• undocumented
  OR
• 4 wk or less before delivery
  OR
• nonpenicillin drug
  OR
• maternal evidence of reinfection/relapse (4-fold or greater increase in maternal titers)[c]

Maternal penicillin treatment during pregnancy AND >4 wk before delivery AND no evidence of maternal reinfection or relapse

Adequate maternal treatment before pregnancy with stable low titer (serofast)[d] AND infant examination normal; if infant examination is abnormal, proceed with evaluation[e]

Evaluate[e]

Infant RPR/VDRL 4-fold or greater than maternal RPR/VDRL titer[c]

Infant RPR/VDRL same or <4-fold the maternal RPR/VDRL titer[c]

Infant physical examination normal; evaluation normal; infant RPR/VDRL same or <4-fold the maternal RPR/VDRL titer[c]

Infant physical examination abnormal; OR evaluation abnormal or incomplete; OR RPR/VDRL at least 4-fold greater than maternal RPR/VDRL titer[c]

Infant physical examination abnormal

Infant physical examination normal

Treatment[f]

Treatment (Option 1)

Evaluation[e] and treatment (Option 1)

No evaluation; treatment (Option 2)

No evaluation; no treatment[g]

FTA-ABS, flourescent treponemal antibody adsorption; MHA-TP, microhemagglutination test for antibodies to *Treponema pallidum*; RPR, rapid plasma reagin; TP-EIA, *T. pallidum* enzyme immunoassay; TP-PA, *T. pallidum* particle agglutination; VDRL, Venereal Disease Research Laboratory.

[a]TP-PA, FTA-ABS, TP-EIA, or MHA-TP.

[b]Test for human immunodeficiency virus (HIV) antibody. Infants of HIV-infected mothers do not require different evaluation or treatment.

[c]A 4-fold change in titer is the same as a change of 2 dilutions. For example, a titer of 1:64 is 4-fold greater than a titer of 1:16, and a titer of 1:4 is 4-fold lower than a titer of 1:16.

[d]Women who maintain a VDRL titer 1:2 or less or an RPR 1:4 or less beyond 1 year after successful treatment are considered serofast.

[e]Complete blood cell (CBC) and platelet count; cerebrospinal fluid (CSF) examination for cell count, protein, and quantitative VDRL; other tests as clinically indicated (eg, chest radiographs, long-bone radiographs, eye examination, liver function tests, neuroimaging, and auditory brainstem response).

[f]Treatment (Option 1 or Option 2, below), with many experts recommending Treatment Option 1. If a single dose of benzathine penicillin G is used, then the infant must be fully evaluated, full evaluation must be normal, and follow-up must be certain. If any part of the infant's evaluation is abnormal or not performed, or it the CSF analysis is rendered uninterpretable, then a 10-day course of penicillin is required.

[g]Some experts would consider a single intramuscular injection of benzathine penicillin (Treatment Option 2), particularly if follow-up is not certain.

Treatment options:

(1) Aqueous penicillin G 50,000 U/kg, intravenously, every 12 hours (1 week of age or younger) or every 8 hours (>1 week); or procaine penicillin G, 50,000 U/kg, intramuscularly, as a single daily dose for 10 days. If 24 or more hours of therapy is missed, the entire course must be restarted.

(2) Benzathine penicillin G, 50,000 U/kg, intramuscularly, single dose.

FIGURE 138–1. Algorithm for evaluation and treatment of infants born to mothers with reactive serologic tests for syphilis. (*Used with the permission of the American Academy of Pediatrics. Syphilis. In: Pickering LK, Baker CJ, Kimberlin DW, Long SS, eds. Red Book: 2012 Report of the Committee on Infectious Diseases. 29th ed. Elk Grove Village, IL: American Academy of Pediatrics; 2012:695.*)

guidelines is **aqueous crystalline penicillin G** 100,000–150,000 U/kg/d, administered as 50,000 U/kg/dose intravenously every 12 hours during the first 7 days of life and every 8 hours thereafter for a total of 10 days *or* **procaine penicillin G,** 50,000 U/kg/dose intramuscularly (IM) in a single daily dose for 10 days. If >1 day of therapy is missed, the entire course should be restarted. Data are insufficient regarding the use of other antimicrobial agents (eg, ampicillin). A full 10-day course of penicillin is needed, even if ampicillin was initially provided for possible sepsis. These patients always should be treated with penicillin, even if desensitization for penicillin allergy is necessary (extremely rare in the newborn period).

2. Asymptomatic infants who have normal physical examination and a serum quantitative NTA titer ≤4-fold the maternal titer should be managed according to the status of maternal treatment:

a. Maternal treatment *uncertain.* The mother was not treated, inadequately treated, or has no documentation of having received treatment; the mother was treated with erythromycin or other nonpenicillin regimen; or the mother received treatment <4 weeks before delivery. These infants should be fully evaluated and treated as described in Section VII.B.1. Alternatively, **benzathine penicillin G,** 50,000 U/kg as a single **IM** dose, is acceptable provided adequate follow-up is ensured.

b. Maternal treatment *during* pregnancy is adequate. (Penicillin therapy given >4 weeks before delivery and the mother has no evidence of infection or relapse.) No evaluation is needed; however, a single **IM** dose of **benzathine penicillin G,** 50,000 U/kg, is recommended.

       c. Maternal treatment *before* pregnancy is adequate, and mother's NTA titer remained low and stable during pregnancy and at delivery. No evaluation or therapy is needed for the infant.

    C. **Isolation procedures.** Precautions regarding drainage, secretions, and blood and body fluids are indicated for all infants with suspected or proven CS until therapy has been given for 24 hours.

    D. **Follow-up care.** The infant should have repeated quantitative NTA tests at 3, 6, and 12 months. Most infants have a negative titer with adequate treatment. A rising titer requires further investigation and retreatment.

VIII. **Prognosis.** Infants infected early in the pregnancy are usually stillborn. Infants infected in the second and third trimester are at risk for premature delivery, low birthweight, neonatal death, and symptomatic congenital infection. Infants infected through the birth canal and treated early have excellent prognosis.

Selected References

American Academy of Pediatrics. Syphilis. In: Pickering LK, Baker CJ, Kimberlin DW, Long SS, eds. *Red Book: 2012 Report of the Committee on Infectious Diseases.* 29th ed. Elk Grove Village, IL: American Academy of Pediatrics; 2012:690–703.

Caddy SC. Pregnancy and neonatal outcomes of women with reactive syphilis serology in Alberta, 2002 to 2006. *J Obstet Gynaecol Can.* 2011;33:453–459.

Centers for Disease Control and Prevention; Workowski KA, Berman SM. Sexually transmitted diseases treatment guidelines, 2010. *MMWR Recomm Rep.* 2010;59:36–39.

Centers for Disease Control and Prevention. Congenital syphilis: United States, 2003–2008. *MMWR Morb Mortal Wkly Rep.* 2010;59:413–417.

Herremans T, Kortbeek L, Notermans DW. A review of diagnostic tests for congenital syphilis in newborns. *Eur J Clin Microbiol Infect Dis.* 2010;29:495–501.

Kamb ML, Newman LM, Riley PL, et al. A road map for the global elimination of congenital syphilis. *Obstet Gynecol Int* (Epub head of print on July 14, 2010).

Reyna-Figueroa J, Esparza-Aguilar M, Hernández-Hernández Ldel C, Fernández-Canton S, Richardson-Lopez Collada VL. Congenital syphilis, a reemergent disease in Mexico: its epidemiology during the last 2 decades. *Sex Transm Dis.* 2011;38:798–801.

Tridapalli E, Capretti MG, Reggiani ML, et al. Congenital syphilis in Italy: a multicentre study. *Arch Dis Child Fetal Neonatal Ed.* 2012;97:F211–F213.

Woods CR. Congenital syphilis-persisting pestilence. *Pediatr Infect Dis J.* 2009;28:536–537.

139 Thrombocytopenia and Platelet Dysfunction

  I. **Definition.** Thrombocytopenia is defined as a platelet count $<150,000/\mu L$ and is classified as **mild** ($100–149,000/\mu L$), **moderate** ($50–99,000/\mu L$), or **severe** ($<50,000/\mu L$). One percent of normal neonates may have mild thrombocytopenia.

 II. **Incidence. Thrombocytopenia is the most common hematologic abnormality among sick newborn infants (when admitted to the neonatal intensive care unit [NICU], incidence is as high as 35%).** Its incidence reaches 70% in newborn infants with birthweight <1000 g.

III. Pathophysiology
  A. **Normal platelets.** Similar to older children and adults, the platelet life span in neonates is 7–10 days, and the mean platelet count is >200,000/μL.
  B. **Etiology of thrombocytopenia.** See Figure 139–1.
    1. **Maternal disorders causing thrombocytopenia in infant**
      a. **Chronic intrauterine hypoxia** is the most frequent cause of thrombocytopenia in preterm neonates in the first 72 hours of life. This is seen in cases of placenta insufficiency such as diabetes and pregnancy-induced hypertension.
      b. **Preeclampsia** (in particular with HELLP syndrome [*h*emolysis, *e*levated *l*iver enzymes, *l*ow *p*latelet count]). Thrombocytopenia is present at birth,

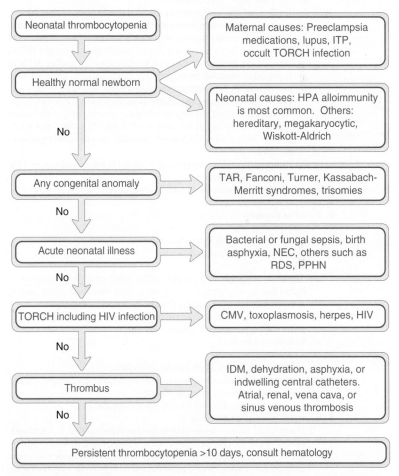

FIGURE 139–1. Algorithm for the evaluation of neonatal thrombocytopenia. CMV, cytomegalovirus; HIV, human immunodeficiency virus; HPA, human platelet antigen; IDM, infant of diabetic mother; ITP, idiopathic thrombocytopenic purpura; NEC, necrotizing enterocolitis; PPHN, persistent pulmonary hypertension of the newborn; RDS, respiratory distress syndrome; TAR, thrombocytopenia and absent radius; TORCH, *t*oxoplasmosis, *o*ther infections, *r*ubella, *c*ytomegalovirus, and *h*erpes simplex virus.

is usually associated with neutropenia, and should recover by the second week of life.

c. Drug use (eg, heparin, quinine, hydralazine, tolbutamide, and thiazide diuretics).

d. Infections (eg, TORCH [*t*oxoplasmosis, *o*ther infections, *r*ubella, *c*ytomegalovirus, and *h*erpes simplex virus] infections, bacterial or viral infections).

e. Disseminated intravascular coagulation (DIC).

f. Antiplatelet antibodies

   i. Antibodies against maternal and fetal platelets (autoimmune thrombocytopenia)

     (a) Idiopathic thrombocytopenic purpura (ITP)

     (b) Drug-induced thrombocytopenia

     (c) Systemic lupus erythematosus

   ii. Antibodies against fetal platelets (isoimmune thrombocytopenia)

     (a) Neonatal alloimmune thrombocytopenia is the most common cause of severe thrombocytopenia, seen mostly in term infants <72 hours of age. It is due to an incompatibility in human platelet antigen (HPA) between the newborn infant and its HPA-negative mother. HPA-1a is the most common incompatibility in Caucasians, while HPA-4b incompatibility is mostly seen in Asians. Only 10% of HPA-1a–negative women become sensitized after being exposed to HPA-1a because this immunological response occurs in the presence of specific human leukocyte antigens (HLAs) such as HLA-B8, HLA-DR3, and HLA-DR52a. HLA antibodies, though common, do not cause significant thrombocytopenia.

     (b) Immune thrombocytopenia can be found in some cases of hemolytic disease of the newborn.

2. Placental disorders causing thrombocytopenia in infant (rare)

  a. Chorioangioma

  b. Vascular thrombi

  c. Placental abruption

3. Neonatal disorders causing thrombocytopenia

  a. Decreased platelet production

   i. Isolated.

   ii. Thrombocytopenia and absent radius syndrome (TAR syndrome) is characterized by normal neutrophil and red blood cell counts; absent radii, usually bilateral; and the presence of a normal thumb.

   iii. Fanconi anemia is characterized by pancytopenia and the presence of abnormal (hypoplastic or aplastic) thumb.

   iv. Rubella syndrome.

   v. Congenital leukemia.

   vi. Trisomies 13, 18, or 21 or Turner syndrome.

   vii. Inherited metabolic disorders include methylmalonic, propionic, and isovaleric acidemia; ketotic glycinemia.

   viii. Congenital amegakaryocytic thrombocytopenia.

  b. Increased platelet destruction

   i. Many "sick" newborns develop thrombocytopenia that is not associated with any specific pathologic state. About 20% of newborns admitted to the NICU have thrombocytopenia, and 20% of those counts are <50,000/μL. This form of thrombocytopenia generally improves after the primary sickness (respiratory distress syndrome [RDS], persistent pulmonary hypertension of the newborn [PPHN], etc.) resolves.

   ii. Pathologic states associated with thrombocytopenia

     (a) Sepsis. Bacterial and *Candida* sp.

     (b) Congenital infections. TORCH infections, especially cytomegalovirus (CMV). Neonates with human immunodeficiency virus (HIV) and Enterovirus frequently have thrombocytopenia.

      (c) **Thrombosis** (renal vein, intracardiac, vascular).
      (d) **DIC.**
      (e) **Intrauterine growth restriction.**
      (f) **Birth asphyxia.**
      (g) **Necrotizing enterocolitis (NEC) or bowel ischemia.**
      (h) **Platelet destruction** associated with giant hemangioma (Kasabach-Merritt syndrome).

  C. **Platelet dysfunction**
    1. **Drug-induced platelet dysfunction**
      a. **Maternal use of aspirin**
      b. **Indomethacin**
    2. **Metabolic disorders**
      a. **Phototherapy-induced metabolic abnormalities**
      b. **Acidosis**
      c. **Fatty acid deficiency**
      d. **Maternal diabetes**
    3. **Inherited thrombasthenia (Glanzmann disease)**

IV. **Risk factors.** Low birthweight; low gestational age; small for gestational age; hypoxia at birth (Apgar score <5 at 5 minutes); umbilical line placement; respiratory assistance; hyperbilirubinemia; phototherapy; respiratory distress syndrome; sepsis, especially by *Candida* infection; meconium aspiration; NEC; mother with ITP; preterm infants of hypertensive mothers.

V. **Clinical presentation**
  A. **Symptoms and signs.** It is important to assess the general condition of the infant carefully. A "sick"-appearing newborn implies a very different approach for the investigation and treatment of thrombocytopenia (such as sepsis) than the infant who otherwise appears healthy (such as with most cases of alloimmune thrombocytopenia).
    1. **Generalized superficial petechiae** are often present, particularly in response to minor trauma or pressure, or increased venous pressure. Platelet counts are usually <60,000/μL. *Note:* Petechiae in normal infants tend to be clustered on the head and upper chest, do not recur, and are associated with normal platelet counts. They are a result of a transient increase in venous pressure during birth.
    2. **Gastrointestinal bleeding, mucosal bleeding, or spontaneous hemorrhage** in other sites may be occurring with platelet counts <20,000/μL.
    3. **Intracranial hemorrhage** may occur with severe thrombocytopenia.
    4. **Large ecchymoses and muscle hemorrhages** are more likely to be due to coagulation disturbances than to platelet disturbances.
  B. **History**
    1. There may be a **family history** of thrombocytopenia or a history of intracranial hemorrhage in a sibling.
    2. **Maternal drug ingestion** may be a factor.
    3. A **history of infection** should be noted.
    4. **Previous episodes of bleeding** may have occurred.
  C. **Placental examination.** The placenta should be carefully examined for evidence of chorioangioma, thrombi, or abruptio placentae.
  D. **Physical examination**
    1. **Petechiae and bleeding sites** should be noted.
    2. **Physical malformations** may be present. TAR syndrome, rubella syndrome, giant hemangioma, or trisomy syndromes.
    3. **Hepatosplenomegaly** may be caused by viral or bacterial infection or congenital leukemia.

VI. **Diagnosis**
  A. **Laboratory studies**
    1. **For all newborns**

a. Neonatal platelet count. Thrombocytopenia diagnosed from a capillary sample should be confirmed by a repeated count from a sample obtained from a venous sample and by careful examination of peripheral blood smear.
b. Complete blood count (CBC) and differential.
c. Blood typing.
2. For healthy newborns without congenital anomalies
a. Coombs test.
b. Maternal serum and whole blood sample for rapid HPA-1a (Pl^{A1}) phenotyping plus screen for anti-HPA alloantibodies. These antibodies are not detected in 10% of sensitized mothers.
c. Maternal, paternal, and infant genotyping of HPA 1–5 and 15 are required for diagnosis and for matching platelet donors.
d. TORCH evaluation and rapid HIV test.
e. Test for maternal thrombocytopenia. A low maternal count suggests autoimmune thrombocytopenia or inherited thrombocytopenia (X-linked recessive thrombocytopenia or autosomal dominant thrombocytopenia).
f. In cases of unexplained and severe thrombocytopenia, a bone marrow study is indicated. However, because of its technical difficulties in neonates, new blood tests are being developed to evaluate platelet production. Many have shown promising results (serum thrombopoietin [Tpo] concentrations, megakaryocyte progenitors, reticulated platelet percentages [RP%], and glycocalicin concentrations). An immature platelet fraction (IPF) test is similar to RP%, is already available, and is being used in some institutions. Bone marrow studies are still indicated in selected patients (marrow cellularity or megakaryocyte morphology).
3. For healthy newborns with congenital anomalies
a. Chromosome analysis for trisomies and Turner syndrome
b. "DEB/MMC" (diepoxybutane/mitomycin C) stress test to establish DNA breakage in peripheral blood lymphocytes
4. For "sick" newborns
a. Differential of white blood count, serum C-reactive protein, bacterial and fungal blood cultures
b. Coagulation studies. Prothrombin time, activated partial thromboplastin time, fibrinogen, and D-dimer level
c. TORCH titers. Culture of cytomegalovirus from urine samples, and other viruses if indicated (coxsackie, echovirus)
VII. Management
A. Obstetric management of maternal autoimmune thrombocytopenia
1. The occurrence of fetal hemorrhage (in utero) is very rare compared with the risk of such hemorrhage in alloimmune thrombocytopenia (10%).
2. Treatment is aimed at prevention of an intracranial hemorrhage during vaginal delivery.
3. There is an increased risk of severe neonatal thrombocytopenia and intracranial hemorrhage if antibody is present in the maternal plasma or if fetal scalp platelet counts are <50,000/µL.
4. Cesarean delivery may be indicated.
B. Management of maternal alloimmune thrombocytopenia
1. After a pregnancy has been affected by alloimmune thrombocytopenia, the proportion of subsequent pregnancies affected mostly depends on the father's genotype. If the father is heterozygous (HPA-1a/HPA-1b), the risk is 50%, and the risk is close to 100% if he is homozygous (HPA-1a/HPA-1a). The history of intracranial hemorrhage in a previous sibling is predictive of the presence of severe thrombocytopenia for the next fetus. In subsequent pregnancies, administering corticosteroids and intravenous immune globulin (IVIG) during

the third trimester coupled with transfusions of platelets to the fetus using ultrasound-guided intraumbilical cord infusion has been described.

2. **Instrumental vaginal delivery, fetal scalp electrodes,** and fetal scalp blood sampling should be avoided. Vaginal delivery is allowed when fetal platelet count is known to be >50,000/μL and presentation and labor are normal. Otherwise cesarean delivery is indicated.

C. **Treatment of infants with thrombocytopenia**

1. **Treat the underlying cause (eg, sepsis).** If drugs are the cause, stop their administration.

2. **Platelet transfusions**

   a. **Platelet transfusions** are indicated if active bleeding is occurring with any degree of thrombocytopenia or if there is no active bleeding but platelet counts are <20,000/μL. It may be desirable to transfuse premature infants with a greater risk of hemorrhage "those that are sick or in the first week of life" if the platelet count is <50,000/μL. Leukocyte-reduced, irradiated, random donor platelets are given in a dosage of 10–20 mL/kg of standard platelet concentrates. The plasma in platelets should be ABO and Rh compatible with the infant's red blood cells. The platelet count should increase to >100,000/μL. Platelet count should be repeated 1 hour posttransfusion. Failure to achieve or sustain a rise in platelet count suggests a destructive process. Washed and irradiated maternal platelets or platelets from an HPA-compatible donor (in general HPA-1a–negative platelets) need to be used for infants with alloimmune thrombocytopenia. When not available, a random donor platelet transfusion combined with IVIG may achieve a transient rise.

   b. **Harmful effects related to platelet transfusions** have been raised, such as an increased incidence of bacterial infection and an exacerbation of inflammatory injury. In addition, mortality rate in thrombocytopenic NICU patients who received platelet transfusions increased dramatically with the increase in the number of platelet transfusions.

3. **IVIG.** 400 mg/kg/d for 3–5 consecutive days, or a single dose of 1000 mg/kg on 2 consecutive days is given for immune thrombocytopenia.

4. **Prednisone.** 2 mg/kg/d may also be beneficial in immune thrombocytopenia.

VIII. **Prognosis.** Etiology of the thrombocytopenia dictates the outcome and prognosis.

Selected References

Baer VL, Lambert DK, Henry E, Snow GL, Sola-Visner MC, Christensen RD. Do platelet transfusions in the NICU adversely affect survival? *J Perinatol.* 2007;27:790–796.

Chakravorty S, Murray N, Roberts I. Neonatal thrombocytopenia. *Early Hum Dev.* 2005;81:35.

Roberts I, Stanworth S, Murray NA. Thrombocytopenia in the neonate. *Blood Rev.* 2008;22(4):173–186.

Sola-Visner M, Sallmon H, Brown R. New insights into the mechanisms of nonimmune thrombocytopenia in neonates. *Semin Perinatol.* 2009;33(1):43–51.

Sola-Visner M, Saxonhouse MA, Brown RE. Neonatal thrombocytopenia: what we do and we don't know. *Early Hum Dev.* 2008;84:499–506.

van den Akker E, Oepkes D, Brand A, Kanhai HH. Vaginal delivery for fetuses at risk of alloimmune thrombocytopenia? *BJOG.* 2006;113(7):781–783.

140 Thyroid Disorders

Disorders of thyroid function in neonates often present a diagnostic dilemma. The initial clinical signs and symptoms are often subtle or misleading. A good understanding of the unique thyroid physiology, the assessment of thyroid function, and a sense of urgency are necessary to recognize, diagnose, and treat thyroid disorders early.

GENERAL CONSIDERATIONS

I. **Fetal and neonatal thyroid function**
   A. **Embryogenesis** begins in the third week of gestation, with thyroglobulin synthesis detected by 4–6 weeks, thyrotropin-releasing hormone (TRH) synthesis by 6–8 weeks, and iodine trapping at 8–10 weeks through 12 weeks' gestation. At that time, thyroxine (T_4), triiodothyronine (T_3), and thyroid-stimulating hormone (TSH) secretion can be detected. Thyroid activity remains low until midgestation and then increases slowly until term.
   B. **Thyroid hormones** undergo rapid and dramatic changes in the immediate postnatal period.
      1. **An acute release of TSH occurs within minutes after birth.** Peak values of 60–80 mU/L are seen at 30–90 minutes attributed to clamping of the cord and the stress of delivery. Levels decrease to <10 mU/L by the end of the first postnatal week.
      2. **Stimulated by the TSH surge,** T_4, free T_4 (FT_4), and T_3 rapidly increase, reaching peak levels by 24 hours. Levels decrease slowly over the first 1–2 weeks of life to levels typically seen in the infant.
   C. **Thyroid function in the premature infant.** Identical changes in TSH, T_4, and T_3 are seen in premature infants; however, absolute values are lower in proportion to the gestational age and birthweight. TSH levels return to normal by 3–5 days of life.
II. **Physiologic action of thyroid hormones.** Thyroid hormones have profound effects on growth and neurologic development. They also influence oxygen consumption, thermogenesis, and the metabolic rate of many processes. Maternal T_4 is critical for normal central nervous system maturation in the fetus.
III. **Biochemical steps to thyroid hormone synthesis.** Thyroid hormone production includes the stages of iodide transport, thyroglobulin synthesis, organization of iodide, monoiodotyrosine and diiodotyrosine coupling, thyroglobulin endocytosis, proteolysis, and deiodination.
IV. **Assessment of thyroid function.** Thyroid tests are intended to measure the level of thyroid activity and to identify the cause of thyroid dysfunction.
   A. **T_4 concentration** is an important parameter in the evaluation of thyroid function. More than 99% of T_4 is bound to thyroid hormone–binding proteins. Therefore, changes in these proteins may affect T_4 levels. Serum levels for term newborn infants range between 6.4 and 23.2 mcg/dL.
   B. **Free T_4** reflects the availability of thyroid hormone to the tissues. Serum levels vary widely by gestational age: newborn term infants (2.0–5.3 ng/dL) and infants of 25–30 weeks' gestation (0.6–3.3 ng/dL).
   C. **TSH measurement** is a valuable test in evaluating thyroid disorders, particularly primary hyperthyroidism. Serum levels over all gestational ages of 25–42 weeks range from 2.5 to 18.0 mU/L.
   D. **T_3 concentration** is particularly useful in the diagnosis and treatment of hyperthyroidism. Serum levels of T_3 are very low in the fetus and cord blood samples (20–75 ng/dL). Shortly after birth, levels exceed 100 ng/dL to ~400 ng/dL. In hyperthyroid states, levels may exceed 400 ng/dL. In sick preterm infants, a very low T_3

(hypothyroid range) may signal the euthyroid sick syndrome, also known as the nonthyroidal illness syndrome.

E. **Thyroid-binding globulin (TBG)** can be measured directly by radioimmunoassay.

F. **The thyrotropin-releasing hormone (TRH) stimulation test** can assess pituitary and thyroid responsiveness. It is used to differentiate between secondary and tertiary hypothyroidism.

G. **Thyroid imaging**

   1. Thyroid scanning with ^{123}I (preferred isotope) is performed to identify functional thyroid tissue.

   2. **Color Doppler ultrasonography** has shown improved sensitivity in detecting ectopic thyroid tissue in recent studies.

CONGENITAL HYPOTHYROIDISM

   I. **Definition.** Congenital hypothyroidism (CH) is defined as a significant decrease in, or the absence of, thyroid function present at birth. Unrecognized CH leads to mental retardation without treatment within 2 weeks of birth.

  II. **Incidence.** The overall incidence is 1 in 3000 to 1 in 4000 newborn infants. Sporadic cases account for 85% of patients diagnosed; 15% are hereditary. The incidence of CH is higher in Hispanic individuals and lower in black individuals. There is a 2:1 incidence in females compared with males, and there is an increased risk in infants with Down syndrome. The incidence of CH has been found to be 4–5 times more common than phenylketonuria.

 III. **Pathophysiology**

   A. **Primary hypothyroidism**

      1. **Developmental defects** such as ectopic thyroid (most common), thyroid hypoplasia, or agenesis.

      2. **Inborn errors** of thyroid hormone synthesis including total and partial iodide organification defects.

      3. **Maternal exposure** to radioiodine, propylthiouracil, or methimazole during pregnancy.

      4. **Iodine deficiency** (endemic cretinism).

   B. **Secondary hypothyroidism.** TSH deficiency.

   C. **Tertiary hypothyroidism.** TRH deficiency.

   D. **Hypopituitary hypothyroidism.** Associated with other hormonal deficiencies.

  IV. **Risk factors.** Genetic or family history, birth defects, female sex, and gestational age >40 weeks.

   V. **Clinical presentation.** Symptoms are usually absent at birth; however, subtle signs may be detected during the first few weeks of life. Obtain a serum-free thyroxine and TSH for any clinical signs, even if the newborn screening is negative. CH can occur even after a normal newborn screening.

   A. **Early manifestations.** Signs at birth include prolonged gestation, large size for gestational age, large fontanelle, and respiratory distress syndrome. Manifestations that may be seen by 2 weeks include hypotonia, umbilical hernia, lethargy, constipation hypothermia, prolonged jaundice, and feeding difficulty.

   B. **Late manifestation.** Classic features usually appear after 6 weeks and include puffy eyelids, coarse hair, large tongue, myxedema, and hoarse cry. Late manifestations in borderline hypothyroidism detected in screening programs can present as significant hearing impairment with speech delay.

  VI. **Diagnosis**

   A. **Screening.** Newborn screening for CH in addition to the profound clinical benefit is cost-effective.

      1. **Methods.** The screening strategies include primary TSH, backup T_4 (may miss TBG deficiency, hypothalamic-pituitary hypothyroidism, and hypothyroxinemia

with delayed TSH elevation), primary T_4, backup TSH (will miss delayed TSH elevation with initial normal T_4), and **primary T_4 and TSH (ideal screening approach)**. In the Netherlands, the measurement of T_4/TBG ratio in newborns with low T_4 and nonelevated TSH levels and TRH stimulation tests are used to identify central congenital hypothyroidism.

2. Timing. The ideal time for screening is by 48 hours to 4 days of age. Infants discharged before 48 hours should be screened before discharge; however, this increases the number of false-positive TSH elevations. A repeat test at 2–6 weeks identifies ~10% of cases.

3. American Academy of Pediatrics (AAP) recommended screening.
   a. Term delivery in hospital. Filter paper collection at 2–4 days of age or at discharge.
   b. Neonatal intensive care unit/preterm birth/home birth. Within 7 days of birth.
   c. Mother on thyroid medication/family history of CH. Screen cord blood.

4. Results. Accurate screening results depend on good quality of blood spots. A low T_4 level and TSH concentrations >40 mU/L are indicative of CH. Normal TSH at 2–12 weeks is 9.1 mU/L. **The update of newborn screening and therapy for congenital hypothyroidism (June 2006, reaffirmed December 2011) by the AAP, American Thyroid Association, and Lawson Wilkins Pediatric Endocrine Society provides a useful algorithm.**
   a. Low T_4, TSH > 40 mU/L. Check T_4, FT_4, and TSH immediately to confirm results. If T_4 low and TSH elevated, start treatment. See further management later.
   b. Low T_4, TSH slightly elevated but <40 mU/L. Do another newborn screen immediately. Check T_4, FT_4, and TSH.
      i. Low T_4 and increased TSH. Start treatment. See further management later.
      ii. Normal T_4 and TSH. **Transient hypothyroidism** is rare and can be secondary to prenatal/postnatal exposure to iodides, intrauterine exposure to maternal antithyroid drugs, maternal thyrotropin receptor antibody (TRAb), mutation in TSH-R, endemic iodide deficiency, or heterozygous thyroid oxidase 2 deficiency. No treatment is necessary.
   c. Low T_4, Normal TSH. Check serum T_4, FT_4, and TSH again. Rule out transient hypothyroxinemia, TBG deficiency, and central hypothyroidism.
      i. Central hypothyroidism. Start treatment. See further management later.
      ii. Isolated lo T_4. Monitor monthly.
   d. Normal T_4, increased TSH. This can be transient, permanent mild congenital hypothyroidism, TH resistance, delayed maturation of hypothalamic/pituitary axis, or Down syndrome.
      i. Check TSH again at 2–4 weeks.
         (a) Normal TSH. No treatment necessary.
         (b) Persistent increased TSH (>10 mU/L). Start treatment. Stop therapy at 3 years of age and recheck FT_4 and TSH at 30 days. See further management later.
   e. Persistent increased TSH (6–10 mU/L at 1 month). Check TSH, T_4, and FT_4 in 2 weeks.
      i. Normal TSH. No treatment necessary.
      ii. Persistent increased TSH (>10 mU/L). Start treatment. Stop therapy at 3 years of age and recheck FT_4 and TSH at 30 days. See further management later.
   f. Low T_4 (<3 mcg/dL), delayed increased TSH in a sick term newborn, preterm low birthweight or very low birthweight infant. Check serum T_4, FT_4, and TSH at 2 weeks.

      i. Persistent decreased T_4 and increased TSH. Start treatment and see further management later.

    5. Continued monitoring of thyroid function by serum specimens in ill newborns with prolonged intensive care unit care regardless of birthweight will help identify late rise of TSH.

  B. Diagnostic studies

    1. Serum for confirmatory measurements of T_4 and TSH concentrations. If an abnormality of TBG is suspected, FT_4 and TBG concentrations should also be evaluated.

    2. Ultrasonography is used to separate a structural defect from a normal or enlarged gland.

    3. Thyroid scan (scintigraphy) with radioactive iodine or technetium remains the most accurate diagnostic modality to determine the cause of congenital hypothyroidism.

VII. Management

  A. Consultation. Consult with a pediatric endocrinologist is recommended.

  B. Goal of therapy. The goal of the therapy is to ensure normal growth and development and normalize TSH and maintain T_4 or FT_4 in upper half of reference range.

  C. Treatment. Levothyroxine (L-T_4) is the treatment of choice. The average starting dose is 10–15 mcg/kg/d orally. Customization of the doses based on underlying cause and severity may result in more rapid normalization of values of TSH and T_4. The pill, universally available, should be crushed and suspended in breast milk, formula, or water. Care should be taken to avoid concomitant administration of soy, fiber, or iron. In Europe, liquid preparations with 5 mcg/drop concentration are licensed. The goal of therapy is to maintain T_4 concentration in the upper normal range (10–16 mcg/dL), FT_4 (1.4–2.3 ng/dL), and low-normal serum TSH (0.5–2 mU/L).

  D. Follow-up. Clinical examination, including assessment of growth and development, should be performed every few months during the first 3 years of life. Infants with CH are at risk of other congenital anomalies. Cardiovascular anomalies, including pulmonary stenosis, atrial septal defect, and ventricular septal defect, are the most common. Infants need to undergo frequent laboratory and clinical evaluations of thyroid function, growth, and development to ensure optimal T_4 dosage and adherence to their therapy regimen. **Serum T_4 and TSH measurements should be performed as follows:**

    1. 2 and 4 weeks after initiation of therapy.

    2. Every 1–2 months during the first 6 months of life.

    3. Every 3–4 months between 6 months and 3 years.

    4. Every 6–12 months until growth is completed.

    5. More frequent intervals with dose change, abnormal values, and compliance concerns.

    6. Monitoring more intensely during puberty is recommended to prevent unwanted cardiovascular dysfunction.

VIII. Assess permanence of CH

  A. If initial thyroid scan shows an ectopic or absent gland, CH is a permanent condition.

  B. If initial TSH is <50 mU/L and there is no increase in TSH after newborn period, then a trial off therapy at 3 years of age may be considered.

  C. If TSH increases off therapy, consider CH a permanent condition.

IX. Prognosis. CH can adversely influence growth, intelligence, cardiovascular function, and quality of life in the long term. The more severe the thyroid dysfunction at diagnosis, the lower is their performance IQ later in life. Early initiation of therapy within the first 2 weeks of life, at doses of 10–15 mcg/kg of L-T_4 (levothyroxine), and subsequent management through puberty may help to mitigate these deficits and promote optimal somatic growth.

NEONATAL THYROTOXICOSIS

I. **Definition.** Neonatal thyrotoxicosis is defined as a hypermetabolic state resulting from excessive thyroid hormone activity in the newborn.

II. **Incidence.** This is a rare disorder occurring in only ~1 of 70 thyrotoxic pregnancies (autoimmune disease). The incidence of maternal thyrotoxicosis in pregnancy is 1–2 per 1000 pregnancies.

III. **Pathophysiology**
   A. **Usually results from transplacental passage** of thyroid-stimulating immunoglobulin from a mother with Graves disease or Hashimoto thyroiditis.
   B. **Congenital nonautoimmune hyperthyroidism** has been identified as a result of activating mutations in the TSH receptor, stimulatory G protein, and the McCune-Albright syndrome.

IV. **Risk factors.** Mother with active or inactive Graves disease or Hashimoto thyroiditis.

V. **Clinical presentation.** Fetal tachycardia in the third trimester may be the first manifestation. Signs are usually apparent within hours after birth to the first 10 days of life. Delayed presentation up to 45 days may occur in the presence of coexisting maternal blocking and stimulating antibodies. Thyrotoxic signs include irritability, tachycardia, hypertension, flushing, tremor, poor weight gain, thrombocytopenia, hepatomegaly, and arrhythmias. A goiter is usually present and may be large enough to cause tracheal compression. Eye signs such as lid retraction and exophthalmos, as well as craniosynostosis, may also be present.

VI. **Diagnosis**
   A. **History and physical examination.** A maternal past history of thyrotoxicosis and presence of maternal thyroid-stimulating antibodies in the last trimester correlate well the development of neonatal thyrotoxicosis. At birth, the infant may be euthyroid or even hypothyroid by laboratory values; however, paradoxically, the presence of goiter may be the only abnormal finding in addition to the clinical features of thyrotoxicosis on physical examination, as discussed earlier.
   B. **Laboratory studies.** Diagnosis is confirmed by demonstrating increased levels of T_4, FT_4, and T_3 with suppressed levels of TSH.

VII. **Management.** Although the disorder is usually self-limited, therapy depends on the severity of the symptoms and is a life-threatening emergency in its most severe form. Care should be exercised not to induce hypothyroidism with excessive medication.
   A. **Mild.** Close observation is required. Therapy is not necessary.
   B. **Moderate.** Administer one of the following antithyroid medications:
      1. **Lugol solution.** To inhibit thyroid hormone release and decrease vascularity: (8.3 mg iodide/drop), 1 drop every 8 hours.
      2. **Propylthiouracil (PTU).** To inhibit organification and block peripheral conversion of T_4 to more active T_3: 5–10 mg/kg/d in 3 divided doses.
      3. **Methimazole.** Mode of action is the same as PTU: 0.5–1 mg/kg/d in 3 divided doses. (Total dose not to exceed 40 mg/d.)
   C. **Severe.** In addition to the medications just listed:
      1. **Prednisone.** To inhibit thyroid hormone secretion and inhibit conversion of T_4 to T_3: 2 mg/kg/d.
      2. **Propranolol.** To control tachycardia, 1–2 mg/kg/d in 2–4 divided doses; and digitalis (to guard against cardiovascular decompensation).
      3. **Human intravenous immunoglobulin.** Used with success in refractory neonatal thyrotoxicosis.
   D. **Nonautoimmune hyperthyroidism.** Requires thyroid gland ablation or near-total thyroidectomy.

VIII. **Prognosis.** The disorder is usually self-limited and disappears spontaneously within 2–4 months. Mortality in affected infants is ~15% if the disorder is not recognized and treated properly. Potential long-term morbidity includes hyperactivity, impaired intellect, advanced bone age, and craniosynostosis.

TRANSIENT DISORDERS OF THYROID FUNCTION IN THE NEWBORN

I. **EUTHYROID SICK SYNDROME**
   A. **Definition.** Transient alteration in thyroid function associated with a severe non-thyroidal illness.
   B. **Incidence.** The syndrome is frequently seen in premature infants because of their increased susceptibility to neonatal morbidity. Preterm infants with respiratory distress syndrome have been the most frequently reported patients with this disorder.
   C. **Diagnosis.** A low T_3 level is usually present, associated with low or normal T_4 and normal TSH. Infants are euthyroid (normal TSH).
   D. **Treatment.** Treatment has not been shown to be beneficial. Abnormal thyroid functions return to normal as the sick infant improves. However, preterm infants at risk should be monitored by serial determinations of FT_4 and TSH, and treatment should be initiated if there is progressive increase in TSH and decrease in FT_4. Treatment should be initiated if the illness state is expected to be persistent and TSH remains elevated for a month or longer.

II. **TRANSIENT HYPOTHYROXINEMIA OF PREMATURITY**
   A. **Definition.** Decreased thyroid levels without elevated TSH, but not as low as congenital hypothyroidism.
   B. **Incidence.** All preterm infants have some degree of hypothyroxinemia (>50% have T_4 levels <6.5 mcg/dL).
   C. **Pathophysiology.** The condition is presumed to be related to immaturity of the hypothalamic-pituitary axis that cannot compensate for the loss of maternal thyroid hormone.
   D. **Diagnosis.** The biochemical profile of transient hypothyroxinemia in premature infants (before 30–32 weeks' gestation) comprises low T_4 and FT_4 levels with normal or low TSH levels.
   E. **Treatment.** Therapy has not been consistently effective in improving neurologic outcome or reducing morbidity. Therapy is only recommended when low T_4 is accompanied by TSH elevation.

Selected References

American Academy of Pediatrics, Rose SR; Section on Endocrinology and Committee on Genetics, American Thyroid Association, et al. Update of newborn screening and therapy for congenital hypothyroidism. *Pediatrics.* 2006;117:2290–2303. (Reaffirmed December 2011)

Bollepalli S, Rose SR. Disorders of the thyroid gland. In: Gleason CA, Devaskar SU, eds. *Avery's Diseases of the Newborn.* 9th ed. Philadelphia, PA: Elsevier Saunders; 2012:1307–1319.

Djemli A, Van Vliet G, Delvin EE. Congenital hypothyroidism: from paracelsus to molecular diagnosis. *Clin Biochem.* 2006;39:511–518.

Fisher DA. Thyroid function and dysfunction in premature infants. *Pediatr Endocrinol Rev.* 2007;4:317–328.

Olney RS, Grosse SD, Vogt RF Jr. Prevalence of congenital hypothyroidism: current trends and future directions. *Pediatrics.* 2010;125:S31–S36.

Rose SR. Thyroid disorders. In: Martin RJ, Fanaroff AA, Walsh MC, eds. *Fanaroff and Martin's Neonatal-Perinatal Medicine.* 9th ed. St. Louis, MO: Mosby; 2011:1556–1583.

141 TORCH Infections

TORCH is an acronym that denotes a chronic nonbacterial perinatal infection. It stands for *t*oxoplasmosis, *o*ther infections, *r*ubella virus, *c*ytomegalovirus (CMV), and *h*erpes simplex virus (HSV). "Other" infections include syphilis, hepatitis B, coxsackievirus, Epstein-Barr virus, varicella-zoster virus (VZV), enteroviruses, human immunodeficiency virus (HIV), tuberculosis, and parvovirus B-19. Herpetic disease in the neonate does not fit the pattern of chronic intrauterine infection but is traditionally grouped with the others. This group of infections may present in the neonate with similar clinical and laboratory findings (ie, small for gestational age, hepatosplenomegaly, rash, central nervous system [CNS] manifestations, early jaundice, and low platelets), hence the usefulness of the TORCH concept. However, because the "other infections" category of responsible pathogens is growing and becoming diverse, the validity of indiscriminate screening of neonates presenting with findings compatible with congenital infection using "TORCH titers" has been questioned. Additionally, some of this serological testing yields both false-positive and false-negative results. An alternative approach involves testing of infants with suspected congenital infections for specific pathogens based on their clinical presentation (see Table 141–1 and individual chapters on each pathogen). A high index of suspicion for congenital infection and awareness of the prominent features of the most common congenital infections help to facilitate early diagnosis and possible therapy. Clinicians are getting away from the acronym TORCH; therefore, each of these chapters has been separated and listed as a single chapter. See Chapter 142 for toxoplasmosis, Chapter 128 for rubella, Chapter 90 for cytomegalovirus, Chapter 96 for herpes simplex viruses, and other disease-specific chapters. See Appendix F for isolation precautions for all infectious diseases, including maternal and neonatal precautions, breast-feeding, and visiting issues.

Table 141–1. SIGNS SUGGESTIVE OF A SPECIFIC CONGENITAL INFECTION IN THE NEONATE

Toxoplasmosis	Intracranial calcifications (diffuse), hydrocephalus, chorioretinitis
Syphilis	Snuffles, maculopapular rash (on palms and soles), skeletal abnormalities (osteochondritis and periostitis)
Rubella	Blueberry muffin lesions, eye findings (cataracts, congenital glaucoma, pigmentary retinopathy), congenital heart disease (most commonly patent ductus arteriosus), radiolucent bone disease
Cytomegalovirus	Periventricular intracranial calcifications, microcephaly
Herpes simplex virus	Mucocutaneous vesicles or scarring, conjunctivitis or keratoconjunctivitis, elevated liver transaminases

142 Toxoplasmosis

I. **Definition.** Toxoplasmosis is caused by *Toxoplasma gondii*, an intracellular parasitic protozoan capable of causing intrauterine infection.
II. **Incidence.** The incidence of congenital infection is 1–10 per 10,000 live births. An estimated number of 400–4000 cases of congenital toxoplasmosis occur each year in the United States. Serologic surveys demonstrate that worldwide exposure to *T. gondii* is high (30% in the United States and 50–80% in Europe).

III. **Pathophysiology.** *T. gondii* is a coccidian parasite ubiquitous in nature. Members of the feline family are definitive hosts. The organism exists in 3 forms: **oocyst, tachyzoite,** and **tissue cyst** (bradyzoites). Cats generally acquire the infection by feeding on infected animals such as mice or uncooked household meats. The parasite replicates sexually in the feline intestine. Cats may begin to excrete **oocysts** in their stool for 7–14 days after infection. During this phase, the cat can shed millions of oocysts daily for 2 weeks. After excretion, oocysts require a maturation phase (sporulation) of 24–48 hours before they become infective by oral route. Intermediate hosts (sheep, cattle, and pigs) can have tissue cysts within organs and skeletal muscle. These cysts can remain viable for the lifetime of the host. The pregnant woman usually becomes infected by consumption of raw or undercooked meat that contains cysts or by the accidental ingestion of sporulated oocysts from soil or contaminated food. Ingestion of oocysts (and cysts) releases sporozoites that penetrate the gastrointestinal mucosa and later differentiate into **tachyzoites.** Tachyzoites are ovoid unicellular organisms characteristic of the acute infection. Tachyzoites spread throughout the body via the bloodstream and lymphatics. It is during this stage that vertical transmission from mother to the fetus occurs. In the immunocompetent host, the tachyzoites are sequestered in **tissue cysts** and form bradyzoites. Bradyzoites are indicative of the chronic stage of infection and can persist in the brain, liver, and skeletal tissue for the life of the individual. There are reports of transmission of toxoplasmosis through contaminated municipal water, blood transfusion, organ donation, and occasionally as a result of a laboratory accident.

Acute infection in the adult is often **subclinical** (90% of the cases). If symptoms are present, they are generally nonspecific: mononucleosis-like illness with fever, painless lymphadenopathy, fatigue, malaise, myalgia, fever, skin rash, and splenomegaly. The vast majority of congenital toxoplasmosis cases are a result of acquired maternal primary infection during pregnancy; however, toxoplasmic reactivations can occur in immunosuppressed pregnant women and result in fetal infection. Approximately 84% of women of childbearing age in the United States are seronegative and thereby are at risk to acquire *T. gondii* infection during gestation. Placental infection occurs and persists throughout pregnancy. The infection may or may not be transmitted to the fetus. The later in pregnancy that infection is acquired, the more likely is transmission to the fetus (**first trimester, 17%; second trimester, 25%; and third trimester, 65% transmission**). Infections transmitted earlier in gestation are likely to cause more severe fetal effects (abortion, stillbirth, or severe disease with teratogenesis). Those transmitted later are more likely to be subclinical. Infection in the fetus or neonate usually involves the central nervous system (CNS) or the eyes with or without disseminated systemic infection. Approximately 70–90% of infants with congenital infection are asymptomatic at birth; however, visual impairment, learning disabilities, or mental impairment becomes apparent in a large percentage of children months to several years later.

IV. **Risk factors.** Several epidemiologic studies have identified some risk factors for acquiring toxoplasmosis during pregnancy. These risk factors include eating or contact with raw or undercooked meat, cleaning the cat litter box, eating unwashed raw vegetables or fruits, exposure to soil, and travel outside the United States, Europe, or Canada. Interestingly, cat ownership by itself is not linked to toxoplasmosis (except having ≥3 kittens). One study found that eating raw oysters, clams, or mussels was a novel risk factor for acquiring toxoplasmosis. Premature infants have a higher incidence of congenital toxoplasmosis than term infants (25–50% of cases in most series).

V. **Clinical presentation.** Congenital toxoplasmosis may be subclinical (identified only during screening) or may manifest as clinical neonatal disease, disease in the first few months of life, or as late sequelae or relapsed infection. Subclinical disease occurs in the majority of cases.

A. **Antenatal detection.** Fetuses that are infected early in pregnancy may become symptomatic in utero with abnormalities detected on fetal ultrasound. These include intracranial hyperechogenic foci or calcifications and ventricular dilatation. Other abnormalities include anemia, hydrops, and ascites.

B. **Subclinical neonatal infection.** Occurs in 70–90% of infected newborns, where no manifestations are found on routine physical examination. These infants are typically identified by routine maternal or newborn screening. When more specific tests are performed (eg, cerebrospinal fluid [CSF] tap, CNS imaging, and retinal eye examinations), up to 40% have abnormalities such as macular retinal scars, focal cerebral calcifications, and elevations of CSF protein and mononuclear cell count.

Infants born to mothers known to be infected with both human immunodeficiency virus and *T. gondii* should be tested for congenital toxoplasmosis. There is an increased risk for intrauterine reinfection after maternal reactivated *T. gondii* disease (see National Collaborative Chicago Based Congenital Toxoplasmosis Study: http://www.uchospitals.edu/specialties/infectious-diseases/toxoplasmosis/).

C. **Clinical neonatal disease.** Those with evident clinical disease may have disseminated illness or isolated CNS or ocular disease. Late sequelae are primarily related to ocular or CNS disease. **Obstructive hydrocephalus, chorioretinitis, and diffuse intracranial calcifications** form the **classic triad** of toxoplasmosis, which is found in <10% of the cases. **Prominent features** in **symptomatic** infants include chorioretinitis, abnormalities of CSF (high protein), anemia, seizures, intracranial calcifications, direct hyperbilirubinemia, fever, hepatosplenomegaly, lymphadenopathy, hydrocephalus, eosinophilia, bleeding diathesis, hypothermia, rash, and pneumonitis. Some of these symptoms may develop in the first few months of life.

D. **Late manifestations.** May develop in congenitally infected infants, especially in those who do not receive extended antiparasitic therapy. **Chorioretinitis** is the most common late manifestation. The lifetime incidence for the untreated infants approaches 90%, and the risk extends into adulthood. Treated patients may have episodic recurrences of chorioretinitis. Associated ophthalmologic findings may include microphthalmia, strabismus, cataract, glaucoma, and nystagmus. These complications can lead to vision loss and retinal detachment. Other late CNS manifestations include microcephaly, seizures, motor and cerebellar dysfunction, mental retardation, and sensorineural hearing loss. In addition, toxoplasmosis is associated with other systemic sequelae such as congenital nephrosis, various endocrinopathies (secondary to hypothalamic or pituitary effects), and myocarditis.

VI. **Diagnosis.** Congenital toxoplasmosis should be suspected in infants born to mothers who had primary infection during pregnancy, infants born to women who are immunosuppressed, infants who have suggestive clinical findings, and infants who test positive (toxoplasma IgM) through universal newborn screening (in regions where it is done). Infants suspected of the disease should undergo detailed evaluation that includes eye examination, CNS imaging, spinal tap, and detailed laboratory evaluation.

A. **Laboratory studies.** The maternal diagnosis of toxoplasmosis during pregnancy is primarily made by the use of serologic tests. Polymerase chain reaction (PCR) assay of body fluids (eg, amniotic fluid) is valuable for confirming the diagnosis of toxoplasmosis. Presence or absence of symptoms or a detailed epidemiologic history suggesting exposures to *T. gondii* are not useful tools for deciding whether laboratory testing should be performed. The diagnosis of congenital toxoplasmosis in the newborn is most often based on clinical suspicion plus serologic tests. However, most cases of neonatal disease are asymptomatic and, therefore, without a screening test, will be missed. Many hospital-based and commercial laboratories' serologic tests are inaccurate and frequently misinterpreted.

Therefore, establishing the diagnosis of congenital toxoplasmosis can be challenging. This is particularly true of the indirect fluorescence test for immunoglobulin IgG and IgM antibodies and of enzyme-linked immunosorbent assay (ELISA) systems for quantitation of IgM-specific antibodies. In 1997, a Food and Drug Administration warning was issued about the misinterpretation of IgM serologies. **The recommendation is that all IgM-positive results be confirmed by a toxoplasma reference laboratory** such as the Palo Alto Medical Foundation (PAMF-TSL; **http://www.pamf.org/serology**).

1. **Direct isolation of the organism from body fluids or tissues** requires inoculating blood, body fluids, or placental tissue into mice or tissue culture and is not readily available. Isolation of the organism from placental tissue correlates strongly with fetal infection.

2. **Serologic tests.** Tests with toxoplasma-specific IgG and IgM are usually done through commercial labs. IgG peaks at 1–2 months after infection and is positive indefinitely. IgM is positive within 1–2 weeks of infection and persists for months or years, especially when very sensitive assays are used. Negative results in IgG and IgM tests indicate that the patient has not been exposed. If IgG is positive and IgM is negative, it usually indicates past exposure without current active infection.

   Rarely, IgM titers can normalize if the infection happened early in the first trimester and the test was not done until late in the third trimester of pregnancy. If IgM is positive, it may indicate acute infection, especially if titers are high (needs confirmation with multiple markers [IgM, IgA, IgE] by reference lab). A toxoplasma serologic profile (TSP), which consists of the dye test, IgM ELISA, IgA ELISA, IgE ELISA, and AC/HS (differential agglutination) test is commonly used. The TSP has been successfully used at the PAMF-TSL to establish whether a pregnant woman has been infected with the parasite. Researchers at PAMF-TSL have shown the ability to decrease the rate of unnecessary abortions by ~50% among women with initial positive IgM done by outside laboratories. Sometimes, when IgM results are equivocal, more specialized tests such as the IgG avidity test are used to help discriminate between past and recently acquired infection.

3. **Perinatal diagnosis** can be made by PCR amplification of *T. gondii* DNA in a sample of amniotic fluid. Cordocentesis has been largely abandoned (higher risk for fetal injury and lower yield for diagnosis of congenital infection compared with amniotic PCR). Because IgM and IgA antibodies do not cross the placenta, they form the basis of serodiagnosis of congenital infection in the live newborn. Toxoplasma-specific IgM and IgA should be done in a reference laboratory as discussed earlier. **PCR and *T. gondii*-specific immunoperoxidase** staining can be attempted in virtually any body fluid or tissue, depending on the clinical scenario. Specimens on which PCR can be performed include vitreous fluid, aqueous humor, CSF, bronchoalveolar lavage fluid, peritoneal fluid, pleural fluid, peripheral blood, amniotic fluid, bone marrow, and urine. **A positive test result for presence of *T. gondii* DNA in any body fluid is diagnostic of toxoplasmosis.**

4. **CSF examination** should be performed in suspected cases. The most characteristic abnormalities are xanthochromia, mononuclear pleocytosis, and a very high protein level (sometimes >1 g/L). Tests for PCR and CSF IgM to toxoplasmosis should also be performed.

B. **Imaging and other studies**

1. **A cranial ultrasonogram or computed tomography (CT) of the head** may demonstrate characteristic diffuse intracranial calcifications (speckled throughout the CNS, including the meninges), hydrocephalus, and/or brain atrophy. **CT is the radiologic technique of choice**, because it is the most sensitive for calcifications.

2. **Long-bone films** may show abnormalities, specifically metaphyseal lucency and irregularity of the line of calcification at the epiphyseal plates without periosteal reaction.

3. **Ophthalmologic examination** characteristically shows chorioretinitis.

VII. **Management.** **Congenital toxoplasmosis** is a treatable infection, although at present it is not curable. Therapeutic agents are effective in killing the tachyzoite phase of the parasite but are not capable of eradicating encysted bradyzoites.

A. **Treatment.** Antiparasitic therapy is indicated for infants in whom a diagnosis of congenital toxoplasmosis is confirmed or probable based on serology, PCR, or clinical symptoms. The typical course consists of **sulfadiazine** (50 mg/kg, twice daily), **pyrimethamine** (2 mg/kg/d for 2 days, then 1 mg/kg/d for 2–6 months, then 1 mg/kg/d 3 times a week), and **folinic acid** (10 mg, 3 times weekly) for a minimum of 12 months. Serial follow-up to gauge the response of the infant to therapy should include neuroradiology, ophthalmologic examinations, and CSF analysis if indicated. A follow-up study of a cohort of 120 children with severe congenital *T. gondii* infection found an improved outcome in children receiving 1 year of treatment with sulfadiazine and pyrimethamine compared with historical controls. Most experts recommend adding corticosteroids in the form of **prednisone** (1 mg/kg/d in 2 divided doses) when CSF protein is >1g/dL and when active chorioretinitis threatens vision. Prednisone is continued until resolution of CSF protein elevation and active chorioretinitis. Infants treated with pyrimethamine and sulfadiazine require weekly blood counts (including platelets) and urine microscopy to detect any adverse drug effects.

B. **Prevention.** **Primary prevention** should be done through education. Pregnant women should be counseled that toxoplasma infection can be prevented in large part by cooking meat to a safe temperature (152°F); peeling or thoroughly washing fruits and vegetables before eating; avoid drinking unfiltered water in any setting; cleaning cooking surfaces and utensils after they have contacted raw meat, poultry, seafood, or unwashed fruits or vegetables; avoiding changing cat litter or, if necessary, using gloves, then washing hands thoroughly; not feeding raw or undercooked meat to cats; and keeping cats inside to prevent acquisition of toxoplasma by eating infected prey.

C. **Secondary prevention.** Secondary prevention by serologic screening of the pregnant woman and the newborn infant is done in some countries but is not widely used in the United States. However, treatment of confirmed primary *T. gondii* infection in pregnant women, including women with HIV infection, is recommended. Appropriate specialists should be consulted for management. **Spiramycin** treatment during gestation is used in an attempt to decrease transmission of *T. gondii* from the mother to the fetus. Spiramycin treatment in pregnant women may reduce congenital transmission but does not treat the fetus if in utero infection has already occurred. Maternal therapy may decrease the severity of sequelae in the fetus once congenital toxoplasmosis has occurred. A recent European prospective cohort study showed prenatal maternal treatment to reduce the risk of postnatal death and serious neurologic sequelae by two-thirds. Spiramycin is available only as an investigational drug in the United States. The drug may be obtained from the manufacturer, at no cost, following the advice of PAMF-TSL and with authorization from the U.S. Food and Drug Administration. If fetal infection is confirmed at or after 18 weeks of gestation or if the mother acquires infection during the third trimester, consideration should be given to starting therapy with pyrimethamine and sulfadiazine.

VIII. **Prognosis.** Maternal toxoplasmosis acquired during the first and second trimesters is associated with stillbirth (35%) and perinatal death (7%). Infants with congenital toxoplasmosis have a mortality rate as high as 12% and are at risk for many other problems later in life (seizures, visual impairment, learning disabilities, deafness, mental retardation, and spasticity). Adults who were treated as infants for congenital toxoplasmosis appear to have reasonable quality of life and visual function.

Selected References

American Academy of Pediatrics. *Toxoplasma gondii* infections. In: Pickering LK, Baker CJ, Kimberlin DW, Long SS, eds. *Red Book: 2012 Report of the Committee on Infectious Diseases.* 29th ed. Elk Grove Village, IL: American Academy of Pediatrics; 2012:720–728.

Berger F, Goulet V, Le Strat Y, Desenclos JC. Toxoplasmosis among pregnant women in France: risk factors and change of prevalence between 1995 and 2003. *Rev Epidemiol Sante Publique.* 2009;57:241–248.

Berrébi A, Assouline C, Bessiéres MH, et al. Long-term outcome of children with congenital toxoplasmosis. *Am J Obstet Gynecol.* 2010;203:552.e1–6.

Cortina-Borja, M, Tan HK, Wallon M, et al. Prenatal treatment for serious neurological sequelae of congenital toxoplasmosis: an observational prospective cohort study. *PLoS Med.* 2010;7:pii: e1000351.

Jones JL, Dargelas V, Roberts J, Press C, Remington JS, Montoya JG. Risk factors for *Toxoplasma gondii* infection in the United States. *Clin Infect Dis.* 2009;49:878–884.

Remington J, McLeod R, Wilson CB, Desmonts G. Toxoplasmosis. In: Remington JS, Klein JO, Wilson CB, Nizet V, Maldonado Y, eds. *Infectious Diseases of the Fetus and Newborn Infant.* 7th ed. Philadelphia, PA: Elsevier Saunders; 2011:918–1041.

Sterkers Y, Ribot J, Albaba S, Issert E, Bastien P, Pratlong F. Diagnosis of congenital toxoplasmosis by polymerase chain reaction on neonatal peripheral blood. *Diagn Microbiol Infect Dis.* 2011;71:174–176.

Villena I, Ancelle T, Delmas C, et al. Congenital toxoplasmosis in France in 2007: first results from a national surveillance system. *Euro Surveill.* 2010;15:pii: 19600.

143 Transient Tachypnea of the Newborn

I. **Definition. Transient tachypnea of the newborn (TTN) is a benign self-limited respiratory distress syndrome of term and late preterm infants related to delayed clearance of lung liquid.** The distress appears shortly after birth and usually resolves within 3–5 days. **Synonymous terms** include wet lung, type II respiratory distress syndrome (type II RDS), transient respiratory distress syndrome, retained fetal lung liquid syndrome, and benign unexplained respiratory distress in the newborn.

II. **Incidence.** It is the most common perinatal respiratory disorder, responsible for 40% of respiratory distress after birth. Incidence varies in the literature from 4 to 11 cases per 1000 singleton live births.

III. **Pathophysiology.** A delayed resorption of liquid from the lungs is believed to be the central mechanism for TTN. The lung liquid inhibits gas exchange, leading to an increased work of breathing. Tachypnea develops to compensate for that. Hypoxia develops because of poorly ventilated alveoli. The following factors are involved:

   A. **Inactivated/immature amiloride-sensitive sodium channels.** During gestation the pulmonary epithelium actively secretes fluid and chloride into the air spaces. **During labor** a surge of fetal catecholamines (adrenaline, glucocorticoids) are released and the lung switches from active chloride and fluid secretion to active sodium absorption. However, when during labor sodium channels are inactivated or ineffective, this will result in a larger volume of lung liquid at birth, leading to a reduced postnatal respiratory function. Infants born by elective cesarean section have a higher risk of TTN as they are not exposed to the stress (catecholamines) during labor before birth.

Whatever mechanism is responsible for the liquid remaining in the lung, at birth the transpulmonary pressure created during inspiration is for a major part responsible for the direct lung aeration and clearance of lung liquid (seconds). The pressure moves the column of liquid distally toward the alveolus, where it is transferred passively through the membrane into the interstitium. Then the liquid in the interstitium is slowly absorbed by the lymph and blood vessels (hours), leading to temporarily positive pressure in the interstitium. The role of the activated Na transport from alveolus to interstitium after birth is to prevent the liquid from going back into the alveolus as a consequence of the positive pressure in the interstitium. When the sodium channels are immature or ineffective, liquid will fill the air spaces, leading to a decrease in compliance and diffusion problems, and respiratory distress will occur.

B. **Uterine contractions.** Infants delivered by elective cesarean miss the lung liquid efflux via the trachea by high transpulmonary pressures caused by uterine contractions. Infants delivered by cesarean and breech deliveries miss the fetal trunk flexion when the head first goes through the birth canal, which increases abdominal pressure, elevates the diaphragm, and increases transpulmonary pressure, thereby forcing liquid out via the nose and mouth.

C. **Pulmonary immaturity.** One study noted that a mild degree of pulmonary immaturity is a central factor in the cause of TTN. The authors found a mature lecithin-sphingomyelin (L-S) ratio but negative phosphatidylglycerol (the presence of phosphatidylglycerol indicates completed lung maturation) in infants with TTN. Infants who were closer to 36 weeks' gestation than to 38 weeks had an increased risk of TTN. One study demonstrated that a relative surfactant deficiency may play a role in prolonged TTN. Surfactant deficiency leads to an increased surface tension and lowers the compliance of the lung. A layer of surfactant also plays a role in preventing lung liquid from going back to the alveoli.

D. **Genetic predisposition.** Because of familial clustering of some cases, there is speculation that there may be a genetic predisposition.
   1. Some propose that there may be a genetic predisposition for β-adrenergic hyporesponsiveness, and this plays a role in TTN.
   2. Studies have also revealed that polymorphisms in the β-adrenergic receptor (ADRB)-encoding genes, β 1 Gly 49 homozygosity and TACC haplotype of ADRB2 gene, may predispose to TTN.
   3. Maternal and fetal mutated alleles of the PROGINS progesterone receptor polymorphism reduce the risk for TTN.

IV. **Risk factors**
   A. **Cesarean delivery** (with or without labor). Labor prior to a cesarean delivery is not protective for TTN.
   B. **Male gender.**
   C. **Prematurity/late preterm.**
   D. **Macrosomia** (birthweight ≥4500 g).
   E. **Multiple gestations.**
   F. **Prolonged labor with long intervals.**
   G. **Negative amniotic fluid phosphatidylglycerol.**
   H. **Perinatal/birth asphyxia.**
   I. **Fluid overload in the mother,** especially with oxytocin infusion.
   J. **Family history of asthma** (especially history in the mother).
   K. **Breech delivery.**
   L. **Infant of a diabetic mother** (2–3 times more common). Reasons could be the increased rate of cesarean sections in this group or the decreased fluid clearance in the diabetic fetal lung.
   M. **Infant of drug-dependent mother** (narcotics).

N. Exposure to B-mimetic agents.

O. Precipitous delivery (rapid vaginal delivery)/absence of exposure to labor.

P. Urban location.

Q. Nulliparity.

R. History of infertility therapy.

S. Augmentation of labor/vacuum/forceps delivery.

T. Low Apgar score (<7) at 1 and 5 minutes. A low Apgar at 1 minute was associated the most with TTN.

U. Absence of premature rupture of membranes (PROM).

V. Increased risk of prolonged TTN/increased severity of TTN

A. Grunting, maximum respiratory rate >90/min, and an FIO_2 >0.40 within 6 hours of life were associated with an increase in prolonged TTN.

B. Peak respiratory rate in the first 36 hours of life >90/min caused a 7 times increased risk of prolonged tachypnea. This group with prolonged tachypnea had longer hospitalization and antibiotic treatment. The white blood cell count and hematocrit levels were lower in the group with prolonged tachypnea than the group with tachypnea that lasted <72 hours.

C. Absence of labor contractions or reduced labor duration is associated with a more severe course of TTN at term, requiring longer oxygen supplementation.

D. Long-distance land-based transport in neonates with TTN. They required increased respiratory support in the neonatal intensive care unit (NICU) and incidence of pulmonary air leak syndrome was higher.

VI. Clinical presentation. The infant is usually near term, term, or large and premature, and shortly after delivery has tachypnea (>60 breaths/min and can be up to 100–120 breaths/min) or within the first 6 hours of delivery. The infant may also have grunting, nasal flaring, rib retraction, and varying degrees of cyanosis (uncommon, usually mild and responsive to oxygen). The infant often appears to have the classic "barrel chest" secondary to the increased anteroposterior diameter (hyperinflation). One can hear crackles on auscultation. The liver and spleen are palpable because of the hyperinflation. There are usually no signs of sepsis. Some infants may have edema and a mild ileus on physical examination. One can also see tachycardia with usually a normal blood pressure. Neurologically normal and no signs of sepsis. **Some clinicians differentiate transitional delay, transient tachypnea, and prolonged tachypnea.**

A. Transitional delay. Tachypnea right after birth for usually <6 hours (but can be for 2–12 hours). Grunting can occur right after birth with transitional delay and usually subsides by 2 hours (93%). Transitional delay usually subsides within 6 hours and infants are able to feed orally.

B. Transient tachypnea of the newborn (TTN). Tachypnea that lasts from after birth usually <72 hours. It typically resolves by 12–24 hours. One study found that 74% of infants had resolution of their symptoms by 48 hours.

C. Prolonged tachypnea of the newborn (PTTN). Some infants have prolonged tachypnea, lasting >72 hours. Some have classified this as prolonged tachypnea of the newborn.

VII. Diagnosis. TTN is a clinical diagnosis. It is based on clinical and radiologic findings.

A. Laboratory studies

1. Prenatal testing. A mature L-S ratio with the presence of phosphatidylglycerol in the amniotic fluid may help rule out RDS.

2. Amniotic fluid sampling at delivery. **Amniotic lamellar body counts** can predict the occurrence of TTN. It is lower than controls and higher than in infants with RDS.

3. Postnatal testing

a. Arterial blood gas on room air shows some degree of mild to moderate hypoxemia. Partial carbon dioxide is usually normal because of the tachypnea.

Hypocarbia is usually present. Hypercarbia, if it exists, is usually mild (Pco$_2$ >55 mm Hg). A mild respiratory acidosis is seen, which can be a sign of fatigue and impending respiratory failure or complication such as a pneumothorax.

b. **Pulse oximetry** should be monitored continuously.

c. **Complete blood count (CBC) with differential** is normal in TTN but should be obtained if one is considering an infectious process. The hematocrit will also rule out polycythemia.

d. **Other promising tests. Plasma endothelin-1 levels** may be higher in RDS compared with those in TTN. This test may prove useful in differentiating RDS from TTN. **Interleukin-6 (IL-6)** may distinguish proven and clinical sepsis from TTN. This may make it possible to avoid antibiotics in this group of infants. **Serum atrial natriuretic peptide levels** were lower for infants with TTN than normal infants in one study.

B. **Imaging and other studies**

1. **Chest radiograph.** (See example in Figure 11–16A and B.) The chest radiograph is the diagnostic standard. The typical findings in TTN are as follows:

   a. **Hyperexpansion (hyperinflation)** of the lungs is a hallmark of TTN.

   b. **Prominent perihilar streaking** (secondary to engorgement of periarterial lymphatics). Engorgement of the lymphatic system with retained lung fluid and fluid in the fissures.

   c. **Mild to moderately cardiomegaly.**

   d. **Depression (flattening) of the diaphragm** is best seen on a lateral view of the chest.

   e. **Fluid in the minor fissure** and perhaps fluid in the pleural space (pleural effusions), laminar effusions.

   f. **Prominent pulmonary vascular markings.** "Fuzzy vessels," a sunburst pattern, peripheral air trapping resulting in increased lung volumes.

   g. **Air leaks** are rarely seen.

   h. There should be **no areas of consolidation.**

2. **Lung ultrasonography.** An ultrasound sign (**"double lung point"**) was found to be diagnostic of TTN. Lung ultrasound shows a difference in lung echogenicity between the upper and lower lung areas. It was also noted that very compact comet-tail artifacts in the inferior fields and not in the superior fields (the **"double lung point"**) was seen in infants **with TTN** and not seen in other lung pathology or in healthy infants.

C. **Other tests.** Any infant who is hypoxic on room air must have a **hyperoxia test** to rule out heart disease. This test is described on pages 606–608.

D. **Confirm the diagnosis.** TTN is often a **diagnosis of exclusion**, and other causes of tachypnea should be excluded first. There are many causes of tachypnea and usually the history, physical examination, and initial radiograph will help to narrow down the differential. If still uncertain, the clinical course can help guide you. **An infant who does not improve, who worsens, and whose radiograph pattern changes, not following the typical pattern, should alert you that the diagnosis may not be TTN.**

1. **Causes of tachypnea are extensive in the newborn.** Use the mnemonic **TRACHEA** to help remember some of the causes of tachypnea in a newborn: **T. transient tachypnea of the newborn; R, respiratory infections (pneumonia); A, aspiration syndromes (meconium, blood, or amniotic fluid); C, congenital malformations; H, hyaline membrane disease (now known as respiratory distress syndrome); E, edema; A, air leaks and acidosis.**

   a. **Respiratory infections (pneumonia)/sepsis.** If the infant has pneumonia/sepsis, the prenatal history usually suggests infection. There may be maternal chorioamnionitis, PROM, and fever. The blood cell count may show evidence of infection (neutropenia or leukocytosis with abnormal numbers of immature cells). The urine antigen test may be positive if the infant has group B streptococcal infection. Remember that it is best to give broad-spectrum antibiotics if there is any suspicion or evidence of infection. The antibiotics can always be discontinued if the cultures are negative in 48 hours.

b. **Sepsis.**

c. **Congenital cyanotic heart disease.** Infants with hypoplastic right and left heart syndromes, tetralogy of Fallot, and transposition of the great arteries can all present after birth. Usually these infants present with cyanosis with few respiratory symptoms. Cardiomegaly may be seen on chest x-ray. The hyperoxia test should be done to rule out heart disease (see pages 606–608). An echocardiogram should also be done if cyanotic heart disease is suspected.

d. **Respiratory distress syndrome (RDS).** (See also Chapter 124.) The infant is normally premature (<34 weeks) or has some reason for delayed lung maturation, such as maternal diabetes. The infant presents with respiratory distress after birth that continues to worsen. The chest radiograph is helpful because it shows the typical RDS reticulogranular pattern with air bronchograms and underexpansion (atelectasis) of the lungs.

e. **Aspiration syndromes (meconium, blood, or amniotic fluid).** Infants with meconium aspiration syndrome (most common syndrome) are usually fully or post mature. Blood and amniotic fluid can also be aspirated. All of these aspiration syndromes can present at birth or several hours after birth. Infants usually have more severe respiratory distress than in TTN. The x-ray can be similar to that in TTN but usually has perihilar infiltrates/opacities. TTN can have patchy opacities from fluid in the alveoli. Infants usually require more oxygen and have increased tachypnea and retractions. The blood gases usually show more hypoxemia, hypercapnia, and acidosis. These infants can progress and develop pulmonary hypertension.

f. **Cerebral hyperventilation.** This disorder is seen when central nervous system (CNS) lesions (eg, subarachnoid hemorrhage, meningitis, hypoxic ischemic encephalopathy) cause overstimulation of the respiratory center, resulting in tachypnea. Arterial blood gas measurements show respiratory alkalosis. Chest x-ray may show cardiomegaly, normal lungs.

g. **Metabolic disorders.** Infants with hypothermia, hyperthermia, or hypoglycemia may have tachypnea.

h. **Polycythemia and hyperviscosity.** This syndrome may present with tachypnea with or without cyanosis.

i. **Congenital malformations.** (Congenital diaphragmatic hernia, cystic adenomatoid malformations.) These can present with respiratory distress. A chest x-ray will help make the diagnosis.

j. **Pulmonary hypertension.**

k. **Pulmonary edema.** Secondary to patent ductus arteriosus (PDA) (left-to-right shunt with failure, anomalous venous drainage).

l. **Air leaks (pneumothorax, pneumomediastinum).** A chest x-ray is diagnostic.

m. **Primary pulmonary hypoplasia.** This can cause persistent tachypnea.

n. **Metabolic acidosis.**

VIII. **Management**

A. **Preventive**

1. An elective cesarean section (CS) scheduled at a gestational age (GA) of 39 weeks or later may decrease the frequency of TTN. Labor prior to CS did not prevent TTN. Vaginal birth appears to be protective against TTN (even after 37 weeks of gestation).

2. **Establish fetal maturity** prior to elective CS.

3. **Antenatal betamethasone prior to elective CS at term** reduced the incidence of respiratory morbidity in infants (reduced TTN from 4% of elective CS to 2.1%). The steroids encourage the expression of the epithelial channel gene and allow the lung to switch from fluid secretion to fluid absorption. It induces lung Na^+ reabsorption by increasing the number and activity of channels even in hypoxia. Also, antenatal glucocorticoids induce maturation of the surfactant system.

4. **Prevent low Apgar scores.** A low Apgar score <1 minute is strongly associated with TTN. Improved obstetric surveillance may decrease low Apgar scores.

B. **General.** Management is supportive.

1. **Oxygenation.** Initial management consists of providing adequate oxygenation. Start with extra **oxygen via hood or nasal cannula** and deliver enough to maintain normal arterial saturation. If there is increased work of breathing and oxygen need >30%, then **nasal continuous positive airway pressure** (NCPAP) is an effective alternative treatment. CPAP gives a continuous positive pressure on the airways, helping to oppose the reentry of liquid and maintaining functional residual capacity. **Intubation** criteria vary per center, but we intubate when oxygen need is >40% when on a CPAP of 8 cm H_2O. Other diseases should be considered, but administration of exogenous surfactant promotes a dramatic clinical response in infants with TTN needing intubation and mechanical ventilation, underlining the role of surfactant deficiency in severe TTN.

2. **Maintain a neutral thermal environment.**

3. **Antibiotics.** Most infants are initially treated with broad-spectrum antibiotics (usually ampicillin and gentamicin) for 48 hours until the diagnosis of sepsis or pneumonia is excluded (*controversial*). In a randomized controlled trial of restrictive fluid management in TTN, all 73 infants with TTN were not treated with antibiotics and none of the infants manifested neonatal pneumonia or bacteremia.

4. **Feeding.** Because of the risk of aspiration, an infant should not be fed by mouth if the respiratory rate is >60 breaths/min. If the respiratory rate is <60 breaths/min, oral feeding is permissible. If the rate is 60–80 breaths/min, feeding should be by nasogastric tube. If the rate is >80 breaths/min, IV nutrition is indicated.

5. **Fluid and electrolytes.** Should be monitored and hydration maintained. Fluid management is *controversial*. A small randomized trial in restrictive fluid management in infants with severe TTN showed a reduced duration of respiratory support and hospitalization cost. However, the control group in this trial received a more liberal fluid intake than currently recommended, and although significant, the differences were small.

6. **Diuretics are not recommended.** Diuretics have been used in practice in some centers with the rationale of accelerating lung liquid absorption with an immediate diuresis-independent lung liquid resorption and a delayed increase in urine output. Furosemide also causes pulmonary vasodilatation, leading to an improved ventilation/perfusion (V/P) match. However, trials investigating the oral or aerosolized administration of furosemide in infants with TTN have shown no differences in the course of disease.

7. **Inhaled epinephrine.** Infants with TTN have low levels of epinephrine, and epinephrine helps to mediate fetal lung fluid absorption. However, inhaled racemic epinephrine did not increase the rate of resolution of tachypnea in one study.

8. **β_2-Agonist salbutamol.** Stimulation of β-adrenergic receptors with salbutamol upregulates the activity of the sodium channels. A small randomized controlled trial in aerosolized salbutamol versus saline in infants with TTN showed significant improvement in clinical and laboratory findings. Larger studies are needed before this can be recommended as standard therapy.

IX. Prognosis
   A. TTN is usually self-limited and usually lasts only 2–5 days.
   B. Asthma/wheezing syndromes. Asthma is a multifactorial disease. Recent studies
      have revealed that TTN is associated with the development of wheezing syndromes
      (bronchiolitis, acute bronchitis, chronic bronchitis, asthma, or prescription for
      asthma medication) in early childhood and subsequent diagnosis of childhood
      asthma. The risk of TTN is increased in babies born to mothers with asthma. In one
      study the risk was found to be greatest in males of nonwhite race whose mothers
      lived at an urban address and did not have asthma. Some believe TTN may be a
      marker for deficient pulmonary function, increasing the (inherited) susceptibility
      to the development of asthma. Liem et al proposed that environmental and genetic
      interactions predispose these infants to asthma.
   C. Complications (rare). **If these occur, it is best to reevaluate the infant.**
      1. Some infants can develop prolonged tachypnea (>72 hours) and can progress
         to respiratory failure (hypoxia, respiratory fatigue with acidosis) and require
         intubation and mechanical ventilation.
      2. It is very rare, but a few infants may develop air leaks (usually a pneumothorax
         or pneumomediastinum). There is a higher risk of air leak if the infant is
         on CPAP. Familial neonatal pneumothorax has been associated with TTN in
         siblings of 2 families.
      3. Some may develop pulmonary hypertension with right-to-left shunting across
         the ductus arteriosus or foramen ovale. This may be present because of possible
         elevation in the pulmonary vascular resistance associated with retained fetal
         lung fluid and hyperinflation of the lungs and require extracorporeal membrane
         oxygenation/extracorporeal life support (ECMO/ECLS). (See Chapter 120.)

Selected References

Armangil D, Yurdaköök M, Korkmaz A, Yiğit S, Tekinalp G. Inhaled beta-2 agonist salbutamol
   for the treatment of transient tachypnea of the newborn. *J Pediatr.* 2011;159:398–403.

Copetti R, Cattarossi L. The 'double lung point': an ultrasound sign diagnostic of transient
   tachypnea of the newborn. *Neonatology.* 2007;91(3):203–209.

Hooper SB, te Pas AB, Lewis RA, Morley CJ. Establishing functional residual capacity at birth.
   NeoReviews. 2010;9:e1–e8.

Kao B, Stewart de Ramirez SA, Belfort MB, Hansen A. Inhaled epinephrine for the treatment
   of transient tachypnea of the newborn. *J Perinatol.* 2008;28(3):205–210.

Levine EM, Ghai V, Barton JJ, Strom CM. Mode of delivery and risk of respiratory diseases in
   newborns. *Obstet Gynecol.* 2001;97:439.

Liem JJ, Huq SI, Ekuma O, Becker AB, Kozyrskyj AL. Transient tachypnea of the newborn
   may be an early clinical Manifestation of wheezing symptoms. *J Pediatr.* 2007;151:
   29–33.

Machado LU, Fiori HH, Baldisserotto M, et al. Surfactant deficiency in transient tachypnea of
   the newborn. *J Pediatr.* 2011;159(5):750–754.

Miller MJ, Fanaroff AA, Martin RJ. Respiratory disorders in preterm and term infants. In: Fanaroff AA, Martin RJ, eds. *Neonatal-Perinatal Medicine: Diseases of the Fetus and Infant.*
   7th ed. St. Louis, MO: Mosby; 2002.

Newman B. Neonatal imaging. *Radiol Clin North Am.* 1999;37:1049.

Schatz M, Zeiger RS, Hoffman CP, Saunders BS, Harden KM, Forsythe AB. Increased transient tachypnea of the newborn in infants of asthmatic mothers. *Am J Dis Child.* 1991;
   145:156.

Stroustrup A, Trasande L, Holzman IR. Randomized controlled trial of restrictive fluid management in transient tachypnea of the newborn. *J Pediatr.* 2012;160(1):38–43; e1.

144 Tuberculosis

I. **Definition.** Tuberculosis (TB) is an infection caused by the organism *Mycobacterium tuberculosis.* TB is a global disease that has important implications for affected neonates who can acquire the disease in either the postnatal period or, more rarely, through congenital transmission from an infected mother.

II. **Incidence.** The World Health Organization (WHO) estimates that there were 9.4 million incident and 14 million prevalent cases of TB in 2009. A total of 3.3 million (35%) of the new cases in 2009 occurred in women. The majority of incident cases in 2009 occurred in Asia (55%) and Africa (30%). An estimated 1.1 million (12%) of cases occurred in human immunodeficiency virus (HIV)–positive individuals. Approximately 1.7 million people died of TB in 2009. The Centers for Disease Control and Prevention (CDC) reports 11,545 incident cases of TB in the United States in 2009, with 59% of cases occurring in foreign-born individuals. Although the exact incidence of neonatal cases is unknown, <200 cases of congenital TB have been reported in the English literature.

III. **Pathophysiology.** *M. tuberculosis* is transmitted via inhalation of airborne droplet nuclei. Alveolar macrophages engulf *M. tuberculosis*, which then spreads through the lymphatic system to hilar lymph nodes. The infection can either be contained or lead to primary progressive TB. Granulomas containing the mycobacterium form via cell-mediated immunity within 2–8 weeks in most individuals. Infected macrophages interact with T lymphocytes to release cytokines that promote phagocytosis of *M. tuberculosis* and granuloma formation. Children under the age of 5 years and immunosuppressed individuals lack host immunity and therefore develop active primary progressive disease in the lung parenchyma and hilar lymph nodes. In these individuals, the characteristic fibrous granuloma capsule is disrupted, and liquefactive necrosis of the central caseous material occurs. The necrotic material can then flow into adjacent vasculature and disseminate systemically or to adjacent bronchi and spread externally via respiratory droplets. Immunosuppression and malnutrition are risk factors for reactivation of latent infection.

Vertical transmission to the fetus can occur hematogenously or transplacentally. Hematogenous spread results in lesions in the liver and periportal lymph nodes or lungs. The increase in oxygenation and circulation in the postnatal period activate the replication of the bacilli. *M. tuberculosis* has been identified in amniotic fluid, and transmission of TB can occur via aspiration of infected fluid.

IV. **Risk factors.** The highest risk of transmission to newborns occurs via respiratory transmission from untreated mothers during the postnatal period. Maternal extrapulmonary TB, such as miliary TB or tuberculous endometritis, increases the risk of congenital infection. Maternal treatment for 2–3 weeks in the antenatal period reduces the risk of postnatal infection. HIV is a risk factor for maternal TB, which in turn increases the risk of mother to child transmission of HIV. Living in endemic areas or crowded conditions also increases the risk of TB.

V. **Clinical presentation**
   A. **Pregnancy.** Pregnant women with TB tend to have fewer of the typical symptoms associated with TB. Active TB symptoms and signs include fever, cough, night sweats, anorexia, weight loss, general malaise, and weakness. Extrapulmonary TB can affect the genitourinary tract, bones and joints, meninges, lymph nodes, pleural lining, and peritoneum. Extrapulmonary TB is more common when there is coinfection with HIV. The natural history of TB is thought to be unaffected by pregnancy. Maternal TB, especially extrapulmonary disease, does increase pregnancy and perinatal complications such as preeclampsia, vaginal bleeding, early pregnancy loss, preterm labor, and low birthweight.

B. **Neonatal period.** Neonates with congenital infection can present with symptoms at any time from birth up to 4 months of age but usually present by the second or third week of life. As neonates tend to present with atypical signs, the diagnosis of TB must be considered in the differential diagnosis of other congenital infections (eg, syphilis, cytomegalovirus, toxoplasmosis) or neonatal sepsis. Congenital TB can present with hepatosplenomegaly, respiratory distress, fever, lymphadenopathy, abdominal distention, lethargy or irritability, ear discharge, and papular skin lesions. Less common symptoms and signs include vomiting, apnea, cyanosis, jaundice, seizures, and petechiae. The clinical presentation of infants <3 months with either congenital or postnatal acquired TB include respiratory signs such as cough, wheezing, tachypnea, stridor, and crepitations and are thought to result from obstruction of bronchi by enlarged hilar lymph nodes. Other signs include failure to thrive, hepatosplenomegaly, prolonged jaundice, meningitis, and cervical lymphadenopathy. Young infants are at increased risk for disseminated or miliary TB due to their immature immune systems. They are also at increased risk for meningeal presentations including meningoencephalitis, basal arachnoiditis, and intracranial tuberculomas. TB of the spine (Pott disease) has also been described in congenital infection. Clinical signs of congenital or postnatally acquired TB are typically occult and delayed in presentation because of the immaturity of the newborn and infant immune system. Only *M. tuberculosis* meningitis is known to present clinically as early as 2 weeks of age.

VI. **Diagnosis**
   A. **Clinical criteria.** Congenital infection is diagnosed if the infant has the primary criteria and meets one of the secondary criteria for congenital TB (also known as Cantwell's criteria). Otherwise, postnatally acquired TB is diagnosed on the basis of known exposure and a proven tuberculous lesion as per Cantwell's secondary criteria.
      1. **Primary criteria.** The infant must have proven tuberculous lesions.
      2. **Secondary criteria**
         a. **Lesions in the first week of life.**
         b. **A primary hepatic complex** or caseating hepatic granulomas.
         c. **Tuberculous infection of the placenta** or the maternal genital tract.
         d. **Exclusion of the possibility of postnatal transmission** by a thorough investigation of contacts, including the infant's hospital attendants, and by adherence to existing recommendations for treating infants exposed to tuberculosis.
   B. **Acid-fast bacillus (AFB) smear and culture.** *M. tuberculosis* can be identified by culture from the following specimens: gastric aspirates, sputum, bronchial washings, pleural fluid, cerebrospinal fluid (CSF), urine, or other body fluids. A biopsy specimen can also be obtained from lymph node, pleura, mesentery, liver, bone marrow, or other tissues. **The best specimen in neonates and infants who may have an absent or nonproductive cough is an early-morning gastric aspirate, obtained by a nasogastric tube before feeding.** Aspirates should be collected on 3 separate days. Gastric aspirates usually yield negative AFB smears, with an overall diagnostic yield of <50%. Fluorescent staining methods increase the sensitivity of gastric aspirates. The presence of nontuberculous mycobacteria can result in a false-positive smear. Liquid media culture facilitates growth of *M. tuberculosis*, which can take between 3 and 6 weeks to grow.
   C. **Polymerase chain reaction (PCR).** PCR assays are currently available for AFB-positive respiratory tract specimens as well as any respiratory tract specimen, but they have low sensitivity with gastric aspirates, CSF, and tissue specimens. False-positive and false-negative results have also been reported.
   D. **Tuberculin skin testing (TST).** **A negative TST result should be considered unreliable in infants <3 months of age.** The definition of a positive Mantoux skin test is as follows:

1. Reaction ≥5 mm
   a. Infants in close contact with known or suspected infectious cases of TB
   b. Infants suspected to have TB disease based on clinical evidence or abnormal chest radiograph
   c. Infants with an immunosuppressive condition, including HIV or receiving immunosuppressive therapy
2. Reaction ≥10 mm
   a. Age <4 years
   b. Medical risk factors such as chronic renal failure or malnutrition
   c. Increased environmental exposure
E. **Chest radiograph.** Although chest imaging may be normal early in the course of disease, most infants present with abnormal imaging findings, including miliary TB, multiple pulmonary nodules, lobar pneumonia, bronchopneumonia, interstitial pneumonia, and mediastinal adenopathy. The upper lobes and posterior lung segments are thought to be the most common sites for TB in infants.
F. **Imaging.** Other imaging modalities include abdominal sonography for hepatic involvement and thoracic computed tomography (CT) for adenopathies. Central nervous system (CNS) imaging includes ultrasonography, CT, and magnetic resonance imaging (MRI).
G. **Laboratory markers.** Increased blood leukocyte count with neutrophil predominance and elevation of C-reactive protein has been reported in congenital TB due to the inflammatory response associated with *M. tuberculosis.* Thrombocytopenia has also been observed, although it is a nonspecific finding.
H. **CSF.** A lumbar puncture should promptly be performed when congenital or postnatally acquired TB is suspected. CSF findings can include lymphocytic pleocytosis, increased protein levels, and decreased CSF/serum glucose ratio.
I. **HIV testing.** All individuals with TB should be evaluated for HIV infection due to the increased incidence of TB coinfection.
J. **Placental pathology.** The placenta may demonstrate evidence of granulomas, and an AFB smear and culture should be sent from a specimen of suspected congenital tuberculosis.
VII. **Management**
A. **Antimicrobial therapy during pregnancy**
   1. **Latent infection.** The CDC recommends deferring treatment of pregnant women with latent infection until the postpartum period except in high-risk situations. Isoniazid therapy for 9 months should be considered for latent TB (positive TST and normal chest radiographic findings) in pregnant women with HIV, recent contagious contact, and skin test conversion within the prior 2 years. Pyridoxine supplementation should be administered for the duration of pregnancy and breast-feeding.
   2. **Active infection.** The CDC recommends an initial treatment regimen with isoniazid, rifampin, and ethambutol for 2 months, followed by isoniazid and rifampin for a total of 9 months. **Isoniazid, rifampin, and ethambutol are considered relatively safe for the fetus. Streptomycin should not be administered to the mother due to ototoxic effects in the fetus.** Although pyrazinamide is used in some regiments, its safety during pregnancy has not been established.
B. **Antimicrobial therapy during the neonatal period**
   1. **Active maternal and congenital or neonatal acquired infection.** In cases in which the maternal physical examination and chest radiographic findings are diagnostic of active TB, **the infant should be treated promptly with isoniazid, rifampin, pyrazinamide, and an aminoglycoside such as amikacin.** Pyridoxine supplementation in infants receiving isoniazid therapy is recommended in the following instances: exclusively breast-fed infants, malnourished infants, and those with symptomatic HIV infection. Hepatotoxic effects of isoniazid therapy are rare but can be life-threatening.

2. **Active maternal infection without congenital infection.** If the mother has active TB disease but the neonate is not affected, isoniazid should be given until 3 or 4 months of age. If a negative TST result is obtained at the end of therapy and the mother demonstrates successful response to therapy, the infant's isoniazid can be discontinued. A positive TST at 3–4 months of age necessitates a reevaluation for TB disease in the infant and continued isoniazid therapy for a total of 9 months with monthly evaluation.

3. **Latent maternal infection.** Neonatal evaluation and therapy are not required in cases where the mother is asymptomatic and is diagnosed with latent TB infection.

4. **Postnatal TB infection.** For infants with pulmonary disease, pulmonary disease with hilar adenopathy, and hilar adenopathy disease, a 6-month 4-drug regimen is recommended as follows: isoniazid, rifampin, pyrazinamide, and ethambutol for 2 months followed by isoniazid and rifampin for 4 months. The duration of therapy is extended to 9 months if there is evidence of cavitary pulmonary lesions or sputum culture remains positive after 2 months of therapy. The risks and benefits of using ethambutol in infants need to be considered due to a dose and duration dependent risk of optic neuritis. An infectious disease consultation is essential for managing infants who are coinfected with HIV due to drug interactions and overlapping drug toxicities, especially between antiretrovirals and rifampin.

5. **Extrapulmonary TB.** For tuberculous meningitis, treatment is initiated with isoniazid, rifampin, pyrazinamide, and ethambutol/aminoglycoside. Pyrazinamide is given for a total of 2 months, and isoniazid and rifampin are given for a total of 9–12 months. Ethambutol or aminoglycoside is discontinued after drug susceptibility is established. Corticosteroids should be added in confirmed cases of TB meningitis as they reduce mortality rates and long-term neurologic impairment. A regimen of isoniazid, rifampin, pyrazinamide, and streptomycin for 1–2 months, followed by isoniazid and rifampin for another 10 months, is recommended for skeletal and miliary TB. Corticosteroids can also be considered for pleural and pericardial effusions, severe miliary disease, endobronchial disease, and abdominal tuberculosis. Surgical therapy for lymphadenitis, bone and joint abscesses, and hydrocephalus complicating CNS disease may be indicated.

C. **Isolation precautions/breast-feeding**

1. **Maternal latent infection.** No separation or restrictions on breast-feeding are required.

2. **Maternal active disease.** In suspected or proven cases of maternal TB, the mother and infant should be separated pending evaluation and appropriate maternal and infant therapy. Separation is not necessary once the infant begins isoniazid; the mother adheres to treatment, wears a mask, and follows infection control measures. In cases of multidrug-resistant TB or maternal nonadherence to therapy, the infant should be separated, and bacille Calmette-Guerin (BCG) vaccine should be considered in consultation with an infectious disease specialist. Breast-feeding restrictions can be removed after the mother has been treated appropriately for ≥2 weeks and is not considered contagious.

D. **Hospital control measures.** Restriction to an airborne infection isolation room is indicated in the following cases: neonates with congenital or acquired TB undergoing manipulation of the oropharyngeal airway, infants with cavitary lesions, positive sputum AFB smears, and laryngeal or extensive pulmonary involvement. Nosocomial transmission from infants to health care workers and between infants via contaminated respiratory equipment has been reported.

E. **Prevention.** The BCG vaccine contains a live attenuated strain of *Mycobacterium bovis.* The WHO recommends that a single dose of BCG vaccine should be given to all infants soon after birth in countries with a high TB burden. BCG vaccine should not be given to symptomatic HIV-positive or immunosuppressed infants. If the neonate is exposed to smear-positive pulmonary TB shortly after birth, BCG vaccine should be delayed pending completion of isoniazid therapy. The CDC does not recommend routine use of BCG vaccine in the United States due to the low burden of disease and interference of the vaccine with TST reactivity.

VIII. **Prognosis.** Information on prognostic factors are not well defined for infants of either congenital or acquired disease. Survival rate is not influenced by the following factors: specific signs or symptoms, birthweight, the nature or severity of maternal disease, timing of maternal diagnosis, prematurity, hepatic dysfunction, or thrombocytopenia. An improved survival rate was seen in all infants with the following: presentation of symptoms after 3 weeks of age, no CNS TB disease, appropriate anti-TB therapy, higher leukocyte count, absence of a military pattern on chest radiographs, and multiple pulmonary nodules on chest radiograph.

Selected References

American Academy of Pediatrics. Tuberculosis. In: Pickering LK, Baker CJ, Kimberlin DW, Long SS, eds. *Red Book: 2012 Report of the Committee on Infectious Diseases*. 29th ed. Elk Grove Village, IL: American Academy of Pediatrics; 2012:736–759.

Cantwell MF, Shehab ZM, Costello AM, et al. Brief report: congenital tuberculosis. *N Engl J Med*. 1994;330:1051–1054.

Crockett M, King SM, Kitai I, et al. Nosocomial transmission of congenital tuberculosis in a neonatal intensive care unit. *Clin Infect Dis*. 2004;39:1719–1723.

Frieden TR, Sterling TR, Munsiff SS, Watt CJ, Dye C. Tuberculosis. *Lancet*. 2003;362:887–899.

Gupta A, Bhosale R, Kinikar A, et al. Maternal tuberculosis: a risk factor for mother-to-child transmission of human immunodeficiency virus. *J Infect Dis*. 2011;203:358–363.

Nhan Chang C, Jones TB. Tuberculosis in pregnancy. *Clin Obstet Gynecol*. 2010;53:311–321.

Peng W, Yang J, Liu E. Analysis of 170 cases of congenital TB reported in the literature between 1946 and 2009. *Pediatr Pulmonol*. 2011;46:1215–1224.

Skevaki CL, Kafetzis DA. Tuberculosis in neonates and infants: epidemiology, pathogenesis, clinical manifestations, diagnosis, and management issues. *Paediatr Drugs*. 2005;7:219–234.

World Health Organization. Global tuberculosis control: WHO report 2010. Geneva, Switzerland: WHO; 2010. http://www.who.int/tb/publications/global_report/en.

145 *Ureaplasma* Infection

I. **Definition.** *Ureaplasma* belongs to the Mycoplasmataceae family. These are small pleomorphic bacteria that characteristically lack a cell wall. The genus *Ureaplasma* contains 2 species capable of causing human infection, *U. urealyticum* and *U. parvum*.

II. **Incidence.** *Ureaplasma* species are frequently present in the lower genital tract of sexually active women with a colonization rate ranging between 40 and 80%. Vertical transmission to the newborn is high, especially in premature infants <1000 g birthweight where transmission rate approaches 90%.

III. **Pathophysiology.** *U. urealyticum* has been implicated in a variety of obstetric and neonatal diseases including **preterm labor, preterm premature rupture of membranes (PPROM), chorioamnionitis, postpartum fever and endometritis, congenital pneumonia, bacteremia, meningitis, and bronchopulmonary dysplasia/chronic lung disease (BPD/CLD).** The presumed mechanisms of infection include fetal exposure to ascending intrauterine infection, passage through an infected birth canal, and hematogenous dissemination through the placenta into umbilical vessels. This exposure leads to colonization of the skin, mucosal membranes, and respiratory tract, and sometimes leads to dissemination into the bloodstream and central nervous system (CNS). Phospholipases and cytokines produced through the inflammatory response can trigger uterine contractions and premature birth. Ureaplasmal infection of the respiratory tract in the newborn promotes a proinflammatory cytokine cascade with increase in tumor necrosis factor α, interleukin (IL)-1β, and IL-8. These cytokines recruit neutrophils to the lungs and intensify the inflammatory cascade, which damages the premature lung and impairs future alveolar development.

IV. **Risk factors.** *Ureaplasma* colonization is associated with preterm labor, chorioamnionitis, birthweight <1000 g, and gestational age <30 weeks.

V. **Clinical presentation**

A. **Preterm labor, PPROM, and chorioamnionitis.** Ureaplasmas can invade the amniotic fluid early in pregnancy and are the single most common organisms that can be isolated from inflamed placentas. Ureaplasmas can persist in the amniotic fluid subclinically for several weeks. Detection of *Ureaplasma* in second-trimester amniotic fluid by polymerase chain reaction (PCR) correlates with subsequent preterm labor and delivery (58.6% for those with positive PCR vs 4.4% for those with negative results). In addition, *Ureaplasma* cord blood infections (identified by cultures) are far more common in spontaneous than indicated preterm deliveries and are strongly associated with markers of acute placental inflammation. Positive cord cultures are also associated with neonatal systemic inflammatory response syndrome.

B. **Congenital pneumonia.** Evidence that suggests *Ureaplasma* as a cause of congenital pneumonia includes isolation of the organism in pure culture from amniotic fluid and tracheal aspirate of neonates <24 hours after birth with specific immunoglobulin M (IgM) response in the midst of an acute inflammatory reaction and radiographic changes. These infants develop early interstitial pulmonary infiltrates with cystic/dysplastic changes as early as 10–14 days of age.

C. **Meningitis.** Multiple studies have shown *Ureaplasma* to be isolated from cerebrospinal fluid (CSF) of premature infants with meningitis, intraventricular hemorrhage, and hydrocephalus. The contribution of *Ureaplasma* to the outcome of these newborns is uncertain.

D. **Predisposition to chronic lung disease.** Multiple cohort studies have linked the development of BPD/CLD with colonization of the airways with *Ureaplasma*.

VI. **Diagnosis**

A. **Laboratory studies**

1. **Culture.** Specimens for culture require specific transport media with refrigeration at 4°C. Dacron or calcium alginate swabs should be used instead of cotton swabs.

2. **Other tests.** Several sensitive PCR assays have been developed, but they are not available routinely. Serologic assays are of limited value.

VII. **Management.** Isolation precautions for all infectious diseases, including maternal and neonatal precautions, breast-feeding, and visiting issues, can be found in Appendix F.

A. **Treatment of the colonized pregnant mother.** Treatment of pregnant women who present with PPROM with a 10-day course of **erythromycin** has been shown in a large randomized study to prolong pregnancy, reduce neonatal treatment with surfactant, decrease infant oxygen dependency at ≥28 days of age, and result in fewer major cerebral abnormalities on ultrasonography before discharge. Those same benefits were not accrued if the mother presented with preterm labor but with intact membranes.

B. **Treatment of the colonized newborn infant is** *controversial.* Limited current evidence does not demonstrate a reduction in BPD/CLD or other long-term neonatal morbidities when *Ureaplasma*-colonized and intubated preterm infants are treated with erythromycin. For infants with congenital pneumonia, some experts recommend treatment with erythromycin if there is radiographic evidence of early interstitial pneumonitis and when *Ureaplasma* is the only microorganism isolated from the respiratory tract. Antimicrobial treatment may also be considered when *Ureaplasma* is isolated from a normally sterile site such as the bloodstream or CSF.

The macrolide azithromycin is being considered to treat colonized infants at risk for BPD/CLD as it has both anti-inflammatory and anti-infective properties.
VIII. **Prognosis.** In utero exposure to *Ureaplasma* is associated with increased rate of intraventricular hemorrhage and BPD/CLD in preterm infants. It is also associated with adverse neuromotor outcome at 1 and 2 years adjusted age in these infants.

Selected References

American Academy of Pediatrics. *Ureaplasma urealyticum* infections. In: Pickering LK, Baker CJ, Kimberlin DW, Long SS, eds. *Red Book: 2012 Report of the Committee on Infectious Diseases.* 29th ed. Elk Grove Village, IL: American Academy of Pediatrics; 2012:772–774.

Berger A, Witt A, Haiden N, et al. Intrauterine infection with *Ureaplasma* species is associated with adverse neuromotor outcome at 1 and 2 years adjusted age in preterm infants. *J Perinat Med.* 2009;37:72–78.

Clifford V, Tebruegge M, Everest N, Curtis N. *Ureaplasma*: pathogen or passenger in neonatal meningitis? *Pediatr Infect Dis J.* 2010;29:60–64.

Goldenberg RL, Andrews WW, Goepfert AR, et al. The Alabama Preterm Birth Study: umbilical cord blood *Ureaplasma urealyticum* and *Mycoplasma hominis* cultures in very preterm newborn infants. *Am J Obstet Gynecol.* 2008;198:43.e1–e5.

Kasper DC, Mechtler TP, Böhm J, et al. In utero exposure to *Ureaplasma* spp. is associated with increased rate of bronchopulmonary dysplasia and intraventricular hemorrhage in preterm infants. *J Perinat Med.* 2011;39:331–336.

Turner MA, Jacqz-Aigrain E, Kotecha S. Azithromycin, *Ureaplasma* and chronic lung disease of prematurity: a case study for neonatal drug development. *Arch Dis Child.* 2012;97:573–577.

Viscardi RM. *Ureaplasma* species: role in diseases of prematurity. *Clin Perinatol.* 2010;37:393–409.

Waites KB, Schelonka RL, Xiao L, Grigsby PL, Novy MJ. Congenital and opportunistic infections: *Ureaplasma* species and *Mycoplasma hominis*. *Semin Fetal Neonatal Med.* 2009;14:190–199.

146 Urinary Tract Infection

I. **Definition.** Urinary tract infection (UTI) is the presence of pathogenic bacteria or fungus in the urinary tract.
II. **Incidence.** Various series report an incidence of 0.5–1.0% in term infants weighing >2500 g and higher rates (3–5%) in premature infants or infants weighing <2500 g. *Escherichia coli* remains the most common pathogen, followed by other gram-negative rods.
III. **Pathophysiology.** Inoculation of the normally sterile urinary tract is thought to occur via fecal-perineal contamination, instrumentation, or spread from an infectious process outside of the urinary tract.
IV. **Risk factors.** Any altered anatomy (ie, posterior urethral valves, vesicoureteral reflux, ureteropelvic junction obstruction) or derangement in normal bladder function predispose to UTI. For hospital-acquired infections, indwelling Foley catheters or recent instrumentation are the most common risk factors. In addition, uncircumcised males and patients with systemic infectious processes or immunosuppression are at greater risk.
V. **Clinical presentation.** Infants may appear acutely toxic (respiratory distress, apnea, bradycardia, hypoglycemia, poor perfusion) or present with nonspecific findings of lethargy, irritability, poor feeding, vomiting, jaundice, or failure to thrive.
VI. **Diagnosis**
   A. **Laboratory studies**

1. **Urine culture.** Suprapubic aspiration or bladder catheterizations are the only 2 methods of obtaining a reliable urine culture in a neonate (see Chapters 25 and 26). Cultures obtained from a suprapubic bladder aspiration or urethral catheterization that grow >50,000 colony-forming units of a single organism and have evidence of pyuria on urinalysis are interpreted as positive. Clean-catch or collection bag specimens often are inaccurate due to contamination and are only clinically reliable if the culture demonstrates no growth. Urine culture is no longer recommended in infants <72 hours of age in an early-onset sepsis workup and is more appropriately done for late-onset sepsis workup.

2. **Urinalysis.** Leukocyte esterase is the most sensitive (83%) finding on a urinalysis and has a specificity of 78%. The presence of nitrites is 98% specific but is only has a sensitivity of 53%. Detection of bacteria by microscopy has high interexaminer variability, but is as high as 81% sensitive and 83% specific in some hands. No single finding is diagnostic; however, when there is microscopic bacteriuria or pyuria in addition to the presence of leukocyte esterase or nitrites, a urinalysis is >99% sensitive and 70% specific.

VII. **Management**
   A. **Initial antibiotic treatment.** For the majority of neonatal cases, initial treatment with broad-spectrum intravenous (IV) antibiotics is appropriate (usually Ampicillin and Gentamicin). In nontoxic infants over a month of age, oral therapy has been found to be as efficacious as IV therapy. (For dosages and other pharmacologic information, see Chapter 148.)
   B. **Further investigations.** All neonates with a febrile UTI or suspected anatomic abnormality require renal/bladder ultrasonography, and voiding cystourethrogram (VCUG). The **American Academy of Pediatrics guidelines** no longer recommend VCUG at the time of a first febrile urinary tract infection in infants >2 months of age. Until a national prospective randomized trial (RIVUR [Randomized Intervention for Children With Vesicoureteral Reflux]; estimated completion late 2013) clarifies the effectiveness or lack thereof of prophylactic antibiotics in infants, we feel that a VCUG at the time of the first febrile UTI during infancy is still warranted to evaluate urinary tract anatomy and VUR. Within the next few years, data from the RIVUR study will be available, providing further insight into the role of prophylactic antibiotics and thus VCUG in children with UTI.

Selected References

Hoberman A, Wald ER, Hickey RW, et al. Oral versus initial intravenous therapy for urinary tract infections in young febrile children. *Pediatrics.* 1999;104:79–86.

Hoberman A, Wald ER, Reynolds EA, Penchansky L, Charron M. Pyuria and bacteriuria in urine specimens obtained by catheter from young children with fever. *Pediatrics.* 1994;124:513–519.

Ma JF, Shortliffe LM. Urinary tract infection in children: etiology and epidemiology. *Urol Clin North Am.* 2004;31:517–526.

Subcommittee on Urinary tract infection, Steering Committee on Quality Improvement and Management. Urinary tract infection. Clinical practice guideline for the diagnosis and management of the initial UTI in febrile infants and children 2 to 24 months. *Pediatrics.* 2011;128;595.

To T, Agha M, Dick PT, Feldman W. Cohort study on circumcision of newborn boys and subsequent risk of urinary-tract infection. *Lancet.* 1998;352:1813–1816.

147 Varicella-Zoster Infections

Varicella-zoster virus (VZV) is a member of the herpesvirus family. Primary maternal VZV infection (chickenpox) can result in fetal or neonatal infection. Other rare complications include spontaneous abortion, fetal demise, and premature delivery. Reactivation infection (zoster) does not result in fetal infection. Primary maternal VZV infection during the last trimester can cause pneumonia with significant morbidity and mortality. The overall incidence of maternal and neonatal varicella has decreased over the past 10–15 years, presumably due to varicella vaccination. Active surveillance among adults has shown that the incidence of varicella declined 74% during 1995–2005, despite vaccination rates among adults of only 3%. Herd immunity is the likely explanation for this phenomenon. Varicella immunization is recommended for all nonimmune women as part of prepregnancy and postpartum care. Varicella vaccine should not be administered to pregnant women, because the possible effects on fetal development are unknown, although no cases of congenital varicella syndrome or patterns of malformation have been identified after inadvertent immunization of pregnant women. When postpubertal females are immunized, pregnancy should be avoided for at least 1 month after immunization. Reporting of instances of inadvertent immunization with a varicella-zoster–containing vaccine during pregnancy is encouraged (1-800-986-8999, **www.merckpregnancyregistries.com/varivax.html**).

There are **three forms of varicella-zoster infections involving the neonate: fetal, congenital (early neonatal), and postnatal.**

FETAL VARICELLA SYNDROME

I. **Definition.** This form occurs when the mother has her first exposure to VZV during the first half of pregnancy. It is also recognized in the literature as **congenital varicella syndrome (CVS).**

II. **Incidence.** This form is fortunately rare; only ~5% of women of childbearing age are susceptible to VZV. The incidence of varicella during pregnancy is estimated at 1–5 cases per 10,000 pregnancies. The incidence of embryopathy and fetopathy after maternal varicella infection in the first 20 weeks is ~1%. Recent evidence suggests that the incidence is much lower than previously estimated.

III. **Pathophysiology.** Maternal transmission of the virus probably occurs via respiratory droplets or direct contact with chickenpox or zoster lesions. The virus replicates in the oropharynx, and viremia results, before the onset of rash, with transplacental passage to the fetus. Almost all cases reported have involved exposure between the 8th and 20th weeks of pregnancy. The pathogenesis of fetal varicella syndrome (FVS) may reflect disseminated infection in utero or as a consequence of failure of virus–host interaction to result in establishment of latency, as normally occurs in postnatal VZV infection. Since VZV is a lymphotropic virus, it has the potential to spread to all fetal organs by the hematogenous route. Pathology specimens from aborted fetuses with VZV infection have shown the virus to be distributed throughout fetal tissues. Microcephaly can be attributed to VZV encephalitis and irreversible damage to growth of the developing brain. Of interest, the virus does not appear to cause intrauterine damage to the lungs or liver in infants with FVS, as it can in perinatal varicella or in other immunocompromised hosts. Fulminant infection involving these organs may result in fetal demise, rather than birth of an infant with FVS. VZV is also a neurotropic virus; many of the defects have been postulated to be a direct result of spinal cord and ganglia infection, which causes destruction of the plexi during embryogenesis, leading to denervation of the limb bud and subsequent hypoplasia. Failure of muscle development has consequences for limb bone formation. The cutaneous defects are also likely to reflect VZV infection of sensory nerves. VZV infection of cells in developing optic tracts also explains the optic atrophy and chorioretinitis. From the pattern of dermatomal distribution of the skin defects seen in FVS, particularly the scarring and limb hypoplasia, it has been suggested that FVS is the result of intrauterine herpes zoster.

The extremely short latent period between fetal infection and reactivation, if latency is established at all, is the consequence of the lack of cell-mediated immunity in the fetus before 20 weeks' gestation. Infants exposed to VZV in utero also can develop unapparent varicella and subsequent zoster early in life without having had extrauterine varicella.

IV. **Risk factors.** A pregnant woman with no history of varicella infection or vaccination who becomes exposed to VZV between the 8th and 20th weeks of gestation is at risk.

V. **Clinical presentation.** The main symptoms of FVS are:
   A. **Skin lesions (60–70%).** Cicatricial scars and skin loss.
   B. **Central nervous system defects or disease (60%).** Microcephaly, seizures, encephalitis, cortical atrophy and spinal cord atrophy, mental retardation, and cerebral calcifications.
   C. **Ocular abnormalities (60%).** Microphthalmia, chorioretinitis, cataracts, optic atrophy, nystagmus, and Horner syndrome (ptosis, miosis, and enophthalmos).
   D. **Limb hypoplasia and other skeletal defects (50%).**
   E. **Prematurity and intrauterine growth restriction (35%).**

VI. **Diagnosis.** Alkalay et al proposed the following criteria for the diagnosis of FVS in the newborn:
   A. **Appearance of maternal varicella during pregnancy.**
   B. **Presence of congenital skin lesions** in dermatomal distribution and/or neurologic defects, eye disease, or limb hypoplasia.
   C. **Proof of intrauterine VZV infection** by detection of viral DNA in the infant by polymerase chain reaction (PCR), presence of VZV-specific immunoglobulin (Ig)M, persistence of VZV IgG beyond 7 months of age, or appearance of zoster during early infancy. VZV DNA PCR (both from fetal blood or amniotic fluid) appears to be sensitive and accurate in detecting fetal infection; however, most of the "infected" fetuses are morphologically normal (ie, not affected by FVS). Prenatal diagnosis is most often done by detailed ultrasound, searching for typical anomalies and VZV-specific PCR in amniotic fluid. At least a 5-week interval is advised between onset of maternal rash and obtaining of the ultrasound. An initial ultrasound is recommended at 17–21 weeks' gestation with a follow-up study done 4–6 weeks later. The role of prenatal magnetic resonance imaging for assessment of the fetus after maternal varicella is only beginning to be delineated, but it may provide improved specificity, particularly for central nervous system damage.

VII. **Management.** Isolation precautions for all infectious diseases, including maternal and neonatal precautions, breast-feeding, and visiting issues, can be found in Appendix F.
   A. **Mother.** If the mother is exposed to VZV infection in the first or second trimester, treat the mother with **varicella-zoster immune globulin (VZIG)** if her past history of varicella infection or vaccination is negative or uncertain. For dosage, see Chapter 148. VZIG should be given within 72–96 hours and appears to protect both mother and fetus. In 2012, the U.S. Food and Drug Administration (FDA) extended the period for administration of VZIG from 96 hours to 10 days after exposure. The only U.S.-licensed VZIG was discontinued by the manufacturer in 2004. Since February 2006, an investigational (not licensed) VZIG called **VariZIG** has become available under an investigational new drug (IND) protocol and can be requested by calling FFF Enterprises, 24-hour toll-free, at 800-843-7477. If VariZIG is not available, intravenous immunoglobulin (IVIG) can be used. If chickenpox is diagnosed during pregnancy, antiviral therapy with acyclovir should be strongly considered. Acyclovir therapy during pregnancy appears to be safe; it has not been associated with increased congenital abnormalities compared with the general population.
   B. **Infant.** Supportive care of the infant is required because there is usually profound neurologic impairment. Acyclovir therapy may be helpful to stop the progression of eye disease or to treat recurrent zoster (shingles), which is common in the first 2 years of life.
   C. **Isolation.** Isolation is not necessary.

VIII. **Prognosis.** Approximately 30% of these infants die in the first months of life, often because of intractable gastroesophageal reflux, severe recurrent aspiration pneumonia, and respiratory failure. Survivors usually suffer profound mental retardation and major neurologic disabilities. These infants are also at risk for developing zoster (shingles) in the first 2 years of life.

CONGENITAL (EARLY NEONATAL) VARICELLA INFECTION

I. **Definition.** This is the form of the disease that occurs when a pregnant woman suffers chickenpox during the last 3 weeks of pregnancy or within the first few days postpartum. Disease begins in the neonate just before delivery or within the first 10–12 days of life.

II. **Incidence.** Although the congenital form is more common than the teratogenic form, it is still rare, with recent estimates of 0.7 per 100,000 live births per annum. The introduction of varicella vaccination in 1995 greatly reduced the incidence of varicella infection in all age groups (herd immunity).

III. **Pathophysiology.** Maternal chickenpox near term or soon after delivery may cause severe or fatal illness in the newborn. Maternal varicella can affect the baby through transplacental viremia, ascending infection during birth, or respiratory droplet/direct contact with infectious lesions after birth. Neonatal chickenpox occurring in the first 10–12 days of life is typically caused by intrauterine transmission of VZV (incubation period 10–21 days). Chickenpox after the 10th to 12th day of the neonatal period is most likely acquired by postnatal VZV infection. If the onset of maternal disease is between 5 days before delivery or 2 days postpartum, there is a high attack rate (up to 50%) with significant associated mortality (up to 30%). Those babies present with the classic skin lesions, but can disseminate with pneumonia, hepatitis, meningoencephalitis, and severe coagulopathy (disseminated intravascular coagulation [DIC]) resulting from liver failure and thrombocytopenia. If the maternal rash happens >5 days before delivery, there is enough maternal anti-VZV IgG production with subsequent transplacental transfer that protects the newborn and results in a milder case of chickenpox.

IV. **Risk factors.** Primarily a mother with chickenpox during the last 3 weeks of pregnancy or within the first few days postpartum. There is a higher risk of mortality if the onset of maternal disease is 5 days before delivery or 2 days postpartum. Premature infants, especially those <28 weeks, are extremely susceptible.

V. **Clinical presentation** is variable. There may be only mild involvement of the infant, with vesicles on the skin, or the following may be seen:

A. **Skin.** A centripetal rash (beginning on the trunk and spreading to the face and scalp, sparing the extremities) begins as red macules and progresses to vesicles and encrustation. Lesions are more common in the diaper area and skin folds. There may be 2 or 3 lesions or thousands of them. The differential diagnosis includes herpes simplex virus and enterovirus. The main complication is staphylococcal and streptococcal secondary skin infections.

B. **Lungs.** Lung involvement is seen in all fatal cases. It usually appears 2–4 days after the onset of the rash but may be seen up to 10 days after. Signs include fever, cyanosis, rales, and hemoptysis. Chest radiograph shows a diffuse nodular-miliary pattern, especially in the perihilar region.

C. **Other organs.** Focal necrosis may be seen in the liver, adrenals, intestines, kidneys, and thymus. Glomerulonephritis, myocarditis, encephalitis, and cerebellar ataxia are sometimes seen.

VI. **Diagnosis.** The diagnosis of varicella usually is made clinically based on the characteristic appearance of skin lesions.

A. **Polymerase chain reaction (PCR).** The most sensitive and specific method for detection of VZV DNA in clinical specimens. This is the diagnostic method of choice for investigation of vesicular fluid or scabs, biopsies, and amniotic fluid. This testing also can be used to distinguish between wild-type and vaccine-strain VZV (genotyping). Viral culture and direct fluorescent antibody (DFA) assay are less sensitive than PCR and are not usually recommended.

B. **Serum testing of VZV antibody.** Serologic tests may help to document acute infection in confusing cases. IgM antibody may be detected as soon as 3 days after the appearance of VZV symptoms, but the test may not be reliable.

VII. **Management**
   A. **VariZIG**
      1. **Perinatal infection.** Infants of mothers who develop VZV infection (rash) within 5 days before or 2 days after delivery should receive 125 U of **VariZIG** as soon as possible and not later than 10 days. Intravenous immunoglobulin (**IVIG**) (400 mg/kg) should be used if VariZIG is not available. Infants treated with immune globulins should be placed in strict respiratory isolation for 28 days because immunoglobulin treatment may prolong the incubation period. VariZIG is not expected to reduce the clinical attack rate in treated newborns; however, these infants tend to develop milder infections than the untreated neonates. Prophylactic administration of oral **acyclovir** beginning 7 days after exposure also may prevent or attenuate varicella disease in exposed infants.
      2. **Maternal rash occurring >7 days before delivery.** These infants do not need VZIG. It is believed that infants will have received antibodies via the placenta.
   B. **Acyclovir** therapy 15 mg/kg/dose every 8 hours for 7 days should be considered for postexposure prophylaxis as well as a treatment in symptomatic neonates.
   C. **Antibiotics.** Use antibiotics if secondary bacterial skin infections occur.
VIII. **Prognosis.** Prognosis is good if the onset of maternal varicella occurs >5 days before delivery, because the mother has enough time to develop antibodies and pass these to the infant. In these cases, the infant has a mild case of varicella with excellent prognosis. If the mother has onset of disease within 5 days before delivery or 2 days after, the infant is exposed with no antibodies. In these cases the disease is usually severe with dissemination. Overwhelming sepsis and multiple organ failure can lead to a mortality rate as high as 30%. The usual causes of death are pneumonia, fulminant hepatitis, and DIC. With the use of VZIG, the mortality rate is reduced to 7%. There is an increased risk of developing zoster (shingles) in the first 2 years of life.

POSTNATAL CHICKENPOX

   I. **Definition.** This form of the disease presents on days 12–28 of life. It does not represent transplacental infection from the mother.
   II. **Incidence.** There has been a significant decline in the incidence since the introduction of the vaccine in 1995 (by 85–90%). The incidence of neonatal varicella in the vaccine era is ~0.7 per 100,000 live births.
   III. **Pathophysiology.** Postnatal VZV infection occurs by droplet transmission. This disease is usually mild because of passive protection from maternal antibodies. Placental antibody transfer is lower in preterm infants, which makes them more susceptible compared with term infants. Horizontal transmission in Neonatal Intensive Care Units has been well documented. Neonatal vaccine-strain VZV infection after maternal postpartum vaccination has been reported.
   IV. **Risk factors.** Seronegative mother, delivery before 28 weeks, birthweight <1.5 kg, postnatal age >2 months (maternal transplacental immunity has waned), immunocompromised neonates (sepsis, steroids, etc.).
   V. **Clinical presentation.** The typical chickenpox rash is seen with centripetal spread, beginning on the trunk and spreading to the face and scalp and sparing the extremities. All stages of the rash may appear at the same time, from red macules to clear vesicles to crusting lesions. Complications of this form of the disease are rare but may include secondary infections and varicella pneumonia. In older children, necrotizing fasciitis secondary to group A streptococcal infections is particularly worrisome and may be associated with ibuprofen use (Plate 13).
   VI. **Diagnosis.** Same as for congenital varicella (see the previous section). Diagnosis is usually made based on clinical grounds.
   VII. **Management.** For the full-term infant in community setting, the disease is usually mild. Therefore, acyclovir therapy is **controversial**. For nosocomial chickenpox in the intensive care nursery (exposure):

A. **VariZIG.** Recommended for all exposed infants of **<28 weeks'** gestational age or weighing **≤1000 g regardless of the maternal history**. It is also recommended in premature infants whose mothers do not have a history of chickenpox or varicella vaccination **(seronegative)**.

B. **Infants >28 weeks' gestation.** These infants should have sufficient transplacental antibodies, if the mother is immune to protect them from the risk of complications.

C. **Isolation.** Exposed infants should be placed in strict isolation for 10–21 days after the onset of the rash in the index case. Exposed infants who receive VariZIG should be in strict respiratory isolation for 28 days.

D. **Acyclovir.** Recommended for infants who develop breakthrough lesions or prophylactically beginning 7 days after exposure. Therapy should be continued for 7 days (if used prophylactically) or for 48 hours after the last new lesions have appeared.

VIII. **Prognosis.** This form of the disease is mild, and death is extremely rare. Normal-term infants who develop postnatal chickenpox have the same risk of complications of chickenpox as older children. Premature infants are at increased risk for nosocomial acquisition of VZV. The risk of complications for infants <28 weeks who develop postnatal chickenpox is unknown.

Selected References

Alkalay AL, Pomerance JJ, Rimoin DL. Fetal varicella syndrome. *J Pediatr.* 1987;111:320–323.

American Academy of Pediatrics. Varicella-zoster infections. In: Pickering LK, Baker CJ, Kimberlin DW, Long SS, eds. *Red Book: 2012 Report of the Committee on Infectious Diseases.* 29th ed. Elk Grove Village, IL: American Academy of Pediatrics; 2012:774–789.

Gardella C, Brown ZA. Managing varicella zoster infection in pregnancy. *Cleve Clin J Med.* 2007;74:290–296.

Gershon AA. Chickenpox, measles, and mumps. In: Remington JS, Klein JO, Wilson CB, Nizet V, Maldonado YA, eds. *Infectious Diseases of the Fetus and Newborn Infant.* 7th ed. Philadelphia, PA: Elsevier Saunders; 2011:661–705.

Gibson CS, Goldwater PN, MacLennan AH, et al. Fetal exposure to herpesviruses may be associated with pregnancy-induced hypertensive disorders and preterm birth in a Caucasian population. *Br J Obstet Gynaecol.* 2008;115:492–500.

Kellie SM, Makvandi M, Muller ML. Management and outcome of a varicella exposure in a neonatal intensive care unit: lessons for the vaccine era. *Am J Infect Control.* 2011 (Epub ahead of print).

Khandaker G, Marshall H, Peadon E, et al. Congenital and neonatal varicella: impact of the national varicella vaccination programme in Australia. *Arch Dis Child.* 2011;96:453–456.

Lamont RF, Sobel JD, Carrington D, et al. Varicella-zoster virus (chickenpox) infection in pregnancy. *BJOG* 2011;118:1155–1162.

Marin M, Watson TL, Chaves SS, et al. Varicella among adults: data from an active surveillance project, 1995–2005. *J Infect Dis.* 2008;197(suppl 2):S94–S100.

Pasternak B, Hviid A. Use of acyclovir, valacyclovir, and famciclovir in the first trimester of pregnancy and the risk of birth defects. *JAMA* 2010;304:859–866.

Rodríguez-Fanjul X, Noguera A, Vicente A, González-Enseñat MA, Jiménez R, Fortuny C. Herpes zoster in healthy infants and toddlers after perinatal exposure to varicella-zoster virus: a case series and review of the literature. *Pediatr Infect Dis J.* 2010;29:574–576.

Sanchez MA, Bello-Munoz JC, Cebrecos I, et al. The prevalence of congenital varicella syndrome after a maternal infection, but before 20 weeks of pregnancy: a prospective cohort study. *J Matern Fetal Neonatal Med.* 2011;24:341–347.

Smith CK, Arvin AM. Varicella in the fetus and newborn. *Semin Fetal Neonatal Med.* 2009;14:209–217.

Wilson E, Goss MA, Marin M, et al. Varicella vaccine exposure during pregnancy: data from 10 years of the pregnancy registry. *J Infect Dis.* 2008;197(suppl 2):S178–S84.

148 Medications Used in the Neonatal Intensive Care Unit[a]

This section provides a description of medications used in the contemporary care of sick newborn infants. It is not intended to be an exhaustive list of all drugs available for infants, nor is it intended to be an in-depth source of information about neonatal pharmacology. Readers are encouraged to consult with their institutional pharmacists regarding issues of pharmacokinetics, drug interactions, drug elimination and metabolism, and monitoring drug serum levels. Information on medications and breast-feeding and pregnancy can be found in Chapter 149.

When the designations of neonate/newborn or infant are used for medication doses, it refers to the following:

Neonate/Newborn: Birth to 28 days postnatal age.
Infant: >28 days (1 month) to 1 year of age.

ACETAMINOPHEN (APAP) (LIQUIPRIN, TEMPRA, TYLENOL)

INDICATIONS AND USE: Analgesic, antipyretic.
ACTIONS: Analgesic effect—inhibition of prostaglandin synthesis in the central nervous system (CNS) and peripherally, blocking pain impulse generation. Antipyretic effect—inhibition of hypothalamic heat-regulating center.
DOSAGE: PO, PR.

- **Preterm infants 28–32 weeks:** 10–12 mg/kg/dose PO every 6–8 hours or 20 mg/kg/dose PR every 12 hours. Maximum daily dose: 40 mg/kg.
- **Preterm infants 33–37 weeks; term neonates <10 days:** 10–15 mg/kg/dose PO every 6 hours or 30 mg/kg PR loading dose; then 15 mg/kg/dose every 8 hours. Maximum daily dose: 60 mg/kg.
- **Term infants ≥10 days:** 10–15 mg/kg/dose PO every 4–6 hours or 30 mg/kg PR loading dose; then 20 mg/kg/dose every 6–8 hours. Maximum daily dose: 90 mg/kg.

ADVERSE EFFECTS: Rash, blood dyscrasias (neutropenia, leukopenia, and thrombocytopenia), and hepatic necrosis with overdose; renal injury may occur with chronic use.
PHARMACOLOGY: Extensively metabolized by the liver primarily by sulfonation, and by glucuronidation to a much lesser extent. Excretion by the kidney with elimination half-life: term infants—~3 hours, preterm infants >32 weeks—5 hours, and in premature infants <32 weeks—up to 11 hours. Prolonged elimination with liver dysfunction.
COMMENTS: Rectal administration may result in inaccurate dosing. Prophylactic use during vaccination may result in potential reduction in antibody response. Beginning 2011 into 2012—transition to one pediatric concentration 160 mg/5 mL and elimination of 80 mg/0.8 mL infant drops per U.S. Food and Drug Administration (FDA) recommendations. *N*-acetylcysteine is the antidote of choice for acetaminophen poisoning.

ACETAZOLAMIDE (DIAMOX)

INDICATIONS AND USE: Reduce intraocular pressure in glaucoma; an anticonvulsant in refractory neonatal seizures; decrease cerebrospinal fluid (CSF) production in posthemorrhagic hydrocephalus; treatment of renal tubular acidosis.
ACTIONS: Competitive, reversible, carbonic anhydrase inhibitor; increases renal excretion of sodium, potassium, bicarbonate, and water, resulting in the production of acidosis. Decreases the production of aqueous humor and reduces abnormal discharge from central nervous system (CNS) neurons.
DOSAGE: IV, PO.

- **Glaucoma:** 8–30 mg/kg/day PO divided every 8 hours or IV 20–40 mg/kg/day divided every 6 hours; maximum 1 gram/day.
- **Anticonvulsant:** 4–16 mg/kg/day PO divided every 6–8 hours not to exceed 30 mg/kg/day or 1 gram/day.
- **Alkalinize urine:** 5 mg/kg/dose PO 2–3 times over 24 hours.

---

[a]Edited Black Box "Warnings" are provided for select medications. Readers should review the entire package insert for each medication. Selected brand names are provided in addition to the generic name.

• **Decrease CSF production:** 5 mg/kg/dose IV/PO every 6 hours; increased by 25 mg/kg/day to a maximum of 100 mg/kg/day. Furosemide has been used in combination.

ADVERSE EFFECTS: Gastrointestinal (GI) irritation, transient hypokalemia, hyperchloremic metabolic acidosis, growth retardation, bone marrow suppression, thrombocytopenia, hemolytic anemia, pancytopenia, agranulocytosis, leukopenia, drowsiness, and paresthesia.

PHARMACOLOGY: Unchanged in urine. Half-life is 4–10 hours.

COMMENTS: Currently, rarely used in neonates; a 1998 study failed to show efficacy in slowing the progression of posthemorrhagic hydrocephalus in neonates and infants. In neonates, use is limited to the treatment of glaucoma. Used as an adjunct to other medications in refractory seizures. Tolerance to diuretic effect may occur with long-term use. Oral solution may be compounded by using tablets.

ACYCLOVIR (ZOVIRAX)

ACTION AND SPECTRUM: Treatment and prophylaxis of herpes simplex virus (HSV-1 and HSV-2) infections, herpes simplex encephalitis, herpes zoster infections, and varicella-zoster infections.

DOSAGE: **PO, IV**.

Herpes simplex (based on AAP *Red Book*, 2012):

• **Neonatal:** 20 mg/kg/dose IV every 8 hours for 14–21 days. Treat central nervous system (CNS) infections for 21 days and all other infections for 14 days. Reduce dosing interval to every 12 hours in neonates <30 weeks' gestational age.
• **Dosing in renal impairment:**
   • **Serum creatinine 0.8–1.1 mg/dL:** 20 mg/kg IV every 12 hours.
   • **Serum creatinine 1.2–1.5 mg/dL:** 20 mg/kg IV every 24 hours.
   • **Serum creatinine >1.5 mg/dL:** 10 mg/kg IV every 24 hours.

Herpes zoster (shingles):

• **Infants and children:** 10 mg/kg/dose IV every 8 hours for 7–10 days. In immunocompromised host, the AIDS information guidelines recommend duration of therapy of 10–14 days.

Varicella-zoster (chickenpox) in immunocompromised host:

• **Infants <1 year:** 10 mg/kg/dose IV every 8 hours for 7–10 days.

ADVERSE EFFECTS: Generally well tolerated. Thrombophlebitis and inflammation of injection site. Acute renal failure/acute kidney injury, increased blood urea nitrogen (BUN) and serum creatinine, nephrotoxicity. Increased liver transaminases. Neutropenia, thrombocytopenia, anemia, thrombocytosis, leukocytosis, and neutrophilia. Neutropenia may necessitate reduction in dose or treatment with granulocyte colony-stimulating factor (G-CSF) if absolute neutrophil count (ANC) remains <500/mm^3. Adequate hydration and infusion rate of at least 1 hour reduces risk of transient renal impairment and crystalluria.

PHARMACOLOGY: Inhibits DNA synthesis and viral replication. Oral absorption is 15–30%, cerebrospinal fluid (CSF) concentrations are 50% of serum and primarily excreted by the kidneys.

COMMENTS: Infuse over at least 1 hour; concentration <7 mg/mL, 5 mg/mL is preferred. Do not refrigerate. Monitor complete blood cell count (CBC) and renal and liver function.

ADENOSINE (ADENOCARD)

INDICATIONS AND USE: Acute treatment of sustained paroxysmal supraventricular tachycardia for conversion to normal sinus rhythm.

ACTIONS: A purine nucleoside that slows conduction time through the atrioventricular (AV) node and interrupts reentry pathways through the AV node to restore normal sinus rhythm. Effects are mediated by depression of calcium slow-channel conduction, an increase in potassium conductance, and possibly indirect antiadrenergic effects.

DOSAGE: **IV**.

• 0.05–0.2 mg/kg by rapid IV push over 1–2 seconds. Repeat bolus doses at 2-minute intervals by increasing increments of 0.05–0.1 mg/kg until sinus rhythm is achieved or until a maximum dose of 0.3 mg/kg is reached. Infuse as close as possible to IV site and immediately flush IV with saline to ensure dose enters circulation. For doses <0.2 mL, prepare dilution using normal saline (NS) to final concentration of 300 mcg/mL.

ADVERSE EFFECTS: Contraindicated in heart block. Transient arrhythmias, flushing, dyspnea, and hypotension. May cause bronchoconstriction; use with caution in patients with history of bronchospasm.

PHARMACOLOGY: Rapid onset of action; half-life is <10 seconds; duration is 20–30 seconds.

COMMENTS: Methylxanthines (caffeine and theophylline) are competitive antagonists; larger adenosine doses may be required.

ALBUMIN, HUMAN

INDICATIONS AND USE: Treatment of hypovolemia, maintenance of cardiac output in shock, plasma volume expansion, hypoproteinemia associated with generalized edema or decreased intravascular volume; acute nephrotic syndrome in premature infants. Not recommended for initial volume expansion; use isotonic crystalloid solutions—0.9% NaCl or lactated Ringer's (Pediatric Advanced Life Support [PALS] and Neonatal Resuscitation Program [NRP] guidelines).

ACTIONS: Increases intravascular oncotic pressure, which results in a mobilization of fluid from the interstitial spaces into the intravascular space.

DOSAGE: IV.

• **Neonates, infants, and children:** 0.5–1 gram/kg IV (or 10–20 mL/kg of 5% IV bolus) repeated as necessary. Maximum: 6 grams/kg/day. Five percent solutions should be used in hypovolemic or intravascularly depleted patients; 25% solutions should be used in cases of fluid or sodium restriction.

• **Hypoproteinemia in neonates:** Dose may be added to hyperalimentation solutions; however, may increase potential for growth of bacteria or fungi.

ADVERSE EFFECTS: Rapid infusion may cause vascular overload and precipitation of congestive heart failure or pulmonary edema. The 25% solution should be used with extreme caution in premature neonates due to increased risk of intraventricular hemorrhage.

PHARMACOLOGY: Duration of volume expansion is ~24 hours.

COMMENTS: Refer to individual product information for use of correct in-line IV filter. A 5% concentration is osmotically equivalent to equal volume of plasma, and 25% concentration is osmotically equivalent to 5 times its volume of plasma. If unavailable, 5% solutions can be prepared by diluting the 25% solution with normal saline (NS) or 5% dextrose in water (D5W). Do not use sterile water to prepare dilution; this may cause hypotonic-associated hemolysis, which can be fatal.

ALBUTEROL (PROVENTIL, VENTOLIN)

INDICATIONS AND USE: Prevention and treatment of bronchospasm; bronchodilator in respiratory distress syndrome (RDS) and bronchopulmonary dysplasia/chronic lung disease (BPD/CLD). Used for treatment of hyperkalemia.

ACTIONS: Primarily β_2-adrenergic stimulation (bronchodilation and vasodilation) with minor β_1 stimulation (increased myocardial contractility and conduction).

DOSAGE: Inhalation, nebulization.

• **Nebulization:** 0.1–0.5 mg/kg/dose (minimum of 2.5 mg) every 2–6 hours as needed.

• **Inhalation:** Metered dose inhaler (MDI) 90 mcg/spray: 1–2 puffs every 2–6 hours as needed.

ADVERSE EFFECTS: Tachycardia, tremors, central nervous system (CNS) stimulation, hypokalemia, hyperglycemia, and hypertension.

COMMENTS: Duration of action is ~2–5 hours. Titrate dose according to the effect on heart rate and improvement in respiratory symptoms.

ALPROSTADIL (PROSTAGLANDIN E₁) (PROSTIN VR)

> **WARNING:** Apnea is experienced by about 10–12% of neonates with congenital heart defects treated with alprostadil injection, USP. Apnea is most often seen in neonates weighing <2 kg at birth and usually appears during the first hour of drug infusion. Therefore, respiratory status should be monitored throughout treatment, and alprostadil should be used where ventilatory assistance is immediately available.

INDICATIONS AND USE: Any clinical condition in which blood flow must be maintained through the ductus arteriosus to sustain either pulmonary or systemic circulation until corrective or palliative surgery can be performed. Examples are pulmonary atresia, pulmonary stenosis, tricuspid atresia, transposition of the great arteries, aortic arch interruption, coarctation of the aorta, and severe tetralogy of Fallot (TOF).

ACTIONS: Causes vasodilation of all vascular smooth muscle including the ductus arteriosus.

DOSAGE: IV.

• **Initial:** 0.05–0.1 mcg/kg/minute by continuous infusion. Gradually titrate to maintain acceptable oxygen levels without adverse effects. Use the lowest rate to maintain improved oxygenation response.

• **Maintenance:** 0.01–0.4 mcg/kg/minute.

ADVERSE EFFECTS: See black box warning. May cause gastric outlet obstruction and reversible cortical proliferation of the long bones after prolonged treatment. Hypotension, cutaneous vasodilation, bradycardia, inhibits platelet aggregation, hypoventilation, seizure-like activity, jitteriness, temperature elevation, hypocalcemia, hypoglycemia.

COMMENTS: Decreased response after 96 hours of infusion. Maximal improvement in Pao₂, usually within 30 minutes in cyanotic infants and 1.5–3 hours in acyanotic infants. Use cautiously in infants with bleeding tendencies.

ALTEPLASE, RECOMBINANT (ACTIVASE, CATHFLO ACTIVASE, TISSUE PLASMINOGEN ACTIVATOR [tPA])

INDICATIONS AND USE: Used to restore patency of occluded central venous catheters and for the dissolution of large-vessel thrombus (systemic use). (See also Chapters 79 and 87.)

ACTIONS: Alteplase is a thrombolytic. It enhances conversion of plasminogen to plasmin, which then cleaves fibrin, fibrinogen, factor V, and factor VIII, resulting in clot dissolution.

DOSAGE: IV.

Occluded central venous catheter:

- **Manufacturer's recommendations (CathFlo, Activase):** Postnatal age ≥14 days, use 1 mg/mL; instill a volume equal to 110% of the internal lumen volume; do not exceed 2 mg in 2 mL; leave in lumen for up to 2 hours and then aspirate out of catheter. May repeat process if lumen is still occluded. Check the catheter product literature or manufacturer for catheter volume.
- *Chest*, **2008 dosing recommendations (Monagle et al, 2008):** 0.5 mg diluted in a volume of normal saline (NS) equal to the catheter lumen internal volume; instill over 1–2 minutes; dwell time is 1–2 hours. Aspirate solution from catheter and then flush catheter with NS.

Dissolution of large vessel thrombus (systemic use):

- **Dose is *controversial*** and optimal dose has not been established. May consider fresh frozen plasma (FFP) prior to administration of alteplase.
- *Chest*, **2008 recommendations (Monagle et al, 2008):** 0.1–0.6 mg/kg/hour for 6 hours. Dose must be titrated to effect; some patients require longer or shorter duration of therapy.

ADVERSE EFFECTS: The risk of complications increases at rates >0.4 mg/kg/hour. Systemic use is not recommended with preexisting intraventricular hemorrhage or cerebral ischemic changes. Bleeding from venipuncture sites may occur. During the treatment of occluded central venous catheter, bleeding may occur if excess alteplase is inadvertently injected into the systemic circulation. Excessive pressure during instillation may force clot into systemic circulation.

COMMENTS: Increases risk of bleeding in infants concurrently on heparin, warfarin, or indomethacin. Monitor prothrombin time (PT), activated partial thromboplastin time (aPTT), fibrinogen, and fibrin split products prior to the initiation of therapy and at least daily through the duration of therapy. Fibrinogen levels should be maintained >100 mg/dL and platelets >50,000/mm^3.

AMIKACIN SULFATE (AMIKIN)

ACTION AND SPECTRUM: Active against gram-negative bacteria, including most *Pseudomonas, Klebsiella, Enterobacter, Proteus, Escherichia coli*, and *Serratia* spp. No activity against anaerobic organisms. Reserve for treatment of gram-negative organisms resistant to gentamicin and tobramycin. Treatment of susceptible mycobacterial organisms.

DOSAGE: IM, IV. Infuse over 30 minutes. Dosage should be monitored and adjusted by use of pharmacokinetics. Initial empirical dosing based on body weight:

- **Neonates 0–4 weeks and <1.2 kg:** 7.5 mg/kg/dose every 18–24 hours.
- **Postnatal age <7 days:**
  - **1.2–2 kg:** 7.5 mg/kg/dose every 12 hours.
  - **>2 kg:** 7.5–10 mg/kg/dose every 12 hours.
- **Postnatal age ≥7 days:**
  - **1.2–2 kg:** 7.5–10 mg/kg/dose every 8–12 hours.
  - **>2 kg:** 10 mg/kg/dose every 8 hours.
- **Infants and children:** 15–22.5 mg/kg/day divided every 8 hours; some patients may require higher doses of 30 mg/kg/day divided every 8 hours.
- **Treatment of nontuberculous mycobacterial infection:** 15–30 mg/kg/day divided every 12–24 hours as a part of a multidrug regimen.

PHARMACOLOGY: Displays concentration-dependent killing; bactericidal activity. Renal elimination (glomerular filtration); half-life is 4–8 hours; volume of distribution is 0.6 L/kg.

ADVERSE EFFECTS: Possible nephrotoxicity and ototoxicity. Toxicities may be potentiated when used with furosemide or vancomycin, and neuromuscular blockade is increased if used with pancuronium or with coexisting hypermagnesemia.

COMMENTS: Monitor serum levels when treating >48 hours, in patients with decreased or changing renal function, with signs of nephrotoxicity or ototoxicity, with concomitant use of other nephrotoxic agents, and in patients who may require higher doses. Adjust the dosage according to serum peak and trough levels. **Therapeutic peak level** is 15–40 mcg/mL depending on type of infection, and trough level is <5–8 mcg/mL. Nephrotoxicity is associated with serum trough concentrations >10 mcg/mL; ototoxicity, with serum peak concentrations >35–40 mg/mL (more cochlear damage than vestibular).

AMINOPHYLLINE-THEOPHYLLINE

INDICATIONS AND USE: To reduce frequency and severity of apnea of prematurity, following extubation or during alprostadil administration. A bronchodilator in the treatment of bronchopulmonary dysplasia/chronic lung disease. Caffeine is more effective and safer for the treatment of apnea of prematurity. Caffeine also has the advantage of once-a-day dosing. Aminophylline/theophylline has greater bronchodilator effects.

ACTIONS: Theophylline (the active component of aminophylline) causes relaxation of bronchial smooth muscle; increases the force of contraction of the diaphragmatic muscles; dilates the pulmonary, coronary, and renal arteries; causes mild diuretic action; causes increased sensitivity of the central nervous system (CNS) medullary respiratory centers to CO_2; stimulates central respiratory drive and peripheral chemoreceptors; and increases sensitivity to catecholamines resulting in increased cardiac output and improved oxygenation. Aminophylline is ~80% theophylline. Neonates have a unique ability to convert theophylline to caffeine in a ratio of 1:0.3. Caffeine may account for as much as 50% of the theophylline level.

DOSAGE: PO, IV.

- **IV loading dose:** 5–8 mg/kg, slowly over 30 minutes. IV maintenance dosage is 1.5–3.0 mg/kg/dose every 8–12 hours starting 8–12 hours after loading dose.
- **PO (use immediate-release dosage form) loading dose:** Same as IV. PO maintenance dose as theophylline is 4–22 mg/kg/day divided every 6–8 hours. Older infants may need higher doses as clearance rate increases with increased postnatal age, possibly up to 25–30 mg/kg/day.

ADVERSE EFFECTS: Hyperglycemia, dehydration, diuresis, and feeding intolerance. CNS effects include jitteriness, hyperreflexia, and seizures. Most common side effects are cardiovascular with tachycardia (heart rate ≥180 beats/min) and other tachyarrhythmias.

COMMENTS: Therapeutic levels—apnea 6–14 mcg/mL; bronchospasm 10–20 mcg/mL. Toxicity usually >20 mcg/mL. Monitor serum levels at a peak 1 hour after IV dosing or 2 hours after PO dosing. Take trough levels 30 minutes before next dose. Serum levels should be monitored any time toxicity is suspected or when apneic episodes are increased.

AMIODARONE (CORDARONE)

INDICATIONS AND USE: Treatment of resistant life-threatening ventricular arrhythmias unresponsive to other agents; prevention and suppression of supraventricular arrhythmias (especially those associated with Wolff-Parkinson-White [WPW] syndrome) and postoperative junctional ectopic tachycardia (JET).

ACTIONS: An iodinated benzofuran that prolongs the action potential and increases the effective refractory period. It decreases afterload (causes peripheral and coronary vasodilation), and demonstrates α- and β-blocking properties and calcium channel inhibition. It slows the heart rate (decreases A-V node and sinus node conduction–negative inotropic effects).

DOSAGE: IV. Limited data are available. Generally not first line due to high incidence of adverse effects. Recommend consultation with pediatric cardiologist prior to use.

- **IV loading dose:** 5 mg/kg over 30–60 minutes; do not exceed 0.25 mg/kg/minute unless clinically indicated; central venous access is recommended. May repeat dose up to total loading dose of 15 mg/kg.
- **Maintenance:** 5 mcg/kg/minute gradually increasing as needed to 15 mcg/kg/minute.
- **PO loading dose:** 10–20 mg/kg/day divided into 2 doses per day for 7–10 days or until adequate control of arrhythmia is achieved or significant adverse effects occur. Reduce dose to 5–10 mg/kg/day given once daily for several weeks. Attempt to reduce dose to lowest possible without the recurrence of arrhythmia: 2.5 mg/kg/day.

ADVERSE EFFECTS: Bradycardia and hypotension (may be related to rate of infusion), proarrhythmias (including torsade de pointes), heart block, congestive heart failure (CHF), and paroxysmal ventricular tachycardia. Amiodarone may cause hypo/hyperthyroidism (may partially inhibit the peripheral conversion of T_4 to T_3; serum T_4, and rT3 concentrations may be increased, and serum T_3 may be decreased). Amiodarone HCl contains 37% iodine by weight and is a potential source of iodine; ~3 mg of inorganic iodine/100 mg of amiodarone is released into the circulation. Elevated liver enzymes, elevated bilirubin. Phlebitis and local injection site irritation: avoid concentrations >2 mg/mL, administer through central vein.

PHARMACOLOGY: Adult data: onset of oral antiarrhythmic effects may take up to 3–6 weeks. Duration of antiarrhythmic effects may persist for 30–90 days or longer following discontinuation of therapy. Protein binding: 96%. Metabolized in liver.

COMMENTS: Potential drug interactions may occur. Amiodarone inhibits certain cytochrome P450 enzymes and may increase serum levels of digoxin, flecainide, lidocaine, theophylline, procainamide, quinidine, warfarin, and phenytoin. To avoid toxicities with these agents, dosage reduction and serum concentration monitoring is recommended. Dosage reductions of 30–50% have been recommended. Concurrent administration of amiodarone with β-blockers, digoxin, or calcium channel blockers may result in bradycardia, sinus arrest, and heart block.

AMPHOTERICIN B (AMPHOCIN); AMPHOTERICIN B, LIPOSOMAL (AMBISOME); AMPHOTERICIN B LIPID COMPLEX (ABELCET)

ACTION AND SPECTRUM: Antifungal agent that acts by binding to sterols and disrupting the fungal cell membranes. Broad spectrum of activity against *Candida* spp. and other fungi.

DOSAGE: IV, intrathecal, intraventricular.

Conventional amphotericin B:

- **Initial dose:** 0.5 mg/kg IV over 2–6 hours. Use a 0.1 mg/mL concentration in 5% dextrose in water (D5W). Incompatible with NaCl.
- **Maintenance:** 1–1.5 mg/kg IV every 24 hours for 2–6 weeks or longer, but a lower dose may suffice. Infuse over 2–6 hours, but infusion over 1–2 hours may be used if tolerated.

- **Intrathecal or intraventricular:** Reconstitute with sterile water at 0.25 mg/mL; dilute with cerebrospinal fluid (CSF) and reinfuse. Usual dose: 25–100 mcg every 48–72 hours; increase to 500 mcg as tolerated.

Liposomal amphotericin B:
- Concentrates in liver and spleen, but penetrates the central nervous system (CNS) less than conventional amphotericin B. Used when refractory to or intolerant of conventional amphotericin B.
- 5–7 mg/kg/dose IV infused over 2 hours. May be diluted with D5W, D10W, or D20W to a final concentration of 1–2 mg/mL; concentrations of 0.2–0.5 mg/mL may be needed to provide sufficient volume for infusion.

Amphotericin B lipid complex:
- Used when refractory to or intolerant of conventional amphotericin B. Less nephrotoxic.
- 5 mg/kg/dose IV every 24 hours infused over 2 hours. Dilute with D5W to final concentration of 1 mg/mL; a maximum concentration of 2 mg/mL. Manufacturer recommends that an in-line filter should *not* be used.

PHARMACOKINETICS: Slow renal excretion.

ADVERSE EFFECTS: Fewer adverse effects in neonates as compared to adults. May cause fever, chills, vomiting, thrombophlebitis at injection sites, renal tubular acidosis, renal failure, hypomagnesemia, hypokalemia, bone marrow suppression with reversible decline in hematocrit, hypotension, hypertension, wheezing, and hypoxemia.

COMMENTS: Protect the solution from light. Monitor serum potassium, magnesium, blood urea nitrogen (BUN), creatinine, and urine output at least every other day until the dosage is stabilized, then every week. Monitor complete blood cell count (CBC) and liver function every week. Discontinue if BUN is >40 mg/dL, serum creatinine is >3 mg/dL, or liver function tests are abnormal.

AMPICILLIN (POLYCILLIN, OTHERS)

ACTION AND SPECTRUM: Semisynthetic penicillinase-sensitive penicillin that is bactericidal and acts by inhibiting the late stages of cell wall synthesis. Treatment of susceptible bacterial infections caused by streptococci, pneumococci, enterococci, nonpenicillinase-producing staphylococci, *Listeria*, meningococci; some strains of *Haemophilus influenzae, Proteus mirabilis, Salmonella, Shigella, Escherichia coli, Enterobacter,* and *Klebsiella*; used in combination with an aminoglycoside or cefotaxime in neonates for prevention and treatment of infections due to group B streptococci, *Listeria*, and *E. coli*.

DOSAGE: IM, IV, PO (only for children).

Postnatal age ≤7 days:
- **≤2 kg:** 50 mg/kg/day IM, IV divided every 12 hours. Meningitis: 100 mg/kg/day divided every 12 hours.
- **>2 kg:** 75 mg/kg/day IM, IV divided every 8 hours. Meningitis: 150 mg/kg/day divided every 8 hours.
- **Group B streptococcal meningitis:** 200–300 mg/kg/day IM, IV divided every 8 hours.

Postnatal age >7 days:
- **<1.2 kg:** 50 mg/kg/day IM, IV divided every 12 hours. Meningitis: 100 mg/kg/day divided every 12 hours.
- **1.2–2 kg:** 75 mg/kg/day IM, IV divided every 8 hours. Meningitis: 150 mg/kg/day divided every 8 hours.
- **>2 kg:** 100 mg/kg/day IM, IV divided every 6 hours. Meningitis: 200 mg/kg/day divided every 6 hours.
- **Group B streptococcal meningitis:** 300 mg/kg/day IM, IV divided every 6 hours.

Infants and children:
- 100–200 mg/kg/day IM, IV divided every 6 hours.
- **Meningitis:** 200–400 mg/kg/day IM, IV divided every 6 hours. Maximum dose: 12 grams/day.
- **Oral dosing in children:** 50–100 mg/kg/day PO divided every 6 hours. Maximum dose: 2–3 grams/day.

ADVERSE EFFECTS: Hypersensitivity, rash, abdominal discomfort, nausea, vomiting, diarrhea, hemolytic anemia, thrombocytopenia, neutropenia, prolongation of bleeding time, interstitial nephritis, and eosinophilia. Large doses may cause central nervous system (CNS) excitation or seizures.

AMPICILLIN SODIUM/SULBACTAM SODIUM (UNASYN)

ACTION AND SPECTRUM: Combination β-lactamase inhibitor and β-lactam. The bactericidal spectrum of ampicillin that is extended by the addition of sulbactam, a β-lactamase inhibitor; includes organisms producing β-lactamases such as *Staphylococcus aureus, Haemophilus influenzae, Escherichia coli, Klebsiella, Acinetobacter, Enterobacter,* and anaerobes.

DOSAGE: IV, IM. Dose based on ampicillin component.

Preterm infants and neonates during the first week of life (0–7 days):
- 100 mg ampicillin/kg/day IM/IV divided every 12 hours.

Neonates >7 days:
- 100 mg ampicillin/kg/day IM/IV divided every 6–8 hours.

Infants ≥1 month:
- 100–150 mg ampicillin/kg/day IM/IV divided every 6 hours.

Meningitis
- 200–300 mg ampicillin/kg/day IM/IV divided every 6 hours.

ADVERSE EFFECTS: Elevated blood urea nitrogen (BUN) and serum creatinine. See Ampicillin.
COMMENTS: Modify dosage in patients with renal impairment.

ARGININE HCL (R-GENE)

INDICATIONS AND USE: Treatment of severe metabolic alkalosis after other treatment has failed, pituitary function test (stimulant for the release of growth hormone), and treatment of certain neonatal-onset urea cycle disorders.
ACTIONS: Corrects severe hypochloremic metabolic alkalosis resulting from the high chloride content of arginine. Arginine stimulates pituitary release of growth hormone and prolactin and the pancreatic release of glucagon and insulin.
DOSAGE: **IV.**
Metabolic alkalosis in infants and children:
- Arginine HCl dose (mEq) = 0.5 × weight (kg) × [HCO_3^- − 24] where HCO_3^- = the patient's serum bicarbonate concentration in mEq/L; give one-half to two-thirds of calculated dose and reevaluate.

Correct hypochloremia in infants and children:
- Arginine HCl dose (mEq) = 0.2 × weight (kg) × [103 − Cl^-] where Cl^- = the patient's serum Cl^- concentration in mEq/L; give one-half to two-thirds of the calculated dose, then reevaluate.
- IV: May use undiluted (irritating to tissues) or dilute with normal saline (NS) or dextrose. Administer through a central line. Infuse over at least 30 minutes or over 24 hours in maintenance IV. Maximum: 1 gram/kg/hour (= 10 mL/kg/hour of 10% solution). PO: May use the injectable form, diluted.

Growth hormone reserve test:
- IV 500 mg/kg (= 5 mL/kg of the 10% solution) infused IV over 30 minutes. (Use only IV, not PO administration, for this test.)

Urea cycle disorders
- Consult specialists in metabolic disorders if a urea cycle disorder is suspected.

ADVERSE EFFECTS: Not a first-line treatment for metabolic alkalosis and should never be used as initial therapy; try sodium, potassium, or ammonium chlorides first. May be toxic in infants with arginase deficiency. Do not use in patients sensitive to arginine HCl or in those with hepatic or renal failure. May cause hyperchloremic metabolic acidosis, elevated gastrin, glucagon, and growth hormone; flushing and gastrointestinal (GI) upset with rapid IV administration; hyperglycemia, hypoglycemia, hyperkalemia; tissue necrosis on extravasation, vein irritation; allergic reactions; elevated blood urea nitrogen (BUN) and creatinine.
COMMENTS: Monitor IV site, blood glucose, chloride, and blood pressure.

ATROPINE SULFATE

INDICATIONS AND USE: Sinus bradycardia, in conjunction with neostigmine for the reversal of nondepolarizing neuromuscular blockade. Used preoperatively to inhibit salivation and reduce excessive secretions of the respiratory tract.
ACTIONS: A competitive antagonist of acetylcholine at parasympathetic sites in smooth muscle, cardiac muscle, and various glandular cells, leading to increased heart rate, increased cardiac output, reduced gastrointestinal (GI) motility and tone, urinary retention, cycloplegia, and decreased salivation and sweating.
DOSAGE: **IM, IV, ETT, PO.**
Bradycardia in infants and children:
- 0.02 mg/kg/dose; may repeat once in 3–5 minutes; reserve use for those patients unresponsive to improved oxygenation and epinephrine. **No longer part of AHA neonatal resuscitation algorithm.**

Preanesthetic:
- 0.02 mg/kg/dose 30–60 minutes preoperatively, then every 4–6 hours as needed.

Reversal of neuromuscular blockade:
- Neostigmine 0.06 mg/kg/dose with atropine 0.02 mg/kg/dose.

Intubation, nonemergent (preferred vagolytic):
- 0.02 mg/kg/dose IM/IV.

Endotracheal tube (ETT):
- 0.04–0.06 mg/kg/dose; may repeat once if needed. Flush with 1–5 mL normal saline (NS) based on patient size.

Oral:
- Initial dose: 0.02 mg/kg/dose given every 4–6 hours. May increase gradually to 0.09 mg/kg/dose.

ADVERSE EFFECTS: Xerostomia, blurred vision, mydriasis, tachycardia, palpitations, constipation, urinary retention, ataxia, tremor, and hyperthermia. Toxic effects are especially likely in children receiving low doses.
COMMENTS: Contraindicated in thyrotoxicosis, tachycardia secondary to cardiac insufficiency, and obstructive GI disease. In low doses, it may cause paradoxic bradycardia secondary to its central actions.

AZITHROMYCIN

ACTION AND SPECTRUM: Treatment of upper respiratory tract infections due to *Haemophilus influenzae, Moraxella catarrhalis, Streptococcus pyogenes, Chlamydophila pneumoniae, Mycoplasma pneumoniae, Streptococcus pneumoniae,*

Chlamydia trachomatis, Neisseria gonorrhoeae, Staphylococcus aureus, Mycobacterium avium complex, *Chlamydophila psittaci,* and *Mycoplasma hominis.* Has also been used for treatment of pertussis.
DOSAGE: PO.
Infants <6 months:
- **Pertussis:** 10 mg/kg/dose PO once daily for 5 days (based on AAP *Red Book,* 2012). Azithromycin is drug of choice for age <1 month because of idiopathic hypertrophic pyloric stenosis with erythromycin.
Children ≥6 months:
- **Respiratory tract infections:** 10 mg/kg on day 1 (maximum dose 500 mg) followed by 5 mg/kg/day (maximum dose 250 mg) once daily on days 2–5.
- **Pertussis:** 10 mg/kg on day 1 (maximum dose 500 mg) followed by 5 mg/kg/day (maximum dose 250 mg) once daily on days 2–5 (based on AAP *Red Book,* 2012).
ADVERSE EFFECTS: Diarrhea, vomiting, irritability, rash.
PHARMACOLOGY: Macrolide antibiotic; half-life of ~80 hours.
COMMENTS: Limited data in neonates.

AZTREONAM (AZACTAM)

ACTION AND SPECTRUM: Monobactam antibiotic that is bactericidal against most Enterobacteriaceae, *Pseudomonas aeruginosa, Escherichia coli, Klebsiella pneumoniae, Proteus mirabilis, Serratia, Haemophilus influenzae,* and *Citrobacter* spp., but essentially no activity against gram-positive aerobic or anaerobic bacteria.
DOSAGE: IV, IM.
Neonates postnatal age <7 days:
- **≤2 kg:** 30 mg/kg/dose every 12 hours.
- **>2 kg:** 30 mg/kg/dose every 8 hours.
Neonates postnatal age ≥7 days:
- **<1.2 kg:** 30 mg/kg/dose every 12 hours.
- **1.2–2 kg:** 30 mg/kg/dose every 8 hours.
- **>2 kg:** 30 mg/kg/dose every 6 hours.
Children >1 month:
- 90–120 mg/kg/day divided every 6–8 hours.
ADVERSE EFFECTS: Diarrhea, nausea, vomiting, rash, hypoglycemia, irritation at the infusion site. May cause transient eosinophilia, leukopenia, thrombocytopenia, hypoglycemia, and elevated liver enzymes.
PHARMACOLOGY: Renal elimination as unchanged drug. Half-life is 3–9 hours in neonates. Widely distributed into body tissues, cerebrospinal fluid, bronchial secretions, peritoneal fluid, bile, bone.
COMMENTS: Demonstrates synergistic activity with aminoglycosides against most strains of *P. aeruginosa,* many strains of Enterobacteriaceae, and other gram-negative aerobic bacilli.

BERACTANT (SURVANTA)

INDICATIONS AND USE: Prevention and treatment of respiratory distress syndrome in preterm infants.
ACTIONS: A natural bovine lung extract containing phospholipids, neutral lipids, fatty acids, and surfactant-associated proteins to which dipalmitoylphosphatidylcholine (DPPC), palmitic acid, and tripalmitin are added to mimic the surface tension–lowering properties of natural lung surfactant. Surfactant lowers surface tension on alveolar surfaces during respiration and stabilizes the alveoli against collapse.
DOSAGE: ETT.
- 4 mL/kg (100 mg of phospholipids/kg) birthweight. Divide dose into 4 aliquots, repositioning the infant with each dose. Inject each aliquot gently into the catheter over 2–3 seconds. Ventilate the infant after each one-quarter dose for at least 30 seconds or until stable. Four doses of 4 mL/kg can be given in the first 48 hours of life, no more frequently than every 6 hours. Wean ventilator settings rapidly after administration.
ADVERSE EFFECTS: Most adverse effects are associated while administering the beractant to the infant: transient bradycardia, oxygen desaturation, endotracheal tube (ETT) reflux, pallor, vasoconstriction, hypotension, endotracheal blockage, hypertension, hypocarbia, hypercarbia, and apnea. Pulmonary hemorrhage has been reported, especially in very low birthweight infants.

BUMETANIDE (BUMEX)

> **WARNING:** Bumetanide is a potent diuretic that, if given in excessive amounts, can lead to a profound diuresis with water and electrolyte depletion. Therefore, careful medical supervision is required, and dose and dosage schedule have to be adjusted to the individual patient's needs.

INDICATIONS AND USE: A potent loop diuretic used for the management of edema associated with congenital heart disease, congestive heart failure, and hepatic or renal disease.

ACTIONS: Inhibition of sodium and chloride in the ascending loop of Henle and proximal renal tubule. Urinary excretion of sodium, chloride, potassium, hydrogen, calcium, magnesium, ammonium, phosphate, and bicarbonate increases with bumetanide-induced diuresis. Renal blood flow increases substantially as a result of renovascular dilation and increases prostaglandin secretion.

DOSAGE: IV, IM, PO.

- **Neonates:** 0.005–0.1 mg/kg/dose every 12–24 hours.
- **Infants and children:** 0.015 mg/kg/dose up to 0.1 mg/kg/dose every 6–24 hours (maximum dose is 10 mg/kg/day).

ADVERSE EFFECTS: Hypokalemia, hypochloremia, hyponatremia, metabolic alkalosis, and hypotension. Potentially ototoxic but less so than furosemide.

COMMENTS: Patients refractory to furosemide may respond to bumetanide for diuretic therapy. Although patients may respond differently, bumetanide is ~40 times more potent on a milligram-per-milligram basis than furosemide. Follow electrolytes.

CAFFEINE CITRATE

INDICATIONS AND USE: Treatment of apnea of prematurity; postextubation and postanesthesia apnea.

ACTIONS: Similar to other methylxanthine drugs (eg, aminophylline and theophylline). Caffeine appears to be more active on and less toxic to the central nervous system (CNS) and the respiratory system. Proposed mechanisms of action include increased production of adenosine $3',5'$-cyclic monophosphate (cAMP) alterations of intracellular calcium concentrations. Stimulates the CNS, which increases the medullary respiratory center sensitivity to carbon dioxide, stimulates central inspiratory drive, and improves diaphragmatic contractility. Caffeine exerts a positive inotropic effect on the myocardium, increases renal blood flow and glomerular filtration rate, and stimulates glycogenolysis and lipolysis.

DOSAGE: IV, PO.

- **Loading dose:** 20–25 mg/kg of caffeine citrate IV or PO (equivalent to 10–12.5 mg of caffeine base).
- **Maintenance:** 5–10 mg/kg/day caffeine citrate IV or PO every 24 hours, starting 24 hours after loading dose (equivalent to 2.5–5 mg of caffeine base).

ADVERSE EFFECTS: Nausea, vomiting, gastric irritation, agitation, tachycardia (if heart rate >180 beats/min may consider holding dose), and diuresis. Symptoms of overdosage include arrhythmias and tonic-clonic seizures.

PHARMACOLOGY: Therapeutic serum trough levels 5–25 mcg/mL; severe toxicity is with levels >50 mcg/mL. Draw trough on day 5 of treatment. The serum half-life in neonates ranges from 40 to 230 hours and decreases with increased postnatal age; in infants >9 months half-life is ~5 hours. Half-life is prolonged with cholestasis.

CALCIUM CHLORIDE (VARIOUS)

INDICATIONS AND USE: Acute treatment of symptomatic hypocalcemia, treatment of hypermagnesemia, cardiac disturbances of hyperkalemia, hypocalcemia, or calcium channel blocker toxicity and prevention of hypocalcemia.

ACTIONS: Calcium is essential for the functional integrity of the nervous, muscular, skeletal, and cardiac systems and for clotting function.

DOSAGE: IV. Dosage expressed in milligrams of calcium chloride.

- **Acute treatment of symptomatic hypocalcemia:** 10–20 mg/kg per dose, dilute in appropriate fluid and infuse IV over 10 minutes.
- **Cardiac arrest in the presence of hyperkalemia or hypocalcemia, magnesium toxicity, or calcium antagonist toxicity:** 20 mg/kg/dose IV every 10 minutes as needed. If effective, consider IV infusion 20–50 mg/kg/hour.
- **Tetany:** IV: 10 mg/kg over 5–10 minutes; may repeat after 6 hours or follow with an infusion with a maximum dose of 200 mg/kg/day.

ADVERSE EFFECTS: Arrhythmias (in particular, bradycardia) and deterioration of cardiovascular function; may potentiate digoxin-related arrhythmias; may increase risk of metabolic acidosis. Calcium chloride is contraindicated in ventricular fibrillation or hypercalcemia. Extravasation may cause severe tissue damage (sloughing and necrosis).

COMMENTS: Supplied as a 10% solution (10 mL) (equivalent to elemental calcium 27 mg [1.36 mEq]/mL). Chloride salt is preferred to the gluconate form in cardiac arrest because it may be more bioavailable. Calcium chloride precipitates when mixed with sodium bicarbonate. *Warning:* Multiple salt forms of calcium exist; when ordering and administering calcium, incorrect selection or substitution of one salt for another without proper dosage adjustment may result in serious over- or under-dosing. There is a 3-fold difference in the primary cation concentration between calcium chloride (1 gram = 13.6 mEq [270 mg] of elemental Ca^{++}) and calcium gluconate (1 gram = 4.65 mEq [90 mg] of elemental Ca^{++}).

CALCIUM GLUCONATE

INDICATIONS AND USE: Treatment and prevention of hypocalcemia and prevention of hypocalcemia during exchange transfusion.

ACTIONS: See Calcium Chloride. Calcium gluconate must be metabolized to release calcium ion.

DOSAGE: **IV, PO** (dosage expressed in milligrams of calcium gluconate).

- **Acute treatment of symptomatic hypocalcemia:** 100–200 mg/kg/dose IV diluted in appropriate fluid and administered over 10–30 minutes.
- **Maintenance IV:** 200–800 mg/kg/day divided every 6 hours or as infusion; maximum rate: 50–100 mg/ minute of calcium gluconate. Continuous infusion is more efficacious than intermittent infusion due to less renal calcium loss.
- **Maintenance PO:** 200–800 mg/kg/day divided every 6 hours, mixed in feedings.
- **Exchange transfusion:** 100 mg calcium gluconate/100 mL of citrated blood exchanged infused IV over 10 minutes.

ADVERSE EFFECTS: See Calcium Chloride. Oral administration may cause gastrointestinal (GI) irritation; dilute and use with caution in infants at risk for necrotizing enterocolitis.

CALFACTANT (INFASURF)

INDICATIONS AND USE: Prevention and treatment of neonatal respiratory distress syndrome (RDS).

ACTIONS: Natural, preservative-free calf lung extract that contains phospholipids, neutral lipids, fatty acids, and surfactant-associated proteins B and C. Each milliliter of calfactant contains 35 mg of total phospholipids and 0.65 mg of proteins (0.26 mg of protein B). Calfactant decreases the surface tension on alveolar surfaces, stabilizing the alveoli and preventing collapse. This results in improved ventilation, lung compliance, and gas exchange.

DOSAGE: **ETT.**

- **Prophylactic initial dose for RDS:** As soon as possible after birth, give 3 mL/kg/dose, divided into two 1.5–mL/kg aliquots. After the instillation of each aliquot, position infant either on the right or left side. Ventilation is continued during administration over 20–30 seconds. The 2 aliquots should be separated by a pause to evaluate respiratory status and reposition the patient.
- The initial dose may be followed by 3 subsequent doses of 3 mL/kg/dose at 12-hour intervals, if necessary.

ADVERSE EFFECTS: Bradycardia, cyanosis, airway obstruction, pneumothorax, pulmonary hemorrhage, and apnea. Most adverse effects occur during administration of dose.

COMMENTS: Following administration, lung compliance and oxygenation often rapidly improve. Patients should be closely monitored and appropriate changes in ventilatory support should be made as clinically indicated.

CAPTOPRIL (CAPOTEN)

INDICATIONS AND USE: Moderate to severe congestive heart failure (reduction of afterload) and hypertension.

ACTIONS: Competitive inhibitor of angiotensin-converting enzyme. Causes a decrease in angiotensin II and aldosterone levels; increases plasma and tissue renin activity; decreases systemic vascular resistance without reflex tachycardia and augmentation of cardiac output.

DOSAGE: **PO.**

- **Premature and term neonates, postnatal age (PNA) ≤7 days:** Initial dose: 0.01 mg/kg/dose every 8–12 hours; titrate dose and interval based on response.
- **Term neonates, PNA >7 days:** Initial dose: 0.05–0.1 mg/kg/dose every 8–24 hours; titrate dose up to maximum 0.5 mg/kg/dose given every 6–24 hours.
- **Infants:** Initial dose: 0.15–0.3 mg/kg/dose; titrate dose up to 6 mg/kg/day divided in 2–4 doses.

ADVERSE EFFECTS: Hypotension, rash, fever, eosinophilia, angioedema, neutropenia, gastrointestinal (GI) disturbances, and hyperkalemia. Significant decreases in cerebral and renal blood flow have occurred in premature infants who have chronic hypertension and received higher doses (0.15–0.3 mg/kg/dose); may result in neurologic complications including seizures, apnea and lethargy, and oliguria.

COMMENTS: Administer 1 hour before or 2 hours after feedings if possible; food decreases absorption. Contraindicated in patients with bilateral renovascular disease. Use with caution in patients with low renal perfusion pressure. Reduce the dose with renal impairment and in sodium- and water-depleted patients (use with caution if on concurrent diuretic therapy).

CARBAMAZEPINE (TEGRETOL)

WARNING: Serious dermatologic reactions associated with HLA-B*1502 allele (mostly Asian ancestry). Aplastic anemia and agranulocytosis have been reported.

INDICATIONS AND USE: Anticonvulsant. Treatment of partial (especially complex partial), primary generalized tonic-clonic seizures and mixed partial or generalized seizures.

ACTIONS: Decrease synaptic transmission, limits influx of sodium ions across cell membrane.

DOSAGE: **PO.**

- 10–20 mg/kg/day of oral suspension, initially divided 4 times a day; may increase weekly to optimal response, then to a maximum of 35 mg/kg/day. Administer daily dose in 3–4 divided doses with feedings.

ADVERSE EFFECTS: Nausea, vomiting, leukopenia, thrombocytopenia, aplastic anemia and agranulocytosis, congestive heart failure (CHF), heart block, dystonia, drowsiness, and behavioral changes, syndrome of inappropriate antidiuretic hormone secretion (SIADH), hyponatremia, hepatitis and cholestasis, rash and Stevens-Johnson syndrome, urine retention, azotemia, oliguria, and anuria. Monitor complete blood cell count (CBC), liver function, and urinalysis; perform periodic eye examination. Do not discontinue abruptly because seizures may result in epileptic patients.

PHARMACOLOGY: Metabolized in liver by cytochrome P450 3A4. Induces liver enzymes and increases its own metabolism. Half-life in neonates is 8–28 hours. Therapeutic range is 4–12 mcg/mL.

COMMENTS: Avoid switching between Tegretol and generic carbamazepine; changes in serum concentration and seizure activity may result; monitor serum concentrations. Interactions are numerous. Erythromycin, isoniazid, and cimetidine may inhibit hepatic metabolism of carbamazepine, resulting in increased carbamazepine serum concentrations. Concurrent phenobarbital may lower carbamazepine serum levels. Carbamazepine may induce metabolism of warfarin, phenytoin, theophylline, benzodiazepines, and corticosteroids.

CASPOFUNGIN

ACTION AND SPECTRUM: Treatment of invasive aspergillosis that is refractory to other antifungal agents or in patients intolerant of other agents; infections caused by susceptible *Candida* species.

DOSAGE: IV.

- **Preterm neonates—infants <3 months:** 25 mg/m^2 (or equivalent to ~2 mg/kg)/dose IV every 24 hours; infuse over at least 1 hour via syringe pump.
- **Infants ≥3 months:** Initial dose of 70 mg/m^2/dose IV followed by 50 mg/m^2/dose IV every 24 hours starting day 2. May increase to 70 mg/m^2/dose IV every 24 hours if clinical response is inadequate. Maximum dose is 70 mg/day.
- **Length of therapy:** At least 14 days after last positive culture.

ADVERSE EFFECTS: Hypokalemia, hypercalcemia, elevated liver enzymes, thrombocytopenia, direct hyperbilirubinemia, thrombophlebitis, hypotension, fever, and rash.

PHARMACOLOGY: An echinocandin acts by inhibiting the synthesis of β-(1,3)-D-glucan, an important component of the fungal cell wall. Fungicidal against *Candida* species and fungistatic against *Aspergillus*. Metabolized by the liver, not cytochrome P450 enzymes; results in fewer drug-drug interactions than the azole class of antifungal agents. Serum concentrations of caspofungin may be lower if concomitant therapy with dexamethasone, phenytoin, carbamazepine, nevirapine, and rifampin. Caspofungin clearance is induced and higher doses may be required: 70 mg/m^2/dose.

COMMENTS: *Note:* Dosing information based on very limited pharmacokinetic data of 18 neonates and infants (Saez-Llorens, 2009). Do not use diluents containing dextrose for reconstitution.

CEFAZOLIN SODIUM (ANCEF, KEFZOL)

ACTION AND SPECTRUM: First-generation cephalosporin; a broad-spectrum semisynthetic β-lactam antibiotic with bactericidal activity. Activity against susceptible gram-positive cocci (except enterococci), including penicillinase-producing staphylococci; some gram-negative coverage of susceptible *Escherichia coli*, *Klebsiella*, and *Proteus*. Primarily used in neonates for urinary tract infections, perioperative prophylaxis, and soft tissue infections.

DOSAGE: IV.

Neonates:

- **Postnatal age ≤7 days:** 40 mg/kg/day divided every 12 hours.
- **Postnatal age >7 days:** ≤2 kg: 40 mg/kg/day divided every 12 hours; >2 kg: 60 mg/kg/day divided every 8 hours.

Infants and children:

- 50–100 mg/kg/day divided every 8 hours; maximum dose: 6 grams/day.

ADVERSE EFFECTS: Infrequent; fever, rash, and urticaria. May cause eosinophilia, leukopenia, neutropenia, and thrombocytopenia. Excessive dosage (especially in renal impairment) may result in central nervous system (CNS) irritation with seizure activity.

PHARMACOLOGY: 80–100% excreted unchanged in urine. Half-life is 3–5 hours in neonates.

COMMENTS: Dosage reduction is required in moderate to severe renal failure.

CEFEPIME

ACTION AND SPECTRUM: Fourth-generation cephalosporin used for treatment of infections caused by susceptible gram-negative bacteria: *Escherichia coli*, *Haemophilus influenzae*, *Enterobacter*, *Klebsiella*, *Providencia*, *Serratia*, *Proteus*, *Morganella*, *Neisseria*, *Pseudomonas aeruginosa*, *Acinetobacter*, and *Citrobacter*. Treatment of infections caused by susceptible gram-positive bacteria: *Staphylococcus aureus*, *Streptococcus pyogenes*, *Streptococcus pneumoniae*, and *Streptococcus agalactiae*.

DOSAGE: IV.

- **Neonates and infants ≤8 days of age:** 30 mg/kg/dose IV every 12 hours.
- **Infants >28 days of age:** 50 mg/kg/dose every 12 hours.
- **For meningitis or infections due to *Pseudomonas* or *Enterobacter*:** 50 mg/kg/dose every 12 hours.

ADVERSE EFFECTS: Rash, elevated hepatic transaminase enzymes, prothrombin time (PT), partial thromboplastin time (PTT), thrombocytopenia, leukopenia, neutropenia, eosinophilia, and hypophosphatemia.

PHARMACOLOGY: Distributes well into body tissues and fluids. Low protein binding; primarily excreted in urine unchanged.

COMMENTS: Manufacturer does not recommend use for treatment of serious infections due to *H. influenzae* type b for suspected meningitis.

CEFOTAXIME SODIUM (CLAFORAN)

ACTION AND SPECTRUM: Third-generation cephalosporin with bactericidal activity against susceptible gram-negative organisms (except *Pseudomonas*), including *Escherichia coli*, *Enterobacter*, *Klebsiella*, *Haemophilus influenzae* (including ampicillin-resistant strains), *Proteus*, *Serratia*, *Neisseria gonorrhoeae*, and *Neisseria meningitidis*. Generally poor activity against gram-positive aerobic organisms.

DOSAGE: IV, IM.

Neonates:

- **0–4 weeks and <1.2 kg:** 100 mg/kg/day divided every 12 hours.

Postnatal age ≤7 days:

- **1.2–2 kg:** 100 mg/kg/day divided every 12 hours.
- **>2 kg:** 100–150 mg/kg/day divided every 8–12 hours.

Postnatal age >7 days:

- **1.2–2 kg:** 150 mg/kg/day divided every 8 hours.
- **>2 kg:** 150–200 mg/kg/day divided every 6–8 hours.

Infants and children 1 month to 12 years:

- **<50 kg:** 100–200 mg/kg/day divided every 6–8 hours.
- **Meningitis:** 200 mg/kg/day divided every 6 hours; 225–300 mg/kg/day divided every 6–8 hours has been used to treat invasive pneumococcal meningitis.

Disseminated gonococcal infection and scalp abscesses: The Centers for Disease Control and Prevention (CDC) recommends cefotaxime as an alternative to ceftriaxone in the treatment of disseminated gonococcal infection and gonococcal scalp abscesses in newborns. The dose of cefotaxime is 25 mg/kg in a single daily dose IM or IV for 7 days; duration is 10–14 days for meningitis.

Gonococcal ophthalmia prophylaxis in newborns of mothers with gonorrhea at delivery: 100 mg/kg IV or IM as a single dose (topical antibiotic therapy alone is inadequate).

ADVERSE EFFECTS: Arrhythmias; transient neutropenia, thrombocytopenia, eosinophilia, leukopenia; transient hepatic and renal dysfunction.

PHARMACOLOGY: Excreted principally unchanged in the urine. Half-life in neonates is 1–4 hours.

COMMENTS: Reserved for suspected or documented gram-negative meningitis or sepsis. When used as empiric therapy, combine with ampicillin or penicillin to provide gram-positive coverage (ie, group B streptococci, pneumococci, and *Listeria monocytogenes*). Third-generation cephalosporins induce the emergence of multidrug-resistant bacteria or fungal infection when used excessively and without proper clinical indications.

CEFOXITIN (MEFOXIN)

ACTIONS AND SPECTRUM: Second-generation cephalosporin used for infections from gram-negative enteric organisms *Escherichia coli*, *Klebsiella*, and *Proteus*; active against many strains of *Neisseria gonorrhoeae*, ampicillin-resistant *Haemophilus influenzae*, and anaerobic bacteria, including *Bacteroides* species of the gastrointestinal (GI) tract.

DOSAGE: IV.

Neonates:

- 90–100 mg/kg/day divided every 8 hours.

Infants ≥3 months and children:

- **Mild-moderate infection:** 80–100 mg/kg/day divided every 6–8 hours.
- **Severe infection:** 100–160 mg/kg/day divided every 4–6 hours; maximum dose: 12 grams/day.

PHARMACOLOGY: Highly protein bound and renally excreted essentially unchanged.

ADVERSE EFFECTS: Usually well tolerated. May cause rash, thrombophlebitis; transient leukopenia, thrombocytopenia, neutropenia, anemia, and eosinophilia, and transient elevation of blood urea nitrogen (BUN), serum creatinine, and liver enzymes.

COMMENTS: Not inactivated by β-lactamase. Has poor central nervous system (CNS) penetration. The safety and efficacy in infants <3 months have not been established.

CEFTAZIDIME (FORTAZ, TAZIDIME)

ACTION AND SPECTRUM: Third-generation cephalosporin with bactericidal activity against gram-negative aerobic bacteria, including *Neisseria*, *Haemophilus influenzae*, some Enterobacteriaceae, and *Pseudomonas*. Pseudomonal infections in patients at risk of developing aminoglycoside-induced nephrotoxicity and/or ototoxicity. Poor gram-positive activity. Aminoglycosides act synergistically with ceftazidime.

DOSAGE: IV.
Neonates:

- **0–4 weeks and <1.2 kg:** 100 mg/kg/day divided every 12 hours.

Postnatal age <7 days:

- **1.2–2 kg:** 100 mg/kg/day divided every 12 hours.
- **>2 kg:** 100–150 mg/kg/day divided every 8–12 hours.

Postnatal age ≥7 days and ≥1.2 kg:

- 150 mg/kg/day divided every 8 hours.

Infants and children 1 month to 12 years:

- 100–150 mg/kg/day divided every 8 hours; maximum dose: 6 grams/day.

Meningitis:

- 150 mg/kg/day divided every 8 hours; maximum dose: 6 grams/day.

ADVERSE EFFECTS: Infrequent except for fever, rash, urticaria. May cause transient leukopenia, neutropenia, thrombocytopenia, and hemolytic anemia; transient elevation in liver enzymes, hyperbilirubinemia, transient elevation of blood urea nitrogen (BUN) and serum creatinine.

PHARMACOLOGY: Renally excreted 80–90% unchanged. Half-life is 2.2–4.7 hours; penetrates well into cerebrospinal fluid (CSF).

CEFTRIAXONE SODIUM (ROCEPHIN)

ACTION AND SPECTRUM: Third-generation cephalosporin with activity against gram-negative aerobic bacteria, *Haemophilus influenzae*, Enterobacteriaceae, and *Neisseria*, and activity against gram-positive cocci, methicillin-susceptible *Staphylococcus* and *Streptococcus*. No activity against *Pseudomonas aeruginosa*, *Chlamydia trachomatis*, methicillin-resistant staphylococci, and enterococci.

DOSAGE: IV, IM.
Neonates:

- **Postnatal age <7 days:** 50 mg/kg/day every 24 hours.
- **Postnatal age ≥7 days:**
  - **≤2 kg:** 50 mg/kg/day every 24 hours.
  - **>2 kg:** 50–75 mg/kg/day every 24 hours.

Gonococcal prophylaxis:

- 25–50 mg/kg as a single dose (dose not to exceed 125 mg).

Gonococcal infection:

- 25–50 mg/kg/day (maximum dose 125 mg) every 24 hours for 7 days; up to 10–14 days if meningitis is documented. (**Note**: Use cefotaxime in place of ceftriaxone in hyperbilirubinemic neonates.)

Ophthalmia neonatorum:

- 25–50 mg/kg as a single dose (maximum dose 125 mg).

Infants and children:

- 50–75 mg/kg/day divided every 12–24 hours.

Meningitis:

- 80–100 mg/kg/day divided every 12–24 hours; loading dose of 75 mg/kg may be administered at the start of therapy; maximum dose 4 grams/day.

ADVERSE EFFECTS: Diarrhea, cholelithiasis, gallbladder sludging. May also cause neutropenia, eosinophilia, hemolytic anemia, increased prothrombin times, rash, thrombophlebitis, elevated liver enzymes, jaundice, hyperbilirubinemia; use with caution in infants with hyperbilirubinemia.

PHARMACOLOGY: Biliary and renal excretion. Half-life is 5–19 hours.

COMMENTS: *Warning:* Ceftriaxone is incompatible with calcium-containing solutions. Calcium-containing solutions or products must not be administered within 48 hours of the ceftriaxone dose due to the fatal reaction involving calcium-ceftriaxone precipitates in the lungs and kidneys of neonates. Dosage reduction is required only in patients with both renal and hepatic dysfunction.

CEFUROXIME SODIUM (KEFUROX, ZINACEF)

ACTION AND SPECTRUM: Second-generation cephalosporin with activity against susceptible staphylococci, group B streptococci, pneumococci, *Haemophilus influenzae* (type A and B), *Escherichia coli*, *Enterobacter*, and *Klebsiella*.

DOSAGE: IM, IV.

- **Neonates:** 50–100 mg/kg/day divided every 12 hours.
- **Children:** 75–150 mg/kg/day divided every 8 hours; maximum dose 6 grams/day.
- **Meningitis:** Not recommended due to reports of treatment failures and slower bacteriologic response time.

ADVERSE EFFECTS: Fever, seizures, rash, thrombophlebitis, diarrhea, hemolytic anemia, transient neutropenia and leukopenia, eosinophilia, increased prothrombin time. Transient elevation in liver enzymes, hepatitis, and cholestasis; elevation in blood urea nitrogen (BUN) and serum creatinine.

PHARMACOLOGY: Primarily excreted unchanged in the urine. Half-life is 5.1–5.8 hours in infants <3 days old and 1–4.2 hours in infants >8 days of age.

COMMENTS: Decrease the dosage in renal failure. Limited experience in neonates. Safety and efficacy in infants <3 months of age have not been established.

CHLORAL HYDRATE (NOCTEC)

INDICATIONS AND USE: Short-term sedative and hypnotic; central nervous system (CNS) depressant.

DOSAGE: PO, PR. Use the lowest effective dose.

- Usual dose 25–50 mg/kg/dose PO or PR every 6–8 hours as needed.
- Sedation prior to electroencephalography and other procedures: 25–75 mg/kg/dose once PO or PR. Typical dose: 50 mg/kg/dose once; repeat 25 mg/kg/dose once if needed.

ADVERSE EFFECTS: Gastrointestinal irritation resulting in nausea, vomiting, and diarrhea; paradoxic excitation; and respiratory depression, particularly if administered with opiates and barbiturates. May cause direct hyperbilirubinemia with chronic use (active metabolite 2,2,2-trichloroethanol [TCE]); competes with bilirubin for glucuronide conjugation in the liver); overdose can be lethal.

COMMENTS: Contraindicated with marked renal or hepatic impairment. Syrup may contain sodium benzoate; benzoic acid (benzoate) is a metabolite of benzyl alcohol.

CHLORAMPHENICOL (CHLOROMYCETIN)

> WARNING: Bone marrow hypoplasia including aplastic anemia and death have been reported following topical application of chloramphenicol. Chloramphenicol should not be used when less potentially dangerous agents would be expected to provide effective treatment.

ACTION AND SPECTRUM: Broad-spectrum bacteriostatic agent, reserved for serious infections due to organisms resistant to other less toxic agent due to *Haemophilus influenzae*, *Neisseria meningitides*, and *Escherichia coli*; *Klebsiella*, *Serratia*, *Enterobacter*, *Salmonella*, *Shigella*, *Neisseria gonorrhoeae*, staphylococci, *Streptococcus pneumoniae*, and *Bacteroides*; active against many vancomycin-resistant enterococci.

DOSAGE: IV.

Neonates:

- **Loading dose:** 20 mg/kg IV.
- **Maintenance dose:** 12 hours after the loading dose.
  - **≤7 days:** 25 mg/kg/day IV once every 24 hours.
  - **>7 days, ≤2 kg:** 25 mg/kg/day IV once every 24 hours.
  - **>7 days, >2 kg:** 50 mg/kg/day IV divided every 12 hours.

Infants and children:

- **Meningitis:** 75–100 mg/kg/day IV divided every 6 hours.
- **Other infections:** 50–75 mg/kg/day IV divided every 6 hours. Maximum daily dose 4 grams/day.

ADVERSE EFFECTS: Idiosyncratic reactions result in aplastic anemia (irreversible and rare), reversible bone marrow suppression (dose related), allergy (rash and fever), diarrhea, vomiting, stomatitis, glossitis, fungal overgrowth, "gray baby" syndrome (early signs are hyperammonemia and unexplained metabolic acidosis; other signs are abdominal distention, hypotonia, gray skin color, and cardiorespiratory collapse), and cardiotoxicity due to left ventricular dysfunction. Use with extreme caution in neonates.

PHARMACOLOGY: Metabolized by hepatic glucuronyl transferase. Half-life is 10–24 hours in neonates.

COMMENTS: Must monitor serum levels. Desired peak is 10–25 mcg/mL; levels >50 mcg/mL are strongly associated with "gray baby" syndrome. Monitor complete blood cell count (CBC) with differential, platelet count, and reticulocyte count every 3 days.

CHLOROTHIAZIDE (DIURIL)

INDICATIONS AND USE: Mild to moderate edema, and hypertension.

ACTIONS: Thiazide diuretic; inhibits sodium reabsorption in the distal renal tubules. Sodium, potassium, bicarbonate, magnesium, phosphate, and chloride excretion are increased, whereas calcium excretion is decreased.

DOSAGE: PO, IV. *Note:* IV dosage in infants and children has not been established. IV doses in infants and children are based on anecdotal reports. The IV dosing regimens have been extrapolated from oral dosing regimens considering only 10–20% of an oral dose is absorbed.

Neonates and infants <6 months:

- **Oral:** 20–40 mg/kg/day PO divided every 12 hours; maximum 375 mg/day.
- **IV:** 2–8 mg/kg/day IV divided every 12 hours; doses up to 20 mg/kg/day have been used.

Infants >6 months and children:

- **Oral:** 20 mg/kg/day PO divided every 12 hours; maximum 1 gram/day.
- **IV:** 4 mg/kg/day IV divided in 1–2 doses; doses up to 20 mg/kg/day have been used.

ADVERSE EFFECTS: Hypokalemia, hypochloremic alkalosis, dehydration and prerenal azotemia, hyperuricemia, hyperglycemia, hypermagnesemia, hyperlipidemia.

PHARMACOLOGY: Duration of action 6–12 hours; onset of action is within 2 hours.

COMMENTS: Do not use in patients with anuria or severe hepatic dysfunction.

CHOLESTYRAMINE RESIN (QUESTRAN)

INDICATIONS AND USE: A resin-binding agent in patients with chronic diarrhea and short-gut syndrome to decrease fecal output.

ACTION: Cholestyramine resin binds to bile acids in the intestine, forms a nonabsorbable complex preventing the reabsorption and enterohepatic recirculation of bile salts, and releases chloride ions in the process.

DOSAGE: PO.

- **Children:** 240 mg/kg/day in 3 divided doses. Titrate dose depending on the indication.

ADVERSE EFFECTS: Constipation. High doses can cause hyperchloremic acidosis and increase urinary calcium excretion.

PHARMACOKINETICS: Not absorbed; excreted in the feces.

COMMENTS: May bind concurrent oral medications, in particular levothyroxine.

CIMETIDINE (TAGAMET)

INDICATIONS AND USE: Prevention and treatment of duodenal and gastric ulcers, gastroesophageal reflux, esophagitis, and hypersecretory conditions.

ACTIONS: A histamine (H_2)-receptor antagonist; competitively inhibits the action of histamine on the gastric parietal cells, decreasing gastric acid secretion.

DOSAGE: PO.

- **Neonates:** 5–10 mg/kg/day PO divided every 8–12 hours.
- **Infants:** 10–20 mg/kg/day PO divided every 6–12 hours.
- **Children:** 20–40 mg/kg/day PO divided every 6 hours.

ADVERSE EFFECTS: Central nervous system (CNS) toxicity such as agitation and alterations in consciousness, neutropenia, agranulocytosis, thrombocytopenia, antiandrogenic effects; elevated aspartate transaminase (AST), alanine transaminase (ALT), and creatinine levels.

PHARMACOLOGY: Cimetidine reduces the hepatic metabolism of drugs metabolized by the cytochrome P450 pathway, which may result in decreased elimination of diazepam, theophylline, phenytoin, propranolol, and carbamazepine. Doses of these drugs may need to be decreased.

COMMENTS: Limited use in neonates.

CITRATE AND CITRIC ACIDS SOLUTIONS (BICITRA, ORACIT, POLYCITRA-K)

INDICATIONS AND USE: Treatment of metabolic acidosis or as a urinary alkalinizing agent for conditions that require the maintenance of alkaline urine.

ACTIONS: Sodium and potassium citrate salts have the capability to buffer gastric acidity (pH >2.5) and are metabolized to bicarbonate to act as systemic alkalinizers.

DOSAGE: PO.

- 2–3 mEq/kg/day of bicarbonate in divided doses 3–4 times per day with water.

ADVERSE EFFECTS: Metabolic alkalosis, hypernatremia (if sodium salt used), hypocalcemia, hyperkalemia (if potassium salt used), diarrhea, nausea, vomiting.

COMMENTS: Supplied as oral solutions: **Bicitra** and **Oracit** contain 1 mEq of sodium and 1 mEq of bicarbonate equivalent per milliliter; **Polycitra** contains 1 mEq of sodium and 1 mEq of potassium and 2 mEq of bicarbonate equivalents per milliliter; **Polycitra-K** contains 2 mEq of potassium and 2 mEq of bicarbonate equivalents per milliliter. Conversion to bicarbonate may be impaired in patients with hepatic failure.

CLINDAMYCIN (CLEOCIN)

ACTION AND SPECTRUM: Bacteriostatic agent active against most aerobic gram-positive staphylococci and streptococci (except enterococci); *Fusobacterium*, *Bacteroides* spp., *Actinomyces*, and certain anaerobic gram-positive organisms.

DOSAGE: IM, IV.

Neonates

- **Postnatal age <7 days:**
  - **≤2 kg:** 10 mg/kg/day IM/IV divided every 12 hours.
  - **>2 kg:** 15 mg/kg/day IM/IV divided every 8 hours.
- **Postnatal age ≥7 days:**
  - **<1.2 kg:** 10 mg/kg/day IM/IV divided every 12 hours.
  - **1.2–2 kg:** 15 mg/kg/day IM/IV divided every 8 hours.
  - **>2 kg:** 20–30 mg/kg/day IM/IV divided every 6–8 hours.

Infants and children:

- 25–40 mg/kg/day IM/IV divided every 6–8 hours; doses as high as 4.8 grams/day have been given IV in life-threatening situations or 10–30 mg/kg/day PO divided every 6–8 hours; maximum dose 1.8 grams/day.

ADVERSE EFFECTS: Diarrhea, colitis, pseudomembranous colitis rash, pruritus, neutropenia, granulocytopenia and thrombocytopenia, hypersensitivity reactions, and elevated liver enzymes. Sterile abscess formation at the IM injection site.

PHARMACOLOGY: Primarily hepatic metabolism, highly protein bound.

COMMENTS: Does not cross the blood-brain barrier; therefore, do not use to treat meningitis.

CLONAZEPAM (KLONOPIN)

INDICATIONS AND USE: For the treatment of petit mal, Lennox-Gastaut, infantile spasms, and akinetic and myoclonic seizures, either as a single agent or as adjunctive therapy.

ACTIONS: Depresses all areas of the central nervous system (CNS) including the limbic and reticular formation by binding to the benzodiazepine site on the γ-aminobutyric acid (GABA) receptor complex; suppresses the spike-and-wave discharge in absence seizures by depressing nerve transmission in the motor cortex.

DOSAGE: **PO.**

Seizure disorders

- **Infants and children <10 years or 30 kg.**
- **Initial daily dose:** 0.01–0.03 mg/kg/day PO (maximum 0.05 mg/kg/day) given in 2–3 divided doses; increase by no more than 0.5 mg every third day until seizures are controlled or adverse effects occur.
- **Maintenance:** 0.1–0.2 mg/kg/day PO divided into 3 doses; do not exceed 0.2 mg/kg/day.

ADVERSE EFFECTS: Hypotension, drowsiness, hypotonia, thrombocytopenia, anemia, leukopenia, eosinophilia, tremor, choreiform movements, bronchial hypersecretion, respiratory depression.

PHARMACOLOGY: Cytochrome P450 isoenzyme CYP3A3/4 substrate. CNS depressants increase sedation; phenytoin, carbamazepine, rifampin, and barbiturates increase clonazepam clearance; drugs that inhibit cytochrome P450 isoenzyme CYP3A3/4 may increase levels and effects of clonazepam (monitor for altered benzodiazepine response); concurrent use with valproic acid may result in absence status.

COMMENTS: Caution in patients with chronic respiratory disease, hepatic disease, or impaired renal function. Abrupt discontinuation of clonazepam may precipitate withdrawal symptoms, status epilepticus, or seizures. (Withdraw gradually when discontinuing therapy in children. Safely reduce by ≤0.04 mg/kg/week and discontinue when the daily dose is ≤0.04 mg/kg/day.) Worsening of seizures may occur when clonazepam is added to patients with multiple seizure types.

CLONIDINE (CATAPRES; CATAPRES-TTS)

INDICATIONS AND USE: Adjunctive treatment of neonatal abstinence syndrome (NAS) and iatrogenic narcotic dependency.

ACTIONS: Stimulates central nervous system (CNS) α_2-adrenergic receptors which results in decreased sympathetic outflow, peripheral vascular resistance, systolic and diastolic blood pressure, and heart rate. Clonidine reduces circulating plasma renin levels.

DOSAGE: **PO.**

Neonatal abstinence syndrome (opioid withdrawal):

- **Preterm neonate:** 0.5–1 mcg/kg/dose PO every 6 hours. Taper dose when stabilized by 0.25 mcg/kg/dose PO every 6 hours (Leikin et al, 2009).
- **Full-term neonate:** 1 mcg/kg/dose PO every 4 hours in combination with diluted opium tincture. A randomized, controlled, comparative trial in 80 neonates (gestational age [GA]: ≥35 weeks) with NAS demonstrated a decreased length of therapy and opioid doses in the combination treatment (clonidine plus diluted opium tincture) as compared to diluted tincture of opium alone (Agthe et al, 2009).
- **Alternate dosing:** Initial dose of 0.5–1 mcg/kg/dose every 3–6 hours; maximum dose 1 mcg/kg/dose every 3 hours (AAP Clinical Report—Neonatal Drug Withdrawal, 2012).

ADVERSE EFFECTS: Very few side effects reported when used to treat NAS. Observe for hypotension and bradycardia and avoid abrupt discontinuation.

COMMENTS: More experience is needed before clonidine is routinely used to treat opioid withdrawal in infants.

COSYNTROPIN (CORTROSYN)

INDICATIONS AND USE: Aid in the diagnosis of adrenocortical insufficiency; used in the diagnosis of congenital adrenal hyperplasia.

ACTIONS: Stimulates the adrenal cortex to secrete cortisol (hydrocortisone and cortisone), androgenic substances, and a small amount of aldosterone.

DOSAGE: **IM/IV.** Diagnostic test doses.

Adrenocortical insufficiency:

- **Preterm neonates:** Not well defined; 0.1 mcg/kg, 0.2 mcg/kg, 1 mcg/kg, and 3.5 mcg/kg have been used.
- **Neonates:** 15 mcg/kg (1 dose only).
- **Children ≤2 years:** 0.125 mg.

Congenital adrenal hyperplasia evaluation:
- 1 mg/m^2/dose up to a maximum of 1 mg.

COMMENTS: Plasma cortisol concentrations should be measured immediately before and exactly 30 minutes after administration of cosyntropin; dose should be given in early morning; 0.25 mg of cosyntropin = 25 USP units of corticotropin.

CYCLOPENTOLATE

INDICATIONS AND USE: For diagnostic and therapeutic ophthalmologic procedures that require mydriasis and cycloplegia.

ACTIONS: Causes pupillary dilatation by inhibition of the cholinergic response of the ciliary body muscle and sphincter muscle of iris.

DOSAGE: Ocular.
- One to two drops into the eye 10–30 minutes prior to procedure; usually used in conjunction with phenylephrine 2.5%. The 0.5% concentration is recommended for neonates.

ADVERSE EFFECTS: Tachycardia, vasodilatation, restlessness, delayed gastric emptying, urinary retention.

PHARMACOLOGY: Maximal effect occurs 30–60 minutes after administration, with pharmacologic effects lasting 6–24 hours.

COMMENTS: Consider holding feeds for 4 hours after procedure.

DEXAMETHASONE (DECADRON)

INDICATIONS: Treatment of airway edema prior to extubation. Used in infants with bronchopulmonary dysplasia/ chronic lung disease to facilitate weaning from the ventilator.

ACTIONS: Long-acting, potent glucocorticoid without mineralocorticoid properties; prevents or suppresses inflammatory and immune responses in pharmacologic doses. Inhibits leukocyte infiltration at site of inflammation, interferes in function of mediators of inflammatory response, and suppresses humoral immune responses. May reduce edema and scar tissue formation; reversal of increased capillary permeability, and general suppression in immune response.

DOSAGE: IV, PO.
Neonates:
- **Airway edema or extubation:** Usual dose: 0.25 mg/kg/dose IV given ~4 hours prior to scheduled extubation and then every 8 hours for 3 doses total. Range: 0.25–1 mg/kg/dose for 1–3 doses. Maximum dose: 1 mg/kg/day. *Note:* A longer duration of therapy may be needed in more severe cases.
- **Bronchopulmonary dysplasia/chronic lung disease (facilitate ventilator weaning):**
  - **Numerous dosing schedules proposed:** Range: 0.5–0.6 mg/kg/day given in divided doses PO or IV every 12 hours for 3–7 days, then taper over 1–6 weeks.
  - **DART trial protocol (Doyle et al, 2006):** 0.075 mg/kg/dose every 12 hours for 3 days, 0.05 mg/kg/dose every 12 hours for 3 days, 0.025 mg/kg/dose every 12 hours for 2 days, 0.01 mg/kg/dose every 12 hours for 2 days.

ADVERSE EFFECTS: With long-term use, increased susceptibility to infection, osteoporosis, growth retardation, hyperglycemia, fluid and electrolyte disturbances, cataracts, myopathy, gastrointestinal perforation and hemorrhage, hypertension, and acute adrenal insufficiency. Dexamethasone use for low birthweight infants has come under close scrutiny because of increasing numbers of reports indicating neurodevelopmental compromise (see Comments).

COMMENTS: Please review the important statement from the American Academy of Pediatrics, Committee on Fetus and Newborn, and Canadian Pediatric Society, Fetus and Newborn Committee (2002).

DIAZEPAM (VALIUM)

INDICATIONS: Alternative choice to lorazepam for status epilepticus. Treatment of seizures refractory to other combined anticonvulsant agents. Reduces anxiety, and can use for preoperative or preprocedural sedation.

ACTIONS: Exact action is unknown; acts as a central nervous system (CNS) depressant. Like other benzodiazepines, diazepam increases the activity of the inhibitory neurotransmitter γ-aminobutyric acid (GABA) by binding the benzodiazepine receptor sites in the CNS.

DOSAGE: IV, PO.
Status epilepticus:
- **Neonates:** 0.1–0.3 mg/kg/dose IV given over 3–5 minutes, every 15–30 minutes to a maximum total dose of 2 mg. (Not recommended as first line; injection contains benzoic acid, benzyl alcohol, and sodium benzoate.)
- **Infants >30 days and children <5 years:** 0.1–0.3 mg/kg/dose given over 3–5 minutes, every 5–10 minutes to a maximum total dose of 5 mg, or 0.2–0.5 mg/dose every 2–5 minutes to a maximum total dose of 5 mg; repeat in 2–4 hours as needed.

Conscious sedation for procedures:

- **IV:** Initial: 0.05-0.1 mg/kg over 3–5 minutes, titrate slowly to effect (maximum total dose 0.25 mg/kg) (Krauss and Green, 2006).
- **PO:** 0.2–0.3 mg/kg (maximum dose 10 mg) 45–60 minutes prior to procedure.

Sedation or muscle relaxation or anxiety:

- **Oral:** 0.12–0.8 mg/kg/day in divided doses every 6–8 hours.
- **IV:** 0.04–0.3 mg/kg/dose every 2–4 hours to a maximum of 0.6 mg/kg within an 8-hour period if needed.

ADVERSE EFFECTS: May cause rash, vasodilation, bradycardia, respiratory arrest, and hypotension. Use with caution in patients receiving other CNS depressants; may have additive CNS and respiratory depressant effects.
COMMENTS: Observe for and be prepared to manage respiratory arrest. Rapid IV push may cause sudden respiratory depression, apnea, or hypotension. Use of the rectal gel formulation in infants <6 months is not recommended; for use in children <2 years, the safety and efficacy have not been studied; contains benzoic acid, benzyl alcohol, ethanol 10%, propylene glycol, and sodium benzoate.

DIAZOXIDE (HYPERSTAT IV, PROGLYCEM)

INDICATIONS AND USE: Persistent hyperinsulinemic neonatal hypoglycemia (oral).
ACTIONS: Nondiuretic thiazide with antihypertensive and hyperglycemic effects. Inhibits the release of insulin from the pancreas and reduces total peripheral vascular resistance by direct relaxation of arteriolar smooth muscle, which results in a decrease in blood pressure and reflex increase in heart rate and cardiac output.
DOSAGE: PO.

Hyperinsulinemic hypoglycemia:

- **Neonates:** Initial: 10 mg/kg/day PO in divided doses every 8 hours; usual range: 5–15 mg/kg/day in divided doses every 8 hours.
- **Infants:** Initial: 10 mg/kg/day in divided doses every 8 hours; usual range: 5–20 mg/kg/day in divided doses every 8 hours (Hussain et al, 2004; Kapoor et al, 2009).

ADVERSE EFFECTS: Tachycardia; sodium and fluid retention is common; congestive heart failure (CHF) may cause bilirubin displacement from albumin, hypotension, hyperglycemia, hyperuricemia, rash, fever, leukopenia, thrombocytopenia, and ketosis.
COMMENTS: Oral solution contains propylene glycol and sodium benzoate.

DIGIBIND (DIGOXIN IMMUNE FAB)

INDICATIONS AND USE: Treatment of potentially life-threatening digoxin or digitoxin toxicity in carefully selected patients; use in life-threatening ventricular arrhythmias secondary to digoxin, acute digoxin ingestion (ie, >4 mg in children), and hyperkalemia (serum potassium >5 mEq/L) in the setting of digoxin toxicity.
ACTIONS: Binds with molecules of free (unbound) digoxin or digitoxin and then is removed from the body by renal excretion.
DOSAGE: IV.

Dose determination:

- Determine the dose by determining the total body-loading dose of digoxin (TBL) using either method 1 or method 2.
- **Method 1:** An approximation of the amount ingested:
  - TBL of digoxin (in mg) = C (in ng/mL) × 5.6 × body weight (in kg)/1000 or TBL = mg of digoxin ingested (as tablets or elixir) × 0.8.
  - Dose of Digibind (in mg) IV = TB × 76.
  - Dose of digoxin immune Fab (Digibind) (number of vials) IV = TBL/0.5.
- **Method 2:** A postdistribution serum digoxin concentration C determination (Table 148–1).

Table 148–1. DOSE ESTIMATES OF DIGOXIN IMMUNE FAB BASED ON SERUM ON DIGOXIN CONCENTRATION

Patient Weight 1 kg and Serum Digoxin Concentration	Patient Weight 3 kg and Serum Digoxin Concentration	Patient Weight 5 kg and Serum Digoxin Concentration
1 ng/mL: 0.4 mg	1 ng/mL: 1 mg	1 ng/mL: 2 mg
2 ng/mL: 1 mg	2 ng/mL: 2–2.5 mg	2 ng/mL: 4 mg
4 ng/mL: 1.5 mg	4 ng/mL: 5 mg	4 ng/mL: 8 mg
8 ng/mL: 3 mg	8 ng/mL: 9–10 mg	8 ng/mL: 15–16 mg
12 ng/mL: 5 mg	12 ng/mL: 14 mg	12 ng/mL: 23–24 mg
16 ng/mL: 6–6.5 mg	16 ng/mL: 18–19 mg	16 ng/mL: 30–32 mg
20 ng/mL: 8 mg	20 ng/mL: 23–24 mg	20 ng/mL: 38–40 mg

Acute digoxin toxicity:
- **Ingestion of known amount of digoxin:** Each vial (38 mg) IV binds ~0.5 mg digoxin. Bioavailability of digoxin is 0.8 for 0.25 mg tablets *or* 1 for 0.2 Lanoxicaps.
- **Use the following formula:** Dose (in vials) = digoxin ingested (mg) × bioavailability/0.5 mg of digoxin bound/vial.

Chronic digoxin toxicity:
- **Infants and small children:** Single vial (38 mg) IV initially.
- **Or use the following formula:** Number of vials needed = (serum digoxin concentration in ng/mL) × (wt in kg)/100, then dose (in mg) = number of vials × 38 mg/vial.

ADVERSE EFFECTS: Caution in renal or cardiac failure; allergic reactions possible; epinephrine should be immediately available; patients may deteriorate due to withdrawal of digoxin and may require IV inotropic support (eg, dobutamine) or vasodilators. Hypokalemia reported following reversal of digitalis intoxication; monitor serum potassium levels.

PHARMACOLOGY: Volume of distribution: Digibind—0.3 L/kg; half-life: Digibind—15–20 hours; renal impairment prolongs the half-life of both agents. Improvement in signs and symptoms occurs within 2–30 minutes following IV infusion.

DIGOXIN (LANOXIN)

INDICATIONS AND USE: Treatment of congestive heart failure, atrial fibrillation or flutter, and supraventricular tachycardia.

ACTIONS: Exerts a positive inotropic effect (increased myocardial contractility). Its negative chronotropic effects (antiarrhythmic actions/decrease in heart rate) are due to the slowing of conduction through the sinoatrial (SA) and atrioventricular (AV) nodes caused by vagal stimulation.

DOSAGE: IV, PO. Total digitalizing dose (TDD) to be divided one-half, one-fourth, and one-fourth every 8 hours. *Note:* Oral doses (elixir) are ~25% higher than IV doses listed in the following.

Preterm neonates:
- **TDD:** 15–25 mcg/kg IV or 20–30 mcg/kg PO.
- **Daily maintenance:** 4–6 mcg/kg/dose IV every 24 hours or 5–7.5 mcg/kg/dose PO every 24 hours.

Full-term neonates:
- **TDD:** 20–30 mcg/kg IV, 25–35 mcg/kg PO.
- **Daily maintenance:** 5–8 mcg/kg/day IV divided every 12 hours or 6–10 mcg/kg/day PO divided every 12 hours.

1 month to 2 years:
- **TDD:** 30–50 mcg/kg IV or 35–60 PO mcg/kg.
- **Daily maintenance:** 7.5–12 mcg/kg/day IV or 10–15 mcg/kg/day PO divided every 12 hours.

ADVERSE EFFECTS: Sinus bradycardia may be a sign of digoxin toxicity. Any dysrhythmias (paroxysmal ventricular contractions, bradycardia, tachycardia) in a child on digoxin should be considered as digoxin toxicity. The gastrointestinal (GI) and central nervous system (CNS) symptoms are not frequently seen in children. To manage toxicity, see Digibind.

COMMENTS: Therapeutic levels: 0.5–2.0 ng/mL. Considerable overlap exists between toxic and therapeutic serum levels. Digoxin-like immunoreactive substance (DLIS) may cross-react with digoxin immunoassay and falsely increases serum concentrations; DLIS has been found in neonates. Use with caution and reduce dosage in patients with renal impairment; use with caution in patients with sinus nodal disease (may worsen condition). Correct electrolyte disturbances, especially hypokalemia or hypomagnesemia, prior to use and throughout therapy. Hypercalcemia may increase the risk of digoxin toxicity. Contraindicated in second- and third-degree block, idiopathic hypertrophic subaortic stenosis, and atrial flutter or fibrillation with slow ventricular rates.

DOBUTAMINE HCL (DOBUTREX)

INDICATIONS AND USE: To increase cardiac output during states of depressed contractility, such as septic shock, organic heart disease, or cardiac surgical procedures. Treat hypotension and hypoperfusion related to myocardial dysfunction.

ACTIONS: A direct β_1-agonist that increases myocardial contractility, oxygen delivery, and oxygen consumption; actions on β_2- and α-adrenergic receptors are much less marked than those of dopamine. Unlike dopamine, dobutamine does not cause release of endogenous norepinephrine, nor does it have any effect on dopaminergic receptors.

DOSAGE: IV.
- 2–20 mcg/kg/minute by continuous infusion and titrate to desired response. Maximum: 40 mcg/kg/minute.

ADVERSE EFFECTS: Tachycardia and arrhythmias at higher doses, hypotension if patient is hypovolemic, ectopic heartbeats, and elevated blood pressure.

PHARMACOLOGY: Has more prominent effect on cardiac output than dopamine and less effect on blood pressure. Onset of action 1–2 minutes; peak effect in 10 minutes. Serum half-life is several minutes. Metabolized in liver and renally excreted.

COMMENTS: Correct hypovolemia prior to initiation of therapy; contraindicated in idiopathic subaortic stenosis and atrial fibrillation.

DOPAMINE HCL (DOPASTAT, INTROPIN)

INDICATIONS AND USE: To increase cardiac output, blood pressure, renal perfusion, and glomerular filtration rate (GFR) (low dosages), which persists despite volume resuscitation.

ACTIONS: Actions are dose dependent. Low doses act directly on dopaminergic receptors to produce renal and mesenteric vasodilation. In moderate doses, β_1-adrenergic effects become prominent, resulting in a positive inotropic effect on the myocardium. High doses stimulate α-adrenergic receptors, producing increased peripheral resistance (vasoconstriction and increased blood pressure) and renal vasoconstriction.

DOSAGE: **IV.** *Note:* Dose-effect relationship is speculative in neonates.

Continuous IV infusion:

- 1–20 mcg/kg/minute; titrate to desired response.
- **Low:** 1–5 mcg/kg/minute may increase renal perfusion and urine output.
- **Moderate:** 5–15 mcg/kg/minute facilitates increased cardiac output, renal blood flow, heart rate, cardiac contractility, blood pressure.
- **High:** >15 mcg/kg/minute causes systemic vasoconstriction and blood pressure.

ADVERSE EFFECTS: Dopamine may cause ectopic heartbeats, tachycardia, ventricular arrhythmias, hypertension, and azotemia. Gangrene of the extremities has occurred with high doses over prolonged periods. **Extravasation may cause tissue necrosis and sloughing of surrounding tissues; if this occurs,** infiltrate area with a small amount (1 mL) of phentolamine, made by diluting 2.5–5 mg in 10 mL preservative-free normal saline (NS); do not exceed 0.1 mg/kg or 2.5 mg total for neonates and 0.1–0.2 mg/kg or 5 mg total for infants (see Chapter 31).

PHARMACOLOGY: Rapidly metabolized; serum half-life 2–5 minutes, variable clearance. Individual developmental differences in endogenous norepinephrine stores; α-adrenergic, β-adrenergic, and dopaminergic receptor function and the ability of the neonatal heart to increase stroke volume will affect response to different dopamine doses.

COMMENTS: Administration of phenytoin IV to patients receiving dopamine may result in severe hypotension and bradycardia; therefore, use with extreme caution. Do not infuse through umbilical arterial catheter or other arterial catheter.

DORNASE ALPHA

INDICATIONS AND USE: Reduce frequency of pulmonary infections and improve pulmonary function in cystic fibrosis patients; treatment of atelectasis as a result of mucous plugging that has failed to respond to conventional therapies.

ACTIONS: Selectively cleaves DNA resulting in a reduction of the viscosity of mucus in pulmonary secretions.

DOSAGE: **ETT.**

- 1.25–2.5 mL/dose administered once or twice daily nebulized; instillation into endotracheal tube.

ADVERSE EFFECTS: Airway obstruction secondary to mobilization of secretions in airway, desaturations, fever, cough, dyspnea, wheezing.

PHARMACOLOGY: Recombinant human DNA enzyme; hydrolyzes DNA released by degenerating leukocytes from purulent pulmonary secretions resulting in decreased viscosity.

COMMENTS: Not approved for use in infants and children ≤5 years of age; however, studies with small numbers of children as young as 3 months have shown efficacy and similar side effect profile.

DOXAPRAM HCL (DOPRAM)

INDICATIONS AND USE: Apnea of prematurity unresponsive to methylxanthine therapy.

ACTIONS: Stimulates respiration through action on central respiratory centers and reflex stimulation of carotid, aortic, or other peripheral chemoreceptors; decreases Pco_2 and increases minute ventilation and tidal volume without changing respiratory rate or inspiratory and expiratory times.

DOSAGE: **IV.**

- **Loading dose:** 2.5–3 mg/kg IV over 30 minutes followed by maintenance dose.
- **Continuous IV infusion:** 0.5–1.5 mg/kg/hour (maximum 2.5 mg/kg/hour); decrease the infusion rate when control of apnea is achieved.

ADVERSE EFFECTS: Hypertension, QT prolongation with heart block, tachycardia, skeletal muscle hyperactivity, abdominal distention, increased gastric residuals, bloody stools, necrotizing enterocolitis, vomiting, jitteriness, hyperglycemia, and glycosuria.

PHARMACOLOGY: **Therapeutic range:** 1.5–3 mcg/mL (<5 mcg/mL). Onset of respiratory stimulation is 20–40 seconds; maximum effect is 1–2 minutes; duration is 5–12 minutes.

COMMENTS: Use cautiously in premature neonates because of its side effects. Avoid use during the first few days of life, when hypertensive episodes may be associated with increased risk of intraventricular hemorrhage; contraindicated in cardiovascular and seizure disorders. Doxapram contains benzyl alcohol.

ENALAPRIL (PO)/ENALAPRILAT (IV) (VASOTEC)

> **WARNING:** When used in pregnancy during the second and third trimesters, ACE inhibitors can cause injury and even death to the developing fetus. When pregnancy is detected, enalaprilat injection should be discontinued as soon as possible.

INDICATIONS AND USE: Treatment of moderate to severe hypertension and heart failure by reducing left ventricular preload and afterload.

ACTIONS: An angiotensin-converting enzyme (ACE) inhibitor that acts by inhibiting the conversion of angiotensin I to angiotensin II and results in lower levels of angiotensin II, which causes an increase in plasma renin activity and a reduction in aldosterone secretion and the breakdown of bradykinin, causing vasodilation. Enalapril increases sodium and fluid loss, and serum potassium.

DOSAGE: IV, PO.

- **IV:** 5–10 mcg/kg/dose every 8–24 hours. The frequency depends on blood pressure response. Monitor patient closely.
- **PO:** Initial: 0.04–0.1 mg/kg/day given every 24 hours; initiate at the lower end of the range and titrate to effect as required every few days; may need to dose every 6 hours. Maximum dose is typically 0.15 mg/kg/dose as frequently as every 6 hours.

ADVERSE EFFECTS: Hypotension, hyperkalemia, decreased renal function, oliguria, cough, anemia, neutropenia, and angioedema.

PHARMACOLOGY: Onset of action after oral dose is 1–2 hours. The duration of action is variable (8–24 hours).

COMMENTS: Use with extreme caution in renal dysfunction; reduce dose. Use a low initial dose to avoid a profound drop in blood pressure, especially in patients on diuretics who are hyponatremic or hypovolemic. Monitor blood pressure hourly for the first 12 hours. Note that the IV dose is much smaller than the PO dose; use caution to adjust the dose when changing route of administration.

ENOXAPARIN (LOVENOX)

INDICATIONS AND USE: Prophylaxis and treatment of thromboembolic disorders. (See Chapter 87.)

ACTIONS: Low molecular weight heparin that potentiates the action of antithrombin III and inactivates coagulation factor Xa and factor IIa (thrombin).

DOSAGE: Subcutaneous.

Initial treatment:

- **Infants <2 months:** 1.5 mg/kg subcutaneous every 12 hours.
- **Infants >2 months and children ≤18 years:** 1 mg/kg subcutaneous every 12 hours.
- **Maintenance:** Adjust dose to maintain antifactor Xa level between 0.5 and 1.0 units/mL. It may take several days to reach target range. Preterm infants may require higher doses to maintain antifactor Xa levels in target range: mean dose of 2 mg/kg every 12 hours, range of 0.8–3 mg/kg every 12 hours.

Initial prophylaxis:

- **Infants <2 months:** 0.75 mg/kg subcutaneous every 12 hours.
- **Infants >2 months and children ≤18 years:** 0.5 mg/kg subcutaneous every 12 hours.
- **Maintenance:** Adjust to maintain antifactor Xa level between 0.1 and 0.4 units/mL.

ADVERSE EFFECTS: Bleeding, intracranial hemorrhage, thrombocytopenia (incidence of heparin-induced thrombocytopenia is less than that with heparin therapy). Hematoma, irritation, ecchymosis, and erythema can occur at the injection site.

PHARMACOLOGY: Measure antifactor Xa levels 4 hours after a dose. After target level is reached, dosage adjustments may be required once or twice a month. Preterm infants and infants with hepatic or renal dysfunction may require more frequent adjustments.

COMMENTS: Compared with standard heparin, enoxaparin has much less activity against thrombin. Low antithrombin plasma concentration reduces the efficacy in neonates. Enoxaparin is less likely to cause thrombocytopenia and osteoporosis.

EPINEPHRINE

INDICATIONS AND USE: Bradycardia, cardiac arrest, cardiogenic shock, anaphylactic reactions, and bronchospasm.

ACTIONS: Acts directly on both α- and β-adrenergic receptors; β_2 effects predominate at lower doses. Exerts both positive chronotropic and inotropic effects on the heart, and relaxes bronchial smooth muscle. The α-adrenergic stimulation increases systolic blood pressure and constricts renal blood vessels.

DOSAGE: IV, ETT.

- **IV bolus:** (1:10,000) 0.01–0.03 mg/kg (0.1–0.3 mL/kg) every 3–5 minutes PRN. Follow administration with a flush of 0.5–1 mL of normal saline (NS).
- **IV infusion:** Initial rate: 0.1 mcg/kg/minute; titrate to desired response to a maximum of 1 mcg/kg/minute.

- **Endotracheal:** 0.05–0.1 mg/kg (0.5–1 mL/kg of 1:10,000 solution) every 3–5 minutes until IV access is established or return of spontaneous circulation; immediately followed by 1 mL NS.
- **Nebulization:** 0.25–0.5 mL of 2.25% racemic epinephrine diluted in 3 mL of NS.

ADVERSE EFFECTS: Hypertension, tachycardia, nausea, pallor, tremor, cardiac arrhythmias, increased myocardial oxygen consumption, and decreased renal and splanchnic blood flow.

ERYTHROMYCIN (ILOSONE, OTHERS)

ACTION AND SPECTRUM: Macrolide antibiotic; bactericidal or bacteriostatic depending on the tissue concentration of drug and the microorganism. Spectrum of activity is broad and includes susceptible streptococci and staphylococci; also *Mycoplasma, Legionella,* pertussis, *Chlamydia,* and *Campylobacter* gastroenteritis.
DOSAGE: **PO, IV, ocular.**
Neonates:
- **Oral ethylsuccinate form, postnatal age:**
  - **<7 days:** 20 mg/kg/day PO divided every 12 hours.
  - **>7 days:**
    - <1.2 kg: 20 mg/kg/day PO divided every 12 hours.
    - 1.2–2 kg: 30 mg/kg/day PO divided every 8 hours.
    - >2 kg: 30–40 mg/kg/day PO divided every 6–8 hours.
- **IV lactobionate form:** 5–10 mg/kg/dose every 6 hours for severe infections or when PO route is unavailable.
- **Chlamydial conjunctivitis or pneumonia:** Oral: ethylsuccinate—50 mg/kg/day divided every 6 hours for 14 days (based on AAP *Red Book*, 2012).

Infants and children:
- **Oral base and ethylsuccinate:** 30–50 mg/kg/day PO divided every 6–8 hours; do not exceed 2 grams/day (as base) or 3.2 grams/day (as ethylsuccinate). *Note:* 200 mg erythromycin ethylsuccinate produces the same serum levels as 125 mg erythromycin base due to absorptive differences.
- **IV lactobionate:** 15–50 mg/kg/day IV divided every 6 hours, not to exceed 4 grams/day.
- **Stearate:** 30–50 mg/kg/day PO divided every 6 hours; maximum 2 grams/day.
- *Chlamydia trachomatis:* Child <45 kg: 50 mg/kg/day PO divided every 6 hours for 14 days; maximum 2 grams/day.
- **Pertussis treatment or postexposure prophylaxis:** Ethylsuccinate: 40 mg/kg/day divided every 6 hours for 14 days. *Note:* Azithromycin considered first-line agent in infants <1 month of age; erythromycin is associated with infantile hypertrophic pyloric stenosis in neonates (based on AAP *Red Book.* 2012).

Ophthalmic prophylaxis: 0.5 to 1-cm ribbon in each eye once.
Ophthalmic for acute infection: 0.5 to 1-cm ribbon in each eye every 6 hours.
Gastrointestinal motility disorders: 10 mg/kg/dose PO every 8 hours, 30 minutes before feedings; in neonates up to 2 weeks old, exposure to high doses (30–50 mg/kg/day) for ≥14 days has been associated with a 10-fold increase in the risk of hypertrophic pyloric stenosis. May be given IV 1–3 mg/kg infused over 60 minutes, but PO is preferred route.
ADVERSE EFFECTS: Infantile hypertrophic pyloric stenosis, stomatitis, epigastric distress, transient cholestatic hepatitis, and allergic reactions occur rarely. Cardiac toxicity requiring cardiopulmonary resuscitation (CPR) may occur with IV erythromycin; reduce risk of arrhythmias by slowly infusing over 1 hour.
PHARMACOLOGY: Hepatic metabolism, excreted via the bile and kidneys. Half-life is 1.5–3 hours (prolonged in renal failure). May cause increased serum levels of theophylline, digoxin, and carbamazepine.
COMMENTS: Parenteral forms are painful and irritating; dilute to 5 mg/mL and infuse >60 minutes. Do not use IM.

ERYTHROPOIETIN/EPOETIN ALFA (EPOGEN, PROCRIT) [EPO, rEpo]

INDICATIONS AND USE: To stimulate erythropoiesis and decrease the need for erythrocyte transfusions (rEpo) in preterm infants; treatment of anemia of prematurity.
ACTIONS: Epoetin alfa (EPO) induces erythropoiesis by stimulating division and differentiation of committed erythroid progenitor cells; induces release of reticulocytes from the bone marrow into the bloodstream where they mature to erythrocytes (dose-response relationship).
DOSAGE: **Subcutaneous.**
- 200–400 units/kg/dose, 3–5 times per week, for 2–6 weeks. Total dose per week: 600–1400 units/kg/week. Short course: 300 units/kg/dose daily × 10 days.

ADVERSE EFFECTS: May cause hypertension, edema, fever, rash, possible seizures, transient early thrombocytosis and late neutropenia, polycythemia, and local skin reaction at injection site.
PHARMACOLOGY: Noticeable effects on hematocrit and reticulocyte counts occur within 2 weeks. Half-life in neonates: subcutaneous—17.6 hours on day 3 of therapy, 11.2 hours on day 10 of therapy.
COMMENTS: Supplement with oral iron therapy 3–8 mg/kg/day; optimal response is achieved when iron stores are adequate. EPO should be used in conjunction with restrictive transfusion guidelines and minimizing

of phlebotomy losses. EPO is not a substitute for emergency blood transfusion. Do not use in patients with uncontrolled hypertension.

ESMOLOL

INDICATIONS AND USE: Treatment of supraventricular tachycardia (SVT); acute management of postoperative tachycardia and hypertension.
ACTIONS: Competitively blocks response to β_1-adrenergic stimulation with little or no effect on β_2-receptors except at high doses.
DOSAGE: IV.
Neonatal (limited data available):
- **SVT:** 100 mcg/kg/minute by continuous infusion; adjust dose based on individual clinical response and tolerance. Increase by 50–100 mcg/kg/minute every 5 minutes until ventricular rate is controlled.
- **Postoperative tachycardia and hypertension:** 50 mcg/kg/minute by continuous infusion; increase by 25–50 mcg/kg/minute every 5 minutes until target blood pressure is reached.
- **Maximum dosage:** 200 mcg/kg/minute.

Infants and children (limited data available):
- **SVT:** 100–500 mcg/kg over 1 minute; titrate infusion rate by 50–100 mcg/kg/minute every 5–10 minutes until ventricular rate is controlled.
- **Postoperative tachycardia and hypertension:** Loading dose of 500 mcg/kg/minute over 1 minute followed by continuous infusion of 50–250 mcg/kg/minute; titrate infusion rate by 50 mcg/kg/minute every 10 minutes until target blood pressure is reached.
- **Maximum dose:** 1000 mcg/kg/minute.

ADVERSE EFFECTS: Hypotension and bradycardia at higher doses; peripheral ischemia, agitation, local induration, inflammation phlebitis, and skin necrosis after extravasation.
PHARMACOLOGY: Ultra-short-acting β_1-selective blocking agent with half-life of 2.8–4.5 minutes and duration of action of 10–30 minutes. Onset of action ranges from 2 to 10 minutes; shorter if loading dose is given.
COMMENTS: Monitor IV site for infiltration, especially with the use of concentrations >10 mg/mL.

ETHACRYNIC ACID (EDECRIN)

WARNING: Ethacrynic acid is a potent diuretic that, if given in excessive amounts, may lead to profound diuresis with water and electrolyte depletion. Therefore, careful medical supervision is required, and dose and dose schedule must be adjusted to the individual patient's needs.

INDICATIONS AND USE: Reserved for use only when other diuretics have failed to produce effective diuresis due to toxicities.
ACTIONS: Loop diuretic that inhibits reabsorption of sodium and chloride in ascending loop of Henle and distal tubules, resulting in increased excretion of water, sodium, chloride, magnesium, and calcium. The inhibition of sodium reabsorption is greater than that of other diuretics. Also, there is not a direct effect on the pulmonary vasculature, as seen with furosemide.
DOSAGE: IV, PO.
- **IV:** 0.5–1 mg/kg/dose. Repeat doses are not routinely recommended; however, if indicated, repeat doses every 8–12 hours.
- **PO:** 1 mg/kg/dose once daily; increase at intervals of 2–3 days to a maximum of 3 mg/kg/day.

ADVERSE EFFECTS: Inject IV dose slowly over several minutes; may cause hypotension, dehydration, electrolyte depletion, diarrhea, gastrointestinal (GI) bleeding, hearing loss, rash, local irritation and pain, hematuria, and, rarely, hypoglycemia and neutropenia.
COMMENTS: Close medical supervision and dose evaluation is required; may increase risk of gastric hemorrhage associated with corticosteroid treatment.

FAMOTIDINE (PEPCID)

INDICATIONS AND USE: Prevention and short-term treatment of gastroesophageal reflux disease (GERD), stress, gastric and duodenal ulcers, and gastrointestinal (GI) hemorrhage.
ACTIONS: Inhibits gastric acid secretion by reversible, competitive antagonism of histamine on the H_2 receptor of the gastric parietal cells.
DOSAGE: IV, PO.
- **Neonates and infants <3 months:** 0.25–0.5 mg/kg/dose every 24 hours slow IV push.
- **GERD:** <3 months: 0.5 mg/kg PO once daily for up to 8 weeks; 3–12 months: 0.5 mg/kg PO twice daily for up to 8 weeks.

ADVERSE EFFECTS: Hypotension and cardiac arrhythmias with rapid IV administration; bradycardia, tachycardia, hypertension, thrombocytopenia, elevated liver enzymes, cholestatic jaundice, elevated blood urea nitrogen (BUN) and creatinine, and proteinuria.

PHARMACOLOGY: Onset of GI effect is within 1 hour. Duration is 10–12 hours. Elimination 65–70% unchanged in urine.

COMMENTS: Limited experience in infants and children. Famotidine does not inhibit cytochrome P450.

FENTANYL (SUBLIMAZE)

INDICATIONS AND USE: Analgesia, anesthesia, and sedation.

ACTIONS: A synthetic opiate agonist that binds to the opioid μ-receptors within the central nervous system, (CNS), increases the pain threshold, alters pain reception, and inhibits ascending pain pathway. Acts similarly to morphine and meperidine but without the cardiovascular effects of those drugs and with shorter respiratory depressant effects.

DOSAGE: IV.

Neonates:

- **Analgesia:** International Evidence-Based Group for Neonatal Pain recommendations (Anand et al, 2001).
  - **Intermittent doses:** Slow IV push: 0.5–3 mcg/kg/dose.
  - **Continuous infusion:** 0.5–2 mcg/kg/hour.

Neonates and younger infants:

- **Analgesia/sedation:** 1–4 mcg/kg/dose slow IV push every 2–4 hours as needed.

Continuous analgesia/sedation: Initial 1–2 mcg/kg IV bolus then 0.5–1mcg/kg/hour; titrate upward.

Continuous sedation/analgesia during extracorporeal membrane oxygenation/extracorporeal life support (ECMO/ ECLS): Initial IV bolus: 5–10 mcg/kg slow IV push over 10 minutes, then 1–5 mcg/kg/hour; titrate upward; tolerance may develop; higher doses (up to 20 mcg/kg/hour) may be needed by day 6 of ECMO/ECLS.

Anesthesia: 5–50 mcg/kg/dose.

ADVERSE EFFECTS: CNS and respiratory depression; bradycardia; skeletal muscle and chest wall rigidity with reduced pulmonary compliance, apnea, and laryngospasm, which is reversible with naloxone. Tolerance and withdrawal symptoms reported with continuous use. Urinary retention, gastrointestinal symptoms, and biliary spasms may occur.

PHARMACOLOGY: Metabolized in liver by CYP3A4 enzyme and excreted by kidneys. Liver failure prolongs serum half-life; 80–85% protein bound; lipid soluble. The volume of distribution and half-life are highly variable.

COMMENTS: Synthetic opioid narcotic analgesic that is 50–100 times more potent on a weight basis than morphine. Concurrent ventilatory assistance is suggested with its use. Tachyphylaxis occurs after several days of therapy. Adheres to ECMO/ECLS filter membranes; may have to adjust the dose.

FERROUS SULFATE (20% ELEMENTAL IRON)

INDICATIONS AND USE: Treatment and prevention of iron deficiency anemia; supplemental therapy for patients receiving epoetin alfa.

ACTIONS: Iron is required for production of heme proteins. Iron is released from the plasma to replenish the depleted stores in the bone marrow where it is incorporated into hemoglobin.

DOSAGE: PO. Recommendations of the American Academy of Pediatrics (AAP) for treatment and prevention of iron deficiency; dosages are for elemental iron.

- **Term infants:** 1 mg elemental iron/kg/day divided every 12–24 hours. Begin at 4 months of age.
- **Preterm infants:** 2–4 mg elemental iron/kg/day divided every 12–24 hours. Begin therapy by 1 month of age.
- **Iron deficiency anemia:** 6 mg/kg/day in 3 divided doses.
- **Iron supplementation with erythropoietin:** 6 mg/kg/day in 1 or 2 divided doses.

ADVERSE EFFECTS: Gastrointestinal irritation (vomiting, diarrhea, constipation, and darkened stool color).

COMMENTS: The use of iron-fortified formulas during the first year of life usually prevents iron deficiency anemia in both preterm and term infants. Iron-fortified formulas can be fed safely to preterm infants. Of the ferrous salts available (sulfate, fumarate, and gluconate), sulfate is preferred. *Note:* Multiple concentrations of ferrous sulfate oral liquid exist. Caution parents to guard against iron poisoning from accidental ingestion. Antidote is chelation with deferoxamine; consult specialized references and regional Poison Control Center for further information.

FILGRASTIM (GRANULOCYTE COLONY-STIMULATING FACTOR [G-CSF])

INDICATIONS AND USE: For the reduction of neutropenia in neonates with sepsis.

ACTIONS: Stimulates the production, maturation, and activation of neutrophil granulocytes and activates neutrophils to enhance both their migration and cytotoxicity.

DOSAGE: IV or subcutaneous.

- **Neonates:** 5–10 mcg/kg/day IV/subcutaneous once daily for 3–5 days has been administered to neutropenic neonates with sepsis. Refer to individual protocols.

ADVERSE EFFECTS: Thrombocytopenia, leukocytosis, transient decrease in blood pressure.

PHARMACOLOGY: There is an immediate transient leukopenia with nadir occurring 5–15 minutes after an IV dose or 30–60 minutes after a subcutaneous dose followed by a sustained elevation in neutrophil levels within the first 24 hours, which plateaus in 3–5 days. Following discontinuation of G-CSF, absolute neutrophil count (ANC) decreases by 50% within 2 days and returns to pretreatment levels within 1 week; white blood cell (WBC) counts return to normal range in 4–7 days.

FLECAINIDE

WARNING: Should only be used for sustained, life-threatening arrhythmias that have not responded to conventional therapies.

INDICATIONS AND USE: Prevention and treatment of sustained, life-threatening ventricular arrhythmias; prophylaxis of paroxysmal atrial flutter and fibrillation and supraventricular tachycardia. Contraindicated in patients with structural heart disease.
ACTIONS: Class 1C antiarrhythmic that slows conduction throughout the myocardium, with the greatest effect on the His-Purkinje system.
DOSAGE: PO.
• Initial dose: 1–3 mg/kg/day divided into 2 or 3 doses; maintenance dose of 3–6 mg/kg/day up to 8 mg/kg/day divided into 2 or 3 doses. Titrate dose based on response. Higher doses have been associated with increased risk of pro-arrhythmias.
ADVERSE EFFECTS: May cause new or worsening ventricular arrhythmias, heart block, bradycardia, torsade de pointes, dizziness, blurred vision, headache, blood dyscrasias, and hepatic dysfunction.
PHARMACOLOGY: Demonstrates both local anesthetic and moderate inotropic effects. Reduction in conduction throughout the myocardium results in increased PR, QRS, and QT intervals. Infant formula and milk products may inhibit absorption. Elimination half-life in children <1 year of age is ~11–12 hours and in newborns and after maternal administration is ~29 hours. Half-life increased with congestive heart failure (CHF) or renal impairment.
COMMENTS: Therapeutic levels: 0.2–1 mcg/mL.

FLUCONAZOLE (DIFLUCAN)

INDICATIONS AND USE: Antifungal agent for treatment of susceptible fungal infections including oropharyngeal and esophageal candidiasis; treatment of systemic candidal infections including urinary tract infection, peritonitis, cystitis, and pneumonia. There continues to be an increased number of strains of *Candida* isolated with decreased susceptibility to fluconazole. Fluconazole is more active against *C. albicans* than other candida strains like *C. parapsilosis*, *C. glabrata*, and *C. tropicalis*; alternative to amphotericin B in patients with preexisting renal impairment or when requiring concomitant therapy with other potentially nephrotoxic drugs.
ACTIONS: Interferes with fungal cytochrome P450 and sterol C-14 α-demethylation, resulting in a fungistatic effect.
DOSAGE: IV, PO.
Systemic infections, including meningitis:
• **≤29 weeks' gestation:**
  • **Postnatal age 0–14 days:** 12–25 mg/kg loading dose, then 6–12 mg/kg IV/PO every 48 hours.
  • **Postnatal age >14 days:** 12–25 mg/kg loading dose, then 6–12 mg/kg IV/PO every 24 hours.
• **30 weeks' gestation and older:**
  • **Postnatal age 0–7 days:** 12–25 mg/kg loading dose, then 6–12 mg/kg IV/PO every 48 hours.
  • **Postnatal age >7 days:** 12–25 mg/kg loading dose, then 6–12 mg/kg IV/PO every 24 hours.
• **Neonates >14 days, infants, and children:**
  • **Oropharyngeal candidiasis IV or PO:** Day 1: 6 mg/kg IV/PO, then 3 mg/kg IV/PO minimum 14 days.
  • **Esophageal candidiasis IV or PO:** As above but 21-day minimum.
• **Candidiasis prophylaxis:** 3–6 mg/kg/dose IV infusion twice weekly has been used in extremely low birthweight (ELBW) infants at increased risk of invasive fungal infection. Dose of 6 mg/kg may be used if targeting *Candida* strains with higher minimal inhibitory concentrations (MICs) of 4–8 mcg/mL.
ADVERSE EFFECTS: Usually well tolerated. Vomiting, diarrhea, rash, and elevations in liver transaminases. Eosinophilia, leukopenia, thrombocytopenia, neutropenia.
PHARMACOLOGY: Good oral bioavailability; absorption not affected by food with peak serum concentrations achieved within 1 hour; good penetration into tissues and body fluids including cerebrospinal fluid (CSF). Less than 12% protein bound, primarily excreted unchanged in urine.
COMMENTS: Reduce dose in renal dysfunction. Use caution in preexisting renal dysfunction. Monitor liver function tests. Cimetidine and rifampin decrease fluconazole levels. Hydrochlorothiazide increases fluconazole area under the curve (AUC). Fluconazole interferes with the metabolism of barbiturates, theophylline, midazolam, phenytoin, and zidovudine. Contraindicated in patients receiving cisapride.

FLUCYTOSINE (ANCOBON)

ACTION AND SPECTRUM: Antifungal agent that penetrates fungal cells and is converted to fluorouracil, which competes with uracil interfering with fungal RNA and protein synthesis. Used in combination with amphotericin B in the treatment of serious candida or cryptococcal pulmonary or urinary tract infections, sepsis, meningitis, or endocarditis (resistance emerges if flucytosine is used as a single agent); used in combination with another antifungal agent for treatment of chromomycosis and aspergillosis.

DOSAGE: PO. Administer in combination with amphotericin B due to development of resistance.

• **Neonates:** Initial: 25–100 mg/kg/day PO in divided doses every 12–24 hours.

• **Infants and children:** 50–150 mg/kg/day PO divided every 6 hours.

• **Renal impairment:** Use lower initial dose.

  • **Creatinine clearance 20–40 mL/minute:** Usual dose every 12 hours.

  • **Creatinine clearance 10–20 mL/minute:** Usual dose every 24 hours.

  • **Creatinine clearance <10 mL/minute:** Usual dose every 24–48 hours.

ADVERSE EFFECTS: Vomiting, diarrhea, rash, anemia, leukopenia, thrombocytopenia, elevated liver enzymes and bilirubin, increased blood urea nitrogen (BUN) and creatinine, and central nervous system (CNS) disturbances.

PHARMACOLOGY: Desired peak serum concentrations: 25–100 mcg/mL. Half-life, neonates: 4–34 hours. Renal elimination.

COMMENTS: Toxicities related to serum concentration >100 mcg/mL and usually reversible when drug is discontinued or dose is reduced. Amphotericin B may increase toxicity by decreasing renal excretion.

FLUDROCORTISONE (FLORINEF)

INDICATIONS AND USE: Used for partial replacement therapy for adrenocortical insufficiency and treatment of salt-losing forms of congenital adrenogenital syndrome, usually used with concurrent hydrocortisone in patients with salt-losing forms of congenital adrenogenital syndrome.

ACTIONS: Fludrocortisone is a potent mineralocorticoid with glucocorticoid activity that acts on the distal tubule to increase loss of potassium and hydrogen ion and increases reabsorption of sodium with subsequent water retention.

DOSAGE: PO.

• **Usual:** 0.05–0.1 mg/day (50–100 mcg/day) as a single daily dose. (**Note:** Doses are the same regardless of patient weight or age. Newborns are insensitive to the drug and may require larger doses than adults). May administer with feedings.

• **Congenital adrenal hyperplasia (salt losers):** Maintenance: 0.05–0.3 mg/day (American Academy of Pediatrics, Section on Endocrinology and Committee on Genetics, 2000).

ADVERSE EFFECTS: Hypertension, congestive heart failure, gastrointestinal upset, hypokalemia, growth suppression, hyperglycemia, salt and water retention, edema, hypothalamic-pituitary-adrenal suppression, osteoporosis, and muscle weakness resulting from excessive potassium loss. Monitor serum electrolytes (particularly sodium and potassium).

COMMENTS: Fludrocortisone 0.1 mg has a sodium retention activity equal to deoxycorticosterone acetate (DOCA) 1 mg.

FLUMAZENIL

> WARNING: Flumazenil has been associated with the occurrence of seizures. These are most frequent in patients who have been on benzodiazepines for long-term sedation or in overdose cases where patients are showing signs of serious cyclic antidepressant overdose. Individualize the dosage of flumazenil injection and be prepared to manage seizures.

INDICATIONS AND USE: Reversal of benzodiazepine sedative effect; management of benzodiazepine overdose.

ACTIONS: Competitive inhibition of effects of benzodiazepines on the γ-aminobutyric acid (GABA)/benzodiazepine receptor complex.

DOSAGE: IV.

• 5–10 mcg/kg/dose IV over 15 seconds; may repeat every 45 seconds until patient is awake. The maximum total cumulative dose is 50 mcg/kg (0.05 mg/kg) or 1 mg, whichever is lower. Administer IV through a large vein to minimize pain on injection and phlebitis. Monitor injection site for extravasation.

ADVERSE EFFECTS: Very limited data in neonates; hypotension, arrhythmias reported in adults. Use with caution in patients with preexisting seizure disorders. May precipitate acute withdrawal in patients with long-term benzodiazepine exposure.

PHARMACOLOGY: Highly lipid soluble. In children, peak concentration is achieved in 3 minutes and half-life is 20–75 minutes. There are very limited data in neonates.

FOLIC ACID (FOLATE, FOLVITE)

INDICATIONS AND USE: Treatment of anemia due to nutritional deficit, prematurity, megaloblastic anemia, or macrocytic anemia.

ACTIONS: Required for formation of a number of coenzymes in many metabolic systems, specifically for purine and pyrimidine synthesis, nucleoprotein synthesis, and maintenance of erythropoiesis. Also stimulates white blood cell (WBC) and platelet production in folate deficiency anemia.

DOSAGE: PO, IM, IV, subcutaneous.

Recommended daily allowance:

- **Premature neonates:** 50 mcg/day PO (~15 mcg/kg/day).
- **Neonates to 6 months:** 25–35 mcg/day PO.
- **Children 6 months to 3 years:** 150 mcg/day PO.

Folic acid deficiency (PO, IM, IV, subcutaneous):

- **Infants:** 0.1 mg/day.
- **Children <4 years:** Up to 0.3 mg/day.

ADVERSE EFFECTS: Generally well tolerated.

PHARMACOLOGY: Absorbed in the proximal portion of small intestine; metabolized in the liver.

FOLINIC ACID (LEUCOVORIN, LEUCOVORIN CALCIUM)

CAUTION: May be confused with folic acid.

INDICATIONS: Adjunctive treatment with sulfadiazine and pyrimethamine to prevent hematologic toxicity; antidote for folic acid antagonist overdosage.

ACTIONS: Folinic acid is a derivative of tetrahydrofolic acid, a reduced form of folic acid; enables purine and thymidine synthesis, required for normal erythropoiesis.

DOSAGE: PO, IV.

Folic acid antagonist overdosage (eg, pyrimethamine, trimethoprim):

- 5–15 mg PO/IV per day for 3 days or until blood counts are normal or 5 mg PO/IV every 3 days; doses of 6 mg/day are needed for patients with platelet counts <100,000/mm^3.

Adjunctive treatment with sulfadiazine to prevent hematologic toxicity (for toxoplasmosis):

- **Infants and children:** 5–10 mg PO/IV once daily; repeat every 3 days.

ADVERSE EFFECT: Thrombocytosis.

PHARMACOLOGY: Onset of action following oral dose is within 30 minutes; IV administration is within 5 minutes. Metabolism: Folinic acid is rapidly converted to 5-methyl-tetrahydrofolate (5MTHF), an active metabolite, in the intestinal mucosa and the liver.

FOSPHENYTOIN (CEREBYX)

INDICATIONS AND USE: Management of generalized convulsive status epilepticus; used for short-term parenteral administration of phenytoin, prevention and management of seizures.

ACTIONS AND SPECTRUM: Fosphenytoin is a water-soluble prodrug of phenytoin that is rapidly converted by phosphatases in blood and tissues.

DOSAGE: IM, IV (fosphenytoin 1 mg phenytoin equivalent [PE] = phenytoin 1 mg).

- **Loading dose:** 15–20 mg PE/kg IM or IV infusion over at least 10 minutes.
- **Maintenance dose:** 4–8 mg PE/kg every 24 hours IM or IV slow push. Start maintenance dose 24 hours after loading dose.
- **Term infants >1 week of age:** May require doses up to 8 mg PE/kg/dose every 8–12 hours.

ADVERSE EFFECTS: Hypotension (with rapid IV administration), vasodilation, tachycardia, bradycardia, drowsiness.

PHARMACOLOGY: Conversion to phenytoin half-life is ~7 minutes. Fosphenytoin is highly protein bound. (Caution in neonates with hyperbilirubinemia: Both fosphenytoin and bilirubin displace phenytoin from protein-binding sites, which results in increased serum-free phenytoin concentrations.)

COMMENTS: Dilute with 5% dextrose in water (D5W) or normal saline (NS) to 1.5–25 mg PE/mL. Maximum rate of infusion is 1.5 mg PE/kg/minute. Flush IV with saline pre- and postadministration. Monitor blood pressure during infusion.

FUROSEMIDE (LASIX)

INDICATIONS AND USE: Fluid overload, pulmonary edema, congestive heart failure, and hypertension.

ACTIONS: Inhibits reabsorption of sodium and chloride in the ascending limb of the loop of Henle and distal rental tubule. Furosemide-induced diuresis results in enhanced excretion of sodium, chloride, potassium, calcium, magnesium, bicarbonate, ammonium, hydrogen, and possibly phosphate. Nondiuretic effects include decreased pulmonary transvascular fluid filtration and improved pulmonary function.

DOSAGE: PO, IM, IV.

Neonates, premature:

- **PO:** 1–4 mg/kg/dose 1–2 times a day as initial dose has been used, and increase slowly if needed; highly variable oral bioavailability.
- **IV or IM:** 1 mg/kg/dose every 12–24 hours.

Infants and children:

- **Oral:** 2 mg/kg PO once daily; if effective, may increase in increments of 1–2 mg/kg/dose every 6–8 hours; not to exceed 6 mg/kg/dose. In most cases, it is unnecessary to exceed individual doses of 4 mg/kg or a dosing frequency of once or twice daily.
- **IM, IV:** 1–2 mg/kg/dose every 6–12 hours.
- **Continuous infusion:** 0.05–0.2 mg/kg/hour; titrate in 0.1 mg/kg/hour increments every 12–24 hours to a maximum infusion rate of 0.4 mg/kg/hour.

ADVERSE EFFECTS: Hypokalemia, hypocalcemia, hyponatremia, and hypercalciuria and with prolonged use nephrocalcinosis and hypochloremic metabolic alkalosis. Ototoxicity is possible especially in association with concurrent use of aminoglycosides.

PHARMACOLOGY: Onset of action: oral within 30–60 minutes; IV: 5 minutes. Duration of action: oral dose is 6–8 hours; IV dose is 2 hours.

GANCICLOVIR

INDICATIONS AND USE: Symptomatic congenital cytomegalovirus (CMV) infection for the prevention of progressive hearing loss decreased developmental delay.

ACTIONS AND SPECTRUM: An acyclic nucleoside structurally related to acyclovir, possesses antiviral activity against herpes viruses. Ganciclovir is a prodrug that is phosphorylated to a substrate that inhibits viral DNA synthesis by competitive inhibition of viral DNA polymerases and incorporation into viral DNA resulting in eventual termination of viral DNA elongation. Ganciclovir is preferentially metabolized in virus-infected cells.

DOSAGE: IV.

- **Neonates:** 6 mg/kg/dose every 12 hours IV, infused over 1 hour. Treat for a minimum of 6 weeks. Reduce dose by half for significant neutropenia (<500 cells/mm³).

ADVERSE EFFECTS: Edema, arrhythmias, hypertension; seizures, sedation; vomiting, diarrhea; neutropenia, thrombocytopenia, leukopenia, anemia, eosinophilia; elevated liver enzymes; phlebitis; retinal detachment in patients with CMV retinitis; hematuria, elevated blood urea nitrogen (BUN), and serum creatinine and dyspnea.

PHARMACOLOGY: Oral bioavailability is poor. Renal excretion is the major route of elimination; primarily excreted unchanged in the urine via glomerular filtration and active tubular secretion.

COMMENTS: Handle and dispose according to guidelines issued for cytotoxic drugs; avoid direct contact of skin or mucous membranes with the powder contained in capsules or the IV solution. Dosage adjustment or interruption of ganciclovir therapy may be necessary in patients with neutropenia and/or thrombocytopenia and patients with impaired renal function.

GENTAMICIN SULFATE (GARAMYCIN)

ACTION AND SPECTRUM: Aminoglycoside with bactericidal activity against gram-negative aerobic bacteria, including most *Pseudomonas*, *Proteus*, and *Serratia*. Some activity against coagulase-positive staphylococci, but ineffective against anaerobes and streptococci.

DOSAGE: IV, IM, intrathecal, intraventricular. Base the initial dose on body weight, then monitor levels and adjust using pharmacokinetics. Many dosing strategies exist such as extended interval, age based, weight based, and traditional.

Age based:

- **≤29 weeks postmenstrual age (PMA):**
  - **0–7 days:** 5 mg/kg/dose IV/IM every 48 hours.
  - **8–28 days:** 4 mg/kg/dose IV/IM every 36 hours.
  - **≥29 days:** 4 mg/kg/dose IV/IM every 24 hours.
- **30–34 weeks PMA:**
  - **0–7 days:** 4.5 mg/kg/dose IV/IM every 36 hours.
  - **>7 days:** 4 mg/kg/dose IV/IM every 24 hours.
- **≥35 weeks PMA:** 4 mg/kg/dose IV/IM every 24 hours.

Intrathecal or intraventricular (use preservative-free):

- **Newborns:** 1 mg/day.
- **Infants >3 months and children:** 1–2 mg/day.

Ophthalmic solution: 1 drop into each eye every 4 hours.

Ophthalmic ointment: Apply 2–3 times a day.

ADVERSE EFFECTS: Ototoxicity (may be associated with high serum aminoglycoside concentrations persisting for prolonged periods) with tinnitus, hearing loss; early toxicity usually affects high-pitched sound; nephrotoxicity (high trough levels) with proteinuria, elevated serum creatinine, oliguria, and macular rash.

PHARMACOLOGY: Renal excretion by glomerular filtration. Half-life is 3–11.5 hours initially. Volume of distribution is increased in neonates and with fever, edema, ascites, fluid overload.

COMMENTS: Desired serum peak is 4–12 mcg/mL (sample obtained 30 minutes after infusion has been completed), and desired serum trough is 0.5–2 mcg/mL (sample obtained 30 minutes to just before next dose). Obtain serum levels if treating for >48 hours. Monitor serum creatinine. Aminoglycosides should not be used alone against gram-positive pathogens.

GLUCAGON

INDICATIONS AND USE: Management of hypoglycemia unresponsive to routine treatment.

ACTIONS: Glucagon, a hormone produced by the alpha cells of the pancreas, stimulates synthesis of adenosine $3',5'$-cyclic monophosphate (cAMP), hepatic glycogenolysis, and gluconeogenesis, causing an increase in blood glucose levels; it inhibits small bowel motility and gastric acid secretion; produces both positive inotropic and chronotropic effects.

DOSAGE: IV, IM, subcutaneous.

Persistent hypoglycemia:

- 0.02–0.30 mg/kg/dose IV, IM, subcutaneous; may repeat in 20 minutes as needed. Maximum single dose: 1 mg.
- Continuous infusion: Initial: 10–20 mcg/kg/hour (0.5–1 mg) infused in 24 hours.

Congenital hyperinsulinism; hyperinsulinemic hypoglycemia:

- Continuous IV infusion: 0.005–0.02 mg/kg/hour.

ADVERSE EFFECTS: Tachycardia, ileus, hyponatremia, thrombocytopenia, nausea, and vomiting.

COMMENTS: Incompatible with electrolyte-containing solutions, precipitates with chloride solutions; compatible with dextrose solutions. *Caution:* Do not delay initiation of glucose infusion while observing for glucagon effect.

HEPARIN SODIUM

INDICATIONS AND USE: Prophylaxis and treatment of thromboembolic disorders and to maintain patency of arterial or venous catheters. (See Chapter 87.)

ACTIONS: Activates antithrombin III (heparin cofactor) and inactivates coagulation factors IX, X, XI, and XII and thrombin, inhibiting the conversion of fibrinogen to fibrin. Heparin also stimulates release of lipoprotein lipase (lipoprotein lipase hydrolyzes triglycerides to glycerol and free fatty acids).

DOSAGE: IV.

Treatment of thrombosis:

- **Loading dose:** 75 units/kg as IV bolus given over 10 minutes, followed by 28 units/kg/hour as continuous infusion; adjust dose to maintain activated partial thromboplastin time (aPTT) of 60–85 seconds (assuming this reflects an antifactor Xa level of 0.3–0.7).

Maintain catheter patency:

- Heparinized fluid with a usual final concentration of 0.5–1 unit/mL; may use concentration as low as 0.25 unit/mL.

Line flushing:

- Daily flushes of heparin to maintain patency of central catheters: 10 unit/mL is commonly used for younger infants (eg, <10 kg); 100 unit/mL is used for older infants and children. May need to flush every 6-8 hours for some catheters.

ADVERSE REACTIONS: Thrombocytopenia, bleeding tendency, hemorrhage, fever, rash, and abnormal liver function tests (LFTs). Follow platelet counts every 2–3 days.

PHARMACOLOGY: Clearance in neonates is more rapid than in children or adults; half-life is dose dependent, but the average is 1–3 hours.

COMMENTS: Antidote: Protamine Sulfate; refer to monograph for dosing.

HEPATITIS B IMMUNE GLOBULIN (HBIG)

INDICATIONS AND USE: Provide prophylactic passive immunity to hepatitis B infection.

ACTIONS: Passive immunization agent. Immune serum provides protection against the hepatitis B virus by directly providing specific antibody to hepatitis B surface antigen (HBsAg). The duration of immunity is short (3–6 months).

DOSAGE: IM.

Neonates born to HBsAg-positive mothers:

- 0.5 mL IM as soon after birth as possible (within 12 hours; efficacy decreases significantly if treatment is delayed >48 hours); hepatitis B vaccine series to begin at the same time; if this series is delayed for as long as 3 months, the HBIG dose may be repeated.

Neonates born to mothers with unknown HBsAg status at birth:

- **Birthweight <2 kg:** 0.5 mL within 12 hours of birth (along with hepatitis B vaccine) if unable to determine maternal HBsAg status within 12 hours.
- **Birthweight ≥2 kg:** 0.5 mL within 7 days of birth while awaiting maternal HBsAg result.

ADVERSE EFFECTS: Swelling, warmth, erythema, and soreness at the injection site. Rash, fever, and urticaria are rare.

COMMENTS: Administer with caution in patients with immunoglobulin (Ig) A deficiency, thrombocytopenia, or coagulopathy. Do not administer IV.

HEPATITIS B VACCINE (HEPTAVAX-B, RECOMBIVAX HB, ENGERIX-B)

INDICATIONS AND USE: Immunization against infection caused by all known subtypes of hepatitis B virus in individuals considered at high risk of potential exposure to hepatitis B virus.

ACTIONS: Promotes immunity to hepatitis B virus by inducing the production of specific antibodies to the virus.
DOSAGE: IM. Recommended schedule: 0.5 mL/dose in 3 total doses.

Infants born to hepatitis B surface antigen (HBsAg)-positive mothers:

• First dose within the first 12 hours of life, even if premature and regardless of birthweight (hepatitis immune globulin should also be administered at the same time/different site); second dose at 1–2 months of age; and third dose at 6 months of age. Check anti-HBs and HBsAg at 9–15 months of age. If anti-HBs and HBsAg are negative, reimmunize with 3 doses 2 months apart and reassess. *Note:* Premature infants <2000 grams should receive 4 total doses at 0, 1, 2–3, and 6–7 months of chronological age.

Infants born to HBsAg-negative mothers:

• First dose prior to discharge; however, the first dose may be given at 1–2 months of age. Another dose is given 1–2 months later, and a final dose at 6 months of age. A total of 4 doses of vaccine may be given if a "birth dose" is administered and a combination vaccine is used to complete the series. *Note:* Premature infants <2000 grams may have the initial dose deferred up to 30 days of chronological age.

Infants born to mothers whose HBsAg status is unknown at birth:

• First dose within 12 hours of birth even if premature, regardless of birthweight; second dose following 1–2 months later; the third dose at 6 months of age; if the mother's blood HBsAg test is positive, the infant should receive hepatitis immune globulin as soon as possible (no later than age 1 week). Due to possible decreased immunogenicity, premature neonates <2 kg who received an initial dose within 12 hours of birth should receive 4 total doses at 0, 1, 2–3, and 6–7 months of chronological age.

ADVERSE EFFECTS: Swelling, warmth, erythema, soreness at the injection site, and, rarely, vomiting, rash, and low-grade fever.
COMMENTS: Do not give IV or intradermally.

HYALURONIDASE

INDICATIONS AND USE: Treatment of extravasation injuries.
ACTIONS: An enzyme that temporarily hydrolyses hyaluronic acid (one of the chief components of tissue cement) and thereby allows the infiltrated drug or solution to be absorbed over a larger surface area. This speeds absorption and reduces tissue contact time with the irritant substance.
DOSAGE: **Subcutaneous.**

• Using a 25- or 26-gauge needle, inject 5 separate 0.2-mL subcutaneous injections around the periphery of the extravasation site. Change the needle after each injection. Elevate the extremity. Do not apply heat. Repeat as needed. Some use 5 separate 0.2-mL subcutaneous injections of 15 units/mL dilution.

ADVERSE EFFECTS: Usually well tolerated. Urticaria occurs rarely. Administer hyaluronidase within 1 hour of the extravasation, if possible.

HYDRALAZINE HCL (APRESOLINE HCL)

INDICATIONS AND USE: For the management of moderate to severe hypertension and as an afterload reducing agent to treat congestive heart failure.
ACTIONS: Causes direct relaxation of smooth muscle in the arteriolar resistance vessels; decreases systemic vascular resistance and increases cardiac output; increases renal, coronary, cerebral, and splanchnic blood flow.
DOSAGE: **IM, IV, PO.**

• IM or IV: 0.1–0.5 mg/kg/dose every 6–8 hours (maximum 2 mg/kg/dose).
• PO: 0.25–1 mg/kg/dose every 6–8 hours; increase over 3–4 weeks to maximum of 5 mg/kg/day in infants.

ADVERSE EFFECTS: Most frequent are tachycardia and hypotension; most serious is a reversible lupus-like syndrome. Tachyphylaxis often occurs on chronic therapy. Gastrointestinal (GI) bleeding or diarrhea.
COMMENTS: Contraindicated in mitral valve rheumatic heart disease.

HYDROCHLOROTHIAZIDE (VARIOUS)

INDICATIONS AND USE: Mild to moderate edema and hypertension.
ACTIONS: Inhibits sodium reabsorption in the distal tubules causing increased excretion of sodium and water as well as potassium, hydrogen, magnesium, phosphate, calcium, and bicarbonate ions.
DOSAGE: **PO.**

Neonates:

• 1–4 mg/kg/day divided in 2 doses.

Edema:

• **Infants <6 months:** 2–3.3 mg/kg/day in 2 divided doses; maximum dose 37.5 mg/day.
• **Infants >6 months and children:** 2 mg/kg/day in 2 divided doses; maximum dose 200 mg/day.

Hypertension:

• **Infants and children:** Initially, administer 1 mg/kg/day once daily; increase to maximum 3 mg/kg/day if needed; not to exceed 50 mg/day.

ADVERSE EFFECTS: Hypokalemia, hyperglycemia, hyperuricemia, hypochloremic metabolic alkalosis.

HYDROCORTISONE

INDICATIONS AND USE: Management of acute adrenal insufficiency, congenital adrenal hyperplasia, and vasopressor-resistant hypotension. Adjunctive treatment for persistent hypoglycemia.

ACTIONS: The short-acting adrenal corticosteroid that possesses glucocorticoid activity, anti-inflammatory activity, and some mineralocorticoid effects; most effects probably result from modification of enzyme activity, thus affecting almost all body systems. Promotes protein catabolism, gluconeogenesis, renal excretion of calcium, capillary wall permeability and stability, and red blood cell production; suppresses immune and inflammatory responses.

DOSAGE: IV, IM, PO.

Acute adrenal insufficiency:

- 1–2 mg/kg/dose IV bolus, then 25–150 mg/day divided every 6–8 hours.

Congenital adrenal hyperplasia (AAP recommendations):

- **Initial:** 10–20 mg/m^2/day PO in 3 divided doses.
- **Usual requirement:**
  - **Infants:** 2.5–5 mg 3 times per day.
  - **Children:** 5–10 mg 3 times per day.

Physiologic replacement:

- **Oral:** Usual dose is 20–25 mg/m^2/day or 0.5–0.75 mg/kg/day divided and administered every 8 hours. IM: 0.25–0.35 mg/kg/day or 12–15 mg/m^2/day once daily.
- **Stress doses (treatment-resistant hypotension):** 20–30 mg/m^2 IV divided into 2 or 3 doses; alternatively 1 mg/kg/dose every 8 hours.

Refractory hypoglycemia (refractory to continuous glucose infusion rates >12–15 mg/kg/minute):

- **IV, PO:** 5 mg/kg/day divided every 8–12 hours or 1–2 mg/kg/dose every 6 hours. Consider consultation with pediatric endocrinologist for treatment guidance.

ADVERSE EFFECTS AND COMMENTS: Hypertension, hypothalamic-pituitary-adrenal axis (HPA) suppression, hypokalemia, hyperglycemia, growth suppression, sodium and water retention, decreased bone mineral density, and immunosuppression. *Note:* Morning dose should be administered as early as possible; tablets may result in more reliable serum concentrations than oral liquid formulation; individualize dose by monitoring growth, hormone levels, and bone age; mineralocorticoid (eg, fludrocortisone) and sodium supplement may be required in salt losers.

IBUPROFEN (MOTRIN, OTHERS)

INDICATIONS AND USE: Treatment of mild to moderate pain, fever, and inflammatory diseases. Oral ibuprofen may be a safe alternative for patent ductus arteriosus (PDA) closure; recent studies have shown this, but larger studies are needed.

ACTIONS: Inhibits prostaglandin synthesis by decreasing the activity of the enzyme cyclooxygenase.

DOSAGE: PO.

Infants and children:

- **Analgesic:** 4–10 mg/kg/dose PO every 6–8 hours; maximum daily dose is 40 mg/kg/day.
- **Antipyretic:** 6 months to 12 years, maximum daily dose is 40 mg/kg/day.
  - **Temperature <102.5°F (39°C):** 5 mg/kg/dose every 6–8 hours.
  - **Temperature ≥102.5°F (39°C):** 10 mg/kg/dose every 6–8 hours.
- **PDA closure:** 10 mg/kg body weight for the first dose, followed at 24 hours intervals by 2 doses of 5 mg/kg each on the second and third day of life.

ADVERSE EFFECTS: Edema, hypertension, fluid retention, gastrointestinal (GI) bleed, GI perforation, neutropenia, anemia, inhibition of platelet aggregation, elevated liver enzymes, acute renal failure/acute kidney injury.

PHARMACOLOGY: Hepatic metabolism. Primarily renally excreted.

COMMENTS: To reduce the risk of adverse cardiovascular and GI effects, use the lowest effective dose for the shortest period of time. May increase risk of GI irritation, ulceration, bleeding, and perforation; may compromise existing renal function; use with caution in patients with decreased liver function.

IBUPROFEN LYSINE (NEOPROFEN)

INDICATIONS AND USE: Pharmacologic closure of patent ductus arteriosus. Not indicated for intraventricular hemorrhage prophylaxis.

ACTIONS: Nonsteroidal anti-inflammatory drug (NSAID) with analgesic and antipyretic properties. Action is principally by inhibition of prostaglandin synthesis, thus inhibiting cyclooxygenase, an enzyme that catalyzes the formation of prostaglandin precursors (endoperoxides) from arachidonic acid.

DOSAGE: IV.

- 10 mg/kg initially, followed by 2 doses of 5 mg/kg at 24- and 48-hour intervals after the initial dose.

ADVERSE EFFECTS: Anemia, fluid retention, edema, tachycardia, hepatic dysfunction, decreased urine output, elevated blood urea nitrogen (BUN) and serum creatinine (renal effects are less severe and less frequent than those with indomethacin); may inhibit platelet aggregation; monitor for signs of bleeding. Use with caution in infants when total bilirubin is elevated (ibuprofen may displace bilirubin from albumin-binding sites). Feeding intolerance, gastrointestinal irritation, ileus.

COMMENTS: NeoProfen is contraindicated in preterm neonates with infection, active bleeding, thrombocytopenia or coagulation defects, necrotizing enterocolitis (NEC), significant renal dysfunction, and congenital heart disease with ductal-dependent systemic blood flow.

IMIPENEM/CILASTATIN

ACTION AND SPECTRUM: Treatment of noncentral nervous system (CNS) infections caused by multidrug-resistant gram-negative organisms.

DOSAGE: IV.

Neonates:

- **0–4 weeks, <1.2 kg:** 20 mg/kg/dose every 18–24 hours.
- **Postnatal age ≤7 days, 1.2–1.5 kg:** 20 mg/kg/dose every 12 hours.
- **Postnatal age ≤7 days, >1.5 kg:** 25 mg/kg/dose every 12 hours.
- **Postnatal age >7 days, 1.2–1.5 kg:** 20 mg/kg/dose every 12 hours.
- **Postnatal age >7 days, >1.5 kg:** 25 mg/kg/dose every 8 hours.

Infants 4 weeks to 3 months:

- 25 mg/kg/dose every 6 hours.

Infants ≥3 months and children:

- 60–100 mg/kg/day divided every 6 hours; maximum dose 4 grams/day.

ADVERSE EFFECTS: Irritation, pain, phlebitis at injection site, elevated liver transaminases; diarrhea and seizures in patients with meningitis.

PHARMACOLOGY: Broad-spectrum carbapenem combines with cilastatin (renal dipeptidase inhibitor that prevents renal metabolism of imipenem). Inhibits cell wall synthesis. Half-life is prolonged with renal insufficiency.

IMMUNE GLOBULIN, INTRAVENOUS (IVIG)

INDICATIONS AND USE: Neonatal alloimmune thrombocytopenia, hemolytic jaundice, adjuvant treatment of fulminant neonatal sepsis (*controversial*) and immunodeficiency syndromes.

ACTIONS: The pooled, heterogeneous immunoglobulin G (IgG) present in IVIG provides a plethora of antibodies capable of opsonization and neutralization of many toxins and microbes, as well as complement activation. Although the amount of each IgG subclass in the parenteral products is similar to that of human plasma, the titers against specific antigens vary from manufacturer to manufacturer. The passive immunity imparted by IVIG is capable of attenuating or preventing infectious diseases or deleterious reactions from toxins, *Mycoplasma*, parasites, bacteria, and viruses. IVIG is thought to promote blockade of Fc receptors in macrophages (preventing phagocytosis of circulating opsonized platelets or cells tagged with autoantibodies).

DOSAGE: IV.

- **Usual dosage:** 400 mg to 1 gram/kg/dose infused over 2–6 hours. Many different products available; consult specific product insert for dosing details.

ADVERSE EFFECTS: Hypotension, transient tachycardia, and anaphylaxis. If either occurs, the rate of infusion should be decreased or stopped until resolved, then resumed at a slower rate as tolerated. Contraindicated in IgA deficiency (except with the use of Gammagard S/D or Polygam S/D).

INDOMETHACIN (INDOCIN IV)

INDICATIONS AND USE: Pharmacologic closure of patent ductus arteriosus (PDA). May provide prophylaxis for intraventricular hemorrhage (IVH) in low birthweight infants.

ACTIONS: Nonsteroidal anti-inflammatory drug (NSAID) with analgesic and antipyretic properties. Inhibits prostaglandin synthesis by decreasing cyclooxygenase activity, an enzyme that catalyzes the formation of prostaglandin precursors (endoperoxides) from arachidonic acid. Decreases cerebral blood flow.

DOSAGE: IV.

Patent ductus arteriosus:

- **Neonates:** Initially, 0.2 mg/kg IV, followed by 2 doses depending on postnatal age (PNA):
  - **PNA at first dose <48 hours:** 0.1 mg/kg at 12- to 24-hour intervals.
  - **PNA at first dose 2–7 days:** 0.2 mg/kg at 12- to 24-hour intervals.
  - **PNA at first dose >7 days:** 0.25 mg/kg at 12- to 24-hour intervals.
- **Dosing interval:**
  - **12-hour dosing interval** if urine output is >1 mL/kg/hour after prior dose.
  - **24-hour dosing interval** if urine output is <1 mL/kg/hour but >0.6 mL/kg/hour.
  - **Hold dose if patient has oliguria** (urine output <0.6 mL/kg/hour) or anuria.

Prophylaxis for IVH: 0.1 mg/kg/dose IV every 24 hours for 3 doses; give first dose at 6–12 hours of age.

ADVERSE EFFECTS: May cause decreased platelet aggregation, transient oliguria (decreased glomerular filtration rate), increased serum creatinine, and increased serum concentration of renally excreted drugs such as gentamicin. May also cause hyponatremia, hyperkalemia, and hypoglycemia. Gastrointestinal perforations are known to occur if used concurrently with corticosteroids.

COMMENTS: Contraindicated in premature neonates with necrotizing enterocolitis (NEC), severe renal impairment (urine output <0.6 mL/kg/hour or creatinine ≥1.8 mg/dL), thrombocytopenia, active bleeding, or if there has been intraventricular bleeding within the preceding 7 days (*controversial*).

INSULIN, REGULAR

INDICATIONS AND USE: Hyperglycemia, hyperkalemia, and increasing caloric intake in infants with glucose intolerance on parenteral nutrition (PN).

ACTIONS: Hormone derived from the β cells of the pancreas and the principal hormone required for glucose utilization. In skeletal and cardiac muscle and adipose tissue, insulin facilitates transport of glucose into these cells. Insulin stimulates lipogenesis and protein synthesis and inhibits lipolysis and release of free fatty acids from adipose cells. Promotes intracellular shift of potassium and magnesium.

DOSAGE: IV, **subcutaneous.**

Hyperglycemia:

- **Continuous IV infusion:** 0.01–0.1 unit/kg/hour (titrate with hourly determinations of blood glucose until stable, then every 4 hours).
- **Intermittent:** 0.1–0.2 unit/kg/dose subcutaneous every 6–12 hours.

Hyperkalemia:

- **Continuous IV infusion:** 0.1–0.2 unit/kg/hour in combination with a continuous infusion of 0.5 gram/kg/hour of dextrose. Adjust infusion rates based on serum glucose and potassium concentrations.

ADVERSE EFFECTS: Hypoglycemia (may cause coma and severe central nervous system [CNS] injury), hyperglycemic rebound (Somogyi effect), urticaria, and anaphylaxis.

COMMENTS: To minimize absorption of insulin to IV solution bag or tubing: If new tubing is not needed, wait a minimum of 30 minutes between the preparation of the solution and the initiation of the infusion. If new tubing is needed, after receiving the insulin continuous infusion solution, the administration set should be attached to the IV container and the line should be flushed with the insulin solution; wait 30 minutes, then flush the line again with the insulin solution prior to initiating the infusion. Because of adsorption, the actual amount of insulin being administered could be substantially less than the apparent amount. Therefore, adjustment of the insulin drip rate should be based on the effect and not solely on the apparent insulin dose.

IPRATROPIUM BROMIDE (ATROVENT)

INDICATIONS AND USE: Bronchodilator for adjunctive treatment of acute bronchospasm.

ACTIONS: Anticholinergic drug that acts by antagonizing the action of acetylcholine at the parasympathetic receptor sites, thereby producing bronchodilation.

DOSAGE: **Inhalation.**

- **Neonates:** 25 mcg/kg/dose nebulized every 8 hours.
- **Infants:** 125–250 mcg/dose nebulized every 8 hours. Dilute to 3 mL with normal saline (NS) or concurrent albuterol.
- **Metered inhaler:** 2–4 puffs as needed every 6–8 hours.

ADVERSE EFFECTS: Rebound airway hyperresponsiveness after discontinuation. Nervousness, dizziness, nausea, blurred vision, dry mouth, exacerbation of symptoms, airway irritation, cough, palpitations, rash, and urinary retention. Use with caution in narrow-angle glaucoma or bladder neck obstruction.

COMMENTS: Compatible when admixed with albuterol if given within 1 hour. Bronchodilator effect may be potentiated when given with β_2-agonist (ie, albuterol).

IRON DEXTRAN

INDICATIONS AND USE: Used to treat iron deficiency anemia, as an iron supplement for infants on epoetin, and for infants on long-term parenteral nutrition (PN). Oral iron is much safer than the parenteral form; the parenteral form is usually reserved for patients who cannot take oral iron.

ACTIONS: Iron is a component in the formation of hemoglobin, and adequate amounts are necessary for erythropoiesis and oxygen transport capacity of blood.

DOSAGE: IV. *Note:* Multiple parenteral iron forms exist.

Total replacement dosage of iron dextran for iron deficiency anemia:

- Dose (mL) = $0.0442 \times$ LBW (kg) $\times$ (Hbn – Hbo) + [$0.26 \times$ LBW (kg)]
  - LBW = lean body weight
  - Hbn = desired hemoglobin (grams/dL) = 12 if <15 kg or 14.8 if >15 kg
  - Hbo = measured hemoglobin (grams/dL)

Total iron replacement dosage for acute blood loss (assumes 1 mL of normocytic, normochromic red cells = 1 mg elemental iron):

- Iron dextran (mL) = $0.02 \times$ blood loss (mL) $\times$ hematocrit (expressed as a decimal fraction)

Anemia of prematurity:

- 0.2–1 mg/kg/day IV or 20 mg/kg/week with epoetin alfa therapy.

Parenteral nutritional addition:
- Admixed in the PN solution (solution must contain at least 2% amino acids): 0.4–1 mg/kg/day (or 3–5 mg/kg as a single weekly dose).

ADVERSE EFFECTS: Iron accumulation in patients with serious liver dysfunction; anaphylaxis, fever, and arthralgia. IV use: Pain and redness at IV site, rash, shivering; hypotension and flushing with rapid infusion.

ISONIAZID (INH)

INDICATIONS AND USE: Treatment of susceptible *Mycobacterium* spp. (eg, *M. tuberculosis, M. kansasii,* and *M. avium*) and for prophylaxis for individuals exposed to tuberculosis.

ACTION AND SPECTRUM: Antimycobacterial agent that is bactericidal for both extracellular and intracellular organisms. Inhibits mycolic acid synthesis resulting in disruption of the bacterial cell wall.

DOSAGE: PO.
- **Perinatal tuberculosis:** 10–15 mg/kg/day PO divided every 12 hours with rifampin (see Rifampin for dosage) for 3–12 months. If skin test conversion is positive, treat with 10–15 mg/kg/day PO every 24 hours for 9–12 months.

ADVERSE EFFECTS: Peripheral neuropathy, seizures, encephalopathy, blood dyscrasias, nausea, vomiting, and diarrhea (associated with administration of syrup formulation) and hypersensitivity reactions. May be hepatotoxic; follow liver function tests at regular intervals during treatment.

ISOPROTERENOL (ISUPREL, OTHERS)

INDICATIONS AND USE: Low cardiac output or vasoconstrictive shock states, cardiac arrest, ventricular arrhythmias resulting from atrioventricular (AV) block.

ACTIONS: Stimulates both β_1- and β_2-adrenergic receptors with minimal or no effect on α-receptors in therapeutic doses. Relaxes bronchial smooth muscle, cardiac stimulation (inotropic and chronotropic), and peripheral vasodilation (reduces cardiac afterload).

DOSAGE: IV.
- 0.05–0.5 mcg/kg/minute IV continuous infusion; maximum dose is 2 mcg/kg/minute. Correct acidosis before initiating therapy.

ADVERSE EFFECTS: Tremor, vomiting, hypertension, tachycardia, cardiac arrhythmias, hypotension, and hypoglycemia.

COMMENTS: Contraindicated in hypertension, hyperthyroidism, tachycardia caused by digoxin toxicity, and preexisting cardiac arrhythmias. Increases cardiac oxygen consumption disproportional to the increase in cardiac oxygen output. Not considered an inotropic agent of choice.

KANAMYCIN SULFATE

> WARNING: Neurotoxicity/ototoxicity/nephrotoxicity possible with increased risk in those with renal impairment, high dose, and prolonged treatment. Neuromuscular blockade including respiratory paralysis is possible.

ACTION AND SPECTRUM: Aminoglycoside indicated for treatment of serious infections caused by susceptible strains of *Escherichia coli, Proteus* spp., *Enterobacter aerogenes, Klebsiella pneumoniae, Serratia marcescens,* and *Acinetobacter* spp.; second-line treatment of *Mycobacterium tuberculosis.* Not considered first-line therapy.

DOSAGE: IV, IM. Base the initial dose on body weight, then monitor levels and adjust using pharmacokinetics.

0–4 weeks of age and <1.2 kg:
- 7.5 mg/kg/dose every 18–24 hours.

1.2–2 kg:
- **0–7 days old:** 7.5 mg/kg/dose every 12–18 hours.
- **>7 days old:** 7.5 mg/kg/dose every 8–12 hours.

>2 kg:
- **0–7 days old:** 10 mg/kg/dose every 12 hours.
- **>7 days old:** 10 mg/kg/dose every 8 hours.

ADVERSE EFFECTS: Discontinue treatment if signs of nephrotoxicity occur; renal damage is usually reversible. Ototoxicity (auditory and vestibular) is proportional to the amount of drug given and the duration of treatment. Tinnitus or vertigo may be indications of vestibular injury and impending bilateral irreversible damage. Discontinue treatment if signs of ototoxicity occur.

PHARMACOLOGY: Primarily renally excreted by glomerular filtration. Half-life is 4–8 hours.

COMMENTS: **Serum levels:** ideal peak 15–30 mcg/mL (sample 30 minutes after infusion is complete), and serum trough is 5–10 mcg/mL (sample 30 minutes prior to next dose). Obtain levels at about the fourth maintenance dose. Monitor serum creatinine every 3–4 days. Excessive peak levels are associated with ototoxicity; excessive trough levels, nephrotoxicity.

KETOCONAZOLE (NIZORAL)

> **WARNING:** Ketoconazole has been associated with hepatic toxicity. Coadministration of cisapride or astemizole with ketoconazole is contraindicated. Serious cardiovascular adverse events have occurred.

ACTION AND SPECTRUM: A broad-spectrum antifungal agent that acts by disrupting cell membranes. Fungicidal against susceptible candidiasis, blastomycosis, coccidioidomycosis, histoplasmosis, paracoccidioidomycosis, chronic mucocutaneous candidiasis, as well as certain recalcitrant cutaneous dermatophytoses (U.S. Food and Drug Administration [FDA] approved in those ≥2 years of age).
DOSAGE: PO.

- 3.3–6.6 mg/kg/day PO once daily with food to decrease nausea and vomiting; administer 2 hours prior to antacids, proton pump inhibitors, or H_2-receptor antagonists to prevent decreased ketoconazole absorption; shake suspension well before use.

ADVERSE EFFECTS: Gastric distress is the most common side effect. Check periodic liver function tests; caution in patients with impaired hepatic function; high doses of ketoconazole may depress adrenocortical function and decrease serum testosterone concentrations.
PHARMACOLOGY: Hepatic metabolism. Penetration into cerebrospinal fluid (CSF) is poor.
COMMENTS: Not indicated for treatment of fungal meningitis. Minimum period of treatment for candidiasis is 1–2 weeks, but duration should be based on clinical response. Limited experience in neonates.

KETAMINE HYDROCHLORIDE (KETALAR)

INDICATIONS AND USE: Ketamine is a rapid-acting general anesthetic agent for short diagnostic and minor surgical procedures that do not require skeletal muscle relaxation.
ACTIONS: Produces dissociative anesthesia by direct action on the cortex and limbic system; does not usually impair pharyngeal or laryngeal reflexes. Induces coma, analgesia, and amnesia. Increases cerebral blood flow and cerebral oxygen consumption; improves pulmonary compliance and relieves bronchospasm.
DOSAGE: IV, IM, PO.

- **IV:** 0.5–2 mg/kg/dose; use smaller doses (0.5–1 mg/kg) for sedation for minor procedures.
- **Usual induction dose:** 1–2 mg/kg IV. Reduce dose in hepatic dysfunction.

ADVERSE EFFECTS: Avoid use of ketamine in patients with increased intracranial pressure, increased cerebral blood flow, increased cerebrospinal fluid (CSF) pressure, increased cerebral metabolism, or if a significant elevation in blood pressure may present a risk to the patient. Elevated blood pressure (frequent), tachycardia, arrhythmia, hypotension, bradycardia, increased cerebral blood flow, and decreased cardiac output may occur. Respiratory depression, and apnea after rapid IV administration of high doses; laryngospasm; and hypersalivation. Increased airway resistance, cough reflex may be depressed, decreased bronchospasm. Nystagmus and increased intraocular pressure. Emergence reactions (psychic disturbances such as hallucinations and delirium lasting up to 24 hours). Minimize by reducing verbal, tactile, and visual simulation in the recovery period. These occur less commonly in pediatric patients than in adults. Severe reactions can be treated with a benzodiazepine. Increased muscle tone that may resemble seizures and extensor spasm with opisthotonos may occur in infants receiving high, repeated doses. Rash as well as pain and redness at the IM injection site.
PHARMACOLOGY: IV acts in 30 seconds and lasts 5–10 minutes. Amnesia lasts for 1–2 hours. Concurrent narcotics or barbiturates prolong recovery time.
COMMENTS: Pretreatment with a benzodiazepine 15 minutes before ketamine may reduce side effects such as psychic disturbances, increased intracranial pressure and cerebral blood flow, tachycardia, and jerking movements. Monitor heart rate, respiratory rate, blood pressure, and pulse oximetry. Observe for CNS side effects during the recovery period. Have equipment for resuscitation available.

LABETALOL (NORMODYNE)

INDICATIONS AND USE: Treatment of mild to severe hypertension. IV form for hypertensive emergencies.
ACTIONS: Dose-related decrease in blood pressure through α-, β_1-, and β_2-adrenergic receptor blockade without causing significant reflex tachycardia or a decrease in heart rate. Reduces elevated renin levels.
DOSAGE: PO, IV. Limited experience in neonates; labetalol should be initiated cautiously; carefully monitor blood pressure, heart rate, and electrocardiogram, and adjust the dose accordingly. Use the lowest effective dose.
IV intermittent bolus:

- 0.2–0.5 mg/kg/dose over 2–3 minutes every 4–6 hours with a range of 0.2–1 mg/kg/dose has been suggested; maximum dose 20 mg/dose.

Treatment of pediatric hypertensive emergencies:

- **Continuous IV infusion:** 0.4–1 mg/kg/hour with a maximum of 3 mg/kg/hour.
- **Alternate dosing:** Bolus 0.2–1 mg/kg followed by a continuous infusion of 0.25–1.5 mg/kg/hour.

Oral:

- **Initial:** 1–2 mg/kg/day in 2 divided doses. Maximum dose 10–20 mg/kg/day.

ADVERSE EFFECTS: Orthostatic hypotension, bronchospasm, nasal congestion, edema, congestive heart failure, bradycardia, myopathy, and rash. Intensifies atrioventricular (AV) block. Reversible hepatic dysfunction (rare).
PHARMACOLOGY: Peak effect with PO is 1–4 hours after the dose, while peak effect with IV is 5–15 minutes. Metabolized in the liver by glucuronidation. Oral labetalol has a bioavailability of only 25% because of extensive first-pass effect. Oral absorption is improved by taking with food. Concomitant oral cimetidine may increase the bioavailability of oral labetalol.
COMMENTS: Do not discontinue chronic labetalol abruptly; taper over 1–2 weeks. Contraindicated in patients with asthma, overt cardiac failure, heart block, cardiogenic shock, or severe bradycardia. May cause a paradoxic increase in blood pressure in patients with pheochromocytoma. Use with caution in hepatic dysfunction. Incompatible with sodium bicarbonate.

LAMIVUDINE (EPIVIR)

ACTION AND SPECTRUM: Antiretroviral agent that inhibits reverse transcription by viral DNA chain termination. Used for the prevention of mother-to-child transmission of human immunodeficiency virus (HIV); treatment of HIV infection.
DOSAGE: PO. Use in combination with other antiretroviral agents—regimen containing 3 antiretroviral agents is strongly recommended.
Prevention of maternal-child HIV transmission:

- 2 mg/kg/dose every 12 hours for 7 days; given from birth to 1 week of age. Given to neonate in combination with nevirapine and 6 weeks of zidovudine in certain maternal situations, such as no treatment prior to labor or during labor, only intrapartum therapy; inadequate viral suppression at time of delivery or known drug-resistant virus.

Treatment of HIV infection:

- **Neonates <30 days:** 2 mg/kg/dose every 12 hours.
- **Infants 1–3 months:** 4 mg/kg/dose every 12 hours.
- **Infants >3 months and children <16 years:** 4 mg/kg/dose every 12 hours; maximum dose 150 mg every 12 hours.

ADVERSE EFFECTS: Very limited data in neonates; black box warning of lactic acidosis and severe hepatomegaly in adults; some fatal cases.
PHARMACOLOGY: Synthetic nucleoside analogue that is converted to active metabolite; oral solution is well absorbed with 66% bioavailability. Resistance develops rapidly with monotherapy.
COMMENTS: Blood levels/effects may be increased by ganciclovir, valganciclovir, ribavirin, and trimethoprim.

LANSOPRAZOLE (PREVACID)

INDICATIONS AND USE: Short-term treatment of gastroesophageal reflux disease (GERD); erosive esophagitis.
ACTIONS: Suppression of gastric acid secretion by selective inhibition of parietal cell membrane enzyme hydrogen-potassium adenosine triphosphatase (ATPase) or proton pump.
DOSAGE: PO.
Neonatal:

- 0.2–0.3 mg/kg/dose once daily (Zhang et al, 2008) based on pharmacokinetic data; patients <10 weeks of age have decreased clearance.
- Alternate dosing has been used: 0.5–1 mg/kg/dose once daily (Springer, 2008).

Infants >4 weeks:

- 1–1.5 mg/kg/dose once daily (Springer, 2008).

Infants ≥10 weeks:

- 1–2 mg/kg/dose once daily (Orenstein et al, 2009; Springer, 2008; Zhang et al, 2008).

ADVERSE EFFECTS: Limited data; proteinuria, abdominal pain, mild elevation of serum transaminases.
PHARMACOLOGY: Degrades in acid pH of stomach; extensively metabolized in liver by CYP2C19 and CYP3A4; the absorption of weakly acidic drugs such as digoxin and furosemide is increased and weakly basic drugs inhibited.
COMMENTS: Recent clinical trial (Orenstein, 2009) did not demonstrate efficacy in the treatment of GERD in patients <12 months of age, and the use in this patient population is ***controversial***.

LEVETIRACETAM (KEPPRA)

INDICATIONS AND USE: Adjunctive therapy in the treatment of partial onset seizures in patients 1 month of age and older. It is only approved for use in combination with other seizure medications.
ACTIONS: Mechanism of action unknown; studies suggest that one or more of these central pharmacologic effects may be involved: inhibition of voltage-dependent N-type calcium channels; blockade of γ-aminobutyric acid (GABA)-ergic inhibitory transmission through displacement of negative modulators; reversal of the inhibition of glycine currents; reduction of delayed rectifier potassium current; and/or binding to synaptic proteins that modulate neurotransmitter release.

DOSAGE: IV, PO. (*Note:* When switching from oral to IV formulation, the total daily dose should be the same.)
Neonatal dosing:

- **Initial dose:** 10 mg/kg/day IV given in 2 divided doses; may increase over 3 days to 30 mg/kg/day, if tolerated, to maximum of 45–60 mg/kg/day. Loading doses of 20–30 mg/kg have been used. (Dosing information is from studies with very small sample size.)
- **Oral:** 10 mg/kg/day PO in 1 to 2 divided doses; increase daily by 10 mg/kg to 30 mg/kg/day (maximum dose used: 60 mg/kg/day).

Infant (U.S. Food and Drug Administration [FDA] approved):

- **1 month to <6 months:** 7 mg/kg twice daily; increase in increments of 7 mg/kg twice daily every 2 weeks to recommended dose of 21 mg/kg twice daily.

ADVERSE EFFECTS: Somnolence, nervousness. Use with caution in patients with renal dysfunction; decrease dose.
PHARMACOLOGY: Oral absorption is rapid and complete; oral bioavailability 100%.
COMMENTS: Do not abruptly discontinue therapy; gradually decrease dose to reduce risk of increased seizure activity.

LEVOTHYROXINE SODIUM (T_4) (SYNTHROID, LEVOXYL, OTHERS)

INDICATIONS AND USE: Replacement or supplemental therapy in congenital or acquired hypothyroidism.
ACTIONS: The exact mechanism of action is unknown; however, it is believed the thyroid hormone exerts its many metabolic effects through control of DNA transcription and protein synthesis. Thyroid hormones increase the metabolic rate of body tissues, noted by increases in oxygen consumption; respiratory rate; body temperature; cardiac output; heart rate; blood volume; rates of fat, protein, and carbohydrate metabolism; and enzyme system activity, growth, and maturation. Thyroid hormones are very important in central nervous system (CNS) development. Deficiency in infants results in growth retardation and failure of brain growth and development.
DOSAGE: PO, IV, IM (use 50–75% of the oral dose).

- **0–3 months:** 10–15 mcg/kg PO; if the infant is at risk for development of cardiac failure, use a lower starting dose, ~25 mcg/day; if the initial serum T_4 is very low (<5 mcg/dL), begin treatment at a higher dosage, ~50 mcg/day.
- **>3–6 months:** 8–10 mcg/kg or 25–50 mcg PO.
- **>6–12 months:** 6–8 mcg/kg or 50–75 mcg PO.
- **Alternate dosing:** 8–10 mcg/kg/day PO for infants from birth to 1 year.

ADVERSE EFFECTS: Adverse effects are usually due to excessive dose. If the following occur, discontinue and reinstitute at a lower dose: tachycardia, cardiac arrhythmias, tremors, diarrhea, weight loss, and fever.
PHARMACOLOGY: Onset of action—oral: 3–5 days; IV: 6–8 hours. Maximum effect occurs in 4–6 weeks. Protein binding >99%.

LIDOCAINE (XYLOCAINE, OTHERS)

INDICATIONS AND USE: IV lidocaine is used almost exclusively for the short-term control of ventricular arrhythmias (premature beats, tachycardia, and fibrillation) or for prophylactic treatment of such arrhythmias. Also used as a local anesthetic or for the treatment of severe recurrent or prolonged seizures that fail to respond to first-line therapies.
ACTIONS: Class IB antiarrhythmic agent, suppresses spontaneous depolarization of the ventricles during diastole by a direct action on the tissues; blocks both the initiation and conduction of nerve impulses by decreasing the neuronal membrane's permeability to sodium ions; inhibits depolarization and results in blockade of conduction.
DOSAGE: IV, ETT.
Antiarrhythmic:

- **Initial:** 0.5–1 mg/kg/dose as IV bolus over 5 minutes. May repeat dose every 10 minutes as necessary to control arrhythmia; maximum total bolus dose is 5 mg/kg.
- **Maintenance IV infusion:** 10–50 mcg/kg/minute. Use lowest possible dose for preterm infants.
- **Endotracheal:** 2–3 mg/kg; flush with 5 mL of normal saline (NS) and follow with 5 assisted manual ventilations.

Anticonvulsant in term, normothermic neonates:

- **Loading dose** of 2 mg/kg IV over 10 minutes, immediately followed by
- **Maintenance infusion** of 6 mg/kg/hour for 6 hours, then 4 mg/kg/hour for 12 hours, then 2 mg/kg/hour for 12 hours.

ADVERSE EFFECTS: Drowsiness, dizziness, tremulousness, paresthesias, muscle twitching, seizures, and coma; respiratory depression and/or arrest. Hypotension and heart block can occur.
PHARMACOLOGY: Onset of action 1–2 minutes after IV bolus; half-life in neonates is 3 hours; primarily metabolized by the liver.
COMMENTS: Therapeutic levels: 1.5–5 mcg/mL; toxic levels >6 mcg/mL. Adjust dosage in liver failure. Contraindicated in sinoatrial or atrioventricular (AV) nodal block and Wolff-Parkinson-White syndrome. Avoid using with epinephrine.

LIDOCAINE/PRILOCAINE CREAM (EMLA)

INDICATIONS AND USE: Topical anesthetic for use on intact skin for minor procedures such as insertion of intravenous catheters, venipuncture, and lumbar puncture in infants ≥37 weeks' gestational age.
ACTIONS: EMLA (eutectic mixture of local anesthetics) contains 2 local anesthetics: lidocaine and prilocaine. Local anesthetics inhibit conduction of nerve impulses from sensory nerves by changing the cell membrane's permeability to ions.
DOSAGE: Topical.
Maximum EMLA dose, application area, and application time:

- **0–3 months or <5 kg:** Maximum 1 gram over 10 cm^2 for 1 hour.
- **3–12 months and >5 kg:** Maximum 2 grams over 20 cm^2 for 4 hours.
- **1–6 years and >10 kg:** Maximum 10 grams over 100 cm^2 for 4 hours.

ADVERSE EFFECTS: Not for use on mucous membranes or for ophthalmic use. May cause methemoglobinemia. Not for use in infants <37 weeks' gestational age or infants <12 months old receiving concurrent methemoglobin-inducing agents (sulfonamides, acetaminophen, nitroprusside, nitric oxide, phenobarbital, phenytoin). Reduce amounts if infant has hepatic and/or renal dysfunction.
COMMENT: Do not rub into skin; cover with occlusive dressing.

LINEZOLID (ZYVOX)

ACTIONS AND SPECTRUM: Oxazolidinone agent for treatment of pneumonia; complicated and uncomplicated skin and soft tissue infections; bacteremia caused by susceptible vancomycin-resistant *Enterococcus faecium* (VREF), *Enterococcus faecalis*, *Streptococcus pneumoniae* including multidrug-resistant strains, *Staphylococcus aureus* including methicillin-resistant *S. aureus* (MRSA), *Streptococcus pyogenes*, or *Streptococcus agalactiae*. *Note:* There have been reports of vancomycin-resistant *E. faecium* and MRSA developing resistance to linezolid during its clinical use.
DOSAGE: PO, IV.
Neonates 0–4 weeks and <1.2 kg:

- **Oral, IV:** 10 mg/kg/dose every 8–12 hours. (*Note:* Use every 12 hours in patients <34 weeks' gestation and <1 week of age.)

Neonates <7 days and ≥1.2 kg:

- **Oral, IV:** 10 mg/kg/dose every 8–12 hours. (*Note:* Use every 12 hours in patients <34 weeks' gestation and <1 week of age.)

Neonates ≥7 day and ≥1.2 kg (infants and children):

- 10 mg/kg/dose PO/IV every 8 hours.

Complicated skin and skin structure infections, and nosocomial or community-acquired pneumonia including concurrent bacteremia: Treat for 10–14 days.
VREF: Treat for 14–28 days.
ADVERSE EFFECTS: Thrombocytopenia, anemia, leukopenia, and pancytopenia have been reported in patients receiving linezolid—may be dependent on duration of therapy (generally >2 weeks of treatment); monitor patients' complete blood cell count (CBC) weekly during linezolid therapy; discontinuation of therapy may be required in patients who develop or have worsening myelosuppression. *Clostridium difficile*–associated colitis has been reported; fluid and electrolyte management, protein supplementation, antibiotic treatment, and surgical evaluation may be indicated. Peripheral and optic neuropathy with vision loss has been reported primarily in patients treated for >28 days with linezolid. Cases of lactic acidosis in which patients experienced repeated episodes of nausea and vomiting, acidosis, and low bicarbonate levels have been reported. Elevated transaminases, rash, and diarrhea.
PHARMACOLOGY: Orally well absorbed; low protein binding; metabolized in the liver.
COMMENTS: Therapeutic linezolid concentrations inconsistently achieved in the cerebrospinal fluid (CSF) of pediatric patients with ventriculoperitoneal shunts; not recommended for the empiric treatment of pediatric central nervous system (CNS) infections. Not approved for the treatment of catheter-related bloodstream, catheter-site, or gram-negative infections. Linezolid is a reversible, nonselective inhibitor of monoamine oxidase: enhanced vasopressor effects if used with sympathomimetic agents such as dopamine, epinephrine; myelosuppressive drugs (may increase risk of myelosuppression with linezolid).

LORAZEPAM (ATIVAN)

INDICATIONS AND USE: Treatment of status epilepticus resistant to conventional anticonvulsant therapy; sedation.
ACTIONS: A benzodiazepine that binds to the γ-aminobutyric acid (GABA)-receptor complex and facilitates the inhibitory effect of GABA on the central nervous system (CNS).
DOSAGE: IV.
Status epilepticus:

- **Neonates:** 0.05 mg/kg/dose IV over 2–5 minutes. If no response after 10–15 minutes, repeat the dose; dilute with an equal volume of sterile water, normal saline (NS), or 5% dextrose in water (D5W).

- **Infants and children:** 0.05–0.1 mg/kg slow IV over 2–5 minutes; do not exceed 4 mg per single dose; may repeat second dose of 0.05 mg/kg slow IV in 10–15 minutes if needed; dilute with an equal volume of sterile water, NS, or D5W.

Sedation, anxiety:

- 0.02–0.1 mg/kg/dose IV or PO every 4–8 hours as needed; not to exceed 2 mg/dose.

ADVERSE EFFECTS: May cause respiratory depression, apnea, hypotension, bradycardia, cardiac arrest, and seizure-like activity. Paradoxic CNS stimulation may occur, usually early in therapy. Some preterm infants may exhibit myoclonic activity; discontinue if any CNS effect occurs. Overdose may be reversed using flumazenil (Romazicon), 5–10 mcg/kg/dose IV. Reversal agent may trigger seizures.

COMMENTS: *Note:* IV preparations contain benzyl alcohol, propylene glycol, and polyethylene glycol. Contraindicated for infants with preexisting CNS, hepatic, or renal disease.

LUCINACTANT (SURFAXIN)

INDICATIONS AND USE: Prevention of respiratory distress syndrome (RDS) in premature infants at high risk for RDS.

ACTIONS: A synthetic pulmonary surfactant that acts like an endogenous surfactant by lowering the surface tension at the air-liquid interface of alveolar surfaces and stabilizes the alveoli. The synthetic formulation consists of phospholipids, a fatty acid, and sinapultide (KL4 peptide), a 21–amino acid hydrophobic synthetic peptide.

DOSAGE: ETT.

- 5.8 mL/kg birthweight divided into 4 aliquots and administered by intratracheal administration. Up to 4 doses of Surfaxin can be administered in the first 48 hours of life. Doses should be given no more frequently than every 6 hours. Prior to administration, each vial of lucinactant must be warmed for 15 minutes in a preheated dry block heater set at 44°C (111°F). Remove vial from heater and shake vigorously until suspension is uniform and free flowing. Warmed vials should not be refrigerated after warming and may be stored at room temperature for no more than 2 hours.

ADVERSE EFFECTS: Bradycardia, hypoxemia, airway obstruction, and reflux of drug into the endotracheal tube (ETT). **COMMENTS:** Treatment may need to be interrupted if adverse effects occur. Suctioning of the ETT or reintubation may be necessary if airway obstruction persists. Rapid changes in respiratory status may occur with administration; frequent assessment of oxygen and ventilatory support is recommended so appropriate changes can be made.

MAGNESIUM SULFATE

INDICATIONS AND USE: Treatment and prevention of hypomagnesemia and refractory hypocalcemia.

ACTIONS: Magnesium is an important cofactor in many enzymatic reactions. In the central nervous system (CNS), magnesium prevents or controls seizures by blocking neuromuscular transmission and decreasing the amount of acetylcholine liberated. It also has a depressant effect on the CNS. In the heart, magnesium acts as a calcium channel blocker and acts on cardiac muscle to slow sinoatrial nodal impulse formation and prolong conduction time. Magnesium is necessary for the maintenance of serum potassium and calcium levels through its effect on the renal tubule.

DOSAGE: IV, IM (1 gram of magnesium sulfate = 98.6 mg elemental magnesium = 8.12 mEq magnesium).

Hypomagnesemia:

- **Neonates:** 25–50 mg/kg/dose (0.2–0.4 mEq/kg/dose) IV every 8–12 hours for 2–3 doses until magnesium level is normal or symptoms resolve.
- **Maintenance:** 0.25–0.5 mEq/kg every 24 hours IV (add to infusion or give IV).
- **Children:** 25–50 mg/kg/dose (0.2–0.4 mEq/kg/dose) IM/IV every 4–6 hours for 3–4 doses; maximum single dose 2000 mg (16 mEq).

ADVERSE EFFECTS: Primarily related to magnesium serum level; hypotension, bradycardia, flushing, depression of reflexes, depressed cardiac function, and CNS and respiratory depression.

COMMENTS: Contraindicated in renal failure. Monitor serum magnesium, calcium, and phosphate levels. For intermittent infusion: dilute to a concentration of 0.5 mEq/mL (60 mg/mL) of magnesium sulfate; maximum concentration 1.6 mEq/mL (200 mg/mL) of magnesium sulfate; infuse magnesium sulfate over 2–4 hours and do not exceed 1 mEq/kg/hour.

MEROPENEM (MERREM)

ACTIONS AND SPECTRUM: Broad-spectrum carbapenem that penetrates well into cerebrospinal fluid (CSF) and most body tissues; specifically active against pneumococcal and pseudomonas meningitis, extended-spectrum β-lactamase–producing *Klebsiella pneumoniae*. Treatment of serious infections caused by multidrug-resistant gram-negative organisms and gram-positive aerobic and anaerobic pathogens susceptible to meropenem.

DOSAGE: IV.

Neonatal sepsis:

- **Gestational age <32 weeks and ≤14 days postnatal:** 20 mg/kg/dose IV every 12 hours; >14 days postnatal, dosing interval is every 8 hours.

- **Gestational age ≥32 weeks and ≤7 days postnatal:** 20 mg/kg/dose IV every 12 hours; >7 days postnatal, dosing interval is every 8 hours.

Neonatal meningitis caused by *Pseudomonas* species:

- 40 mg/kg/dose IV every 8 hours for all ages.

Children ≥3 months:

- **Complicated skin and skin structure infection:** 10 mg/kg/dose IV every 8 hours; maximum dose 500 mg.
- **Intra-abdominal infection:** 20 mg/kg/dose IV every 8 hours; maximum dose 1 gram.
- **Meningitis:** 40 mg/kg/dose IV every 8 hours; maximum dose 2 grams.

ADVERSE EFFECTS: Gastrointestinal effects such as diarrhea, vomiting, and rarely pseudomembranous colitis; fungal infections are a risk. Thrombocytosis and eosinophilia have been noted. Monitoring liver enzymes is recommended. Some cautionary reports have noted seizure-like episodes in a few preterm infants.

COMMENT: Serum half-life of meropenem is relatively short in infants (3 hours or less).

METHADONE HCL (DOLOPHINE)

> **WARNING:** Deaths have been reported during initiation of methadone treatment for opioid dependence. Respiratory depression is the chief hazard associated with methadone hydrochloride administration. Cases of QT interval prolongation and serious arrhythmia (torsade de pointes) have been observed.

INDICATIONS AND USE: Long-acting narcotic analgesic used for the treatment of neonatal abstinence syndrome and opioid dependence.

ACTIONS: Central nervous system (CNS) opiate receptor agonist resulting in analgesia and sedation; produces generalized CNS depression.

DOSAGE: PO, IV.

Neonatal abstinence syndrome:

- 0.05–0.2 mg/kg/dose PO/IV every 12–24 hours or 0.5 mg/kg/day divided every 8 hours. Individualize dose and tapering schedule to control symptoms of withdrawal; usually taper dose by 10–20% per week over 1 to 1-1/2 months. ***Note:*** Due to long elimination half-life, tapering is difficult; consider alternate agent like morphine.

ADVERSE EFFECTS: Respiratory depression, gastric residuals, abdominal distension, constipation, hypotension, bradycardia, prolongation of QT interval, torsade de pointes, CNS depression, sedation, increased intracranial pressure, urinary tract spasm, urine retention, biliary tract spasm, and dependence with prolonged use.

COMMENTS: *Caution:* Methadone may accumulate; reassess for the need to adjust the dose downward after 3–5 days to avoid overdose. Smaller doses or less frequent administration may be required in renal and hepatic dysfunction. Rifampin and phenytoin increase metabolism of methadone and may precipitate withdrawal symptoms. Methadone 10 mg IM = morphine 10 mg IM.

METHICILLIN SODIUM (STAPHCILLIN)

ACTION AND SPECTRUM: Activity primarily against penicillinase-positive and penicillinase-negative staphylococci and less effective than penicillin G against other gram-positive cocci; does not demonstrate any activity against enterococci. Other antistaphylococcal penicillins such as nafcillin and oxacillin are used more commonly in the United States.

DOSAGE: IV.

Meningitis:

- **<2 kg and 0–7 days old:** 100 mg/kg/day divided every 12 hours.
- **<2 kg and >7 days old:** 150 mg/kg/day divided every 8 hours.
- **>2 kg and 0–7 days old:** 150 mg/kg/day divided every 8 hours.
- **>2 kg and >7 days old:** 200 mg/kg/day divided every 6 hours.

Other indications:

- **<2 kg and 0–7 days old:** 50 mg/kg/day divided every 12 hours.
- **<2 kg and >7 days old:** 75 mg/kg/day divided every 8 hours.
- **>2 kg and 0–7 days old:** 75 mg/kg/day divided every 8 hours.
- **>2 kg and >7 days old:** 100 mg/kg/day divided every 6 hours.

ADVERSE EFFECTS: Nephrotoxicity (interstitial nephritis) occurs more often with methicillin than with other penicillins. Hypersensitivity reactions, anemia, leukopenia, thrombocytopenia, phlebitis at the infusion site, and hemorrhagic cystitis (in poorly hydrated patients).

PHARMACOLOGY: Renal excretion. Half-life is variable (60–120 minutes or longer).

COMMENTS: In cases of methicillin resistance, vancomycin becomes the antistaphylococcal drug of choice. Dosage adjustment is necessary in renal impairment. Monitor serum urea nitrogen and creatinine.

METOCLOPRAMIDE HCL (REGLAN)

INDICATIONS AND USE: In neonates and infants, the drug is used to facilitate gastric emptying and gastrointestinal (GI) motility. May improve feeding intolerance and gastroesophageal reflux.

ACTIONS: Dopamine-receptor antagonist acting on the central nervous system (CNS). Metoclopramide improves GI motility by releasing acetylcholine from the myenteric plexus resulting in contraction of the smooth muscle. Metoclopramide's effects on the GI tract include the following: increased resting esophageal sphincter tone, improved gastric tone and peristalsis, relaxed pyloric sphincter, and augmented duodenal peristalsis, which leads to increased gastric emptying and a decrease in the transit time through the duodenum, jejunum, and ileum.

DOSAGE: PO, IM, IV.

Gastroesophageal reflux in neonates:

- 0.1–0.15 mg/kg/dose PO/IM/IV every 6 hours, 30 minutes before feedings.

Infants and children:

- 0.4–0.8 mg/kg/day PO/IM/IV divided into 4 doses.

ADVERSE EFFECTS: CNS effects include restlessness, drowsiness, and fatigue. Extrapyramidal reactions may occur, generally manifested as acute dystonic reactions within the initial 24–48 hours of use (increased with higher doses). May cause tardive dyskinesia, which is often irreversible; duration of treatment and total cumulative dose are associated with an increased risk.

COMMENTS: Therapy durations >12 weeks should be avoided (except in rare cases where benefit exceeds risk). Contraindicated with bowel obstruction and seizure disorders.

METRONIDAZOLE (FLAGYL)

ACTION AND SPECTRUM: Treatment of meningitis, ventriculitis, and endocarditis due to *Bacteroides fragilis* and other anaerobes that are resistant to penicillin; serious intra-abdominal infections; treatment of *Clostridium difficile* colitis.

DOSAGE: PO, IV.

Neonates, anaerobic infections:

- **0–4 weeks and <1.2 kg:** 7.5 mg/kg PO/IV every 24–48 hours.
- **Postnatal age <7 days:**
  - **1.2–2 kg:** 7.5 mg/kg/day PO/IV given every 24 hours.
  - **>2 kg:** 15 mg/kg/day PO/IV in divided doses every 12 hours.
- **Postnatal age ≥7 days:**
  - **1.2–2 kg:** 15 mg/kg/day PO/IV in divided doses every 12 hours.
  - **>2 kg:** 30 mg/kg/day PO/IV in divided doses every 12 hours.

Infants and children:

- **Anaerobic infections:** 30 mg/kg/day PO/IV in divided doses every 6 hours; maximum dose 4 grams/day.
- **Antibiotic-associated pseudomembranous colitis:** 30 mg/kg/day PO divided every 6 hours for 7–10 days.

ADVERSE EFFECTS: Occasional vomiting, diarrhea, insomnia, irritability, seizures, rash, discoloration of urine (dark or reddish brown), phlebitis at the injection site, and (rarely) leukopenia.

PHARMACOLOGY: Hepatic metabolism with final excretion via the urine and feces. Large volume of distribution (penetrates into all body tissues and fluids).

COMMENTS: Some recommend an initial loading dose of 15 mg/kg, with the first maintenance dose either 48 hours later (for premature infants <2 kg) or 24 hours later (for infants >2 kg at birth). Effectively penetrates the cerebrospinal fluid (CSF) (indicated for meningitis). *Note:* Some centers use metronidazole for empiric coverage with ampicillin and gentamicin for necrotizing enterocolitis (NEC). Use of metronidazole in NEC remains *controversial.*

MICAFUNGIN

ACTION AND SPECTRUM: Treatment of fungal septicemia, peritonitis, and disseminated infections due to *Candida* species, including *C. albicans* and non-albicans species—*C. krusei, C. glabrata, C. tropicalis,* and *C. parapsilosis.*

DOSAGE: IV.

Neonates:

- **<1 kg:** 10 mg/kg/dose every 24 hours; doses as high as 15 mg/kg/dose have been used in extremely low birthweight neonates.
- **≥1 kg:** 7 mg/kg/dose every 24 hours.

Infants and children:

- 2–4 mg/kg/dose every 24 hours.

ADVERSE EFFECTS: Limited data in neonates; in adults—vomiting, diarrhea, hypokalemia, thrombocytopenia.

PHARMACOLOGY: Echinocandin agent with broad-spectrum fungicidal activity. The volume of distribution in extremely premature infants is very high; therefore, higher doses are required. Highly protein bound to albumin but does not displace bilirubin. Metabolized in the liver.

COMMENTS: Infuse over at least 1 hour. Not U.S. Food and Drug Administration (FDA) approved for use in children, and data are limited.

MIDAZOLAM HCL (VERSED)

> **WARNING:** Intravenous midazolam has been associated with respiratory depression and respiratory arrest, especially when used for sedation in noncritical care settings. In some cases, where this was not recognized promptly and treated effectively, death or hypoxic encephalopathy has resulted.

INDICATIONS AND USE: Anxiolytic and antiepileptic agent. Used as a sedative before procedures and given IV continuously to sedate intubated patients.

ACTIONS: Short-acting benzodiazepine; depresses central nervous system (CNS) by binding to the benzodiazepine site on the γ-aminobutyric acid (GABA)-receptor complex and increasing GABA, which is a major inhibitory neurotransmitter in the brain.

DOSAGE: IM, IV, PO, intranasal, sublingual.

Intermittent:
- 0.05–0.15 mg/kg/dose IV/IM over at least 5 minutes every 2–4 hours as needed.

Continuous infusion:
- **<32 weeks:** Initial 0.03 mg/kg/hour (0.5 mcg/kg/minute).
- **>32 weeks:** Initial 0.06 mg/kg/hour (1 mcg/kg/minute).
- Dosage ranges from 0.01 to 0.06 mg/kg/hour. May need to increase dose after several days due to tolerance or increased clearance. *Note:* Do not use IV loading doses in neonates; for faster sedation effect, infuse the continuous infusion at a faster rate for the first several hours; use the smallest dose possible.

Antiepileptic:
- **Loading dose:** 0.06–0.15 mg/kg/dose IV followed by a continuous infusion of 0.06–0.4 mg/kg/hour (1–7 mcg/kg/minute). Start with lower end of dosing range.

Oral sedation:
- 0.25–0.5 mg/kg/dose using oral syrup.

Intranasal:
- 0.2–0.3 mg/kg/dose using 5-mg/mL injectable form; may repeat in 5–15 minutes.

Sublingual:
- 0.2 mg/kg/dose using 5-mg/mL injectable form mixed with small amount of flavored syrup.

ADVERSE EFFECTS: Respiratory depression and cardiac arrest with excessive doses or rapid IV infusions. May cause hypotension and bradycardia. Myoclonic activity has been reported in preterm infants as well as other seizure-like activity.

COMMENT: Infuse IV slowly. Benzodiazepine withdrawal may occur if abruptly discontinued in patients receiving prolonged IV continuous infusions; doses should be tapered slowly with prolonged use. Contraindicated if preexisting CNS depression.

MILRINONE (PRIMACOR)

INDICATIONS AND USE: Short-term (<72 hours) treatment of acute low cardiac output due to septic shock or following cardiac surgery.

ACTIONS AND SPECTRUM: Inhibits phosphodiesterase III (PDE III), which increases adenosine 3′5′-cyclic monophosphate (cAMP) and potentiates the delivery of calcium to myocardial contractile systems; results in a positive inotropic effect. Inhibition of PDE III in vascular tissue results in relaxation of vascular muscle and vasodilatation. Unlike catecholamines, milrinone does not increase myocardial oxygen consumption.

DOSAGE: IV, intraosseous.

NEONATES, INFANTS, AND CHILDREN: A limited number of studies have used different dosing schemes. Further pharmacodynamic studies are needed to define pediatric milrinone guidelines. Several centers use the following guidelines:
- **Loading dose:** 50 mcg/kg over 15 minutes followed by a continuous infusion of 0.5 mcg/kg/minute; range: 0.25–0.75 mcg/kg/minute; titrate to effect.
- **IV, IO (PALS Guidelines, 2010):** Loading dose 50 mcg/kg over 10–60 minutes followed by a continuous infusion of 0.25–0.75 mcg/kg/minute; titrate dose to effect.

ADVERSE EFFECTS: Hypokalemia, thrombocytopenia, abnormal liver function tests, ventricular arrhythmias, and hypotension.

PHARMACOLOGY: Excreted in urine as unchanged drug (83%) and glucuronide metabolite (12%). With renal impairment, half-life is prolonged and clearance is decreased.

COMMENTS: Use with caution and modify dosage in patients with impaired renal function; adequate intravascular volume is necessary prior to initiating therapy.

MORPHINE SULFATE (VARIOUS)

INDICATIONS AND USE: Analgesia, preoperative sedation, supplement to anesthesia, treatment of opioid withdrawal, and relief of dyspnea associated with pulmonary edema.

ACTIONS: A pure opioid agonist, selective to the μ-receptor in the central nervous system (CNS). The interaction with these opioid receptors results in effects that mimic the actions of enkephalins, β-endorphin, and other exogenous ligands.

DOSAGE: **IM, IV, PO, subcutaneous.**

Neonates (use preservative-free form):

- **Initial:** 0.05 mg/kg IM, IV, subcutaneous every 4–8 hours; titrate carefully to effect; maximum dose 0.1 mg/kg/dose.
- **Continuous infusion:** Initial: 0.01 mg/kg/hour (10 mcg/kg/hour); do not exceed infusion rates of 0.015–0.02 mg/kg/hour due to decreased elimination, increased CNS sensitivity, and adverse effects; may need to use slightly higher doses, especially in neonates who develop tolerance.
- **International evidence-based group for neonatal pain recommendations (Anand et al, 2001):**
  - **Intermittent dose:** 0.05–0.1 mg/kg/dose.
  - **Continuous infusion:** Range: 0.01–0.03 mg/kg/hour.
- **Neonatal narcotic abstinence:** 0.03–0.1 mg/kg/dose PO every 3–4 hours. Taper dose by 10–20% every 2–3 days based on abstinence scoring.

Infants and children:

- **Oral:** 0.2–0.5 mg/kg/dose every 4–6 hours as needed.

ADVERSE EFFECTS: Dose-dependent side effects include miosis, respiratory depression, drowsiness, bradycardia, and hypotension. Constipation, sedation, gastrointestinal upset, urinary retention, histamine release, and sweating may occur. Causes physiologic dependence; taper the dose gradually after long-term use to avoid withdrawal.

PHARMACOLOGY: Metabolized in the liver via glucuronide conjugation to morphine-6-glucuronide (active) and morphine-3-glucuronide (inactive). Morphine is 20–40% bioavailable when administered orally. Metabolites are renally excreted.

COMMENTS: When changing routes of administration in chronically treated patients, oral doses are ~3–5 times the parenteral dose.

MUPIROCIN (BACTROBAN)

INDICATIONS AND USE: Topical treatment of impetigo resulting from *Staphylococcus aureus* (including methicillin-resistant strains), β-hemolytic *Streptococcus*, and *Streptococcus pyogenes*. Used for minor bacterial skin infections resulting from susceptible organisms and eradication of *S. aureus* from nasal and perineal carriage sites.

ACTIONS: Inhibits protein and RNA synthesis by binding to bacterial isoleucyl-tRNA synthetase.

DOSAGE: **Intranasal, topical.**

Intranasal:

- Apply sparingly 2–3 times a day for 5–14 days. Reevaluate in 5 days if no response.

Topical:

- **Cream:** Apply small amount 3 times a day for 10 days.
- **Ointment:** Apply a small amount 3–5 times a day for 5–14 days.

ADVERSE EFFECTS: Burning, rash, erythema, and pruritus.

COMMENTS: Use with caution in burn patients and patients with impaired renal function. Avoid contact with eyes; not for ophthalmic use. When applied to extensive open wounds or burns, the possibility of absorption of the polyethylene glycol vehicle, resulting in serious renal toxicity, should be considered.

NAFCILLIN SODIUM (UNIPEN)

ACTION AND SPECTRUM: Semisynthetic penicillinase-resistant penicillin with bactericidal activity against susceptible bacteria; treatment of bacterial infections such as osteomyelitis, septicemia, endocarditis, and central nervous system (CNS) infections due to susceptible penicillinase-producing strains of *Staphylococcus*.

DOSAGE: **IM, IV.** Consider higher doses when treating CNS infections.

Neonates:

- **0–4 weeks and <1.2 kg:** 50 mg/kg/day IM/IV in divided doses every 12 hours.
- **<7 days:**
  - **1.2–2 kg:** 50 mg/kg/day IM/IV in divided doses every 12 hours.
  - **>2 kg:** 75 mg/kg/day IM/IV in divided doses every 8 hours.
- **≥7 days:**
  - **1.2–2 kg:** 75 mg/kg/day IM/IV in divided doses every 8 hours.
  - **>2 kg:** 100–140 mg/kg/day IM/IV in divided doses every 6 hours.

Children:

- **Mild to moderate infections:** 50–100 mg/kg/day IM/IV in divided doses every 6 hours; maximum dose 4 grams/day.
- **Severe infections:** 100–200 mg/kg/day IM/IV in divided doses every 4–6 hours; maximum dose 12 grams/day.

ADVERSE EFFECTS: Thrombophlebitis, hypersensitivity, granulocytopenia, and agranulocytosis. Severe tissue injury after IV extravasation.
PHARMACOLOGY: Hepatic metabolism; concentrated in bile. Has better CNS penetration than methicillin.
COMMENTS: Avoid IM use if possible.

NALOXONE HCL (NARCAN)

INDICATIONS AND USE: Narcotic antagonist that reverses central nervous system (CNS) and respiratory depression in suspected narcotic overdose; neonatal opiate depression; adjunct in the treatment of septic shock.
ACTIONS: An opiate antagonist that competes with and displaces narcotics at narcotic receptor sites. It has little to no agonistic activity.
DOSAGE: IV. May be given IM if perfusion is adequate.
Opioid intoxication:
- **Usual dose:** 0.1 mg/kg IV and may repeat in 3–5 minutes, or
- **Alternative dosing to reverse opioid-induced depression:** 0.01–0.03 mg/kg and repeat every 2–3 minutes PRN.

ADVERSE EFFECTS: Hypertension, hypotension, tachycardia, and ventricular arrhythmias.
PHARMACOLOGY: Onset of action is within 1–2 minutes after IV injection and 2–5 minutes after IM injection. Duration of action is generally 20–60 minutes.
COMMENTS: Avoid use in infants of narcotic-addicted mothers and infants with physical dependence to opiates (may precipitate acute withdrawal syndrome). Infants must be monitored for reappearance of respiratory depression and the need for repeated doses. Naloxone is not recommended as part of initial resuscitation in the delivery room for newborns with respiratory depression.

NEOMYCIN SULFATE

ACTION AND SPECTRUM: Aminoglycoside indicated in the treatment of diarrhea resulting from enteropathogenic *Escherichia coli* and as preoperative prophylaxis before intestinal surgery; an adjunct therapy in hepatic encephalopathy. Neomycin is inactive against anaerobic organisms.
DOSAGE: PO.
- 50–100 mg/kg/day PO divided every 6–8 hours.

ADVERSE EFFECTS: Diarrhea, colitis, and malabsorption; nephrotoxicity and ototoxicity.
PHARMACOLOGY: Renal excretion if systemic absorption occurs; otherwise, eliminated unchanged in feces. Poorly absorbed from the gastrointestinal tract.

NEOSTIGMINE METHYLSULFATE (PROSTIGMIN)

INDICATIONS AND USE: Improvement of muscle strength in the treatment of myasthenia gravis; may be used to reverse nondepolarizing neuromuscular-blocking agents.
ACTIONS: Neostigmine competitively inhibits hydrolysis of acetylcholine by acetylcholinesterase, facilitating transmission of impulses across the myoneural junction and producing cholinergic activity.
DOSAGE: IV, IM, subcutaneous.
Myasthenia gravis:
- **Diagnostic testing:** 0.025–0.04 mg/kg/dose IM once. (Discontinue all cholinesterase medications at least 8 hours before; atropine should be administered IV immediately prior to or IM 30 minutes before neostigmine.)
- **Treatment:** 0.01–0.04 mg/kg/dose IM, IV, or subcutaneous every 2–4 hours as needed or 1 mg PO given 2 hours prior to feeding.

Reversal of nondepolarizing neuromuscular blockade:
- 0.025–0.1 mg/kg/dose. (Use with atropine: 0.01–0.04 mg/kg, or 0.4 mg of atropine for each 1 mg of neostigmine.)

ADVERSE EFFECTS: Cholinergic crisis, which may include bronchospasm, increased bronchial secretions and salivation, vomiting, diarrhea, bradycardia, respiratory depression, and seizures.
COMMENTS: Does not antagonize and may prolong the phase I block of depolarizing muscle relaxants.

NETILMICIN SULFATE (NETROMYCIN)

ACTION AND SPECTRUM: Aminoglycoside used for the treatment of infections caused by aerobic gram-negative bacilli such as *Pseudomonas*, *Klebsiella*, and *Escherichia coli*. Usually used in combination with a β-lactam antibiotic.
DOSAGE: IV, IM. Monitor and adjust by pharmacokinetics. Initial empiric dosing is based on body weight.
Neonates, premature, and normal gestational age (0–1 week of age):
- 3 mg/kg IV or IM every 12 hours.

Neonates over 1 week of age and infants:
- 2.5–3 mg/kg IV or IM every 8 hours.

Children:
- 2–2.5 mg/kg IV or IM every 8 hours.

ADVERSE EFFECTS: Transient, reversible renal tubular dysfunction that may result in increased urinary losses of sodium, calcium, and magnesium. Vestibular and auditory ototoxicity with serum peak concentrations >12 mcg/mL; nephrotoxicity with serum trough >4 mcg/mL. The addition of other nephrotoxic and/or ototoxic medications may increase these adverse effects.

PHARMACOLOGY: Renal excretion. Half-life is 4–8 hours.

COMMENTS: Therapeutic range is 5–12 mcg/mL (sample 30 minutes after the infusion is completed); trough concentrations are 0.5–2 mcg/mL (sample 30 minutes to just before the next dose). Obtain an initial set of serum peak and trough levels at about the fourth maintenance dose. Monitor serum creatinine every 3–4 days. Limited experience in neonates.

NEVIRAPINE

> **WARNING:** Reports of fatal hepatotoxicity even after short-term use; severe life-threatening skin reactions (Stevens-Johnson, toxic epidermal necrolysis, and allergic reactions); monitor closely during first 8 weeks of treatment.

ACTION AND SPECTRUM: Nonnucleoside antiretroviral agent that inhibits HIV-1 replication by selectively interfering with viral reverse transcriptase. Acts synergistically with zidovudine. Used for the prevention of maternal-fetal human immunodeficiency virus (HIV) transmission and HIV treatment.

DOSAGE: PO (based on aidsinfo.nih.gov/guidelines, 2012).

Prevention of maternal-fetal HIV transmission:
- Three doses given in the first week of life as follows: First dose within 48 hours of birth, second dose 48 hours after first dose, and third dose 96 hours after second dose. Give in combination with **zidovudine**. Used in select situations such as infants born to HIV-infected mothers with no antiretroviral therapy prior to labor or during labor; infants born to mothers with only intrapartum therapy; infants born to mothers with suboptimal viral suppression at delivery or infants born to mothers with known antiretroviral drug–resistant virus.
- **Birthweight 1.5–2 kg:** 8 mg/dose PO.
- **Birthweight >2 kg:** 12 mg/dose PO.

Treatment of HIV infection (in combination with other antiretroviral agents):
- **Neonates ≥15 days, infants, and children:**
  - **Initial dose:** 200 mg/m^2/dose once daily for the first 14 days of treatment; increase to 200 mg/m^2/dose every 12 hours if no rash or adverse effects. Maximum dose is 200 mg every 12 hours.

ADVERSE EFFECTS: Limited data in neonates; rash, elevated liver enzymes, hepatotoxicity, liver failure, cholestatic hepatitis, hepatic necrosis, jaundice.

PHARMACOLOGY: Metabolized by cytochrome P450 isoenzymes 3A4 and 2B6 and has potential for drug interactions; more rapidly metabolized in pediatric patients.

COMMENTS: Please note manufacturers' black box warning regarding severe life-threatening and fatal skin reactions and hepatotoxicity.

NICARDIPINE

INDICATIONS AND USE: Short-term treatment of severe hypertension.

ACTIONS: Inhibits calcium ions from entering select voltage-sensitive channels in vascular smooth muscle and myocardium during depolarization; produces relaxation of coronary vascular smooth muscle and coronary vasodilatation.

DOSAGE: IV.

Neonates:
- **Initial dose:** 0.5 mcg/kg/minute by continuous infusion. Titrate to desired response; blood pressure will decrease within minutes of starting infusion. Maintenance doses 0.5–2 mcg/kg/minute.

Infants and children:
- **Initial dose:** 0.5–1 mcg/kg/minute by continuous infusion. Titrate increasing rate of infusion every 15–30 minutes to a maximum dose of 4–5 mcg/kg/minute.

ADVERSE EFFECTS: Hypotension, tachycardia, peripheral edema, hypokalemia.

PHARMACOLOGY: Extensively metabolized by the liver and is highly protein bound. Experience in neonates is very limited, and there is no pharmacokinetic data.

COMMENTS: Use with caution in the presence of cardiac, renal, and hepatic disease.

NITRIC OXIDE (INOMAX FOR INHALATION; INHALED NITRIC OXIDE [iNO])

INDICATIONS AND USE: iNO is indicated for the treatment of term and near-term (≥34 weeks) neonates with hypoxic respiratory failure associated with clinical or echocardiographic evidence of persistent pulmonary hypertension of the newborn (PPHN).

ACTIONS: iNO is a selective pulmonary vasodilator without significant effects on the systemic circulation that decreases extrapulmonary right-to-left shunting. Nitric oxide relaxes vascular smooth muscle by binding to the heme moiety of cytosolic guanylate cyclase, activating guanylate cyclase, and increasing intracellular levels of cyclic guanosine $3'5'$-monophosphate, which leads to vasodilation and an increase in the partial pressure of arterial oxygen.

DOSAGE: Inhalation.

Term infants or >34 weeks' gestation:

- **Begin at 20 ppm.** Reduce dose to lowest possible level. Doses >20 ppm are usually not used due to increased risk of methemoglobinemia and elevated NO_2. Maintain treatment up to 14 days or until the underlying oxygen desaturation has resolved and the infant is ready to be weaned from iNO. Abrupt discontinuation may lead to worsening hypotension, oxygenation, and increasing pulmonary artery pressure (PAP). Further diagnostic testing should be sought for infants who are unable to be weaned off iNO after 4 days of therapy.

ADVERSE EFFECTS: Do not use in neonates dependent on right-to-left shunting of blood. Direct pulmonary injury from excess levels of NO_2 and ambient air contamination may occur. May cause methemoglobinemia and elevated NO_2. Risk of adverse effects increases when iNO is given at doses >20 ppm. Conflicting data have been published on whether or not iNO inhibits platelet aggregation and prolongs bleeding time. Monitor methemoglobin levels, iNO, NO_2, and O_2 levels. iNO therapy should be directed by physicians qualified by education and experience in its use and offered only at centers that are qualified to provide multisystem support, generally including on-site extracorporeal membrane oxygenation/extracorporeal life support (ECMO/ECLS) capability or with a collaborating ECMO/ECLS center. Consult the manufacturer's product literature and specialized references for complete information on the use of iNO.

NITROPRUSSIDE SODIUM (NIPRIDE, NITROPRESS)

> **WARNING:** Nitroprusside is not suitable for direct injection and must be further diluted in sterile 5% dextrose in water (D5W) before infusion. Nitroprusside can cause precipitous decreases in blood pressure. In patients not properly monitored, these decreases can lead to irreversible ischemic injuries or death. Nitroprusside can give rise to cyanide ion, which can reach toxic, potentially lethal levels. If blood pressure has not been adequately controlled after 10 minutes of infusion at the maximum rate, stop the infusion. Review package insert before administration.

INDICATIONS AND USE: Severe hypertension and hypertension crisis; acute reduction of afterload in patients with refractory congestive heart failure.

ACTIONS: Direct-acting vasodilator (arterial and venous) that reduces peripheral vascular resistance (afterload). Venous return is reduced (preload); increases cardiac output by decreasing afterload.

DOSAGE: IV. Infuse through a large vein.

- **Initial:** 0.25–0.5 mcg/kg/minute; titrate dose every 20 minutes to the desired response.
- **Usual dose:** 3 mcg/kg/minute; rarely need >4 mcg/kg/minute; maximum dose 8–10 mcg/kg/minute.

ADVERSE EFFECTS: Generally related to a very rapid reduction in blood pressure. Thiocyanate may accumulate, especially in patients receiving high doses or those who have impaired renal function. Cyanide toxicity can develop abruptly if large doses are administered rapidly. Cyanide causes early persistent acidosis. Thiocyanate toxicity appears at plasma levels of ~35–100 mcg/mL; levels >200 mcg/mL are associated with death. Thiocyanate levels should be monitored in any patient receiving 3 mcg/kg/minute or more of nitroprusside or prolonged infusion (>3 days), especially those with renal impairment. Toxicity is treated with IV sodium thiosulfate.

PHARMACOLOGY: Acts within seconds to lower blood pressure; when discontinued, the effect dissipates within minutes. Rapidly metabolized to thiocyanate, which is eliminated by the kidneys.

COMMENTS: Contraindicated with decreased cerebral perfusion, hypertension secondary to arteriovenous shunts, or coarctation of the aorta. May add sodium thiosulfate to infusion solution at a 10:1 ratio to minimize thiocyanate toxicity; however, this has not been studied. Protect from light.

NOREPINEPHRINE BITARTRATE (LEVARTERENOL BITARTRATE) (LEVOPHED)

> **WARNING:** Antidote for extravasation ischemia. To prevent sloughing and necrosis, the area should be infiltrated as soon as possible with saline solution containing phentolamine, an adrenergic blocking agent (see Comments).

INDICATIONS AND USE: Treatment of shock, which persists after adequate fluid volume replacement; severe hypotension; cardiogenic shock.

ACTIONS: Stimulates β_1-adrenergic receptors and α-adrenergic receptors causing increased contractility and heart rate as well as vasoconstriction, resulting in an increase in systemic blood pressure and coronary blood flow; clinically, α-adrenergic effects (vasoconstriction) are greater than β_1-adrenergic effects (inotropic and chronotropic effects).

DOSAGE: IV.

- 0.02–0.1 mcg/kg/minute initially, titrated to desired perfusion; maximum dose 2 mcg/kg/minute.

ADVERSE EFFECTS: Respiratory distress, arrhythmias, bradycardia or tachycardia, hypertension, chest pain, headache, and vomiting. Organ ischemia (due to vasoconstriction of renal and mesenteric arteries).

COMMENTS: Ischemic necrosis may occur after extravasation. Administer phentolamine, 0.1–0.2 mg/kg subcutaneous, infiltrated into the area of extravasation within 12 hours to minimize damage. (See Chapter 31.)

NYSTATIN (MYCOSTATIN, NILSTAT)

ACTION AND SPECTRUM: May be fungistatic or fungicidal, which acts by disrupting fungal cell membranes. Treatment of susceptible cutaneous, mucocutaneous, and oral cavity fungal infections normally caused by the *Candida* species.

DOSAGE: PO, topical.

Oral thrush:

- **Therapeutic:** Continue for 3 days after symptoms have resolved.
    - **Neonates:** 0.5–1 mL to each side of the mouth 4 times a day after feedings.
    - **Infants:** 1–2 mL to each side of mouth 4 times a day after feedings.
- **Prophylaxis:** 1 mL divided to each side of mouth or 1 mL orally or via oral gavage tube 3–4 times a day.

Diaper rash:

- Topical cream/ointment/powder applied 3–4 times a day for 7–10 days.

ADVERSE EFFECTS: Side effects are uncommon but may cause diarrhea, local irritation, contact dermatitis, rash, pruritus, and Stevens-Johnson syndrome.

PHARMACOLOGY: Poorly absorbed orally. Most is passed unchanged in the stool.

OCTREOTIDE (SANDOSTATIN)

INDICATIONS AND USE: Short-term management of persistent hyperinsulinemic hypoglycemia of the newborn. Useful in the management of chylothorax. Chyle accumulation usually decreases after 24 hours of continuous infusion. Has also been used to treat hypersecretory diarrhea and fistulas in infants. Significant reductions in stool or ileal output were achieved with this drug.

ACTIONS: A synthetic polypeptide that mimics natural somatostatin by inhibiting serotonin release, and the secretion of gastrin, vasoactive intestinal peptide (VIP), insulin, glucagon, secretin, motilin, thyrotropin, cholecystokinin; reduces splanchnic blood flow, decreases gastrointestinal motility, and inhibits intestinal secretion of water and electrolytes.

DOSAGE: IV, subcutaneous.

Persistent hyperinsulinemic hypoglycemia of infancy:

- **Initial dose:** 2–10 mcg/kg/day divided every 6–12 hours; up to 40 mcg/kg/day divided every 6–8 hours. Adjust to maintain symptomatic control.

Diarrhea:

- 1–10 mcg/kg/dose IV/subcutaneous given every 12 hours. Adjust the dose to maintain symptomatic control.

Chylothorax:

- 0.5–4 mcg/kg/hour IV continuous infusion; titrate dose to response; case reports of effective dosage ranging between 0.3 and 10 mcg/kg/hour; treatment duration is usually 1–3 weeks but may vary with clinical response.

ADVERSE EFFECTS: Possible growth retardation during long-term treatment, flushing, hypertension, insomnia, fever, chills, seizures, Bell's palsy, hair loss, bruising, rash, hypoglycemia, hyperglycemia, galactorrhea, hypothyroidism, diarrhea, abdominal distention, vomiting, constipation, hepatitis, jaundice, local injection site pain, thrombophlebitis, muscle weakness, increased creatine kinase, muscle spasm, tremor, oliguria, shortness of breath, and rhinorrhea.

PHARMACOLOGY: Duration of action (subcutaneous) is 6–12 hours with immediate-release formulation; excreted unchanged in the urine.

COMMENTS: Tachyphylaxis may occur.

OMEPRAZOLE (PRILOSEC)

INDICATIONS AND USE: Short-term (<8 weeks) treatment of reflux esophagitis, duodenal ulcer refractory to conventional therapy.

ACTIONS: Inhibits gastric acid secretion by inactivating the parietal cell membrane enzyme (H^+/K^+)-adenosine triphosphatase (ATPase) or proton pump.

DOSAGE: PO.

• **Neonates:** 0.5–1.5 mg/kg once daily in the morning.
• **1 month to 2 years:** 0.7 mg/kg once daily; increase to 3 mg/kg once daily if necessary (maximum dose 20 mg).

ADVERSE EFFECTS: Mild elevation of liver enzymes, diarrhea.

PHARMACOLOGY: Cytochrome P450 isoenzyme CYP1A2 inducer; isoenzyme CYP2C8, CYP2C18, CYP2C19, and CYP3A3/4 substrate; isoenzyme CYP2C9, CYP3A3/4, CYP2C8, and CYP2C19 inhibitor. Maximum secretory inhibition is 4 days. Extensive first-pass metabolism in the liver. Bioavailability: 30–40%; improves slightly with repeated administration.

ADVERSE EFFECTS: Mild elevation of liver enzymes, diarrhea.

COMMENTS: Lack of data regarding the safety of long-term use in children.

OPIUM TINCTURE

HIGH ALERT MEDICATION: May also be confused with camphorated tincture of opium (Paregoric). Opium tincture is 25 times as potent as paregoric. Avoid the use of the abbreviation "DTO."

INDICATIONS AND USE: A 25-fold dilution with water (final concentration 0.4 mg/mL) can be used to treat neonatal abstinence syndrome (opiate withdrawal).

ACTIONS: Contains many narcotic alkaloids including morphine; inhibition of gastrointestinal (GI) motility due to morphine content; decreases digestive secretions; increases GI muscle tone.

DOSAGE: PO.

Neonates (full-term):

• **Neonatal abstinence syndrome (opiate withdrawal):** Use a 25-fold dilution with water of opium tincture (final concentration 0.4 mg/mL morphine).
    • **Initial dose:** Give 0.04 mg/kg/dose of a 0.4 mg/mL solution with feedings every 3–4 hours; increase as needed by 0.04 mg/kg/dose of a 0.4 mg/mL solution every 3–4 hours until withdrawal symptoms are controlled.
    • **Usual dose:** 0.08–0.2 mg/dose of a 0.4 mg/mL solution given every 3–4 hours; it is rare to exceed 0.28 mg/dose of a 0.4 mg/mL solution; stabilize withdrawal symptoms for 3–5 days, then gradually decrease the dosage (keeping the same dosage interval) over a 2- to 4-week period.

ADVERSE EFFECTS: Hypotension, bradycardia, peripheral vasodilation, central nervous system (CNS) depression, drowsiness, sedation, urinary retention, constipation, respiratory depression, and histamine release.

PHARMACOLOGY: Metabolized in liver and eliminated in urine and bile.

COMMENTS: Observe for excessive sedation and respiratory depression. Do not abruptly discontinue. Monitor for the resolution of withdrawal symptoms (such as irritability, high-pitched cry, stuffy nose, rhinorrhea, vomiting, poor feeding, diarrhea, sneezing, yawning, etc.), and signs of overtreatment (such as bradycardia, lethargy, hypotonia, irregular respirations, respiratory depression, etc.). An abstinence scoring system (eg, Finnegan abstinence scoring system) should be used to more objectively assess neonatal opiate withdrawal symptoms and the need for dosage adjustment (see Chapter 103). Use 25-fold dilution with water for the treatment of neonatal abstinence syndrome.

OXACILLIN SODIUM (BACTOCILL, PROSTAPHLIN)

ACTION AND SPECTRUM: Semisynthetic penicillinase-resistant penicillin; bactericidal activity used for the treatment of bacterial infections such as osteomyelitis, septicemia, endocarditis, and central nervous system (CNS) infections due to susceptible penicillinase-producing strains of *Staphylococcus*.

DOSAGE: IM, IV.

Neonates:

• **<1.2 kg and ≤4 weeks old:** 50 mg/kg/day IM/IV divided every 12 hours.
• **1.2–2 kg and <7 days old:** 50–100 mg/kg/day IM/IV divided every 12 hours.
• **1.2–2 kg and ≥7 days old:** 75–150 mg/kg/day IM/IV divided every 8 hours.
• **>2 kg and <7 days old:** 75–150 mg/kg/day divided IM/IV every 8 hours.
• **>2 kg and ≥7 days old:** 100–200 mg/kg/day divided IM/IV every 6 hours.

Infants and children:

• **Mild to moderate infections:** 100–150 mg/kg/day IM/IV in divided doses every 6 hours; maximum 4 grams/day.
• **Severe infections:** 150–200 mg/kg/day IM/IV in divided doses every 4–6 hours; maximum 12 grams/day.

ADVERSE EFFECTS: Hypersensitivity reactions (rash), thrombophlebitis, mild leukopenia, acute interstitial nephritis, hematuria, azotemia, and elevation in aspartate transaminase (AST). *Clostridium difficile* colitis has been reported.

PHARMACOLOGY: Metabolized chiefly in the liver and excreted in bile; dosage modification required in patients with renal impairment.

COMMENTS: Avoid IM injection.

PALIVIZUMAB (SYNAGIS)

INDICATIONS AND USE: Immunoprophylaxis against severe respiratory syncytial virus (RSV) lower respiratory tract infections in high-risk infants and children:

The American Academy of Pediatrics recommends RSV prophylaxis with palivizumab during RSV season for:

- Infants <3 months of age who were born between gestational age 32 weeks 0 days and 34 weeks 6 days and have one of the following:
  - Daycare attendance.
  - ≥1 sibling who is <5 years of age living in the same household.
- Infants <6 months of age who were born between gestational age 29 weeks and ≤31 weeks 6 days.
- Infants <12 months of age who were born gestational age ≤28 weeks.
- Infants <12 months of age with congenital airway abnormality or neuromuscular disorder that decreases the ability to manage airway secretions.
- Infants and children <24 months of age with chronic lung disease (CLD) necessitating medical therapy within 6 months of age prior to the beginning of RSV season.
- Infants and children <24 months with congenital heart disease and one of the following:
  - Receiving medication to treat congestive heart failure.
  - Moderate to severe pulmonary hypertension.
  - Cyanotic heart disease.

ACTION: Humanized monoclonal antibody directed to an epitope in the A-antigenic site of the respiratory syncytial virus F protein, resulting in neutralizing and fusion-inhibitory activity against RSV.

DOSAGE: IM.

- 15 mg/kg/dose IM once a month during the RSV season. The first dose should be administered before the start of the RSV season.

ADVERSE EFFECTS: Upper respiratory tract infection, otitis media, fever, and rhinitis. Rash, injection site reaction, erythema, induration. Rare cases of anaphylaxis (<1 case/100,000 patients) and severe hypersensitivity reactions (<1 case/1000 patients) have been reported.

PHARMACOLOGY: The mean half-life of palivizumab is ~20 days and adequate antibody titers are maintained for 30 days. Time to achieve adequate serum antibody titers is 48 hours.

COMMENTS: Palivizumab is not indicated for the treatment of RSV infections. Palivizumab does not interfere with the response to routine childhood vaccines and therefore may be administered concurrently.

PANCURONIUM BROMIDE (PAVULON)

INDICATIONS AND USE: Skeletal muscle relaxation during surgery; increases pulmonary compliance during assisted mechanical ventilation, and facilitates endotracheal intubation.

ACTIONS: Nondepolarizing neuromuscular-blocking agent that produces skeletal muscle paralysis by blocking acetylcholine binding at the receptor at the myoneural junction. Pancuronium may cause an increase in heart rate and changes in blood pressure.

DOSAGE: IV.

Neonates and infants:

- 0.05–0.1 mg/kg IV every 30–60 minutes as needed; maintenance 0.04–0.15 mg/kg IV every 1–4 hours as needed to maintain paralysis, or as continuous IV infusion 0.02–0.04 mg/kg/hour or 0.4–0.6 mcg/kg/minute.

ADVERSE EFFECTS: Tachycardia, hypertension, hypotension, excessive salivation, and bronchospasm may occur. Potentiation of neuromuscular blockade may result from aminoglycosides, electrolyte abnormalities, severe hyponatremia, severe hypocalcemia, severe hypokalemia, hypermagnesemia, neuromuscular diseases, acidosis, renal failure, and hepatic failure. Antagonism of neuromuscular blockade may result from alkalosis, hypercalcemia, hyperkalemia, and epinephrine.

PHARMACOLOGY: The onset of action is generally 1–2 minutes, with duration of action of ~40–60 minutes, but is variable and may be prolonged in neonates.

COMMENTS: Neonates are particularly sensitive to its actions; prolonged paralysis may be noted. Ventilation must be supported during neuromuscular blockade. Neostigmine and atropine are used for reversal. Sensation remains intact; analgesia should be used with painful procedures.

PAPAVERINE HCL

INDICATIONS AND USE: Reduce peripheral arterial spasms in efforts to prolong arterial catheter patency.

ACTIONS: Directly relaxes vascular smooth muscle and results in vasodilation.

DOSAGE: IV.

Peripheral arterial catheter patency in full-term neonates:

- Add 30 mg preservative-free papaverine to 250 mL of arterial catheter solution that contains heparin 1 unit/mL; infuse at a rate of ≤1 mL/hour. Not recommended for use in preterm neonates <3 weeks of age due to potential risk of developing or extending an intracranial hemorrhage.

COMMENTS: IV infusion should be performed under a physician's supervision because arrhythmias and fatal apnea may result from rapid injection. *Note:* Not U.S. Food and Drug Administration (FDA) approved for use in children. Limited experience in neonates.

PENICILLIN G (AQUEOUS), PARENTERAL

ACTION AND SPECTRUM: Treatment of infection due to gram-positive cocci (except *Staphylococcus aureus*), including all susceptible strains of streptococci (non-enterococcal). However, penicillin G–resistant *Streptococcus pneumoniae* strains have been isolated. Gram-positive bacilli are usually sensitive to penicillin G (*Clostridium tetani, Corynebacterium diphtheriae*). Penicillin G is effective for some gram-negative organisms including *Neisseria meningitides, Haemophilus influenzae,* and *Neisseria gonorrhoeae.* The Enterobacteriaceae are resistant to penicillin G therapy, and resistance of many gram-negative organisms such as *Escherichia coli* is a result of the ability to produce β-lactamase. Used for the treatment of congenital syphilis.

DOSAGE: IM, IV.

Neonates postnatal age <7 days:

- ≤2 kg: 50,000 units/kg/day IM/IV in divided doses every 12 hours. Meningitis: 100,000 units/kg/day IM/IV in divided doses every 12 hours.
- >2 kg: 75,000 units/kg/day IM/IV in divided doses every 8 hours. Meningitis: 150,000 units/kg/day IM/IV in divided doses every 8 hours.
- **Congenital syphilis:** 100,000 units/kg/day IM/IV in divided doses every 12 hours.
- **Group B streptococcal meningitis:** 250,000–450,000 units/kg/day IM/IV in divided doses every 8 hours.

Neonates postnatal age ≥7 days:

- <1.2 kg: 50,000 units/kg/day IM/IV in divided doses every 12 hours. Meningitis: 100,000 units/kg/day IM/IV in divided doses every 12 hours.
- 1.2–2 kg: 75,000 units/kg/day IM/IV in divided doses every 8 hours. Meningitis: 150,000 units/kg/day IM/IV in divided doses every 8 hours.
- >2 kg: 100,000 units/kg/day IM/IV in divided doses every 6 hours. Meningitis: 200,000 units/kg/day IM/IV in divided doses every 6 hours.
- **Congenital syphilis:** 150,000 units/kg/day IM/IV in divided doses every 8 hours.
- **Group B streptococcal meningitis:** IV: 450,000 units/kg/day IV in divided doses every 6 hours.

Infants and children:

- **Usual dose:** 100,000–250,000 units/kg/day IM/IV in divided doses every 4–6 hours.
- **Severe infections:** 250,000–400,000 units/kg/day IM/IV in divided doses every 4–6 hours; maximum dose 24 million units/day.

ADVERSE EFFECTS: Allergic reactions, rash, fever, alterations in bowel flora, *Candida* superinfection, diarrhea, and hemolytic anemia. Acute interstitial nephritis. Bone marrow suppression with granulocytopenia. Very large doses may cause seizures. Rapid IV push of potassium penicillin G may cause cardiac arrhythmias and arrest because of the potassium component. Infuse slowly over 30 minutes.

PHARMACOKINETICS: Penetration across the blood-brain barrier is poor with normal meninges; excreted in urine mainly by tubular secretion.

COMMENTS: Good activity against anaerobes. Drug of choice for tetanus neonatorum.

PENICILLIN G BENZATHINE (BICILLIN L-A)

ACTION AND SPECTRUM: See Penicillin G (Aqueous), Parenteral. Treatment of asymptomatic congenital syphilis.

DOSAGE: IM.

- **Asymptomatic congenital syphilis:** Single dose of 50,000 units/kg IM.

ADVERSE EFFECTS: See Penicillin G (Aqueous).

PHARMACOLOGY: Renally excreted over a prolonged interval owing to slow absorption from the injection site.

COMMENTS: See Penicillin G (Aqueous). Not often used. For IM injection only.

PENICILLIN G PROCAINE (WYCILLIN)

ACTION AND SPECTRUM: See Penicillin G (Aqueous), Parenteral. Treatment of symptomatic or asymptomatic congenital syphilis.

DOSAGE: IM.

- 50,000 units/kg/dose IM every 24 hours for 10 days; if more than 1 day of therapy is missed, the entire course should be restarted.

ADVERSE EFFECTS: See Penicillin G (Aqueous), Parenteral. May also cause sterile abscess formation at the injection site. Contains 120 mg of procaine per 300,000 units, which may cause allergic reactions, myocardial depression, or systemic vasodilation. There is cause for much greater concern about these effects in the neonate than in older patients, and therefore it is not recommended for use in neonates.

COMMENTS: Not often used.

PENTOBARBITAL SODIUM (NEMBUTAL)

INDICATIONS AND USE: Sedative/hypnotic. Used for agitation, for preprocedure sedation, or as an anticonvulsant.
ACTIONS: Short-acting barbiturate.
DOSAGE: IV.
Procedural sedation:
- 1–2 mg/kg/dose IV slow push <50 mg/minute; additional doses of 1–2 mg/kg may be given every 3–5 minutes to desired effect. Total dose: 1–6 mg/kg.

Hypnotic:
- 2–6 mg/kg/dose IM. Maximum 100 mg/dose.

ADVERSE EFFECTS: Observe the IV site closely during administration for extravasation injury. Tolerance and physical dependence may occur with continued use. May cause somnolence, bradycardia, rash, pain on IM injection (solutions are highly alkaline), thrombophlebitis, osteomalacia from prolonged use (rare), and excitability.
COMMENTS: Rapid IV administration may cause respiratory depression, apnea, laryngospasm, bronchospasm, and hypotension; administer over 10–30 minutes.

PHENOBARBITAL

INDICATIONS AND USE: Treatment of neonatal seizures; used to treat neonatal abstinence symptoms; may also be used for prevention and treatment of neonatal hyperbilirubinemia and lowering of bilirubin in chronic cholestasis.
ACTIONS: Anticonvulsant activity by increasing the threshold for electrical stimulation of the motor cortex and depresses central nervous system (CNS) activity by binding to barbiturate site at γ-aminobutyric acid (GABA)-receptor complex enhancing GABA activity.
DOSAGE: PO, IV.
Anticonvulsant, status epilepticus:
- **Neonates and infants:**
  - **Loading dose:** 15–20 mg/kg IV in a single or divided dose. *Note:* In select patients, may give additional 5 mg/kg/dose every 15–30 minutes until seizure controlled or a total dose of 40 mg/kg; be prepared to provide respiratory support.
  - **Maintenance:** Begin 12–24 hours after loading dose:
    - **Neonates:** 3–4 mg/kg/day PO/IV given once daily; assess serum concentrations; increase to 5 mg/kg/day if needed.
    - **Infants:** 5–6 mg/kg/day in 1–2 divided doses.

Hyperbilirubinemia:
- 3–8 mg/kg/day PO in 2–3 divided doses up to 12 mg/kg/day have been used; dose not clearly established.

Neonatal abstinence syndrome:
- 2–8 mg/kg/day in 1–4 divided doses. Monitor serum concentrations coincident to abstinence scores. Loading dose is optional: 16 mg/kg IV as a single dose or PO in divided into 2 doses.

ADVERSE EFFECTS: Sedation, lethargy, paradoxic excitement, hypotension, gastrointestinal distress, ataxia, rash, and phlebitis (pH of IV solution is 10). Drug accumulation may occur if treating concurrently with phenytoin. Monitor drug levels. Respiratory depression can occur at levels exceeding 60 mcg/mL or with rapid IV administration.
PHARMACOLOGY: Initial half-life in neonates is 40–200 hours or longer, gradually declining to about 20–100 hours at 3–4 weeks of age. Reduction in serum bilirubin levels is attributed to increased levels of glucuronyl transferase; stimulates bile flow and increases the concentration of the Y-binding protein involved in the uptake of bilirubin by hepatocytes. Observed reductions usually require 2–3 days of treatment.
COMMENTS: Contraindicated if porphyria suspected. Maintenance serum levels usually fall between 15 and 40 mcg/mL. Abrupt withdrawal may precipitate status epilepticus.

PHENTOLAMINE (REGITINE)

INDICATIONS AND USE: Treatment of extravasation from IV α-adrenergic drugs (dobutamine, dopamine, epinephrine, norepinephrine, or phenylephrine). Helps prevent dermal necrosis and sloughing. (See also Chapter 31.)
ACTIONS: Phentolamine blocks α-adrenergic receptors and reverses the severe vasoconstriction from the extravasation of α-adrenergic drugs.
DOSAGE: Subcutaneous.
Neonate:
- Infiltrate area with small amount of solution (~1 mL) made by diluting 2.5–5 mg in 10 mL of preservative-free normal saline (NS); treat within 12 hours of extravasation. Do not exceed 0.1 mg/kg or 2.5 mg total.

Infants and children:
- Infiltrate area with small amount of solution (~1 mL) made by diluting 5–10 mg in 10 mL of preservative-free NS; treat within 12 hours of extravasation; do not exceed 0.1–0.2 mg/kg or 5 mg maximum.

ADVERSE EFFECTS: Hypotension, tachycardia, cardiac arrhythmias, and flushing.

PHENYLEPHRINE (OPHTHALMIC)

INDICATIONS AND USE: A mydriatic for ophthalmic procedures.
ACTIONS: α-Adrenergic stimulation and weak β-adrenergic activity. Causes pupils to contract by activation of dilator muscle of the pupil. Causes vasoconstriction of the arterioles of the nasal mucosa and conjunctiva; produces systemic arterial vasoconstriction.
DOSAGE: Ophthalmologic.
• **Infants <1 year:** Instill 1 drop of 2.5% solution 15–30 minutes before ophthalmic procedure.
• **Children:** Instill 1 drop of 2.5% or 10% solution 15–30 minutes before ophthalmic procedure, may repeat in 10–60 minutes as needed.
ADVERSE EFFECTS: Arrhythmias, hypertension, lacrimation, respiratory distress.
PHARMACOLOGY: Mydriasis within 15–30 minutes of instillation; duration of mydriasis is 1–2 hours.
COMMENTS: Apply pressure to the lacrimal sac during and for 2 minutes after instillation to minimize systemic absorption.

PHENYTOIN (DILANTIN)

INDICATIONS AND USE: Management of generalized convulsive status epilepticus; prevention and management of seizures.
ACTIONS: Stabilizes neuronal membranes and decreases seizure activity by increasing efflux or decreasing influx of sodium ions across cell membranes in the motor cortex during generation of nerve impulses.
DOSAGE: PO, IV. Phenytoin should be administered IV directly into a large vein through a large-gauge needle or IV catheter. IV injections should be followed by normal saline (NS) flushes through the same needle or IV catheter to avoid local irritation of the vein. Highly unstable in any IV solution. Avoid infusion through central line due to risk of precipitation. Avoid IM use due to erratic absorption, pain on injection, and precipitation of drug at injection site. pH: 10.0–12.3.
• **Loading dose:** 15–20 mg/kg IV at a rate not to exceed 0.5 mg/kg/minute.
• **Maintenance:** 12 hours after loading dose, 4–8 mg/kg/day PO/IV divided every 12 hours; some patients may require dosing every 8 hours.
ADVERSE EFFECTS: Local tissue damage if extravasation occurs. High serum levels can precipitate seizures. Other central nervous system (CNS) complications included drowsiness, lethargy, ataxia, and nystagmus. Cardiovascular affects can be arrhythmias, hypotension, or cardiovascular collapse with too rapid an infusion. Reactions also include hypersensitivity rash or Stevens-Johnson syndrome. Other complications include hepatic dysfunction, pancreatic dysfunction with hyperglycemia and hypoinsulinemia, and blood dyscrasias.
PHARMACOLOGY: Bilirubin displaces phenytoin from albumin-binding sites, thereby increasing unbound drug levels and complicating dosage to serum level interpretations. Neonates absorb phenytoin poorly from gastrointestinal tract; separate tube feedings and oral phenytoin by 2 hours.
COMMENTS: Therapeutic levels 10–20 mcg/mL; lower levels preferred for preterm infants. Multiple drug interactions include corticosteroids, carbamazepine, cimetidine, digoxin, furosemide, phenobarbital, and heparin (especially in central lines causing precipitation).

PHOSPHATE

INDICATIONS AND USE: Treatment of hypophosphatemia, provision of maintenance phosphorus in parenteral nutrition (PN) solutions, and treatment of nutritional rickets of prematurity.
ACTIONS: Phosphorus is an intracellular ion required for formation of energy-transfer enzymes such as adenosine diphosphate (ADP) and adenosine triphosphate (ATP). Phosphorus is also needed for bone metabolism and mineralization.
DOSAGE: IV, PO.
Treatment of hypophosphatemia:
• 0.15–0.33 mmol/kg/dose IV over 6 hours, with repeat doses to maintain serum phosphorus >2 mg/dL. Potassium or sodium phosphate should be diluted in IV fluids and infused at a rate not >0.2 mmol/kg/hour.
• **Maintenance:** IV dose is 0.5–1.5 mmol/kg/24 hours; oral maintenance is 2–3 mmol/kg/24 hours.
Maintenance in hyperalimentation:
• 0.5–2 mmol/kg/day. May use parenteral solution for oral dose; give in divided doses and dilute in feedings.
ADVERSE EFFECTS: Hyperphosphatemia, hypocalcemia, and hypotension. Gastrointestinal discomfort may occur with oral administration. Rapid IV bolus of potassium phosphates can cause cardiac arrhythmias.
COMMENTS: Supplied as injection, sodium phosphates: 3 mmol of elemental phosphorus/mL and 4 mEq of sodium/mL; and potassium phosphates: 3 mmol of elemental phosphorus/mL and 4.4 mEq of potassium/mL. The amount of sodium and potassium must be considered when ordering phosphate. The most reliable method of ordering IV phosphate is by millimoles, then specify the potassium or sodium salt.

PIPERACILLIN SODIUM (PIPRACIL)

ACTION AND SPECTRUM: Semisynthetic extended-spectrum penicillin with increased activity against *Pseudomonas aeruginosa* and many strains of *Klebsiella, Serratia, Escherichia coli, Enterobacter, Citrobacter,* and *Proteus.* Also demonstrates activity against Group B *Streptococcus.*
DOSAGE: IV.
Neonates, gestational age <36 weeks:
- **0–7 days:** 75 mg/kg/dose every 12 hours.
- **8–28 days:** 75 mg/kg/dose every 8 hours.

Neonates, gestational age ≥36 weeks:
- **0–7 days:** 75 mg/kg/dose every 8 hours.
- **8–28 days:** 75 mg/kg/dose every 6 hours.

Infants and children:
- 200–300 mg/kg/day in divided doses every 4–6 hours; maximum dose 24 grams/day.

ADVERSE EFFECTS: Hemolytic anemia, eosinophilia, neutropenia, prolonged bleeding time, thrombocytopenia; elevated liver enzymes, cholestatic hepatitis; acute interstitial nephritis, thrombophlebitis, and hypokalemia.
PHARMACOLOGY: Inactivated by β-lactamase–producing bacteria; synergistic with aminoglycosides. Good penetration into bone. Excreted unchanged in the urine.

PIPERACILLIN-TAZOBACTAM (ZOSYN)

ACTION AND SPECTRUM: Treatment of sepsis, intra-abdominal infections, infections involving the skin and skin structure, lower respiratory tract and urinary tract infections caused by β-lactamase–producing strains that are susceptible, including *Staphylococcus aureus, Haemophilus influenza, Bacteroides fragilis, Klebsiella, Pseudomonas, Proteus mirabilis, Escherichia coli,* and *Acinetobacter.*
DOSAGE: IV. Based on the piperacillin component.
- **Infants <6 months of age:** IV: 150–300 mg of piperacillin component/kg/day in divided doses every 6–8 hours.
- **Infants and children ≥6 months:** IV: 240 mg of piperacillin component/kg/day in divided doses every 8 hours.
- **Higher doses have been used for serious pseudomonal infections:** 300–400 mg of piperacillin component/kg/day in divided doses every 6 hours; maximum dose 16 grams of piperacillin component/day.

ADVERSE EFFECTS: Elevations in blood urea nitrogen (BUN), serum creatinine; interstitial nephritis, renal failure; leukopenia, thrombocytopenia, neutropenia, decrease in hemoglobin/hematocrit, eosinophilia, elevations in aspartate transaminase (AST) and alanine transaminase (ALT), hyperbilirubinemia, cholestatic jaundice, hypokalemia.
PHARMACOLOGY: Widely distributed into tissues and body fluids including lungs, intestinal mucosa, interstitial fluid, gallbladder, and bile; penetration into cerebrospinal fluid (CSF) is poor when meninges are not inflamed.
COMMENTS: When used to treat hospital-acquired pneumonia caused by *Pseudomonas aeruginosa,* consider the addition of an aminoglycoside.

PNEUMOCOCCAL 13-VALENT CONJUGATE VACCINE (PREVNAR)

INDICATIONS AND USE: For active immunization of infants and toddlers against *Streptococcus pneumoniae* invasive disease caused by the 13 capsular serotypes in the vaccine for all children 2–23 months of age. It is also recommended for certain children 24–59 months of age. *S. pneumoniae* causes invasive infections such as bacteremia and meningitis, pneumonia, otitis media, and sinusitis (see Advisory Committee on Immunization Practices [ACIP] guidelines for the most current recommendations).
ACTIONS: A vaccine of saccharides of the capsular antigens of *S. pneumoniae* serotypes 1, 3, 4, 5, 6A, 6B, 7F, 9V, 14, 18C, 19A, 19F, and 23F conjugated to diphtheria CRM197 protein. CRM197 protein is a nontoxic variant of diphtheria toxin.
DOSAGE: IM.
- 0.5 mL/dose as a single dose IM at 2, 4, 6, and 12–15 months of age. Shake well before administration. Refer to the current American Academy of Pediatrics (AAP)/ACIP immunization recommendations. The schedule usually begins at 2 months of age, but 6 weeks of age is acceptable. Three doses of 0.5 mL each are ideally given at ~2-month intervals, but a dosing interval of 4–8 weeks is acceptable, followed by a fourth dose of 0.5 mL at 12–15 months of age. Give the fourth dose at least 2 or more months after the third dose.

ADVERSE EFFECTS: Decreased appetite, drowsiness, irritability, fever, and injection site local tenderness, redness, and edema. Not a treatment of active infection. Do not give if patient is hypersensitive to any component of the vaccine. Use of this vaccine does not replace the use of the 23-valent pneumococcal polysaccharide vaccine in children ≥24 months old with sickle cell disease, chronic illness, asplenia, human immunodeficiency virus (HIV), or those who are immunocompromised. May be administered simultaneously with other vaccines as part of the routine immunization schedule.

PORACTANT ALFA (CUROSURF)

INDICATIONS AND USE: Treatment of neonatal respiratory distress syndrome (RDS).

ACTIONS: An extract of natural porcine lung surfactant, contains phospholipids, neutral lipids, fatty acids, and surfactant-associated proteins B and C. It replaces deficient or ineffective endogenous lung surfactant in neonates with RDS; surfactant prevents the alveoli from collapsing during expiration by lowering surface tension between air and alveolar surfaces.

DOSAGE: ETT.

• **Initial 2.5 mL/kg intratracheally**, divided into 2 aliquots, followed by up to 2 doses of 1.25 mL/kg administered at 12-hour intervals as needed to infants who continue to require mechanical ventilation and oxygen supplementation. Administer intratracheally through a side port adapter or through a 5F feeding catheter inserted into the endotracheal tube. Allow to warm to room temperature prior to administration. Do not shake or swirl vial to resuspend particles. Inspect for discoloration; normal color is creamy white. Discard unused drug.

ADVERSE EFFECTS: Transient bradycardia, hypotension, endotracheal tube blockage, and oxygen desaturation. Pulmonary hemorrhage has been reported.

COMMENTS: Following administration, lung compliance and oxygenation often improve rapidly. Patients should be closely monitored and appropriate changes in ventilation support should be made as clinically indicated.

POTASSIUM ACETATE

INDICATIONS AND USE: Treatment and prevention of hypokalemia in clinical situations where the use of chloride is not desirable. Also for correction of metabolic acidosis through the conversion of acetate to bicarbonate.

ACTIONS: Potassium acetate is metabolized to bicarbonate on an equimolar basis, which neutralizes hydrogen ion concentration and raises the blood and urine pH. Potassium is the major intracellular cation that is essential for neural conduction and muscular contraction.

DOSAGE: IV.

• **Normal daily requirement (based on mEq of potassium):** 2–6 mEq/kg/day. Dose should be added to maintenance IV fluids.
• **Intermittent IV administration for severe hypokalemia (based on mEq of potassium):** 0.5–1 mEq/kg/dose, infused at a rate of 0.3–0.5 mEq/kg/hour, not to exceed 1 mEq/kg/hour.

ADVERSE EFFECTS: Hyperkalemia, metabolic acidosis, arrhythmias; with rapid IV infusion—heart block, hypotension, and cardiac arrest.

PHARMACOLOGY: 1 mEq of acetate is equivalent to the alkalinizing effect of 1 mEq of bicarbonate.

COMMENTS: Continuous monitoring should be used for the infusion of intermittent doses >0.5 mEq/kg/hour. Do *not* administer undiluted or IV push. Potassium must be diluted prior to IV administration. Maximum recommended concentration for peripheral line is 80 mEq/L and for a central line is 150 mEq/L.

POTASSIUM CHLORIDE (KCL)

INDICATIONS AND USE: Treatment of hypokalemia and as a supplement to maintain adequate serum potassium levels. Also corrects hypochloremia.

ACTIONS: Potassium is the major intracellular cation. Potassium is essential for maintaining intracellular tonicity; transmission of nerve impulses; contraction of cardiac, skeletal, and smooth muscle; and maintenance of normal renal function.

DOSAGE: IV, PO. Monitor serum potassium levels and adjust dose as needed.

Acute treatment of hypokalemia:

• 0.5–1 mEq/kg/dose IV over 1 hour. Maximum dose/rate: 1 mEq/kg/hour; continuous electrocardiographic monitoring should be used for intermittent doses >0.5 mEq/kg/hour.

Maintenance:

• 2–6 mEq/kg/day (usually 2–3 mEq/kg/day) diluted in 24-hour maintenance IV solution. Higher doses are often required in infants receiving diuretics.

Oral supplementation:

• 2–6 mEq/kg/day (usually 2–3 mEq/kg/day) in divided doses and diluted with feedings. The injectable form of the drug may be given in divided doses PO and diluted in the infant's formula.

ADVERSE EFFECTS: Avoid rapid IV injection. Excessive dose or rate of infusion may cause cardiac arrhythmias (peaked T waves, widened QRS, flattened P waves, bradycardia, and heart block), respiratory paralysis, and hypotension. Monitor renal function, urine output, and serum potassium levels; hyperkalemia may result with renal dysfunction.

COMMENTS: Causes severe vein irritation; do not give undiluted in a peripheral vein. Dilute to 0.04 mEq/mL for a peripheral line, maximum of 0.08 mEq/mL. For a central line, dilute to 0.08 mEq/mL with maximum of 0.15 mEq/mL.

PREDNISONE (LIQUID PRED, PREDNISONE INTENSOL CONCENTRATE)

INDICATIONS AND USE: Used chiefly as an anti-inflammatory or immunosuppressive agent. Prednisone is an intermediate-acting glucocorticoid that has 4 times the anti-inflammatory potency of hydrocortisone and half the mineralocorticoid potency.
DOSAGE: PO.
- 0.25–2 mg/kg/day as a single daily dose or divided every 6–12 hours. Many different dosing regimens have been used.

ADVERSE EFFECTS: Cataracts, leukocytosis, peptic ulcer, nephrocalcinosis, myopathy, osteoporosis, diabetes, growth failure, hyperlipidemia, hypocalcemia, hypokalemic alkalosis, sodium retention and hypertension, and increased susceptibility to infection. Withdraw the dose gradually after prolonged therapy to prevent acute adrenal insufficiency.

PROCAINAMIDE HCL

> **WARNING:** The prolonged administration of procainamide often leads to the development of a positive antinuclear antibody (ANA) test, with or without symptoms of a lupus erythematosus-like syndrome. If a positive ANA titer develops, the benefit versus risks of continued procainamide therapy should be assessed.

INDICATIONS AND USE: Treatment of ventricular tachycardia, premature ventricular contractions, paroxysmal atrial tachycardia, and atrial fibrillation; to prevent recurrence of ventricular tachycardia, paroxysmal supraventricular tachycardia, atrial fibrillation or flutter. *Note:* Due to proarrhythmic effects, use should be reserved for life-threatening arrhythmias.
ACTIONS: Class I antiarrhythmic agent that increases the effective refractory period of the atria and ventricles of the heart. Partially metabolized by the liver to the active metabolite N-acetylprocainamide (NAPA).
DOSAGE: IV. Consider consult with pediatric cardiologist prior to use.
- **Initial bolus dose (monitor electrocardiogram [ECG], heart rate, and blood pressure):** 7–10 mg/kg (dilute to 20 mg/mL) IV over 10–30 minutes, then infusion of 20–80 mcg/kg/minute; maximum dose is 2 grams/day. Use lowest dose in preterm neonates.

ADVERSE EFFECTS: Toxic effects if given rapidly IV, including asystole, myocardial depression, ventricular fibrillation, hypotension, and reversible lupus-like syndrome. May cause nausea, vomiting, diarrhea, anorexia, skin rash, tachycardia, agranulocytosis, and hepatic toxicity. Potentially fatal blood dyscrasias have occurred with therapeutic doses.
PHARMACOLOGY: Therapeutic levels—procainamide: 4–10 mcg/mL, toxicity with levels >10 mcg/mL; NAPA: 6–20 mcg/mL, toxicity with levels >30 mcg/mL.
COMMENTS: Contraindicated in second- or third-degree heart block, bundle-branch block, digitalis intoxication, and allergy to procaine. Do not use in atrial fibrillation or flutter until the ventricular rate is adequately controlled to avoid a possible paradoxic increase in ventricular rate. Do not administer with amiodarone; may cause severe hypotension and prolongation of QT interval.

PROPRANOLOL (INDERAL)

INDICATIONS AND USE: Hypertension; supraventricular tachycardia, especially if associated with Wolff-Parkinson-White syndrome; tachyarrhythmias; and tetralogy of Fallot spells. Adjunctive therapy for neonatal thyrotoxicosis. Treatment of infantile hemangiomas.
ACTIONS: Nonselective β-adrenergic blocking agent that inhibits adrenergic stimuli by competitively blocking β-adrenergic receptors within the myocardium and bronchial and vascular smooth muscle. Propranolol decreases heart rate, myocardial contractility, blood pressure, and myocardial oxygen demand.
DOSAGE: IV, PO.
Arrhythmias:
- **Intravenous:** 0.01–0.15 mg/kg/dose IV to a maximum of 1 mg/dose as slow push over 10 minutes; may repeat every 6–8 hours as needed; increase slowly to maximum (neonates) of 0.15 mg/kg/dose every 6–8 hours; maximum dose 1 mg (infants) and 3 mg (children).
- **Neonates, PO:** 0.25 mg/kg/dose PO every 6–8 hours. Increase slowly as needed to 5 mg/kg/day.
- **Children, PO:** Initially 0.5–1 mg/kg/day in divided doses every 6–8 hours; titrate dosage upward every 3–5 days. Usual dose: 2–4 mg/kg/day; higher doses may be needed; do not exceed 16 mg/kg/day or 60 mg/day.

Hypertension:
- **Neonates:** 0.25 mg/kg/dose PO every 6–8 hours. Increase slowly as needed to 5 mg/kg/day.
- **Children:** 0.5–1 mg/kg/day PO in divided doses every 6–12 hours. May increase gradually every 5–7 days; usual dose is 1–5 mg/kg/day PO; maximum dose is 8 mg/kg/day PO.

Tetralogy spells:
- **IV:** 0.01–0.02 mg/kg/dose IV over 10 minutes; titrate to effect, up to 0.1–0.2 mg/kg/dose. Some centers use 0.15–0.25 mg/kg/dose slow IV; may repeat in 15 minutes; maximum initial dose is 1 mg.

- **Oral palliation:** Initial: 0.25 mg/kg/dose every 6 hours; if ineffective within first week, may increase by 1 mg/kg/day every 24 hours to maximum of 5 mg/kg/day; if patient is refractory may increase slowly to a maximum of 10–15 mg/kg/day but must carefully monitor heart rate, heart size, and cardiac contractility. Some centers use an initial 0.5–1 mg/kg/dose every 6 hours.

Thyrotoxicosis:

- **Neonates:** 2 mg/kg/day PO in divided doses every 6–12 hours; occasionally higher doses may be required.

ADVERSE EFFECTS: Generally dose-related hypotension and related to β-adrenergic blockage; nausea, vomiting, bronchospasm, increased airway resistance, heart block, depressed myocardial contractility, hypoglycemia, and inhibition of warning signs of hypoglycemia.

COMMENTS: Contraindicated in obstructive pulmonary disease, asthma, heart failure, shock, second- or third-degree heart block, and hypoglycemia. Use with caution in renal or hepatic failure.

PROTAMINE SULFATE

> WARNING: Severe hypotension, cardiovascular collapse, pulmonary edema, pulmonary vasoconstriction/hypertension possible. Risk factors: high dose/overdose, repeat doses, rapid administration, prior protamine use, current or prior protamine-containing products (NPH [isophane] or protamine zinc insulin, some β-blockers), severe left ventricular dysfunction, abnormal pulmonary hemodynamics. Vasopressors and resuscitation equipment must be available in case of reaction.

INDICATIONS AND USE: Treatment of heparin overdose, neutralize heparin during surgery.
ACTIONS: Combines with heparin, forming a stable salt complex and neutralizing the anticoagulation activity of both drugs. Effect on heparin is rapid (~5 minutes) and persists for ~2 hours.
DOSAGE: IV.

Heparin overdosage:

- Blood heparin concentrations decrease rapidly after heparin administration is stopped; adjust the protamine dosage depending on the duration of time since heparin administration as follows:
- **Time since last heparin <30 minutes:** 1 mg neutralizes 100 units heparin.
- **Time since last heparin 30–60 minutes:** 0.5–0.75 mg neutralizes 100 units heparin.
- **Time since last heparin >60–120 minutes:** 0.375–0.5 mg neutralizes 100 units heparin.
- **Time since last heparin >120 minutes:** 0.25–0.375 mg protamine neutralizes 100 units heparin.

Low molecular weight heparin (LMWH) overdosage:

- Most recent LMWH dose has been administered within the last 4 hours, use 1 mg protamine/1 mg (100 units) LMWH; a second dose of 0.5 mg protamine/1 mg (100 units) LMWH may be given if activated partial thromboplastin time (aPTT) remains prolonged 2–4 hours after the first dose.

ADVERSE EFFECTS: May cause hypotension, bradycardia, dyspnea, and anaphylaxis. Excessive administration beyond that needed to reverse a heparin effect may cause bleeding as a paradoxical coagulopathy.

PYRIDOXINE (VITAMIN B_6)

INDICATIONS AND USE: Treatment of pyridoxine-dependent seizures; to prevent or treat vitamin B_6 deficiency; treatment of drug-induced deficiency (eg, isoniazid or hydralazine); treatment of acute intoxication of isoniazid or hydralazine.
ACTIONS: Vitamin B_6 is essential in the synthesis of γ-aminobutyric acid (GABA), an inhibitory neurotransmitter in the central nervous system (CNS); GABA increases the seizure threshold. Pyridoxine is also required for heme synthesis and protein, carbohydrate, and fat metabolism.
DOSAGE: PO, IV.

Pyridoxine-dependent seizures:

- 50–100 mg IV single test dose, followed by a 30-minute observation period. If a response is seen, begin maintenance of 50–100 mg PO daily; range: 10–200 mg.

Dietary deficiency:

- **Children:** 5–25 mg/day PO for 3 weeks, then 1.5–2.5 mg/day in multivitamin product.

ADVERSE REACTIONS: Sensory neuropathy (after chronic administration of large doses), seizures (following IV administration of very large doses), acidosis, nausea, decreased serum folic acid concentration, respiratory distress.

PYRIMETHAMINE (DARAPRIM)

ACTION AND SPECTRUM: Inhibits parasitic dihydrofolate reductase resulting in inhibition of tetrahydrofolic acid synthesis.
DOSAGE: PO.

Newborns and infants:

- **Toxoplasmosis:** 2 mg/kg/day divided every 12 hours for 2 days, then 1 mg/kg/day daily together with sulfadiazine for 6 months, followed by 1 mg/kg/day 3 times weekly with sulfadiazine and leucovorin (oral folinic acid) (5–10 mg 3 times per week) should be administered to prevent hematologic toxicity for the next 6 months.

Infants and children ≥1 month of age:
- **Prophylaxis for first episode of *Toxoplasma gondii*:** 1 mg/kg/day once daily with dapsone plus oral folinic acid (5 mg every 3 days); maximum 25 mg/day.
- **Prophylaxis for recurrence of** *T. gondii:* 1 mg/kg/day once daily given with sulfadiazine or clindamycin, plus oral folinic acid (5 mg every 3 days); maximum 25 mg/day.

ADVERSE EFFECTS: Anorexia, vomiting, abdominal cramps, megaloblastic anemia, leukopenia, thrombocytopenia, pancytopenia, atrophic glossitis, rash, seizures, and shock.

COMMENTS: Administer with feedings if vomiting persists. Upon discontinuation of pyrimethamine, leucovorin should be continued for another week (due to long half-life of pyrimethamine). Dose reduction is necessary in hepatic dysfunction.

RANITIDINE (ZANTAC)

INDICATIONS AND USE: Short-term treatment of duodenal and gastric ulcers, gastroesophageal reflux disease (GERD), upper gastrointestinal bleed, and hypersecretory conditions.

ACTIONS: Histamine (H_2)-receptor antagonist; competitively inhibits the action of histamine on the gastric parietal cells; inhibits gastric acid secretion.

DOSAGE: PO, IV.

IV dosing:
- **Loading dose:** 1.5 mg/kg/dose IV then maintenance 12 hours later. Maintenance 1.5–2 mg/kg/day divided every 12 hours IV.
- **Continuous infusion:** 1.5 mg/kg/dose loading dose then 0.04–0.08 mg/kg/hour infusion (or 1–2 mg/kg/day).

Oral dosing:
- **Neonatal:** 2–4 mg/kg/day divided every 8–12 hours; maximum 6 mg/kg/day.
- **Infants >1 month:** GERD: 4–10 mg/kg/day divided twice daily.
- **Gastric/duodenal ulcer: Treatment:** 4–8 mg/kg/day PO divided twice daily.

Maintenance: 2–4 mg/kg/day once daily.

ADVERSE EFFECTS: Constipation, abdominal discomfort, sedation, malaise, leukopenia, thrombocytopenia, elevated serum creatinine, bradycardia, and tachycardia.

COMMENTS: Use of H_2 blockers in preterm infants is associated with increased risk for late-onset sepsis and fungal sepsis. Routine use of gastric acid suppression in neonates should be avoided. Dose adjustment needed in renal dysfunction. May add the daily dose to the total parenteral nutrition (PN) regimen and infuse over 24 hours to avoid the need for intermittent dosing.

RIFAMPIN

ACTION AND SPECTRUM: Broad-spectrum antibiotic with bacteriostatic activity against mycobacteria, *Neisseria meningitidis*, and gram-positive cocci; used to eliminate meningococci from asymptomatic carriers; for prophylaxis in contacts of patients with *Haemophilus influenzae* type B infection; management of active tuberculosis (TB) in combination with other agents; and used in combination with other antibiotics for the treatment of staphylococcal infections.

DOSAGE: PO, IV.

Synergy for staphylococcal infections:
- **Neonates:** 5–20 mg/kg/day PO/IV in divided doses every 12 hours with other antibiotics.

H. influenzae **prophylaxis:**
- **Neonates <1 month:** 10 mg/kg/day PO/IV every 24 hours for 4 days.
- **Infants and children:** 20 mg/kg/day PO/IV every 24 hours for 4 days, not to exceed 600 mg/dose.

Nasal carriers of *Staphylococcus aureus*:
- **Children:** 15 mg/kg/day PO/IV divided every 12 hours for 5–10 days in combination with at least 1 other systemic antistaphylococcal antibiotic. Not recommended for first-line therapy.

Meningococcal prophylaxis:
- **<1 month:** 10 mg/kg/day PO/IV in divided doses every 12 hours for 2 days.
- **Infants and children:** 20 mg/kg/day PO/IV in divided doses every 12 hours for 2 days, not to exceed 600 mg/dose.

Tuberculosis:
- **Active infection:** A 4-drug regimen (isoniazid, rifampin, pyrazinamide, and ethambutol) is preferred for the initial, empiric treatment of TB. Alter therapy regimen when drug susceptibility results are available.
- **Infants and children:** 10–20 mg/kg/day PO/IV in divided doses every 12–24 hours.

ADVERSE EFFECTS: Anorexia, vomiting, and diarrhea; rash, pruritus, and eosinophilia; drowsiness, ataxia, blood dyscrasias (leukopenia, thrombocytopenia, and hemolytic anemia), hepatitis (rare), and elevation of serum urea nitrogen and uric acid levels. Causes red-orange discoloration of body fluids.

PHARMACOLOGY: Highly lipophilic; crosses the blood-brain barrier and is widely distributed into body tissues and fluids; hepatic metabolism, undergoes enterohepatic recycling. Half-life is ~1–3 hours.

COMMENTS: Rifampin should always be used in combination with other agents; if used as monotherapy, resistance develops rapidly. Administer by slow IV infusion over 30 minutes to 3 hours at 6 mg/mL concentration. Extravasation may cause local irritation and inflammation. *Note:* A potent enzyme inducer of hepatic metabolism. Patients receiving digoxin, phenytoin, phenobarbital, or theophylline may have a substantial decrease in the serum concentration of these drugs after starting rifampin. Careful monitoring of serum drug concentrations is necessary.

ROCURONIUM

HIGH ALERT MEDICATION: To be administered only by experienced clinicians or adequately trained individuals supervised by an experienced clinician familiar with the use and actions, characteristics, and complications of neuromuscular blocking agents.

INDICATIONS AND USE: Produces skeletal muscle relaxation and paralysis to facilitate endotracheal intubation or increase pulmonary compliance in patients who are mechanically ventilated.

ACTIONS: Nondepolarizing neuromuscular blocking agent; blocks neural transmission at myoneural junction at cholinergic receptor sites.

DOSAGE: IV.

- 0.3–0.6 mg/kg/dose IV push over 5–10 seconds for tracheal intubation.

ADVERSE EFFECTS: Hypotension, hypertension, arrhythmias, tachycardia, bronchospasm. Neuromuscular blockade may be potentiated by severe hyponatremia, severe hypokalemia, severe hypokalemia, acidosis, renal failure, and liver failure.

PHARMACOLOGY: Onset of clinical effect is within 2 minutes, and the duration of effect ranges from 20 minutes to 2 hours.

COMMENTS: Adequate sedation/analgesia should be provided with the use of rocuronium.

SILDENAFIL (VIAGRA, REVATIO)

INDICATIONS AND USE: (Revatio) Treatment of persistent pulmonary hypertension of the newborn (PPHN) refractory to treatment with inhaled nitric oxide; to facilitate weaning from nitric oxide (by attenuating rebound effects after discontinuing inhaled nitric oxide); secondary pulmonary hypertension following cardiac surgery.

ACTIONS: Selective phosphodiesterase-type 5 (PDE-5) inhibitor found in the pulmonary vascular smooth muscle, vascular and visceral smooth muscle, corpus cavernosum, and platelets, and is responsible for the degradation of cyclic guanosine monophosphate (cGMP). Normally, nitric oxide (NO) activates the enzyme guanylate cyclase, which increases the levels of cGMP; cGMP produces smooth muscle relaxation. Inhibition of PDE-5 by sildenafil increases the cellular levels of cGMP that potentiate vascular smooth muscle relaxation, particularly in the lung where there are high PDE-5 concentrations. Sildenafil causes vasodilation in the pulmonary vasculature and, to a lesser extent, in the systemic circulation.

DOSAGE: PO, IV. Limited pediatric information exists; most pediatric literature consists of case reports or small studies and a wide range of doses have been used; further studies are needed.

Oral dosing:

- **Full-term neonates:** 0.3–1 mg/kg/dose PO every 6–12 hours. Usual range: 0.5–3 mg/kg/dose every 6–12 hours.
- **Infants and children:** Initial: 0.25–0.5 mg/kg/dose PO every 4–8 hours; increase if needed and tolerated to 1 mg/kg/dose every 4–8 hours; doses as high as 2 mg/kg/dose every 4 hours have been used in several case reports.

IV dosing:

- **Neonates >34 weeks' gestation and <72 hours:** Loading dose of 0.4 mg/kg over 3 hours followed by continuous infusion of 1.6 mg/kg/day or 0.067 mg/kg/hour.

ADVERSE EFFECTS: Use in neonatal and pediatric patients should be limited and considered experimental. The safety and efficacy in pediatric patients have not been established. There is short-term concern for worsening oxygenation and systemic hypotension; concern for increased risk of retinopathy of prematurity and platelet dysfunction.

PHARMACOLOGY: Metabolism is via the liver via cytochrome P450 isoenzyme CYP3A4 (major) and CYP2C9 (minor). Major metabolite is formed via N-demethylation pathway and has 50% of the activity of sildenafil.

COMMENTS: Significant increases in sildenafil concentrations may occur when used concurrently with CYP3A4 inhibitors such as azole antifungal agents, cimetidine, and erythromycin. Concurrent use with heparin may have an additive effect on bleeding time.

SODIUM ACETATE

INDICATIONS AND USE: Correction of metabolic acidosis through the conversion of acetate to bicarbonate; sodium replacement.

ACTIONS: Sodium acetate is metabolized to bicarbonate on an equimolar basis, which neutralizes hydrogen ion concentration and raises the blood and urine pH. Sodium is the primary extracellular cation.

DOSAGE: **IV.** If sodium acetate is desired over sodium bicarbonate (dosing similar to sodium bicarbonate).

• **Neonates, infants, and children:** IV 3–4 mEq/kg/day, maintenance sodium requirements.

ADVERSE EFFECTS: Hypernatremia, hypokalemic metabolic alkalosis, hypocalcemia, edema.

COMMENTS: Use with caution with hepatic failure, congestive heart failure (CHF).

SODIUM BICARBONATE

INDICATIONS AND USE: Management of metabolic acidosis; alkalinization of urine; stabilization of acid-base status in cardiac arrest, and treatment of life-threatening hyperkalemia.

ACTIONS: Alkalinizing agent that dissociates to provide bicarbonate ion, which neutralizes hydrogen ions, and raises the pH of the blood and urine.

DOSAGE: **IV.**

• **Initial dose:** 1–2 mEq/kg IV slowly over 30 minutes.

ADVERSE EFFECTS: Rapid correction of metabolic acidosis with sodium bicarbonate can lead to intraventricular hemorrhage, hyperosmolality, metabolic alkalosis, hypernatremia, hypokalemia, and hypocalcemia.

COMMENTS: Use with close monitoring of arterial blood pH. Use only when adequate ventilation is confirmed. Routine use in cardiac arrest is not recommended. Avoid extravasation; tissue necrosis can occur due to the hypertonicity of $NaHCO_3$. For direct IV administration: in neonates and infants, use the 0.5 mEq/mL solution or dilute the 1 mEq/mL solution 1:1 with sterile water for injection (SWI); administer slowly (maximum rate in neonates and infants: 10 mEq/minute); for infusion, dilute to a maximum concentration of 0.5 mEq/mL in dextrose solution and infuse over 2 hours (maximum rate of administration: 1 mEq/kg/hour).

SODIUM POLYSTYRENE SULFONATE

INDICATIONS AND USE: Treatment of hyperkalemia.

ACTIONS: Cation exchange resin that removes potassium by exchanging sodium ions for potassium ions in the intestine before the resin is passed from the body.

DOSAGE: **PO, PR** (1 gram of resin will exchange 1 mEq of sodium for 1 mEq of potassium).

• **Infants and children:** 1 gram/kg/dose PO every 6 hours or every 2–6 hours PR.

ADVERSE EFFECTS: Large doses may cause fecal impaction. Hypokalemia, hypocalcemia, hypomagnesemia, and sodium retention may occur.

COMMENTS: Due to complications of hypernatremia and necrotizing enterocolitis (NEC), use in neonates is not recommended. Small amounts of magnesium and calcium may also be lost in binding. When using the powder for oral administration, dilute in 3–4 mL fluid per gram of resin; 10% sorbitol, water, or syrup may be used as diluent. When using powder for rectal administration, dilute in water or 25% sorbitol at a concentration of 0.3–0.5 gram/mL; retain enema in colon for at least 30–60 minutes or several hours, if possible.

SPIRONOLACTONE (ALDACTONE)

> WARNING: Aldactone has been shown to be a tumorigenic in chronic animal studies. Unnecessary use of this drug should be avoided.

INDICATIONS AND USE: Primarily used in conjunction with other diuretics for the treatment of hypertension, congestive heart failure (CHF), and edema with prolonged diuretic therapy.

ACTIONS: Competes with aldosterone for receptor sites in the distal renal tubules; increases sodium chloride and water excretion while conserving potassium and hydrogen ions; it also may block the effect of aldosterone on arteriolar smooth muscle.

DOSAGE: **PO.**

• 1–3 mg/kg/day divided every 12–24 hours.

ADVERSE EFFECTS: Hyperkalemia, dehydration, hyponatremia, hyperchloremic metabolic acidosis, rash, vomiting, diarrhea, and gynecomastia in males.

COMMENTS: Contraindicated in hyperkalemia, anuria, and rapidly deteriorating renal function. Monitor potassium closely when giving potassium supplements.

SUCROSE

INDICATIONS AND USE: Mild analgesia in neonates during minor procedures, such as heelstick, eye examination for retinopathy of prematurity, circumcision, immunization, venipuncture, endotracheal tube (ETT) intubation and suctioning, nasogastric (NG) tube insertion, IM or subcutaneous injection. (See also Chapter 76.)

ACTIONS: Exact mechanism of action is unknown; sucrose may induce endogenous opioid release.

DOSAGE: PO.

• **Neonates:** 0.5–1 mL of 24% solution placed on the tongue or buccal surface 2 minutes prior to procedure; various regimens reported (maximum dose 2 mL). Term: 2 mL of 24% solution. May be administered directly into baby's mouth or via a pacifier dipped into solution.

ADVERSE EFFECTS: Avoid in patients with gastrointestinal tract abnormalities—use only in patients with functioning gastrointestinal (GI) tract; necrotizing enterocolitis (NEC) has not been reported with sucrose administration. Avoid use in patients at risk for aspiration. Do not use in patients requiring ongoing analgesia.
PHARMACOLOGY: Time to maximum effect is 2 minutes; duration of effect is 5–10 minutes.
COMMENTS: Sucrose 24% solution has an osmolarity of 1000 mosmol/L.

SULFACETAMIDE SODIUM

ACTION AND SPECTRUM: Interferes with bacterial growth by inhibiting bacterial folic acid synthesis. Used for the treatment and prophylaxis of conjunctivitis caused by susceptible strains of gram-positive and gram-negative bacteria such as *Staphylococcus aureus*, *Streptococcus pneumoniae*, *Haemophilus influenzae*, and *Moraxella*.
DOSAGE: Ocular.

• Instill 1–2 drops into each eye every 1–3 hours initially, then increase the time interval as the condition responds; apply ointment to each eye 1–4 times per day and at bedtime; treatment duration is usually 7–10 days.

ADVERSE EFFECTS: May cause burning and stinging sensation of eyes, increased sensitivity to light, blurred vision, and pruritus.
COMMENTS: Contraindicated in infants <2 months of age or with hypersensitivity to sulfonamides.

SULFADIAZINE

ACTION AND SPECTRUM: Acts via competitive antagonism of p-aminobenzoic acid, an essential factor in bacterial folic acid synthesis; used as adjunctive treatment for *Toxoplasma gondii* in combination with pyrimethamine.
DOSAGE: PO. See also Pyrimethamine (page 994) for dosing information.
Congenital toxoplasmosis:

• **Newborns:** 100 mg/kg/day divided every 12 hours for 12 months in conjunction with pyrimethamine.
• **Infants:** 100 mg/kg/day divided every 12 hours for 12 months in conjunction with pyrimethamine.

Acquired toxoplasmosis:

• **Infants ≥2 months and children:** 100–200 mg/kg/day divided every 6 hours in conjunction with pyrimethamine (maximum dose 6000 mg/day).

ADVERSE EFFECTS: Hypersensitivity (fever, rash, hepatitis, vasculitis, and lupus-like syndrome), neutropenia, agranulocytosis, thrombocytopenia, aplastic anemia, Stevens-Johnson syndrome, and crystalluria (keep urine alkaline, maintain adequate hydration and urine output high). Kernicterus may occur. Caution in patients with G6PD deficiency.
COMMENTS: Avoid use in neonates, except for treatment of congenital toxoplasmosis. Concurrent folinic acid supplementation is necessary to prevent folic acid deficiency.

TICARCILLIN DISODIUM

ACTION AND SPECTRUM: Semisynthetic extended-spectrum penicillin used to treat infections caused by susceptible strains of *Pseudomonas aeruginosa*, *Proteus*, *Escherichia coli*, *Enterobacter*, and *Streptococcus faecalis*.
DOSAGE: IV.
Neonates, postnatal age ≤7 days:

• ≤2 kg: 150 mg/kg/day IV in divided doses every 12 hours.
• >2 kg: 225 mg/kg/day IV in divided doses every 8 hours.

Neonates, postnatal age >7 days:

• ≤2 kg: 225 mg/kg/day IV in divided doses every 8 hours.
• >2 kg: 300 mg/kg/day IV in divided doses every 6–8 hours.

Infants and children:

• 50–100 mg/kg/day IV in divided doses every 6–8 hours.
• 200–300 mg/kg/day IV in divided doses every 4–6 hours; doses as high as 400 mg/kg/day divided every 4–6 hours have been used in acute pulmonary exacerbations of cystic fibrosis. Maximum dose is 24 grams/day.

ADVERSE EFFECTS: Hypersensitivity reactions with eosinophilia; hypernatremia and hypokalemia; inhibition of platelet aggregation; hyperbilirubinemia, elevation of aspartate transaminase (AST), alanine transaminase (ALT), blood urea nitrogen (BUN), and serum creatinine. Thrombophlebitis and pain on injection.
PHARMACOLOGY: Mostly excreted in urine as unchanged drug.

TICARCILLIN DISODIUM AND CLAVULANATE POTASSIUM

ACTION AND SPECTRUM: Combination antibiotic of ticarcillin, a carboxypenicillin, and clavulanic acid, a β-lactamase inhibitor. Clavulanate expands activity of ticarcillin to include β-lactamase–producing strains of *Staphylococcus aureus, Haemophilus influenzae, Moraxella catarrhalis, Bacteroides fragilis, Klebsiella, Prevotella, Pseudomonas aeruginosa, Escherichia coli,* and *Proteus* species.

DOSAGE: IV. Timentin (ticarcillin/clavulanate) is a combination product; dosage is based on ticarcillin component.

Postnatal age 0–28 days and <1.2 kg:
- 150 mg/kg/day IV divided every 12 hours.

Postnatal age <7 days and 1.2–2 kg:
- 150 mg/kg/day IV divided every 12 hours.

Postnatal age <7 days and >2 kg:
- 225 mg/kg/day IV divided every 8 hours.

Postnatal age ≥7 days and 1.2–2 kg:
- 225 mg/kg/day IV divided every 8 hours.

Postnatal age ≥7 days and >2 kg:
- 300 mg/kg/day IV divided every 8 hours.

Term neonates and infants <3 months:
- 200–300 mg ticarcillin component/kg/day IV divided every 6 hours.

Infants ≥3 months and children <60 kg:
- **Mild to moderate infections:** 200 mg/kg/day IV divided every 6 hours.
- **Severe infections outside the central nervous system (CNS):** 300 mg/kg/day IV divided every 4–6 hours.

ADVERSE EFFECTS: Eosinophilia, leukopenia, inhibition of platelet aggregation, prolongation of bleeding time, neutropenia, hemolytic anemia, thrombocytopenia, hypernatremia, hypokalemia, elevations in aspartate transaminase (AST), alanine transaminase (ALT), blood urea nitrogen (BUN), and serum creatinine, and thrombophlebitis.

PHARMACOLOGY: Ticarcillin, renal (tubular secretion); clavulanic acid, hepatic and renal.

COMMENTS: Use with caution and modify dose in patients with renal impairment.

TOBRAMYCIN SULFATE

ACTION AND SPECTRUM: Aminoglycoside antibiotic used for documented or suspected infections caused by susceptible gram-negative bacilli including *Pseudomonas aeruginosa* and non-pseudomonal enteric bacillus infection, which is more sensitive to tobramycin than gentamicin based on susceptibility tests; usually used in combination with a β-lactam antibiotic.

DOSAGE: IV, IM, ocular, inhalation. Base the initial dose on body weight, then monitor levels and adjust using pharmacokinetics. Many dosing strategies exist such as extended interval, age based, weight based, and traditional. Monitor serum levels after 2 days of therapy.

Age based:
- **≤29 weeks postmenstrual age (PMA):**
  - **0–7 days:** 5 mg/kg/dose IV/IM every 48 hours.
  - **8–28 days:** 4 mg/kg/dose IV/IM every 36 hours.
  - **≥29 days:** 4 mg/kg/dose IV/IM every 24 hours.
- **30–34 weeks PMA:**
  - **0–7 days:** 4.5 mg/kg/dose IV/IM every 36 hours.
  - **>7 days:** 4 mg/kg/dose IV/IM every 24 hours.
- **≥35 weeks PMA:** 4 mg/kg/dose IV/IM every 24 hours.

Infants and children <5 years:
- 2.5 mg/kg/dose IM/IV every 8 hours.

Ophthalmic:
- Instill 1–2 drops into each eye every 4 hours or more often if infection is severe, or apply a small amount of ointment into each eye 2–3 times per day or for severe infections every 3–4 hours.

Inhalation:
- 150 mg twice daily nebulized has been used for difficult to manage neonatal intensive care unit (NICU) patients.

ADVERSE EFFECTS: See Gentamicin (page 966).

COMMENTS: Reserve for cases resistant to gentamicin. Obtain serum peak and trough concentrations at about the third maintenance dose. **Desired peak** is 4–12 mcg/mL (sample 30 minutes after the infusion is complete); desired trough is 0.5–2 mcg/mL (sample 30 minutes to just before the next dose).

TROMETHAMINE (THAM ACETATE)

INDICATIONS AND USE: Treatment of metabolic acidosis in mechanically ventilated patients with significant hypercarbia or hypernatremia. Not indicated for the treatment of metabolic acidosis due to bicarbonate deficiency.

ACTIONS: Alkalinizing agent that acts as a proton (hydrogen ion) acceptor; combines with hydrogen ions and their associated anions of acids (lactic, pyruvic, carbonic, and other metabolic acids) to form bicarbonate and buffer to correct acidosis. It buffers both metabolic and respiratory acids, limiting carbon dioxide generation. The resulting salts are then renally excreted.

DOSAGE: **IV.**

- **Method 1:** 3.3–6.6 mL/kg (1–2 mmol/kg) of undiluted solution infused in a large vein over 1 hour.
- **Method 2:** Dose (mL) = weight (kg) × 1.1 × base deficit (mEq/L).
- **Maximum dose in neonates with normal renal function:** ~5–7 mmol/kg/24 hours.

ADVERSE EFFECTS: Respiratory depression, apnea, thrombophlebitis, venospasm, alkalosis, hypoglycemia, and hyperkalemia. Avoid infusion via low-lying umbilical venous catheters due to associated risk of hepatocellular necrosis; severe local tissue necrosis and sloughing may occur if solution extravasates; administer via central line or large vein slowly.

COMMENTS: Contraindicated in anuria, uremia, salicylate toxicity, and chronic respiratory acidosis. For short-term use only; administration beyond 24 hours is not recommended. Monitor for hyperkalemia and pH, especially with renal dysfunction.

TROPICAINAMIDE

INDICATIONS AND USE: Mydriasis and cycloplegia for diagnostic and therapeutic ophthalmic procedures.
ACTIONS: Anticholinergic activity produces pupillary dilation.
DOSAGE: **Ocular.**

- One drop of 0.5% ophthalmic solution instilled into eye at least 10 minutes prior to procedure. Apply pressure to lacrimal sac during and for 2 minutes after instillation to reduce systemic absorption.

ADVERSE EFFECTS: Fever, tachycardia, vasodilatation, restlessness, decreased gastrointestinal (GI) motility, urinary retention.
PHARMACOLOGY: Onset of mydriasis is 5 minutes; cycloplegia 20–40 minutes.
COMMENTS: Consider holding feeds for 4 hours after procedure.

URSODIOL

INDICATIONS AND USE: Facilitate bile excretion in infants with biliary atresia; treatment of cholestasis secondary to parenteral nutrition (PN); improve the hepatic metabolism of essential fatty acids in patients with cystic fibrosis.
ACTIONS: A hydrophobic bile acid that decreases the cholesterol content of bile and bile stones by reducing the secretion of cholesterol from the liver and decreases the fractional reabsorption of cholesterol by the intestines.
DOSAGE: **PO.**

Biliary atresia:
- **Infants:** 10–15 mg/kg/day PO once daily.

Total parenteral nutrition–induced cholestasis:
- **Infants and children:** 30 mg/kg/day PO in 3 divided doses.

Improvement in the hepatic metabolism of essential fatty acids in cystic fibrosis:
- **Children:** 30 mg/kg/day PO in 2 divided doses.

ADVERSE EFFECTS: Rash, diarrhea, biliary pain, constipation, stomatitis, flatulence, nausea, vomiting, abdominal pain, elevated liver enzymes.
PHARMACOKINETICS: Absorbed well orally. Metabolism: Undergoes extensive enterohepatic recycling; following hepatic conjugation and biliary secretion, the drug is hydrolyzed to the unconjugated form and it is recycled or transformed to lithocholic acid by colonic microbial flora.
COMMENTS: Use with caution in patients with nonvisualizing gallbladder and patients with chronic liver disease.

VALGANCICLOVIR

ACTION AND SPECTRUM: Prodrug of ganciclovir that is converted to ganciclovir by the liver and intestinal esterases. Used to treat symptomatic congenital cytomegalovirus (CMV) infection.
DOSAGE: **PO.**

- 16 mg/kg/dose PO every 12 hours for a minimum of 6 weeks; longer treatment duration may be necessary. Use commercially available product only.

ADVERSE EFFECTS: Neutropenia is frequent; if absolute neutrophil count (ANC) is <500 cells/mm³, hold dose until ANC is >750 cells/mm³. If ANC falls below 750 cells/mm³, reduce dose by 50%; if ANC falls again to below 500 cells/mm³, discontinue drug. Also, granulocytopenia, anemia, thrombocytopenia; acute renal failure/ acute kidney injury, dysuria, increased serum creatinine; hyperglycemia, hyper/hypokalemia, hypocalcemia, hypomagnesemia, hypophosphatemia, and edema.
PHARMACOLOGY: Excreted unchanged by the kidney; elimination half-life is 3 hours—dosing adjustment necessary with renal impairment.

VANCOMYCIN HCL

ACTION AND SPECTRUM: Bactericidal action with activity against most gram-positive cocci and bacilli, including streptococci, staphylococci (including methicillin-resistant staphylococci), clostridia (including *Clostridium difficile*), *Corynebacterium*, and *Listeria monocytogenes*. Bacteriostatic against enterococci.

DOSAGE: PO, IV, intrathecal, intraventricular.
Neonates:
- **Postnatal age <7 days:**
  - **<1.2 kg:** 15 mg/kg/day IV every 24 hours.
  - **1.2–2 kg:** 10–15 mg/kg/dose IV every 12–18 hours.
  - **>2 kg:** 10–15 mg/kg/dose IV every 8–12 hours.
- **Postnatal age ≥7 days:**
  - **<1.2 kg:** 15 mg/kg/day given IV 24 hours.
  - **1.2–2 kg:** 10–15 mg/kg/dose IV every 8–12 hours.
  - **>2 kg:** 15–20 mg/kg/dose IV every 8 hours.

Infants >1 month and children:
- 40 mg/kg/day IV in divided doses every 6–8 hours.

Intrathecal/intraventricular:
- **Neonates:** 5–10 mg/day.

Serious infection or organisms with a minimal inhibitory concentration (MIC) = 1 mcg/mL:
- **Initial:** 15-20 mg/kg/dose every 6-8 hours.
- **Methicillin-resistant *Staphylococcus aureus* (MRSA) infections/bacteremia:** 15 mg/kg/dose every 6 hours for 2–6 weeks depending on severity.
- **Complicated skin and skin structure infections:** Treat for 7–14 days.
- **Meningitis:** Treat for 2 weeks (± rifampin).
- **Osteomyelitis:** Treat for minimum of 4–6 weeks.
- **Pneumonia:** Treat for 7–21 days.

Antibiotic-associated pseudomembranous colitis:
- (*Note:* Metronidazole is the drug of initial choice based on 2012 AAP *Red Book* recommendations). Children: 30 mg/kg/day in divided doses every 6 hours for 10 days, not to exceed 2 grams/day.

ADVERSE EFFECTS: Allergy (rash and fever), ototoxicity (with prolonged peak >40 mcg/mL), nephrotoxicity (higher incidence with trough >10 mcg/mL), and thrombophlebitis at the site of injection. Rapid infusion may cause rash, chills, and fever ("red-man" syndrome), mimicking anaphylactic reaction. Apnea and bradycardia without other signs of "red-man" syndrome have also been associated with rapid infusion. Infuse dose over at least 60 minutes.
PHARMACOLOGY: Renally excreted. Half-life is 6–10 hours.
COMMENTS: Therapeutic: Peak 25–40 mcg/mL; 30–40 mcg/mL when treating meningitis (sample 60 minutes after the infusion is completed) and trough level of 5–15 mcg/mL; experts recommend 15–20 mcg/mL for organisms with an MIC = 1 mcg/mL when treating MRSA pneumonia, endocarditis, or bone/joint infections (sample drawn 30 minutes prior to scheduled dose). Draw serum peak and trough around the fourth maintenance dose. Monitor serum creatinine, blood urea nitrogen (BUN), and urine output. If staphylococci exhibit tolerance to the drug, combine with an aminoglycoside, with or without rifampin. Oral doses are poorly absorbed.

VARICELLA-ZOSTER IMMUNE GLOBULIN (VZIG)

INDICATIONS AND USE: For protection of infants of mothers with varicella-zoster infections (chickenpox) within 5 days before or 48 hours after delivery, of postnatally exposed preterm infants ≤1 kg or <28 weeks' gestation regardless of maternal history, and of postnatally exposed premature infants ≥28 weeks' gestation whose maternal history is negative for varicella.
ACTIONS: Passive immunity through infusion of immunoglobulin G (IgG) antibodies. Protection lasts 1 month or longer and does not reduce the incidence, but acts to decrease the risk of complications.
DOSAGE: IM.
- **<10 kg:** 125 units = 1 × 125-unit vial, minimum dose: 125 units; do not give fractional doses. Maximum dose is 625 international units.

ADVERSE EFFECTS: Pain, erythema, swelling, rash at the site of injection, and, rarely, anaphylaxis.
COMMENTS: Best results are achieved if given within 96 hours after exposure. VZIG was discontinued in the United States in 2005. It is currently available as **VariZIG** under an Investigational New Drug Application Expanded Access protocol. Inventory for anticipated patients may be obtained by contacting FFF Enterprises at 800-843-7477. Additional information may be found at: http://www.fffenterprises.com/Products/VariZIGINDProtocolPre.aspx.

VECURONIUM BROMIDE

HIGH ALERT MEDICATION: To be administered only by experienced clinicians or adequately trained individuals supervised by an experienced clinician familiar with the use and actions, characteristics, and complications of neuromuscular-blocking agents.
INDICATIONS AND USE: Skeletal muscle relaxation and paralysis in infants requiring mechanical ventilation or surgery, or to facilitate endotracheal intubation.
ACTIONS: Nondepolarizing muscle relaxant that competitively antagonizes autonomic cholinergic receptors.

DOSAGE: IV.
Neonates:
- 0.1 mg/kg/dose, then maintenance 0.03–0.15 mg/kg IV push every 1–2 hours as needed.

Infants >7 weeks to 1 year:
- 0.1 mg/kg/dose; repeat every hour as needed; may be administered as a continuous infusion at 1–1.5 mcg/kg/minute (0.06–0.09 mg/kg/hour).

ADVERSE EFFECTS: May cause hypoxemia with inadequate mechanical ventilation; bronchospasm, apnea, arrhythmias, tachycardia, hypotension, hypertension. See Pancuronium.

PHARMACOLOGY: Onset of action is 1–2 minutes with a duration that varies with dose and age.

COMMENTS: Causes less tachycardia than pancuronium bromide. When used with narcotics, decreases in heart rate and blood pressure have been observed.

VITAMIN A

INDICATIONS AND USE: Treatment and prevention of vitamin A deficiency; to reduce the risk of chronic lung disease in high-risk premature neonates with vitamin A deficiency.

ACTIONS: Vitamin A is required for growth and bone development, vision, reproduction, and differentiation and maintenance of epithelial tissue. The pulmonary histopathologic changes seen in patients with bronchopulmonary dysplasia/chronic lung disease (BPD/CLD) are similar to those seen with vitamin A deficiency. Retinol metabolites exhibit potent and site-specific effects on gene expression as well as lung growth and development.

DOSAGE: PO, IM.
Prevention of bronchopulmonary dysplasia/chronic lung disease in premature infants:
- 5000 units IM 3 times a week for 4 weeks; start within first 4 days of life.

Prophylactic therapy for children at risk for developing deficiency:
- **Infants ≤1 year:** 100,000 units PO every 4–6 months.

Adequate intake:
- **1 to <6 months:** 400 mcg (1330 units).
- **6 to <12 months:** 500 mcg (1670 units).

Daily dietary supplement:
- **Infants up to 6 months:** 1500 units PO.
- **Children 6 months to 3 years:** 1500–2000 units.

ADVERSE EFFECTS: Concomitant use with glucocorticoids should be avoided, as it significantly raises plasma vitamin A concentrations; seen only with doses that exceed physiologic replacement. Monitor for signs of toxicity: full fontanel, lethargy, irritability, hepatosplenomegaly, edema, and mucocutaneous lesions.

VITAMIN D$_3$ (CHOLECALCIFEROL)

INDICATIONS AND USE: Prevention and treatment of vitamin D deficiency and/or rickets; dietary supplement.

ACTIONS: Stimulates calcium and phosphate absorption from the small intestine; promotes secretion of calcium from bone to blood; promotes renal tubule phosphate resorption; acts on osteoblasts to stimulate skeletal growth and on the parathyroid glands to suppress parathyroid hormone synthesis and secretion.

DOSAGE: PO.
Prevention of vitamin D deficiency:
- **Premature infants:** 400–800 international units per day or 150–400 international units per kilogram per day.
- **Breast-fed neonates (fully or partially):** 400 international units per day beginning in first few days of life. Continue supplementation until infant is weaned to ≥1000 mL/day or 1 quart per day of vitamin D–fortified formula or whole milk (after 12 months of age).
- **Formula-fed neonates ingesting <1000 mL of vitamin D–fortified formula:** 400 international units per day.

Treatment of vitamin D deficiency and/or rickets:
- 1000 international units per day for 2–3 months together with calcium and phosphorus supplementation; once radiologic evidence of healing is observed, decrease to 400 international units per day.

ADVERSE EFFECTS: Hypercalcemia, azotemia, vomiting, and nephrocalcinosis.

PHARMACOLOGY: 25(OH)-D concentration >250 nmol/L may be associated with risk of vitamin D intoxication.

COMMENTS: For detailed information see the 2008 American Academy of Pediatrics (AAP) statement, *Prevention of Rickets and Vitamin D Deficiency in Infants, Children and Adolescents* (Wagner et al, 2008). Excessive doses may lead to hypervitaminosis D, manifested by hypercalcemia and its associated complications. (See also Chapter 116.)

VITAMIN E (DL-α-TOCOPHEROL ACETATE)

INDICATIONS AND USE: Treatment or prevention of vitamin E deficiency.

ACTIONS: Antioxidant that prevents oxidation of vitamins A and C; protects polyunsaturated fatty acids in membranes from attack by free radicals and protects red blood cells against hemolysis by oxidizing agents.

DOSAGE: PO.
Prevention of vitamin E deficiency:
- **Premature or low birthweight neonates:** 5 units PO per day diluted with feedings. Do not give simultaneously with iron; will decrease iron absorption.

Vitamin E deficiency:
- 25–50 units per day.

COMMENTS: Physiologic serum vitamin E levels are 0.8–3.5 mg/dL. Serum levels should be monitored when pharmacologic doses of vitamin E are administered. Liquid preparation is very hyperosmolar (3620 mosmol/kg H_2O) and should be diluted (1 mg of DL-α-tocopherol acetate = 1 unit).

VITAMIN K$_1$ (PHYTONADIONE)

INDICATIONS AND USE: Prevention and treatment of hemorrhagic disease of the newborn and vitamin K deficiency.
ACTIONS: Required for the synthesis of blood coagulation factors II, VII, IX, and X. Because vitamin K$_1$ may require 3 hours or more to stop active bleeding, fresh-frozen plasma, 10 mL/kg, may be necessary when bleeding is severe. The drug has no antagonistic effects against heparin.
DOSAGE: PO, IM, IV.
Neonatal hemorrhagic disease:
- **Prevention:** 1 mg IM at birth.
  - **Preterm infant <32 weeks' gestation:**
    - **Birthweight >1000 grams:** 0.5 mg IM at birth.
    - **Birthweight <1000 grams:** 0.3 mg/kg IM at birth.
- **Treatment:** 1–2 mg IM per day.

Vitamin K deficiency (drugs, malabsorption, or decreased synthesis of vitamin K):
- **Infants and children:** 2.5–5 mg/day PO per day or 1–2 mg subcutaneous, IM, IV, as a single dose.

Oral anticoagulant overdose:
- 0.5–2 mg/dose IV every 12 hours as needed. (Monitor the serial prothrombin time and partial thromboplastin time for response.)

ADVERSE EFFECTS: Relatively nontoxic. Hemolytic anemia and kernicterus have been reported in neonates given greater than recommended dose. Severe hypersensitivity or anaphylactic reactions have been associated with IV administration of vitamin K$_1$. Efficacy of treatment with vitamin K$_1$ is decreased in patients with liver disease.

ZIDOVUDINE (AZT, ZDV)

INDICATIONS AND USE: Chemoprophylaxis to reduce perinatal human immunodeficiency virus (HIV) transmission; prophylactic treatment of neonates born to HIV-infected mothers; treatment of HIV infection in combination with other antiretroviral agents.
ACTIONS: Nucleoside reverse transcriptase inhibitor (NRTI) that inhibits HIV viral polymerases and DNA replication.
DOSAGE: IV, PO (aidsinfo.nih.gov/guidelines, 2011).
Prevention of maternal-fetal HIV transmission:
- Dosing should begin as soon as possible after birth (by 6–12 hours after delivery) and continue for the first 6 weeks of life. Use IV route only until oral therapy can be administered.
  - **≥35 weeks' gestation:** 4 mg/kg/dose PO twice daily; or if unable to tolerate oral medications, 1.5 mg/kg/dose IV every 6 hours.
  - **<35 to ≥30 weeks' gestation:** 2 mg/kg/dose PO every 12 hours; or if unable to tolerate oral medications, 1.5 mg/kg/dose IV every 12 hours. Advance to every 8 hours at 2 weeks postnatal age.
  - **<30 weeks' gestation:** 2 mg/kg/dose PO every 12 hours; or if unable to tolerate oral medications, 1.5 mg/kg/dose IV every 12 hours. Advance to every 8 hours at 4 weeks postnatal age.

HIV infection, treatment:
- Use in combination with other antiretroviral agents:
  - **Infants <6 weeks:** 2 mg/kg/dose PO every 6 hours.
  - **Infants ≥6 weeks and children:** 160 mg/m^2/dose PO every 8 hours. Maximum: 200 mg every 8 hours. 180–240 mg/m^2/dose every 12 hours to improve compliance; data on this dose in children are limited.
  - **IV continuous infusion:** 20 mg/m^2/hour.
  - **IV intermittent infusion:** 120 mg/m^2/dose every 6 hours.

ADVERSE EFFECTS: The most frequent are granulocytopenia and severe anemia. Others include thrombocytopenia, leukopenia, diarrhea, fever, seizures, insomnia, cholestatic hepatitis, and lactic acidosis.
COMMENTS: Use with caution in patients with impaired hepatic function, bone marrow compromise, or folic acid or vitamin B$_{12}$ deficiency.
INTERACTIONS: Concurrent acetaminophen, probenecid, cimetidine, indomethacin, morphine, and benzodiazepines may increase toxicity as a result of decreased glucuronidation or reduced renal excretion of zidovudine. Concomitant acyclovir may cause neurotoxicity; ganciclovir and flucytosine may cause severe hematologic toxicity as a result of synergistic myelosuppression. Ribavirin and zidovudine are antagonistic and should not be used concurrently.

Selected References

Agthe AG, Kim GR, Mathias KB, et al. Clonidine as an adjunct therapy to opioids for neonatal abstinence syndrome: a randomized, controlled trial. *Pediatrics.* 2009;123(5):e849–e856.

American Academy of Pediatrics. In: Pickering LK, Baker CJ, Kimberlin DW, Long SS, eds. *Red Book: 2012 Report of the Committee on Infectious Diseases.* 29th ed. Elk Grove Village, IL: American Academy of Pediatrics; 2012.

American Academy of Pediatrics, Committee on Drugs, and Committee on Fetus and Newborn. Neonatal drug withdrawal. *Pediatrics.* 2012;129:e540–e560.

American Academy of Pediatrics, Committee on Fetus and Newborn, and Canadian Pediatric Society, Fetus and Newborn Committee. Postnatal corticosteroids to treat or prevent chronic lung disease in preterm infants. *Pediatrics.* 2002;109:330–338.

American Academy of Pediatrics, Committee on Substance Abuse. Tobacco, alcohol, and other drugs: the role of the pediatrician in prevention and management of substance abuse. *Pediatrics.* 1998;101(1 Pt 1): 125–128.

American Academy of Pediatrics, Section on Endocrinology and Committee on Genetics. Technical report: congenital adrenal hyperplasia. *Pediatrics.* 2000;106(6):1511–1518. Reaffirmed May 1, 2005.

Anand KJ; International Evidence-Based Group for Neonatal Pain. Consensus statement for the prevention and management of pain in the newborn. *Arch Pediatr Adolesc Med.* 2001;155(2):173–180. Review: http://dailymed.nlm.nih.gov/dailymed/, http://www.accessdata.fda.gov. Accessed September, 2012.

Doyle LW, Davis PG, Morley CJ, McPhee A, Carlin JB; DART Study Investigators. Low-dose dexamethasone facilitates extubation among chronically ventilator-dependent infants: a multicenter, international, randomized, controlled trial. *Pediatrics.* 2006;117:75–83.

Hussain K, Aynsley-Green A, Stanley CA. Medications used in the treatment of hypoglycemia due to congenital hyperinsulinism of infancy (HI). *Pediatr Endocrinol Rev.* 2004;2 (suppl):163–167.

Kapoor RR, Flanagan SE, James C, Shield J, Ellard S, Hussain K. Hyperinsulinaemic hypoglycaemia. *Arch Dis Child.* 2009;94(6):450–457 (Epub 2009 Feb 4).

Kleinman ME, Chameides L, Schexnayder SM, et al. Part 14: pediatric advanced life support 2010 American Heart Association Guidelines for cardiopulmonary resuscitation and emergency cardiovascular care. *Circulation.* 2010;122(18 suppl 3):S893.

Krauss B, Green MG. Procedural sedation and analgesia in children. *Lancet.* 2006;367:766–780.

Leikin JB, Mackendrick WP, Maloney GE, et al. Use of clonidine in the prevention and management of neonatal abstinence syndrome. *Clin Toxicol (Phila).* 2009;47(6):551–555.

MICROMEDEX® 2.0, Thomson Reuters Healthcare, 2012.

Monagle P, Chalmers E, Chan A, et al. Antithrombotic therapy in neonates and children: American College of Chest Physicians Evidence-Based Clinical Practice Guidelines (8th Edition). *Chest.* 2008; 133(suppl 6):S887–S968.

NeoFax 2012, A Manual of Drugs Used in Neonatal Care. 25th ed. AnnArbor, MI: Thomson Reuters; 2012.

Orenstein SR, Hassall E, Furmaga-Jablonska W, Atkinson S, Raanan M. Multicenter, double-blind, randomized, placebo-controlled trial assessing the efficacy and safety of proton pump inhibitor lansoprazole in infants with symptoms of gastroesophageal reflux disease. *J Pediatr.* 2009;154(4):514–520.e4.

Springer M. Safety and pharmacodynamics of lansoprazole in patients with gastroesophageal reflux disease aged <1 year. *Paediatr Drugs.* 2008;10(4):255–263.

Sáez-Llorens X, Macias M, Maiya P, et al. Pharmacokinetics and safety of caspofungin in neonates and infants less than 3 months of age. *Antimicrob Agents Chemother.* 2009;53(3):869–875.

Taketomo CK, Hodding JH, Kraus DM. *Pediatric and Neonatal Dosage Handbook.* 18th ed. Hudson, OH: Lexicomp; 2011.

Wagner CL, Greer FR; American Academy of Pediatrics Section on Breastfeeding; American Academy of Pediatrics Committee on Nutrition. Prevention of rickets and vitamin D deficiency in infants, children and adolescents. *Pediatrics.* 2008;122(5):1142–1152.

Zhang W, Kukulka M, Witt G, Sutkowski-Markmann D, North J, Atkinson S. Age-dependent pharmacokinetics of lansoprazole in neonates and infants. *Paediatr Drugs.* 2008;10(4):265–274.

149 Effects of Drugs and Substances on Lactation and Infants

The chapter provides some summary data on medications and substances that may be taken by the mother during pregnancy and/or breast-feeding. Regardless of the designated risk category or presumed safety, no drug or substance should be used during pregnancy and/or breast-feeding unless it is clearly needed and the potential benefits clearly outweigh the risks. The table lists the generic medication name and, in parentheses, the Food and Drug Administration (FDA) fetal risk category followed by the breast-feeding compatibility. At the present time there is no formally FDA-sanctioned breast-feeding category, and the system used here is discussed later. Lastly, any reported effects on lactation or on infant effects based on breast milk consumption are noted. The editorial board has made an attempt to summarize the data based on the best information available for an individual agent where sources disagree. These data are subject to change as new information becomes available. The reader is advised to consult the FDA (www.fda.gov) and manufacturer's web site for the latest information concerning risks of these medications.

U.S. FDA FETAL RISK CATEGORIES

CATEGORY A
Adequate studies in pregnant women have not demonstrated a risk to the fetus in the first trimester of pregnancy; there is no evidence of risk in the last two trimesters.

CATEGORY B
Animal studies have not demonstrated a risk to the fetus, but there are no adequate studies in pregnant women.

or

Animal studies have shown an adverse effect, but adequate studies in pregnant women have not demonstrated a risk to the fetus during the first trimester of pregnancy, and there is no evidence of risk in the last two trimesters.

CATEGORY C
Animal studies have shown an adverse effect on the fetus, but there are no adequate studies in humans. The benefits from the use of the drug in pregnant women may be acceptable despite its potential risks.

or

There are no animal reproduction studies and no adequate studies in humans.

CATEGORY D
There is evidence of human fetal risk, but the potential benefits from the use of the drug in pregnant women may be acceptable despite its potential risks.

CATEGORY X
Studies in animals or humans or adverse reaction reports, or both, have demonstrated fetal abnormalities. The risk of use in pregnant women clearly outweighs any possible benefit.

BREAST-FEEDING COMPATIBILITY

As noted, no formal system exists for categorizing drugs or substances and their effect on breast-feeding, lactation, and effects on the infant. The following system is used in this book:

CATEGORY (+): Generally compatible with breast-feeding.
CATEGORY (–): Avoid with breast-feeding. Toxicity can be seen.
CATEGORY (CI): Contraindicated.

Drug (FDA Fetal Risk Category/ Breast-Feeding Compatibility)	Effect on Lactation and Adverse Effects on Infant
Abacavir (C/–)	CDC recommends HIV-infected mothers to not breast-feed.
Acarbose (B/–)	No human lactation data available. Avoid breast-feeding until safety data available.
Acebutolol (B/–)	Associated with adverse effects in nursing infants.
Acetaminophen (B/+)	AAP classifies as compatible with breast-feeding.
Acetylcysteine (B/+)	No human lactation data available. Probably compatible.
Acyclovir (B/+)	AAP classifies as compatible with breast-feeding.
Adenosine (C/+)	IV drug, used in acute care situations, short half-life.
Albendazole (C/+)	Probably compatible. Low oral bioavailability suggests excretion into breast milk not clinically significant. Avoid ingestion with high-fat meal.
Albuterol (C/+)	Monitor nursing infant for agitation and spitting up. Use inhaled form to decrease maternal absorption.
Alendronate (C/+)	Probably compatible. Low plasma concentrations and rapid plasma clearance suggest minimal amounts excreted into breast milk.
Alfentanil (C/+)	Limited human lactation data available. Probably compatible.
Allopurinol (C/+)	Limited human lactation data available. Probably compatible. AAP classifies as compatible with breast-feeding.
Almotriptan (C/+)	No human lactation data available. Probably compatible. Low molecular weight of drug suggests excretion into breast milk but effect on nursing infant is unknown.
Alprazolam (D/–)	Excreted into breast milk. Because of the potent effects on neurodevelopment, probable withdrawal, lethargy, and weight loss in infant, use should be avoided during breast-feeding.
Amantadine (C/CI)	Causes release of levodopa in CNS.
Amikacin (D/+)	Low concentrations in breast milk because of poor oral absorption.
Amiloride (B/+)	Excreted into breast milk of lactating rats at higher concentrations than in blood. No human lactation data available. Probably compatible.
Amitriptyline (C/–)	Milk plasma ratio of 1.0. Use in breast-feeding may be of concern.
Amlodipine (C/+)	No human lactation data available. Low molecular weight suggests excretion into breast milk. Effects on nursing infant are unknown. Probably compatible.
Amoxapine (C/–)	Active metabolites in milk. Use in breast-feeding may be of concern.
Amoxicillin (B/+)	Monitor nursing infant for diarrhea.

Drug (FDA Fetal Risk Category/ Breast-Feeding Compatibility)	Effect on Lactation and Adverse Effects on Infant
Amphetamine (C/CI)	AAP classifies as contraindicated during breast-feeding. Monitor nursing infant for irritability and poor sleeping pattern.
Amphotericin B (B/+)	No human lactation data available. Probably compatible.
Amphotericin B lipid complex (B/+)	No human lactation data available. Probably compatible.
Ampicillin (B/+)	Monitor nursing infant for diarrhea.
Amprenavir (C/CI)	CDC recommends HIV-infected mothers to not breast-feed.
Aripiprazole (C/−)	No human lactation data available. Potential for toxicity. The low molecular weight of drug combined with the prolonged half-life and the active metabolite suggest that one or both will be excreted into breast milk. However, the extensive protein binding should limit the excretion. If mother breast-feeds while taking drug, observe nursing infant for potent CNS effects, orthostatic hypotension, seizures, dysphasia, nausea, and vomiting. Long-term evaluation is warranted.
Aspirin (C, D/−)	Use with caution. Monitor nursing infant for spitting up or bleeding. May affect platelet function. Increased risk with high doses used for rheumatoid arthritis (3–5 grams/day). Metabolic acidosis may occur.
Atazanavir (B/CI)	CDC recommends HIV-infected mothers to not breast-feed.
Atenolol (D/−)	Use with caution. Monitor nursing infant for signs of β-blockade such as bradycardia. Has been associated with significant effects in nursing infants (cyanosis and bradycardia).
Atorvastatin (X/CI)	Some excretion into breast milk is expected; therefore, the potential for adverse effects in nursing infants exists and breast-feeding should be avoided.
Atropine (C/+)	No adverse effects reported. AAP classifies as compatible with breast-feeding.
Azathioprine (D/−)	Potential for toxicity with the active metabolites of the drug.
Azithromycin (B/+)	Accumulates in breast milk. Limited human lactation data available. Probably compatible.
Aztreonam (B/+)	Excreted into breast milk in low amounts, and with the acidic nature of the drug and low lipid solubility, oral absorption is poor. Systemic effects in nursing infants are unlikely.
Bacitracin (C/+)	No human lactation data available. Topical use compatible.
Baclofen (C/+)	Limited human lactation data available. AAP classifies as compatible with breast-feeding.
Beclomethasone (C/+)	Limited human lactation data available. Probably compatible. May be excreted into breast milk.
Belladonna (C/+)	No human lactation data available. Probably compatible.
Benazepril (C 1st tri; D 2nd, 3rd tri/+)	No human lactation data available. Probably compatible. Other ACE inhibitors are excreted into breast milk in low amounts with no adverse effects on nursing infants.
Benztropine (C/−)	No human lactation data available. Probably compatible.
Betamethasone (C, D/+)	No human lactation data available. Molecular weight suggests excretion into breast milk. Probably compatible.
Bethanechol (C/−)	Limited human lactation data available. Low molecular weight suggests excretion into breast milk. Abdominal pain and diarrhea reported in nursing infant exposed to bethanechol.

(Continued)

Drug (FDA Fetal Risk Category/ Breast-Feeding Compatibility)	Effect on Lactation and Adverse Effects on Infant
Bisacodyl (C/+)	No human lactation data available. Although molecular weight is low enough for excretion into breast milk, only minimal amounts are absorbed into maternal circulation. Therefore, effects on nursing infant would be negligible.
Bismuth subsalicylate (C/–)	Use with caution because of potential for adverse effects from salicylates. Should be avoided.
Bisoprolol (C/–)	No human lactation data available. Excreted into milk of lactating rats. If used during breast-feeding, nursing infant should be observed for hypotension, bradycardia, and other signs and symptoms of β-blockade.
Botulinum toxin type A (C/+)	No human lactation data available. Probably compatible. Toxin not expected to appear in circulation and therefore will not appear in breast milk.
Brompheniramine (C/+)	Monitor nursing infant for agitation, poor sleeping pattern, and feeding problems. Probably compatible.
Budesonide (oral/inhaler/nasal) (B, inhaler; C, oral/+)	Systemic bioavailability of inhaled budesonide is low, so the actual amount in breast milk may also be low. Oral potency is 25 times more glucocorticoid activity than hydrocortisone; however, the clinical significance is unknown. Manufacturer suggests that mother who must use the PulmicortTurbuhaler stop breast-feeding.
Bumetanide (C/+)	No human lactation data available. Probably compatible. Diuretics may suppress lactation.
Buprenorphine (C/–)	Excreted into breast milk. May suppress milk production and result in lower amounts of weight gain in nursing infant. Mothers should avoid breast-feeding if taking buprenorphine.
Bupropion (B/–)	Excreted into breast milk. Effect on nursing infant is unknown but may be of concern.
Buspirone (B/–)	Limited human lactation data available. Potential toxicity exists. Buspirone and its metabolites are excreted into the milk of lactating rats. Potential exists for CNS impairment in nursing infant. May be of concern because of effects on the developing brain that may not be known until later in life.
Butorphanol (C/+)	Limited human lactation data available. Probably compatible. Excreted into breast milk at levels that are probably not clinically significant.
Caffeine (B/+)	Monitor nursing infant for irritability and poor sleeping pattern. No effect with moderate intake (2–3 cups/day).
Calcitonin—salmon (C/+)	May inhibit lactation.
Calcitriol (C/+)	High-dose supplementation in mothers can lead to elevated levels of vitamin D_2 in breast milk and subsequently lead to hypercalcemia in breast-fed infants. Caution is advised.
Candesartan (C 1st tri; D 2nd, 3rd tri/+)	No human lactation data available. Low molecular weight suggests that drug would be excreted into breast milk. Effects on nursing infant unknown.
Captopril (C 1st tri; D 2nd, 3rd tri/+)	Excreted into breast milk in low concentrations. Available data showed no effects on nursing infants. AAP classifies as compatible with breast-feeding.
Carbamazepine (D/+)	Risk of bone marrow suppression if taken chronically.

(Continued)

Drug (FDA Fetal Risk Category/ Breast-Feeding Compatibility)	Effect on Lactation and Adverse Effects on Infant
Carisoprodol (C/+)	Limited human lactation data available. Probably compatible. Observe nursing infant for sedation and other behavioral changes.
Carvedilol (C/−)	No human lactation data available. Excreted into milk of lactating rats. If used during breast-feeding, nursing infant should be observed for hypotension, bradycardia, and other signs and symptoms of β-blockade.
Casanthranol (C/+)	Limited human lactation data available. Probably compatible. Observe nursing infant for diarrhea.
Cascara sagrada (C/+)	Limited human lactation data available. Probably compatible. Observe nursing infant for diarrhea.
Cefaclor (B/+)	Excreted into breast milk in low concentrations. The bowel flora of nursing infants may be altered and there is the potential for interference with the interpretation of an infectious workup. Observe nursing infants for possible allergic reaction. Compatible with breast-feeding.
Cefadroxil (B/+)	Excreted into breast milk in low concentrations. The bowel flora of nursing infants may be altered and there is the potential for interference with the interpretation of an infectious workup. Observe nursing infants for possible allergic reaction. Compatible with breast-feeding.
Cefazolin (B/+)	Excreted into breast milk in low concentrations. The bowel flora of nursing infants may be altered and there is the potential for interference with the interpretation of an infectious workup. Observe nursing infants for possible allergic reaction. Compatible with breast-feeding.
Cefdinir (B/+)	Probably excreted into breast milk in low concentrations. The bowel flora of nursing infants may be altered and there is the potential for interference with the interpretation of an infectious workup. Observe nursing infants for possible allergic reaction. Compatible with breast-feeding.
Cefepime (B/+)	Excreted into breast milk in low concentrations. The bowel flora of nursing infants may be altered and there is the potential for interference with the interpretation of an infectious workup. Observe nursing infants for possible allergic reaction. Compatible with breast-feeding.
Cefixime (B/+)	Probably excreted into breast milk in low concentrations. The bowel flora of nursing infants may be altered and there is the potential for interference with the interpretation of an infectious workup. Observe nursing infants for possible allergic reaction. Compatible with breast-feeding.
Cefotaxime (B/+)	Excreted into breast milk in low concentrations. The bowel flora of nursing infants may be altered and there is the potential for interference with the interpretation of an infectious workup. Observe nursing infants for possible allergic reaction. Compatible with breast-feeding.
Cefotetan (B/+)	Excreted into breast milk in low concentrations. The bowel flora of nursing infants may be altered and there is the potential for interference with the interpretation of an infectious workup. Observe nursing infants for possible allergic reaction. Compatible with breast-feeding.

(*Continued*)

Drug (FDA Fetal Risk Category/ Breast-Feeding Compatibility)	Effect on Lactation and Adverse Effects on Infant
Cefoxitin (B/+)	Excreted into breast milk in low concentrations. The bowel flora of nursing infants may be altered and there is the potential for interference with the interpretation of an infectious workup. Observe nursing infants for possible allergic reaction. Compatible with breast-feeding.
Ceftazidime (B/+)	Excreted into breast milk in low concentrations. The bowel flora of nursing infants may be altered and there is the potential for interference with the interpretation of an infectious workup. Observe nursing infants for possible allergic reaction. Compatible with breast-feeding.
Ceftriaxone (B/+)	Excreted into breast milk in low concentrations. The bowel flora of nursing infants may be altered and there is the potential for interference with the interpretation of an infectious workup. Observe nursing infants for possible allergic reaction. Compatible with breast-feeding.
Cefuroxime (B/+)	Excreted into breast milk in low concentrations. The bowel flora of nursing infants may be altered and there is the potential for interference with the interpretation of an infectious workup. Observe nursing infants for possible allergic reaction. Compatible with breast-feeding.
Celecoxib (C/−)	Excreted into breast milk. Safest course of action is to avoid use during breast-feeding.
Cephalexin (B/+)	Excreted into breast milk in low concentrations. The bowel flora of nursing infants may be altered and there is the potential for interference with the interpretation of an infectious workup. Observe nursing infants for possible allergic reaction. Compatible with breast-feeding.
Cerivastatin (X/CI)	Excreted into breast milk. Because of potential for adverse effects, avoid use if breast-feeding.
Cetirizine (B/+)	Manufacturer states drug excreted into breast milk. Effects on nursing infant unknown but observe for sedation.
Chloral hydrate (C/+)	Monitor nursing infant for sedation and rash.
Chlordiazepoxide (D/−)	No human lactation data available. Low molecular weight suggests excretion into breast milk should be expected. Other benzodiazepines have produced adverse effects in nursing infants. Use should be avoided during breast-feeding.
Chlorhexidine (B/+)	No reports of excretion into breast milk available. Rinse nipples if chlorhexidine is used to cleanse them. Compatible with breast-feeding.
Chloroquine (C/+)	Insufficient amounts excreted in breast milk to provide adequate protection against malaria.
Chlorothiazide (C/+)	May suppress lactation, especially in the first month of lactation. Adverse effects have not been reported, but infant's electrolytes and platelets should be monitored.
Chlorpromazine (C/−)	Excreted into breast milk in low amounts. Observe nursing infant for sedation. AAP classifies it as a drug that is a concern for nursing infants because of drowsiness and lethargy and because of galactorrhea induced in adults.
Chlorpheniramine (B/+)	Monitor nursing infant for agitation, poor sleeping pattern, and feeding problems.

(Continued)

Drug (FDA Fetal Risk Category/ Breast-Feeding Compatibility)	Effect on Lactation and Adverse Effects on Infant
Cholecalciferol (C, D/+)	Compatible with breast-feeding. Excreted into breast milk in limited amounts. The Committee on Nutrition of the AAP recommends vitamin D supplementation in breast-fed infants if maternal intake is low or exposure to ultraviolet light is insufficient. Monitor serum calcium levels of nursing infant if mother is taking pharmacologic doses of vitamin D.
Cholestyramine (B/+)	Nonabsorbable resin. No human lactation data available. Drug binds fat-soluble vitamins, and prolonged use may result in deficiencies of these vitamins in mother and nursing infant.
Cimetidine (B/+)	Use with caution. May suppress gastric acidity in infant, inhibit drug metabolism, and cause CNS stimulation.
Ciprofloxacin (C/+)	Data are limited and the amount of drug in breast milk does not appear to represent significant risk to nursing infant. AAP classifies as compatible with breast-feeding. However, the manufacturer recommends that mother should wait 48 hours after last dose before breast-feeding.
Citalopram (C/–)	Doses >20 mg/day or concurrent use of other sedative agents may increase risk of adverse effects to nursing infants. Observe for toxicity. Long-term effects on neurobehavioral development are unknown. Avoid nursing around peak maternal concentrations—about 4 hours after a dose.
Clarithromycin (C/+)	No human lactation data available. Passage of drug into breast milk should be expected. Based on experience with other antibiotics such as erythromycin, risk to nursing infant is probably minimal.
Clavulanate (B/+)	No human lactation data available. Molecular weight suggests excretion into breast milk. Effects of β-lactamase inhibitors on nursing infants are unknown.
Clindamycin (B/+)	Excreted into breast milk. The bowel flora of nursing infants may be altered and there is the potential for interference with the interpretation of an infectious workup. Observe nursing infants for possible allergic reaction. AAP classifies as compatible with breast-feeding.
Clonazepam (D/–)	Monitor nursing infant for respiratory and CNS depression.
Clonidine (C/+)	Excreted in breast milk. Hypotension was not observed in nursing infants, although clonidine was found in the serum of these nursing infants. Long-term significance of this exposure is unknown.
Clopidogrel (B/+)	No human lactation data available. Low molecular weight suggests excretion into breast milk. Effects on nursing infants are unknown.
Clotrimazole (B/+)	Absorption from skin and vagina is minimal. Unlikely that the levels of this antifungal agent appear in breast milk.
Clozapine (B/–)	Concentrated in breast milk. Avoid breast-feeding.
Cocaine (C/CI)	Causes cocaine intoxication in infant from maternal intranasal use (hypertension, tachycardia, mydriasis, and apnea) and from topical use on mother's nipples (apnea and seizures).

(Continued)

Drug (FDA Fetal Risk Category/ Breast-Feeding Compatibility)	Effect on Lactation and Adverse Effects on Infant
Codeine (C, D/−)	Short-term therapy (1 or 2 days) with close monitoring is compatible; however, long-term therapy is not compatible with breast-feeding. Monitor nursing infant for sedation. Milk ejection reflex (letdown) may be inhibited.
Colchicine (D/+)	Excreted into breast milk. No adverse effects on nursing infants have been observed. Waiting 8–12 hours after dose to breast-feed minimizes exposure of nursing infant.
Cortisone (C, D/+)	No reports of the excretion of exogenous cortisone into human milk. Unlikely that it poses risk to nursing infant. Compatible with breast-feeding.
Cromolyn sodium (B/+)	No human lactation data available.
Cyclobenzaprine (B/−)	No reports of excretion into breast milk available. Low molecular weight suggests excretion should occur.
Dactinomycin (C/−)	No human lactation data available. Despite the high molecular weight, women receiving the drug should avoid breast-feeding because of the potential risk of severe adverse effects.
Dalteparin (B/+)	No human lactation data available. Based on the molecular weight and because the drug would be inactivated in the GI tract, the risk to the nursing infant would be negligible.
Darbepoetin alfa (C/+)	No human lactation data available. Passage into breast milk is not expected. Risk to nursing infant appears to be negligible.
Deferasirox (B/−)	No human lactation data available. Molecular weight and long elimination half-life suggest excretion into breast milk. Amount of oral absorption in infants unknown; in adults oral bioavailability is 70%. With the potential to deplete infant's iron stores, breast-feeding should be avoided during therapy.
Deferoxamine (C/+)	No human lactation data available. Molecular weight is low enough for some excretion into breast milk to be expected. Effects, if any, on nursing infant are unknown.
Delavirdine (C/CI)	No human lactation data available. Molecular weight suggests excretion into breast milk should be expected. Effect on nursing infant is unknown. CDC recommends HIV-infected mothers in developed countries to not breast-feed.
Desloratadine (C/+)	No human lactation data available. Desloratadine and loratadine are excreted into breast milk. Probably compatible.
Dexamethasone (C, D/+)	No human lactation data available. Excretion into breast milk should be expected. Probably compatible.
Dextroamphetamine (C/−)	May cause infant stimulation.
Dextromethorphan (C/+)	No human lactation data available. Low molecular weight suggests excretion into breast milk. Probably compatible. Use alcohol-free preparation.
Diatrizoate (C/+)	In one study, not detected in breast milk. Probably compatible.
Diazepam (D/−)	May cause infant sedation. May accumulate in breast-fed infants.
Diclofenac (B/+)	No human lactation data available. Manufacturer states that drug excreted into breast milk. Short half-life in adults. Probably compatible.

(Continued)

Drug (FDA Fetal Risk Category/ Breast-Feeding Compatibility)	Effect on Lactation and Adverse Effects on Infant
Dicloxacillin (B/+)	No human lactation data. However, other penicillins are excreted into breast milk in low concentrations. Adverse effects rare. The bowel flora of nursing infants may be altered and there is the potential for interference with the interpretation of an infectious workup. Observe nursing infants for possible allergic reaction.
Didanosine (B/CI)	No human lactation data available. Molecular weight suggests excretion into breast milk should be expected. Effect on nursing infant is unknown. CDC recommends HIV-infected mothers in developed countries to not breast-feed.
Diethylstilbestrol (DES) (X/CI)	No human lactation data available. Possible decreased milk volume and decreased nitrogen and protein content could occur.
Digoxin (C/+)	Excreted into breast milk in small amounts. Monitor nursing infant for spitting up, diarrhea, and heart rate changes. Compatible with breast-feeding.
Dihydroergotamine (X/CI)	No human lactation data available. Molecular weight and long half-life suggests excretion into breast milk, but high protein binding will limit this. Concern for symptoms of ergotism—vomiting, diarrhea, and convulsions in nursing infants. Breast-feeding is contraindicated.
Diltiazem (C/+)	Excreted into breast milk. Two nursing infants were not affected. Probably compatible.
Dimenhydrinate (B/+)	No human lactation data available. Molecular weight suggests excretion into breast milk should be expected. Probably compatible. Caution—newborns and premature infants have increased sensitivity to antihistamines.
Diphenhydramine (B/+)	Excreted into breast milk but levels are thought not to be in sufficiently high amounts to affect nursing infant. Monitor nursing infant for agitation, poor sleeping pattern, and feeding problems. Probably compatible.
Diphenoxylate (C/–)	Active metabolite probably excreted into breast milk. Potential toxicity.
Dipyridamole (B/+)	Excreted into breast milk. Effect unknown on nursing infant. Probably compatible.
Diphtheria and tetanus vaccine (C/+)	No human lactation data. Probably compatible.
Docusate (calcium, potassium, sodium) (C/+)	Probably compatible. Monitor nursing infant for diarrhea.
Dolasetron (B/+)	No human lactation data available. Low molecular weight of drug suggests excretion into breast milk should be expected. Effects on nursing infant are unknown.
Dornase alfa (B/+)	No human lactation data available. Inhaled drug does not increase endogenous serum concentration of drug. Not expected to be excreted into breast milk. Negligible risk to nursing infant.
Doxycycline (D/+)	Excreted into breast milk in low concentrations. Theoretical dental staining and inhibition of bone growth is remote. The bowel flora of nursing infants may be altered and there is the potential for interference with the interpretation of an infectious workup. Observe nursing infants for possible allergic reaction. AAP classifies as compatible with breast-feeding.

(Continued)

Drug (FDA Fetal Risk Category/ Breast-Feeding Compatibility)	Effect on Lactation and Adverse Effects on Infant
Echinacea (C/–)	Avoid use during breast-feeding.
Efavirenz (C/CI)	No human lactation data available. Molecular weight suggests excretion into breast milk should be expected. Effect on nursing infant is unknown. CDC recommends HIV-infected mothers in developed countries to not breast-feed.
Eletriptan (C/+)	Excreted into breast milk. Effects of exposure to nursing infants are unknown but low concentration not thought to be significant. Compatible with breast-feeding.
Emtricitabine (B/CI)	No human lactation data available. Molecular weight, low plasma protein binding, and long half-life suggest excretion into breast milk should be expected. Effect on nursing infant is unknown. CDC recommends HIV-infected mothers in developed countries to not breast-feed.
Enalapril (C 1st tri; D 2nd, 3rd tri/+)	Enalapril and enalaprilat are excreted into breast milk in small amounts such that risk to nursing infant appears negligible/ clinically insignificant. AAP classifies as compatible with breast-feeding.
Enfuvirtide (B/CI)	No human lactation data available. Molecular weight and high plasma protein binding should inhibit but not prevent excretion into breast milk. Effect on nursing infant is unknown. CDC recommends HIV-infected mothers in developed countries to not breast-feed.
Enoxaparin (B/+)	No human lactation data available. Based on high molecular weight and probable inactivation by GI tract, the passage of drug into breast milk and its risk to nursing infant is considered negligible.
Entecavir (C/CI HIV; C/+ hepatitis B)	No human lactation data available. Molecular weight and half-life suggest drug should be excreted into breast milk. Effects on nursing infants are unknown. Infants of HBsAg-positive or HBeAg-positive mothers should receive HBIG at birth and hepatitis B vaccine soon after birth. Then breast-feeding is permitted. Breast-feeding is contraindicated in HIV-1–positive mothers in the United States.
Ephedrine (C/–)	Limited human lactation data available. Observe nursing infant for irritability, excessive crying, and disturbed sleeping patterns. Avoiding breast-feeding is recommended.
Epoetin alfa (C/+)	No human lactation data available. Excretion into breast milk is not expected and drug would be digested in GI tract. No risk to nursing infant expected.
Epoprostenol (B/+)	No human lactation data available. Based on its rapid degradation, a physiologic pH, and the GI tract, amount of drug nursing infant exposed to would not be clinically significant.
Eprosartan (C 1st tri; D 2nd, 3rd tri/+)	No human lactation data available. Expect excretion into breast milk. Effects on nursing infant are unknown. AAP classifies ACE inhibitors, a similar class of agents, compatible with breast-feeding.
Ergotamine (X/CI)	Causes vomiting, diarrhea, and convulsions in the nursing infant. May hinder lactation. Breast-feeding is contraindicated.

(*Continued*)

Drug (FDA Fetal Risk Category/ Breast-Feeding Compatibility)	Effect on Lactation and Adverse Effects on Infant
Ertapenem (B/+)	Excreted into breast milk in low concentrations. Effects on nursing infant unknown but probably are not clinically significant. The bowel flora of nursing infants may be altered and there is the potential for interference with the interpretation of an infectious workup. Observe nursing infants for possible allergic reaction. Compatible with breast-feeding.
Erythromycin (B/+)	Excreted into breast milk in low concentrations. No reports of adverse effects in nursing infants. The bowel flora of nursing infants may be altered and there is the potential for interference with the interpretation of an infectious workup. Observe nursing infants for possible allergic reaction. Compatible with breast-feeding.
Escitalopram (C/−)	No human lactation data available. Expect excretion into breast milk. Effects on nursing infant unknown. Adverse effects have been seen with similar agent (citalopram), expect similar effects. Closely monitor nursing infants. AAP classifies other SSRIs as drugs for which effect on nursing infants is unknown but may be of concern.
Esomeprazole (B/−)	No human lactation data available. Expect excretion into breast milk. Effects on nursing infant unknown. Potential for toxic effects: headache, diarrhea and abdominal pain, suppression of gastric acid secretion. Half-life is short, 1–1.5 hours. Waiting 5–7.5 hours after dose should eliminate 97% of drug from plasma.
Estrogens, conjugated (X/+)	No adverse effects in nursing infants reported. May decrease milk volume, and nitrogen and protein content.
Ethambutol (B/+)	Excreted into breast milk. AAP classifies as compatible with breast-feeding.
Ethanol (D, X/−)	Passes freely into breast milk in levels similar to those in maternal serum. Because of risk of toxicity in nursing infant, safest course is to hold breast-feeding for 1–2 hours for each ounce of alcohol consumed.
Ethinyl estradiol (X/+)	No adverse effects in nursing infants reported. May decrease milk volume, and nitrogen and protein content. Monitor weight gain of infant and use lowest dose.
Famciclovir (B/−)	No human lactation data available. Expect excretion into breast milk. Avoid breast-feeding.
Famotidine (B/+)	Excreted into breast milk but to lesser extent than cimetidine and ranitidine. Effects on nursing infant are unknown. Potential risk for adverse effects; however, AAP classifies cimetidine as compatible with breast-feeding. Famotidine may be preferred because of lesser amount in breast milk.
Flecainide (C/+)	Excreted into breast milk but effects on nursing infant are unknown. Probably not toxic. AAP classifies as compatible with breast-feeding.
Fluconazole (C/+)	Excreted into breast milk. No drug-associated toxicity has been reported. AAP classifies as compatible with breast-feeding.
Flucytosine (C/−)	No human lactation data available. Because of potential serious adverse effects in nursing infant, breast-feeding should be avoided.

(*Continued*)

Drug (FDA Fetal Risk Category/ Breast-Feeding Compatibility)	Effect on Lactation and Adverse Effects on Infant
Fluoxetine (C/−)	Long-term effects on neurobehavioral development from exposure to potent serotonin reuptake blocker during period of rapid CNS development have not been adequately studied. Manufacturer recommends breast-feeding should be avoided during fluoxetine therapy. AAP classifies as effects on nursing infant unknown but may be of concern. Maternal benefits may outweigh risks to nursing infant if treating postpartum depression. Colic, irritability, sleep disorders, and poor weight gain may occur.
Fondaparinux (B/+)	No human lactation data available. Excretion into breast milk should be expected. Effects on nursing infants unknown but not thought to be clinically significant.
Fosamprenavir (C/CI)	No human lactation data available. Molecular weight suggests excretion into breast milk should be expected. Effect on nursing infant is unknown. CDC recommends HIV-infected mothers in developed countries to not breast-feed.
Furosemide (C/+)	Excreted into breast milk. No reports of adverse effects in a nursing infant.
Gabapentin (C/+)	No human lactation data available. Probably compatible. Low molecular weight of drug suggests excretion into breast milk but effect on nursing infant is unknown.
Gadopentetate dimeglumine (MRI contrast) (C/+)	Excreted into breast milk in small amounts. Very little is absorbed systemically. AAP classifies as compatible with breast-feeding.
Ganciclovir (C/−)	No human lactation data available. Potential for serious toxicity in nursing infant. Avoid breast-feeding.
Gentamicin (C/+)	Small amounts excreted into breast milk and absorbed by nursing infants. Observe infant for bloody stools and diarrhea. AAP classifies as compatible with breast-feeding.
Ginkgo biloba (C/−)	No human lactation data available. Herbal product that is not standardized and may contain other compounds. Safest course is to avoid breast-feeding.
Ginseng (B/−)	No human lactation data available. Herbal product that is not standardized and may contain other compounds. Safest course is to avoid breast-feeding.
Glimepiride (C/+)	No human lactation data available. Molecular weight suggests excretion into breast milk should be expected. Risk of neonatal hypoglycemia. Breast-feeding women should consider insulin.
Glipizide (C/+)	Minimal to nondetectable levels in breast milk. Normal glucose levels in nursing infants.
Glucosamine (C/+)	No human lactation data available. Molecular weight and prolonged plasma protein elimination half-life suggest excretion into breast milk should be expected. Unbound drug is undetectable in plasma; therefore, little if any drug will be excreted into milk. Probably compatible.
Glyburide (C/+)	Nondetectable levels in breast milk. Normal glucose levels in nursing infants. Probably compatible.
Guaifenesin (C/+)	No human lactation data available. Probably compatible.
Haemophilus b conjugate vaccine (C/+)	Compatible with breast-feeding.

(Continued)

Drug (FDA Fetal Risk Category/ Breast-Feeding Compatibility)	Effect on Lactation and Adverse Effects on Infant
Haloperidol (C/–)	Excreted into breast milk. Use may be of concern. Effects on nursing infant unknown. Possible decline in developmental score.
Heparin (C/+)	Not excreted into breast milk.
Hepatitis A vaccine (C/+)	No human lactation data available. Probably compatible.
Hepatitis B vaccine (C/+)	No human lactation data available. Probably compatible.
Heroin (B, D/CI)	Crosses into breast milk in sufficient amounts to cause addiction in nursing infant. Breast-feeding is contraindicated.
Human papillomavirus vaccine (B/+)	Compatible with breast-feeding.
Hydralazine (C/+)	Excreted into breast milk. No adverse effects noted in nursing infants. AAP classifies as compatible with breast-feeding.
Hydrochlorothiazide (B/+)	May suppress lactation, especially in the first month of lactation. Adverse effects have not been reported, but infant's electrolytes and platelets should be monitored.
Hydrocodone (C, D/+)	No human lactation data available. Molecular weight suggests excretion into breast milk should be expected. Observe nursing infant for GI effects, sedation, and changes in feeding patterns.
Hydrocortisone (C, D/+)	No human lactation data available. Unlikely that it poses risk to nursing infant. Compatible with breast-feeding.
Hydromorphone (B, D/+)	Excreted into breast milk. Monitor nursing infant for sedation. Milk ejection reflex (letdown) may be inhibited.
Hydroxychloroquine (C/+)	Excreted into breast milk. Slow elimination rate. Breast-feeding during daily therapy should be done with caution. Once-weekly doses significantly reduce amount of drug exposure to nursing infant. AAP classifies as compatible with breast-feeding. Amount in breast milk is not adequate to provide malaria protection for infant.
Hydroxyzine (C/+)	No human lactation data available. Molecular weight suggests excretion into breast milk should be expected. Effects on nursing infant unknown.
Ibuprofen (B/+)	Excreted into breast milk. Amount of drug available to nursing infant is minimal. AAP classifies as compatible with breast-feeding.
Imipenem-cilastatin (C/+)	Small amounts excreted into breast milk in amounts comparable to other β-lactam antibiotics. Effects on nursing infant are unknown.
Indinavir (C/CI)	No human lactation data available. Molecular weight suggests excretion into breast milk should be expected. Effect on nursing infant is unknown. CDC recommends HIV-infected mothers in developed countries to not breast-feed.
Indomethacin (B, D/+)	Excreted into breast milk. One case report of seizure in nursing infant. AAP classifies as compatible with breast-feeding.
Influenza vaccine (C/+)	Maternal vaccination is compatible with breast-feeding.
Iodine (D/+)	May cause goiter.
Isoniazid (C/+)	Isoniazid and its metabolite are excreted into breast milk. Monitor nursing infant for signs and symptoms of peripheral neuritis or hepatitis. AAP classifies as compatible with breast-feeding.

(Continued)

Drug (FDA Fetal Risk Category/ Breast-Feeding Compatibility)	Effect on Lactation and Adverse Effects on Infant
Ivermectin (C/+)	Excreted into breast milk but no human lactation data available. Low drug levels in milk probably not a risk to nursing infant. AAP classifies as compatible with breast-feeding.
Kaolin/pectin (C/+)	No effect on nursing infant.
Ketamine (B/+)	Should be undetectable in maternal plasma ~11 hours after dose. Breast-feeding after this time should not expose the nursing infant to drug.
Ketoconazole (C/+)	Excreted into breast milk. Effects of exposure to nursing infants are unknown but not thought to be significant. AAP classifies as compatible with breast-feeding.
Ketorolac (C; D if used in 3rd tri or near delivery/+)	Excreted into breast milk in amounts that are considered clinically insignificant. AAP classifies as compatible with breast-feeding.
Labetalol (C/+)	Monitor nursing infant for hypotension and bradycardia.
Lactulose (B/+)	No human lactation data. Probably compatible.
Lamivudine (C/CI)	Excreted into breast milk. Effect on nursing infant is unknown. CDC recommends HIV-infected mothers in developed countries to not breast-feed.
Lamotrigine (C/−)	May be of concern. Consider monitoring infant's serum lamotrigine concentration.
Lansoprazole (B/−)	No human lactation data available. Excretion into breast milk is expected. Potential effects on nursing infant—carcinogenicity (animal data) and suppression of gastric acid secretion. Avoid breast-feeding.
Levetiracetam (C/+)	No human lactation data available. Low molecular weight and protein binding suggest excretion into breast milk should be expected. Effects on nursing infant are unknown. AAP classifies as compatible with breast-feeding.
Levofloxacin (C/+)	Excreted into breast milk. Effects on nursing infants are unknown. AAP classifies as compatible with breast-feeding.
Levothyroxine (A/+)	Probably does not interfere with neonatal thyroid screening.
Lindane (B/+)	No human lactation data available. Excreted into breast milk. Small amounts ingested by nursing infant are probably clinically insignificant. Waiting 4 days after discontinuing lotion should prevent exposure to nursing infant.
Linezolid (C/−)	No human lactation data available. Excretion into breast milk is expected. Effects on nursing infant unknown. Potential effects—myelosuppression and reversible thrombocytopenia. Avoid breast-feeding.
Lisinopril (C 1st tri; D 2nd, 3rd tri/+)	No human lactation data available. Excretion into breast milk should be expected. AAP classifies as compatible with breast-feeding.
Lithium (D/−)	Milk levels average 40% of maternal serum concentration. Monitor nursing infant for cyanosis, hypotonia, bradycardia, and other lithium toxicities.
Loperamide (B/+)	No human lactation data available. AAP classifies as compatible with breast-feeding.

(Continued)

Drug (FDA Fetal Risk Category/ Breast-Feeding Compatibility)	Effect on Lactation and Adverse Effects on Infant
Lopinavir (C/CI)	No human lactation data available. Molecular weight and lipid solubility suggest excretion into breast milk should be expected; however, extensive plasma protein binding should limit this. Effect on nursing infant is unknown. CDC recommends HIV-infected mothers in developed countries to not breast-feed.
Loratadine (B/+)	Loratadine and its metabolite are excreted into breast milk. Probably little clinical risk to nursing infant. AAP classifies as compatible with breast-feeding.
Lorazepam (D/−)	Monitor nursing infant for sedation, especially if exposure is prolonged.
Losartan (C 1st tri; D 2nd, 3rd tri/+)	No human lactation data available. Excretion into breast milk is expected. Effects of exposure to nursing infant are unknown. AAP considers compatible with breast-feeding.
Measles vaccine (X, C/+)	Compatible with breast-feeding.
Meclizine (B/+)	No human lactation data available. Molecular weight suggests excretion into breast milk should be expected. Probably compatible. Caution—newborns and premature infants have increased sensitivity to antihistamines.
Medroxyprogesterone (D/+)	AAP classifies as compatible with breast-feeding.
Meningococcal vaccine (C/+)	No human lactation data. Probably compatible.
Meperidine (B, D/+)	Monitor nursing infant for sedation. Milk ejection reflex (letdown) may be inhibited. AAP classifies as compatible with breast-feeding.
Meropenem (B/+)	No human lactation data available. Expect excretion into breast milk. Potential effects on nursing infant are unknown.
Mesalamine (B/−)	Small amount excreted into breast milk. Risk of adverse effect (diarrhea) in nursing infant. AAP classifies as drug that should be used with caution during breast-feeding.
Metformin (B/+)	Excreted into breast milk. Nursing infants had normal blood glucose levels.
Methadone (B, D/+)	Generally compatible with breast-feeding. Monitor nursing infant for sedation, depression, and withdrawal on cessation of methadone treatment. AAP classifies as compatible with breast-feeding.
Methamphetamine (C/CI)	AAP classifies amphetamines as contraindicated during breast-feeding. Monitor nursing infant for irritability and poor sleeping pattern.
Methimazole (D/+)	Potential for interfering with thyroid function.
Methocarbamol (C/+)	Any amounts of drug excreted into breast milk probably not clinically significant.
Methyldopa (B/+)	Risk of hemolysis and increased liver enzymes.
Methylphenidate (C/−)	Excreted into breast milk. Potential toxicity will probably occur in 1st month of life. Observe nursing infant for signs and symptoms of CNS stimulation—decreased appetite, insomnia, and irritability.
Metoclopramide (B/−)	Increases milk production. Effects on nursing infant unknown but may be of concern because it is a dopaminergic-blocking agent.

(Continued)

Drug (FDA Fetal Risk Category/ Breast-Feeding Compatibility)	Effect on Lactation and Adverse Effects on Infant
Metolazone (B/+)	May suppress lactation, especially in the first month of lactation. Adverse effects have not been reported but infant's electrolytes and platelets should be monitored.
Metoprolol (C/−)	Monitor nursing infant for bradycardia and hypotension.
Metronidazole (B/−)	Discontinue during breast-feeding. Do not nurse until 12–24 hours after discontinuing to allow excretion of drug.
Minocycline (D/+)	Excreted into breast milk in low concentrations. Theoretical dental staining and inhibition of bone growth are remote. The bowel flora of nursing infants may be altered and there is the potential for interference with the interpretation of an infectious workup. Observe nursing infants for possible allergic reaction. Compatible with breast-feeding.
Mirtazapine (C/−)	Excreted into breast milk. Long-term effects on neurobehavioral development unknown. AAP classifies other antidepressants as drugs for which effect on nursing infant is unknown but may be of concern.
Montelukast (B/+)	Monitor nursing infant for sedation. Milk ejection reflex (letdown) may be inhibited.
Morphine (C/+)	Excreted into breast milk. AAP classifies as compatible with breast-feeding. Long-term effects on neurobehavioral development are unknown.
Mumps vaccine (C/+)	No human lactation data. Probably compatible.
Nafcillin (B/+)	No human lactation data. Refer to Penicillin.
Nalbuphine (B/+)	No human lactation data available. Expect small amount of drug to be excreted into breast milk. Amounts are clinically insignificant.
Nalorphine (D/+)	No human lactation data available.
Naloxone (B/+)	No human lactation data available.
Naltrexone (C/−)	No human lactation data available. Expect excretion into breast milk. Effects on nursing infant are unknown. Potential adverse effects of drug—alteration of opioid receptors in the brain; altered levels of some hormones of hypothalamic, pituitary, adrenal, and gonadal origin.
Naproxen (B/+)	Passes into breast milk in very small quantities. Effects on nursing infant are unknown. AAP classifies as compatible with breast-feeding.
Naratriptan (C/+)	No human lactation data available. Excretion into breast milk should be expected. Effects on nursing infant are unknown.
Nelfinavir (B/CI)	No human lactation data available. Molecular weight suggests excretion into breast milk should be expected. Effect on nursing infant is unknown. CDC recommends HIV-infected mothers in developed countries to not breast-feed.
Nevirapine (C/CI)	Excreted into breast milk. CDC recommends HIV-infected mothers in developed countries to not breast-feed.
Nicotine (transdermal, others) (D/−)	May be of concern. Excessive amounts may cause diarrhea, vomiting, tachycardia, irritability, decreased milk production, and decreased weight gain.
Nifedipine (C/+)	Manufacturer states significant amounts of drug excreted into breast milk. No human lactation data available.

(Continued)

Drug (FDA Fetal Risk Category/ Breast-Feeding Compatibility)	Effect on Lactation and Adverse Effects on Infant
Nitrofurantoin (B/+)	Excreted in breast milk in small amounts. Monitor nursing infants with G6PD deficiency for hemolytic anemia.
Nortriptyline (C/−)	Excreted into breast milk in low concentrations. No adverse effects noted in breast-feeding infants. Long-term effects of chronic exposure to antidepressants in nursing infants are unknown with concern for effects on the infant's neurobehavioral development. AAP classifies as drug for which effect on nursing infant is unknown but may be of concern.
Nystatin (C/+)	Poorly absorbed if at all. Excretion into breast milk would not occur.
Olanzapine (C/−)	Sedation has occurred in nursing infants. Decreasing dose may eliminate this problem but may affect control of mother's disease. Avoid use during breast-feeding.
Olsalazine (C/−)	Active metabolite, 5-aminosalicylic acid (mesalamine), is excreted into human milk. Diarrhea reported in nursing infant of mother receiving mesalamine.
Omeprazole (C/−)	Limited human lactation data available. Excretion into breast milk is expected. Effects on nursing infant are unknown. Use during breast-feeding should be avoided. Concern for suppression of gastric acid secretion and carcinogenicity observed in animals.
Ondansetron (B/+)	No human lactation data available. Expect excretion into breast milk. Effects on nursing infant are unknown.
Oral contraceptives (all classes) (X/+)	Causes dose-dependent suppression of lactation. Decreased weight gain, milk production, and nitrogen and protein content of human milk have been associated with this drug. Changes probably only significant in malnourished mothers. Use lowest dose possible. AAP classifies drug as compatible with breast-feeding.
Orlistat (B/+)	No human lactation data available. Limited systemic bioavailability would suggest that it would not appear in breast milk.
Oseltamivir (C/+)	No human lactation data available. Molecular weight suggests excretion into breast milk should be expected. Effect on nursing infant is unknown.
Oxacillin (B/+)	Excreted into breast milk in low concentrations. Adverse effects rare. The bowel flora of nursing infants may be altered and there is the potential for interference with the interpretation of an infectious workup. Observe nursing infants for possible allergic reaction.
Oxcarbazepine (C/+)	One report of use during human lactation. No adverse effects reported. AAP classifies carbamazepine as compatible with breast-feeding; oxcarbazepine can be also considered compatible.
Oxycodone (B/+)	Monitor nursing infant for drowsiness.
Pamidronate (D/+)	No human lactation data available. Molecular weight, prolonged half-life, and lack of metabolism suggest drug will be excreted into breast milk. Considering the bioavailability, the amount absorbed by the nursing infant will be clinically insignificant. Probably compatible.

(Continued)

Drug (FDA Fetal Risk Category/ Breast-Feeding Compatibility)	Effect on Lactation and Adverse Effects on Infant
Pantoprazole (B/+)	Excreted into breast milk in small amounts. Has potential for suppression of gastric acid secretion in nursing infant but overall risk of toxicities is low.
Paregoric (B, D/+)	Probably excreted into breast milk. Limited human lactation data available. Probably compatible.
Paroxetine (D/−)	Effect on nursing infant is unknown but may be of concern.
Penicillin G (all forms) (B/+)	All antibiotics are excreted in breast milk in limited amounts. Monitor nursing infant for rash, diarrhea, and spitting up.
Pentamidine (C/CI)	Systemic concentrations reached with aerosolized drug are very low. Breast milk levels would be nil.
Pentobarbital (D/−)	Excreted into breast milk. Effects on nursing infant are unknown.
Permethrin (B/+)	No human lactation data available. Little if any drug expected to be excreted into breast milk. CDC considers permethrin or pyrethrins with piperonyl butoxide treatment of choice for pubic lice during lactation.
Phenobarbital (D/−)	Monitor nursing infant for sucking problems, sedation, rashes, and withdrawal. AAP classifies as drug that has caused major adverse effects in some nursing infants. Use caution if breast-feeding.
Phenytoin (D/+)	Monitor nursing infant for methemoglobinuria (rare). Keep maternal phenytoin in therapeutic range.
Piroxicam (C/+)	Excreted into breast milk in amounts that probably do not present a risk to nursing infant. AAP classifies as compatible with breast-feeding.
Pneumococcal vaccine (C/+)	No human lactation data available. Probably compatible.
Poliovirus inactivated vaccine (C/+)	No human lactation data available. Probably compatible.
Poliovirus live vaccine (C/+)	Compatible with breast-feeding. To prevent inhibition of the vaccine, breast-feeding should be withheld 6 hours before and after administration of vaccine.
Pravastatin (X/CI)	No human lactation data available. Excreted into breast milk. Because of the potential for adverse effects in the nursing infant, avoid use during lactation.
Prednisolone (C, D/+)	Trace amounts have been measured in breast milk. Concentration did not pose clinically significant risk to nursing infant. AAP classifies as compatible with breast-feeding.
Prednisone (C, D/+)	Trace amounts have been measured in breast milk. Concentration did not pose clinically significant risk to nursing infant. AAP classifies as compatible with breast-feeding.
Pregabalin (C/−)	No human lactation data available. Expect excretion into breast milk. Effects on nursing infants are unknown. Monitor nursing infant for dizziness, somnolence, blurred vision, peripheral edema, myopathy, and decreased platelet count. Avoid use during breast-feeding.
Probenecid (C/−)	Excreted into breast milk. Toxicity observed probably related to concurrent antibiotic administered. Observe nursing infant for diarrhea.
Procainamide (C/+)	Excreted in and accumulates in milk. AAP classifies as compatible with breast-feeding. Long-term effects of exposure in nursing infants are unknown.

(Continued)

Drug (FDA Fetal Risk Category/ Breast-Feeding Compatibility)	Effect on Lactation and Adverse Effects on Infant
Prochlorperazine (C/–)	Other phenothiazines excreted into breast milk, so prochlorperazine excretion expected. Sedation in nursing infant a possible side effect.
Propoxyphene (C, D/+)	Monitor nursing infant for withdrawal after long-term high-dose maternal use.
Propranolol (C/–)	Monitor nursing infant for hypotension and bradycardia.
Propylthiouracil (D/+)	Monitor thyroid function of infant periodically.
Pseudoephedrine (C/+)	Monitor nursing infant for agitation.
Pyrazinamide (C/+)	Excreted into human milk in small amounts. Probably compatible.
Pyrimethamine (C/+)	Excreted into breast milk. AAP classifies as compatible with breast-feeding.
Quetiapine (C/–)	Excreted into breast milk. No reports of adverse effects in nursing infants. Long-term effects of this exposure are unknown. Manufacturer recommends avoiding breast-feeding.
Quinidine (C/+)	Monitor nursing infant for rash, anemia, and arrhythmias. Risk of optic neuritis with chronic use.
Quinine (X/+)	Excreted into breast milk. No adverse effects reported in nursing infants. G6PD should be ruled out in infants at risk for the disease. AAP classifies as compatible with breast-feeding.
Quinupristin/dalfopristin (B/–)	No human lactation data available. Probably not excreted into breast milk. Caution—may alter the bowel flora of nursing infants. There is the potential for the development of resistant strains of VRE. Breast-feeding is not recommended.
Ranitidine (B/+)	Excreted into breast milk. Effects on nursing infant are unknown. Decreases gastric acidity but effect on nursing infant has not been studied. AAP classifies similar agent (cimetidine) as compatible with breast-feeding.
Remifentanil (C/+)	No human lactation data available. Expect excretion into breast milk. Very short half-life. Other narcotic agents are classified as compatible with breast-feeding by AAP.
Rifabutin (B/CI)	No human lactation data available. Excretion into breast milk expected. Milk may be stained brown-orange color. Effects on nursing infants are unknown but serious toxicity (leukopenia, neutropenia, rash) are potential adverse effects. Contraindicated if nursing mother is HIV-1 infected.
Rifampin (C/+)	Excreted into breast milk in amounts that pose very little risk to nursing infants. No adverse effects reported. AAP classifies as compatible with breast-feeding.
Rifapentine (C/+)	No human lactation data available. Expect excretion into breast milk. May cause red-orange discoloration. Effects on nursing infants are unknown. AAP classifies rifampin, a similar agent, as compatible with breast-feeding.
Rifaximin (C/+)	No human lactation data available. Expect excretion into breast milk but in very small amounts due to limited systemic absorption. Effects on nursing infants are unknown but probably not clinically significant.
Risperidone (C/–)	Excreted into breast milk. AAP classifies other antipsychotic drugs for which the effects on nursing infants are unknown but may be of concern, especially with long-term use. Could possibly alter short- and long-term CNS function.

(Continued)

Drug (FDA Fetal Risk Category/ Breast-Feeding Compatibility)	Effect on Lactation and Adverse Effects on Infant
Ritonavir (B/CI)	No human lactation data available. Molecular weight suggests excretion into breast milk should be expected. Effect on nursing infant is unknown. CDC recommends HIV-infected mothers in developed countries to not breast-feed.
Rizatriptan (C/+)	No human lactation data available. Expect excretion into breast milk. Effects on nursing infants are unknown.
Rubella vaccine (C/+)	Compatible with breast-feeding. ACOG and CDC recommend vaccination of susceptible women in immediate postpartum period.
Salmeterol (C/+)	No human lactation data available. Expect excretion into breast milk but maternal plasma levels after inhaled dose are very low to undetectable. It is unlikely that clinically significant amounts would appear in breast milk.
Saquinavir (B/CI)	No human lactation data available. Molecular weight suggests excretion into breast milk should be expected. Effect on nursing infant is unknown. CDC recommends HIV-infected mothers in developed countries to not breast-feed.
Scopolamine (C/+)	No human lactation data available. Excreted into breast milk. AAP classifies as compatible with breast-feeding.
Secobarbital (D/+)	Excreted into breast milk. Amount and effects on nursing infants are unknown. AAP classifies as compatible with breast-feeding.
Senna (C/+)	Observe nursing infant for diarrhea. AAP classifies as compatible with breast-feeding.
Sertraline (C/−)	Effect on nursing infant is unknown but may be of concern. Concentrated in human milk.
Simvastatin (X/CI)	No human lactation data available. Expect excretion into breast milk. Because of the potential for adverse effects in the nursing infant, avoid use during lactation.
Smallpox vaccine (X/CI)	CDC recommends breast-feeding women should not routinely be vaccinated; however, if nursing woman is exposed to smallpox or monkeypox, she should be vaccinated and stop breast-feeding.
Sotalol (B/−)	Milk levels 3–5 times maternal serum levels. Could cause bradycardia and hypotension.
Spironolactone (C/+)	Unknown if spironolactone is excreted into breast milk, but metabolite is found in breast milk—probably insignificant amount. Effects on nursing infants unknown. AAP classifies as compatible with breast-feeding.
SSKI (potassium iodide) (D/+)	The significance to nursing infant of chronic ingestion of higher levels of iodine unknown. AAP recognizes maternal use of iodides during lactation may affect infant's thyroid activity by producing elevated iodine levels in breast milk; it classifies as compatible with breast-feeding. Consider monitoring infant's thyroid function.
St. John's wort (C/−)	Unknown if any of the constituents and possible contaminants are excreted into breast milk or if exposure represents risk to nursing infant.

(*Continued*)

Drug (FDA Fetal Risk Category/ Breast-Feeding Compatibility)	Effect on Lactation and Adverse Effects on Infant
Stavudine (C/CI)	No human lactation data available. Molecular weight suggests excretion into breast milk should be expected. Effect on nursing infant is unknown. CDC recommends HIV-infected mothers in developed countries to not breast-feed.
Sucralfate (B/+)	Minimal, if any, drug expected to be excreted into breast milk because only small amounts systemically absorbed.
Sulbactam (B/+)	Excretion into breast milk expected. Effects on nursing infants are unknown. The bowel flora of nursing infants may be altered and there is the potential for interference with the interpretation of an infectious workup. Observe nursing infants for possible allergic reaction. AAP classifies as compatible with breast-feeding.
Sulfamethoxazole (C/–)	Avoid in ill, stressed, or preterm infants and those with hyperbilirubinemia or G6PD deficiency.
Sulfasalazine (B, D/–)	May cause diarrhea in nursing infants. AAP classifies as drug that has been associated with significant effects on some nursing infants and should be given to nursing mother with caution.
Sulindac (B, D/–)	No human lactation data available. Because of prolonged half-life, use safer alternatives—diclofenac, fenoprofen, flurbiprofen, ibuprofen, ketoprofen, ketorolac, or tolmetin—during breast-feeding.
Sumatriptan (C/+)	Excreted into breast milk. Absorption from GI tract is inhibited so amount reaching nursing infant is probably negligible. AAP classifies as compatible with breast-feeding.
Telmisartan (C 1st tri; D 2nd, 3rd tri/+)	No human lactation data available. Molecular weight suggests that excretion into breast milk should be expected. Effects on nursing infant are unknown. AAP classifies as compatible with breast-feeding.
Temazepam (X/–)	Excreted into breast milk. Observe nursing infant for sedation and poor feeding.
Tenofovir (B/CI)	No human lactation data available. Molecular weight suggests excretion into breast milk should be expected. Effect on nursing infant is unknown. CDC recommends HIV-infected mothers in developed countries to not breast-feed.
Terbutaline (B/+)	Monitor nursing infant for agitation and spitting up. Use inhaled form to decrease maternal absorption if available.
Tetanus/diphtheria toxoids and acellular pertussis vaccine (C/+)	Compatible with breast-feeding.
Tetracycline (D/+)	Excreted into breast milk in low concentrations. Theoretical dental staining and inhibition of bone growth is remote. The bowel flora of nursing infants may be altered and there is the potential for interference with the interpretation of an infectious workup. Observe nursing infants for possible allergic reaction. Compatible with breast-feeding.
THC (marijuana) (X/CI)	AAP classifies as drug that should not be used during breast-feeding.
Theophylline (C/+)	AAP classifies as compatible with breast-feeding. Monitor nursing infant for irritability.

(Continued)

Drug (FDA Fetal Risk Category/ Breast-Feeding Compatibility)	Effect on Lactation and Adverse Effects on Infant
Tobramycin (C, D/+)	Excreted into breast milk. No adverse effects reported, and because of poor oral absorption, ototoxicity is not a risk. The bowel flora of nursing infants may be altered and there is the potential for interference with the interpretation of an infectious workup. Observe nursing infants for possible allergic reaction. Compatible with breast-feeding.
Topiramate (C/–)	Excreted into breast milk. No adverse effects noted in limited number of exposed nursing infants. However, potential for adverse effects—fatigue, somnolence, difficulty with concentration/attention, aggressive reaction, confusion, difficulty with memory, ataxia, purpura, epistaxis, infections (viral and pneumonia), anorexia, and weight loss. Observe nursing infants for signs of toxicity.
Tramadol (C/+)	Drug and its active metabolite excreted into breast milk. Effects on nursing infants unknown.
Trazodone (C/–)	Excreted in breast milk. Effects on nursing infant are unknown but may be of concern.
Tretinoin (systemic) (D/+)	Vitamin A and probably tretinoin are natural constituents of breast milk. No human lactation data available on amounts excreted into breast milk after doses for treatment of promyelocytic leukemia or risk to nursing infant. Probably compatible.
Trimethoprim/sulfamethoxazole (C/+)	Excreted into breast milk in low concentrations. Considered negligible risk to nursing infant. AAP classifies as compatible with breast-feeding.
Valacyclovir (B/+)	Lack of adverse effects seen with acyclovir, the primary metabolite of valacyclovir. Considered compatible with breast-feeding.
Valganciclovir (C/CI)	Active metabolite, ganciclovir, has potential to cause serious toxicity. HIV-1–infected mothers in developed countries should not breast-feed. Breast-feeding contraindicated.
Valproic acid (D/–)	Generally compatible with breast-feeding per AAP but carries risk of fatal hepatotoxicity.
Valsartan (C 1st tri; D 2nd, 3rd tri/+)	No human lactation data available. Low molecular weight suggests excretion into breast milk is expected. Effects on nursing infant are unknown. AAP considers compatible with breast-feeding.
Vancomycin (B/+)	Excreted into breast milk. Effects on nursing infant are unknown but vancomycin is poorly absorbed from GI tract. The bowel flora of nursing infants may be altered and there is the potential for interference with the interpretation of an infectious workup. Observe nursing infants for possible allergic reaction. Compatible with breast-feeding.
Varicella vaccine (C/+)	Compatible with breast-feeding.
Venlafaxine (C/–)	Excreted into breast milk. Long-term effects on neurobehavioral and cognitive development from exposure to potent serotonin reuptake inhibitors during a period of rapid CNS development have not been adequately studied. AAP classifies as drug for which effect on nursing infant is unknown but may be of concern.

(Continued)

Drug (FDA Fetal Risk Category/ Breast-Feeding Compatibility)	Effect on Lactation and Adverse Effects on Infant
Verapamil (C/+)	Excreted into breast milk. Limited human lactation data available. Probably compatible.
Voriconazole (D/−)	No human lactation data available. Low molecular weight suggests excretion into breast milk. Potential for toxicity in neonatal period. Avoid breast-feeding.
Warfarin (X/+)	Maternal warfarin therapy does not appear to pose a significant risk to normal full-term infants. Other oral anticoagulants are contraindicated in lactating women.
Zanamivir (C/+)	No human lactation data available. Low molecular weight and pharmacokinetics of drug suggest it will be excreted into breast milk. Effects on nursing infants are unknown but risk of harm is low.
Zidovudine (C/CI)	It is recommended that HIV-1–infected mothers in developed countries to not breast-feed.
Zolmitriptan (C/+)	No human lactation data available. Molecular weight and low protein binding suggest drug and its active metabolite will be excreted into breast milk. Effects on nursing infant are unknown.
Zolpidem (B/+)	Excreted into breast milk in small amounts which would indicate few adverse effects, if any, would occur in nursing infant. Observe for increased sedation, lethargy, and changes in feeding habits.

AAP, American Academy of Pediatrics; ACE, angiotensin-converting enzyme; ACOG, American Congress of Obstetricians and Gynecologists; CDC, Centers for Disease Control and Prevention; CI, contraindicated; CNS, central nervous system; FDA, U.S. Food and Drug Administration; GI, gastrointestinal; HBIG, hepatitis B immune globulin; HIV, human immunodeficiency virus; IV, intravenous; SSRIs, selective serotonin reuptake inhibitors; tri, trimester; VRE, vancomycin-resistant enterococci.

References

Briggs GG, Freeman RK, Yaffe SJ. *Drugs in Pregnancy and Lactation.* 9th ed. Philadelphia, PA: Lippincott Williams and Wilkins; 2011.

Hale TW. *Medications and Mother's Milk.* 14th ed. Amarillo Texas: Hale Publishing; 2010.

LactMed Online. U. S. National Library of Medicine: Bethesda, MD; 2011. http://toxnet.nlm.nih.gov/cgi-bin/sis/htmlgen?LACT. Accessed January, 2012.

Appendix A. Abbreviations Used in Neonatology

A1AT	α_1 antitrypsin	**APTT**	Activated partial thromboplastin time
AaDO$_2$	Alveolar-to-arterial oxygen gradient	**AR**	Autosomal recessive
AAP	American Academy of Pediatrics	**ARA**	Arachidonic acid
a/A ratio	Arterial-to-alveolar oxygen ratio	**ARC**	AIDS-related complex
AATD	α_1-antitrypsin deficiency	**ARD**	Antibiotic removal device, antiretroviral drugs
ABR	Auditory brainstem response		
ABS	Amniotic band syndrome	**AREDFV**	Absent or reversed end-diastolic velocities
A/C	Assist/control		
ACAAI	American College of Allergy, Asthma, and Immunology	**ARF/AKI**	Acute renal failure/acute kidney injury
ACMG	American College of Medical Genetics	**ART**	Assisted reproductive technology
ACOG	American College of Obstetricians and Gynecologists	**ARV**	Antiretroviral
		AS	Aortic stenosis
ACT	Activated clotting time, activated coagulation time	**ASA**	Argininosuccinic aciduria
		ASAP	As soon as possible
ADH	Antidiuretic hormone	**ASD**	Atrial septal defect
ADHD	Attention deficit hyperactivity disorder	**AST**	Aspartate aminotransferase
AE	Adverse effects	**ATN**	Acute tubular necrosis
AED	Automatic external defibrillator	**ATP**	Adenosine triphosphate
aEEG	Amplitude-integrated encephalography	**A-V**	Arteriovenous
AEP	Auditory evoked potential	**AV**	Atrioventricular
AF	Amniotic fluid	**A-VO$_2$**	Arteriovenous oxygen
AFI	Amniotic fluid index	**BAEP**	Brainstem auditory evoked potential
AFP	α-Fetoprotein		
AGA	Appropriate for gestational age	**BAER**	Brainstem audiometric evoked response
AGS	Adrenogenital syndrome		
AHA	American Heart Association	**BAS**	Balloon atrial septostomy
AI	Aortic insufficiency	**BASD**	Bile acid synthetic defect
AIDS	Acquired immunodeficiency syndrome	**BBS**	Bronze baby syndrome
		BD	Base deficit
AIS	Amniotic infection syndrome, arterial ischemic stroke	**BE**	Base excess
		BF	Breast-feeding
ALP	Alkaline phosphatase	**BG**	Babygram (radiograph that includes the chest and abdomen)
ALRI	Acute lower respiratory tract infection		
		β-hCG	Beta human chorionic gonadotropin
ALT	Alanine aminotransferase	**bid**	Twice daily
ALTE	Apparent life-threatening event	**BIND**	Bilirubin-induced neurologic dysfunction
AM	Morning		
Ao	Aortic	**BIOT**	Biotinidase deficiency
AoI	Aortic isthmus	**BLP**	BabyLance preemie
AOI	Apnea of infancy	**BM**	Breast milk
AOP	Apnea of prematurity	**BMC**	Bone mineral content
AP	Anteroposterior	**BOLD**	Blood oxygen level dependent
APGAR	Appearance, pulse, grimace, activity, respirations	**BP**	Blood pressure
		BPD	Biparietal diameter
Apo-A	Apolipoprotein A	**BPD/CLD**	Bronchopulmonary dysplasia/chronic lung disease
APR	Acute-phase reactants		
AP-ROP	Aggressive posterior retinopathy of prematurity	**bpm**	Breaths per minute

BPP	Biophysical profile		**CMTC**	Cutis marmorata telangiectatica congenita
BSEP	Bile salt export pump			
BUN	Blood urea nitrogen		**CMV**	Cytomegalovirus
BW	Birthweight; body weight		**CNS**	Central nervous system; Crigler-Najjar syndrome
BWS	Beckwith-Wiedemann syndrome			
c̄	With (Latin word *cum*)		**CO**	Cardiac output, carbon monoxide
C	Cervical; centigrade		**CO₂**	Carbon dioxide
CA	Community acquired		**CoA**	Coarctation of aorta
CAH	Congenital adrenal hyperplasia		**CO Hb**	Carboxyhemoglobin
CAM	Complementary and alternative medicine; cystic adenomatoid malformation		**CoNS**	Coagulase-negative staphylococci
			cP	Centipoises
CA-MRSA	Community-acquired MRSA		**CPAP, N(n)**	Continuous positive airway pressure,
CANMWG	Chicago Area Neonatal MRSA Working Group		**CPAP**	nasal CPAP
			CPD	Citrate phosphate dextrose
CAVSD	Complete atrioventricular septal defect		**CPIP**	Chronic pulmonary insufficiency of prematurity
CBC	Complete blood count			
CBF	Cerebral blood flow		**CRIES**	*C*rying, *r*equires oxygen, *i*ncreased vital signs, *e*xpression, *s*leepless (Pain scale)
CBG	Capillary blood gases			
CBS	Capillary blood sampling			
CC	Congenital chylothorax		**CRI**	Catheter-related infection
CCAM	Congenital cystic adenomatoid malformation		**CRL**	Crown-rump length
			CRP	C-reactive protein
CCHB	Congenital complete heart block		**CRT**	Capillary refill time
CCHS	Congenital central hypoventilation syndrome		**CRS**	Congenital rubella syndrome
			CRYO-ROP	Cryotherapy for retinopathy of prematurity
CDC	Centers for Disease Control and Prevention			
			C-section	Cesarean section
CDH	Congenital diaphragmatic hernia		**CS**	Congenital syphilis; cesarean section
CDG	Congenital disorders of glycosylation			
cEEG	Conventional EEG		**CSE**	Combined spinal epidural
CF	Cystic fibrosis, clubfoot		**CSF**	Cerebrospinal fluid
CFM	Cerebral function monitor		**CSII**	Continuous subcutaneous insulin infusion
CGH	Comparative genomic hybridization			
CGMS	Continuous glucose monitoring system		**CST**	Contraction stress test
CH	Congenital hydrocephalus, congenital hypothyroidism		**CSVT**	Cerebral sinovenous thrombosis
			CTA	CT angiography
CHARGE	*C*oloboma of the eye, *h*eart defects, *a*tresia of the nasal choanae, *r*etardation of growth and development, *g*enital and urinary abnormalities, and *e*ar anomalies and deafness		**CTG**	Cardiotocography
			CUD	Carnitine uptake deficiency/defect
			CVB	Coxsackievirus B
			CVB3	Coxsackievirus B3
			CVC	Central venous catheters
			CVH	Combined ventricular hypertrophy
			CVP	Central venous pressure
CHD	Congenital hip dislocation, congenital heart disease		**CVS**	Chorionic villus sampling, congenital varicella syndrome
CHF	Congestive heart failure		**CT**	Computed tomography
CHIME	Collaborative home infant monitoring evaluation		**cUS, CUS**	Cranial ultrasound
			CXR	Chest x-ray
CI	Cardiac index		**d**	Day
CID	Cytomegalovirus inclusion disease		**DAT**	Direct antibody test (Coombs test)
CIE	Counterimmunoelectrophoresis		**D25**	25% Dextrose solution
CIT	Citrullinemia		**DBP**	Diastolic blood pressure
CLABSI	Central line–associated bloodstream infections		**DC**	Direct current, differential cyanosis
			D/C	Discharge or discontinue
cm	Centimeter		**DDAVP**	Desmopressin acetate
CMA	Chromosomal microarray analysis			

DDH	Developmental dysplasia of hip	EDC	Estimated date of confinement
DDST	Denver developmental screening test	EDV	End-diastolic velocity
DDx	Differential diagnosis	EEG	Electroencephalogram
DES	Diethylstilbestrol	EFA	Essential fatty acid
DEXA	Dual energy x-ray absorptiometry	EFM	Electronic fetal monitoring
DFA	Direct fluorescent antibody	EHEC	Enterohemorrhagic *Escherichia coli*
DHT	Dihydrotestosterone	EHR	Electronic health records
DI	Drug interactions, diabetes insipidus	EHMF	Enfamil human milk fortifier
DIC	Disseminated intravascular coagulation	EIA	Enzyme immunoassay
		ELBW	Extremely low birthweight
DISIDA	Diisopropyl iminodiacetic acid	ELISA	Enzyme-linked immunosorbent assay
dL	Deciliter	ELSO	Extracorporeal Life Support Organization
DM	Diabetes mellitus	EME	Early myoclonic encephalopathy
DMSA	Dimercaptosuccinic acid	EMG	Electromyelogram
DNPH	2,4-Dinitrophenylhydrazine	EMLA	Eutectic mixture of lidocaine and prilocaine
DNR	Do not resuscitate		
DOA	Dead on arrival	EMR	Electronic medical records
DOCA	Deoxycorticosterone acetate	EN	Enteral nutrition
DORA	Directory of rare analyses	ENNS	Early Neonatal Neurobehavioral Scale
DP	Dorsalis pedis		
DPT	Diphtheria-pertussis-tetanus	ENT	Ear nose throat
DRIFT	Drainage, irrigation, and fibrinolytic therapy	EOS	Early-onset sepsis
		EPO	Erythropoietin
DS	Double strength	ERCP	Endoscopic retrograde cholangiopancreatography
DSD	Disorder of sex development		
DTI	Diffusion tensor imaging	ESR	Erythrocyte sedimentation rate
DTO	Deodorized/diluted tincture of opium (do not use this abbreviation)	ESRD	End-stage renal disease
		ET	Ejection time, expiratory time, exchange transfusion
DTPA	Diethylenetriamine pentaacetic acid		
		ETCOc	End-tidal carbon monoxide (concentration)
DTR	Deep tendon reflexes		
DV	Ductus venosus	$ETCO_2$	End-tidal carbon dioxide (concentration)
DVSNI	Distress scale for ventilated newborn infants		
		ETT	Endotracheal tube
DVT	Deep venous thrombosis	F	French scale (1 F=1/3 mm)
D%W	% Dextrose in water	FAO	Fatty acid oxidation
DWI	Diffusion-weighted (magnetic resonance) imaging	FAS	Fetal alcohol syndrome
		FBG	Fetal blood gas
Dx	Diagnosis	FBS	Fasting blood sugar, fetal blood sample
DXA	Dual energy x-ray absorptiometry		
DXM	Dexamethasone	FD	Forceps delivery
DZ	Disease	FDA	Food and Drug Administration
EA	Esophageal atresia	FDP	Fibrin degradation products
EBL	Estimated blood loss	Fe	Iron
EBV	Epstein-Barr virus	FE	Fractional excretion
ECG	Electrocardiogram	FeNa	Fractional excretion of sodium
ECHO	Echocardiography	FF	Forefoot
ECM	External cardiac massage	FFP	Fresh-frozen plasma
ECP	Eosinophil cationic protein	FFTS	Feto-fetal (twin) transfusion syndrome
ECPR	Extracorporeal cardiopulmonary resuscitation	FGR	Fetal growth restriction
		FH	Fibular hemimelia
ECMO/ECLS	Extracorporeal membrane oxygenation/ extracorporeal life support	FHR	Fetal heart rate
		FHT	Fetal heart tone
ECS	Elective caesarean section	FIO_2	Fraction of inspired oxygen
ECW	Extracellular water	FISH	Fluorescence in situ hybridization

FIRS	Fetal inflammatory response syndrome		**GVHD**	Graft-versus-host disease
FLM	Fetal lung maturity		**HAA**	Hepatitis-associated antigen
FMH	Fetomaternal hemorrhage		**HAART**	Highly active antiretroviral therapy
fMRI	Functional magnetic resonance imaging		**HAV**	Hepatitis A virus
			HBcAg	Hepatitis B core antigen
FOBT	Fecal occult blood testing		**HBeAg**	Hepatitis B e antigen
FRC	Functional residual capacity		**HBIG**	Hepatitis B immune globulin
FSH	Follicle-stimulating hormone		**HBP**	High blood pressure
FSP	Fibrin split products		**HBsAg**	Hepatitis B surface antigen
FTA-Abs	Fluorescent treponemal antibody-absorption		**HBV**	Hepatitis B virus
			HBW	High birthweight
FTT	Failure to thrive		**HC**	Head circumference
FU, F/U	Follow up		**hCG**	Human chorionic gonadotropin
FUO	Fever of unknown origin		**HCM**	Health care maintenance
F-V	Flow-volume		**HC-MRSA**	Health care facilities MRSA
FVC	Forced vital capacity		**HCO$_3$**	Bicarbonate
FVS	Fetal varicella syndrome		**Hct**	Hematocrit
FVZS	Fetal varicella zoster syndrome		**HCTZ**	Hydrochlorothiazide
Fx	Fracture		**HCV**	Hepatitis C virus
Fxn	Function		**HCW**	Health care worker
g, G	Gram, gravida		**HCY**	Homocystinuria
GAI	Glutaric academia type I		**HD**	Hirschsprung disease
GA	Gestational age, general anesthesia, glutaric acidemia		**HDN**	Hemolytic disease of the newborn
			HDV	Hepatitis D virus
GABA	γ-aminobutyric acid		**HEENT**	Head, eyes, ears, nose, and throat
GALE	Galactose-4-epimerase		**HELLP**	Preeclampsia with *h*emolysis, *e*levated *l*iver enzymes, and *l*ow *p*latelet (count)
GALK	Galactokinase			
GALT	Galactose-1-phosphate uridyltransferase, galactosemia			
			HFPPV	High-frequency positive-pressure ventilation
GBS	Group B *Streptococcus*			
GBV-C	Hepatitis G virus		**HEV**	Hepatitis E virus, human enterovirus
G-CSF	Granulocyte colony-stimulating factor		**HF**	Hind foot
GCK	Glucokinase		**HFJV**	High-frequency jet ventilation
GE	Gastroesophageal		**HFNC**	High-flow nasal cannula
GER (GERD)	Gastroesophageal reflux (disease)		**HFO**	High-frequency oscillation
GFR	Glomerular filtration rate		**HFOV**	High-frequency oscillatory ventilation
GGT	γ-Glutamyl transferase		**HFV**	High-frequency ventilation
GGTP	γ-Glutamyl transpeptidase		**Hgb**	Hemoglobin
GI	Gastrointestinal		**HGV**	Hepatitis G virus
GIR	Glucose infusion rate		**HHV**	Human herpes virus
GM-CSF	Granulocyte macrophage colony-stimulating factor		**Hib vaccine**	*Haemophilus influenzae* type b vaccine
GM/IVH	Germinal matrix/intraventricular hemorrhage		**HIDA**	Hepatobiliary iminodiacetic acid
			HIE	Hypoxic ischemic encephalopathy
G$_x$P$_x$Ab$_x$LC$_x$	Shorthand for gravida/para/abortion/living children (subscript variables represent numbers of each)		**HIG**	Hyperimmune globulin
			HIV	Human immunodeficiency virus
			HLA	Human leukocyte antigen
G$_x$P$_x$0000	First zero, full term; second zero, premature; third zero, abortion; fourth zero, living children		**HLHS**	Hypoplastic left heart syndrome
			HMD	Hyaline membrane disease
			HMG	3-Hydroxy-3-methylglutaric aciduria
			HMO	Human milk oligosaccharides
GROW	Gestation-related optimal growth		**H/O**	History of
G6PD	Glucose-6-phosphate dehydrogenase		**H&P**	History and physical examination
gt, gtt	Drop, drops (*gutta*, Latin)		**HPA**	Human platelet antigen
GT	Gastrostomy tubes		**HPeV**	Human parechovirus
GTT	Glucose tolerance test		**HPF**	High-power field
GU	Genitourinary			

HPI	History of present illness	IPPV	Intermediate positive-pressure ventilation
HPLC	High-performance liquid chromatography	IQ	Intelligence quotient
HPS	Hypertrophic pyloric stenosis	IRT	Immunoreactive serum trypsinogen
HR	Heart rate	ISAM	Infant of substance-abusing mother
HSM	Hepatosplenomegaly	ISG	Immune serum globulin
HSV	Herpes simplex virus	IT	Intrathecal, inspiratory time
H/t	Head-to-trunk ratio	I:T	Ratio of immature to total neutrophils
HT	Healing touch	ITP	Idiopathic thrombocytopenic purpura
HTLV	Human T-cell lymphotropic virus	IU	International unit
HTN	Hypertension	IUGR	Intrauterine growth restriction
HCY	Homocystinuria	IUT	Intrauterine transfusion
Hx	History	IV	Intravenous
Hz	Hertz	IVA	Isovaleric academia
IAA	Interrupted aortic arch	IVC	Inferior vena cava, intravenous cholangiogram
IAP	Intrapartum antibiotic prophylaxis	IVH	Intraventricular hemorrhage
IAT	Indirect antiglobulin technique	IVIG	Intravenous immunoglobulin
IC	Incubator care	IVP	Intravenous pyelogram, IV push
ICH	Intracranial hemorrhage	IWL	Insensible water loss
ICN	Intensive care nursery	JEB	Junctional epidermolysis bullosa
ICP	Intracranial pressure	JODM	Juvenile-onset diabetes mellitus
ICPH	Intracerebellar parenchymal hemorrhage	K/K+	Potassium
ICS	Intercostal space	KC	Kangaroo care
ICU	Intensive care unit	KCAL/kcal	Kilocalorie
ICW	Intracellular water	kg	Kilogram
I&D	Incision and drainage	KMC	Kangaroo mother care
ID	Internal diameter	KOH	Potassium hydroxide
IDAM	Infant of drug-abusing mother	KSHV	Kaposi sarcoma–associated herpes virus
IDDM	Insulin-dependent diabetes mellitus	KU	Klobusitzky unit
IDM	Infant of diabetic mother	KUB	Kidneys, ureter, bladder
I:E	Inspiratory-to-expiratory ratio	L	Liter
IEM	Inborn errors of metabolism	LA	Left atrium, lactic acidosis
IFA	Immunofluorescent antibody assay	LAD	Left axis deviation, left atrial diameter, left anterior descending
Ig	Immunoglobulin	LAE	Left atrial enlargement
I/G	Insulin-to-glucose ratio	LAH	Left atrial hypertrophy
IGF	Insulin growth factor	LANE	Mnemonic for meds acceptable thru ETT (lidocaine, atropine, naloxone, epinephrine)
IHPS	Idiopathic hypertrophic pyloric stenosis	LBBB	Left bundle branch block
IL	Interleukin	LBC	Lamellar body count
IM	Intramuscular	LBW	Low birthweight
IMV	Intermittent mandatory ventilation	LBWL	Low birthweight "lytes" (electrolytes)
INF	Intravenous nutritional feedings	LC	Living children
IND	Investigational new drug	LCAD	Long-chain acyl-CoA dehydrogenase
iNO	Inhaled nitric oxide	LCHAD	Long-chain 3-hydroxyacyl CoA dehydrogenase
INR	International normalized ratio	LCPUFAs	Long-chain polyunsaturated fatty acids
INSURE	Intubation surfactant extubation	LDH	Lactate dehydrogenase
I&O	Intake and output	LEDs	Light-emitting diodes
IO₂	Oxygenation index	LFT	Liver function tests
IOI	Intraosseous infusion	LGA	Large for gestational age
IOR	Intraosseous route		
IPPB	Intermittent positive-pressure breathing		
IPV	Inactivated poliovirus vaccine		

LH	Luteinizing hormone	mL	Milliliter
LIDS	Liverpool infant distress scale	mm	Millimeter
LLD	Limb length discrepancy	MMA	Methylmalonic acidemia
LLL	Left lower lobe	MMR	Measles mumps rubella (vaccine)
LLQ	Left lower quadrant	MMWR	Morbidity and Mortality Weekly
LMWH	Low molecular weight heparin		Report
LMA	Laryngeal mask airway	MN	Micronucleus
LMP	Last menstrual period	mOsm	Milliosmole
LMX4	4% Liposomal lidocaine cream	MR	Mitral regurgitation (insufficiency)
LOS	Late-onset sepsis	MRA	Magnetic resonance arteriography
LP	Lumbar puncture	MRCP	Magnetic resonance cholangiopancrea-
LPM	Liters per minute		tography
LPS	Lipopolysaccharide	MRI	Magnetic resonance imaging
LR	Lactated Ringer's solution	MRS	Magnetic resonance spectroscopy
LV	Left ventricle	MRSA	Methicillin-resistant *Staphylococcus*
LVED	Left ventricular end diastolic		*aureus*
LVES	Left ventricular end systolic	MRV	Magnetic resonance venography
LVH	Left ventricular hypertrophy	MS	Mitral stenosis, morphine sulfate,
LVO	Left ventricular output		mass spectrometry
LVOTO	Left ventricular outflow tract	MS/MS	Tandem mass spectrometry
	obstruction	MSAF	Meconium-stained amniotic fluid
L-S ratio	Lecithin-to-sphingomyelin ratio	MSAFP	Maternal serum levels of α-fetoprotein
L3–L4	Third lumbar to fourth lumbar vertebra	MSUD	Maple syrup urine disease
	space	MTCT	Mother-to-child transmission
M, m	Molar, meter	MV	Minute volume, multiple vitamins,
MA	Metatarsus adductus		mechanical ventilation
MAC	Minimum alveolar concentration,	MVI	Multiple vitamin infusion
	Mycobacterium avium complex	MVP	Maximum vertical pocket, mitral valve
MAP	Mean arterial pressure (mean airway		prolapse
	pressure)	MZ	Monozygotic
MAS	Meconium aspiration syndrome	N/A	Not applicable
Max	Maximum	Na/Na+2	Sodium
MBC	Minimum bactericidal concentration	NAA	Nucleic acid amplification
MC	Most common	NACS	Neurologic and adaptive capacity
MCA	Multiple congenital anomaly, middle		score
	cerebral artery	NAIT	Neonatal alloimmune thrombocytopenia
MCAD	Medium-chain acyl-CoA dehydrogenase	NANN	National Association of Neonatal
	deficiency		Nurses
MCD	Multiple carboxylase deficiency	NAT	Nucleic amplification testing
MCH	Mean cell hemoglobin	NAVEL	Mnemonic for groin anatomy (*n*erve,
MCHC	Mean cell hemoglobin concentration		*a*rtery, *v*ein, *e*mpty space,
MCA-PSV	Middle cerebral artery peak systolic		*l*ymphatic)
	velocity	NBAS	Neonatal behavior assessment
MCT	Medium-chain triglyceride		scale
MCV	Mean cell volume	NBS	New Ballard score, newborn screening
MDCT	Multidetector computer tomography	NBW	Normal birthweight
MDT	Metered dose inhaler	NCBI	National Center for Biotechnology and
mEq, meq	Milliequivalent		Information
Mg/Mg+2	Magnesium	NCPAP	Nasal CPAP
MH-TPA	Micro hemagglutination assay for	NCV	Nerve conduction velocity
	Treponema pallidum	NE	Norepinephrine, neonatal
MI	Myocardial infarction, mitral		encephalopathy
	insufficiency, meconium ileus	NEC	Necrotizing enterocolitis
MIC	Mean inhibitory concentration	NEAL	Mnemonic for ETT administered
min	Minute		medications (*n*aloxone, *e*pineph-
			rine, *a*tropine, and *l*idocaine)

NETS	Neonatal emergency transport services	OFC	Occipital frontal circumference
NFCS	Neonatal facial coding system	OG	Orogastric
NG	Nasogastric	17-OHP	17-Hydroxyprogesterone
NGO	Nitroglycerine ointment	OI	Oxygenation index
NHLBL	National Heart Lung and Blood Institute	OM	Otitis media
		ON	Ophthalmia neonatorum
NICHD	National Institute of Child Health and Human Development	OPHTH	Ophthalmic
		OR	Operating room
NICU	Neonatal intensive care unit	OSA	Obstructive sleep apnea
NIDCAP	Newborn Individualized Developmental Care and Assessment Program	Osm	Osmolality
		OTC	Over the counter (nonprescription drug), ornithine transcarbamylase
NIPPV	Nasal intermittent positive pressure ventilation	OU	Both eyes (Latin, *oculus unitas*)
NIPS	Neonatal infant pain scale	OWB	Oscillating waterbed
NIRS	Near infrared spectroscopy	oz	Ounce
NKA	No known allergies	P	Para (the number of viable [>20 weeks] births)
NKDA	No known drug allergy		
NKH	Nonketotic hyperglycinemia	PA	Pulmonary artery, posteroanterior, pulmonary atresia, propionic acidemia
NI	Normal		
NMR	Nuclear magnetic resonance		
NNS	Nonnutritive sucking	PAC	Premature atrial contraction
NORD	National Organization for Rare Disorders	$Paco_2$	Partial pressure of carbon dioxide, arterial
NP	Nasopharyngeal, neonatal pneumothorax, nurse practitioner	PAF	Platelet activating factor
		PAL	Pacifier-activated lullaby
NNP	Neonatal nurse practitioner	Pao_2	Partial pressure of oxygen, arterial
N-PASS	Neonatal pain agitation and sedation scale	PAo_2	Partial pressure of oxygen, alveolar
		PAP	Pulmonary artery pressure
NPCPAP	Nasopharyngeal continuous positive airway pressure	PAPP-A	Pregnancy-associated plasma protein A
NPO	Nothing by mouth	PAPVR	Partial anomalies pulmonary venous return
NRN	Neonatal Research Network		
NRP	Neonatal resuscitation program	PARAM	Paramedic
NS	Normal saline	PAT	Paroxysmal atrial tachycardia
NSAID	Nonsteroidal anti-inflammatory drug	PAT	Path assessment tool
		$P\overline{aw}$	Mean airway pressure
NSR	Normal sinus rhythm	P&PD	Percussion and postural drainage
NST	Nonstress test	PB	Periodic breathing, preterm baby
NSVD	Normal spontaneous vaginal delivery	PBF	Pulmonary blood flow
NT	Nasotracheal, (fetal) nuchal translucency	PBP	Perinatal bereavement program
		PBLC	Premature birth living child
NTA	Nonspecific nontreponemal antibody	PCA	Postconceptional age, primary cutaneous aspergillosis
NTA tests	Nontreponemal antibody tests (VDRL, RPR, ART)		
		PCE	Pericardial effusion
NTB	Necrotizing tracheobronchitis	PCG	Pneumocardiogram
NTDs	Neural tube defects	PCN	Penicillin
NTE	Neutral thermal environment	PCP	*Pneumocystis jiroveci* pneumonia, phencyclidine
NVP	Nevirapine		
O_2	Oxygen	PCR	Polymerase chain reaction
OA	Organic aciduria/acidemia	PCT	Procalcitonin
OAE	Otoacoustic emissions	PCVC	Percutaneous central venous catheter
OB	Obstetrics		
OBSN	Observation	PCWP	Pulmonary capillary wedge pressure
OCP	Oral contraceptive pill		
OCT	Oxytocin challenge test	PD	Peritoneal drainage
OD	Outer diameter	PDA	Patent ductus arteriosus

PDE	Phosphodiesterase, pyridoxine-dependent epilepsy
PDH	Pyruvate dehydrogenase
PE	Pleural effusion, physical examination, pulmonary embolus
PEA	Pulseless electrical activity
PEEP	Positive end expiratory pressure
PET	Partial exchange transfusion
$Petco_2$	Partial pressure of end tidal carbon dioxide
PETS	Pediatric emergency transport service
PF	Purpura fulminans
PFC	Persistent fetal circulation
PFFD	Proximal focal femoral deficiency
PFIC	Progressive familial intrahepatic cholestasis
PFO	Patent foramen ovale
PFT	Pulmonary function test
PG	Phosphatidylglycerol
PGE_1	Prostaglandin E_1
PGI_2	Prostacyclin
PH	Pulmonary hemorrhage
PHH	Posthemorrhagic hydrocephalus
PHN	Pulmonary hypertension
PI	Pulsatility index
PICC	Percutaneous inserted central catheter
PICU	Pediatric intensive care unit
PID	Pelvic inflammatory disease
PIE	Pulmonary interstitial emphysema
PIH	Postinfections hydrocephalus
PIP	Peak inspiratory pressure
PIPP	Premature infant pain profile
PIV	Peripheral intravenous
PKU	Phenylketonuria
PLAST	Percussion, lavage, suction, turn
PLV	Partial liquid ventilation, pressure limited ventilation
PM	At night, pneumomediastinum
PMA	Postmenstrual age
PMH	Past medical history
PMN	Polymorphonuclear neutrophil
PN	Parenteral nutrition
PNA	Postnatal age
PNAC	Parenteral nutrition–associated conjugated hyperbilirubinemia
PNCV	Peripheral nerve conduction velocity
PNIDDM	Permanent neonatal insulin dependent diabetes mellitus
PO	By mouth
P&PD	Percussion and postural drainage
PP	Pneumoperitoneum
PPD	Purified protein derivative
PPH	Persistent pulmonary hypertension
PPHN	Persistent pulmonary hypertension of newborn

PPN	Peripheral parenteral nutrition
PPROM	Preterm premature rupture of membranes
PPS	Peripheral pulmonic stenosis
PPV	Positive-pressure ventilation
PR	Per rectum
PRBC	Packed red blood cells
PRN	As needed
PROM	Premature rupture of membranes
PROP	Propionic acidemia
PS	Pulmonary stenosis, pressure support
PSV	Peak systolic velocity
PT	Prothrombin time
PTB	Preterm birth
PTH	Parathyroid hormone
PTL	Preterm labor
PTNB	Preterm newborn
PTT	Partial thromboplastin time
PTTN	Prolonged transient tachypnea of the newborn
PTX	Pneumothorax
PUBS	Percutaneous umbilical blood sampling
PUFA	Polyunsaturated fatty acids
PUV	Posterior urethral valves
P-V	Pressure volume
PVC	Premature ventricular contraction
PVD	Posthemorrhagic ventricular dilation
PVET	Peripheral vessel exchange transfusion
PVH	Periventricular hemorrhage
PVHI	Periventricular hemorrhagic infarction
PV-IVH	Periventricular (hemorrhage) intraventricular hemorrhage
PVH-IVH	Periventricular hemorrhage-intraventricular hemorrhage
PVL	Periventricular leukomalacia
PVR	Pulmonary vascular resistance
PVS	Percussion, vibration, and suctioning/pulmonary valve stenosis
PVT	Portal vein thrombosis
q	Every (Latin, *quaque*)
qd	Everyday (use not recommended)
qXh	Every X hours
qid	Four times daily
qod	Every other day (Latin, *quaque otram diem*)
Quad screen	Quadruple screen test (maternal serum α-fetoprotein, total human chorionic gonadotropin, unconjugated estriol, inhibin A)
RA	Right atrium
RAD	Right axis deviation
RAE	Right atrial enlargement
RAH	Right atrial hypertrophy
RAST	Radioallergosorbent test
RAT	Right atrial thrombosis
RBBB	Right bundle branch block

RBC	Red blood cell
RCT	Randomized controlled trial
RDA	Recommended dietary allowance
RDC	Reverse differential cyanosis
RDS	Respiratory distress syndrome
rFVIIa	Recombinant factor VII, activated
RFI	Renal failure index
Rh	Rhesus factor
rhAPC	Recombinant human activated protein C
rHuEPO	Recombinant human erythropoietin
RIA	Radioimmunoassay
RIVUR	Randomized intervention for children with vesicoureteral reflux
RL	Ringer's lactate
RLF	Retrolental fibroplasia, retained lung fluid
RLL	Right lower lobe
RLQ	Right lower quadrant
RML	Right middle lobe
RN	Registered nurse
R/O	Rule out
ROM	Range of motion, rupture of membranes
ROP	Retinopathy of prematurity
ROS	Review of systems
RPR	Rapid plasma reagin (test)
RSI	Rapid sequence intubation
RSV	Respiratory syncytial virus
RT	Rubella titer, respiratory therapy, radiation therapy
RTA	Renal tubular acidosis
RTPCR	Reverse transcriptase polymerase chain reaction
RUL	Right upper lobe
RUQ	Right upper quadrant
RV	Right ventricle, residual volume
RVH	Right ventricular hypertrophy
RVT	Renal vein thrombosis
Rx	Treatment
Rxn	Reaction
17-OHP	17-Hydroxyprogesterone
$\bar{s}$	Without (Latin, *sine*)
SA	Sinoatrial
SAE	Serious adverse event
SAH	Subarachnoid hemorrhage
SaO$_2$	Oxygen saturation of arterial blood, arterial oxygen saturation by direct measurement
SBA	Suprapubic bladder aspiration
SBP	Systolic blood pressure
SC	Subcutaneous
SCAD	Short-chain acyl-CoA dehydrogenase deficiency
SCM	Sternocleidomastoid muscle
SD	Standard deviation

SDA	Strand displacement amplification
SDH	Subdural hemorrhage
SEH	Subependymal hemorrhage
SEM	Systolic ejection murmur, skin, eyes, and mouth
SEP	Sensory evoked potential
SIPI	Idiopathic spontaneous intestinal perforation
SGA	Small for gestational age
SGOT	Serum glutamic oxaloacetic transaminase
SGPT	Serum glutamic pyruvic transaminase
SHC	Selective head cooling
SHMF	Similac human milk fortifier
SIADH	Syndrome of inappropriate antidiuretic hormone
SIDS	Sudden infant death syndrome
SIMV	Synchronized intermittent mandatory ventilation
SIP	Spontaneous intestinal perforation
SIRS	Septic inflammatory response syndrome
SK	Streptokinase
SLE	Systemic lupus erythematosus
SHMF	Similac human milk fortifier
SMX	Sulfamethoxazole
Sn	Tin
SNC	Selective neonatal chemoprophylaxis
SNHL	Sensorineural hearing loss
SnMP	Sn (tin)-mesoporphyrin
SOAP	Mnemonic for S (Subjective), O (Objective), A (Assessment), P (Plan)
SOB	Shortness of breath
SOS	Speed of sound
S/P	Status post
SpO$_2$	Pulse oximetry measurement of blood oxygenation saturation
SQ	Subcutaneous
SSEP	Somatosensory evoked potential
SSRI	Selective serotonin reuptake inhibitors
SSSS	Staphylococcal scalded skin syndrome
STAT	Immediately
STD/STI	Sexually transmitted disease/sexually transmitted infection
SU	Shoulder to umbilicus
Supp	Supplement, suppository
Susp	Suspension
SVC	Superior vena cava
SVD	Spontaneous vaginal delivery
SvO$_2$	Venous oxygen saturation
SVR	Systemic vascular resistance
SVT	Supraventricular tachycardia
SWC	Sleep wake cycle

Sx	Symptom
Sz	Seizure
3MCC	3-Methylcrontonyl CoA carboxylase deficiency
T	Testosterone
TA	Tricuspid atresia, truncus arteriosus
TAC	Truncus arteriosus communis
TA-GVHD	Transfusion-associated graft-versus-host disease
TAPVR	Total anomalous pulmonary venous return
TAR	Thrombocytopenia and absent radius (syndrome)
TB	Tuberculosis
TBG	Thyroid-binding globulin
TBLC	Term birth, living child
TBW	Total body water
TcB	Transcutaneous bilirubin
TcPco$_2$	Transcutaneous carbon dioxide tension
TcPo$_2$	Transcutaneous oxygen tension
TD	Transdermal
TD$_x$FLM II	Commercial fetal lung maturity assay
TE	Tracheoesophageal, thromboembolism
TEG	Thromboelastography
TEF	Tracheoesophageal fistula
TENS	Transcutaneous electric nerve stimulation
TEWL	Transepidermal water loss
TFT	Thyroid function test
TGA	Transposition of the great arteries
TGV	Transposition of the great vessels
T&H	Type and hold
THAM	Tris (hydroxymethyl) aminomethane (tromethamine)
THAN	Transient hyperammonemia of the newborn
Ti	Inspiratory time
TI	Tricuspid incompetence (regurgitation)
tid	Three times daily (Latin, *ter in die*)
TIPP	Trial of indomethacin prophylaxis in preterms
TIV	Trivalent inactivated influenza vaccine
TLC	Total lung capacity
TLV	Total liquid ventilation
TM	Tympanic membrane
TMA	Transcription-mediated amplification
TNF	Tumor necrosis factor
TNMG	Transient neonatal myasthenia gravis
TNPM	Transient neonatal pustular melanosis
TOF	Tetralogy of Fallot
TORCH	*T*oxoplasmosis, *o*ther, *r*ubella, *c*ytomegalovirus, *h*erpes simplex virus
TOW	Term optimal weight
tPA	Tissue plasminogen activator
TP-PA	*Treponema pallidum* particle agglutination
TPN	Total parenteral nutrition
TPR	Total peripheral resistance
TPO/THPO	Thrombopoietin
TRH	Thyrotropin-releasing hormone
TRALI	Transfusion-related acute lung injury
TR, TI	Tricuspid regurgitation (incompetence, insufficiency)
TRH	Thyroid/thyrotropin-releasing hormone
TS	Tricuspid stenosis
TSB	Total serum bilirubin
TSH	Thyroid-stimulating hormone
TSP	Toxoplasma serologic profile
TT	Thrombin time
TTN, TTNB	Transient tachypnea of the newborn
TTTS	Twin-twin (feto-fetal) transfusion syndrome
TTV	Torque teno virus, transfusion-transmitted virus
TV	Tidal volume
Type 2 DM	Type 2 diabetes mellitus
TYR1	Tyrosinemia type 1
U	Unit(s) (do not use; dangerous abbreviation; write out "unit")
UA	Umbilical artery
U/A	Urinalysis
UAC	Umbilical artery catheter
UC	Umbilical cord
UDCA	Ursodeoxycholic acid
UDPGT	Uridine diphosphate glucuronyl transferase
UFH	Unfractionated heparin
UGI	Upper gastrointestinal
UK	Urokinase
ULN	Upper limits of normal
UPEP	Urine protein electrophoresis
UPI	Uteroplacental insufficiency
UPJ	Ureteropelvic junction
UPJO	Ureteropelvic junction obstruction
URI	Upper respiratory infection
US	Ultrasound
USPSTF	U.S. Preventive Services Task Force
UTA	Uterine artery
UTI	Urinary tract infection
UV	Umbilical vein
UVC	Umbilical vein catheter
VA	Venoarterial

VATER/	Vertebral defects, anal atresia,
VACTERL	tracheoesophageal fistula, and radial or renal dysplasia/vertebral defects, anal atresia, cardiac malformations, tracheoesophageal fistula, renal dysplasia, and limb abnormalities
VZIG	Varicella zoster immune globulin
VBG	Venous blood gas
VC	Vital capacity
VCUG	Voiding cystourethrogram
VDRL	Venereal disease research laboratory
VE	Vacuum extraction
VEGF	Vascular endothelial growth factor
VEP	Visual evoked potential
VER	Visual evoked response
VF	Ventricular fibrillation
VHBW	Very high birthweight
VISA	Vancomycin intermediate *Staphylococcus aureus*
VLBW	Very low birthweight
VLCAD	Very long-chain acyl-CoA dehydrogenase deficiency
VLCFA	Very long-chain fatty acids
VM	Ventriculomegaly
VMA	Vanillylmandelic acid
V/P	Ventilation perfusion
VP	Ventriculoperitoneal shunt
V/Q	Ventilation-perfusion
VSD	Ventricular septal defect
VSS	Vital signs stable
VT	Ventricular tachycardia, vertical talus
VTV	Volume-targeted ventilation
V_T	Tidal volume (size of breath)
VUE	Villitis of unknown etiology
VUR	Vesicoureteral reflux
VV	Veno-venous
vWD	von Willebrand Disease
vWF	von Willebrand Factor
VZV	Varicella zoster virus
VZIG	Varicella-zoster immune globulin
WBC	White blood cell
WF	White female
WHO	World Health Organization
WM	White male
WNL, wnl	Within normal limits
WNV	West Nile virus
WPW	Wolff-Parkinson-White syndrome
XR	Extended release
ZDV	Zidovudine
ZnMP	Zinc metalloporphyrin

Appendix B. Apgar Scoring

Apgar scores are a numerical expression of the condition of a newborn infant on a scale of 0–10. The scores are recorded at 1 and 5 minutes after delivery and become a permanent part of the health record. If there is a problem, an additional score is given at 10 minutes. A score of 7–10 is normal (10 is very unusual), 4–7 usually requires some resuscitative measures, and <3 requires immediate resuscitation. They have clinical usefulness not only during the nursery stay, but also at later child health visits when clinical status at delivery may have a bearing on current diagnostic assessments. The system was originally described by Virginia Apgar, MD, an anesthesiologist, in 1952 and first published in 1953.

Sign	Score 0	1	2
Appearance (color)	Blue or pale	Pink body with blue extremities	Completely pink
Pulse (heart rate)	Absent	Slow (<100 beats/min)	>100 beats/min
Grimace (reflex irritability)	No response	Grimace	Cough or sneeze
Activity (muscle tone)	Limp	Some flexion	Active movement
Respirations	Absent	Slow, irregular	Good, crying

Appendix C. Blood Pressure Determinations

Table C–1. **BLOOD PRESSURE MEASUREMENTS IN PRETERM AND FULL-TERM NEONATES (DAYS 1–7 AND DAY 30)**

Postnatal Day	Gestational Age (Noncritically Ill Infants)			
	≤28 Weeks	29–32 Weeks	33–36 Weeks	37 Weeks
1	Systolic: 38–46 Diastolic: 23–29 Mean: 29–35	Systolic: 42–52 Diastolic: 26–38 Mean: 33–43	Systolic: 51–61 Diastolic: 32–40 Mean: 39–47	Systolic: 57–69 Diastolic: 35–45 Mean: 44–52
2	Systolic: 38–46 Diastolic: 24–32 Mean: 29–37	Systolic: 46–56 Diastolic: 29–39 Mean: 35–45	Systolic: 54–62 Diastolic: 34–42 Mean: 42–48	Systolic: 58–70 Diastolic: 36–46 Mean: 46–54
3	Systolic: 40–48 Diastolic: 25–33 Mean: 30–38	Systolic: 47–59 Diastolic: 30–35 Mean: 37–47	Systolic: 54–64 Diastolic: 35–43 Mean: 42–50	Systolic: 58–71 Diastolic: 37–47 Mean: 46–54
4	Systolic: 41–49 Diastolic: 26–36 Mean: 31–41	Systolic: 50–62 Diastolic: 32–42 Mean: 39–49	Systolic: 56–66 Diastolic: 36–44 Mean: 44–50	Systolic: 61–73 Diastolic: 38–48 Mean: 46–56
5	Systolic: 42–50 Diastolic: 27–37 Mean: 32–42	Systolic: 51–65 Diastolic: 33–43 Mean: 40–50	Systolic: 57–67 Diastolic: 37–45 Mean: 44–52	Systolic: 62–74 Diastolic: 39–49 Mean: 47–57
6	Systolic: 44–52 Diastolic: 30–38 Mean: 35–43	Systolic: 52–66 Diastolic: 35–45 Mean: 41–51	Systolic: 59–69 Diastolic: 37–45 Mean: 45–53	Systolic: 64–76 Diastolic: 40–50 Mean: 48–58
7	Systolic: 47–53 Diastolic: 31–39 Mean: 37–45	Systolic: 53–67 Diastolic: 36–44 Mean: 43–51	Systolic: 60–70 Diastolic: 37–45 Mean: 45–53	Systolic: 66–76 Diastolic: 40–50 Mean: 50–58
30	Systolic: 59–65 Diastolic: 35–49 Mean: 42–56	Systolic: 67–75 Diastolic: 43–53 Mean: 52–60	Systolic: 68–76 Diastolic: 45–55 Mean: 53–60	Systolic: 72–82 Diastolic: 46–54 Mean: 55–63

Data from Pejovic B, Peco-Antic A, Marinkovic-Eric J. Blood pressure in non-critically ill preterm and full-term neonates. *Pediatr Nephrol.* 2007;22:249–257.

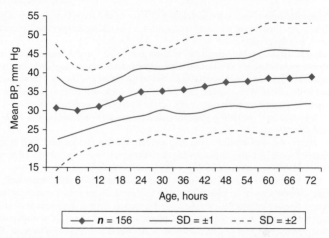

APPENDIX FIGURE C–1. Mean blood pressure of all infants 401–1000 g during the first 72 hours of life. (*Reproduced, with permission, from Fanaroff JM, Wilson-Costello DE, Newman NS, Montpetite MM, Fanaroff AA. Treated hypotension is associated with neonatal morbidity and hearing loss in extremely low birth weight infants.* Pediatrics. *2006;117;1131–1135*).

Appendix D. Chartwork

Many hospitals are now using EMR (electronic medical records) or EHR (electronic health records). These are often in a preformatted template to be completed electronically. Because there are many different formats, there isn't an all-inclusive EMR example. The following section provides an overview of the basic history, progress note, admission orders, and discharge summary. Chapter 6 outlines the newborn physical examination.

ADMISSION HISTORY

A. **Identification (ID).** State the name, age, sex, and weight of the infant. Include whether the patient or mother was transported from another facility or whether the infant was born at home or within the hospital.

   Infant James, a 3-hour-old 1800-g white male, is an inborn patient from Baltimore, Maryland.

B. **Chief complaint (CC).** The major problems of the patient are usually listed in the order of severity of disease process or occurrence.
   1. *Respiratory distress syndrome*
   2. *Suspected neonatal sepsis*
   3. *Premature birth living child* (*PBLC*)

C. **Referring physician.** Include the name, address, and telephone number of the referring physician.

   Dr. Macaca Mulatta, Benjamin Franklin Medical Center, Chadds Ford, PA;(946) 854-8881

D. **History of present illness (HPI).** The HPI is more helpful if it is divided into 4 separate paragraphs.
   1. **Initial statement.** This part of the HPI includes the patient's name, gestational age, birthweight, sex, age of the mother, and the number of times she has been pregnant along with the number of her living children.

2. **Prenatal history.** Discuss the maternal prenatal care and record the number of prenatal clinic visits. Include any medications the mother was taking, any pertinent prenatal tests done, and the results.

3. **Labor and delivery.** Include a detailed history of the labor and delivery: type of delivery, type of anesthesia, any medication used, and any fetal monitoring (including results).

4. **Infant history.** Discuss the initial condition of the infant and the need for resuscitation, and write a detailed description of what occurred. Include the Apgar scores and discuss when the infant became symptomatic or when problems were first noted.

Infant James is an 1800-g white male delivered to a 19-year-old G₂ now P₂, LC₂ married white female.

The mother had excellent prenatal care. She had her first prenatal visit at approximately 8 weeks' gestation and then saw her obstetrician routinely. She was on no medications nor does she have any history of alcohol or cigarette abuse.

She had rupture of membranes (ROM) at 33 weeks with some mild contractions. At that time, she was seen by her obstetrician, who confirmed the premature rupture of the membranes. She was admitted to the hospital and started on tocolytic treatment in an attempt to stop the labor. Vaginal–rectal swab for GBS cultures were obtained. IV penicillin was initiated. Because of a positive GBS culture, penicillin was continued during tocolysis. External fetal monitoring had been normal until 4 hours after the tocolytic therapy, at which time it showed persistent late decelerations. At this point, an emergency cesarean delivery was performed. General anesthesia was used, and the infant was delivered within 6 minutes.

The infant was delivered depressed at birth, with 1-minute Apgar of 4. He required bag-mask ventilation with 100% oxygen. No medications were needed. The 5-minute Apgar was 7. The infant appeared poorly perfused and had poor color without oxygen. He was stabilized and transported on 100% oxygen to the NICU.

E. **Family history (FH).** The family history should include any previous complicated births and their history, miscarriages, neonatal deaths, or premature births. Also include any major family medical problems (eg, hemophilia, sickle cell disease).

Mrs. James had 1 prior uncomplicated vaginal delivery that went to term. There is a history of myelodysplasia in infant James's maternal first cousin.

F. **Social history (SH).** In the social history, include a brief statement discussing the parent's age, marital status, siblings, occupation, and where they are from.

The parents live in Chadds Ford. Mother is a 19-year-old mushroom farm worker and cares for their 2-year-old daughter; the father is 24 years and works in the local museum as a custodial worker.

G. **Physical examination.** See Chapter 6.

H. **Laboratory data.** List the admission laboratory and radiology results.

I. **Assessment.** State your evaluation of the infant's problems. It can include a list of suspected and potential problems as well as a differential diagnosis.

1. *Respiratory distress syndrome: Because the infant is premature, hyaline membrane disease must be considered. Pneumonia is also a likely cause because of the maternal history of suspected chorioamnionitis.*

2. *Suspected neonatal sepsis: Because of the positive GBS culture and the premature onset of labor, there is an increased septic risk in this infant. Certain pathogens need to be ruled out. Group B* Streptococcus *is the most common pathogen in this age group, but* Listeria monocytogenes *and Gram-negative pathogens should be considered.*

3. *Premature birth living child: The infant is at 33 weeks' gestation by Ballard examination.*

J. **Plan.** Include the therapeutic and diagnostic plans for the infant. (See Section on "Admission Orders.")

PROGRESS NOTES

The most commonly used format for daily progress notes is the *SOAP* method. *SOAP* is an acronym; *S* = subjective, *O* = objective, *A* = assessment, and *P* = plan. Each problem should be discussed in this format. First, state the problems you are to discuss in the order of severity or occurrence and assign a number to them. Then discuss each problem in the *SOAP* format as outlined next.

A. **Subjective (S).** Include an overall subjective view of the patient by the physician.

B. **Objective (O).** Include data that can be objectively gathered, usually in 3 areas:
   1. Vital signs (temperature, respiratory rate, pulse, blood pressure).
   2. Pertinent physical examination.
   3. Laboratory data and other test results.

C. **Assessment (A).** Include evaluation of the preceding data.

D. **Plan (P).** Discuss the medication changes, laboratory orders, and any other new orders as well as the treatment plan.

E. **Example.** The following is an example of part of a progress note using the SOAP format.

   Problem 1. Respiratory distress syndrome.
   S: Infant James is now 4 days old and doing much better. He has been able to wean down to 30% oxygen with good arterial gases.
   O: Vital signs: temperature 98.7, respirations 52, pulse 140, blood pressure 55/35.
   Physical examination: The peripheral perfusion appears good with no obvious cyanosis. There is no grunting or nasal flaring, but the infant has mild substernal and intercostal retractions. The chest sounds slightly wet. Laboratory data and other test results: Arterial blood gases on 30% oxygen—pH 7.32, CO_2 48, O_2 67, 97% saturation. Chest radiograph shows mild haziness in both lung fields.
   A: Infant James has resolving mild respiratory distress syndrome.
   P: The plan is to wean the oxygen as long as his arterial Pao_2 is maintained between >55–70.
   Problem 2. Suspected neonatal sepsis—Follow with "SOAP" note.
   Problem 3. Premature birth living child (PBLC)—Follow with "SOAP" note.

ADMISSION ORDERS

The following format is useful for writing admission orders. It involves the mnemonic *A.D.C. VAN DISSEL:* Admit, Diagnosis, Condition, Vital signs, Activity, Nursing procedures, Diet, Input and Output, Specific drugs, Symptomatic drugs, Extras, and Laboratory data. Most centers now have online physician ordering templates.

A. **Admit.** Specify the location of the patient (neonatal intensive care unit, newborn nursery) and the attending physician in charge and the house officer along with their paging numbers.

B. **Diagnosis.** List the admitting diagnoses.
   1. *Respiratory distress syndrome*
   2. *Suspected neonatal sepsis*
   3. *Premature birth living child*

C. **Condition.** Note whether the patient is in stable or critical condition.

D. **Vital signs.** State the desired frequency of monitoring of vital signs. Specify rectal or axillary temperature. Rectal temperature is usually done initially to obtain a core temperature and also to rule out imperforate anus. Then, monitor axillary temperature. Other parameters include blood pressure, pulse, and respiratory rate. Weight, length, and head circumference should also be obtained on admission.

E. **Activity.** All are at bed rest, but one can specify "minimal stress or hands-off protocol" here. This notation is used for infants who react poorly to stress by dropping their oxygenation, as in patients with persistent pulmonary hypertension. At most centers, it means to handle the infant as little as possible and record all vital signs off the monitor.

F. **Nursing procedure.** Respiratory care (ventilator settings, chest percussion and postural drainage orders, endotracheal suctioning with frequency). Also require that a daily weight and head circumference be recorded. The frequency of Dextrostix (or Chemstrip-bG) testing is included in this section because it is a bedside procedure.

G. **Diet.** All infants admitted to the neonatal intensive care unit are usually made NPO (nothing by mouth) for at least 6–24 hours until they are accessed and stabilized. When appropriate, write specific diet orders.

H. **Input and output (I and O).** Request that the nursing staff record accurate input and output of each infant. This record is especially important for infants on intravenous fluids and those just starting oral feedings. Specify how often you want the urine tested for specific gravity and glucose.

I. **Specific drugs.** State drugs to be administered, giving specific dosages and routes of administration. It is useful to also include the milligrams-per-kilogram-per-day dose of the drug to allow cross-checking and verification of the dose ordered. An example is as follows: *Ampicillin 90 mg IV every 12 hours (100 mg/kg/d divided every 12 hours).*

For all infants, order the following medications at the time of admission.

1. Vitamin K (see Chapter 148) is given to prevent hemorrhagic disease of the newborn.
2. Erythromycin eye drops (see Chapter 148) are given to prevent gonococcal ophthalmia.

J. **Symptomatic drugs.** These drugs are not routinely used in a neonatal intensive care unit and would include such items as pain and sleep medications.

K. **Extras.** Any other orders required but not included previously, such as roentgenography, electrocardiography, and ultrasonography.

L. **Laboratory data.** Include laboratory data drawn on admission, plus routine laboratory orders with frequency (eg, arterial blood gases every 2 hours, sodium and potassium bid).

DISCHARGE SUMMARY

The following information is written at the time of discharge and provides a summary of the infant's illness and hospital stay.

A. **Date of admission.**

B. **Date of discharge.**

C. **Admitting diagnosis.**

D. **Discharge diagnosis.** List in order of occurrence or severity.

E. **Attending physician and service caring for the patient.**

F. **Referring physician and address.**

G. **Procedures.** Include all invasive procedures.

H. **Brief history, physical examination, and laboratory data on admission.** Use the admission history, physical examination, and laboratory data as a guide.

I. **Hospital course.** The easiest way to approach this section of the discharge summary is to discuss each problem in paragraph form.

J. **Condition at discharge.** A complete physical examination is done at the time of discharge and included in this section. It is important to include the discharge weight, head circumference, and length so that growth can be assessed at the time of the patient's initial checkup. Also include the type and amount of formula the patient is on and any pertinent discharge laboratory values.

K. **Discharge medications.** Include the name(s) of medication(s), the dosage(s), and length of treatment. If the patient is being sent home on an apnea monitor, it is helpful to include the monitor settings and the planned course of treatment.

L. **Disposition.** Note where the patient is being sent (outside hospital, home, foster home).

M. **Discharge instructions and follow-up.** Include instructions to the parents on medications and when the patient is to return to the clinic (and exact location). It is helpful to indicate tests that need to be done on follow-up and any results that need to be rechecked (eg, bilirubin, repeat phenylketonuria screen).

N. **Problem list.** Same list as the discharge diagnosis list.

Appendix E. Immunization Tables

For most up to date changes, see http://www.cdc.gov/vaccines/schedules/and Pickering LK, Baker CJ, Kimberlin DW, Long SS, eds. *Red Book: 2012 Report of the Committee on Infectious Diseases.* 29th ed. Elk Grove Village, IL: American Academy of Pediatrics; 2012.

IMMUNIZATIONS FOR TERM INFANTS

Term infants follow the recommended immunization schedule for persons aged 0–6 years (http://www.cdc.gov/vaccines/schedules/downloads/child/0-6yrs-schedule-pr.pdf).

IMMUNIZATIONS FOR PRETERM INFANTS

Misconceptions about the safety and efficacy of vaccinations for preterm infants have led to delays in immunization for these infants. It is important that preterm infants with prolonged hospital stays begin necessary immunizations prior to neonatal intensive care unit (NICU) discharge to allow development of early protection from infectious agents prevalent in the community, especially pertussis. The American Academy of Pediatrics current recommendations can be summarized as follows:

"Preterm infants born at less than 37 weeks gestation and infants of low birthweight (<2500 grams) should, with few exceptions, receive all routinely recommended childhood vaccinations at the same chronologic age as term infants" even if they are still hospitalized. "Gestational age and birthweight are not limiting factors when deciding whether a clinically stable preterm infant is to be immunized." In addition, "vaccine doses given to term infants should not be reduced or divided when given to preterm or low birth weight infants."

Effectiveness of Immunizations

For the majority of premature infants, their protective antibody responses to immunizations are comparable to those seen in term infants. However, studies have shown that preterm infants weighing <2000 g may not respond as well to hepatitis B vaccine given at birth. Therefore, the hepatitis B immunization schedule has been altered for preterm infants or low birthweight <2000 g.

Complications of Immunization

Adverse events have been reported after vaccine administration and historically have led to concern limiting immunization of premature infants. Adverse events may be caused by the vaccine or may occur by chance after immunization. Any event that is considered **serious** or **unexpected** and possibly related to the vaccination should be reported. Serious adverse events include **anaphylaxis** (see Chapter 65), **abscess formation, encephalitis, acute flaccid paralysis, fever** (>40.5°C), **persistent screaming, severe local reactions, and seizures**.

Preterm infants are not at higher risk for these types of adverse reactions as compared with term infants. Premature infants generally tolerate immunizations as well as term infants and experience fewer febrile and local reactions to immunizations because of their more immature immune systems. Contraindications to immunizations are the same for all infants and include a significant febrile illness, active seizure disorder or encephalopathy, or any known allergies to the vaccine components (ie, eggs).

Table E–1. IMMUNIZATIONS FOR PRETERM INFANTS

Age	Infection Prevented	Recommended Vaccine
Birth	Hepatitis B[a]	**>2000 g** birthweight, medically stable, mom Hep B antigen negative: Hep B monovalent vaccine[b] at birth or shortly thereafter **>2000 g** birthweight, medically unstable, mom Hep B antigen negative: defer Hep B immunization until stable clinical condition
		<2000 g birthweight, ≥30 days of chronologic age: Hep B monovalent vaccine,[b] dose 1 at 30 days chronologic age, if medically stable **<2000 g** birthweight, <30 days chronologic age at hospital discharge, give Hep B monovalent vaccine[b] at discharge
1–2 months	Hepatitis B[a]	Give the second dose of Hep B vaccine at 1–2 months of age[c]
2 months[d]	Diphtheria, Pertussis, Tetanus	DTaP[e]
	Haemophilus influenzae type b	Hib
	Inactivated polio	IPV
	Pneumococcus	PCV
	Rotavirus	Rotavirus vaccine can be given to preterm infants as follows: medically stable, between 6 weeks and <15 weeks, with first dose given **at hospital discharge**, or after discharge—series should not be started after 15 weeks of age[f]
4 months	All of those listed for 2 months	All of those listed for 2 months except Hep B: if using monovalent Hep B, no vaccine at 4 months. If using a combination vaccine with Hep B, then acceptable to have baby receive a total of 4 doses of Hep B vaccine
6 months	All of those listed for 2 months	All of those listed for 2 months, except: if PedvaxHIB or Comvax is administered at 2 and 4 months, a dose at 6 months for Hib not necessary
	Influenza	Inactivated influenza vaccine, 2 doses beginning at 6 months of age, with second dose 1 month later
Hospital discharge	RSV	Appropriately selected preterm infants may benefit from immunoprophylaxis with palivizumab beginning at hospital discharge and then monthly during RSV season. Refer to yearly regional recommendations for guidelines

[a]Infants whose mothers are hepatitis B surface antigen positive (HbsAg +ve) should receive the hepatitis B vaccine on the day of delivery. In addition, they should also be given hepatitis B immunoglobulin (HBIG 100 U, 0.5 mL intramuscularly) within 12 hours of birth.
[b]Only monovalent Hep B vaccine should be used from birth until 6 weeks of age.
[c]The hepatitis B series can be completed with either monovalent Hep B or a combination vaccine containing Hep B.
[d]Combination vaccines can be given starting at 2 months of age to minimize the number of injections.
[e]Wherever possible, the same brand of DTaP should be used at 2, 4, and 6 months.
[f]Preterm infants may be immunized for rotavirus if the infant is at least 6 weeks' chronologic age and clinically stable. They should be immunized on the same schedule and with the same precautions as term infants. The first dose should be given at discharge from the NICU or after NICU discharge. Severe combined immune deficiency (SCID) and history of intussusception are contraindications for use of the rotavirus vaccine.

An increased incidence of apnea with or without bradycardia after immunization with whole cell DTP was recognized in extremely low birthweight infants <1000 g, but has not been reported with DTaP. Cardiorespiratory events (apnea and bradycardia with desaturations) can be seen in preterm infants given combination DTaP, IPV, HepB, and Hib conjugate vaccines, but are not reported to have a detrimental effect on the clinical course of immunized infants according to the AAP *Red Book*.

Special Circumstances

There is little data regarding the immunologic responses of extremely preterm infants receiving steroids for the treatment of bronchopulmonary dysplasia/chronic lung disease (BPD/CLD). Live vaccines should not be administered to babies receiving prednisolone (2 mg/kg/d for more than 1 week or 1 mg/kg/d for more than 1 month) or the equivalent dose of dexamethasone. Live vaccines should not be administered while babies are hospitalized in the NICU.

Premature infants over 6 months but less than 2 years of age with a history of BPD/CLD or reactive airway disease should be considered for vaccination against influenza.

Select premature infants are eligible to receive prophylaxis against the respiratory syncytial virus (RSV) as a monthly injection given during RSV season. Eligibility requirements can change yearly. It is recommended that physicians use local references at the beginning of the RSV season for guidance on dosing.

Reference

Pickering LK, Baker CJ, Kimberlin DW, Long SS, eds. *Red Book: 2012 Report of the Committee on Infectious Diseases*. 29th ed. Elk Grove Village, IL: American Academy of Pediatrics; 2012.

Appendix F. Isolation Guidelines

The following table, Transmission-Based Precautions for Perinatal/Neonatal Patients in conjunction with Standard Precautions, is based on current knowledge and practices in the fields of epidemiology, pediatrics, and perinatology. Published resource references are listed immediately after the table.

Instructions for Using Precautions for Perinatal/Neonatal Patients Table

- Each disease is considered individually so that only precautions indicated to interrupt transmission for that disease are recommended.
- The column "Maternal Precautions" describes the precautions to be used by staff providing care to the mother.
- The column "Neonatal Precautions" describes the precautions to be used by staff, patients, or visitors in contact with the neonate.
- Staff should assess the mother's ability to wash hands correctly and comply with precautions when determining the appropriateness of permitting rooming in.

Precautions shall be initiated for suspected as well as confirmed infectious diseases/conditions.

Infection/Disease	Maternal Precautions	Neonatal Precautions	Room-In	Mother May Visit in Nursery	Breast-Feeding	Additional Considerations
AIDS/HIV positive	Standard	Standard Bathe baby ASAP when stable	Yes	Yes	No HIV may be transmitted through breast milk.	Recommend tuberculosis testing for mother. Due to constant HIV antiretroviral (ARV) treatment option changes, consult with neonatology expert and refer to http:// aidsinfo.nih.gov for current ARV treatment options. Report AIDS to health department.
Chickenpox (see Varicella)						
Chlamydia trachomatis	Standard	Standard	Yes	Yes	Yes	Topical prophylaxis is ineffective for *Chlamydia* ophthalmic disease. Treatment for *Chlamydia* conjunctivitis and pneumonia is systemic erythromycin for 14 days.
Cytomegalovirus (CMV)	Standard	Standard	Yes	Yes	Yes	No additional precautions for pregnant health care workers.
Gastroenteritis	Contact precautions for diapered or incontinent persons for the duration of illness or to control outbreaks for gastroenteritis caused by infectious agents such as *Clostridium difficile*	Contact precautions for the duration of illness to control outbreaks for gastroenteritis/diarrhea caused by infectious agents such as *C. difficile*	Yes	Yes	Yes	The most effective method to remove *C. difficile* spores from contaminated hands is through meticulous hand hygiene with soap and water. Alcohol-based hand hygiene products do not inactivate *C. difficile* spores. Because *C. difficile* spores are difficult to kill, most surface disinfectants are ineffective. When outbreaks of *C. difficile* diarrhea are not controlled by other measures, it is recommended to use a disinfectant with sporicidal activity (eg, hypochlorite).

Gonococcal ophthalmia neonatorum	Standard	Standard	Yes After 24 hours of maternal treatment with antibiotics	Yes After 24 hours of maternal treatment with antibiotics	Yes After 24 hours of maternal treatment with antibiotics	Prophylactic use of topical 0.5% erythromycin ophthalmic or 1% tetracycline ointment at birth should be performed to prevent ophthalmic neonatorum. Prophylaxis may be delayed for as long as 1 hour after birth to facilitate parent infant bonding. Newborns born to mothers with active gonorrhea should receive a single dose of ceftriaxone 125 mg IV or IM. For low birthweight neonates, the dose is 25–50 mg/kg of body weight. Cefotaxime (100 mg/kg) in a single does is an alternative. Refer to *Perinatal Guidelines* (AAP/ACOG), 2012.
Group B streptococcal infections	Standard	Standard	Yes	Yes	Yes	Follow Centers for Disease Control and Prevention (CDC) guidelines for laboratory testing and antibiotic treatment recommendations.
Hepatitis A, B, C	Standard	Standard	Yes	Yes	Yes	Early hepatitis B immunization is recommended for all medically stable infants with birthweight >2 kg, regardless of maternal status. The American Academy of Pediatrics recommends that infants born to HBsAg-positive mothers, including preterm and low birthweight infants, receive the initial dose of hepatitis B vaccine within 12 hours of birth. Report to health department.

(Continued)

Infection/Disease	Maternal Precautions	Neonatal Precautions	Room-In	Mother May Visit in Nursery	Breast-Feeding	Additional Considerations
Herpes simplex virus (HSV) **Neonatal infection or positive culture in absence of disease**		Contact gown and gloves	Yes If baby is at low risk of infection.	Yes	Yes If no vesicular herpetic lesion in the breast area and all active skin lesions are covered.	Cultures obtained from mouth swab, naso-pharynx, conjunctiva, anus or skin vesicles, CSF, and whole blood samples 12–24 hours after birth are more likely to identify neo-natal infection. A positive culture obtained ≥24 hours after birth needs immediate antiviral treatment, even in the absence of symptoms. Neonates with HSV should be managed in a facility that provides level III subspecialty care and consultation. A mother with HSV infection should be taught to wash her hands carefully and use a clean barrier to ensure that the neonate does not come in contact with the lesions. A mother with herpes labialis (cold sore) should wear a disposable surgical mask when touching her newborn and not kiss or nuzzle her newborn infant until the lesions have crusted and dried. Refer to *Perinatal Guidelines* (AAP/ACOG), 2012 and the *Red Book*, 2012.

Lice (see Pediculosis)

Measles (Rubeola)	Airborne Masks for those susceptible. Labor, delivery, and postpartum recovery should take place in a private room with negative pressure, non-recirculating air with door closed. If mother is transferred to the delivery room for the actual delivery, she should wear mask during transfer and delivery.	No	No	No Until mother is noncontagious.	Contagious during prodrome and for 4 days after onset of rash. Report to health department. Maintain isolation for the duration of illness in immune compromised
Methicillin-resistant *S. aureus* (MRSA)	Contact Gown and gloves	Yes	Yes Follow contact precautions.	Yes	Apply contact precautions for infection or known colonization.
Mumps (infectious parotitis)	Droplet Masks within 3 ft of patient. Private room.	No	No	No Until mother is noncontagious.	Contagious for 5 days after onset of swelling. Report to health department.

(Continued)

Infection/Disease	Maternal Precautions	Neonatal Precautions	Room-In	Mother May Visit in Nursery	Breast-Feeding	Additional Considerations
Pediculosis (lice)	Contact For 24 hours after treatment, gown and gloves.	Contact For 24 hours after treatment, gown and gloves.	Yes	Yes	Yes	Exposed individuals and household contacts should be examined and treated if infected. Instruct mother to clean breasts before feeding, if medication is applied to that area. Stress good hand hygiene with special attention to area under fingernails.
Pertussis (whooping cough)	Droplet Masks within 3 ft of patient. Private room.	Droplet Masks within 3 ft of patient. Private room.	No	No	No Until mother is noncontagious.	Contagious for 5 days after start of effective therapy. Treatment with antimicrobial agents if available for newborns <1 and 2 months of age if the risk of developing severe pertussis and life-threatening complications outweighs the potential risk of developing infantile hypertrophic pyloric stenosis. See *Red Book*, 2012. Depending on the county, it may be reportable to the public health department.
Respiratory syncytial virus (RSV)	Contact Gown, gloves, mask within 3 ft of the patient.	Contact Gown, gloves, mask within 3 ft of the patient.	Yes	Yes May visit private room or cohort.	Yes	Parent education is essential to avoid transmission of the virus. The importance of hand hygiene should be emphasized in all settings. Prophylaxis to prevent RSV in newborns at increased risk for severe disease, particularly those with bronchopulmonary dysplasia/chronic lung disease receiving medical management on a long-term basis is available. Refer to *Perinatal Guidelines* (AAP/ACOG), 2012 and the *Red Book*, 2012. Contagious for duration of illness.

Rubella (German Measles) Postnatal	Droplet	Masks within 3 ft of patient. Private room, masks for those susceptible.	Yes	No	No	Contagious for 7 days after onset of rash. Susceptible persons stay out of room, if possible.
Maternal						Report to health department.
Congenital	Contact	Gown and gloves	Yes	Yes	Yes	Contagious until at least 1 year of age, unless 2 cultures or clinical specimens obtained 1 month apart after 3 months of age are negative for rubella virus. Susceptible persons stay out of room, if possible. Report to health department.
Scabies	Contact	For 24 hours after treatment, gown and gloves.	Yes	Yes	Yes	Treatment of exposed individuals and household contacts is recommended. Instruct mother to clean breasts before feeding, if medication is applied to that area. Stress good hand hygiene.
***Staphylococcus aureus* (not MRSA)**	Standard	Standard	Yes	Yes	Yes	Two or more concurrent cases of impetigo related to a nursery or a single case of breast abscess in a nursing mother or infant is presumptive evidence of an epidemic; report immediately to attending physician and Infection Control.

(Continued)

Infection/Disease	Maternal Precautions	Neonatal Precautions	Room-In	Mother May Visit in Nursery	Breast-Feeding	Additional Considerations
Syphilis	Standard	Standard	Yes	Yes	Yes	Treatment for congenital syphilis is available for infants in the first month of age. See *Red Book*, 2012. Health care workers and parents should wear gloves when handling the neonate until 24 hours of treatment with antibiotics. Report to health department.
Tuberculosis (TB) **1. Mother with recent positive purified protein derivative (PPD) and no evidence of active TB.**	Standard	Standard	Yes	Yes	Yes	If the mother is asymptomatic no separation is required. The newborn infant needs no special evaluation or therapy.
2. Mother with minimal disease, or disease has been treated for ≥2 weeks and is determined by Pulmonary or Infectious Disease to be noncontagious at delivery.	Standard	Standard	Yes	Yes	Yes	Management of the newborn infant suspected of congenital TB is based on categorization of the maternal infection. See testing and treatment in the *Red Book*, 2012. Report to health department.

3. Mother with current pulmonary or laryngeal active TB and suspected of being contagious at time of delivery.	Airborne N95 respirator for health care workers. Labor, delivery, and postpartum care in private room with negative pressure, nonrecirculating air with door closed. If mother is transferred to the delivery room for the actual delivery, she should wear mask during transfer and delivery.	Standard (airborne for intubated neonate with congenital TB)	No Until mother is determined to be noncontagious.	No Until mother is determined to be noncontagious.	No Until mother is determined to be noncontagious.	Management of the newborn infant suspected of congenital TB is based on categorization of the maternal infection. See testing and treatment in the *Red Book*, 2012. Report to health department.
4. Mother has extrapulmonary spread of TB (ie, miliary, bone, meningitis, etc.)	Standard	Standard	No Until mother is determined to be noncontagious.	No Until mother is determined to be noncontagious.		Management of the newborn infant suspected of congenital TB is based on categorization of the maternal infection. See testing and treatment in the *Red Book*, 2012. Report to health department.

(Continued)

Infection/Disease	Maternal Precautions	Neonatal Precautions	Room-In	Mother May Visit in Nursery	Breast-Feeding	Additional Considerations
Varicella (Chickenpox) or Herpes Zoster in immunocompromised mother or if disseminated maternal infection	Airborne/contact Labor, delivery and postpartum care in private room with negative pressure, nonrecirculating air with door closed. If mother is transferred to the delivery room for the actual delivery, she should wear mask during transfer and delivery.		No Until mother's lesions have crusted.	No Until mother's lesions have crusted.	No Until mother's lesions have crusted.	Continue airborne/contact precautions minimal 5 days after onset of rash and until all lesions are crusted. In an immunocompromised patient it may take a week or longer. May be contagious 1–2 days before the onset of rash. Hospitalized patients should be discharged prior to the 10th day after exposure, if possible. Exposed susceptible patients should be placed on airborne precautions beginning 10 days after exposure and continue until 21 days after last exposure, or until 28 days if varicella–zoster immune globulin (VZIG) given. Consider immunologic titer for neonates <28 weeks' gestational age.
Varicella—newborn or exposure to varicella	Airborne Masks for those susceptible. Private room with negative pressure, nonrecirculating air with door closed.		Yes	Yes May visit private room or cohort.	Yes Unless mother has lesions.	Hospitalized patients should be discharged prior to the 10th day after exposure, if possible. Begin precautions 10 days after exposure and continue until 21 days after last exposure, or until 28 days if VZIG given.

Modified from guidelines issued by Kaiser Permanente Hospital, Fontana, CA.

References

American Academy of Pediatrics and The American College of Obstetricians and Gynecologists. *Guidelines for Perinatal Care.* 6th ed. Atlanta, GA: AAP/ACOG; 2007.

Pickering LK, Baker CJ, Kimberlin DW, Long SS, eds. *Red Book: Report of the Committee on Infectious Diseases.* 29th ed. Elk Grove Village, IL: American Academy of Pediatrics; 2012.

Centers for Disease Control and Prevention. *Guidelines for Isolation Precautions in Hospitals.* Atlanta, GA: U.S. Department of Health and Human Services; 2007.

Centers for Disease Control and Prevention. *Guidelines for Infection Control in Health Care Personnel.* Atlanta, GA: U.S. Department of Health and Human Services; 1998.

Young TE, Magnum B. Neofax®: *A Manual of Drugs Used in Neonatal Care.* 20th ed. Montvale, NJ: Thomson Healthcare; 2007.

Appendix G. Temperature Conversion Table

Celsius	Fahrenheit	Celsius	Fahrenheit
34.0	93.2	37.6	99.6
34.2	93.6	37.8	100.0
34.4	93.9	38.0	100.4
34.6	94.3	38.2	100.7
34.8	94.6	38.4	101.1
35.0	95.0	38.6	101.4
35.2	95.4	38.8	101.8
35.4	95.7	39.0	102.2
35.6	96.1	39.2	102.5
35.8	96.4	39.4	102.9
36.0	96.8	39.6	103.2
36.2	97.1	39.8	103.6
36.4	97.5	40.0	104.0
36.6	97.8	40.2	104.3
36.8	98.2	40.4	104.7
37.0	98.6	40.6	105.1
37.2	98.9	40.8	105.4
37.4	99.3	41.0	105.8

Celsius = (Fahrenheit − 32) × 5/9.
Fahrenheit = (Celsius × 9/5) + 32.

Appendix H. Weight Conversion Table[a]

Ounces	1 lb	2 lb	3 lb	4 lb	5 lb	6 lb	7 lb	8 lb
				Grams				
0	454	907	1361	1814	2268	2722	3175	3629
1	482	936	1389	1843	2296	2750	3204	3657
2	510	964	1418	1871	2325	2778	3232	3686
3	539	992	1446	1899	2353	2807	3260	3714
4	567	1021	1474	1928	2381	2835	3289	3742
5	595	1049	1503	1956	2410	2863	3317	3771
6	624	1077	1531	1985	2438	2892	3345	3799
7	652	1106	1559	2013	2466	2920	3374	3827
8	680	1134	1588	2041	2495	2948	3402	3856
9	709	1162	1616	2070	2523	2977	3430	3884
10	737	1191	1644	2098	2552	3005	3459	3912
11	765	1219	1673	2126	2580	3033	3487	3941
12	794	1247	1701	2155	2608	3062	3515	3969
13	822	1276	1729	2183	2637	3090	3544	3997
14	851	1304	1758	2211	2665	3119	3572	4026
15	879	1332	1786	2240	2693	3147	3600	4054

[a]Values represent weight in grams.
To convert from kilograms to pounds, multiply kilograms by 2.2.
To convert from pounds to grams, multiply pounds by 454.

Index

Entries denoted by an italic *f* and *t* indicate figures and tables, respectively. When a drug trade name is listed, the reader is referred to the generic name.

premature delivery, 716, 730, 931
premature infant pain profile (PIPP), 173
premature rupture of membranes (PROM), 169
prematurity, 793–794, 831. *See also* AOP;
 osteopenia of prematurity; ROP
 borderline, 677
 complication of, 359
 correction for, 212–213
 delayed stool passage relating to, 463, 464, 466
 extreme, 448
 in hyperbilirubinemia, 682–683, 683*t*
 iatrogenic, 171
 in NEC, 770
 in PDA, 800
 pulmonary hemorrhage relating to, 502, 503
 risk of sepsis in, 866
 and SIP, 875
 transient hypothyroxinemia of, 913
 in TTN, 920
 in twins, 764
 in VZV, 935
premedications, for nonemergency intubation,
 259, 260*t*–262*t*
prenatal gestational age, 29–30
prenatal hydronephrosis, 895–896
prenatal spasticity, 603
prenatal vitamins, 779
pre-plus disease, 845
preputial skin, 893
prerenal failure, 830–831, 833
 in delayed urine output, 470–471
pressor agents, 818
pressure-passive cerebral circulation, 728
pressure-volume (P-V), 74
preterm birth, 210, 910
preterm delivery, 897
preterm infants, 913
 apnea and bradycardia in, 334, 336
 counseling parents about, 358
 delayed stool passage in, 461*t*
 developmental disability in, 359
 extreme prematurity in, 448
 fluid, and electrolytes of, 89–97
 fluid therapy for, 435
 and gastric intubation, 274
 gestational age of, 35*t*, 358
 growth chart, 39*f*
 IUGR in, 741
 jaundice in, 170
 late, management of, 169–171
 NEC in, 770
 PDA in, 800
 pertussis in, 823
 postnatal growth failure in, 116
 shock in, 453–454
 temperature regulation in, 65
 thrombocytopenia in, 904
 thyroid function in, 908
preterm labor, 169, 712, 926, 931
preterm premature rupture of membranes
 (PPROM), 921, 930, 931

Prevacid. *See* lansoprazole
preventive measures, 486
Prevnar. *See* pneumococcal 7-valent conjugate
 vaccine
priapism, 59
Prilosec. *See* omeprazole
Primacor. *See* milrinone
primary cutaneous aspergillosis (PCA), 509
primary energy failure, 805
primary hypothyroidism, 909
primiparity, 735
probenecid, 1022*t*
probiotics and milk, 122, 774
procainamide, 993, 1022*t*
procaine penicillin G, 901
procalcitonin, 497, 869
procedural pain, acute, 173
prochlorperazine, 1023*t*
Procrit. *See* erythropoietin/epoetin alfa
Proglycem. *See* diazoxide
prognosis
 in ABO incompatibility, 549
 in acute renal failure, 833
 in air leak syndromes, 551
 in ambiguous genitalia, 626
 in apnea, 569
 in BPD, 575
 CMV infection, 618
 in ECLS infants, 208
 of HIV, 656
 in HSV, 648
 of hydrocephalus, 662–663
 in IDMs, 714
 in ISAMs, 723
 in IVH, 731
 in meconium aspiration, 753
 of NEC, 775
 in neonatal seizures, 864
 for neonatal thyrotoxicosis, 912
 in osteopenia of prematurity, 796
 for parvovirus B19 infection, 799
 in perinatal asphyxia, 813–814
 in pertussis, 825
 for postnatal chickenpox, 938
 in PPHN, 822
 in Rh incompatibility, 853–854
 for ROP, 848
 in RSV, 843
 in rubella, 857
 for sepsis, 873
 for SIP, 876
 for TB, 930
 for thyroid disorders, 911
 in TNMG, 769
 for toxoplasmosis, 918
 for TTN, 925
 for VZV, 935–936
progressive familial intrahepatic cholestasis
 (PFIC), 666
progressive panencephalitis, 855
prolonged tachypnea of the newborn (PTTN), 921

respiratory distress syndrome (RDS) (*Cont.*):
  in PPHN, 816
  in thrombocytopenia, 905
  in thyroid disorders, 909
  in TTN, 919, 923
respiratory failure, 210–211, 772, 808
respiratory insufficiency, 888
respiratory management, 71–89, 751–753
respiratory rate, 88, 921
respiratory support, 876
  in apnea, 569
  in BPD, 573
  in ELBW infants, 163–165
  in hypermagnesemia, 748
  in hypotension, 451
  in NEC, 773
  pharmacologic, 78–82
  in sepsis, 867, 872
  strategies of, 82–84
respiratory syncytial virus (RSV), 171, 840–843
resuscitation
  discontinuation of, 225
  of ELBW infants, 157–158
  with IUGR, 740–741
  with NEC, 885
  noninitiation of, 225
  with PPHN, 817
  Rh incompatibility and, 852
  risk of sepsis and, 867
retarded growth and development, 604
reticulocyte count
  in ABO incompatibility, 548
  in anemia, 561
  in hospital discharge criteria, 458
  in hyperbilirubinemia
    conjugated, 397
    unconjugated, 404, 678
  in Rh incompatibility, 850
reticulocytosis, 829, 849
retinal hemorrhage, 531, 536, 823
retinal reattachment, 848
retinoblastoma, 635
retinoic acid, 211
retinopathy of prematurity (ROP), 211, 844–848, 846f
retractions, 912, 923
retrograde pyelography, 878
retrolental fibroplasia (RLF), 844
retroperitoneal tumors, 890–891
Retrovir. *See* zidovudine
Revatio. *See* sildenafil
Rh immunoglobulin (RhoGAM), 849, 851, 853
Rh incompatibility, 269, 674–675, 678, 849–854
Rh isoimmunization, 402
Rh (D) type, 189
rhabdomyolysis, 699
rhAPC. *See* recombinant human activated protein C
Rh-negative mother, 849
RhoGAM. *See* Rh immunoglobulin
rHuEPO. *See* recombinant human erythropoietin therapy

ribavirin, 843
rickets, 794
Rieger syndrome, 622
rifabutin, 1023t
Rifadin. *See* rifampin
rifampin (Rifadin, Rofact), 671, 759, 928, 929, 995–996, 1023t
rifapentine, 1023t
rifaximin, 1023t
right atrial thrombosis (RAT), 593
right upper quadrant sign, 475
right ventricular hypertrophy (RVH), 608
Rigler sign, 475
ring chromosomes, 777
risperidone, 1023t
ritodrine, 429, 719
ritonavir, 1024t
rizatriptan, 1024t
R_L. *See* resistance
RLF. *See* retrolental fibroplasia
Rocephin. *See* ceftriaxone sodium
rocker bottom feet, 61
rocuronium, 519, 996
Rofact. *See* rifampin
rooting reflex, 63
ROP. *See* retinopathy of prematurity
rotavirus, 770
Rotor syndrome, 395
RPR. *See* rapid plasma reagin
RRT. *See* renal replacement therapy
RSI. *See* rapid sequence intubation; rectosigmoid index
RSV. *See* respiratory syncytial virus
rubella, 506, 509, 514, 605, 633, 638, 734, 800, 854–857, 859, 904, 905
rubella vaccine, 1024t
Rubinstein-Taybi syndrome, 800
rupture of membrane, 716, 800, 866
ruptured sac, 880
RVH. *See* right ventricular hypertrophy
RVT. *See* renal vein thrombosis

S
sacral lesions, 782
saddle bag sign, 476
saddle nose, 898
SAE. *See* systemic air embolism
SAH. *See* subarachnoid hemorrhage
Salbutamol. *See* albuterol
salmeterol, 1024t
salt loss, 620
Sandifer syndrome, 521
Sandostatin. *See* octreotide
Sao_2. *See* pulse oximetry
sapropterin dihydrochloride, 707
saquinavir, 1024t
satyr ear, 52
scabies, 509, 514
SCAD. *See* short-chain acyl-CoA dehydrogenase deficiency
scaling, 509–510, 514